KT-482-840

Clinical Medical-Surgical Nursing

A Decision-Making Reference

Beverly George-Gay, RN, MSN, CCRN
Nurse Educator
Medical College of Virginia Hospitals and
Virginia Commonwealth University Health Systems
Richmond, Virginia

Cynthia C. Chernecky, RN, CNS, AOCN, PhD
Associate Professor, School of Nursing
Medical College of Georgia
Augusta, Georgia

W.B. SAUNDERS COMPANY
An Imprint of Elsevier Science
Philadelphia   London   Toronto   Montreal   Sydney   Tokyo

W.B. SAUNDERS COMPANY
An Imprint of Elsevier Science

The Curtis Center
Independence Square West
Philadelphia, Pennsylvania 19106

Library of Congress Cataloging-in-Publication Data

Clinical medical-surgical nursing: a decision-making reference/[edited by] Beverly
George-Gay, Cynthia C. Chernecky.

p.;   cm.

ISBN 0–7216–8532–3

1. Nursing—Handbooks, manuals, etc.   2. Surgical nursing—Handbooks,
   manuals, etc.   3. Decision making—Handbooks, manuals, etc.
   I. George-Gay, Beverly.   II. Chernecky, Cynthia C.
   [DNLM: 1. Perioperative Nursing—Handbooks.   2. Decision Making—
   Handbooks.   3. Nursing—Handbooks. WY 49 C6415 2002]

RT51.C645 2002   610.73—dc21   2001032000

Vice President and Publishing Director, Nursing: Sally Schrefer

Acquisitions Editor: Robin Carter

Developmental Editor: Barbara Cicalese

Illustration Specialist: Peg Shaw

Book Designer: Andy Johnson

CLINICAL MEDICAL-SURGICAL NURSING: ISBN 0–7216–8532–3
A Decision-Making Reference

Copyright © 2002 by W.B. Saunders Company.

All rights reserved. No part of this publication may be reproduced or transmitted
in any form or by any means, electronic or mechanical, including photocopy,
recording, or any information storage and retrieval system, without permission in
writing from the publisher.

Printed in the United States of America.

Last digit is the print number: 9   8   7   6   5   4   3   2   1

To those of you who have helped us with life's lessons in both our personal lives and professional careers—our families, our students and their preceptors, our colleagues and mentors, and our nursing leaders—who have encouraged us and had faith in our abilities and supported our dedication to clinical nursing care—you have made such a difference in our lives, and this book would not be possible without all of you.

To the memory of Donna Fair, Lore Wright, and Una Barker

Contributors

Jan A. Addy, RN, MS
Associate Professor and
Nursing Coordinator of Medical-Surgical Nursing
Baltimore City Community College
Baltimore, Maryland

Lorie Arata, BSN, MN, FNP
Staff Nurse/Charge Nurse, Intensive Care
Athens Regional Medical Center
Athens, Georgia

Selma F. Brophy, RN, MSN, PhD
Associate Professor, College of Nursing
University of Wisconsin
Oshkosh, Wisconsin

Joanne M. Bullard, BSN, MN
Assistant Professor, Division of Nursing
Our Lady of Holy Cross College
New Orleans, Louisiana

Patricia A. Catalano, RN, MSN
Nurse Manager, Intensive Care Unit
St. Joseph Hospital
Augusta, Georgia

Cynthia C. Chernecky, RN, CNS, AOCN, PhD
Associate Professor, School of Nursing
Medical College of Georgia
Augusta, Georgia

Pamela P. Cook, ASN, BSN, MS
Instructor, School of Nursing
Medical College of Georgia
Augusta, Georgia

Karen Crawford, RN, MSN, CNF, ANP-C
Nurse Practitioner and Clinical Nurse Specialist
Novartis Pharmaceuticals, Inc.
Savannah, Georgia

Lee Farris, BSN, MSN
Assistant Professor, School of Nursing
Medical College of Georgia
Athens, Georgia

Christopher R. Friese, RN, MS, OCN
NRSA Pre-Doctoral Fellow and Staff Nurse
University of Pennsylvania School of Nursing and
Hospital of the University of Pennsylvania
Philadelphia, Pennsylvania

Kitty Garrett, BSN, MSN, CCRN
Critical Care Clinical Nurse Specialist
St. Joseph Hospital
Augusta, Georgia

Deborah L. Gentile, RN, MSN
Clinical Instructor and Lecturer, College of Nursing
University of Wisconsin
Oshkosh, Wisconsin

Beverly George-Gay, RN, MSN, CCRN
Nurse Educator
Medical College of Virginia Hospitals and
Virginia Commonwealth University Health Systems
Richmond, Virginia

Mary Jo Gerlach, RN, MSNEd
Assistant Professor, Retired, School of Nursing
Medical College of Georgia
Athens, Georgia

Patricia B. Graham, RN, PhD
Assistant Professor and Director, Retired
Learning Resources Center
Medical College of Georgia
Augusta, Georgia

Judy Graham-Garcia, RN, MN, FNP, ACNP
Nursing Anesthesia Student, School of Nursing
Medical College of Georgia
Augusta, Georgia

Mikel Gray, CUNP, CCCN, FAAN, PhD
Professor and Nurse Practitioner, Department of Urology
University of Virginia
Charlottesville, Virginia

Richard E. Haas, BSN, EdM, MS, CRNA
Assistant Professor, School of Nursing
Medical College of Georgia
Augusta, Georgia

Karen Harris, RN, MSN
Instructor, School of Nursing
Medical College of Georgia
Augusta, Georgia

Rebecca K. Hodges, RN, CCRN
Critical Care Clinician
St. Joseph Hospital
Augusta, Georgia

Vallire Hooper, RN, MSN, CPAN
Clinical Nurse Specialist
St. Joseph Hospital and
Clinical Assistant Professor, School of Nursing
Medical College of Georgia
Augusta, Georgia

Judy Kaye, RN, ACNP, ANP, GNP, CCRN, CNRN, PhD
Assistant Professor, College of Nursing
University of South Carolina
Columbia, South Carolina

Ann M. Kolanowski, RN, MS, PhD
Associate Professor, School of Nursing
The Pennsylvania State University
University Park, Pennsylvania

Linda U. Krebs, RN, MS, AOCN, PhD
Assistant Professor
University of Colorado School of Nursing and
University of Colorado Comprehensive Cancer Center
Denver, Colorado

Linda McCuistion, RN, MN, CNS, PhD
Professor, Division of Nursing
Our Lady of Holy Cross College
New Orleans, Louisiana

Collette McKinney, MSN
Officer in Charge, Urgent Care Clinic
Bassett Army Community Hospital
Fort Wainwright, Alaska

Ethlyn McQueen-Gibson, RN, MSN
Assistant Professor
Tacoma Community College
Tacoma, Washington

Charlotte Harrison Mackey, RN, MSN
Assistant Professor, Department of Nursing
West Chester University
West Chester, Pennsylvania

Denise Macklin, BSN, RNC, CRNI
President
Professional Learning Systems, Inc.
Marietta, Georgia

Diane Anthony Manghram, CCRN, MS, APRN, BC
Clinical Nurse Intensivist, Intensive Care Unit
Medical College of Georgia Hospital & Clinics
Augusta, Georgia

Suzanne K. Marnocha, RN, MSN, CCRN
Assistant Professor, College of Nursing
University of Wisconsin
Oshkosh, Wisconsin

Robert A. Mead, Pharm D
Senior Medical Science Manager
Bristol-Myers Squibb Company
Princeton, New Jersey

Regina Simione Medeiros, RN, MHSA, CCRN
Trauma Nurse Coordinator
Medical College of Georgia
Augusta, Georgia

Veronica P.S. Njie, RN, MSN, CS
Assistant Professor
Baltimore City Community College
Baltimore, Maryland

Debora Burkett Nutt, RN, MN
Clinical Nurse Specialist
Memorial Health University Medical Center
Savannah, Georgia

Bridget Shoulders-Odom, ARNP, MS, CS, CCRN
Acute Care Clinical Nurse Specialist and Nurse Practitioner
West Palm Beach VA Medical Center
West Palm Beach, Florida

Adjunct Faculty
Florida Atlantic University
Boca Raton, Florida

Phyllis G. Peterson, RN, MN
Assistant Professor, Division of Nursing
Our Lady of Holy Cross College
New Orleans, Louisiana

Patricia Preston-Bowman, BSN, MSN
Instructor, School of Nursing
Medical College of Georgia
Augusta, Georgia

Sue Putnam, RN, EMT
Paramedic Instructor and Chief Flight Nurse
LifeNet Georgia
Jefferson, Georgia

Kathy Benton Ravenell, RN, MS
Instructor, School of Nursing
Medical College of Georgia
Augusta, Georgia

Patricia Revolinski, MSN
Instructor, School of Nursing
Medical College of Georgia
Augusta, Georgia

Susan Rick, RN, MSN, DNS, CNS
Assistant Professor, Health Sciences Center
Louisiana State University
New Orleans, Louisiana

Patricia Rikli, RN, MSN, PhD
Assistant Professor, Department of Nursing
State University of West Georgia
Carrollton, Georgia

Jeanene (Gigi) Robison, MSN, RN, AOCN, OCN
Oncology Clinical Nurse Specialist
The Christ Hospital
Cincinnati, Ohio

Diana Davis Rovira, RN, CCRN
Gamma Knife Nurse Coordinator, School of Nursing
Medical College of Georgia
Augusta, Georgia

Rebecca Rule, BSN, MPH, MN, CS-FNP
Assistant Professor, School of Nursing
Medical College of Georgia
Augusta, Georgia

Lori Schumacher, MS
Instructor, School of Nursing
Medical College of Georgia
Augusta, Georgia

Brenda K. Shelton, RN, MS, CCRN
Critical Care Clinical Nurse Specialist
The Johns Hopkins Oncology Center
Baltimore, Maryland

Mia K. Smitt, RN, MS, FNP
Nurse Practitioner
Millen, Georgia

Christine Stackhouse, RN, MSN
Assistant Professor, Department of Nursing
West Chester University
West Chester, Pennsylvania

Nancy L. Stark, BSN, MSN
Director of Nursing
Medical College of Georgia Hospital and Clinics
Augusta, Georgia

Denise Weaver Thompson, RN, MSN
PeriAnesthesia Nurse Manager
Athens Regional Medical Center
Athens, Georgia

Cecilia M. Tiller, RNC, DSN, WHNP
Dean and Professor
Abilene Intercollegiate School of Nursing
Abilene, Texas

Kathleen R. Wren, CRNA, PhD
Assistant Professor, School of Nursing
Medical College of Georgia
Augusta, Georgia

Timothy L. Wren, RN, MS
Assistant Professor, School of Nursing
Louisiana State University Health Sciences Center
New Orleans, Louisiana

Eden Zabat, RN, MSN
Instructor, Department of Nursing
West Chester University
West Chester, Pennsylvania

Reviewers

Suzanne K. Beltz, RN, CS, CNS, PhD
University of Mary Hardin-Baylor
Belton, Texas

Wendy Blackburn, MEd, RN, BScN, CRRN
Parkwood Hospital
London, Ontario, Canada

Michelle Bott, RN, BSN, MN
Sunnybrook & Women's College Health Sciences Centre
Toronto, Ontario, Canada

Karen L. Byrd, MSN, RN, GNP C, OCN
Wake Forest University Baptist Medical Center
Winston-Salem, North Carolina

Deborah H. Cantero, MS, ARNP C
University of South Florida
Tampa, Florida

Rebecca Sue Cate, RN, BSN
IHC LDS Hospital
Respiratory Special Care Unit
Salt Lake City, Utah

Lola A. Coke, MSN, RN, CS
Rush University College of Nursing
Chicago, Illinois

Nancy Eisemon, MPH, RN, CGRN
Northwestern Memorial Hospital
Chicago, Illinois

Patti G. Eisenberg, MSN, RN, CS
Community Hospitals
Indianapolis, Indiana

Mary M. Fabick, MSN, MEd, RN
Milligan College
Milligan College, Tennessee

Margaret M. Gingrich, MSN, RN
Harrisburg Area Community College
Harrisburg, Pennsylvania

Jacqueline L. Harris, MN, RN, ONC
Harding University
Searcy, Arkansas

Kimberly A. Hathaway, MSN, BSN, MHA
Mobile Infirmary Medical Center
Mobile, Alabama

Margie Hesson, MSN, RN, BSN
South Dakota State University
Rapid City, South Dakota

Patricia A. Kelly, RN, CS-FNP
Veterans Administration Medical Center
Outpatient Clinic
Middletown, Ohio

Barbara S. Levine, CRNP, CS, PhD
BSL Consulting Services
Wayne, Pennsylvania

Patrick J. Lilley, RN, MSN
North Central Texas College
Gainesville, Texas

Sue Ann Lopez, MSN, RN
South Plains College
Levelland, Texas

Sheila M. Marquart, MSN, RN, EdS
Middle Tennessee State University
Murfreesboro, Tennessee

Mary Judith Masiak, MSN, RNC
Gwynedd-Mercy College
Gwynedd Valley, Pennsylvania

Jane V. McCloskey, MSN, RN
Carolinas College of Health Sciences
Charlotte, North Carolina

Edwina McConnell, RN, FRCNA, PhD
Independent Nurse Consultant
Madison, Wisconsin

Mary Ann S. McLaughlin, MSN, RN
Freelance Editor
Magnolia, New Jersey

Michelle M. Montpas, RN, MSN, OCN
C.S. Mott Community College
Flint, Michigan

Carrie Morgan, MSN, CFNP
Western Kentucky University
Bowling Green, Kentucky

Judith L. Myers, MSN, RN
St. Louis University School of Nursing
St. Louis, Missouri

Phyllis G. Peterson, RN, MN
Our Lady of Holy Cross College
New Orleans, Louisiana

Linda Polacheck, RN, MSN, MSEd
Milwaukee Area Technical College
Milwaukee, Wisconsin

Ruthie Robinson, MSN, RN, CCRN, CEN
Lamar University
Beaumont, Texas

June Hart Romeo, NP C, PhD
Cleveland State University
Cleveland, Ohio

Victoria S. Seng, RN, PhD
University of Tennessee at Martin
Martin, Tennessee

Cynthia Taylor Smith, MSN, RN
Middle Georgia College
Cochran, Georgia

Susan B. Stillwell, MSN, RN
Arizona State University
Tempe, Arizona

Jacqueline Sullivan, RN, CCRN, CNRN, PhD
Thomas Jefferson University Hospital
Philadelphia, Pennsylvania

Lyn A. Tepper, MS, RN
Northwest Community Hospital
Arlington Heights, Illinois

Susan C. Vaughn, RN, BSN
Carolinas Medical Center
Charlotte, North Carolina

Joanne Venturella, RN, BA, TNCC
Franklin Square Hospital
Baltimore, Maryland

Joyce S. Willens, RN, PhD
Villanova University
Villanova, Pennsylvania

Lynn Wimett, EdD, MSN, RN, ANP
Regis University
Denver, Colorado

Deirdre D. Wipke-Tevis
University of Missouri/Columbia
MU Sinclair School of Nursing
Columbia, Missouri

Preface

The purpose of this book is to serve as a clinical resource that can quickly provide answers to common clinical questions for nursing students and practicing nurses in the medical-surgical practice areas, including hospitals and ambulatory surgery centers, and in the community. The book has two major parts, and the format for each part is consistent.

Part I includes 12 chapters that provide information about critical concepts in the areas of assessment, laboratory and diagnostic procedures, and pharmacology. This information can be applied to a wide variety of diagnoses. Each chapter is divided into sections to more easily find information. The format headings are as follows:

1. Overviews briefly describe the sections
2. Principles of Care provide the background for the topic
3. Decision-Making gives the information needed to provide care and to help nurses elucidate why they are doing what they are doing, and if it is the correct thing to do
4. Resources list the associations or World Wide Web sites that can be helpful to the nurse and the patient
5. Clinical Pearls dispense clinical tips on care.

Part II provides information about the most common patient diagnoses. This part is divided into 14 chapters and is system based. Each chapter is further divided into sections with individual topics. Not all diagnoses are included because of the pocket-sized nature of the book; however, care concepts should provide the information that is needed. For example, pneumothorax is not an individual section, but information on pneumothorax is provided in the section on chest drainage systems. The format for each section in Part II is as follows:

1. Overviews, with a description and an incidence of the disorder
2. Pathophysiology
3. Signs and Symptoms, a universal and patient-friendly term
4. Diagnostic Criteria
5. Interventions, including management of the patient with the disorder. Terminology is chosen to maintain a common language between health care providers working as a team
6. Community Care, providing information on essentials of care for the nurse working in the community, as well as patient education, home care, and illness prevention
7. Prognosis
8. Clinical Pearls, clinical tips on care and important things to remember.
   The major features of this book are as follow:
- A total of 130 medical-surgical conditions or procedures that reflect real-world nursing practice to provide a comprehensive reference
- Tips for the clinical setting not learned in medical-surgical courses or units
- Key information to plan care and anticipate guidance in a concise, pocket-sized book
- Helping students to think critically based on the book's clinical content, critical concepts, diagnosis, and system-based approach
- Highlighting the top priority nursing diagnoses/problems with their associated Nursing Intervention Classification (NIC) to assist in focusing on basic care. NIC, from the Iowa Interventions Project, provides a standard-

ized language to describe nursing treatments that are more compatible with other disciplines.

- Promoting collaboration between nursing and medicine. Interventions are not divided by discipline as the boundaries between nursing and medicine are less rigid.
- Management for nursing care in the community
- Strong clinical expertise provided from authoritative contributors
- Clinical Pearls that summarize key clinical practice tips.

Acknowledgments

I would like to acknowledge the nursing students and bedside nurses who inspired me to write this book. We frequently forget to recognize and thank them for their contributions to the growth of nursing practice. I would especially like to honor my mother, Agnes George, who inspires, supports, loves, and protects me in ways that cannot be described. Thanks Cinda Chernecky for your confidence, Barbara Cicalese for your patience, and Robin Carter for your support. To my husband and best friend, Mantovina Gay, I could not have done this without you.

BG-G

The ability to be blessed with a coeditor like Bev has been a most wonderful experience. She believes in clinical competence, has a zest for student learning, and exemplifies excellence as a practitioner. It has been my pleasure to work with such a dedicated colleague. I also know that there are always a number of people to thank for a project as massive as this one: my family, who have supported me in numerous ways and who never say a negative word when I say YES to yet another book project. Thanks to my mother Olga, brother Richard, godmother Helen, nieces Ellie and Annie, nephew Michael, godsons Jonathon and Vincent, goddaughter Dawn, and cousins Paula, Tom, Karen, and Philip. To the people who care about me and who pray for me and to those who are trying to teach me the word NO out of love and friendship, I thank Mother Thecla and Mother Helena of Saints Mary and Martha Orthodox Monastery in Wagener, South Carolina, Dr. Ann Marie Kolanowski, Dr. Joyceen Boyle, Dr. Katherine Nugent, Dr. Linda Sarna, Dr. Kathleen Wren, and Professors Lori Schumacher and Tim Wren. I want to thank all the contributors who worked so hard and gave so much time to share their expertise so that others may benefit, I truly thank them for their caring spirit. To the personnel at W.B. Saunders Company, who believe in high quality and clinical competence in publishing, I thank Barbara Cicalese and Robin Carter. And, finally, thanks to the best executive secretary one could ever hope for, Kimberly Black, who not only kept my head on my shoulders but kept me focused and organized and shared her skills so this project could become a reality. And, of course, I just have to mention my three dogs, Sasha, Josh, and Buffy, who keep me grounded and who have learned throughout the years that manuscripts are not to be eaten or shredded for play!

CCC

NOTICE

Nursing is an ever-changing field. Standard safety precautions must be followed, but as new research and clinical experience broaden our knowledge, changes in treatment and drug therapy become necessary or appropriate. Readers are advised to check the product information currently provided by the manufacturer of each drug to be administered to verify the recommended dose, the method and duration of administration, and the contraindications. It is the responsibility of the treating licensed prescriber, relying on experience and knowledge of the patient, to determine dosages and the best treatment for the patient. Neither the publisher nor the editor assumes any liability for any injury and/or damage to persons or property arising from this publication.

THE PUBLISHER

Contents

Part I   Decision-Making

Chapter 1   Basic Decision-Making   2
Section 1   Standards of Nursing, 2
Section 2   Vital Parameters, 7
Section 3   Expedited Physical Assessment, 17
Section 4   First Aid for Injuries, 24

Chapter 2   Decision-Making for Fluid Therapy   39
Section 1   Intravenous Fluids, 39
Section 2   Venous Access Devices, 48
Section 3   Blood and Blood Product Administration, 64

Chapter 3   Decision-Making for Wounds and Drainage Systems   77
Section 1   Wound Care, 77
Section 2   Wound Drainage Systems, 84
Section 3   Ostomies, 87
Section 4   Gastrointestinal Drainage Systems, 92

Chapter 4   Decision-Making for Bedside Specimen Collection   98
Section 1   Gastric Specimen Collection and Lavage, 98
Section 2   Urine Specimen Collection, 101
Section 3   Sputum Specimen Collection, 105
Section 4   Blood Glucose Specimen Collection and Monitoring, 109

Chapter 5   Decision-Making for Oxygenation Alterations   115
Section 1   Assessment of Oxygenation, 115
Section 2   Oxygen Delivery Devices, 124
Section 3   Tracheostomy Care, 128
Section 4   Chest Drainage Systems, 135

Chapter 6   Decision-Making for Renal Alterations   142
Section 1   Renal Assessment, 142
Section 2   Hemodialysis, 145
Section 3   Peritoneal Dialysis, 154
Section 4   Renal Transplantation, 160

Chapter 7   Decision-Making for Neurologic Alterations   166
Section 1   Neurologic Assessment, 166
Section 2   Increased Intracranial Pressure, 177
Section 3   Pathologic Brain Lesions, 183

Chapter 8   Decision-Making for Cardiovascular Alterations   189
Section 1   Cardiac Assessment, 189
Section 2   Vascular Assessment, 196
Section 3   Basic Electrical Conduction, 200
Section 4   Telemetry Monitoring, 206
Section 5   12-Lead Electrocardiogram, 210

Chapter **9**   Decision-Making for Nutritional Alterations   **221**
        Section 1   Nutritional Assessment, 221
        Section 2   Daily Requirements, 228
        Section 3   Diets and Supplements, 235
        Section 4   Parenteral Nutrition, 242
        Section 5   Enteral Nutrition, 249

Chapter **10**   Decision-Making for Immunologic Alterations   **259**
        Section 1   Assessment, 259
        Section 2   Immunocompromised Host, 265
        Section 3   Isolation Precautions, 269

Chapter **11**   Decision-Making for Common Laboratory Data   **274**
        Section 1   Red Blood Cell Counts, 274
        Section 2   White Blood Cell Count with Differential, 282
        Section 3   Electrolytes, 290
        Section 4   Laboratory Data Related to Infection, 299
        Section 5   Laboratory Data Related to Renal Function, 304

Chapter **12**   Decision-Making for Pharmacology   **312**
        Section 1   Analgesia, 312
        Section 2   Anticoagulants, 320
        Section 3   Antidepressants, 332
        Section 4   Antihypertensives, 336
        Section 5   Anti-Infectives, 348
        Section 6   Antiseizure Medications, 358
        Section 7   Digestive Tract Medications, 365
        Section 8   Diuretics, 375
        Section 9   Insulins, 384
        Section 10 Respiratory Drugs, 392
        Section 11 Sedatives, 403
        Section 12 Adrenocorticosteroids, 408

Part **II**   **Applied Decision-Making**

Chapter **13**   Respiratory   **418**
        Section 1   Asthma, 418
        Section 2   Bronchitis, 423
        Section 3   Emphysema, 428
        Section 4   Pneumonia, 432
        Section 5   Tuberculosis, 438

Chapter **14**   Cardiac   **446**
        Section 1   Angina, 446
        Section 2   Cardiogenic Shock, 451
        Section 3   Heart Failure, 456
        Section 4   Coronary Artery Disease, 467
        Section 5   Myocardial Infarction, 472
        Section 6   Rheumatic Heart Disease, 481

Chapter **15**   Vascular   **487**
        Section 1   Aortic Aneurysm, 487

Section 2   Buerger's Disease, 494
Section 3   Deep Vein Thrombosis, 500
Section 4   Hypertension, 509
Section 5   Hypovolemic Shock, 519
Section 6   Peripheral Vascular Disease, 526
Section 7   Raynaud's Disease, 531
Section 8   Thrombophlebitis, 537
Section 9   Varicose Veins, 541

Chapter **16**   Gastrointestinal—Lower   **547**
Section 1   Appendicitis, 547
Section 2   Cirrhosis, 549
Section 3   Food Poisoning, 556
Section 4   Hepatitis, 560
Section 5   Inflammatory Bowel Disease, 568
Section 6   Hernias, 576
Section 7   Intestinal Obstructions, 580
Section 8   Obesity, 586
Section 9   Peritonitis, 590

Chapter **17**   Gastrointestinal—Upper   **595**
Section 1   Cholelithiasis and Cholecystitis, 595
Section 2   Hiatal Hernia, 602
Section 3   Pancreatitis, 609
Section 4   Peptic Ulcer, 615

Chapter **18**   Endocrine   **624**
Section 1   Diabetes Mellitus, 624
Section 2   Hyperparathyroidism, 631
Section 3   Hyperthyroidism, 634
Section 4   Hypoparathyroidism, 638
Section 5   Hypothyroidism, 640

Chapter **19**   Neurologic   **644**
Section 1   Alzheimer's Disease, 644
Section 2   Cerebrovascular Accident, 649
Section 3   Guillain-Barré Syndrome, 657
Section 4   Meningitis, 662
Section 5   Multiple Sclerosis, 666
Section 6   Myasthenia Gravis, 671
Section 7   Parkinsonism, 675
Section 8   Seizures, 680
Section 9   Spinal Cord Injury, 686

Chapter **20**   Psychosocial Health   **693**
Section 1   Alcohol Withdrawal Syndrome, 693
Section 2   Depression, 696
Section 3   Drug Overdose and Poisoning, 703
Section 4   Mental/Emotional Abuse, 709
Section 5   Suicidal Ideation, 714

Chapter **21**   Musculoskeletal   **720**
Section 1   Arthritis and Joint Replacement, 720

Section 2   Fractures, 729
Section 3   Gout, 742
Section 4   Osteoporosis, 749
Section 5   Systemic Lupus Erythematosus, 753

Chapter **22**   Immunologic   **764**
Section 1   Human Immunodeficiency Virus, 764
Section 2   Allergies, 773
Section 3   Cancer and Solid Tumors, 780

Chapter **23**   Hematologic   **790**
Section 1   Anemia, 790
Section 2   Leukemia, 794
Section 3   Sickle Cell Disease, 799

Chapter **24**   Sensory   **804**
Section 1   Cataracts, 804
Section 2   Conjunctivitis, 809
Section 3   Glaucoma, 815
Section 4   Meniere's Disease, 824

Chapter **25**   Urinary   **830**
Section 1   Neurogenic Bladder, 830
Section 2   Renal Calculi, 840
Section 3   Renal Failure, 847
Section 4   Urinary Tract Infection, 856

Chapter **26**   Reproductive   **860**
Section 1   Benign Prostatic Hypertrophy, 860
Section 2   Pelvic Inflammatory Disease, 866
Section 3   Sexually Transmitted Diseases, 870

Bibliography   **879**

Index   **933**

II

Decision-Making

chapter 1

Basic Decision-Making

Standards of Nursing

Section 1   Linda Krebs

OVERVIEW

Comprehensive standards are essential for professional occupations. Professional standards ensure that all members of that particular profession have common ground rules from which to function and a common foundation on which to base evaluation. Standards of nursing are valuable to the nursing profession because they provide a consistent basis for practice, shape the profession toward attainment of common goals, and can be used as both a legal and an ethical model from which to evaluate actions and interactions between nurses and the consumers of their care.

Standards of nursing apply not only to practice, but also to the way in which nursing practice and the profession as a whole is conceptualized in terms of legal and ethical requirements and responsibilities. In addition, comprehensive and consistent documentation is an essential component of nursing practice and incorporates both legal and ethical principles. These four areas—practice, legal issues, ethics, and documentation—are all important in the nurses' decision-making process.

PRINCIPLES OF CARE
Standards of Practice

According to the American Nurses Association's (ANA) *Standards of Clinical Nursing Practice,* standards of practice are "authoritative statements by which the nursing profession describes the responsibilities for which its practitioners are accountable. Consequently, standards reflect the values and priorities of the profession" (ANA, 1998a, p. 1). These standards focus on the nurse and define the activities and behaviors needed to achieve identified patient outcomes. Standards are essential to the nursing profession because they not only lay the foundation for both general and specialty nursing practice, but also provide consistent direction for practice and a framework for the evaluation of that practice.

Legal Issues
Regulation of Nursing Practice

According to the ANA pamphlet *Nursing's Social Policy Statement,* nursing practice is regulated in three different ways:

1. *Professional regulation.* The profession defines the basis for practice and methods for its expansion, the methods for expanding the knowledge and skills of the practitioner, the means by which care will be delivered, and the methods for ensuring quality and evaluating outcomes (e.g., a code of

ethics, standards of practice, peer review mechanisms, and credentialing strategies).

2. *Legal regulation.* Practice is regulated by legal statutes, which specify that nurses are legally accountable for their actions and for the actions of those to whom they have delegated aspects of nursing care, as well as by formal and informal covenants between the profession and society.

3. *Self-regulation.* Individual nurses regulate their own practices by remaining clinically competent, knowledgeable, and personally accountable for their actions (ANA, 1995).

Malpractice

Standards of care are the measure by which the legal system evaluates the conduct of a nurse. They are designed to ensure appropriate, consistent, comprehensive, high-quality care to all. The nurse is judged against professional standards (both local and national) set for nursing practice by our professional organizations, and the actions taken by a nurse in a given situation are compared with those that would likely be taken by a similar nurse in a similar situation. *Malpractice* is defined as a failure to meet the standards of care that have been identified by the profession.

Negligence "is a general term that denotes conduct lacking in due care . . . [it] is a deviation from the standard of care that a reasonable person would use in a set of circumstances . . . [it] may also include doing something that the reasonable and prudent person would not do" (Guido, 1997, p. 66). Anyone can be deemed to be negligent.

In contrast, malpractice is a more explicit term that relates both to professional standards of care and the status of the provider of that care. Thus, to be deemed liable for malpractice, one must be identified as a professional (e.g., nurse, lawyer, physician) and have been negligent in some aspect of care. In addition, the professional must have committed an act of misconduct or been unreasonably careless in the care provided, the misconduct or wrong must have resulted in an injury of some type, and there must have been a breach in the standard of care that is owed to and expected by the patient.

Good Samaritan Law

Good Samaritan laws were enacted to protect health care personnel and others who voluntarily provide emergency care at the scene of an accident, emergency, or disaster. Although the laws vary between states, all states and the District of Columbia provide some protection for providers of care in such situations; in addition, a federal law protects providers of care on airplanes. In some states, the laws apply not only to health care providers, but also to any individual who provides emergency assistance.

It is important to note that no provider is required to provide assistance (although there may be an ethical duty to do so), unless subject to a state "duty-to-rescue" statute. Specific requirements must be met for an individual to be covered by a Good Samaritan law:

1. The situation must be an emergency. (Nonemergent care is not covered.)
2. Care must be provided at no cost to the recipient.
3. Care provided must be within the scope of the provider's practice, knowledge, and clinical skills.
4. Once care has been offered, the provider must remain with the patient until someone of equal or more advanced training agrees to take over.

5. The care cannot be provided in the setting in which the provider would normally practice. (For example, an emergency room nurse is not covered for care provided routinely in the emergency room.)

Although Good Samaritan laws protect providers, it is important to be aware that they do not cover acts of gross negligence or actions that are outside the care provider's scope of knowledge and skill. In addition, controversy exists over which individuals are covered and the extent to which they are covered.

Ethical Issues

According to Lancaster (1999), ethics is the "formal study of ways of conceptualizing and understanding the moral life" (p. 338), whereas normative ethics is an "area of inquiry that seeks to determine which approach or action is the most ethically desirable in a given situation" (p. 338). Health care ethics is the application of normative ethics to health care situations. Ethical theories include the following:

- *Deontologic theories* derive their norms and rules from the obligations that one individual has to another. These theories examine the intentions of actions rather than the consequences of those actions.
- *Teleologic theories*, also known as *utilitarianism*, derive their norms and rules from the consequences of actions rather than the intentions. If a consequence is good, then the action was right; if a consequence is bad, then the action was wrong. These theories are based on the idea that useful (right) actions bring about the greatest good.
- *Principalism* combines various current ethical principles and attempts to resolve ethical dilemmas through the application of one or more of these principles. This theory is growing in popularity among health care professionals.

Documentation

According to Iyer and Camp (1999), accurate documentation is essential to denote professional responsibility and accountability and is of prime importance in facilitating continuity of care, enhancing patient interventions, and evaluating patient care. Accurate documentation is necessary to ensure communication of the patient's status and care between providers and others, to promote comprehensive care, and to meet legal and professional guidelines. Comprehensive nursing documentation should include an assessment of the patient's current health status, the health care plan devised to meet the patient's needs and goals, the actions of the nurse and the patient responses to those actions, all information that is communicated to other health care personnel and the responses to that information, and any actions that the nurse undertakes on behalf of the patient.

DECISION-MAKING
Standards

Standards of practice may be both internal and external. External standards are those set by national bodies, such as the Joint Commission on the Accreditation of Healthcare Organizations (JCAHO) and the Occupational and Safety Health Administration (OSHA), whereas internal standards are set by the nursing profession (e.g., ANA, specialty nursing organizations). All nurses are responsible for knowing and understanding the standards of nursing practice. Knowledge can be gained through familiarizing yourself with ANA standards, specialty practice standards (as applicable), federal agency guidelines and regulations, and your state nurse practice act, job description, employment contract, and the institution's employment policies and procedures. Standards may apply to both nursing practice/care and professional performance. Standards may be used in clinical nursing practice to assess the quality of nursing care, manage risk associated with the practice of nursing, address issues related to cost of and access to care, evaluate competence, and assess liability, negligence, and malpractice.

Guidelines are "recommendations for patient management that identify and or support the use of a range of patient care interventions and approaches. Individual groups utilize varying definitions of guidelines" (ANA, 1998b, p. 3). They provide the nurse with a means to meet a specific standard of practice. A guideline is not designed to replace a standard, but rather can be used to provide some of the scientific basis for establishing a specific standard. Guidelines may be developed by an institution, an organization, or a specialty component within an organization or institution to identify components of practice for a specific group (such as cancer screening guidelines for advanced practice nurses working in a cancer prevention clinic).

It is often necessary to differentiate standards from guidelines, because this terminology is a common source of confusion. Table 1-1-1 provides clarification.

Legal Issues

It is difficult to keep abreast of all the laws governing nursing practice. General practice guidelines to follow to protect against legal ramifications are given in Table 1-1-2.

Ethical Issues

Important areas for ethical decision-making include informed consent, withholding or withdrawing treatment, and resource allocation. Additional issues include such areas as access to and allocation of managed care and services; end-of-life care, including palliative care, advance directives, and do-not-

Table 1-1-1. Standards Versus Guidelines

STANDARDS	GUIDELINES
1. Describe professional responsibilities.	1. Describe patient management.
2. Provide direction for practice.	2. Provide direction for practice.
3. Base them on professional values and priorities.	3. Based on current scientific evidence and expert opinion.
4. Focus on the provider.	4. Focus on the care of a patient.
5. Focus on the process.	5. Focus on outcomes.
6. Apply to care in all settings.	6. Apply to care in a specific setting.
7. Write in broad terms.	7. Write in specific terms.
8. Apply to general and specialty practice.	8. These may apply only to a specialty practice.
9. Provide a framework for evaluation.	9. Include assessment criteria, parameters for diagnosis and intervention, and expected outcomes.
10. Design standards to endure over time.	10. Update frequently.

Table 1-1-2. Avoiding Legal Troubles

1. Practice within the scope of your knowledge, abilities, and training.
2. Know the nursing standards that apply to your scope of practice (regardless of how remote they may seem to be).
3. Communicate openly and effectively with your patient, his family, your professional colleagues, and all other institutional personnel.
4. Be caring and compassionate while remaining professional.
5. Continually update your skills and knowledge.
6. Treat all patients and family members with respect.
7. Tell the truth/be honest.
8. Share appropriate information with the patient and family.
9. Participate in your professional organization.
10. Document care precisely and concisely and in a timely fashion.
11. Recognize that some individuals are more likely to sue than others (see Guido, 1997).
12. Recognize that you as a nurse may display traits that are more likely to trigger a lawsuit (Guido, 1997).

resuscitate orders; and ethical issues related to the genetic revolution. Each of these issues requires the nurse to examine the ethical principles of autonomy, nonmaleficence, beneficence, justice, veracity, and fidelity; to identify which principles are involved in the ethical dilemma; and to decide which principle takes precedence in the decision-making. There is no definitive set of guidelines on which to base these types of decisions. Table 1-1-3 lists ethical principles, their definitions, and rules of care to assist health care providers in making such decisions.

Documentation

Methods of charting include narrative formats, flow charts and other forms, and methods of organizing elements of care, including interventions and responses to them. Table 1-1-4 lists important issues in documentation.

 CLINICAL PEARLS

○ Standards of nursing practice provide consistent direction for practice and a framework for the evaluation of that practice.

Table 1-1-3. Ethical Principles, Definitions, and Care

PRINCIPLE	DEFINITION	RULES OF CARE
Autonomy	The obligation to respect a competent individual's right to make his or her own decisions	Avoid coercion, be respectful, maintain confidentiality, ensure informed consent/refusal of care.
Nonmaleficence	The obligation to refrain from causing harm	Do no harm.
Beneficence	The obligation to provide positive benefit to another	Be caring, kind, compassionate, and competent.
Justice	The obligation to be fair and just in providing care and allocating resources	Provide appropriate care regardless of individual/personal differences.
Veracity	The obligation to tell the truth	Do not intentionally mislead patients or others.
Fidelity	The obligation to be faithful to commitments	Maintain loyalty to obligations, commitments, and agreements made as a component of professional practice.

Table 1-1-4. Special Issues in Documentation

METHOD	ISSUES
Phone	There is a legal responsibility for any advice given.
	Follow all institution policies/protocols for documentation.
	A telephone log is an essential tool and should include all aspects of the information communicated and to whom it was communicated.
Fax	Need to assure confidentiality of faxed material.
	Contact the recipient before faxing.
	Triple-check the fax number: before dialing, on the fax display, and before sending.
	Have the recipient confirm receipt of materials.
Computer	Computer records are legitimate forms of documentation.
	Double-check all entries.
	Ensure patient confidentiality: log off promptly, do not share passwords, minimize time information is displayed on the computer screen, promptly pick up all printouts.
	Ensure that backup files are maintained.

- Whenever there is a controversy between an institutional standard and a professional standard, it is always safer legally to follow the professional standard.
- A state's Nurse Practice Act is enacted by the state legislature and defines nursing practice and establishes standards for nursing practice within that state only.
- Understanding ethical principles is integral to comprehensive nursing practice.
- Documentation has multiple principles and requirements that must be met to ensure legal compliance.
- Various methods of documentation exist; finding the right method for an institution is essential for quality nursing practice.

Vital Parameters

Section 2

Patricia Graham

OVERVIEW

Vital parameters can provide much important information about a patient's physical and emotional state. The vital parameters discussed in this section include heart rate/pulse, blood pressure, respiration, temperature, and urine output.

PRINCIPLES OF CARE
Heart Rate/Pulse

Heart rate, defined as the number of times that the ventricles contract each minute, governs the frequency with which blood is ejected from the heart. Pulse, a bounding of blood as it is pumped into the arteries, is palpable at various sites in the body. In healthy individuals, heart rate and pulse rate are the same, but variations may occur, particularly when cardiovascular pathology is present. For this reason, on initial assessment, and in persons with known cardiovascular pathology, it is important to compare apical and radial pulse rates. The normal heart rate may vary widely between individuals; the normal range is between 60 and 100 beats/min, with an average of 80 beats/min.

Heart rate is a major determinant of cardiac output. Cardiac output normally ranges from 4 to 8 L/min and is a product of stroke volume times the heart rate. Stroke volume is the amount of blood ejected with each beat; in adults, stroke volume is normally approximately 70 mL. Because an increase or decrease in heart rate usually reflects changes in cardiac output, heart rate must be evaluated frequently.

Various factors influence regulation of heart rate, including actions of the sympathetic and parasympathetic nervous systems, baroreceptors, and stretch receptors. Sympathetic nervous system stimulation, triggered by emotions such as fear, anxiety, and excitement, causes the heart rate to increase. Increased metabolic needs (e.g., as in fever) or decreased nutrients (e.g., oxygen and glucose) to the cells can also trigger sympathetic activity.

Other factors that can increase heart rate include pain, hemorrhage, and certain drugs. Postural changes can cause a variation in heart rate. Parasympathetic stimulation results in decreased heart rate.

The baroreceptors (sensory nerve endings) in the aortic arch and carotid arteries influence heart rate in the following manner. The receptors note changes in blood pressure and transmit this information to the central nervous system. A decrease in blood pressure causes sympathetic activation and parasympathetic inhibition, resulting in increased heart rate. This response is known as the Bainbridge reflex. In contrast, an increase in blood pressure causes parasympathetic stimulation and results in a decreased heart rate.

Stretch receptors in the vena cavae and the right atrium react to pressure or volume changes. Reduced pressure, occurring in hypovolemia, results in sympathetic stimulation, which in turn increases heart rate and causes constriction of the peripheral blood vessels.

Heart rate can be measured by palpation or auscultation. The pulse is usually easily palpated at the radial artery. If the pulse is faint or irregular, then the apical pulse should be auscultated and counted for a full minute.

Blood Pressure

Blood pressure (systemic/arterial) is the lateral force on the walls of an artery by the pulsing blood under pressure from the heart. It represents the interrelationships of cardiac output, peripheral vascular resistance, blood volume, blood viscosity, and arterial elasticity. A change in any of these factors can cause a change in blood pressure. When cardiac output (i.e., heart rate × stroke volume) increases, more blood is pumped against the arterial walls, causing an increase in blood pressure. Cardiac output can be increased from an increase in heart rate, an increase in heart muscle contractility, or an increase in blood volume.

Changes in peripheral vascular resistance can make blood available to the major organs when needed. The smaller the lumen of a vessel, the greater is the peripheral resistance to blood flow. As this resistance rises, arterial blood pressure rises. As vessels dilate and resistance falls, the blood pressure drops.

Blood volume normally remains constant at about 5000 mL in adults.

Increased volume, as can occur during rapid infusion of IV fluids, causes blood pressure to rise. Decreased volume, as in hemorrhage and dehydration, causes blood pressure to fall. Blood viscosity, or thickness, is determined by the percentage of red blood cells (hematocrit) in the blood. When the hematocrit rises, the heart must contract more forcibly to push the more viscous blood through the system, and blood pressure rises. Adequate elasticity causes arteries to be easily distensible, preventing wide fluctuations in blood pressure. With age, the walls of the blood vessels tend to become less elastic, which creates greater resistance to blood flow and a rise in blood pressure.

Blood pressure is measured in millimeters of mercury (mm Hg) and recorded as a fraction. The numerator is the systolic pressure, which is the maximum pressure exerted on arterial walls when the left ventricle pushes blood into the aorta. The denominator, diastolic pressure, represents the point at which the heart rests between beats, thus creating the lowest pressure on arterial walls. Although blood pressure ranges vary in adults, the accepted norm is 120/80 mm Hg. A reading at or above 140/90 mm Hg is classified as stage one hypertension.

Traditionally, diastolic blood pressure has been of greater concern than systolic blood pressure in the assessment of hypertension. However, current research indicates that systolic blood pressure is more important when assessing hypertension in middle-aged and older adults. For more information on hypertension, see Chapter 15, Section 4.

Respiration

Respiration is the process used by the body to exchange gases between the atmosphere and the blood and cells. Four mechanisms are involved in the respiratory process:

1. Ventilation, the movement of gases in and out of the lungs
2. Diffusion, the movement of oxygen and carbon dioxide between the alveoli of the lung and the blood
3. Transport of oxygen and carbon dioxide to and from the cells
4. The regulatory process of breathing

The rate, depth, and rhythm of respiration indicate the quality of ventilation. Diffusion and perfusion can be assessed in part by measuring blood oxygen and carbon dioxide levels. Breathing is an involuntary activity regulated by the respiratory center in the brain. The center is influenced by changes in the oxygen and carbon dioxide levels in the blood. An increase in carbon dioxide in the blood causes an increase in the rate and depth of breathing. This results in the removal of excess carbon dioxide during expiration.

Chemoreceptors in the carotid artery and aorta are sensitive to low levels of arterial oxygen (hypoxemia). When arterial oxygen levels fall, these receptors send a message to the brain to increase the rate and depth of respiration. Persons with chronic lung disease have hypoxemia and hypercarbia (i.e., excessive carbon dioxide). In these persons, the elevated carbon dioxide level does not provide their stimulus to breathe; rather, the stimulus is provided by hypoxemia. For this reason, administration of high levels of oxygen can be fatal to persons with chronic lung disease, because it shuts off their stimulus to breathe.

Physical changes facilitate the process of breathing in the following ways. During inspiration, the respiratory center in the brain sends impulses along the phrenic nerve, causing the diaphragm to contract. The abdominal organs move downward and forward, increasing the length of the chest cavity to move air into the lungs. During expiration, the diaphragm relaxes, allowing the abdominal organs to return to their original positions. In a normal breath, about 500 mL of air is inhaled. This amount is referred to as the *tidal volume*.

Assessment of respiration includes the rate, rhythm, and depth. In healthy adults, respiratory rate ranges from about 12 to 20 breaths/min. Depth is described as shallow or deep. Periodically, it is normal for a person to inhale deeply or sigh, filling the lungs with more air than the amount inhaled in an average breath. The rhythm, or the amount of time between breaths, should be equal under normal conditions. Respirations are easy to assess, even more so if the patient does not know they are being counted. Becoming aware of one's breathing can cause a person to breathe unnaturally (faster, slower, or irregularly).

Changes in respirations can occur under certain conditions and in certain disease states. Factors that cause changes include exercise, anxiety, pain, smoking, and certain medications. Disease states and injuries affecting the respiratory center in the brain inhibit respiratory rate and rhythm. Cardiac and respiratory disorders often cause changes in respiratory status. A person with anemia breathes more rapidly in an attempt to increase oxygen transport to the cells.

Temperature

Body temperature represents the difference between heat production and heat loss. The body's core temperature (temperature of the deep tissues) remains relatively constant through the action of the thermoregulatory center in the hypothalamus. The center receives messages from receptors throughout the body to produce or conserve body heat or to increase heat loss.

Normally, the hypothalamus maintains a setpoint within a range of 96.6°F to 99.3°F (35.9°C to 37.4°C). Body temperature regulation is under behavioral control to some extent; for example, a person sensing cold can put on a warm wrap, and an overheated person can remove clothing or use a fan to hasten evaporation. Those unable to care for themselves are at risk for the effects of extreme environmental temperatures.

Heat is produced by metabolism, the chemical reaction occurring in all body cells. Food is the primary food source for metabolism. The amount of energy used for metabolism is termed the *basal metabolic rate* (BMR). Heat is lost through sweating, vasodilation, and inhibition of heat production. Heat conservation occurs through vasoconstriction, voluntary muscle contraction, and shivering.

Mechanisms of heat loss include radiation, conduction, convection and evaporation. Radiation accounts for about 50% of heat loss from the skin, as heat rays move from a warmer environment (the body) to a cooler room. When a person is overheated, cardiac output increases, causing increased blood flow to the skin and allowing body heat to be lost through radiation. When the surrounding areas are warmer than the skin, the body absorbs heat through radiation.

Conduction is the transfer of heat from one object to another. For example, a person sitting on a cold chair will experience a transfer of body heat to the chair. Convection is the loss of heat through air currents following conduction of body heat to the air. An individual constantly loses heat from evaporation, which accounts for a total fluid loss of 600 to 900 mL/day. When a person is overheated or in a hot environment, increased sweating promotes further evaporation of heat from the body.

Several factors influence body temperature; these include individual factors such as age, body size, diurnal variations, gender, stress, and activity level, as well as environmental factors. Older adults lose some of their thermoregulatory control and are at increased risk for harm from temperature extremes.

A person's size also affects body temperature. Body fat provides insulation, thus an obese person loses less heat in a cool room than a thin person. Most persons experience diurnal fluctuations with lower body temperature in the morning and a higher temperature in the afternoon and evening. Women usually experience greater temperature fluctuation than do men because of hormonal shifts during the menstrual cycle.

Stress can have an effect on temperature as a result of activity in the sympathetic and parasympathetic nervous systems. Physiologic changes increase metabolism, which increases heat production and leads to a rise in body temperature. Physical exercise also increases metabolism, causing increased heat production and a rise in temperature. Prolonged strenuous exercise can raise body temperature to as high as 105.8°F (41°C).

Excessively cold or warm environmental temperatures affect body temperature. Prolonged exposure to cold through air or submersion can lead to hypothermia, defined as core body temperature below 95°F (35°C). Because the metabolic rate slows greatly in hypothermia, in some cases (e.g., during long surgical procedures) hypothermia is intentionally induced, to reduce the body's need for oxygen. Excessive heat exposure will cause an increase in body temperature. High temperatures become increasingly dangerous as humidity increases, making it impossible for individuals to lose heat through sweating and evaporation.

Urine Output

The measurement of urine output is an extremely valuable means of assessing health status. An improperly functioning urinary system will eventually affect all organ systems. In an adult, normal urine output averages about 1 mL/kg of body weight/hour, 40 to 80 mL/hr and 1500 mL/24 hr. Stress may diminish output to 30 to 50 mL/hr. A decrease in normal output can signal kidney, bladder, cardiovascular disease, hypovolemia or dehydration.

The various factors that can alter urine output include:
- Amount of fluid intake
- Blood volume
- Fluid losses from skin, lungs, or gastrointestinal tract
- Renal concentration ability
- Hormonal influences (aldosterone and antidiuretic hormone)

Certain pathologic conditions also affect urine output. Some are temporary and reversible, whereas others are chronic. *Reversible or treatable conditions* include:
- Urinary tract infection
- Hemorrhage
- Shock
- Burns

- Obstruction in the bladder, ureter, or urethra
- Prostatic hypertrophy
- Myocardial infarction
- Congestive heart failure
- Hypertension
  Chronic, irreversible conditions include:
- Renal failure
- Kidney damage as a result of systemic disease, such as diabetes
- Damage from nephrotoxic agents

DECISION-MAKING
Measurement of Vital Parameters
Heart Rate

Heart rate should be assessed frequently to detect early changes in hemodynamics. This can be done by palpating the pulse. If the pulse is irregular, then the apical rate should be auscultated for a full minute.

Measuring Pulse. Pulses are best palpated over the carotid, brachial, radial, femoral, popliteal, dorsalis pedis, and posterior tibial arteries, all sites close to the body surface. Use the distal pads of the second and third fingers for pulse palpation. The thumb can also be used. It is particularly useful in assessing the brachial and femoral pulses, because these have a tendency to move when probed by the fingers. Pulses are most easily palpated over bony prominences. Press firmly, but not so firmly as to occlude the artery.

Pulse rate is determined by counting the pulsations for 30 seconds and then multiplying by 2. *Normal resting pulse rate ranges from 60 to 90 beats/min.* The pulse rhythm should be regular. If it is irregular, assess for a consistent, repeated pattern. If the pattern is consistently irregular (e.g., pulsus bigeminus), document the rhythm as "regularly irregular." If the pulse is patternless and unpredictable, document the rhythm as "irregularly irregular." Irregular, weak, or very slow or fast pulse rates are associated with certain conditions (Table 1-2-1).

In a patient who has sustained shock, the locations in which pulses are palpable can provide information about the patient's blood pressure status. A palpable radial pulse correlates with a systolic blood pressure of at least 80 mm Hg; a palpable femoral pulse (with the loss of the radial pulse) correlates with a systolic blood pressure of 70 mm Hg; and a palpable carotid pulse (with the loss of the femoral and radial pulses) correlates with a systolic blood pressure of 60 mm Hg.

Measuring Apical Rate. With the patient supine or seated, apply the stethoscope over the apex of the heart. Listen for normal S_1 (closure of the mitral and tricuspid valves) and S_2 (closure of the aortic and pulmonic valves) heart sounds. The S_1 sound is described as "lub," and the S_2 as "dub" (with "lub-dub" representing 1 heart beat). Both produce high-pitched sounds, so be sure to use the diaphragm of the stethoscope, which best assesses high-pitched sounds. Count for 1 full minute while simultaneously palpating the radial pulse. If the apical rate is greater than the radial rate, the condition is called a *pulse deficit.* This occurs with cardiac dysrhythmias such as premature ventricular contractions, in which heart contractions are weak and blood flow does not perfuse adequately to the periphery.

Table 1-2-1. Arterial Pulse Abnormalities

ABNORMALITY	DESCRIPTION	ASSOCIATED CONDITION
Bounding pulse	Increased pulse pressure (difference between systolic and diastolic pressure). Reaches a higher intensity than normal.	Due to shortened ventricular systole and reduced peripheral pressure. Seen in atherosclerosis, aortic rigidity, fever, anemia, hyperthyroidism, anxiety, and exercise.
Labile pulse	Normal when resting, but increases on standing or sitting.	May be due to decreases in stroke volume caused by hypovolemia, or left ventricular dysfunction. May be a normal finding.
Bradycardia	Pulse rate <60 beats/minute	Usually reflective of a threat to cardiac output. Seen in hypothermia, drug intoxication, hypothyroidism, and impaired cardiac conduction. A rate of 40–60 is a normal finding in highly conditioned athletes.
Tachycardia	Pulse rate >100 beats/minute	Usually due to an increase in metabolic rate (fever), pain, anxiety, fear, hypoxemia, or anemia. Also due to reductions in stroke volume (in, e.g., shock states and heart disease).
Pulsus alternans	A weak pulse alternating with a strong one, with a regular rate.	Left ventricular failure.
Pulsus biferiens	Two strong beats followed by a pause, in a repeated pattern.	Aortic regurgitation alone or with aortic stenosis.
Pulsus bigeminus	Two pulse beats followed by a pause, in a repeated pattern.	Due to a normal pulsation followed by a premature ventricular contraction.
Pulsus differens	Unequal pulses between the left and right extremities.	A result of impaired circulation, usually from a local unilateral obstruction.
Pulsus paradoxus	Pulse strength decreases on inspiration and increases on expiration.	May be seen with bronchial asthma, emphysema, pericardial effusion, constrictive pericarditis, and cardiac tamponade.
Water-hammer pulse (Corrigan's pulse)	A short powerful, jerky beat that suddenly collapses.	Seen with aortic regurgitation as the force of blood ejected from the enlarged ventricle produces the powerful beat. The collapse is due to the incompetent valve failing to support the blood.

Respiration

The vital parameters are usually measured at the same time. It is common practice to keep the hand on the pulse while counting respirations in an attempt to keep the patient unaware that respirations are being counted. With the fingers on the pulse, after taking the pulse count, note the rise and fall of the patient's chest with each inspiration/expiration.

Count the number of respiratory cycles in 30 seconds and multiply by two to get the rate per minute. Count for 1 full minute if respirations are irregular. Record the rate, quality, and character of respirations according to your agency's policy.

Normal respiratory rate should be between 12 and 20 breaths/min. The ratio of respirations to heartbeats is approximately 1:4. Chest expansion should be symmetrical bilaterally.

Differentiate between dyspnea and orthopnea (shortness of breath that increases or begins when the patient lies back). Also evaluate respiratory rhythm. *Tachypnea* is defined as a persistent rate of 25 breaths/min or greater; *bradypnea*, as a rate below 12 breaths/min. Respiratory rhythms associated with disorders include the following:

- *Hyperpnea*, or *hyperventilation*, describes a respiratory rate exceeding 20 breaths/min but with deep, laborious breathing. Hyperpnea can be caused by exercise or anxiety, as well as by central nervous system and metabolic disorders.
- *Cheyne-Stokes respirations*, or periodic breathing, is a pattern of intervals of apnea followed by crescendo/decrescendo respirations. This pattern may be seen in patients with drug intoxication or serious brain injury.
- *Kussmaul's respirations* are very rapid and deep; associated with metabolic acidosis.
- *Biot's respirations* are irregular in depth with interspersed periods of apnea without pattern. This rhythm is associated with increased intracranial pressure affecting the medulla or with drug intoxication. It is referred to as *ataxic* in a more severe state.

Blood Pressure

Blood pressure should be measured bilaterally (i.e., in both arms) at least on admission. Have the patient rest 5 or more minutes before proceeding. With the patient either seated or supine, position the forearm, supported, at the level of the heart, with the palm facing up.

Choosing and Applying the Cuff. Be sure to choose the correct-size cuff for the patient. The cuff's width should be one third to one half the circumference of the limb; the bladder should be about 80% of the limb circumference, not quite large enough to completely encircle the limb. A too-wide cuff will produce a falsely low measurement, and a too-narrow cuff will produce a falsely high measurement. If a large cuff is unavailable for an obese patient, place a standard cuff around the patient's forearm and auscultate the radial artery.

When applying the blood pressure cuff, place the center of the bladder over the brachial artery with the lower edge 2 to 3 cm above the antecubital crease. Wrap the cuff snugly; a loose-fitting cuff will give an inaccurate diastolic reading.

Taking the Measurement. Palpate systolic blood pressure first, to decrease the risk of inaccuracy when using the stethoscope. To do so, palpate the brachial pulse while inflating the cuff to 30 mm Hg above the point where the pulse disappears. Slowly deflate the cuff until you once again feel the pulse. This point is the palpable systolic blood pressure. Deflate the cuff and wait 30 seconds.

Next, place the bell of the stethoscope over the brachial artery and inflate the cuff to 30 mm Hg above the palpated systolic blood pressure. *The bell is more effective in transmitting the low-pitched sounds of turbulent blood flow (Korotkoff sounds) produced in the arteries.*

Release the valve slowly, allowing the pressure gauge to fall. Note the point at which you hear the first faint, but clear, sound. Record this as the systolic pressure. Continue deflating the cuff until the sound disappears. Record this as the diastolic pressure. Deflate the cuff completely. Wait 30 to 60 seconds, then recheck the readings. Avoid repeated cuff inflations, which can cause venous congestion and produce inaccurate measurements.

Record both measurements. *Normal systolic pressure should be between 100 and 140 mm Hg; normal diastolic pressure, between 60 and 90 mm Hg.* Note that measurements may vary by as much as 10 mm Hg between arms, with readings tending to be higher in the right arm. The higher reading should be accepted as the closest to the true pressure. A difference of 10 to 15 mm Hg may be indicative of arterial compression or obstruction on the side with the lower pressure, reflecting inhibited blood flow.

When Korotkoff sounds are not audible, a *Doppler flowmeter* may be placed over the radial artery to obtain systolic pressure measurements in the same manner as with the bell of the stethoscope.

Patients who are taking antihypertensive medication, exhibiting signs of dehydration, or complaining of fainting or dizziness should be assessed for *postural*, or *orthostatic*, *hypotension*. This is a decrease in systolic blood pressure of 15 to 20 mm Hg or more with an increase in heart rate associated with rising from a supine to a sitting or standing position. The procedure involves taking and comparing blood pressure measurements with the patient supine, then sitting, and then standing, waiting 1 to 3 minutes between position changes.

Mean arterial pressure (MAP) should also be measured, because it is an indicator of organ perfusion. A MAP below 60 mm Hg indicates that the vital organs are not being perfused. The following formula is used to determine MAP:

$$\text{MAP} = [\text{systolic BP} + (2 \times \text{diastolic BP})] \div 3.$$

Diastolic pressure measurements may be undetermined in certain cases, such as in patients with aortic regurgitation where the sounds of regurgitation do not disappear, as well as in patients with artificial valves.

Temperature

Devices for measuring body temperature include mercury in glass, electronic, and disposable thermometers. The mercury in glass thermometer is the oldest type and is highly reliable. Disadvantages include breakability and possible exposure to a toxic substance (mercury). Electronic temperature measurement of the tympanic membrane is currently preferred in many settings. This approach is accessible, noninvasive, and comfortable and provides an accurate core reading when done correctly. The presence of ear infection or cerumen impaction may distort temperature readings; in these cases, an alternate method should be used. Electronic oral thermometers are quick and easy to use; probes are available for oral, axillary, and rectal use. Disposable thermometers designed for one-time oral or axillary measurement are available, as are temperature-sensitive patches for placement on the forehead or abdomen. To convert degrees Celsius (C) (Centigrade) to degrees Fahrenheit (F), multiply the number of degrees C by $\frac{9}{5}$ and add 32 to the result. To convert F to C, subtract 32 from the number of degrees F and multiply the difference by $\frac{5}{9}$.

The body's core temperature remains fairly constant, but surface temperatures vary as heat is lost to the environment. The *average oral temperature is 98.6°F (37°C)*, but normal temperatures vary among individuals. In most clinical settings, an *oral temperature above 101°F (38°C) is defined as fever.* This value detects disorders that produce fever in almost all patients.

Using a Glass Thermometer

Oral Temperature. If the patient has had hot foods or liquids or has smoked, wait 30 minutes or use a different site. Using a strong wrist movement, shake the thermometer down until the mercury reaches 95°F (36°C). Cover the thermometer with a plastic sheath according to your agency's policy. Place the thermometer under the patient's tongue and instruct the patient to keep the mouth closed. Leave the thermometer in place for 3 minutes or according to your agency's policy. Remove the thermometer and discard the plastic sheath. Read the temperature on the thermometer and inform the patient of the reading. Record findings according to your agency's policy.

Axillary Temperature. Temperatures measured in the axillae are approximately 1°F lower than those measured orally. Place the thermometer into the center of the patient's axilla, lower the patient's arm over the axilla, and place the arm across the patient's chest. Instruct the patient to hold the arm in place. Leave the thermometer in place for 5 to 10 minutes or according to your agency's policy.

Rectal Temperature. Rectal temperatures are approximately ½ to 1°F higher than oral temperatures. Assist the patient into Sims position. Keeping the patient covered, expose the anal area. Dip the stubby end of the rectal thermometer into water-soluble lubricant. Separate the patient's buttocks and gently insert the thermometer into the anus. If you feel resistance, do not force the thermometer. Hold the thermometer in place for 3 minutes or according to your agency's policy.

Using an Electronic Thermometer. Remove the thermometer pack from the charging unit. Lift the probe, and slide the plastic cover over the probe until it locks in place. Place the probe at the chosen site in the same manner as for a glass thermometer. Leave the probe in place until the device beeps. The temperature is displayed within 15 to 60 seconds, depending on the model, in both Fahrenheit and Celsius. Remove the probe and discard the plastic sheath.

Using a Tympanic Membrane Thermometer. Tympanic membrane thermometers use infrared technology and are fast, easy and reliable if used correctly. Ear temperature accurately reflects body temperature, as the tympanic membrane shares the same blood supply as the hypothalamus in the brain.

Attach the tympanic probe cover to the thermometer unit. Insert the probe into the external opening of the ear canal with gentle pressure; do not occlude the canal. The temperature reading is obtained in approximately 2 seconds. Remove the thermometer when the reading is displayed, then remove the cover and discard it.

Urine Output

Urine output should be measured every 2 to 4 hours in patients with low cardiac output states, such as hypovolemia, heart failure, and postmyocardial infarction, as well as those with renal insufficiency and acute renal failure. It should be measured more frequently in stable patients who develop vomiting or diarrhea. A gain or loss of 1 lb of body weight is equal to a gain or loss of 500 mL of fluid.

Measurements below 0.5 mL/kg/hr for 2 or more consecutive hours are significant. This is a more precise method of assessing the adequacy of urine output over the standard 30 mL/hr. Because this method takes body size into account, the patient's weight must be known. If you are measuring UOP every 4 hours, on the fourth hour measure the urine in whatever collection device you may be using (e.g., urine hat, Foley bag) and divide the total amount of urine by 4 to determine the patient's hourly output. Report an output below 0.5 mL/kg/hr to the patient's primary care provider.

Urine output below 400 mL/24 hr is called *oliguria*; that below 100 mL/24 hr is *anuria*. These findings are seen in patients with renal insufficiency or failure. Urine output above 200 mL/hr for 2 or more consecutive hours can be significant and should be investigated. An output exceeding 3 L/24 hr, called *polyuria*, is seen in patients with diabetes insipidus and diabetes mellitus and can be caused by excessive intravenous fluid administration.

Output measurements should be closely monitored following removal of an indwelling (Foley) catheter. If the patient has not voided by 6 hours after catheter removal, then recatheterization may be necessary.

CLINICAL PEARLS

○ The thumb can be used to palpate pulses, especially the brachial and femoral pulses, which have a tendency to move.
○ A "regularly irregular" pulse is one that has an irregular but consistently repeating pattern.
○ An "irregularly irregular" pulse is one that is patternless and unpredictable.
○ When determining the correct cuff size for blood pressure measurements, make sure that the cuff bladder encircles at least 80% of the patient's arm.
○ Orthostatic (postural) hypotension is a decrease in systolic blood pressure of more than 15 to 20 mm Hg associated with rising from a supine to sitting or standing position.
○ Axillary temperatures are approximately 1°F lower than oral temperatures.

Expedited Physical Assessment

Section 3   Patricia Catalano

OVERVIEW

Assessment skills play a key role in nursing practice. This is partly because today's patients are more acutely ill and are discharged to outpatient settings much earlier than they were in the past. The expedited physical assessment provides a focused, systematic approach to completing a physical examination.

PRINCIPLES OF CARE

Expedited physical assessment at the bedside focuses on the patient's primary diagnosis and response to the illness. It is the acute care nurse's challenge to identify the patient's individual needs, paying particular attention to those with highest priority. The nurse at the bedside should perform an accurate assessment and document findings according to the agency's policies and procedures, standards of care and practice, and individual unit protocols for patient assessment. Documentation should enhance continuity of care by providing the opportunity for other members of the health care team to evaluate the patient's progression.

DECISION-MAKING
Components of the Expedited Physical Assessment
General Appearance

Begin the assessment by simply looking at the patient. Observe the patient's general appearance and behaviors, noting any changes, such as shortness of breath, restlessness, altered mental status, and complaints of pain. Assessing the patient's orientation to person, place, and time and also short-term memory can provide important clues as to any memory deficit. Investigate any complaints of pain that the patient may express. You can help identify the cause of the pain by assessing pain characteristics. One effective tool in gathering precise information about the patient's pain is the *PQRST* mnemonic (Table 1-3-1).

Systems Review
Integumentary System

In the expedited physical assessment, priorities for integumentary assessment include evaluating skin color, temperature, integrity, turgor, and moisture.
Color. Inspect the pigmentation and general color of the skin, checking for mottling, cyanosis, or jaundice. Keep in mind that irregularities may be difficult to discern in a dark-skinned patient.

Table 1-3-1. PQRST Method for Pain Assessment

P = Provokes
  • What causes the pain?
  • What makes it better?
  • What makes it worse?

Q = Quality
  • What does the pain feel like?
  • Is it sharp?
  • Is it dull?
  • Is it stabbing?
  • Is it burning?
  • Is it crushing?
    (Try to let patients describe the pain; sometimes they say what they think you want to hear.)

R = Radiates
  • Where does the pain radiate?
  • Is it in one place?
  • Does it go anywhere else?
  • Did it start elsewhere and is now localized to one spot?

S = Severity
  • How severe is the pain on a scale of 1–10?
    (This is a difficult one, as the rating will differ from patient to patient.)

T = Time
  • What time did the pain start?
  • How long did it last?

Temperature. Palpate the skin to assess temperature, which can range from cool to warm. *Cool, moist skin* may reflect such changes as increased sympathetic nervous stimulation (i.e., anxiety, pain, stress response). *Warm skin* may reflect an increased metabolic rate related to disorders such as fever (from sepsis) or hyperthyroidism.

Integrity. Skin integrity may be affected by factors such as decreased blood flow to the tissues, edema, immobility, and invasive catheters.

- Evaluate sites of invasive catheters for signs of *infiltration* (inadvertent administration of a nonvesicant solution into surrounding tissue), such as swelling, tightness, discomfort, and burning at the site, and/or *phlebitis* (inflammation of the vein), such as redness, warmth, tenderness, and edema.
- Inspect dressings, wounds, and exposed suture lines for intactness and drainage. Describe drainage in terms of color, consistency, odor, and amount.
- Evaluate pressure sites for redness and breakdown (decubitus ulcers). Pressure points, such as the ears, scalp, scapulae, shoulders, iliac crests, sacrum, and heels, are especially susceptible to breakdown.

Turgor. Assessing turgor, a common method of evaluating hydration, is done by pinching the skin and observing for *tenting,* the tendency of the skin to remain in a "tent-like" position after it is released. Dehydrated skin will tent; hydrated skin should snap back briskly. Because elasticity of the skin decreases with aging, consider other methods of evaluating dehydration, such as intake and output measurement and daily weights, for elderly patients.

Moisture. Observe mucous membranes for moistness. Tacky mucous membranes may be an indication of dehydration, but dry mouth may also be a side effect of certain drugs (i.e., atropine), general anesthesia, or NPO status. In the well-hydrated patient, mucous membranes are moist and glistening.

Respiratory System

In the expedited physical assessment, priorities for respiratory system assessment are airway patency and gas exchange. This includes evaluation of respirations and breath sounds.

Respirations. Assess the rate, depth, and pattern of respiration, as well as the use of accessory muscles. The normal adult respiratory rate is 12 to 20 breaths/min. Breaths are normally even and regular with occasional sighs. Both rate and depth can be affected by pain, apprehension, anxiety, or awareness of being observed. The use of accessory muscles (in the neck, upper rib cage, clavicles, or shoulders) signals respiratory distress related to such conditions as airway obstruction, air trapping, and neuromuscular or respiratory disorders. Other signs and symptoms of respiratory distress include tachycardia, nasal flaring, cyanosis around the mouth, contraction of sternocleidomastoid muscles, and retraction of the suprasternal notch.

Lung Sounds. Lung auscultation is a reliable technique for identifying the presence of fluid, mucus, or obstruction in the respiratory tract. A common mistake made by nurses when auscultating the lungs is to start too low on the patient's chest. The apices of the lungs rise 2 to 4 cm above the level of the clavicles, and this is where auscultation should begin. Auscultate the anterior, lateral, and posterior lung fields to determine the presence of normal breath sounds, diminished or absent sounds, and adventitious sounds.

Diminished or *absent* breath sounds occur with shallow respirations, fluid accumulation, obstruction, or hyperinflation. A mass or fluid consolidation can cause amplified breath sounds.

Adventitious sounds indicate pathologic changes. They are unexpected noises superimposed on breath sounds, caused by air colliding with secretions or deflated airways. Common adventitious sounds include:

- *Crackles.* Caused by collapsed or fluid filled alveoli popping open, crackles are heard primarily on inhalation. They are classified as either fine or coarse and usually do not clear with coughing.
- *Rhonchi.* These low-pitched, snoring, rattling sounds are heard primarily on inhalation and occur when fluid partially blocks large airways.
- *Wheezes.* These high-pitched sounds, heard first on exhalation, occur when airflow is blocked.
- *Pleural friction rub.* This low-pitched, grating, rubbing sound is heard on both inhalation and exhalation. It results from pleural inflammation, which causes layers of pleura to rub together.

When completing the respiratory assessment, keep in mind these six important respiratory symptoms: cough, sputum production, dyspnea, hemoptysis, chest pain, wheezing.

Cardiovascular System

Priorities of cardiovascular system assessment are evaluating cardiac output and blood flow to the tissues. Assessment focuses on the skin and mucous membranes, nails, edema, peripheral pulses, heart sounds, and heart rhythm.

Skin and Mucous Membranes. Observe for cyanosis. *Central cyanosis* is a bluish discoloration resulting from a large amount of deoxygenated hemoglobin in the capillaries. In dark-skinned patients, cyanosis is most reliably observed in the tongue. In persons of light skin, cyanosis is observed in the lips, ear lobes, and oral mucous membranes. Patients with central cyanosis need oxygen. *Peripheral cyanosis* is a bluish discoloration in the extremities resulting from localized hypoxia due to poor circulation, reduced blood flow, congestive heart failure, or shock.

Nails. Assessing capillary refill time in the nails indicates the adequacy of blood flow to the tissues (peripheral perfusion). Normal refill time is less than 2 or 3 seconds; prolonged refill time indicates impaired perfusion.

Edema. Edema may be classified in several ways, including by location (i.e., presacral, pedal, pretibial), by character (i.e., dependent or pitting), and by severity (Table 1-3-2).

- Pitting edema is a common sign of congestive heart failure.
- Presacral edema may be found in bedridden patients and may lead to decubitus ulcers.
- *Anasarca* is severe generalized edema and ascites, as seen in severe congestive heart failure, liver cirrhosis, and nephrotic syndrome.

Table 1-3-2. Grading of Edema

DEPTH OF INDENTATION	GRADE
0–¼ inch	1+
¼–½ inch	2+
½–1 inch	3+
1 inch	4+

olor. Urine color can indicate various conditions:

ale: Dilute urine, overhydration, diuresis, diabetes insipidus

Amber, yellow, orange: Concentrated urine, dehydration, bilirubin

Green: Bacterial infection, some vitamins

Cloudy: Cells, bacteria, leukocytes, catheter sediment

Foamy: Proteinuria

(See Chapter 11, Section 5 for more detailed descriptions.)

Amount. Normal urine output in adults averages about 1 or 2 mL/kg of weight/24 hr. To accurately evaluate urine output, be sure to identify all forms of fluid intake (oral, parenteral) and output, including gastrointestinal system losses (i.e., diarrhea, nasogastric suction) and insensible losses (i.e. respiration, diaphoresis).

prapubic Area. Assess the suprapubic area for distention. In severe urinary tention, a visible bulge may be seen in the suprapubic area. The area will be m on palpation and dull to percussion.

erineum. Inspect the perineal area for rash, swelling, and discharge; infec-on may be linked to an indwelling urinary catheter.

Neurologic System

Priorities in neurologic assessment include mental status, language, motor esponse, and muscle strength.

Mental Status

The mental status assessment actually begins while assessing general appearance. It includes orientation, language, memory, motor response, and muscle strength.

The Conscious Patient

- **Orientation.** Always evaluate the patient's orientation in three spheres: person, place, and time. A patient beginning to have trouble with orientation can tell his or her name and where he or she is; it is the date or the time that tends to "slip away."
- **Language.** Listen to what the patient says, and how he or she says it. Evaluate the rhythm and clarity of speech. Assess comprehension by determining the patient's ability to follow instructions.
- **Memory.** In an expedited physical assessment, quickly evaluate long-term and short-term memory. Very few patients lose long-term memory; evaluate short-term memory by asking a simple question, such as "What did you have for breakfast today?"
- **Motor response.** Motor response provides a great deal of information on neurologic status. First, identify whether the patient moves normally or abnormally. The highest level of normal response is the ability to follow commands.
- **Muscle strength.** If the patient has normal motor movement (i.e., follows commands), the next step is to assess the strength of that movement. An objective description is important. Replace terms such as "some weakness in lower extremities" with a strength scale. Assess each joint's strength based on its active range of motion (ROM). Have the patient repeat each movement as you apply resistance. Grade muscle strength on a scale of 0 to 5: 0 = no contraction; 1 = slight contraction; 2 = full ROM against some resistance; 3 = full ROM; 4 = full ROM against some resistance; 5 = full ROM against full resistance. Grade muscle strength as a fraction, with the denominator always 5 and the numerator from 0 to 5.

Pulses. Palpate and compare pulses in terms of rate, rhyt
bilateral equality (the pulse on one side of the body compare
other side). Evaluate the radial pulses when checking nail
capillary refill time. Besides checking the apical and radial p
check the dorsalis pedis and posterior tibial pulses each shift. B
the pedal pulses (see Chapter 8, Section 2).

Heart Sounds. Auscultate for the normal S_1 and S_2 sounds, as
third or fourth heart sound (S_3 or S_4) (see Chapter 8, Section 1).

Heart Rhythm. Auscultate the apical pulse and palpate the
simultaneously for a full minute to evaluate rate and rhythm
document any regular or irregular irregularities, the latter being t
characteristic of atrial fibrillation.

Gastrointestinal System

The priorities of gastrointestinal system assessment include insp
abdomen; evaluating the gag, cough, and swallowing reflex; auscultat
sounds; and evaluating bowel function.

Abdomen. Inspect the abdomen for distention. Abdominal disten
hallmark of acute intestinal obstruction; a common, but potentially lit
ening illness. Abdominal distention in the presence of an enteral tu
indicate obstruction of the tube or slowed gastric emptying, either o
can lead to regurgitation and aspiration.

Gag, Cough, and Swallowing Reflex. Assess the presence of the gag,
and swallowing reflex in patients with decreased levels of consciousnes
do so, gently touch the back of the pharynx on each side; this should pr
a bilateral reflex response. Unequal or poor response may signal glossoph
geal or vagal nerve damage. Absence of this reflex increases the ri
aspiration and precludes oral feeding (O'Hannon-Nichols, 1998). Swalle
difficulties may result from decreased level of consciousness, oral obstru
and neurologic disorders, such as stroke or Parkinson's disease. Always
form a thorough mouth examination in a patient with an enteral tul
evaluate tube placement and identify possible nasopharyngeal or upper res
tory obstruction.

Bowel Sounds. Bowel sounds are caused by the movement of air and
through the small intestine. It may be sufficient to auscultate for bowel so
in only the right lower abdominal quadrant. Listen in each quadrant for 1
minute if bowel sounds are decreased. Normal bowel sounds vary but
usually high-pitched, gurgling noises, occurring irregularly (5 to 30 times
minute). Bowel sounds are not counted, thus a judgment is made whether
sounds are normal, hypoactive, or hyperactive (borborygmus).

Bowel Elimination/Function. To assess reported changes in bowel funct
inquire about the patient's usual pattern (stool color and consistency)
compare it to the current pattern. Healthy adults have a stool every 1 t
days. Illness may cause an alteration in the usual pattern of elimination. Bl
tarry stools may indicate melena or high iron content; pale stools may p
to liver or gall bladder problems.

Genitourinary System

Priorities of genitourinary system assessment include evaluating the uri
suprapubic area, and perineum.

Urine. Assess the color, amount and characteristics of urine.

Patient with an Altered Level of Consciousness

A change in level of consciousness (LOC) is the earliest and most sensitive indicator of a patient's altered neurologic status. The mental status evaluation for a patient with altered LOC involves assessing spontaneous activity, responses to verbal stimuli, and responses to painful stimuli. The Glasgow Coma Scale (see Neurologic Assessment Chapter 7, Section 1) is useful in assessing altered LOC.

Environmental Assessment

Priorities for environmental assessment include evaluating life support equipment, bedside monitoring techniques, and patient equipment, including tubings, suction, drains, and dressings. The focus is on providing a safe environment and delivering optimal care.

Life-Support Equipment. When administering oxygen by any delivery system, carefully inspect the entire oxygen—patient circuit—supply, flowmeter, tubing connections and patient's airway—each time that you are at the bedside. Supplied oxygen contains no water, and prolonged inhalation of air that is less than 100% humidified can cause mucosal drying and irritation. Therefore, when oxygen is prescribed, humidification should be a part of the oxygen delivery system.

Bedside Monitoring Techniques

Respiratory Monitoring. Pulse oximetry is a noninvasive method of measuring oxygen saturation (Sao_2). Assess whether the patient's Sao_2 is within prescribed parameters, and check the high and low alarm settings.

Cardiac Monitoring. If your patient has been placed on a telemetry monitor, assess for proper lead placement and rhythm analysis.

Patient Equipment. Verify that tubings, indwelling catheters, and drains are connected as ordered, and assess for intactness, security of connections, patency, and drainage. Evaluate peripheral and central lines for intactness, security of connections, expiration dates, patency, drip rate, and prescribed medications and solutions.

Suction Equipment. Evaluate the availability of suction equipment at the bedside, especially for those patients at high risk for the emergent need of suction equipment (e.g., those with aspiration pneumonia or dysphagia).

 CLINICAL PEARLS

○ While assessing the patient's general appearance, help decrease patient anxiety through verbal interactions, including simple explanations and reassurance where appropriate.

○ When assessing the lungs, remember that normal breath sounds vary among individuals.

○ To assess the peripheral pulses, use the third and fourth fingertips and palpate with gentle pressure.

○ If bowel sounds are not readily heard, listen for at least 2 to 5 minutes before declaring that bowel sounds are absent.

○ Before auscultating the abdomen of a patient with a nasogastric tube or another tube connected to suction, briefly clamp the tube or turn off the suction.

○ A change in the patient's LOC is the earliest and most sensitive indicator of altered neurologic status.

First Aid for Injuries

Section 4   Regina Medeiros ■ Sue Putnam

OVERVIEW

Injuries are the leading cause of death in persons age 44 years and under, and the third leading cause of death in all age groups. A seriously injured body responds predictably with compensatory mechanisms to maintain homeostasis. Once these mechanisms fail, a downward spiral toward death ensues.

The work of R. Adams Cowley in his shock trauma unit in Baltimore has clearly demonstrated that a time from injury to surgical intervention of less than 1 hour is associated with the greatest survival rate, approximately 85%. The purpose of first aid is to use this concept of "the golden hour" along with a systematic approach to recognize the presence of serious injury, prevent further injury, move the victim into the emergency medical system (EMS) and stabilize vital functions until EMS personnel take over.

This section discusses identification and care of the most commonly encountered first aid emergencies: altered mental status, anaphylaxis, bites and stings, burns, cervical spine injury, musculoskeletal injury, near-drowning and diving accidents, shock and bleeding, and soft tissue injury.

PRINCIPLES OF CARE
Systematic Approach

The initial actions for a trauma victim are the same for all health care providers regardless of level of education and licensure. The most experienced trauma surgeon will follow the same principles as a first aid provider. A specific diagnosis of the victim's injuries is not indicated at this time. Rather, a systematic, organized, and efficient plan of care will minimize the risk of causing further harm and optimize the likelihood of a positive outcome.

Scene Size-Up

Take the following initial steps before approaching the victim:
- Prepare *emotionally* for what you will see, especially if you do not normally work with trauma victims.
- Initiate appropriate *body substance isolation* (BSI); you may have to improvise.
- Look for *dangers*, such as traffic, gas or chemical leaks, fire, electrical lines, hostile bystanders or assailants, or falling objects. If you get hurt, you cannot help.
- Determine the *number of victims* (e.g., look in crowds, ditches, and vehicles).
- Determine the *mechanism of injury* (i.e., what forces are involved): for example, damage to the vehicle (e.g., steering wheel, windshield, front, back, side, rollover); distance of fall and type of surface that the victim fell on; speed of involved object or vehicle; penetration of knife, bullet, or other object; concentration and duration of exposure to heat or chemicals.
- Determine the need for and immediately call for any needed resources, manpower, or the EMS.

Cervical Spine Protection

Even relatively minor forces can result in a cervical spine injury. Because of the catastrophic potential for serious, possibly permanent impairment from cervical cord damage, any injury that involves impact or forces with the potential to be transmitted to the neck must be considered to be high risk for cervical injury and treated as such. Careful manual application of cervical immobilization should be done immediately to protect the neck (see Cervical Spine Injury in this section).

LOC and ABCDEF

This aspect of first aid is the heart of the early assessment and treatment of the victim. Its purpose is to identify immediate life-threatening problems and stabilize the victim until additional help arrives (Table 1-4-1). The first check of LOC is a rapid overview of the victim's neurologic status and provides a general impression of the seriousness of the situation. This is followed by a quick evaluation of the *airway* (**A**), *breathing* (**B**), and *circulatory status* (**C**), and more in-depth *neurologic* review (**D**, for disability). The victim is then *exposed* (**E**) in a situation involving major trauma so that all injuries can be found, and finally, action is taken to ensure that the victim does not become *hypothermic* (**F**, for Fahrenheit). Reassess the victim frequently for subtle changes.

Treatment

Treatment in first aid is limited to stabilizing vital functions in life-threatening situations. In situations where the victim is stable, take additional actions to enhance comfort (both physical and emotional) and prevent infection (e.g., careful washing of wounds). Specific treatments are addressed later in this section and in Table 1-4-1.

Information Gathering from the Victim and Bystanders

Gather information about the victim's medical history, any allergies, and events of the current situation now, because the victim could become unresponsive and unable to give information later. Valuable information may include any signs and symptoms that the victim is experiencing, current medications used, pertinent past medical history, last food intake, and events leading up to the current problem. If the victim is experiencing pain, ask what happened to cause the pain. What makes it worse? What is the quality of the pain; does it radiate or travel to other areas? On a scale from 1 to 10, what is the severity of the pain and how long has it been hurting?

DECISION-MAKING
Altered Mental Status

Alterations in mental status may range from very subtle and vague to profound. Any alteration is abnormal and should be evaluated for possible illness or injury. Symptoms can be confusing and sometimes even overlooked. Common causes of altered mental status include closed head injury, epilepsy, tumors, respiratory insufficiency, metabolic disturbances, drug toxicity or overdose, poisons, hypertensive encephalopathy, cardiac arrest, stroke, shock (all

Table 1-4-1. Assessment and Treatment of the Victim

STEP	LOOK FOR	WARNING	ACTION
Level of consciousness	*Alert,* confused, combative, lethargic, pain, responsive, unresponsive, painful appearance, agitated, anxious	Anything other than normal is ominous and EMS activation should be considered.	Call 911 if abnormal or if the situation appears serious.
Airway	*Open,* clear, gurgling, snoring, stridor, wheezing, absence of sound	Caution! No sound of air movement may indicate complete airway obstruction.	Manually open the airway with the chin-lift or jaw-thrust technique while maintaining cervical spine control
Breathing	*Equal chest movement, good chest rise,* unilateral chest movement, paradoxical motion, crepitus, grating sounds, inadequate tidal volume, increased effort or respiratory distress, intercostal retractions, abnormal respiratory rate.	Consider calling EMS activation if findings are anything other than normal.	Ensure an open airway. If indicated or if tidal volume or respirations are inadequate, use mouth-to-mask or rescue breathing, or otherwise assist breathing with available equipment and oxygen.
Circulation	*Pink, warm skin and strong pulses;* cool, diaphoretic skin; mottled skin; weak, rapid pulse; absence of radial pulse; weak carotid pulse. Look for bleeding and hemorrhage	Anything other than normal may indicate shock and inadequate tissue perfusion. Blunt injuries to the abdomen and pelvis can cause massive internal bleeding.	Perform CPR if pulseless. Stop any active bleeding using direct pressure. Remember to use BSI precautions.
Disability	Pupil response *equal and reactive to light.* Is the patient alert and oriented to person, place and time?	Be alert to changes in pupils, slurred speech, or disorientation.	
Expose	All areas of the body should be exposed and checked for injury if dealing with a major trauma victim.	Life-threatening injuries can be easily missed in victims of multiple trauma.	Stop major bleeding. Cover wounds.
Fahrenheit (Temperature)	Cool skin, shivering	Hypothermia is common in injured victims even in warm climates.	Cover patient with a blanket.

types), dementia, encephalitis, meningitis, and fever. A successful patient outcome may depend on your astute observational skills and ability to get the victim definitive treatment.

The goals of emergency care are to recognize the presence of neurologic deficit, establish a baseline, protect the victim from further deterioration (as able), and arrange transport to a hospital.

At the scene, survey and ensure victim safety. Initiate BSI and consider cervical spine injury and immobilize if needed. Assess LOC and ABCDEF. If you detect abnormal findings, take immediate action as outlined in Table 1-4-1 and call EMS. If the victim is stable, then continue the assessment, closely observing for the specific findings listed in Table 1-4-2.

If any specific findings are positive and not quickly correctable (except for chronic and stable dementia), *call EMS (911) and support basic life functions until EMS arrives.* Ensure adequate airway, breathing, and circulation. If trauma is ruled out, place the victim in the "recovery position" on his or her side. Treat problems that are treatable; for example, warm (gently) a hypothermic victim and cool a hyperthermic victim, and give a sugar product (if the victim is alert with an intact gag reflex) to a victim with hypoglycemia.

Protect a victim experiencing a seizure from harming himself or herself. Do not place any object in the victim's mouth during a seizure.

Reassess LOC and ABCDEF frequently. Pay special attention to subtle neurologic changes. Comfort and reassure the victim and family.

Anaphylaxis

Anaphylaxis is a true emergency requiring immediate medical intervention. Causes of this extreme allergic reaction include:

- Insect bites or stings
- Inhaled toxins (e.g., chemicals, dusts, molds, pollen)
- Ingested substances (e.g., shellfish, spices, nuts, drugs)
- Absorbed allergens (chemicals through skin or mucosa)

Anaphylaxis is a rapidly progressive emergency. The key to saving a life is early recognition and treatment. The goals of emergency care are to rapidly initiate first aid measures and maintain basic life functions until EMS personnel arrive. At the scene, identify whether the allergen is still present (e.g., pollen, wasp, scorpion, chemical) and assess for safety. Institute BSI. Consider cervical spine injury if a fall was involved and immobilize as appropriate.

Perform a quick assessment of LOC and ABCDEF. If you detect any abnormal findings, take appropriate actions as outlined in Table 1-4-1. If

Table 1-4-2. Specific Findings in Altered Mental Status

LOC	Pupils: Look for size, equality, reactivity to light, extraocular movements, disconjugate gaze, and vision problems such as blurred or double vision.
	Mental: Be specific. Check orientation to person, place, time, events. Are answers normal, sluggish, slurred, confused, or accurate? Look for agitation, inappropriate laughing or crying, aphasia.
	Motor: Does the patient obey commands? Is there symmetry in movement, equal strength, localized pain, withdrawal from pain? Is decorticate or decerebrate posturing present? Is any flaccidity noted?
A/B	Is the airway open? Check for abnormal respiratory patterns such as bradypnea, apnea, Kussmaul's respirations, tachypnea, and shallow respirations.
Circulation	Check for tachycardia, bradycardia, unusually weak or strong pulse, irregularity. Check skin temperature for hypothermia or hyperthermia. Is the skin pale, red, dry, or wet?
Possible causes	A = acidosis, alcohol; E = epilepsy, encephalitis; I = infection; O = overdose; U = uremia (renal insufficiency); T = trauma, toxicity, tumor; I = insulin (diabetic problem); P = psychosis; S = stroke
Miscellaneous	Look for a Medic-Alert bracelet. Assess for signs of trauma, rash. Check the patient's medical history. Look for environmental hints, such as medicine bottles, alcohol containers, unusual odors, extreme hot or cold temperature, and diabetic supplies.

LOC, level of consciousness.

stable, or if the victim has a history of allergic reactions, monitor closely and assess for specific findings, including:

- **LOC.** Progressive decline; restlessness, anxiety, confusion, unresponsiveness
- **Skin.** Hives, pruritus, urticaria, erythema, edema of lips and tongue, cyanosis
- **Airway.** Tightness, wheezing. Stridor is an ominous sign; contact EMS
- **Breathing.** Progressive deterioration; shortness of breath, tachypnea, decreased tidal volume, increased respiratory effort, use of accessory muscles to breathe, apnea
- **Circulation.** Progressively worsening; developing signs of shock; tachycardia; irregular, weak, thready, or absent pulse.

If specific findings are positive and EMS has not been called, then call and initiate the following care:

- **Airway.** *If the victim is apneic,* then manually open airway with head tilt, chin lift. *If the victim is conscious,* then allow him or her to assume a position of comfort. *Do not* reach into the victim's mouth. Be gentle around the airway.
- **Breathing.** If apnea or inadequate air movement is present, begin rescue breathing. Rescue breathing may require greater than normal pressure to force air through edematous and narrowed airways.
- **Circulation.** Monitor continually. If you cannot palpate a pulse, begin CPR.
- **Medication.** If the victim has a history of allergic reactions, check for an emergency anaphylaxis kit. If local regulations allow, help the victim administer his or her own medication. (Laws vary with regard to the administration of medication to victims who are unable to self-administer.)
- **Reassess** LOC and ABCDEF continually.
- **Provide** emotional support for the victim and family.

Bites and Stings

Bites and stings sometimes occur when a human inadvertently enters an animal's or insect's territory. Local first aid treatment is usually all that is indicated. Rarely, a bite or sting can be severe and even life-threatening. The goals of care are to ensure safety, reduce anxiety, delay absorption of venom/toxins, and recognize early symptoms of anaphylaxis. *An anaphylactic reaction may develop.*

At the scene, survey for the attacking creature. Initiate BSI; consider cervical spine injury if a fall occurred and immobilize as necessary. Assess the LOC and ABCDEF. If findings are abnormal, call the EMS and take immediate action (see Table 1-4-1 for specific actions). If the victim is stable, monitor closely and observe for the specific findings listed in Table 1-4-3.

If you observe specific findings, then initiate care (Table 1-4-4). You may need to accompany the victim to the hospital for further care and assessment. If possible, bring the attacking animal with you to the hospital, but *do not touch or kill it yourself unless specifically trained to do so.* Reassess LOC–ABCD frequently. Anticipate deterioration, and support ABCs until EMS personnel arrive. Give emotional support to the victim and family. Assess for any secondary injuries that the victim may have sustained in an attempt to get away from the attacking creature.

Text continued on page 31

Table 1-4-3. Specific Assessment Findings

Bee, wasp, fire ant	Local pain
	Redness
	Edema
	Wheal
	Hives
	Itching
	Anaphylaxis may develop.
	Fire ants will continue biting until removed.
Tick	Often painless
	May find tick imbedded in skin.
	Associated with infection, Lyme Disease, Rocky Mountain spotted fever.
Spider	Brown recluse: Brown spider with violin shape on back
	No pain at first
	Redness, pain in 24 hours
	Blister in center of red area
	Chills
	Cellulitis
	Local necrosis develops after several days, may require skin grafting.
	Black widow: Black spider with red hourglass shape on the abdomen
	Local pain, redness, edema
	Muscle spasm
	Abdominal pain
	Nausea
	Vomiting
	Tachycardia
	Hypertension
	Diaphoresis
	Seizures
	Acetylcholine release
Snake	Pit vipers (rattlesnake, copperhead, water moccasin/cottonmouth):
	Triangular head
	Vertical elliptical eyes, fangs
	Scratch or fang marks
	Pain
	Edema
	Bruising
	Metallic taste
	Weak
	Nausea, vomiting, diarrhea
	Shock
	Death.
	Coral snake:
	Red stripes touch yellow ("red on yellow, kill a fellow, red on black, venom lack")
	Bite usually on finger or toe
	Neurotoxin—slowly developing respiratory and neuromuscular paralysis over 24–48 hr.
Dog, cat	Dogs: Crushing or tearing injuries. Risk for infection, rabies, nerve damage
	Cats: Puncture/scratching injuries. High risk for infection.
Marine sting (Jellyfish, corals, sea urchins, sting rays)	Severe local pain
	Edema
	Weakness
	Nausea, vomiting
	Dyspnea
	Tachycardia
	Shock (rare)

Table 1-4-4. Emergency Management for Bites and Stings

Bee, wasp, fire ant	Remove stinger by scraping gently with a knife or credit card; do not remove with tweezers.
	Wash with soap and water.
	Apply a cold pack.
	Observe for allergic reaction.
	Consider the need for a tetanus booster.
	Consider the need for EMS.
Tick	Remove imbedded head/body with tweezers (use care to get all mouth parts).
	Wash with soap and water.
	Apply antiseptic.
	Consider a tetanus booster.
	Monitor for developing symptoms of Lyme disease/Rocky Mountain spotted fever.
Spider	Medical attention is required.
	Wash the site.
	Reassure the victim.
	Brown Recluse: Antihistamines may reduce reaction.
	Black Widow: Monitor for hypertensive crisis, administer diazepam, calcium gluconate.
Snake	Medical attention is required–consider 911/EMS
	Reassure the victim (only 25% of pit viper bites inject venom).
	Keep the victim still.
	Wash the area with soap and water (copious amounts in coral snake bite).
	Position the bitten limb below the level of the heart.
	Remove watch, rings on the affected limb.
	Consider a loose constricting band proximal to bite only if time to hospital is greater than 5 hours (local protocols vary).
	Do not cut/suck out venom.
	Do not apply ice.
Dog, cat	Wash with soap and water.
	Apply antibiotic ointment in localized injury.
	Consider medical attention, infection risk, rabies.
Marine sting	Monitor LOC-ABC.
	Heat relieves pain and inactivates many marine venoms.
	Scrape off barbs with a knife or credit card
	Vinegar or rubbing alcohol may inactivate jellyfish venom.

Table 1-4-5. Ensuring Safety at the Burn Scene

THERMAL

Ensure scene safety for yourself and the victim. Remove the victim from an unsafe area only if trained to do so.

ELECTRICAL

Ensure scene safety. Do not touch the victim until the electrical power source is removed by person trained to do so.

CHEMICAL

Ensure scene safety. A person knowledgeable in chemical should determine safety. Wear protective clothing.

Burns

More than 2 million burn injuries are seen each year by medical profession-als in the U.S. Thus, the likelihood of encountering a burn victim is high. The severity of a burn is determined by analyzing the type, depth, extent, and comorbidity factors. The goals of emergency care are to ensure safety; stop the burning process; stabilize airway, breathing, and circulation; manage pain; and reduce the risk of infection.

At the scene, survey and identify the burn by type as either thermal, electrical, or chemical. Ensure safety according to the steps outlined in Table 1-4-5. Initiate BSI; consider cervical spine injury and immobilize as needed.

Assess LOC and ABCDEF. If findings are abnormal, intervene with appro-priate action immediately and call EMS. If the victim is stable, continue burn assessment by evaluating depth, extent, and comorbidity factors.

Depth
- Superficial: Involves the epidermis only; produces pain and redness
- Partial thickness: Involves the epidermis and partial dermis; causes pain and blistering
- Full thickness: Involves all skin layers and possible subcutaneous tissue, muscles, bones, and organs; may be painless because of injury to nerves and vessels

Extent
You can quantify the extent of a burn by using the "rule of nines" presented in Table 1-4-6. Extent may also be estimated by using the victim's palm as 1% to measure the burn surface area; for example, if the burn area on the patient's chest is about the size of his palm, then his burn extent is 1%.

Comorbidity Factors
- Age younger than 5 years or older than 55 years
- Burns of the joints, genitalia, face, airway, hands, or feet
- Circumferential burns (burns that encircle the entire body part)
- Preexisting conditions, illnesses
- Trauma with burn

Call EMS for any burn involving full thickness, any comorbidity factor, or any burn of greater than 9% of total body surface area. Initiate emergency burn management as outlined in Table 1-4-6. Also, watch for and prevent hypothermia. Because the victim's protective skin layer is injured, do not break blisters or apply ointments. Provide emotional support for the victim and family.

Cervical Spine Injury

Injuries to the cervical spine can be devastating. These injuries are most common in young adults and can result in restrictions requiring long-term care

Table 1-4-6. Rule of Nines Describing % of Total Surface Area Burned in an Adult

HEAD (FRONT AND BACK)	TRUNK (FROM SHOULDERS TO GROIN)	BACK (FROM SHOULDERS TO TIP OF THIGHS)	ARM EACH	LEG EACH	GENITALIA
9%	18%	18%	9%	18%	1%

at high cost. It is essential that these injuries be promptly recognized and appropriately managed to minimize the risk of spinal cord damage. Therefore, until ruled out through radiography, cervical spine injury should be assumed in injured victims who exhibit any of the following:

- Altered LOC due to injury
- Impaired judgment due to the influence of drugs or alcohol
- Pain or tenderness in the cervical area
- Altered sensorium in extremities (paralysis, paresthesia)
- Forces or impact to the body with the potential for transmission to the neck

The goal of emergency therapy is to minimize neurologic damage and deficits. At the scene, survey and ensure safety. Initiate BSI and immobilize the cervical spine. Assess LOC and ABCDEF. If abnormal, take immediate actions outlined in Table 1-4-7 and call the EMS. If the victim is stable, but you still suspect cervical spine injury, *do not move the victim.* Instead, call EMS and continue the assessment, observing for the following specific findings:

- Respiratory compromise
- Point tenderness or pain on palpation of the neck
- Deformity along the cervical spine
- Tingling, paresthesias, paralysis, numbness, weakness

Table 1-4-8 presents general management for the victim with known or suspected cervical spine injury.

Reassess LOC–ABCDEF periodically, because deterioration may occur. Support airway, breathing, and circulation as necessary and evaluate additional injuries. Look for secondary injuries such as internal or external hemorrhage, shock, and other nonobvious injuries. Reassure the victim and family.

Musculoskeletal Injury

Musculoskeletal injuries are often impossible to diagnose without radiographic studies. Therefore, when edema and/or pain presents after musculoskeletal injury, a fracture or dislocation should be assumed until proven otherwise.

The goals of emergency care are to reduce pain and minimize the risk of neurovascular damage. At the scene, survey and ensure safety. Initiate BSI;

Table 1-4-7. Emergency Burn Management

THERMAL

- Evaluate for smoke inhalation/respiratory burn. Maintain airway.
- Cool burn with water at 2–5 minutes.
- Cover with a dry dressing.

ELECTRICAL

- Check/monitor vital signs. Anticipate cardiopulmonary arrest. Perform CPR if needed.
- Look for entrance/exit sites.
- Cover burns with dry dressings.

CHEMICAL

- Remove all contaminated clothes.
- Flush with water 20 minutes after brushing off powders.
- Apply a dry dressing.

Table 1-4-8. Emergency Management of a Cervical Spine Injury

Call the EMS and do not move the victim if cervical spine injury is suspected.
If airway is compromised, open using the jaw-thrust maneuver with manual spine control.
If breathing is inadequate, give rescue breathing.
Maintain cervical spine control as follows:
• Kneel at the victim's head.
• Place the palm of each hand over the victim's ears. (Your thumbs should be over the occipital region.)
• Place each forefinger just inferior to the angle of the mandible to support the open airway position. (This keeps your other fingers free to palpate the carotid pulse.)
• Maintain firm and steady pressure with the hands in this position so that head and neck movement in all directions is prevented. Do not release until relieved by EMS.

consider cervical spine injury and immobilize as necessary. Assess LOC and ABCDEF. If findings are abnormal, take immediate actions as outlined in Table 1-4-1 and call EMS. If the victim is stable, then continue assessment.

Specific findings associated with musculoskeletal injuries include:
• The five Ps (pain, pallor, paralysis, paresthesia, pulselessness)
• Edema
• Crepitus
• Deformity
• Decreased range of motion
• Guarding of affected area
• Exposed bone fragment
• Amputation

If any of the specific findings are positive, initiate appropriate management as outlined in Table 1-4-9.

If the victim is stable, continue to reassess LOC–ABCDEF and monitor for any deterioration. Support the ABCs and assess for secondary injuries, such as internal or external hemorrhage, shock, impaled objects (do not remove; secure in place), or other nonobvious injuries. Do not move the injured area,

 Table 1-4-9. Emergency Management for Musculoskeletal Injuries

Call the EMS and do not move the victim if injury is suspected proximal to the knees or elbows.
Ensure an adequate airway, breathing, circulation and stop any bleeding.
Immobilize the affected area of injury in the position that it was found. Include joints above and below the injury. (Improvise splints using blankets, pillows, magazines, etc.).
Check neurovascular status of the extremity before and after splinting.
Cover any open wounds with a dry sterile dressing.
Apply a cold pack (not direct ice) to the area.
Place the victim in a position of comfort if dealing with a distal, single-extremity injury.
Arrange for medical treatment.
Provide amputation care as necessary:
• Manage ABCs first. Saving a life has priority over saving a limb.
• Control hemorrhage with direct pressure to the stump with dry gauze or clean towel
• Ensure that the amputated part is located, washed in sterile or clean water or saline, and placed in plastic bag that is placed in iced water. Do not place the part directly on ice.
• Time is vital if to increase the likelihood of successful reattachment.

Table 1-4-10. Types of Drowning

TYPE	DESCRIPTION
Wet drown	This occurs when protective reflexes preventing inspiration of water are lost and the victim aspirates water. Fresh water drowning: Hemodilution across the alveolar walls from diffusion results in surfactant destruction, atelectasis, shunting, hypoxemia, and death. Salt water drowning: Hypertonic water in the lungs draws water from blood into alveoli, resulting in shunting, pulmonary edema, acidosis, hypoxemia, and death.
Dry drown	This occurs when severe laryngospasm occurs on the victim's first inspiration of water. This prevents the entry of any more water into the lungs, resulting in hypoxia and death.
Cold water	The colder the water, the greater the chance of activating the mammalian diving reflex and the greater the chance of successful resuscitation. Handle gently. Attempt resuscitation.

especially a joint, because of the high risk for neurovascular damage. Determine whether the victim needs transportation to the hospital by ambulance or private vehicle. Reassure the victim and family.

Near-Drowning and Diving Accidents

About 8000 people die annually from drowning in the U.S., and many more experience near-drowning, surviving at least 24 hours postsubmersion. Precipitating events may include diving or water-skiing accidents, head injury, cervical spine injury, seizure, and myocardial infarction. Most drownings involve males, nonswimmers and children. Many of these losses could have been prevented with the simple common sense use of personal protective devices and avoidance of alcohol. Types of drowning are listed in Table 1-4-10.

The goals of emergency management are to restore or maintain basic life functions and protect the victim from further harm. At the scene, survey and pull the victim out of the water with an object; throw anything that floats and tow the victim, if possible. Row or swim to victim only if trained in water rescue. Consider cervical spine injury if the victim is in shallow water and immobilize as necessary. Assess LOC and ABCDEF. If findings are abnormal, take immediate actions as outlined in Table 1-4-1 and call the EMS. Assessment findings may include:

- **LOC:** Panic to unresponsive; use caution, because the victim may grab and pull you under
- **Cervical spine**: May be injured; look for pain, deformity, neurologic impairment
- **Airway and breathing:** May be open, gurgling, stridor, apneic, bradypneic or tachypneic.
- **Circulation:** May be present, absent, bradycardic or tachycardic, weak or bounding.
- **Skin:** Pale, cyanotic, cold—look for secondary injuries.

Management for the near-drowning victim is outlined in Table 1-4-11. In addition, frequently reassess LOC and ABCDEF and provide support as needed. Look for precipitating causes—cervical spine injury, seizure, stroke,

Table 1-4-11. Emergency Management for Near-Drowning

General	• Call the EMS (911) and support basic life functions until EMS arrival.
	• Ensure a clear airway and adequate respiratory status.
	• Expose the injured area and carefully remove debris from the wound surface.
	• Control bleeding with direct pressure, then elevation, then use pressure points if needed.
	• In a single, minor injury, wash with soap and water and apply antibiotic ointment.
	• Consider the need for sutures if the wound is deeper than the superficial skin layers, if fatty tissue is noted, or if the wound lines are gaping open.
	• Bandage open wounds after ABCs and major injuries are stabilized.
	• If more than a single minor injury is present, do not move the victim; consider EMS; treat shock (see Table 1–4–9) or prevent shock.
Impaled Object	• Do not remove impaled objects. Stabilize with roll gauze/bulky dressing.
	• Exception: An object through the cheek impairing breathing may be carefully removed. Remember to control bleeding.
Avulsion	• Remove surface debris, return the flap to normal position, and bandage.
Amputation	• Obtain the amputated part, wrap it in sterile dry dressing, place it in a plastic bag and place the bag in a cool container. Do not soak the part in water or place it directly on ice.
Neck Injury	• If major vessels are severed, the potential for air embolism exists. Cover the injury with an occlusive, air-tight dressing.
Chest Injury	• Be alert for possible pneumothorax, tension pneumothorax, and hemothorax.
	• If any of these is present, apply a three-sided occlusive dressing, support respiration.
Evisceration	• Do not move exposed organs. Cover with sterile, moistened dressing. Place a plastic cover over this to conserve heat.

myocardial infarction, or dysrhythmias. Maintain manual cervical spine control if any chance of injury exists. Do not move the victim unless necessary for resuscitation.

Soft Tissue Injury

Injuries to soft tissues are common and range from minor annoyances to major, sometimes life-threatening, trauma. Types of open wounds include abrasions, surgical incisions, lacerations, avulsions, amputations, crush injuries, and burns. Closed soft tissue injuries include contusions, bruises, and hematomas. Because they tend to be obvious because of bleeding, there can be a dangerous tendency to overlook less obvious and sometimes even more serious associated trauma. The potential for associated injuries, such as internal bleeding, organ damage, and fractures, must be recognized and assessed for when soft tissue damage is present.

The goals of therapy are to recognize the presence of soft tissue injuries and any associated injuries, prevent further damage, and initiate treatment geared toward the optimal healing process.

At the scene, survey and ensure safety. Initiate BSI. Consider cervical spine injury and immobilize as necessary. Assess LOC and ABCDEF. Be sure to take a systematic approach, to help reduce the chance of missing an injury. If you suspect more than one isolated soft tissue injury, do a hands-on, head-to-toe physical assessment. If you find any abnormality in LOC or the ABCs,

Table 1-4-12. Emergency Management of Soft Tissue Injuries

General	• Ensure clear airway and adequate respiratory status. • Expose the injured area and carefully remove debris from wound surface. • Control bleeding with direct pressure, then elevation, then use pressure points if needed. • If single, minor injury, wash with soap and water and apply antibiotic ointment. • Consider need for sutures if the wound is deeper than the superficial skin layers, if fatty tissue is noted, or if the wound lines are gaping open. • Bandage open wounds after ABCs and major injuries are stabilized. • If more than a single minor injury is present, do not move the patient, consider EMS, treat for shock (see Table 1-4-9) or to prevent shock.
Impaled Object	• Do not remove impaled objects. Stabilize with roll gauze/bulky dressing. • Exception: An object through the cheek impairing breathing may be carefully removed. Remember to control bleeding.
Avulsion	• Remove surface debris, return the flap to normal position and bandage.
Amputation	• Obtain amputated part, wrap it in sterile dry dressing, place in plastic bag and place in cool container. Do not soak it directly in water or ice.
Neck Injury	• If major vessels are severed, potential for air embolism exists. Cover injury with occlusive, air tight dressing.
Chest Injury	• Be alert for possible pneumothorax, tension pneumothorax, hemothorax. • If above is present, apply three-sided occlusive dressing, support respiration.
Evisceration	• Do not move exposed organs. Cover with sterile, moistened dressing. Place a plastic cover over this to conserve heat.

call EMS and support basic life functions with bleeding control until they arrive. Table 1-4-12 summarizes the management of soft tissue injuries.

 CLINICAL PEARLS

When giving emergency first aid for injuries, remember to play it **SAFE:**

○ **Safety** of the scene and environment must be ensured. Do not become another victim.

○ **Assessment** must be systematic and thorough to prevent missing serious injuries.

○ **First aid** that addresses the basic ABCs must be done before advanced treatment is provided.

○ **EMS** is the vital link to get a seriously injured victim to definitive care. Call 911 early.

Common Abbreviations

Section 5   Cynthia Chernecky

AAA	**abdominal aortic aneurysm**
ABE	acute bacterial endocarditis
AC (or ac)	**before meals**
AIDS	acquired immune deficiency syndrome
ANC	**absolute neutrophil count**
ARF	acute renal failure
ASA	**acetylsalicylic acid (aspirin)**
BID	twice a day
BP	**blood pressure**
BPH	benign prostatic hypertrophy

BS	**blood sugar**
BSA	body surface area
CA	**cancer**
CAD	coronary artery disease
CBC	**complete blood count**
CHF	congestive heart failure
CII	**continuous intravenous infusion**
CNS	central nervous system
CO	**cardiac output**
COPD	chronic obstructive pulmonary disease
Diff	**differential (complete blood count)**
DM	diabetes mellitus
DT	**delirium tremens**
DVT	deep vein thrombosis
ECG (or EKG)	**electrocardiogram**
EEG	electroencephalogram
EMG	electromyelogram
ESR	**erythrocyte sedimentation rate**
GI	gastrointestinal
GSW	**gunshot wound**
GU	genitourinary
HBP	**high blood pressure**
Hct (or HCT)	hematocrit
HF	**heart failure**
Hgb (or HGB)	hemoglobin
HIV	**human immunodeficiency virus**
HS	hour of sleep
ICP	**increased intracranial pressure**
IM	intramuscular
INR	**international normalized ratio**
IV	intravenous
LOC	**level of consciousness *or* laxative of choice**
MI	myocardial infarction
MS	**multiple sclerosis**
MVA	motor vehicle accident
MVI	**multivitamin**
NC	nasal cannula
NG	**nasogastric (tube)**
OD	right eye
OS	**left eye**
OU	both eyes
PC (or pc)	**after meals**
PCP	*Pneumocystis carinii* pneumonia
PEG	**percutaneous enteral gastric (tube)**
PG	pregnant
PID	**pelvic inflammatory disease**
PO	by mouth
PRN	**as needed**
PT	prothrombin time
PTT	**partial thromboplastin time**
PUD	peptic ulcer disease

PVD	**peripheral vascular disease**
QD	once a day
QOD	**every other day**
RA	rheumatoid arthritis
RBC	red blood cell count
REM	**rapid eye movement**
RHD	rheumatic heart disease
SCD	**sickle cell disease**
SCI	spinal cord injury
SL	**sublingual**
SLE	systemic lupus erythematosus
STD	**sexually transmitted disease**
Subq (or SubQ)	subcutaneously
TID	**three times a day**
UA	urinalysis
UTI	**urinary tract infection**
VAD	venous access device
WBC	**white blood cell count**

 RESOURCES

- AHCPR: 1-800-358-9295 or *www.ahcpr.gov*
- ANA: 1-800-274-4262 or *www.ana.org*
- National EMS Information Exchange (database on Good Samaritan laws): *naemt.org/nemsie/immunity.htm*
- Nursing World: www.nursingworld.org
- OSHA: www.osha.gov
- www.meddean.luc.edu/lumen/meded/medicine
- www.medinflo.ufl.edu/year1/bcs
- www.medlib.com
- www.mosby.com/physexam/seidel
- www.nhlbi.nih.gov/guidelines/hypertension/jnc.6.pdf
- www.RALE.CA

Campbell, John Emory and Alabama Chapter of the American College of Emergency Physicians. (1998). In *Basic Trauma Life Support for Paramedics and Advanced EMS Providers*, (3rd ed. update). Brady Prentice-Hall, Upper Saddle River, New Jersey.

chapter 2

Decision-Making for Fluid Therapy

Intravenous Fluids

Section 1
Richard Haas

OVERVIEW

Intravenous (IV) access is often viewed as a "lifeline" for many patients. The administration of IV fluids, either as carriers for other drugs or as a method of replenishing water and electrolytes, requires technical expertise, logical thought processes, and vigilance. The ability to understand the rationale behind the selection of a certain type of IV infusion is invaluable to the practicing nurse. Although infrequently involved in ordering specific IV fluids, nurses are involved in all other aspects of IV therapy. From insertion to management, nurses must aggressively monitor patients who receive IV therapy.

IV fluids are classified as either crystalloid or colloid (Table 2-1-1). This section focuses on crystalloid therapy.

PRINCIPLES OF CARE
Movement of Water

Water is the medium of life, the environment in which all cellular functions occur. The cells must be nourished with water. When we consume water, it moves to various compartments in the body, notably the plasma (the water component of the blood), the interstitial space (water in tissues outside the cells and outside the blood vessels), the intracellular space (water inside the cells), and the transcellular space (e.g., bowel, cerebrospinal fluid). The categories of body water are shown in Figure 2-1-1.

Whether consumed orally or administered IV, water must reach the cell. The movement of water out of the blood vessels and into the cells (through

Table 2-1-1. Classification of Intravenous Fluids

TYPE	DESCRIPTION	SOLUTIONS
Crystalloids	Clear solutions that easily pass through semipermeable membranes	Saline solutions Lactated Ringer's solution Dextrose solutions
Colloids	Contain large proteins or starches and do not easily pass through semipermeable membranes	Albumin Plasmanate Dextran Hetastarch

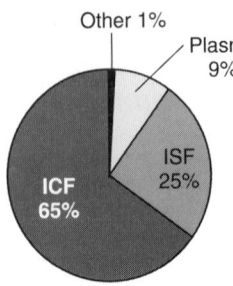

Figure 2-1-1. Body water by compartment.

the interstitial space) is the result of *filtration* across permeable capillaries and osmotic forces. Filtration regulates the movement of fluid (water and electrolytes) between the intravascular space (capillaries) and interstitial space. *Osmosis* regulates the movement of water between interstitial and intercellular spaces.

Filtration

Basically, four pressures regulate filtration. The two forces that move fluid out of the capillary and into the interstitial space are:

- Capillary hydrostatic pressure, the outward push of fluids within the capillary against its wall. This is clinically referred to as *hydrostatic pressure.*
- Interstitial colloid osmotic pressure, the pulling force of particles within the interstitial fluid space.

The two forces that move fluid into the capillary are:

- Interstitial fluid hydrostatic pressure, the push of interstitial fluid against the outside of the capillary walls.
- Capillary colloid osmotic pressure, the pulling force of particles within the capillary.

As these pressures change, so does the movement of water. For instance, if you stand up all day at work, you may notice some swelling in your feet and ankles. This is caused by increased *hydrostatic pressure*, which results in an accumulation of fluid in the interstitial space known as *edema*. Prolonged standing (and the resultant weight of the blood pushing against the walls of the capillaries) causes water to move out of the capillary and into the interstitial spaces, causing the feet to swell. Conditions that contribute to increased hydrostatic pressure are usually related to venous obstruction (e.g., thrombophlebitis, tight clothing around extremities, hepatic obstruction). In a bottleneck effect, as forward flow is impeded, hydrostatic pressure builds, and the water escapes eventually into the interstitial space. If you put your feet up, the *interstitial fluid hydrostatic pressure* becomes higher than that in the capillary, causing the water to move back into the capillary. Water is then carried to the kidneys and removed, and the swelling subsides.

If a person consumes excessive amounts of salt, the sodium eventually enters the bloodstream, increasing *capillary colloid osmotic pressure* (CCOP). In this situation, the blood contains more particles than the interstitial fluid, causing water to be pulled from the tissue spaces into the capillaries to dilute the high sodium level. The water is then carried to the kidneys for excretion. Similarly, the loss of plasma proteins (large particles), especially albumin (which occurs in protein malnutrition, liver disease, and nephrotic syndrome), causes the *interstitial colloid osmotic pressure* to exceed the CCOP. Water is then pulled from the capillary into the interstitial space, also causing edema. If the particles within the capillary are equal to the particles in the interstitial fluid, then the CCOP and the interstitial colloid osmotic pressure are equal, and no water movement should occur.

Osmosis

Water moves between interstitial and intercellular compartments by *osmosis*. Osmosis is the movement of water across a semipermeable membrane to equalize the particle concentrations (osmolality) on both sides of the membrane. *Osmolality* refers to the concentration of solute (particles) to solvent (liquid part) in a solution. Essentially, osmolality controls osmosis. If the solute (particle) concentration (osmolality) of interstitial fluid becomes greater than the solute concentration of intracellular fluid, water will move from the interstitial space to the intracellular space to equalize the osmolality between the two spaces. Osmolality is usually measured in millimoles, or 1/1000th of an osmole (see Formula 1).

Formula 1
1 osmole = 1 gram-molecular weight of an undissociated solute dissolved in 1 kg (1 L) of water
1 osmole of glucose = 180 g of glucose in 1 L of water
1 milliosmole (mOsm) of glucose = 0.180 g of glucose in 1 L of water

The normal osmolality of blood (serum osmolality) is 280 to 300 mOsm/kg. Serum osmolality can be calculated using Formula 2.

Formula 2
Osmolality (mOsm/kg) = [2 × (Na$^+$ + K$^+$)] + (BUN/2.8) + (glucose/18),
where Na$^+$ = serum sodium level, K$^+$ = serum potassium level, BUN = blood urea nitrogen level, and glucose = glucose level
Example:
The patient has a Na$^+$ of 138, a K$^+$ of 4.0, a BUN of 10, and a glucose level of 90.
According to the formula,

$$
\begin{aligned}
\text{mOsm} &= [2 \times (138 + 4) + (10/2.8) + (90/18) \\
&= 284 + 3.57 + 5 \\
&= 292.57
\end{aligned}
$$

In *high serum osmolality* (>300 mOsm/kg), there is an increased concentration of particles in the blood (less volume and more particles, as seen in dehydration). In *low serum osmolality* (<280 mOsm/kg), there is a decreased concentration of particles in the blood (more volume, less particles, as seen in overhydration). Illustrating this concept, in Figure 2-1-2*A*, a semipermeable membrane divides a container of water. There is no movement, because osmolality is equal on both sides of the membrane. A quantity of solute, sodium chloride (NaCl), is placed on one side of this membrane, increasing the particle concentration (osmolality) of the solution (see Fig. 2-1-2*B*). The semipermeable membrane traps the NaCl on one side of the container. Note

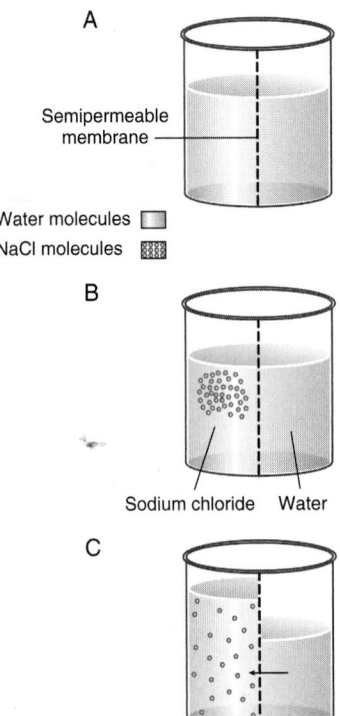

Movement of water toward sodium chloride

Figure 2-1-2. Semipermeable membrane.

the movement of water toward the side of the compartment with the NaCl (see Fig. 2-1-2C). Water will move by osmosis across the semipermeable membrane in an attempt to equalize the osmolality, or particle concentration, of both compartments.

Tonicity

The NaCl/water mix on the left side of the membrane is *hypertonic*, containing more particles of solute than the solution on the right side of the membrane. The solvent (water)-only fluid on the right side of the membrane is *hypotonic*, containing relatively fewer particles. An *isotonic* solution is of equal osmolality on both sides of the semipermeable membrane. Knowledge of a patient's serum osmolality will influence the choice of IV solution to administer.

DECISION-MAKING
Properties of Specific Intravenous Fluids

The osmolality and electrolyte content of IV fluids vary in order to provide for specific patient needs. Patients may have different responses to different types of fluids. Besides providing water for the cells, fluid therapy also provides sodium, glucose in the form of dextrose, and other electrolytes (Table 2-1-2).

Water is needed to maintain circulating volume, to hydrate the cells, and for excretion by the renal system. Daily water intake requirement is approximately 2.5 L, depending on the patient.

Sodium is the most abundant extracellular cation and must be replaced in the absence of oral intake. Serum sodium levels reflect osmolality. As serum sodium level rises, so does serum osmolality, and vice versa. Most IV fluids contain sodium; exceptions include D5W (5% dextrose in water) and D10W (10% dextrose in water).

Dextrose provides a small amount of calories and temporarily increases the osmolality of the IV solution. D5W provides only 200 calories/L. This amount does not provide adequate nutrition alone. For patients with adequate insulin supplies and normally functioning insulin receptors (i.e., patients without diabetes), the small amount of dextrose goes almost immediately to the intracellular space and is metabolized. Once the glucose is gone, the osmolality of the remainder of the IV fluid is significantly lower. For example, D5½ (5% dextrose with one-half normal saline) solution is initially hypertonic but becomes hypotonic once the dextrose is metabolized. For dextrose and water solutions, once the glucose is metabolized, large amounts of water remain in the bloodstream, decreasing serum osmolality and creating "free water."

When water is free, it moves easily from the bloodstream (plasma) into the cells. Thus, D5W is not truly an isotonic solution—rather, it is more like water, which is hypotonic to serum. Too much free water can be dangerous, because it can lead to water intoxication.

Water intoxication is largely related to sodium dilution and decreased serum osmolality. High volumes of water will dilute the blood, decreasing serum sodium and osmolality. This causes water to move from the intravascular space into the cells, making them swell. Cells in the brain and nervous system are most seriously affected. Cerebral edema may manifest as lethargy and headache, progressing to confusion, coma, and death.

Electrolytes can accumulate during rapid fluid resuscitation or additional electrolyte replacement therapy. Various IV fluids provide few or no electrolytes, thus placing the patient at risk for low electrolyte levels. Therefore, sodium, potassium, chloride, and calcium levels should be monitored when these fluids are administered. Magnesium is not provided in any of the solutions and must always be administered additionally.

Tonicity of Intravenous Fluids

The normal osmolality of body fluid is approximately 300 mOsm/kg. In comparison to normal body fluid osmolality, IV fluids are either hypertonic (osmolality of >375 mOsm/L), isotonic (osmolality of 250 to 350 mOsm/L), or hypotonic (osmolality of <250 mOsm/L).

Hypertonic IV fluids (e.g., 3% saline) introduced into the vascular space tend to pull water out of the tissues and cells and into the bloodstream or vascular space. This effect is manifested by increased blood pressure and increased urine output. These solutions must be used with great caution, because the cells can become dehydrated and suffer damage. Some practitioners have used hypertonic solutions, such as 3% saline, in patients with

Table 2-1-2. Contents of Specific Intravenous Fluids (per L)

FLUID	TONICITY	Na+	K+	Cl-	Mg²⁺	Ca²⁺	DEXTROSE (g)	OSMOLARITY (mOsm/kg)	OSMOLARITY MINUS DEXTROSE (mOsm/kg)
D5W	Isotonic						5	252	
D5W + 40 KCl	Isotonic		40	40			5	333	81
D5W + .02% NaCl (D5¼ NS)	Hypotonic	34		34			5	321	69
D5W + .45% NaCl (D5½ NS)	Hypertonic	77		77			5	406	154
D5W + .9% NaCl (D5NS)	Hypertonic	154		154			5	560	308
D5W + LR (D5LR)	Hypertonic	130	4	109		3	5	525	273
LR	Isotonic	130	4	109		3		273	
.45% NaCl (½ NS)	Hypotonic	77		77				154	
.9% NaCl (NS)	Isotonic	154		154				308	
3% NaCl	Hypertonic	513		513				1026	
5% NaCl	Hypertonic	855		855				1710	

D5W, 5% dextrose in water; NaCl, sodium chloride; LR, lactated Ringer's.
Electrolytes are measured in mEq/L.

severe shock to increase circulating volume. This can be done by administering small amounts of the IV solution at slow rates (e.g., 200 mL over 4 hours).

Administration of *hypotonic* solutions (e.g., D5½ NS) will cause water to move from the bloodstream into the tissues and cells. These solutions are given as maintenance fluids to patients who cannot take oral fluids, at rates of about 100 to 125 mL/hr. Hypotonic solutions are very useful for replacing insensible fluid losses (evaporative fluid losses from the skin and respiratory tract) and replacing sodium ions. They are also given to patients who are dehydrated (i.e., patients whose cells lack water).

Isotonic solutions (e.g., NS, lactated Ringer's) are the most commonly administered IV solutions. These solutions initially increase plasma volume but eventually allow water to diffuse into the tissue beds. They may also be used as maintenance fluids to hydrate patients who cannot take oral fluids, at rates of approximately 100 to 125 mL/hr. Isotonic solutions containing sodium are useful for sodium replacement. They are also used to rapidly restore circulating plasma volumes in shock, at rates of up to about 2000 mL/hr. D5W should not be used for rapid fluid replacement.

Fluid Therapy Management

Patients have predictable and unpredictable fluid losses from normal urine output, vomiting, diarrhea, fever, diuretic use, sweating, and drains. Fluid therapy is the primary method of replacing fluids to maintain adequate renal excretion, provide water for the cells, and maintain adequate electrolyte levels and circulatory volumes in the absence or reduction of oral intake (Table 2-1-3).

 CLINICAL PEARLS

○ The free water in D5W may cause water intoxication (because the water leaves the vascular space and enters the intracellular space), resulting in swelling of the cells, especially in the brain, leading to cerebral edema, coma, and death.

○ Normal saline and lactated Ringer's are the preferred solutions for rapid fluid resuscitation.

○ D5W should not be used for rapid fluid replacement and should not be given to patients who have a head injury or undergoing neurosurgery, because it may cause cerebral edema.

○ 3% and 5% saline should never be infused rapidly or given as a bolus. They must be infused slowly and on a pump to prevent severe dehydration of the cells.

○ High serum osmolality (>300 mOsm/kg) is seen in dehydration, where the blood is concentrated.

○ Low serum osmolality (<280 mOsm/kg) is seen in overhydration, where the blood is dilute.

Table 2-1-3. Guidelines for Management of Commonly Used Intravenous Fluids

SOLUTIONS	USES	RATIONALE	PRECAUTIONS/CONSIDERATIONS
ISOTONIC			
0.9% Normal saline (NS) Consists of 85% salt solution Does not contain calories	Replace circulating volume Replacement of sodium ions Treatment of hyponatremia and hypochloremia Treatment of metabolic alkalosis when fluid loss is present. Used to dilute packed cells and whole blood.	NS provides the salt necessary to maintain serum osmolarity and serum sodium levels. NS helps to keep fluid in the intravascular space.	Monitor serum sodium levels. NS may cause hypernatremia, especially in patients who are losing water but not salt, as in the case of profuse watery diarrhea. NS may cause hyperchloremia or it may cause fluid overload in patients with compromised cardiovascular systems.
5% Dextrose in water (D5W) Because the small amount of glucose is metabolized so quickly, this solution may almost be considered hypotonic, because it is mainly water	Treatment of hypernatremia Treatment of dehydration	The water in D5W is free because the dextrose is quickly metabolized. The water will quickly leave the intravascular space, flow into the intracellular space to hydrate the cells, and dilute excess salt as well as other electrolytes.	D5W in excess may cause water intoxication because the water is free; it leaves the intravascular space, flows into the intracellular space, and causes swelling of the cells. This can lead to cerebral edema, coma, and death. D5W may also increase blood pressure and dilute circulating electrolytes. Monitor serum sodium levels. Monitor all electrolytes closely.
10% Dextrose in water (D10W)	D10W replenishes dehydrated patients; assists in the treatment of hyperinsulinemia; and can help drive potassium (K^+) into the cell.	D10W provides free water similar to D5W. Glucose quickly enters the cell for rapid metabolism. Glucose takes potassium into the cell with it, thus decreasing serum K levels.	Same as for D5W. Large amounts of glucose can lead to a hyperosmotic diuresis, resulting in hypotension.

Solution	Use	Action	Nursing Considerations
Lactated Ringer's solution Does not provide calories Closest fluid to plasma in composition	Replacement of fluid and some electrolytes; replaces circulating volume losses; used for patients who may be bleeding	This solution helps to keep fluid in the intravascular space	Do not use this solution to treat lactic acidosis, because during lactic acidosis the body is unable to convert lactate (a precursor to bicarbonate) to bicarbonate. This solution will clot blood and blood products. Monitor all electrolytes closely.
HYPOTONIC			
Half-strength normal saline (½ NS)	Maintenance fluid	This solution hydrates cells as it allows the free water and salt to move from the vascular space to the intracellular space; it does not provide calories.	Monitor all electrolytes closely.
5% Dextrose in 0.45% normal saline (D5½ NS) Initially hypertonic; quickly becomes hypotonic following the rapid metabolism of the dextrose	Most common maintenance IV fluid used Maintenance fluid	This solution rehydrates cells as it allows the free water and salt to move from the vascular space to the intracellular space. It also provides a small amount of calories.	Monitor all electrolytes closely.
HYPERTONIC			
3% Saline	Treatment of symptomatic hyponatremia. May be used cautiously for significant postoperative edema. Used cautiously to replace circulating volume in shock.	3% Saline provides high amounts of sodium. The solution pulls water out of the cells and into the intravascular space.	This solution must be administered slowly on a pump. Monitor serum sodium closely. Monitor all electrolytes closely. This solution may dehydrate the cells.

Venous Access Devices

Section 2   Denise Macklin

OVERVIEW

Vascular access may be divided into two specific categories: peripheral venous access and central venous access. These categories are determined by the location of the distal tip of a vascular access device (VAD) in the vein. The distal tip of a peripheral catheter resides in a peripheral vein. The distal tip of a central catheter dwells in a central vein, usually the superior vena cava. The nurse needs comprehensive knowledge about VADs to maximize their function, minimize nursing time, and reduce the risk of complications associated with their use.

Poor understanding of VADs can lead to inappropriate and delayed choice of an intermediate or long-term VAD, significant pain, permanent damage or loss of veins, permanent disfigurement, life-threatening complications, poor device performance, loss of health care dollars, and emotional and psychosocial damage.

PRINCIPLES OF CARE
Goal of Intravenous Therapy

The goal of IV therapy with a VAD is to maintain the chosen VAD without complications to the completion of therapy. To help achieve this goal, it is important to understand anatomy and physiology of the vein, the basic physical principles that affect VAD function, and the different types of VADs.

Anatomy and Physiology

A single layer of endothelial cells lines the vein wall. VADs reside in veins and depend on the flow of blood to dilute infused substances and provide a buffer between the VAD and the vein wall. Even though VADs are manufactured to be as biocompatible as possible, once placed in a vein, they pose a risk for vein wall damage. Vein wall damage is the major cause of many VAD complications.

Veins increase in size with increasing proximity to the heart. Peripheral veins of the hand and lower forearm are small, major upper arm veins are twice the size of peripheral veins, and the superior vena cava is twice as large as the major vessels of the upper arm. The larger the vein, the greater the rate of blood flow and the greater protection of the vein wall from the VAD. The risk of vein wall damage is greatest in the small veins in the hand and lower forearm.

Physics of Flow

The design of VADs impacts the flow rate of the solution being administered. Flow rate reflects the relationship between resistance and pressure. Resistance is any factor that impedes flow; think of resistance as similar to friction. Variables that impact resistance include:

- **Catheter length.** If the catheter length is doubled, the flow rate is halved. Long central catheters result in slower flow rates than are achieved by short peripheral catheters.

- **Fluid viscosity.** If the viscosity is doubled, the flow rate is halved. Cold solutions are thicker than warm solutions. For example, blood flows slowly when cold and more rapidly as it warms.
- **Internal catheter diameter.** All catheters have a designated gauge size. Gauge size is standardized and reflects the outer circumference of the catheter. The catheter wall thickness impacts internal catheter diameter. Internal diameter has the greatest impact on flow. Catheter flow rate increases 16-fold when the internal catheter radius is doubled. VADs with a similar gauge size may have different internal diameters depending on catheter design and the catheter material.

Peripheral catheters are designed to be either thin-walled or non–thin-walled. Long-term central catheters are made of silicone or polyurethane.

DECISION-MAKING
Peripheral Catheters

In general, peripheral catheters are short and stiff. The stiffness makes them easy to advance into the vein but also prone to damage the vein wall. Select the smallest-gauge catheter possible to achieve the prescribed flow rate. Place this small catheter in the largest vein to ensure the best possible vein-to-catheter ratio and maximum drug hemodilution.

When a large-gauge catheter is successfully inserted into a vein but there is a poor catheter-vein ratio, blood flow is minimized. As a result, hemodilution is limited, and vein wall damage is ensured.

Peripheral catheters come in two configurations: winged steel butterfly and over-the-needle. Steel needles should be used only for single-dose, small bolus therapy or blood collection. Over-the-needle catheters are used for intermittent, continuous, or daily IV access for less than 7 days. Table 2-2-1 presents indications for use and care and maintenance of peripheral catheters.

Central Venous Catheters

Central venous catheters are used to administer medications and solutions that have extreme variations in pH and osmolarity. The increased size of a central vein offers a better catheter/vein ratio and improved hemodilution. Central venous catheters are subdivided into two categories based on length of use:

- Short-term acute central venous catheters, used for therapy less than 30 days in duration.
- Long-term central venous catheters, used for therapy up to 1 year or longer in duration.

Short-Term Acute Central Catheters

These catheters are typically used in the intensive care setting. Insertion is accomplished by a percutaneous venipuncture directly into a central vein. Skin sutures are used to stabilize the catheter at the insertion site. Types of short-term acute central catheters include multilumen subclavian/jugular, dialysis, and hemodynamic catheters. These catheters are softer than peripheral catheters but still much stiffer than a vein. The potential for vein wall trauma limits dwell time to less than 30 days and usually less than 1 week. The direct access into the vein increases the risk of infection. Approximately 90% of

Table 2-2-1. Peripheral Access Devices

	INDICATIONS FOR USE	CARE AND MAINTENANCE POINTERS

Winged needle sets	Patient considerations:
	    Unlimited venous access
	    Well hydrated
	    Has soft, pliable veins and tissue turgor and normal skin
	Uses:
	    Single-dose, small bolus or IVP therapy, 1–20 hour continuous infusion
	    Non-vesicant or irritating medications/solutions
	    Isotonic solutions (280–295 mOsm/L)
	    Normal pH solutions (7.35–7.45)
	    Blood collection
	Cost considerations:
	    Device: less than $0.50
	    Procedure: $15–$80
		Requires an arm board if used for anything beyond IV push
		Not recommended for uncooperative patients
		Dwell time not more than 1–2 hours

Over-the-needle	Patient considerations:
	    Unlimited venous access
	    Activity restrictions
	Uses:
	    Intermittent, continuous, or daily IV access
	    IV fluids, electrolyte solutions, and/or blood products
	    Isotonic solutions (280–295 mOsm/L)
	    Normal pH solutions (7.35–7.45)
	    Dwell time 48–72 hr
	    Therapy duration less than 7 days
	Cost considerations:
	    Device: $1–$15
	    Procedure: $15–$80
		Avoid areas of flexion or bony prominences when inserting.
		Choose the smallest catheter for the best catheter/vein ratio.
		Never place tape over the insertion site.
		Use sterile tape under a transparent dressing.
		Use a stress prevention loop when tubing is in place.
		Flush routinely if not in use with saline in accordance with agency policy.
		Rotate site every 48–72 hours.
		Change administration sets according to the following schedule: q72 hr (CDC); q48 hr (INS)
		Secondary sets—same as above
		Intermittent—q24 hr (INS)
		TPN—q72 hr (CDC)
		Lipid—q24 hr (INS)
		Blood—after each unit or after 4 hr (INS)

IVP, intravenous push.

all bloodstream infections are associated with multilumen subclavian/jugular catheters. Bloodstream infections on average increase length of stay by 6.5 days with a hospital cost of $3200 to $10,000 per episode. Table 2-2-2 presents indications for use and considerations for care and maintenance of short-term acute central catheters.

Long-Term Central Catheters

Long-term central catheters include tunneled, implanted, and peripherally inserted types. These catheters are soft and pliable. Their vein-like quality allows them to remain in place for long periods with minimum trauma to the

Table 2-2-2. Acute Short-Term Central Access Devices

	INDICATIONS FOR USE	CARE AND MAINTENANCE POINTERS
Acute multilumen catheters. (Single lumen, double lumen, triple lumen) Usually placed at bedside by the physician, through the internal jugular or subclavian veins with the catheter tip in the superior vena cava or right atrium. Most common central line inserted in hospital settings. Length: 6–30 cm Gauge: 4F–7F Catheter volumes: 0.3–0.8 mL	Patient selection: Approach for short-term therapy up to 10 days; 3 days for jugular location Uses: Intermittent, continuous, or daily IV access for IV fluids, electrolyte solutions, or blood products Vesicant and irritating medications/solutions, total parenteral nutrition, therapies with extremes of pH and osmolality. Hemodynamic monitoring Cost considerations: Device: $40–$200 Procedure: $100–$500	Change dressing when moist, loose, or soiled. Routine dressing changes vary from every other day (INS) to once every 5–7 days using sterile technique. Change injection caps with the dressing. Change administration set; Table 2–2–1. Flush routinely if not in use with saline and heparin from once a day to every 8 hr. Use 3–5 mL of saline and follow with heparin according to institution policy. Heparin volume minimum should be twice the internal volume of catheter and add-on devices. Flush with 20 mL of saline when drawing blood or after infusing blood. Maintain positive pressure when disconnecting to prevent blood backing up into the catheter. Placement must be confirmed by radiograph before use.
Dialysis Large-gauge catheters used for short-term hemodialysis. Insertion is similar to short-term percutaneously inserted central lines. Length: 13–24 cm Gauge: 13–16 gauge	Patient selection: Need for renal replacement therapy is acute. Renal transplant patient experiencing temporary renal dysfunction associated with rejection Peritoneal dialysis patients with peritonitis Uses: Short-term hemodialysis	Should not be used by nondialysis practitioners

vein. None of these catheters uses an external insertion site directly into a central vein. This indirect entry minimizes the potential for infection. The low infection rate and the vein-like material allow these catheters to safely remain in place for more than 30 days. Table 2-2-3 presents indications for use and considerations for care and maintenance of long-term central catheters.

Nursing Responsibilities

The major nursing responsibilities associated with VADs are appropriate selection, care and maintenance, and troubleshooting problems as they arise (Table 2-2-4).

Selection

Assessment is the cornerstone of VAD selection. The components of a VAD assessment can be specified but not prioritized, because the components are

Text continued on page 60

Table 2-2-3. Long-Term Central Catheters

Tunneled catheters
(Fig. 2-2-1)
Inserted surgically in the operating room (OR). The
catheter tip is advanced into the superior vena cava
(SVC) or right atrium, and the proximal end is
tunneled (threaded under a subcutaneous pocket of the
chest wall and brought through an exit site in upper
chest below the nipple line).
Three types:
Broviac: Smaller lumen, usually used in pediatric
patients. In sizes 2.7–6.6 French.
Catheter volume: 1.0 mL
Hickman, Multiple lumens, Sizes 9–12 French.
Catheter volume: 2 mL
Groshong: Incorporates a valve design that opens
during infusion or aspiration and then closes to
prevent back flow. Omits the need for clamping.
Catheter volume: 0.3–0.8 mL

INDICATIONS FOR USE

Patient selection:
Therapy of 6 months or longer
Uses: Same as short-term catheters
Cost considerations:
Device: $50–$200
Procedure: $500–$2000
Length: 42–80 cm
Gauge: 2.7–19.2

CARE AND MAINTENANCE POINTERS

Dressing changes must be done weekly.
Dressings are required in acute care setting.
Dressing can be omitted 3–5 weeks postinsertion with
granulocyte count above 200 mm.
Change caps with dressing or once weekly and keep
capped at all times.
Tubing should be coiled and secured to prevent pulling.
Clamp when not in use, except the Groshong catheter,
which is never clamped.
Flushing: Same as for central lines.
Repair kits are available for Hickman catheters.
Cuff barrier decreases infection.

52

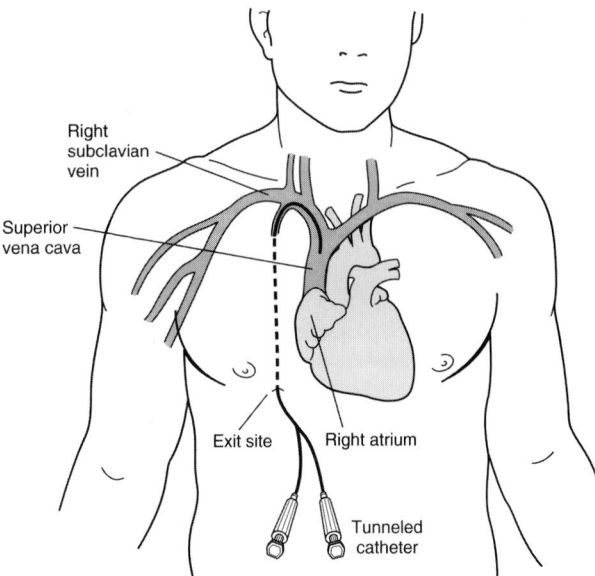

Figure 2-2-1. Tunneled catheter placement.

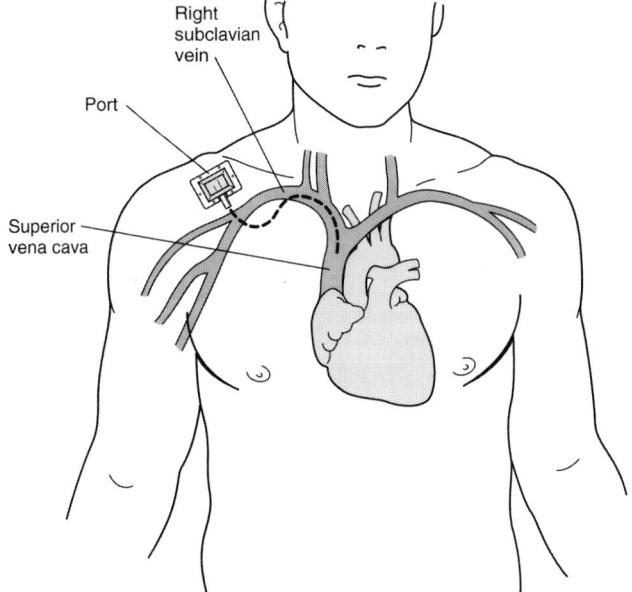

Figure 2-2-2. Implanted port.

Implanted ports
(Fig. 2-2-2)

Surgically inserted in the OR. The catheter tip is inserted into the subclavian vein, internal jugular (IJ) vein, or SVC. An attached port with a self-sealing silicone septum is implanted in a subcutaneous pocket in the chest wall. A small bulge indicates the location of the septum.

Catheter volume: 0.2–1.5 mL

Brands:
- Port-A-Cath
- Mediport
- Infus-A-Port
- Q Port
- Life Port

Patient selection:
Therapy of 6 months or longer
Monthly or cyclic treatments
Unwanted external reminder
Alteration in activities of daily living would negatively impact quality of life
Living conditions increase possibility of infection
Equipment and trained nurses available
Patient has sufficient means for cost of care
Uses: Same as for tunneled catheters
Cost considerations:
Up to $6000

Requires special noncoring needle (Huber) to access septum (Fig. 2-2-3).
Septum can withstand 1000–2000 punctures.
Once accessed, change dressing and needle every 7 days.
Rotate puncture site to maximize life of septum.
Flush every 4 weeks if not in use with 5 mL of heparinized saline.
Provide no interference with activities of daily living and improved body image.
Must be removed by a physician.

Peripherally inserted central catheter (PICC) (Fig. 2-2-4)
Inserted percutaneously by a trained RN at the antecubital fossa or 3 inches above or below, into the cephalic or basilic vein. The tip is then advanced in the SVC.

Patient selection: Therapy lasting several weeks to 6 months
Chest injuries
Radical neck dissection or head/neck cancer
Uses: Same as for tunneled catheters
Dwell time:
6 weeks to 1 year
Cost considerations:
Device: $50–$75
Procedure: $100–$600

Change dressing 24 hours after insertion and then once per week.
Change injection caps with dressing.
Coil and secure external tubing to minimize accidental dislodgement.
Tape applied directly to silicone PICCs can damage the catheter.
Tape applied directly to polyurethane PICCs may be necessary to secure.
Flush using a pulsatile motion.
Maintain positive pressure before disconnecting the syringe.
Never use TB syringes with PICCs.
Placement must be confirmed by x-ray.

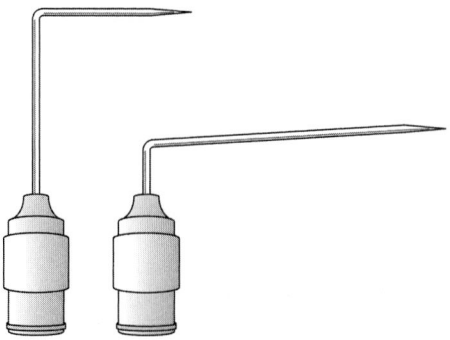

Figure 2-2-3. Huber needle.

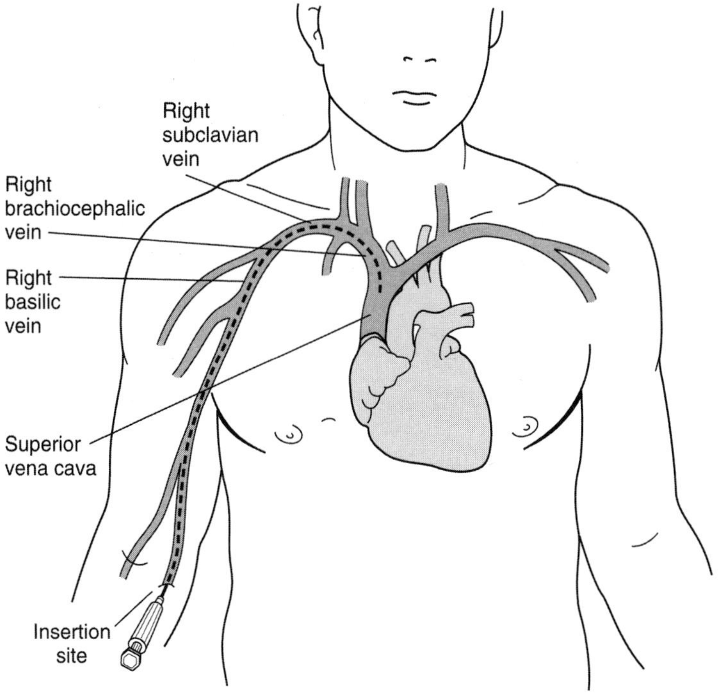

Right
subclavian
vein

Right
brachiocephalic
vein

Right
basilic
vein

Superior
vena cava

Insertion
site

Figure 2-2-4. Peripherally inserted central catheter (PICC).

Table 2-2-4. Complications of VADs

COMPLICATION	SIGNS AND SYMPTOMS	TREATMENT	PREVENTION
Infiltration	Cool skin Blanching Edema Feeling of skin tightness Pain Tenderness Alteration in flow rate Leaking at the insertion site Compare site with same area on opposite extremity Apply pressure above catheter tip, flow rate will continue without slowing	Discontinue IV. Apply a cold compress except with vinca alkaloid, in which case apply heat.	Avoid areas of flexion or bony prominences for insertion. Monitor site q1–2 hr. Teach the patient to observe the IV setup for complications.
Extravasation	Same as infiltration	Same as for infiltration. Administer the appropriate antidote. Notify the physician.	Use central lines for continuous vesicant infusion.
Phlebitis	Redness over catheter or over the vein track Skin warm to touch Swelling Palpable cord (advanced) Pain is the first symptom	Discontinue IV. Apply warm moist heat to site.	Ensure an appropriate vein-catheter ratio. Perform routine site rotation. Choose isotonic solutions for peripheral infusion. Ensure proper drug dilution and infusion rates.
Site infection	Area around insertion site is red and swollen; may or may not have drainage	Discontinue IV. Notify the physician.	Ensure handwashing and proper site preparation with maintenance of aseptic technique. Inspect containers for cracks and leaks. Perform routine fluid and tubing changes.
Venous spasm	Sharp pain at IV site or over vein track Slowing or stopping of flow rate Sudden difficulty with flushing	Apply warm moist heat to site if the solution is cold Slow infusion rate if administering an irritating drug If pain continues, discontinue IV.	Administer irritating medications slowly and if possible through the side port of a running IV. Administer cold infusates slowly. If possible, allow fluids to warm to room temperature before administration.

Complication	Signs and symptoms	Treatment	Prevention
Thrombosis	Sluggish infusion rate Difficulty flushing Leaking at the site Swelling below the insertion site Tender to touch Peripheral: Palpation of vein track above the catheter tip, inability to infuse Central: Patient complaints of pain in the shoulder, neck, or arm	The best treatment is prevention. Discontinue the IV (peripheral). Verify thrombosis before discontinuing the catheter (central). Cold compress may decrease progression of clot formation (peripheral).	Same as for phlebitis. Do not play "catch-up" with infusions. Use all techniques that minimize vein wall trauma.
Sepsis	Chills and abrupt temperature elevation General malaise Headache Nausea and vomiting Vascular collapse Shock Death Identifying patients who have increased susceptibility (e.g., AIDS, cancer, elderly, malnourished, TPN, burns)	Discontinue IV. Notify the physician. If restarting, use new solution and administration setup. Obtain cultures.	Check solution containers for integrity. Change administration sets every 3 days. Change injection caps at least weekly with central lines. Maintain a closed IV system. Ensure handwashing. Maintain aseptic technique. Provide proper dressing management.
Circulatory overload	Rapid weight gain, edema, engorged peripheral veins, distended neck veins, and rise in blood pressure. Wide variance between intake and output Shortness of breath and rales	Slow IV to keep-vein-open rate. Elevated head of bed. Monitor vital signs. Notify the physician. Administer medications and oxygen as ordered.	Never play catch-up with infusions. Maintain prescribed flow rate. Monitor intake and output. Beware of the patient's cardiovascular and renal history.

Table continued on following page

Table 2-2-4. Complications of VADs *Continued*

COMPLICATION	SIGNS AND SYMPTOMS	TREATMENT	PREVENTION

Air embolism	Cyanosis
	Weak, rapid pulse
	Drop in blood pressure
	Churning sound
	Changes in neurologic status
	Advanced symptoms include:
	  Hemiplegia
	  Seizures
	  Coma
	  Cardiac arrest
		Clamp catheter immediately.
		Cover open insertion site immediately.
		Place the patient in Trendelenburg position on the left side.
		Aspiration of air through a right heart catheter or a percutaneous needle and closed chest cardiac massage may be needed.
			Eliminate all air from lines before use.
			Use air-eliminating filters.
			Use electronic infusion devices with air detection alarms.
			Use Luer-Lok connections.
			Attach piggyback solutions to the highest injection port.
			Change solutions before containers are empty.
			Maintain all clamps in the closed position when the central line is not in use.
			Ensure proper suturing and catheter stabilization to prevent catheter dislodgement.

Catheter embolism	Loss of circulation Cyanosis Chest pain Tachycardia Hypotension Cardiac irritability Cardiac arrest	Apply a tourniquet lightly high on the upper extremity (peripheral catheters). Elevate the head of the bed. Notify the physician. Start a new IV in the opposite extremity. For central catheters, stop infusion and get an x-ray.	Never reinsert a stylet. Do not use a TB syringe.

Catheter occlusion	Inability to infuse or withdraw blood Alteration in flow rate	Assess the entire administration setup for closed clamps and air-locked filters. Check to see whether IV fluid flows when disconnected from the patient. (If it does not, then the problem may be with the administration setup.) Assess using direct syringe-to-hub connection. Use a 100 mL syringe with central lines and a 3 mL syringe with peripheral lines and attempt a gentle push-pull technique with normal saline. Do not apply force. With central lines, reposition the patient and have the patient cough or raise the arm. Then attempt to flush again. Maintain a sufficient flow rate to keep the catheter open (usually 50 mL/hr if not using an electronic infusion device). Flush promptly after the infusion of an intermittent medication. Keeping the patients head 36 inches above the patient's heart on gravity flows (even when up walking). With central lines, use a thrombolytic or other suitable declotting agent.	Flushing the catheter with saline is the most important activity in preventing occlusion. Use a pulsating motion to create turbulence. This will "scrub" the catheter wall. Maintain positive pressure on the syringe barrel before removing the syringe to minimize blood reflux into the catheter tip.
Pneumo-, hemo-, hydro-, or chylothorax	Chest pain Shortness of breath Cyanosis Decreased or absent breath sounds on the side of the VAD Confusion Tachycardia	Notify the physician. Obtain an X-ray. Prepare for possible chest tube insertion. Elevate feet. Remove the catheter. Administer oxygen as ordered.	Ensure positioning when the catheter is being inserted. Provide adequate patient teaching before insertion. An active patient may require a sedative before insertion.

interrelated, and it is the patient who determines which factor is most important. Components of VAD assessment include:

- Length of therapy
- Type of therapy
- Diagnosis
- Patient's age
- Secondary risk factors that might affect the incidence of complications
- Limb/mobility restrictions
- Fluid volume status
- Skin assessment findings
- Availability of peripheral veins
- Patient preference
- Mental status

Optimal VAD selection at the beginning of therapy can help ensure maximum function, minimum complications, cost savings, and increased patient satisfaction.

Care and Maintenance

Caring for and maintaining VADs require that the nurse:

- Successfully identify complications when they occur
- Manipulate the catheter (give medications, flush, draw blood)
- Provide care for the insertion site
- Prevent damage to the VAD
- Remove or recognize the need to remove the VAD at the end of therapy or when necessitated by a complication

Complications

The monitoring process provides information regarding the patient's response to therapy, the accurate delivery of fluid and medications, and the detection of complications. Monitoring involves careful inspection of the administration setup including the fluid container, the flow rate, the administration tubing, the dressing, the VAD, and the insertion site. Monitoring the patient's response to therapy is also critical.

Neither the Joint Commission on Accreditation of Healthcare Organizations (JCAHO) nor the National Association of Intravenous Nursing has issued specific guidelines governing the frequency of monitoring VADs. Both organizations recommend that each institution set a policy and procedure governing the frequency of and method for monitoring VADs. Specific intervals should be established. Commonly, IV sites should be inspected at least every 1 to 2 hours. In high-risk environments such as pediatric, geriatric, and critical care, inspection should be more frequent. The insertion site and the affected extremity should be assessed for pain, tenderness, swelling, inflammation, and drainage.

Various complications are associated with VADs.

Infiltration. Infiltration is defined by the Intravenous Nursing Society (INS) as the inadvertent administration of a nonvesicant solution or medication into surrounding tissues as a result of dislodgement of a cannula or perforation of the vein. Veins are elastic and can expand to accommodate increased volume. This elasticity varies from patient to patient and is greatly diminished in elderly patients. When the vein is overextended, it will break even if the catheter is placed correctly inside the vein. (This is why blood return is not an accurate indicator of vein integrity.) Infiltration occurs at a much lower pressure than the occlusion alarm setting on an electronic pump. Thus, electronic infusion devices cannot recognize infiltration. Remember, illnesses such as congestive heart failure can also cause edema in the extremities.

Extravasation. Extravasation is defined as the infiltration of a vesicant solution and/or medication into surrounding tissue. Vesicants cause tissue sloughing. Drugs such as potassium chloride, calcium gluconate, sodium bicarbonate, amphotericin B, contrast media, Phenergan, and dopamine, as well as some cytotoxic drugs, are vesicants.

Phlebitis. This inflammation of the vein wall is classified by causative factor. In *mechanical phlebitis*, the catheter is the causative agent. In *chemical phlebitis*, the infused substance is the causative agent. In *bacterial phlebitis*, a bacterium is the causative agent. The location of the red streak that appears on the extremity provides a clue as to what type of phlebitis has occurred. A streak over the catheter track indicates a mechanical source, whereas a streak over the vein above the tip of the catheter most likely indicates a chemical source. If the patient has a sudden spike in temperature and purulent drainage at the site, bacterial phlebitis should be suspected. (Bacterial phlebitis is rare, however.) Phlebitis is associated with an 18-fold increase in the risk of IV-related septicemia.

Site Infection. Infection may occur at the insertion site. The area around the site may be red and swollen and may or may not have drainage. Site infection is a *local* complication and should not be confused with sepsis, a *systemic* complication.

Sepsis. Sepsis is a catheter-related bloodstream infection. The majority of catheter-related infections result from central venous access, especially with acute short-term multilumen subclavian/jugular catheters. Sepsis occurs when microorganisms or their byproducts invade the bloodstream by way of the IV catheter. In the critical care environment, catheter-related bloodstream infections occur in 3% to 7% of patients with central venous catheters, with an attributable patient mortality of 12% to 25% and associated costs of up to $29,000 per episode.

Venous Spasm. Venous spasm is the sudden involuntary contraction of a vein. Venospasm can cause failure of successful venipuncture.

Thrombosis. A clot may form on the vein wall as a result of injury. With thrombophlebitis, inflammation is also present. Potential consequences of catheter-related venous thrombosis include the inability to administer therapy, inability to recannulate, suppurative thrombophlebitis, catheter entrapment, postthrombotic syndrome, pulmonary embolism, and increased costs. Only 5% of subclavian vein thromboses are symptomatic, because of the development of collateral circulation.

Air Embolism. Sudden obstruction of a blood vessel by a bolus of air entering the circulatory system is associated with central line removal. The short track present when a short-term multilumen central catheter is removed may stay open for a brief moment. A central venous catheter track formed with a 14-gauge catheter can transmit about 200 mL of air in 1 second.

Pneumothorax (Air), Hemothorax (Blood), Hydrothorax (Water), or Chylothorax (Lymph). These complications usually occur when the lung is punctured during central line insertion. Symptoms are often not manifested until after the procedure has been completed. The patient may be asymptomatic for some time afterward, with a gradual onset of symptoms. Pneumothorax is the most common of these complications. Diagnosis is based on radiographic findings.

Catheter Occlusion. Catheters can become occluded by clotted blood or drug precipitates. Deposits can build up on the internal wall of the catheter or the catheter tip, causing narrowing or occlusion of the lumen. With peripheral catheters, removal is usually the recommended course of action. However, with central lines, catheter removal is not always the first choice. Especially with long-term VADs, attempts are made to salvage the catheter.

To successfully declot a VAD, the cause of the occlusion must be determined. If the clot is composed of fibrin, a thrombolytic agent can be used. But if the obstruction is caused by a drug precipitate, a thrombolytic will not work. Usually drug precipitates occur when drugs of different pHs are administered concurrently or in close succession through the same IV line without proper flushing between administrations. For example, vancomycin becomes a solution in an acidic environment. If vancomycin comes into contact with an alkaline IV medication, such as furosemide, then the residual vancomycin cannot stay dissolved, and a precipitate is formed. To remove the precipitate, the vancomycin needs an acidic environment to return to a solution. Tables 2-2-5 and 2-2-6 list agents that will declot drug precipitates and lipid deposits.

Catheter Damage. Catheter damage most often occurs with long-term central catheters. A catheter can be damaged on the external (visible) or internal portion. Damage is more common in long-term central lines made of silicone. The most common cause of catheter damage is the exertion of excessive force on a syringe plunger when flushing a partially occluded catheter. The damage can be a hole, or the entire catheter can break off and become a catheter embolism. Always apply minimal force to the syringe to activate a flush. Do not yield to the natural tendency to apply more pressure with the thumb when resistance is felt. If resistance is felt, stop and evaluate the situation. There are no universal standards available to guide flushing decisions. According to the INS, using a small syringe may exert excessive pressure on the catheter, especially if the catheter is totally or partially occluded.

Catheter Migration/Malposition. Catheter migration or malposition is

Table 2-2-5.   Agents that Alter pH to Solubilize Medication Precipitates

AGENT	HYDROCHLORIC ACID (HCl)	SODIUM BICARBONATE (NaHCO$_3$)
Dose	1 mL of 0.1 N (prepared and filtered by a pharmacist)	1 mL of 8.4% solution (1 mEq/mL is commercially available)
Dwell time	20 minutes, repeat one or two more times.	Precipitate usually clears in 1–2 minutes.
Mechanism	Decreases pH to solubilize acidic drugs or precipitates.	Increase pH to solubilize basic drugs or precipitates.
Cautions	Minimal risk of metabolic acidosis Febrile reaction when infused rather than aspirate	None

TABLE 2-2-6. Agents that Solubilize Lipid Deposits

AGENT	70% ETHANOL (ETHYL ALCOHOL)	SODIUM HYDROXIDE (SODA LYE, NaOH)
Dose	Volume to fill catheter (prepared and filtered by a pharmacist)	Infuse 10 mL of 0.1 N HCl at 1 mL/hr, followed by a 2-hour lock, and then infuse 0.9% NaCl at 1 mL/hour. Quick flush with 20 mL 0.9% NaCl. Repeat one time if necessary.
Dwell time	1–2 minutes	2 hour lock as above
Mechanism	Solvent for lipid	Solvent for both protein and lipid
Cautions	Unpleasant taste when flushing ethanol through the catheter	Solvent for both protein and lipid

seen only with central lines. It occurs when the distal tip that was initially located in the superior vena cava at the time of insertion moves or migrates to another location. Over time, the tip can migrate, especially with vomiting, excessive coughing, or sneezing. Suspect malposition if you are unable to withdraw blood from the catheter or your patient experiences chest pain. Radiographic testing is the only way to determine if the catheter has migrated. **Catheter Manipulations.** Giving intermittent, continuous, or IV push drugs and fluids; flushing the system; and drawing blood samples requires manipulation of the VAD, sometimes numerous times a day. The number of manipulations is an important risk factor for sepsis, especially with multilumen, short-term central catheters. To minimize contamination and the potential for sepsis, clean all entry ports and all vial tops with alcohol, date multidose vials, use a new needle/spike with each multidose vial, apply a new cap to needless adapters that require one, and change IV tubing and injection caps according to your institution's policy.

Site Care And Maintenance

The nurse is responsible for the routine care and maintenance of VADs, including routine changing of the administration set, the IV solution, the IV dressing, and in the case of peripheral catheters, the IV site. This routine care minimizes the risk of complications. Following strict aseptic technique and all applicable infection control guidelines is mandatory when performing routine care. The INS standards specify that administration sets be routinely changed every 72 hours, with sets used with lipids and piggyback medications changed every 24 hours. Blood administration sets are changed after no more than two sequential units have infused. IV sites are routinely rotated every 48 to 72 hours if complication-free.

Dressing management and site care are especially important with central lines. The dressing protects the insertion site and stabilizes the catheter. The INS standards specify that the catheter be stabilized in such a manner that does not interfere with visual site assessment or impede delivery of the prescribed flow rate. The CDC strongly recommends changing dressings when they become damp, soiled, or loose. Changing a nonintact dressing is extremely important with all central lines, because these lines remain in place for extended periods. Peripheral lines require daily dressing changes if gauze and tape are used, but with transparent films, dressings usually remain in place until the IV is discontinued. The insertion site is cleaned with alcohol and iodophor before the dressing is applied. The Centers for Disease Control and Prevention (CDC) strongly advises against routinely applying antimicrobial ointment to any central venous catheter insertion site, because the ointment macerates the skin and increases the risk of catheter contamination.

Discontinuation of Therapy

Because all VADS carry a risk of complications, they are usually removed when they are no longer indicated. However, if there is any question of loss of catheter integrity, the catheter is removed immediately even if the therapy is not complete. With a peripheral VAD, if contamination is suspected, it should be removed immediately. Removing a central line requires special knowledge.

The nurse can minimize the risk of air embolism by taking the following steps:

- Position the patient in the supine position.
- Have the patient hold his or her breath during removal.
- Cover the insertion site with ointment and an occlusive dressing.
- Have the patient remain lying down for 30 minutes.
- Leave the dressing in place for 12 hours.

With jugular venous placement, firm pressure or forceful rubbing of the neck over the carotid artery must be avoided. Massaging the insertion site after VAD removal from an internal jugular (to ensure hemostasis) can dislodge atherosclerotic plaque or thrombus in the carotid artery, causing stroke.

 CLINICAL PEARLS

○ Always choose the smallest-gauge catheter that will accommodate the prescribed therapy. This maximizes hemodilution and minimizes irritation to the vein wall.

○ Antimicrobial ointments should not be applied to the catheter site, as they cause skin maceration and increase the potential for catheter contamination.

○ Although peripheral catheters are the most common, they are not always the best choice for the prescribed therapy. Optimal VAD selection at the beginning of therapy can promote maximum function, minimum complications, cost savings, and increased client satisfaction.

○ Monitoring the IV setup provides information regarding the patient's response to therapy, accurate delivery of fluid and medications, and detection of complications.

○ VAD category is determined by distal tip location.

○ The softer the VAD material, the longer the duration of catheter placement.

Blood and Blood Product Administration

Section 3   Beverly George-Gay ■ Cynthia Chernecky

OVERVIEW

Nurses play a crucial role in the assessment, implementation, evaluation, and administration of blood and blood products/factors. This section discusses the basics of blood administration, as well as the management of the newer blood products and growth factors.

PRINCIPLES OF CARE
Blood Typing

ABO and rhesus (Rh) systems are the major determinants of blood compatibility testing.

ABO Blood Group

Blood is typed according to the antigens found on the surface of the red blood cell (RBC) and the antibodies found in the plasma. Blood type is genetically determined. There are four major blood types, known as ABO groups. International population percentages are A (41%), B (9%), AB (4%), and O (46%). The two major antigens found on RBCs are A and B. The two major antibodies are anti-A antibody and anti-B antibody (Table 2-3-1). If an antigen is mixed with its corresponding antibody, an antigen-antibody reaction occurs in the form of a hemolytic (type II hypersensitivity) reaction.

Universal Donor. Type O is considered the universal donor, because neither antigen A nor B is present. Thus, type O blood can be given to individuals with types A, B, and AB. However, type O does have both A and B antibodies; thus transfusions from types A, B, or AB cause an antigen-antibody reaction in type O persons. For this reason, patients with type O blood can receive only type O blood.

Universal Recipient. Type AB is considered the universal recipient, because there are no antibodies in the plasma. Thus, patients with type AB blood can receive transfusions from any of the four groups.

Rh Blood Group

Developed using the blood of the rhesus monkey, the Rh classification system is also based on a specific antigen, Rh(D), on the surface of RBCs. Persons with the Rh(D) antigen are Rh-positive (encompasses 95% of all African Americans and 85% of all whites), and persons without it are Rh-negative (encompassing 5% of all African Americans and 15% of all whites).

Unlike the ABO group, Rh antibodies do not occur naturally. They develop only when an Rh-negative person is exposed to Rh-positive blood. This can occur only through a natural immune response after blood transfusion or when an Rh-negative woman is pregnant with an Rh-positive child. Once exposed to Rh-positive blood with the Rh(D) antigen, the Rh-negative person will produce antibodies against Rh-positive blood—more specifically, against the Rh(D) antigen. To prevent the production of anti-Rh(D) antibodies, a single dose of immune globulin (RhoGAM) should be administered immediately after each exposure. RhoGAM prevents the formation of natural anti-Rh(D) antibodies. Rh-negative blood can be given to either Rh-negative or Rh-positive recipients.

Type and Crossmatch

Type and crossmatch (T&C) tests the patient's and prospective donor's blood for compatibility. The test involves obtaining a blood sample from the patient as well as pulling a unit of blood from the blood bank inventory for

Table 2-3-1. ABO Typing of Red Blood Cells

TYPE	ANTIGENS	ANTIBODIES	MAY RECEIVE ONLY FROM PERSONS WITH	MAY TRANSFUSE ONLY INTO PERSONS WITH	MAY NOT TRANSFUSE INTO PERSONS WITH
A	A antigen	Anti-B antibody	Types A and O	Types A and O	Types B and AB
B	B antigen	Anti-A antibody	Types B and O	Types B and O	Types A and B
AB (universal recipient)	A and B antigens	None	Types A, B, AB, and O (Because type AB has no antibodies, no antigen antibody reactions should occur.)	Type AB	Types A, B, and O (because these types will interact with the A and/or B antigens in type AB blood)
O (universal donor)	None	Anti-A and anti-B antibodies	Type O (because an antigen-antibody reaction will occur with types A, B, and AB)	Types A, B, AB, and O (Although both A and B antibodies are present, they are so diluted by the recipient's own blood that an antigen-antibody reaction may not occur.)	

Source: Boley & Pulaski, 1997 and Kaye 1997.

compatibility testing. T&C includes ABO, Rh, and Coombs testing. Coombs' test is a blood test to determine the presence or absence of immunoglobulins and complement in the coating of RBCs. The direct Coombs' test detects antibodies on the surface of the RBC; the indirect Coombs' test detects unknown antibodies circulating in the serum. A T&C sample is accurate for only 72 hours, as the patient may develop different antibodies during this time.

Type and Screen

Type and screen (T&S) tests only the patient's blood for ABO group, Rh type, and atypical antibodies. This is a preliminary test that does not deplete units from the blood bank inventory. This test is done if there is a limited possibility that blood would be needed. If the need becomes imminent, then a T&C is necessary. T&S blood samples are reliable for 72 hours.

DECISION-MAKING
ABO Typing

All blood and most blood products require ABO typing before administration. ABO incompatibilities result in significant morbidity and can further result in mortality. Table 2-3-1 gives an overview of ABO typing.

Blood Transfusion Reactions

Several types of transfusion reactions can occur, all of which can be avoided with careful assessment and surveillance. Table 2-3-2 presents information on the onset, manifestations, and management of the different types of blood transfusion reactions.

Blood and Blood Product Administration
General Guidelines
Temperature
- Blood should be administered at room temperature except in cases of massive transfusions. Cold blood may induce dysrhythmias. It takes approximately 30 minutes for blood from the blood bank refrigerator to reach room temperature.
- Blood products administered at rates above 50 mL/kg/hr should be warmed using an electric blood warmer.
- Do not warm blood to >107.6°F (>42°C), because higher temperatures disrupt RBC function.

Intravenous Catheter. A 22-gauge or larger needle is recommended. Although 18-gauge catheters have been preferred historically, current evidence has shown that a 22 gauge is safe and effective.

Filters
- All blood products must be transfused through a filter (standard 170 to 260 μm).
- Change the filter after each unit of blood.
- Leukocyte-poor filters prevent the risk of febrile transfusion reactions. These require a physician's prescription.

Time Limits. All blood products should be infused within 4 hours. If more time is needed, then the blood bank can divide the components into aliquots and keep portions properly refrigerated in a blood bank refrigerator until needed.

Table 2-3-2. Blood Transfusion Reactions

TYPE	ONSET	SIGNS AND SYMPTOMS	MANAGEMENT/CONSIDERATIONS
Allergic or type 1 hypersensitivity: This is a mild allergic reaction due to sensitivity of infused plasma proteins that react with the patient's own IgE proteins.	Occurs during transfusion or 1 hour posttransfusion. Incidence is 1%.	Include flushing, itching, urticaria and bronchial wheezing but no fever. Persons at high risk are those with a history of blood transfusions.	Slow down or discontinue the transfusion while keeping IV access patent with normal saline. Administer acetaminophen and Benadryl 0.5 mg/kg 30 minutes PO or 10 min IV before transfusion to decrease the risk of type I reactions.
Hemolytic or type II hypersensitivity: Hemolysis of RBCs occurs due to ABO incompatibility between the patient's blood and transfused blood, resulting in hemoglobinemia and hemoglobinuria that may lead to renal failure.	Incidence is 1%, or 1:25,000. Can occur within 5 minutes or after the first 100 mL of blood is transfused (usual) or up to 7 days posttransfusion (rare).	Include chills, fever, headache, dyspnea, flank back pain, chest pain, tachycardia, hypotension, anuria, decreased serum hemoglobin, disseminated intravascular coagulation, and cyanosis.	Discontinue the transfusion immediately, keep IV access patent with normal saline, and perform CPR if needed. Send remainder to the blood bank laboratory.
Febrile nonhemolytic: The most common type of blood transfusion reaction, it results from antileukocyte, antiplatelet antibodies. This reaction accompanies 1% of all transfusions.	Occurs during or shortly after the transfusion. Administer acetaminophen and Benadryl before transfusion if febrile reaction is a possibility.	A temperature increase of 2°F or 1°C occurs with chills, chest or low back pain, dyspnea, apprehension, and hypotension.	Discontinue transfusion immediately, keep IV access patent with NS. Administer acetaminophen and Benadryl. Leukocyte reduced components or leukocyte poor filters will be of benefit for patients with repeated febrile reactions.
Anaphylactic: This is a severe allergic reaction due to antigen-antibody reaction in persons with IgA deficiency who were sensitized to IgA through previous transfusion or pregnancy.	Incidence is 1:150,000. Occurs within minutes of or immediately after transfusion.	Include chest pain, dyspnea, tachycardia, hypotension, anxiety, gastrointestinal disturbances, urticaria, circulatory collapse, and cardiac arrest.	Discontinue transfusion immediately, keep IV access patent with normal saline, perform CPR if needed, and have epinephrine 0.4 mL of 1:1000 solution SQ available. Send remainder to the blood bank laboratory.

Preservatives. Citrate anticoagulant-preservative is a commercially prepared solution placed in bags of whole blood, packed red blood cells (PRBCs), platelets, and plasma to preserve and prevent clotting.

Dilution

- Use only 0.9% sodium chloride (NS) to prime tubing and maintain IV patency.
- Avoid dextrose solutions which may induce hemolysis
- Calcium-containing solutions should never be administered with blood components. Calcium binds with citrate, the preservative in banked blood, which can cause clot formation in the bag and/or administration set.
- Never use lactated Ringer's solution, because it contains calcium.
- Inspect the blood component for clots or change in color. If noted, return it to the blood bank.
- 5% human albumin may be used in special circumstances

Specific Guidelines

Table 2-3-3 gives management guidelines for specific products.

Hematopoietic Growth Factors

Hematopoiesis is simply the production of new blood cells. Blood cell levels are normally maintained by hormonal influences and properly functioning bone marrow. In patients with altered hormone levels or compromised bone marrow, blood cell production is reduced. Hematopoietic growth factors are commercially prepared products that will stimulate blood cell production. These growth factors have been widely accepted as a mainstay of therapy for patients with low RBC and white blood cell counts for various reasons. Administration and management of these factors are discussed in Table 2-3-4.

 CLINICAL PEARLS

- The ABO group that can be transfused to any person is type O. Type O blood is the universal donor because it contains neither antigen A nor antigen B. The lack of these antigens ensures that clumping of RBCs will not occur. Although type O contains A and B antibodies, once these donor antibodies mix with the recipient's blood, they are so diluted that they have no effect.
- T&C is reliable for only 72 hours, because of the possibility that the patient may have developed an irregular antibody (in response to a recent blood transfusion or infection) that may react with the potential donor's blood. Hence, to avoid a reaction, another T&C is done.
- The expected increase in a patient's hemoglobin and hematocrit after receiving 1 unit of PRBCs is a 1-g increase in hemoglobin and a 3% rise in hematocrit for every unit infused. Note: In a patient who is not bleeding, hematocrit can be estimated by multiplying the hemoglobin by the factor of 3 (although the relative values are not equal, because grams are not equal to percent).
- Routes and frequency of administration of colony-stimulating factors or hematopoietic growth factors include subcutaneous or IV routes, with frequency varying from daily to 3 times per week for 10 days to several months.

Table 2-3-3. Blood Product Administration

PRODUCT	PACKAGING	INDICATIONS	ADMINISTRATION	MONITORING
Whole blood: Contains plasma, RBCs, WBCs, no platelets or clotting factors. Minimum hematocrit of 38%.	450–500 mL in 1 unit	Rarely used. Management with specific blood products is recommended. Usually used for massive blood loss due to trauma, when patient is actively bleeding.	T&C is required. An 18- to 22-gauge IV catheter is used to prevent hemolysis. Blood tubing has a standard blood filter. With massive transfusions, blood should be warmed in a dedicated blood warmer to prevent hypothermia. Rate: Start at 4 mL/min for first 15 minutes unless massive transfusion is required, in which case infuse at a rate of 60–80 gtt/min or faster.	In a nonbleeding adult, one unit should increase hemoglobin (Hgb) by 1 g and hematocrit (Hct) by 3%. Closely monitor Hgb and Hct; assess for circulatory overload and for transfusion reactions. Monitor for hypocalcemia (citric acid, a preservative found in banked blood has a tendency to bind with the recipient's serum calcium causing hypocalcemia). Monitor for hypersensitivity, anaphylactic, and hemolytic reactions.
Autologous blood: The patient's own blood recovered from a surgical site. Can be collected preoperatively, intraoperatively and postoperatively. This table focuses on postoperative collection.	Volume varies by patient output.	Used usually following cardiac, thoracic or orthopedic surgery when blood loss is expected to be 500–1000 mL. Reduces or eliminates transfusion reactions and transmission of disease.	Blood is collected via suction tubes into a sterile wound drainage system that contains an anticoagulant. The blood must be reinfused within 6 hours of collection or discarded, as it can become contaminated with bacteria.	Administer with caution in patients with sickle cell disease, because the quality of their RBCs may not be adequate. Clot lysis is a potential complication, because postoperative blood is subject to clotting; thus, fibrin split products should be monitored for elevations, which could lead to coagulation problems.

Blood Product	Volume	Indications	Administration	Nursing Considerations
Packed **RBCs**: Contains RBCs (65–80%), plasma (20–35%) (two-thirds of the plasma is removed compared with whole blood), and some platelets, and WBCs. Hematocrit is 65–80%. Contains no clotting factors.	250–350 mL in 1 unit	Restores oxygen carrying capacity in acute or chronic symptomatic anemia. Is also indicated for blood loss. May anticipate transfusion with Hgb <7 or Hct <21%.	T & C is required. An 18- to 22-gauge IV catheter is used to prevent hemolysis. Blood tubing has a standard blood filter. With massive transfusions, blood should be warmed in a dedicated blood warmer to prevent hypothermia. 0.9% saline may be added with Y-tubing to reduce viscosity. Must be administered within 4 hours of being obtained from blood bank. Rate: Start at 5 mL/min for first 15 minutes unless massive transfusion is required, in which case infusion rates may vary depending on patient status. Usually infused over 2 hours or 100–230 mL/hr.	In a nonbleeding adult, one unit should increase Hgb by 1 g and Hct by 3%. Closely monitor Hgb and Hct and assess for circulatory overload and for transfusion reactions. Monitor for hypocalcemia. Monitor for febrile, hypersensitivity, anaphylactic, and hemolytic reactions.
Fresh frozen plasma (FFP): Contains plasma, all coagulation factors except platelets, 400 mg of fibrinogen, and 1 unit/mL of all other factors.	200–300 mL in 1 unit	Treatment of coagulation factor deficiencies (as reflected by abnormal laboratory results), bleeding complications, and blood loss. For every 5 units of PRBC transfused, 1 unit of FFP should be administered during massive transfusions.	ABO compatibility required. Crossmatch not needed. An 18- to 23-gauge IV catheter and blood tubing with standard blood filter are used. Rate: Infuse over 30–60 minutes or 200–300 mL/hour. Must be infused within 4 hours of preparation.	Each unit of FFP should decrease prothrombin time (PT) by 2 seconds. Each unit should also increase clotting factors by 5%. PT, PTT, fibrinogen and D-Dimer tests should be monitored. Monitor for circulatory overload, transfusion reactions, hypocalcemia, hypersensitivity, and anaphylactic reactions.

Table continued on following page

Table 2-3-3. Blood Product Administration *Continued*

PRODUCT	PACKAGING	INDICATIONS	ADMINISTRATION	MONITORING
Serum albumin: Contains 96% albumin, 4% globulin.	Available in either a 5% solution in 250 or 500 mL or a 25% solution in 50- or 100-mL glass bottles.	Volume expansion.	No compatibilities required. An 18- to 21-gauge IV catheter is used. A filter may be required by some manufacturers; check product insert. Rate: Infusion rates may vary, usually 50–100 mL over 30–60 min.	Monitor blood pressure closely. Blood pressure may increase due to albumin's ability to draw fluid into the intravascular space. Monitor for volume overload.
Platelets: Contains platelets separated from a single unit of whole blood suspended in the original plasma.	40–70 mL in 1 unit	Bleeding from thrombocytopenia or abnormal platelet function. Also indicated during massive transfusions.	ABO and Rh compatibility required. Crossmatch not needed. An 18- to 22-gauge IV catheter is used. Only special platelet concentrate infusion filters should be used, usually obtained from blood bank. Rate: Infuse over 20–30 min or 200–300 mL/hour.	Each unit should increase platelet count by 5000–10,000. Monitor counts at 1 hour and 24 hours after infusion. Monitor for hypersensitivity and anaphylactic reactions.
Cryoprecipitate (Cryo): Contains factor VIII, factor XIII, fibrinogen, and von Willebrand's factor.	10–25 mL in 1 unit.	Correction of factor VIII deficiency (hemophilia A, von Willebrand's disease), factor XIII deficiency, fibrinogen deficiency, and the management of disseminated intravascular coagulation.	ABO compatibility required. Crossmatch not needed. An 18- to 21-gauge IV catheter is used. A concentrate infusion filter is required, obtained from blood bank.	Ten units should increase fibrinogen levels by approximately 50 mg/dL. The goal is to maintain fibrinogen levels at >100 mL/dL. Coagulation factors, PT, and PTT should be monitored. Monitor for hypersensitivity and anaphylactic reactions.

| Intravenous immunoglobulin (IVIG): Sterile concentrated solution of primarily IgG pooled from human plasma. Prepared under the following trade names: Gamimune N, Gamagard, IGIV, Iveegam, Sandoglobulin, and Venoglobulin-I; each preparation is slightly different. | Each preparation is slightly different; refer to the package insert. | For the replacement of IgG (an immunoglobulin specific for fighting bacterial and viral infections). Useful in primary immunodeficiency diseases, as well as some acquired immunodeficiency diseases, such as chronic lymphocytic leukemia and AIDS. Also indicated when rapid elevations in platelet count is required (mechanism of action is unknown), as in patients who are bleeding or require immediate surgery, or in the treatment of idiopathic thrombocytopenic purpura. | Infuse at a very slow rate initially; may increase per physician's order or manufacturer's recommendations if well tolerated. Avoid shaking, to prevent foam formation. Do not mix with other drugs. Discard unused portions. | IVIG may contain antibodies, therefore, hemolytic, hypersensitivity, and/or anaphylactic reactions may occur and should be monitored for some patients. |

Table 2–3–4. Hematopoietic Growth Factors

TYPE	USES	ADMINISTRATION	ADVERSE REACTIONS	CONSIDERATIONS
Erythropoietin (EPO, Epoetin alfa, Epogen): A glycoprotein that stimulates red blood cell production	Primarily used to treat anemia due to chemotherapy, chronic renal failure, and zidovudine-treated persons with HIV. Current research use is preoperatively to harvest and save patient's own blood for possible postoperative autologous transfusion	Given SQ or IV three times a week. Recommended starting dose is 150 U/ kg SQ. Takes 2–4 weeks for Hct to rise.	Side effects include diarrhea, edema, and hypertension (primarily in renal patients) and rarely nausea, vomiting or seizures.	Must have normal serum iron levels or be placed on oral iron supplements for drug to be effective. Monitor hematocrit weekly. Contraindicated in uncontrolled hypertension as the increase in hematocrit further elevates blood pressure.
Granulocyte colony stimulating factor (G-CSF, Filgrastim, Neupogen): A growth factor that stimulates neutrophil production	Treatment for granulocytopenia resulting from chemotherapy, aplastic anemia, myelodysplastic syndrome or AIDS, and before peripheral stem cell harvest transplantation	Given SQ or IV daily in doses of 5–60 μg/kg (usual dose 5–8 μg/kg) or 200–2400 μg/m^2 for 10–20 days. Refrigerate; stable at room temperature for 24 hours. To avoid foaming, do not shake vial. In persons receiving chemotherapy the drug should be started 24 hours after chemotherapy initiated and no later than 4 days after the last dose of chemotherapy	Side effects include musculoskeletal pain, mild elevation of LDH and alkaline phosphatase, and, rarely, exacerbation of preexisting cardiac, dermatologic, or autoimmune conditions. Adult respiratory distress syndrome may occur in septic patients.	Monitor CBC differential daily and discontinue if absolute neutrophil count >10,000/mm^3. Use with caution in persons who have leukemia, as it may promote growth of leukemic cells. This drug is expensive, reimbursement by Medicare only if administered in a physician's office and pharmaceutical companies have excellent resources on reimbursement issues.

74

Granulocyte-macrophage colony stimulating factor (GM-CSF, Leukine, Prokine, Sargramostin): A growth factor that stimulates neutrophils, eosinophils and monocytes and induces the release of two cytokines, interleukin-1 and tumor necrosis factor	Used secondary to intensive chemotherapy or bone marrow transplant and to shorten granulocytopenia seen in aplastic anemia, myelodysplastic syndrome or AIDS.	Given SQ, IV, or IM at doses of 250–500 μg/m² daily up to 21 days. Contraindicated in persons allergic to yeast. IV infusions must be given over at least 2 hours. Use within 6 hours of reconstitution; to avoid foaming, do not shake vial.	General side effects include musculoskeletal complaints, flu-like symptoms, and, rarely, skin rash and vomiting. Pericarditis, fluid retention, and venous thrombosis are dose-related side effects and are uncommon at doses below 32 μg/kg.	Discontinue if neutrophil count >20,000 cells/mm³. Common side effects with first dose are flushing, dyspnea, tachycardia, and nausea. This drug is expensive; reimbursement by Medicare is done only if administered in a physician's office. (Pharmaceutical companies have excellent resources about reimbursement issues.)
Thrombopoietin (c-Mpl ligand, TPO) and pegylated recombinant human megakaryocyte factor (PEG-rHuMGDF): Cytokines and experimental growth factors that regulate the production of platelets from megakaryocytes in the bone marrow.	They stimulate platelet production by up to sixfold without affecting other cell line lineages.	Given SQ daily at doses of 0.3–1.0 μg/kg for 10 days.	Side effects include flu-like symptoms and fatigue.	Following chemotherapy or irradiation, TPO increases erythroid, myeloid, and platelet recovery.

RESOURCES

- Arrow International: 800-523-8446
- Bard Access Systems: 800-4545-0890
- Becton Dickson: 800-453-4538
- B. Braun Medical Inc.: 800-523-9695
- Centers for Disease Control (CDC): 800-311-3435 or *www.cdc.gov*
- Epogen: 800-272-9376 (reimbursement); 800-772-6436 (clinical information)
- Genentech Customer Service: 800-551-2231
- HDC Corporation: 800-227-2918
- Intravenous Nurses Society (INS): 617-441-3008 or *www.ins1.org*
- Johnson & Johnson Medical: *www.jnjmedical.com*
- League of Intravenous Therapy Education (LITE): 412-678-5025 or *www.lite.org*
- National Association of Vascular Access Networks (NAVAN): 888-576-2826 or *www.navannet.org*
- National Cancer Institute (NCI): 800-4CA-NCER or *www.nci.nih.gov*
- National Institutes of Health: www.cc.nih.gov/nursing/bldprodp.html
- Neupogen: 800-272-9376 (reimbursement); 800-772-6436 (clinical information)
- Oncology Nursing Society: 412-921-7373 or *www.ons.org*
- Sims Deltec: 800-426-2448
- Thrombopoietin: *www.gene.com*
- Vygon Corporation: 800-544-4907
- http://www.findarticles.com/cf_0/m3231/n10_v28/21224628/p2/article.jhtml
- http://www.nursefriendly.com/nursing/directpatientcare/intravenous.iv.therapy/intravenous.fluids.htm

chapter 3

Decision-Making for Wounds and Drainage Systems

Wound Care

Section 1

Beverly George-Gay

OVERVIEW

A wound is a break in the continuity of the skin caused by surgery, trauma, or an underlying disorder that robs the skin of its needed nutrients. Most wounds heal rapidly; patients at risk for alterations in healing include the obese, diabetic, elderly, malnourished, and immunocompromised. Delayed healing usually results from compromised wound physiology and occurs most commonly with venous stasis, diabetes, or prolonged local pressure. These frequently progress to chronic wounds. Chronic wounds are a serious health issue. Incidence is 1% to 2% in the general population in western countries, with the elderly at significant risk.

PRINCIPLES OF CARE
Normal Wound Healing

The process of normal wound healing occurs in three phases. The initial phase, *inflammation*, begins immediately with clot formation to stop any bleeding. The clot provides the framework on which the new growth will adhere. Vasodilation with increased capillary permeability and the influx of phagocytic cells (macrophages) to clear debris occurs simultaneously. This phase usually last 1 to 4 days, during which time the wound is edematous, warm, and painful.

The *proliferative* phase follows, with migration of fibroblasts, which attach to the framework and synthesize collagen and elastin. Buds of new blood cells grow from the capillaries surrounding the wound. Collagen (a fibrous insoluble protein) is laid down in the wound bed. The capillary buds and collagen form granulation tissue. Epithelial cells then grow in over the granulation, in a process called epithelialization. For epithelialization to be effective, the underlying tissues must be well nourished. This phase usually takes between 5 and 20 days.

Remodeling, the final phase, can last from 21 days to several months. In this phase, collagen fibers reorganize and tighten, increasing tensile strength.

Wound Classification

Wounds may be classified in terms of the level of tissue injury (partial or full thickness), mechanism of closure (primary, secondary, or tertiary), duration (chronic, acute), and risk of infection by surgical site.

77

Table 3-1-1. Nonviable Tissue

Necrotic tissue	Dead tissue that adheres to viable tissue
Slough	Creamy white-yellow, stringy tissue that loosely adheres to the wound
Eschar	Black or brown, dry, leathery denatured collagen

Level of Tissue Injury

Partial-thickness wounds involve tissue injury through the epidermis, extending into, but not through, the dermis. They are superficial and usually heal in 5 to 7 days in healthy individuals.

Full-thickness wounds involve tissue destruction through the dermis and subcutaneous layers. Muscle and bone may be involved. All nonviable tissue (Table 3-1-1) must be removed from these wounds, or else healing will not occur. In addition, without good blood flow and oxygenation, epithelialization will fail.

Mechanisms of Wound Closure

Wound closure occurs by various mechanisms, depending on the wound's cause and condition. Wounds that close by *primary intention* are those in which the edges can be brought together and skin layers are approximated with sutures, staples, or sterile adhesive strips. No open areas or dead spaces remain; thus, wound healing time is shortened. Closure results in minimal scar tissue. Alterations in primary intention closure usually manifest as infection, dehiscence (separation of all layers of an incision), or evisceration (rupture of an abdominal incision with extrusion of its contents).

Closure by *secondary intention* occurs with deeper injuries that involve tissue loss, resulting in cavities or uneven wound edges that cannot be approximated. Such wounds include chronic wounds (e.g., pressure ulcers, venous stasis ulcers) and infected wounds. The tissue loss with resultant dead space requires that these wounds heal by slow, gradual filling in, delaying the healing phases significantly and producing significant scarring.

Closure by *tertiary intention* occurs when a surgical incision is left open for several days and then closed by sutures after inflammation has subsided and debris and exudate have been removed. This is usually done when there is a significant potential for infection, as in incisions of nonsterile or contaminated body cavities and open traumatic wounds. This type of closure is also called *delayed primary closure.*

Common Wound Types
Clean Surgical Wounds

These wounds may be shallow or deep, depending on the surgical procedure performed. The incision line is well approximated, with mild signs of inflammation (erythema and warmth) and minimal drainage. Drainage subsides after 48 hours; inflammation, within 5 days. Edges unite with a thin scar by 7 to 9 days.

Infection is the most common cause of delayed wound healing in operative patients. All surgical incisions are at some degree of risk for infection, which impairs all phases of wound healing.

Traumatic Wounds

In traumatic wounds, which are usually acute, wound edges are edematous and erythematous, and may be indurated. However, there is scant or no drainage, necrosis, or odor. The duration of the healing process depends on the location and size of the wound, as well as on the patient's comorbidities (e.g., malnutrition).

Skin Tears

Skin tears are traumatic wounds involving separation of the epidermis from the dermis (partial thickness or separation of both the epidermis and dermis from underlying structures [full thickness]). Skin tears are most common in elderly persons due to age-related skin changes, such as loss of dermal thickness and loss of subcutaneous fat. They are usually the result of friction alone or shearing and friction forces combined. They occur most often in the upper extremities, but can also occur on the back and buttocks; the latter are frequently mistaken for stage II pressure ulcers. In a skin tear, the skin flap may remain intact or may be partially or totally lost.

Arterial Ulcers

These wounds are commonly associated with peripheral vascular disease (PVD), diabetes mellitus, and advanced age. Typical sites include between the toes, over the phalangeal heads, at the lateral malleolus, and at sites subjected to trauma or rubbing. The wound bed may appear gray, yellow, or black and necrotic with eschar and no evidence of new growth. The margins are smooth and even. Cellulitis may be present, as may exposed tendons. Exudate is minimal, and surrounding skin is blanched, cool, and hairless. Pain occurring at rest and increasing with elevation is common. Surgical revascularization is required for healing.

Venous Ulcers

These wounds are most common in patients with incompetent valves or deep venous thrombophlebitis or thrombosis, as well as in obese and elderly persons. They usually occur between the knee and ankle, with the medial and lateral malleolus (bony protrusion on either side of the ankle joint) the most common sites. They are typically red and beefy with granular tissue and calcification in the wound base. Exudate may be moderate to heavy. The wound edges are irregular, and the surrounding skin is edematous and may be macerated. Pain varies but decreases with elevation. Healing may be difficult and may take up to 1 year, depending on the degree of insufficiency.

Diabetic Ulcers

These wounds occur in patients with diabetes mellitus who have developed peripheral neuropathy or PVD. They are commonly located along the lower limb and foot, areas subjected to repetitive friction, shear, pressure, and trauma. They are usually dry and may have tracking and undermining. Cellulitis and osteomyelitis may be present. In diabetic ulcers due to neuropathy, granulation tissue will be present. Drainage is low to moderate, and the wound edges are round, smooth, and even, with a calloused elevated rim. The wound may appear small superficially but have large subcutaneous areas. The patient feels either no sensation or numbness or burning that is intermittent or constant.

Proper foot care and compliance with diabetes therapy (Chapter 18, Section 1) are essential aspects of treatment; revascularization may be needed.

Pressure Ulcers

These wounds occur in persons with impaired mobility, decreased level of consciousness, impaired circulation, malnutrition, and incontinence. Common sites include the sacrum, heels, coccyx, occiput, and any bony prominence subjected to pressure, friction, or shearing forces. Friction is the irritation or pulling off of epithelial tissue when external surfaces rub the skin. This occurs with dragging or pulling the patient up in bed. Shearing occurs when the skin remains in place but the underlying fat and bone are displaced, which occurs when the patient slides down in bed.

The severity of pressure ulcers can be staged on a scale of I through IV:

- *Stage I*: Nonblanchable erythema of intact skin; the heralding lesion of skin ulceration
- *Stage II*: Partial-thickness skin loss involving the epidermis or dermis; presents clinically as an abrasion, blister, or shallow crater
- *Stage III*: Full-thickness skin loss involving damage or necrosis of subcutaneous tissue that may extend down to, but not through, underlying fascia. Presents clinically as a deep crater with or without undermining of adjacent tissue.
- *Stage IV*: Full-thickness skin loss with extensive destruction, tissue necrosis, or damage to muscle, bone, or supporting structures (tendon or joint capsule)

Care of pressure ulcers involves eliminating or reducing pressure, friction, and shear, while implementing wound care for healing.

DECISION-MAKING

The goals of management for all wounds are to prevent infection, enhance the healing process, and restore function to the area.

Assessment

Measure and document the size and location of the wound. If the wound is round, note the circumference in centimeters. Measure depth from the wound bed to the skin surface, using a sterile cotton-tipped swab.

Assess the level of tissue injury as erythema of intact skin, partial thickness, or full thickness. If wound closure is by primary intention, document which method was used. If the wound is a pressure ulcer, determine the stage.

Assess the wound bed, describing the type of tissue in percentages (e.g., 30% necrotic, 20% slough, and 50% granulation). Assess the wound edges; identify whether they are approximated, smooth, jagged, indurated, or separated from the wound.

Describe the periwound surface, noting edema, maceration, or erythema. Describe the amount of exudate as scant, small, moderate, or large and the character of the exudate as serous, serosanguineous, or purulent. Assess for undermining or tunneling.

Assess wound pain. Determine whether it is continuous, intermittent, burning, or dull and whether it is relieved with elevation.

Wound Cleansing

Normal saline (NS) is the solution of choice for cleansing wounds. Lactated Ringer's solution also may be used. Wound irrigation removes inflammatory material, necrotic tissue, and wound debris without disturbing granulation tissue. Wounds may be effectively irrigated using a 35-mL syringe with a 19-gauge Silastic catheter. Aim the catheter a few inches from the wound base and irrigate with a steady force. This method will deliver the recommended pressure of 8 psi, which has proved to be effective in decreasing wound inflammation and infection.

Cleansing can also be done by gently patting the wound surface with sterile gauze moistened with NS. Whirlpool therapy provides vigorous irrigation for large wounds with foreign debris or nonviable tissue.

All antiseptics (e.g., povidone-iodine, hydrogen peroxide, acetic acid, Dakin's solution) are cytotoxic to fibroblasts and will delay wound healing. Thus, they should *not* be used in a wound or to clean around a drain; they are designed to cleanse intact skin.

Wound Débridement

Débridement is the removal of nonviable tissue when necessary to promote healing and treat infection. There are four methods of débridement: mechanical, sharp/surgical, chemical, and autolytic.

Mechanical débridement can be done with wet-to-dry dressings. Gauze is soaked with NS, squeezed out fully, and placed loosely in the wound. As the gauze dries, necrotic tissue adheres to it, and when the gauze is removed, the necrotic tissue comes with it. This method should be avoided or used with caution in wounds once granulation begins, because it will also strip the new granulation tissue. Because this technique is painful, pain assessment and adequate pain management are essential. The dressings should be changed two to four times a day. Frequent changes will also prevent infection and desiccation of the surrounding skin.

Sharp débridement, also called surgical débridement, involves removing necrotic tissue from viable tissue with a scalpel or scissors. This technique is usually performed by a physician or health care provider with specialized training.

Chemical débridement is accomplished by applying enzymes that dissolve the nonviable tissue. These must be used with caution, because viable tissue may also be lysed.

Autolytic débridement allows the body's own enzymes and white blood cells (WBCs) to lyse and dissolve necrotic tissue. This is done by placing an occlusive or semiocclusive dressing over the wound, allowing for the normal WBC migration and other immune responses to occur. The dressing may be left in place until accumulated wound drainage disrupts the dressing, which can take several days. This method may not be successful in immunocompromised patients.

Pulsed lavage irrigates and débrides wounds using a pressurized, pulsed solution (usually NS). It simultaneously suctions to remove debris and the used solution. The procedure is performed by the physical therapist in the patient's room.

Infection Management

Débridement and cleansing are usually adequate for treating and preventing infection. If an infection does occur, Silvadene (silver sulfadiazine) or another topical antibiotic is added. Silvadene should be applied in a thin layer after the wound has been cleansed, and the dressing changed every 24 hours. Ensure that use is restricted to the prescribed number of days. Systemic antibiotics are not indicated unless signs of systemic infection are present. If the wound is free of nonviable tissue and infected, débridement is not necessary; topical antibiotic therapy is adequate.

Avoiding Pressure

Identify patients at risk for pressure ulcers. Skin assessment scales are used in most institutions. Turn and reposition the patient at least every 1 to 2 hours. Use pillows or foam wedges to support bony prominences and extremities.

To relieve pressure from the heels of an immobilized patient, place pillows under the lower leg lengthwise to the ankle, allowing the heels to float freely. Do not use doughnut-type devices, which may cause venous congestion. Do not rub bony prominences—this may rupture small capillaries and reduce flow.

Place the patient on a pressure-reducing mattress. Reduce friction and shear by keeping the patient in a low Fowler position, unless contraindicated. Use a lift sheet, pad, or lifting device, when possible, to avoid dragging the patient up in bed.

Wound Dressings

Moist-to-moist dressings, such as sterile saline gauze, provide a moist environment, are absorbent, and provide protection and cushioning. These dressings are very useful when drainage is heavy enough to necessitate dressing changes more frequently than every 24 hours. They are useful for infected wounds; anti-infective agents may be applied with them. Dry gauze may be applied to heavily draining wounds. Change the dressing every 4 to 6 hours if the wound is necrotic or infected, and every 12 to 24 hours if the wound is clean.

Transparent adhesive films (Op-site, Tegaderm, Biocclusive) are semiocclusive see-through dressings that allow for autolytic débridement. They are suitable for noninfected wounds that are dry or have minimal drainage. They do not absorb drainage and can cause maceration if used over a draining wound. The semiocclusive membrane allows for the exchange of oxygen, but not bacteria, between the wound bed and the environment. Transparency allows visual wound monitoring. These dressings are commonly used to protect IV insertion sites. They are also useful for stage I and II pressure ulcers, donor sites, lacerations, and abrasions. When used for skin tears, caution is required on removal. They are very useful for protecting against friction and shear. The dressings should be changed if leakage of exudate occurs or every 24 hours in wounds with nonviable tissue.

Nonadherent dressings (Adaptic, Xeroform) are woven or nonwoven cotton or synthetic dressings impregnated with saline solution, petrolatum, or antimicrobial agents. These dressings require secondary dressings (e.g., gauze, Kling wrap) to secure them in place and retain moisture. They are used to soothe and protect partial- and full-thickness wounds with minimal drainage; they are especially suitable for skin tears.

Hydrocolloids (e.g., Duoderm, Tegasorb, Restore, Cutinovare) are occlusive dressings used to maintain a moist wound base and for autolytic débridement in noninfected, full-thickness wounds with nonviable tissue. The occlusive membrane does not allow oxygen to diffuse from the environment to the wound bed. It absorbs exudate and forms a gel (not to be confused with purulent drainage) without causing maceration of surrounding skin. Thin hydrocolloids are useful for partial-thickness wounds with minimal exudate. They are also useful for skin protectants. *Hydrocolloids are not used over infected wounds.* Hydrocolloids may be changed on leakage of exudate or every 7 days.

Hydrogels (e.g., Curasol, Nu-gel, Vigilon) are used to maintain a moist environment for dry wounds or to provide autolytic débridement. Available in sheets, impregnated gauze, or gel, they are 95% water and cannot accept much drainage. A secondary dressing, such as gauze, is needed to adhere the dressing to the wound and secure it. A hydrocolloid dressing may be used if the wound is not infected. Hydrogels should be changed every 3 days for necrotic or sloughy wounds, or 7 days for clean granulating wounds. If gauze is used to secure the dressing, dressing changes should be done every 8 hours for wounds with a necrotic base and every 24 hours for ones with a clean base. Hydrogels can cause maceration if applied to the periwound area. They are very useful for venous stasis ulcers. The moist environment reduces pain, liquefies crusty exudate, and promotes autolysis.

Polyurethane foams (e.g., Allevyn, Hydrosorb, Lyofoam) are nonadhesive dressings that need secondary dressings to secure them. They provide a poor barrier when used alone. These dressings conform to wound edges and are used to fill deep wounds with drainage. They can be used on infected wounds. These foams absorb moderate to heavy amounts of exudate, and the periwound area must be protected to prevent maceration. The dressings are changed when they are saturated.

Alginate dressings (e.g., Kaltostat, Sorbsand, Tegagen) are fibrous products derived from brown seaweed. Alginates form a gel when they come in contact with fluid and can absorb up to 20 times their weight. They are used to fill in deep wounds with moderate to heavy drainage, and infected wounds. They are the dressings of choice for dehisced, full-thickness surgical wounds, because they eliminate dead space and support débridement. Because they are nonadherent, they require a secondary dressing. If the wound is infected, the secondary dressing should be nonocclusive. Dressings are changed daily for infected wounds. For noninfected wounds, dressings should be changed when they becomes saturated or every 3 to 5 days.

Compression dressings (Unna boot) are used with venous ulcers. The dressing is of zinc oxide–impregnated gauze. The gauze is wrapped around the affected extremity from the toes to the knee, and is then covered with an elastic wrap. The boot hardens into a semi-cast material, promoting venous return while providing a sterile environment. The boot can be changed approximately once a week. Peripheral circulation is closely monitored to identify arterial occlusion, which can occur if the boot is wrapped too tightly.

Growth Factors

Growth factors are used to increase the rate of healing rather than to provide a favorable environment for healing. They are naturally occurring proteins that stimulate growth and wound contraction.

Blood Flow and Oxygenation

Blood flow and oxygenation should be assessed for adequacy. Swelling or vessel damage at the injury site can impede blood flow and the removal of bacteria and debris from the wound site. Ensure adequate hydration and elevate the affected area when indicated. Oxygen at low doses (2 to 4 L) may be administered. Hyperbaric oxygen may be indicated in cases of delayed wound healing.

Nutrition

Nutritional assessment (see Chapter 9, Section 1) and support are essential for adequate healing to occur. Ensure adequate intake of protein, calories, and fluid. Vitamin C and iron promote tissue healing. Vitamin A, topical or systemic, reverses steroids' effects on healing.

 CLINICAL PEARLS

○ Clean superficial wounds and around drains by gently patting the wound surface with sterile gauze moistened with NS.

○ Irrigate contaminated or necrotic wounds using a 35-mL syringe with a 19-gauge angiocatheter by aiming the catheter a few inches from the wound base and applying a steady force. This may need to be repeated for up to 100 to 150 mL.

○ Nutritional assessment should be obtained on admission.

○ Wound débridement can be done by placing an occlusive dressing over the wound, allowing the body's own defenses to eat away at the necrosis.

○ A nonadherent dressing (Adaptic) may be used for patients with multiple skin tears on an extremity. These must be wrapped with a dry dressing.

○ Thin hydrocolloids are useful skin protectants in patients requiring multiple dressing changes.

Wound Drainage Systems

Section 2   Beverly George-Gay

OVERVIEW

Surgical drains are inserted prophylactically to prevent accumulation of fluid and blood in deep wounds, which serve as a culture medium for bacteria, as well as to prevent pressure buildup that can cause circulatory impairment. They are also used to drain existing fluid collections, divert fluids, facilitate monitoring of fluid loss, and provide access for wound irrigation. Surgical drains may also be used to remove air. The entrapment of air and fluid in between tissue spaces ("deadspace") prevents wound edges from approximating and can delay wound healing. Drainage can occur by gravity or by suction as part of a closed drainage system.

PRINCIPLES OF CARE
Placement of Drains

Drains may be placed within the wound through the surgical incision line. Most often, though, they are inserted through a separate small incision (known as a *stab wound*) a few centimeters away from the incision line, so that the incision itself can be kept dry.

Types of Drains

Surgical drains are of two basic types: open (passive) and closed (active). The choice of whether to use an *open* or a *closed* drainage system depends on the site being drained and on the patient's activity level and overall healing capability.

Open Drains

Peritoneal cavity or skin wounds may be drained through an open drain, which allows fluid to escape along the outside surface of the drain through capillary action and gravity. The fluid exits the wound via the open drain catheter and is absorbed by a dressing. Drainage is further facilitated by transient increases in intra-abdominal pressure, as occurs as the patient bears down and coughs.

Open drains range in size from 14 to 34 French and 300 to 400 mm in length. Popular open drains include Penrose and Malecot drains; Foley and Word catheters also may be used as open drains.

The *Penrose drain* is soft and smooth, to minimize trauma during insertion and withdrawal. A safety pin placed at the drain's external end keeps it from sliding back into the wound. Penrose drains are used in various settings that involve large cavities with thick walls.

The *Malecot drain* is a soft opaque tube with four wings that extend in four directions on insertion to secure the catheter position. This drain is used most often in urology, but it can also be used in gastrointestinal and pulmonary (for drainage of empyema) situations.

Closed Drains

Closed drainage systems (e.g., Jackson-Pratt) consist of a drain (or drainage catheter), which is slightly stiffer than the open drain catheters, and a vacuum reservoir. These are self-contained systems in which the drainage tube is connected directly to the reservoir. The *drain* is usually flat but may be round with multiple perforations or ducts to allow fluid entry at any point along the drain. Some newer closed drainage catheters are treated with heparin to inhibit clot formation within the catheter. The *vacuum reservoir* creates negative pressure (suction) to facilitate wound drainage. The reservoir is compressed manually to maintain constant low suction. Fluid is drawn toward the suction source via the path of least resistance.

The reservoir may have both the inlet and the outlet on top, or the inlet at the top and the outlet at the bottom. Inlets have nonreturn valves to prevent the regurgitation of fluid. Reservoirs come in various shapes and sizes. The most commonly used vacuum reservoir is the 100-mL bulb known as the Jackson-Pratt (JP) reservoir (although Jackson-Pratt is actually the brand name of a drain). A larger bulb, the Duval bulb, holds up to 400 mL. The vacuum reservoir may also be a pancake-type collapsible device with an inner spring, such as the Hemovac. Closed systems pose a lower hazard of exposure to blood and body fluids for caregivers and eliminate the portal of entry for pathogens that could infect the wound. They also promote healing by reducing edema and preventing hematoma formation.

DECISION-MAKING

Nursing care focuses on preventing contamination through or around the drain. Care measures include ensuring frequent dressing changes, maintaining drain patency, and preserving the integrity of the skin around the drain site. Drain removal should be done using aseptic technique.

Type and Location

Document the type and location of all drains. The patient may have multiple drains in multiple places. Each must be assessed and labeled to ensure accurate measurement of output.

Skin

Assess the condition of the skin around the drain with each shift assessment and dressing change. Pain, induration, and erythema are indicators of infection in the subcutaneous tissue surrounding the drain. This must be reported; antimicrobial therapy may be necessary.

Dressing Changes

The frequency of dressing changes will depend on the type and location of the drain and the amount of drainage present. Remove the old dressing and cleanse the skin around the drain with normal saline or another prescribed solution. Apply precut 4″ × 4″ gauze pads snugly around the drain. Do not cut standard 4″ × 4″ pads, because these will shred, allowing pieces of lint and thread to enter the wound. If precut pads are not available, then fold standard 4″ × 4″s in half and apply one or two on either side of the drain.

If the skin is irritated or if there is a potential for irritation (as with pancreatic drains, which irritate skin), then transparent adhesive film or a thin hydrocolloid protective dressing (see Section 1) may be applied directly to the clean skin. Apply the 4″ × 4″ dressings on top to accept the drainage and tape them to the protective dressing, further protecting the skin from tape irritation. In an open drain, apply 4″ × 4″s around the end of the drain to absorb drainage. Maintain sterile technique when changing open drain dressings. If the drain is within an open incision, Montgomery straps may be used to hold the dressing in place.

Drain Patency

Assess drain patency at least once per shift by anticipating output. Sudden cessation of drainage may indicate an occlusion of the drain by tissue debris or clot formation. Report increased sanguineous drainage, which may be caused by catheter erosion into a blood vessel.

Character of the Drainage

Assess the character of the drainage fluid. Determine whether it is serous, sanguineous, or purulent, and determine whether the character of the fluid has changed since the previous assessment. Note that drainage may become thick and malodorous in infection.

Output

Record the amount of drainage every 4 hours for the first 24 hours and then once every shift. Output from open drains may have to be estimated, or a one-piece ostomy bag can be applied over the stab wound to collect excessive amounts, which are then measured. Closed drains have outlets from which drainage can be emptied. Wearing clean gloves, cleanse the top of the reservoir with an alcohol sponge to decrease the microorganisms around the opening. Empty secretions into a container and measure them. Because the antiregurgitation valve prevents backflow, squeeze the bulb or pancake reservoir to clear all secretions. Remove any secretions from the tip of the outlet with a clean alcohol sponge. The container can then be compressed and closed.

Drain Manipulation

Penrose drains may be gradually pulled from the wound as the amount of drainage decreases. The drain may be pulled 0.5 inch at a time, with the safety pin reattached close to the patient's skin. Sterile procedure should be maintained during wound irrigation. When removing a closed drain, open the vacuum reservoir, thus releasing the suction before pulling the tube. Pull the tube in an upward direction, applying counterpressure around the insertion site. Assess the drainage catheter for intactness after removal; it is subject to breakage because of inadvertent suturing during placement. Adequate analgesia must be given before drain manipulation begins.

 CLINICAL PEARLS

○ Label multiple drains as 1, 2, and 3 or right upper, left lower, and so on.
○ Use clean gloves and alcohol sponges when emptying reservoir bulbs or pancakes.
○ Do not cut 4″ × 4″ gauze pads to place around drains; the frayed lint may enter the wound.
○ When drainage from an open drain is excessive, apply a one-piece ostomy bag over the stab wound.
○ Before removing a closed drainage system, release the suction by opening the bulb or pancake.
○ The possibility of a latex allergy must be ruled out before surgery.

Ostomies

Section 3

Kathy Ravenell

OVERVIEW

Individuals undergoing ostomy surgery are facing temporary or permanent lifestyle changes. Ostomies are surgically created fissures that allow tube drainage of wastes from the body. Stomas are the actual ends of the ureters or intestines that protrude through the abdominal wall. Ostomies used to divert stool are called bowel diversion ostomies; those used to divert urine, urinary diversion ostomies. These ostomies divert stool or urine away from injured, diseased, or congenital areas of the digestive tract. They can be temporary or permanent, depending on the location and extent of the disease and the health of the patient.

PRINCIPLES OF CARE
Colostomy

The most common type of ostomy, a colostomy, is a surgically constructed opening that connects the colon to the abdomen. This forms a stoma that allows waste to be discharged from the body without passing through the diseased portion of the colon and rectum.

A colostomy may be indicated as part of the treatment regimen for a patient diagnosed with cancer of the colon or rectum. Surgery is usually required to eradicate the cancer. The location of the cancer in the colon or rectum determines the type of surgical procedure as well as the need for an ostomy.

Temporary colostomies are used for short periods up to 1 year. They allow the lower portion of the colon to rest or heal. Temporary colostomies are typically performed on patients with diverticulitis or a traumatic bowel injury, such as a gunshot wound, obstruction, or volvulus.

A *loop colostomy* is a type of temporary colostomy formed by bringing an intact portion of the colon through an abdominal incision and suturing it onto the abdomen in the form of a loop. This loop, which is part of the colon, is held in place by a glass rod or plastic bridge, to ensure that the loop does not slip back into the abdominal cavity. The stomal opening is made on the exterior surface of the segment. The loop is usually opened within 24 to 48 hours after surgery. The stoma has no nerve endings and thus is not sensitive to pain, touch, or heat. The glass rod or plastic bridge is removed within 1 to 3 weeks, depending on the patient's status.

A *double-barreled colostomy* is a temporary colostomy involving removal of part of the large intestine. Two stomas are then formed. The proximal portion of the colon forms a functioning stoma that drains fecal material; the distal portion of the colon forms a nonfunctional stoma that drains mucus. This distal stoma is also called a mucous fistula.

Permanent colostomies involve a loss of part of the colon. The colostomy substitutes for the anus when the anus and rectum are removed because of traumatic injury or cancer of the sigmoid colon or rectum. The end of the remaining colon is brought out to the abdominal wall to form a stoma.

Ileostomy

An ileostomy is a surgically created opening in which the small intestine, usually the ileum, is brought through the abdominal wall to form a stoma. Ileostomies may be temporary or permanent and may involve removal of all or a part of the colon.

Ileoconduit

In this procedure, the most common permanent urinary diversion, a section of the small bowel (ileum) is surgically removed and relocated as a passageway (conduit) for urine to pass from the ureters to the outside of the body via a stoma. Surgery is performed to divert urine away from a diseased or defective bladder.

A patient with a urinary diversion is usually required to wear an external pouch at all times to collect urine. A patient who has a Kock pouch, also known as a continent vesicostomy (in which the bladder wall is sutured to the abdominal wall to form a pouch) can wear a small dressing over the stoma for protection.

DECISION-MAKING
Stoma Assessment

Color. The stoma should be red, similar in color to the mucosal lining of the inner cheek. Darker-colored stomas indicate impaired blood circulation to the area.

Size and Shape. New stomas appear swollen, but generally decrease in size up to 6 weeks after surgery. Failure of swelling to decrease may indicate a problem, such as a blockage.

Bleeding. Slight bleeding when the stoma is touched is normal; report any other bleeding.

Status of Peristomal Skin. Note any redness or irritation of the peristomal skin.

Amount and Type of Feces. For a bowel diversion ostomy, assess the amount, color, odor, and consistency of feces (Table 3-3-1). Inspect for abnormalities, such as pus or blood. For a urinary diversion ostomy, assess the amount, color, clarity, and odor of the urine.

Complaints. Because stomas do not have nerve endings, they are not painful. A patient may complain of burning under the faceplate of the pouch. This may indicate skin breakdown. Carefully assess all complaints of abdominal discomfort or distention.

Table 3-3-1. Location of Bowel Diversion Ostomies

Ileostomy	An opening made in the ileum. The drainage will be liquid and constant. It is necessary to wear an appliance at all times, and special care must be given to protecting the skin. Leaking pouches/wafers must be changed immediately because of the caustic nature of the drainage. The patient is at risk for dehydration and needs to drink lots of fluids to maintain fluid and electrolyte balance.
Cecostomy	An opening made in the cecum. Not common, but used in the treatment of large bowel obstruction. The stool drainage will be liquid to semiliquid. It is very irritating to the peristomal skin.
Ascending colostomy	Located within the ascending colon. Similar to ileostomy drainage in that it cannot be regulated, so skin protection is important. The patient must wear a bag at all times. Pouch odor is a problem; this may be controlled by using deodorant in the ostomy pouch.
Transverse colostomy	Located within the transverse colon. Usually produces semiliquid or very soft stool. Special care must be taken to protect the skin from discharge. The patient must wear a pouch at all times.
Descending colostomy	Located in the descending colon. Produces a more solid fecal drainage. Irrigation may regulate bowel movement in some patients.
Sigmoid colostomy	Located in the sigmoid colon. Stool is of normal consistency. The patient may not need to wear a pouch.

Stoma Irrigation

Colostomy irrigation should be taught to patients with permanent descending or sigmoid colostomies. Irrigation is performed to empty the colon of feces, gas, or mucus. It allows the patient to establish a regular pattern of evacuation so that normal life activities may be resumed and maintained. The irrigation procedure should be performed at the same time each day. Colostomy irrigation is performed daily or every other day, making a pouch unnecessary.

The irrigation procedure is as follows:

1. Place an irrigating sleeve or sheath over the colostomy. Secure the sleeve with the adhesive disk on the sleeve or with a sleeve belt.
2. Fill the irrigation container with 500 to 1000 mL of warm water. Allow some of the solution to flow through the tubing and the catheter/cone.
3. Position the patient sitting on a chair in front of the toilet or on the toilet itself. Position the sleeve so that it hangs in the toilet for emptying.
4. Lubricate the catheter/cone, and gently insert it into the stoma (no more than 3 inches).
5. Allow the water to slowly enter the stoma from the container through the tubing. Water should flow in over 5 to 10 minutes. If the patient complains of cramping and/or nausea while the water is flowing, then stop the flow. Leave the cone in place until the symptoms subside, then resume the flow of water. If the patient continues to complain of cramping, the colon is probably ready to evacuate and should be allowed to do so.
6. Hold the catheter/cone in place for a few seconds after the water has been instilled, then gently remove it. Leave the sleeve in place for about 30 to 45 minutes to allow elimination of the water and stool.
7. When elimination is complete, cleanse the area with mild soap and water. Pat the peristomal area dry.
8. Replace the colostomy dressing or pouch.

Pouching Systems

Various types of ostomy pouching systems are available (Table 3-3-2). The choice of pouching system is a personal one geared to each individual's needs. Enterostomal nurses and physicians should offer patients information about different systems. A poorly performing or uncomfortable pouching system can lead to stomal or skin irritation.

Table 3-3-2. Pouching Systems

POUCH TYPE	DESCRIPTION	ADVANTAGES	DISADVANTAGES
One-piece	Skin barrier and pouch are combined into one unit, which allows for a single one-step application	• Allows for greater flexibility • Very low profile under clothing • Little dexterity needed	• More difficult to rinse out • Must look through pouch to center over stoma, which may affect patients with poor vision
Two-piece	Separate wafer and pouch, pouch snaps onto wafer	• Pouch may be removed for cleansing or disposal • Easier to visualize stoma pouch when applying wafer	• Not flexible • Must have good dexterity to snap pouch to wafer

Basic Pouching Principles

Protect Peristomal Skin. Measure the stoma with a measuring guide. The opening should allow the stoma to protrude while covering approximately 2.5 cm (1 in.) of the skin around the stoma. Trace the opening onto the back of the wafer or pouch. Clean and dry the peristomal skin and stoma with water or cleaning agent.

Skin Barriers. Use of a skin barrier protects the peristomal skin. Skin barriers come in several different forms, including powders, pastes, and wafers.

Powder. A pouch will not adhere to powder, cream, or ointment. Powder is sometimes used in treating skin irritations under a wafer barrier. Dust the irritated skin with powder, and allow it to dry.

Paste. Paste is used around a stoma to fill in creases or dimples. Paste forms a smooth surface that seals the wafer to the skin to prevent leakage under the wafer. It does not add any adhesive properties to the wafer. Paste is not routinely used on ileal conduits, because urine melts it.

Skin Barrier Wafers. Skin barrier wafers are used with various types of pouches to protect the skin from stool. The opening of the wafer is carefully measured to ensure proper fit and prevent rubbing and irritation of the stoma.

Skin Sealants. Sprays, liquids, gels, or wipes are used to coat the skin and prevent skin irritation. Skin sealants are used under all tape applied to the skin.

Pouch Emptying (Reusable Pouch)

Pouches should be emptied when they are one-third to one-half full. This prevents overfilling and disruption of the seal. When emptying a fecal pouch, turn back the edge of the pouch to keep the end of the pouch clean. Wipe off any stool on the edge of the pouch and the clip to decrease odor. Fold the edge of the pouch over the clip only once. Rolling up the pouch several times over the clip may cause it to break.

Pouch Cleansing

Although cleansing the pouch with each emptying may not be necessary, cleansing it once a day may help the patient's self-image. Water or another type of cleansing agent, such as Peri-wash or Sproam, may be used.

To rinse a one-piece pouch, empty the contents, then instill cool tap water around the bottom portion of the pouch. Do not aim water up at the top portion of the pouch, because this may loosen the seal on the skin.

To rinse a two-piece pouch, unsnap the pouch from the wafer. Let the drainage flow into the toilet. Rinse the pouch, dry it, and snap it back onto the wafer.

 CLINICAL PEARLS

○ Be alert for possible allergic reactions to adhesives and other ostomy products.

○ Failure to fit the pouch properly over the stoma can result in injury to the stoma or surrounding skin.

○ A patient who gains or loses weight may need a recheck of pouch fit.

○ Empty an ostomy pouch when it is one-third full. This will prevent bulging of the bag that can be seen through clothing and prevents dislodging of the pouch.

- Gas production may be caused by foods from the cabbage family, onions, beans, cucumbers, radishes, and beer.
- Odor-producing foods include cheese, eggs, fish, beans, onions, cheese, and some vitamins or medications.
- Consuming cranberry juice, buttermilk, and yogurt may reduce fecal odor in ostomy bags.

Gastrointestinal Drainage Systems

Section 4   Kathy Ravenell

OVERVIEW

The primary function of the gastrointestinal (GI), or digestive, system is to convert ingested nutrients and fluids into a form for use by body cells as nourishment. This is accomplished through ingestion, digestion, and absorption. The second major function of the GI system is the storage and final excretion of the solid waste products of digestion. Proper functioning of the GI system is necessary for the maintenance of nutrition and health. Some treatments for patients with problems of the GI system involve the use of gastric or intestinal intubation to supply nutrients or remove contents from the GI tract.

PRINCIPLES OF CARE

Intubation of the GI tract is indicated for diagnostic evaluation and potential treatment of upper GI bleeding, management of small bowel or gastric outlet obstructions, enteral nourishment or medication, and lavage for poisoning or overdose. Most commonly, intubation of the GI tract is indicated for decompression of the stomach or intestines. Intubation of the biliary tract is indicated for biliary obstruction that causes bile to escape into surrounding tissue. Bile is very toxic and may cause peritonitis if allowed to leak into the peritoneal cavity.

There are several ways to intubate the GI or biliary tract. Procedures can be performed surgically or at the bedside for temporary or permanent use.

DECISION-MAKING
Gastrostomy Tubes

A gastrostomy tube, or G-tube, is a surgically created fistula that proceeds through the abdominal wall into the stomach. G-tubes can be either temporary or permanent. They are commonly used in patients who have injuries of the oropharyngeal and esophageal areas. These individuals may not be able to orally consume food for indefinite periods. G-tube feedings allow patients to obtain fluid and nutritional support until oral intake is adequate. Gastrostomy tubes are also used to drain contents out of the GI tract. The insertion and placement are performed in the operating room by a surgeon. Site care is discussed in Table 3-4-1.

G-tubes may be used in patients with transient paralytic ileus, which is common after abdominal surgery because of the manipulation of the intestines.

Table 3-4-1. G-tube Exit Site Care

- Perform daily skin care.
- Assess the exit sites at least once each shift. Examine the area for erythema, drainage, and other skin problems.
- There may be a small amount of clear drainage from the exit site in the first few weeks after insertion.
- Clean the area around the exit site with a mild pH-balanced soap, commercial cleanser, or 0.9% sodium chloride.
- A cotton-tipped applicator can be used to clean close to the tube to remove any crusts or drainage.
- Never place gauze under the retaining device. This can lead to abdominal wall erosion or abscesses.

From O'Brien, B., Davis, S., and Erwin-Toth, P. (1999). G-tube site care: A practical guide. *RN, 62* (2), 52–56.

Transient paralytic ileus is more likely in surgeries that use general anesthesia, which depresses intestinal motility. Preoperative anesthetic medications, such as narcotics, are central nervous system depressants that decrease intestinal motility, and cholinergic blocking agents block the action of acetylcholine in the parasympathetic nervous system, thus decreasing peristalsis. G-tubes are used to decompress the intestines. The nurse may help prevent paralytic ileus in a patient who has undergone abdominal surgery by noting when bowel sounds have not returned within 48 to 72 hours after surgery.

Percutaneous Endoscopic Gastrostomy Tubes

Percutaneous endoscopic gastrostomy (PEG) tubes can be inserted endoscopically without general anesthesia. They are used for long-term tube feedings into the stomach in patients with a functional GI tract. They are frequently used in patients with alterations in swallowing due to neurologic diseases, brain injury, or tumors of the head, neck, or esophagus. PEG tubes are safer and less expensive than traditional G-tubes. PEG tubes can be inserted at bedside with local anesthesia and conscious sedation, usually in only 10 to 30 minutes. Caution should be taken with patients who have medical histories associated with obstructions, previous gastric surgeries, morbid obesity, and ascites. These individuals are at increased risk for postoperative complications.

Nursing Management for PEGs

1. Always check tube placement before administering feedings and medications.
2. Assess for the presence of bowel sounds before administering feedings.
3. Use liquid medications instead of pills. Dilute viscous liquid medications and ensure that the medications can be administered with meals.
4. Elevate the head of the bed, check for residual volume, and flush the tube with water.
5. Monitor for complications, such as aspiration, diarrhea, abdominal distention, hyperglycemia, constipation, and fecal impaction.

T-Tubes (Biliary Drainage Tubes)

T-tubes (biliary drainage tubes) are surgically implanted into the common bile duct after cholecystectomy or choledochostomy to facilitate adequate bile

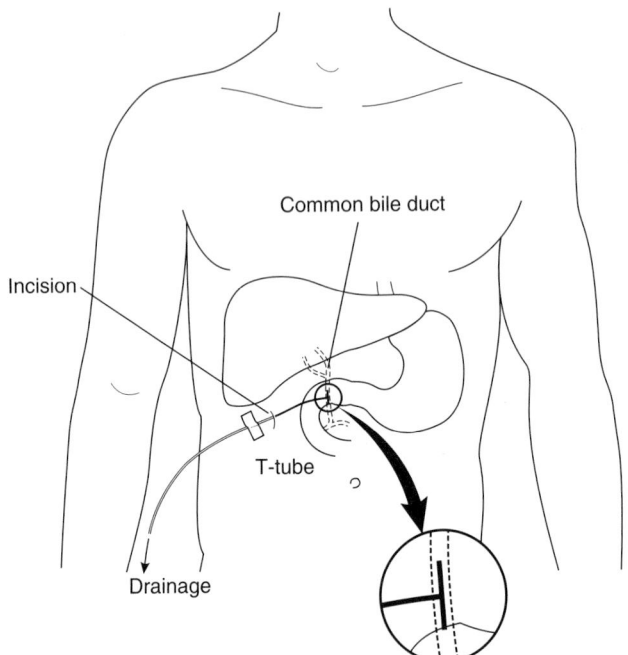

Figure 3-4-1. T-tube placement.

drainage during duct healing. The T-tube remains in place until the common bile duct is no longer edematous and bile flows freely into the ampulla of Vater, which usually occurs 1 to 2 weeks postoperatively.

During surgery, the short end (crossbar) of the T-tube is inserted into the common bile duct, and the long end is drawn through the incision. The T-tube can then be connected to a continuous-gravity drainage bag (Fig. 3-4-1).

Nursing Management for T-Tubes

1. Normal bile color is greenish-brown. The T-tube usually drains blood-tinged bile in the first 24 hours after surgery. The amount of drainage ranges from 500 to 1000 mL/day for the first 4 days and then decreases thereafter. Note and record the color, amount, odor, and consistency of drainage. Closely monitor fluid and electrolyte status.

2. Secure the T-tube drainage system to the abdominal area. This prevents excessive bile loss and/or backflow contamination. If ordered, return excessive bile drainage to the patient mixed with chilled fruit juice or, if possible, through a nasogastric tube.

3. Provide frequent skin care. Monitor for signs of infection at the tube insertion site. Observe for bile leakage, which may indicate obstruction. Assess tube patency and site condition every 4 hours until the physician removes the tube. Protect the skin edges and avoid excessive taping to prevent shearing of the skin.

4. Assess the color of the skin, sclera, and stool. If an obstruction is present, the urine may be amber-colored, and the stools will be clay-colored.

Nasogastric Tubes

Nasogastric (NG) tubes are flexible plastic tubes inserted through the nose into the stomach to relieve gastric distention by removing gas, gastric secretions, or food (Fig. 3-4-2). NG tubes are also used to give clients medications, food, or fluids. Table 3-4-2 presents the insertion procedure.

Types of Nasogastric Tubes

Levin Tube. This single-lumen NG tube is unvented and has holes at the tip and along the sides. It may be made of rubber or plastic. The Levin tube is used to instill irrigating fluids, medications, and nourishment on a temporary basis. Because it does not have air vents, it is not recommended for use with suction because of the risk of gastric mucosal damage.

Salem Sump Tube. This is a double-lumen, vented NG tube. The smaller lumen has a blue sump port that allows atmospheric air into the stomach during suctioning. Thus, the Salem sump tube does not adhere to or damage the gastric mucosa. The larger lumen can be used for decompression and irrigation of the stomach. Suction can be discontinued and the tube can also be used for the instillation of medications and nourishment. The Salem sump is made of clear plastic with openings at the sides and the tip, and radiopaque lines used for x-ray identification of tube placement.

Moss Tube. The three-lumen Moss tube has a radiopaque tip that can be used to guide x-ray placement. The first lumen is positioned and inflated at the cardia and used as a balloon- inflation port. The second lumen serves as an esophageal aspiration port, and the third lumen is used for duodenal feedings.

Gastrointestinal Tube Suctioning

The main purposes of GI suctioning are to relieve abdominal distention, maintain gastric decompression after surgery, remove blood and secretions from the GI tract, relieve discomfort, and maintain the patency of the GI tube.

The equipment used to suction GI tubes varies among institutions. Common

Levin tube   Salem sump tube

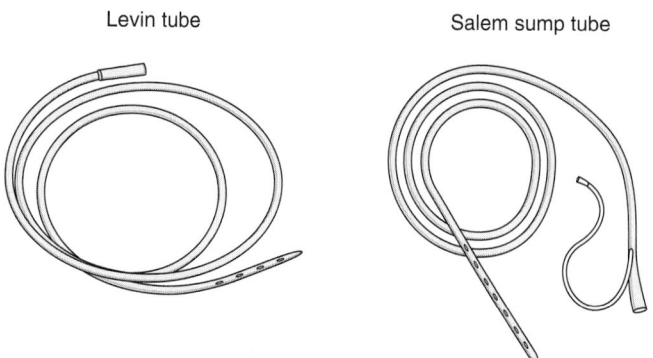

Figure 3-4-2. Types of nasogastric tubes.

Table 3-4-2. Insertion of a Nasogastric Tube

INTERVENTIONS	RATIONALE/SIGNIFICANCE
1. Put on gloves. Measure the length of the tube to be inserted. Measure from the tip of the patient's nose to the tip of the earlobe to the xiphoid process (also called the nose–ear–xiphoid measurement). Mark the tube with pencil, ink, or a piece of tape.	1. The nose–ear–xiphoid process measurement is considered to be equal to the distance for the distal end of the tube to be located in the stomach.
2. If the tube is firm plastic, place it in warm water to soften, if needed.	2. Warm water may or may not be needed to soften the tube.
3. Lubricate the distal 2 to 3 inches of the tube with a water-soluble lubricant (e.g., K-Y jelly).	3. The lubrication allows the tube to pass through the nostril more easily.
4. Instruct the patient to hold the head in a natural position or slightly tilted back while the tube is inserted in the nose. Then have the patient tilt the head forward before the tube is advanced into the throat, so that swallowing is easier.	4. Tilting the head back is avoided, because it is difficult to swallow and it increases the likelihood of introducing the tube into the trachea.
5. If allowed, the patient may take a sip of water through the straw. Insert the tube into a nostril and gently advance it through the nasopharynx to the throat. Ask the patient to take sips of water. Advance the tube into the esophagus as the patient swallows.	5. Swallowing causes the epiglottis to close over the larynx and prevents introduction of the tube into the trachea.
6. If the patient coughs and gags violently and becomes cyanotic, immediately remove the tube from the pharynx but leave it in the nasopharynx and then reinsert it.	6. As the tube enters the pharynx, it stimulates a strong cough and gag reflex in many individuals. It is safer to withdraw the tube, because it may be in the trachea.
7. After the tube is inserted to the marker, check for correct placement in the stomach by: (a) aspirating stomach contents and (b) injecting 20 mL of air into the tube while listening for a gurgle with a stethoscope placed over the stomach or (c) obtaining an x-ray for tube placement. Follow your institution's routine policies and procedures. After confirming placement, mark the tube where it exits the nose. Measure and document the external length.	7. Correct placement must be verified. Marking the exit point of the tube is a reference for the future.
8. Secure, by tape or other specific product, the tube to the patient's nose or upper lip.	8. If the patient is perspiring frequently, the tape may need to be replaced often.
9. Anchor the rest of the tube by placing a piece of tape around a portion of the tube, then pinning the tape to the patient's gown or pajama top.	9. External movement of the tube may cause slight movement of the inserted portion of the tube; this may lead to nausea and irritation of the throat. Anchoring the tube decreases movement.

suction units include portable electric units, Gomco thermotic pumps, and wall suction units. Portable electric motor suction units have an on/off switch, a motor that generates negative pressure, and a drainage bottle that is monitored frequently to prevent overflow drainage into the motor. The Gomco pump is electrically operated and provides intermittent suction. It can be set on high- or low-pressure controls. The setting is prescribed by the physician or set according to institutional protocol. A wall suction unit consists of a pressure regulator and a drainage bottle. This bottle must be checked regularly to prevent overflow.

Suction may be continuous or intermittent. Continuous suction tends to pull the mucosa close to the tip of the suction tube into the tube, causing trauma. Intermittent suction is most commonly used. It is less harmful to the mucous lining at the tip of the suction tube.

Biliary/Pancreatic Stents

Obstruction of the biliary ducts interrupts the flow of bile into the intestines and can be a life-threatening complication. Biliary and pancreatic stents are small, flexible tubes made from medical-grade plastic or wire. They are inserted to hold open bile ducts in the body that have narrowed or become blocked by stones, tumors, or other obstructions. They can be temporary or permanent. They are implanted by a physician, normally a radiologist, during an endoscopic procedure. Early stent-related complications include perforation, pancreatitis, bleeding, and cholangitis.

 CLINICAL PEARLS

○ All tubes must be stabilized to prevent leakage, migration, and dislodgement. This can be done by using a catheter tube holder or placing chevron tape over the nose, applying tincture of benzoin to secure the tape.

○ Always determine whether the NG tube is properly placed before starting any infusion.

○ NG tubes are normally irrigated before and after tube feedings or the installation of medications, and as ordered to prevent clogging. Irrigation may require a physician's order. Check your agency's policy and procedure manual.

○ Secure an NG tube to the patient's nose or to either side of the face, in a position of comfort; avoid pressure on any part of the nostril to prevent ischemia.

○ When inserting an NG in a patient who is unconscious or cannot swallow, stroke the patient's neck to encourage the swallowing reflex and facilitate passage of the tube.

○ To clamp a T-tube, occlude the tube lightly with a clamp or rubber band. Clamping the tube 1 hour before of after meals may aid digestion.

 RESOURCES

- American Cancer Society: 800-ACS-2345
- Continent Ostomy Group, Heartland UOA: 913-856-5679
- ConvaTec: 800-422-8811
- National Pressure Ulcer Advisory Panel: 716-829-3516
- The OLEY Foundation: 800-776-OLEY or web.wizvax.net/oleyfdn
- United Ostomy Association: 800-826-0826 or www.uoa.org/
- Wound, Ostomy and Continence Nurses Society (WOCN): 888-224-WOCN or www.wocn.org
- www.cdc.gov/ncidod/hip/SSI/SSI_guideline.htm
- www.guideline.gov/index.asp

chapter 4

Decision-Making for Bedside Specimen Collection

Gastric Specimen Collection and Lavage

Section 1   Veronica P.S. Njie

OVERVIEW

Gastrointestinal (GI) specimens are routinely obtained to evaluate patients before and after GI procedures and to evaluate the presence of GI disorders or diseases. The nurse is responsible for accurate collection and precise monitoring of these specimens.

An additional nursing intervention involving the GI system is gastric lavage. Gastric lavage is considered an emergent procedure. It is performed to clean or wash the stomach of harmful substances and to arrest hemorrhage.

This section addresses three commonly collected GI specimens: gastric pH; Gastroccult and Hemoccult/fecal occult; and gastric lavage.

PRINCIPLES OF CARE

GI secretions provide information about intestinal motility, acid-base balance, and the mucosal integrity of the GI tract. Indications for obtaining secretions are to assess for bleeding disorders or GI disease, to monitor anticoagulant therapy, to assess unexplained blood loss, to evaluate low hemoglobin and hematocrit levels, to assess for peptic ulcer disease, to confirm NG tube placement, and to screen for colon cancer.

Approximately 7000 mL of fluid is secreted by the GI tract each day. These fluids are composed of gastric juices (1500 to 3000 mL), duodenal juices (1200 to 1500 mL), and fluids produced by the mouth (saliva), liver, gallbladder, and pancreas.

Gastric juice is a slightly viscous, pale-gray, translucent fluid. Saliva is usually present but floats to the top of the sample, appearing frothy. A yellow-green color indicates the presence of bile. A coffee-ground appearance indicates bleeding. The pH of gastric secretions ranges from less than 1.0 to 4.0. Red blood cells (RBCs) and white blood cells (WBCs) should be negative or may be present in very small amounts. Bacteria and yeast should be few to none, and parasites should be absent.

Duodenal juice is a moderately viscous, pearly-gray, translucent fluid. A yellow-green color also indicates the presence of bile. A red, pink, or brown color indicates bleeding. The presence of food particles may indicate intestinal obstruction or duodenal diverticula. The pH of duodenal juice ranges from 8.0

to 8.5. RBCs should be negative. WBCs may be present in very small amounts. Bacteria and parasites should not be present.

Feces should be negative for blood and bile. Black stools are associated with upper GI bleeding; maroon- or red-colored stools, with lower GI bleeding.

DECISION-MAKING
Gastrointestinal pH

Gastric pH determines the acidity or alkalinity of gastric secretions. The acidic gastric secretion protects against the growth of bacteria and aids digestion. Secretion production is increased during meals and with stress. The presence of blood in the stomach increases gastric pH. Gastric pH is low in patients with peptic ulcer disease and Zollinger-Ellison syndrome (a non–beta cell adenoma of the pancreas that causes excessive gastrin production). Elevated gastric pH levels are associated with gastric carcinoma, pernicious anemia, and aplastic anemia. Increased duodenal pH is associated with chronic pancreatitis.

One of the most common uses of bedside gastric pH monitoring is for stress ulcer prophylaxis. Stress ulcers (or stress-erosive gastritis) are acute gastric mucosal erosions that occur in noneating patients with severe physiologic stress, including postsurgical patients, posttrauma patients, and, most commonly, critically ill patients. The cause is thought to be decreased blood supply to the gastric mucosa. Stress ulcers are best managed by prevention. The gastric pH is maintained between 4.0 and 5.0 with the administration of H_2 receptor antagonists, guided by frequent sampling of gastric contents for pH testing. If the gastric pH is below 4.0, then an H_2 receptor antagonist and/or antacid is administered as prescribed. If the patient is receiving continuous tube feedings, the feeding should be stopped 1 hour before obtaining the sample.

Gastric pH testing is also being evaluated as the standard for confirming NG tube placement. The pH in the lung is higher than duodenal pH, which is higher than gastric pH. This method may prove to be more reliable than other non-radiologic methods.

Procedure

Assessing gastric pH requires the aspiration of 1 to 2 mL of gastric contents from an NG tube, nasointestinal tube, gastrostomy tube, or GI tube. Apply one drop of the specimen to the pH test area. Ensure that the entire area is covered. Time for 30 seconds, then compare the color on the pH test area with the colors on the pH strip.

Gastroccult

Nurses conduct the Gastroccult test to assess for the presence of blood in the stomach. The presence of blood might not be readily visible, and the Gastroccult test offers a way to assess occult (hidden) blood in gastric contents. It is most commonly done to monitor patients for active bleeding before and after GI surgeries. False-positive results may be caused by bleeding gums or blood in the nasopharynx, especially following a traumatic intubation.

Procedure

Apply one drop of the gastric specimen to the Gastroccult test slide. Apply two drops of the Gastroccult developer over the sample and one drop between the positive and negative indicators. Read the results within 60 seconds. If the color turns blue, then the test is positive for blood.

Hemoccult/Fecal Occult

The Hemoccult, or fecal occult, test detects hidden blood in the stool. The most frequently performed test on feces, it is done to screen for colon cancer and assess for potential or actual GI bleeding. A diet high in meats, bananas, and certain vegetables (e.g., turnip, horseradish) can cause a false-positive result, as can certain medications, including aspirin, iron preparations, anticoagulants, adrenocorticosteroids, colchicines, and phenylbutazone. Bleeding from the nose and mouth also causes a false-positive result. False-negative results may be caused by ascorbic acid (vitamin C) and tetracycline. If possible, these should be stopped 48 hours before the test. Accidental contamination of the sample with povidone-iodine (Betadine) renders a false-positive result.

Procedure

Collect approximately 1 inch of solid stool or 1 to 2 mL of liquid stool. Open the flap of the specimen card and apply a small amount of feces to box A. Close the flap of the specimen card. Apply another small amount of feces, from a different section of stool sample, to box B. After turning the specimen card over, apply two drops of Hemoccult developer to each box. Read the results in 60 seconds. The color turns blue if blood is present.

Gastric Lavage

Gastric lavage is an emergent procedure performed to cleanse or wash the stomach of poisonous substances before systemic absorption occurs. Lavage of petroleum distillates may require endotracheal intubation to prevent aspiration, because these volatile hydrocarbons may cause severe pulmonary damage. This is contraindicated for strong corrosive agents.

Gastric lavage is also preformed to remove blood and blood clots from the stomach in cases of upper GI bleeding. In this application, lavage allows an ongoing estimation of blood loss. A blood-free lavage suggests that the source of bleeding is the lower GI tract. Lavage is contraindicated in patients without a gag reflex and should be avoided if esophageal varices are suspected, to avoid variceal tearing.

Procedure

Insert a large-bore NG tube and confirm proper placement. The large bore size facilitates evacuation of gastric contents. Aspirate stomach contents before instilling fluids. For an adult, hang 500 mL of room-temperature sterile water or normal saline solution. Run fluid through the tubing to clear out the air, then clamp. Attach the tubing to a Y adapter, and connect the drainage container tubing to the other end of the Y adapter. Clamp the drainage tubing.

Infuse approximately 150 to 200 mL of fluid, then reclamp. After the infusion, unclamp the drainage tubing and allow contents from the stomach to flow out. Another option is to manually aspirate the contents from the stomach. Assess fluid return for amount, color, and consistency. Repeat the procedure until fluid returns clear. Monitor the patient for signs and symptoms of shock or any changes in clinical condition.

CLINICAL PEARLS

○ Use standard precautions at all times when collecting specimens and conducting tests.

○ Ensure the use of the appropriate solution for the required test; keep in mind that some test solutions look identical.

○ Assess the care provider for color blindness, to ensure that the color reported is consistent with the test results.

○ Avoid contaminating the specimen with other fluids or material.

○ Quality control checks on all test equipment is a requirement of the Joint Commission on Accreditation of Healthcare Organizations.

○ Patients with recent GI surgery will have positive occult results. Continuous monitoring is essential to ensure that no new bleeding occurs.

○ Fecal occult tests must be repeated three times on different stool samples over 3 days to obtain accurate results.

Urine Specimen Collection

Section 2   Cynthia Chernecky

OVERVIEW

The examination of a urine sample is an important tool in the diagnosis of urinary disorders, as well as in a multitude of other diseases and conditions. Urine is a product of blood filtration, so much of the information concerning health or disease states carried in the blood can also be found in the urine. Obtaining a urine sample is usually a simple, noninvasive, cost-effective procedure, and most results are available immediately.

PRINCIPLES OF CARE

Urine consists of water and byproducts—urea, uric acid, ammonia, creatinine, salt, minerals, and urochrome (a breakdown product of hemoglobin that gives urine its yellow color). Before urine collection, the patient's history and current medication use should be reviewed.

In an adult, the urge to void occurs after ingestion of about 400 mL of liquids. If the patient has just voided and a sample is needed, encourage fluids to total this amount (if the patient has no fluid restrictions).

Obtaining a urine sample begins with explaining the procedure to the patient. Avoid using jargon and abbreviations (e.g., C&S). Explain the method of specimen collection (i.e., clean versus sterile, standard precautions). This is very important, because the overall contamination rate for specimens is 12.5% for males and 26.3% for females. The contamination rate in emergency rooms is 17.8%, compared with the overall hospital rate of 22.1%. The only factor associated with lower overall urine contamination rates is obtaining cultured specimens from male patients. Higher contamination rates occur in females and infants; rates are even higher for bagged specimens in infants (66%). The contamination rate in infants is lower in pediatric-specific institutions.

Paper cups have a low contamination rate and are virtually sterile. Urine is ready for immediate microscopic examination.

DECISION-MAKING
Urinalysis

Samples for urinalysis require collection of at least 15 mL of urine. The samples may be collected randomly or on awakening in the morning. *Random specimens* can be collected at any time during the day. The *first morning specimen*, the first voided specimen of the day, is preferred, because it is more concentrated from the overnight accumulation of substances that may not be present in dilute urine. *Midstream clean-catch specimens* are preferred to straight-catch samples, because they are less likely to be contaminated with substances such as discharges or menstrual blood.

Handle only the outside of the specimen container. If unable to send the specimen to the lab immediately, refrigerate or place it on ice within 1 hour of collection. If a sample is left at room temperature for longer than 1 hour, the urine will become alkaline, ketones may dissipate, glucose levels will drop, RBCs will break down, and casts will disintegrate, invalidating test results. Prolonged light exposure causes oxidation of bilirubin and urobilinogen. In addition, any bacteria present will begin to multiply, and the urine color will darken. See Chapter 11, Section 5 for normal urinalysis findings.

Reagent Strips

The commercially prepared reagent dipstick is a valuable tool for screening or gathering additional information on numerous disorders. Poor compliance with this tool can result in false and unusable test results. Table 4-2-1 lists common urine tests done by reagent dipsticks and their associated conditions. Standard (universal) precautions should be taken when handling these samples, as with as any body fluid.

When using reagent strips, the nurse needs to check the expiration date, obtain a fresh urine sample, remove excess urine from the dipstick by running the edge of the strip against the urine container, and read the strips at the appropriate time interval. Compare the test pad with the color scale on the box at the specific waiting time recommended by the manufacturer.

False-positive results for ketones can appear if the patient has ingested

Table 4-2-1. Urine Tests for Screening or Gathering Additional Information

URINE TEST	EQUIPMENT NEEDED	IF (+) DISEASE/CONDITION	AMOUNT OF URINE SAMPLE NEEDED
Bilirubin	Reagent	Hepatic, biliary	50 mL
Blood	Reagent	Infection, trauma, tumor, stones	50 mL
Glucose	Reagent	Acute pancreatitis, Cushing's disease, diabetes mellitus, stress	50 mL
Ketones	Reagent	Diabetes mellitus, dieting, starvation	50 mL
Leukocytes	Reagent	Bladder or renal infection	50 mL
Nitrites	Reagent	*E. coli* infection, urinary tract infection	50 mL
Protein	Reagent	Congestive heart failure, hypertension, preeclampsia, renal disease, urinary tract infection	50 mL
Urobilinogen	Reagent	Hemolytic anemia, liver disease	50 mL

phenolphthalein medications (laxatives) or L-dopa medication. False-positive results for blood appear if the reagent becomes contaminated with even an extremely small amount of povidone-iodine (such as from a perineal operative skin scrub). A urine sample of approximately 50 mL is needed to perform all of the tests on the dipstick.

Urine Collection Procedures
Midstream Clean-Catch Collection

Midstream clean-catch specimens are usually used for the collection of urine for *culture and sensitivity (C&S)*. This technique prevents contamination of the sample with microorganisms, urethral cells, and mucus. This technique is also being advocated for urinalysis, as mentioned earlier.

Procedure

Obtain a sterile specimen container/cup. Cleanse the patient's perineum with soap and water or an antibacterial towelette. Wash around the urethra with povidone-iodine. In females, swab over the labia minora and urethra from front to back; in males, swab the meatus and end of the penis, working in a circular motion from inside to outside. Allow the area to dry, then instruct the patient to void. As the patient voids, let some urine pass by the specimen container, then place the container into the urine stream to catch a sample. Obtain 30 to 60 mL.

Handle only the outside of the specimen container. Cap the container and close it tightly. Label and send the specimen to the lab immediately, or refrigerate it or place it on ice within 1 hour after collection. Common organisms found in C&S cultures include *Escherichia coli*, *Streptococcus faecalis*, *Corynebacterium, Lactobacillus*, and coliforms (*Klebsiella, Pseudomonas, Proteus enterobacter, Gardnerella vaginalis*). Yeast and beta streptococci are less common. The C&S test is 98% reliable.

24-Hour Urine Collection

Have the patient void in the toilet and flush. Then begin collecting all urine for a 24-hour period using a urinal (in males) or a toilet hat (in females). The flush time is the start time for the collection period. Offer the patient fluids if no fluid restrictions are in effect. Place all urine in the collection container provided (either with or without preservative) and determine whether or not this container should be put on ice. At the 24th hour, have the patient void, and add this urine to the rest of the sample. Then seal the container and send it to the laboratory for analysis.

This collection technique is used in the assessment of Cushing's syndrome, gout, hyponatremia, renal dysfunction, and urolithiasis. A 24-hour urine for creatinine clearance is a very specific indicator of renal function. It determines the amount of blood cleared of creatinine by the kidneys, which is independent of urine flow. Hence this test indicates impaired glomerular filtration; decreased values indicate damage to more than 50% of the kidneys' nephrons.

12-Hour Urine Collection

This technique follows the same procedure as for 24-hour urine collection. It is used to evaluate for glomerulonephritis, pyelonephritis, and hematuria.

2-Hour Urine Collection

This technique also follows the same procedure as for a 24-hour urine collection. The patient may need to increase fluid intake to produce an adequate amount of urine within the 2-hour collection period. This technique is used in the evaluation of hypertension, kidney disease, nephrolithiasis, and determination of beta-end secretions in late (beyond 36 weeks) gestation.

Indwelling Catheter Specimen Collection

Clamp the tubing just below the catheter's sample port for a maximum of 15 minutes. This is a short enough time to avoid significant backflow of urine into the bladder and prevent bacterial growth. Wipe the sample port with alcohol and allow it to dry for 2 minutes. Then insert a sterile needle (connected to a 10- to 20-mL sterile syringe or needleless syringe) at a 45-degree angle, to avoid passing straight through the tube and creating a needlestick injury. Withdraw the desired amount of urine, then unclamp the tubing.

Suprapubic Catheter Specimen Collection

If the catheter has a sample port, then follow the collection procedure for indwelling catheter specimen collection. If no sample port exists, then replace the collection bag and after 30 minutes open the end of the drainage bag to allow urine to flow into a specimen urine container. Wipe the end of the drainage bag with alcohol before obtaining the specimen.

Straight Catheter Specimen Collection

This procedure is used with incontinent patients or with patients who cannot avoid contaminating the sample. Obtain a sterile specimen container/cup. Cleanse the perineum with soap and water or an antibacterial towelette, and wash around the urethra with povidone-iodine. In females, swab over the labia minora and urethra from front to back. In males, swab over the meatus of the penis in a circular motion from inside to outside, then insert the catheter all the way to the widened section near the catheter hub, and allow to release back. Allow the area to dry.

Lubricate the catheter using sterile technique, then insert the catheter into the urethral orifice slowly until urine return is noted. If no urine returns, then connect the catheter to the closed drainage system and clamp the drainage tube for less than 30 minutes, to allow fresh urine to collect in the catheter. Place the end of the catheter into the sterile collection container and collect a sample of 30 to 60 mL.

After obtaining the sample, either hook up the catheter to the drainage collection bag, if appropriate (ensuring that the clamp at the bottom of the bag is closed), or remove the catheter. Handle only the outside of the specimen container. Cap the container, and close it tightly. Label the container, and either send it to the lab immediately or place it on ice within 1 hour.

Complications
Catheter Encrustation

Encrustation of the catheter can result from alkaline urine due to increased calcium, magnesium, and citrate intake. To acidify the urine, have the patient drink cranberry juice and avoid effervescent tablet medications and alcohol. This is a particularly useful intervention for elderly patients, nursing home clients, and patients with spinal cord injury. Other strategies to prevent catheter encrustation include maintaining a consistent fluid intake (e.g., a glass of water every 3 hours, or 8 to 10 glasses/day), avoiding calcium-containing antacids (which increase calcium intake), avoiding intake of magnesium from sodas and antacids, and avoiding excessive citrate intake from fruit juices and cordials. For a patient taking sulfonamide medications (e.g., Azulfidine, Bactrim, Bleph-10, Sodium Sulamyd, Sulfa), reduce the likelihood of crystalluria by alkalinizing the urine through the administration of sodium bicarbonate.

Urine Sedimentation

Sedimentation can result from antibiotic treatment, urinary stasis, urinary infection, or dehydration. To prevent this problem, increase the patient's fluid intake at regular 2- to 3-hour intervals (if not contraindicated) or begin urinary irrigation as prescribed.

 CLINICAL PEARLS

○ Patient education hint: Throw all toilet paper into the toilet bowl, not into the bedpan or trash containers. Avoid fecal contamination and menstrual contamination (use a tampon).
○ In an adult, the urge to void occurs after ingestion of about 400 mL of liquids.
○ When catheterizing a male patient, insert the catheter to the widened section near the catheter hub, inflate the balloon, then release.
○ Once urine is collected for urinalysis, it must be tested within 1 hour or the sample must be refrigerated. Failure to do so may result in falsely decreased levels of glucose, ketones, bilirubin, and urobilinogen and falsely increased levels of bacteria. A refrigerated sample must be allowed to come back to room temperature before testing is done.
○ Spilled urine should be cleaned up with 1% bleach (sodium hypochlorite).
○ Meatal cleansing in males has no significant impact on contamination rates of urine cultures.
○ Cranberry juice increases the acidity of the urine in older adults, helping prevent UTIs.
○ The presence of nitrites and leukocytes in the urine indicates infection.
○ The herb Barosma betulina, from the buchu leaf, is used as a urinary antiseptic. The herb Arctostaphylos is used to treat UTIs resulting from *E. coli* infection.
○ To prevent calcium oxalate stones in the urine, increase the patient's intake of low-phosphorus-content beverages, such as soft drinks, and avoid milk, coffee, and cocoa.

Sputum Specimen Collection

Section 3   Cynthia Chernecky

OVERVIEW

Sputum is not normally produced in healthy individuals; the lower respiratory tract is normally sterile. Irritating environmental chemicals, tobacco smoke, and infection can lead to sputum production. The examination of sputum constituents and characteristics is very helpful in determining the nature of certain disorders. Sputum examination is a common tool in diagnosing lower respiratory tract infections. For specifics on sputum collection for tuberculosis, see Chapter 13, Section 5.

PRINCIPLES OF CARE

Sputum samples can be collected using various techniques (Table 4-3-1. The different techniques are needed because pulmonary infections do not always produce sputum, and every situation is different.

Collection of an *expectorated sample* should be attempted first for the awake patient. It should be obtained in the early morning, on rising. Instruct the patient to:

1. Cleanse the mouth with water by the swish-and-spit method; this reduces the bacterial content.
2. Take two or three deep breaths, one at a time, and hold the breath each time at maximum inspiration.
3. Using the abdominal muscles, explosively cough several times after each breath is held.
4. Expectorate sputum into a sterile cup.

Samples require 2 to 3 mL of sputum for microscopic analysis and more than 4 mL for C&S. Collecting an adequate specimen may take 30 minutes or longer. If more than 30 minutes is needed, place the specimen container on ice for up to 2 hours more. After a total of 2½ hours, either close the specimen container and send it to the laboratory for analysis or, if insufficient specimen was obtained, discard the specimen as hazardous waste and retry using another method or the same method the next morning.

If this method fails, then *sputum induction* with 3.5 mL of sodium chloride via ultrasonic nebulizer for 10 to 20 minutes may be necessary to obtain a sputum sample. This technique has been found to be 83% sensitive for the detection of *Pneumocystis carinii*.

If the patient is unable to cough, then nasotracheal or orotracheal suctioning may be necessary. In this method, a sputum trap (Lukens trap), a plastic cup-type apparatus that fits onto the suctioning tube, is used to aspirate and collect the sample. Expectorated and aspirated sputum from the upper airway is subject to oropharyngeal bacterial contamination, whereas transtracheal aspiration has a lower contamination rate because of the sterility of the procedure.

If these methods fail, then more invasive collection methods (e.g., bronchoscopy or biopsy) may be necessary.

DECISION-MAKING

The order of sputum examination is first a gross examination, then a wet mount on a slide (under both high and low magnification), and then Gram staining and/or other special staining of the sputum.

The gross examination reveals the **consistency** of the sputum. *Mucoid* sputum (containing mucus and also possibly air bubbles) is seen in patients with chronic inflammation, as in chronic bronchitis, and in some forms of asthma. *Mucopurulent* sputum (containing mucus and pus) indicates acute infection in patients with chronic obstructive pulmonary disease. *Purulent*

Table 4-3-1. Techniques for Obtaining Sputum Samples

TECHNIQUE	PROCEDURE	CONSIDERATIONS
Naso/orotracheal aspiration	Insert the catheter through the mouth or nose into the trachea. Suction for 10 seconds. Withdraw the catheter without suctioning.	May produce laryngospasm or bradydysrhythmias.
Endotracheal (ET) tube aspiration	Insert the catheter through ET tube or tracheotomy tube into the trachea.	Contaminated specimens are possible; bradydysrhythmias may occur.
Bronchoscopic aspiration	Local anesthetic is applied (4% lidocaine) and sedation medication (Midazolam) is given for comfort and to inhibit cough reflex. The bronchoscope is passed through the mouth or nose to the larynx, trachea, and bronchi.	Contaminated specimens are possible. Has the advantage of being able to select the area of lung from which to take a sample. Complications include transient hypoxemia, bradydysrhythmias, bronchial perforation, laryngospasm, and pneumothorax.
Transtracheal aspiration	After skin preparation and anesthetic induction, a large-bore needle is introduced through the cricothyroid membrane, a sterile catheter is introduced into the trachea, and secretions are suctioned.	This technique results in high yield, correlates well with blood culture results, and is useful in diagnosing unusual infections like Legionnaire's disease. Complications include bleeding, esophageal perforation, bradydysrhythmias, and pneumothorax.
Thoracentesis: If this procedure is prescribed, then a sputum sample can be obtained at this time.	With the patient sitting upright, the skin is cleansed, lidocaine is injected into the tissue area, and a 20-gauge or larger needle is inserted. More than 75 mL fluid is extracted. The needle is removed, a pressure dressing is applied, and a chest x-ray is obtained.	Useful for pleural effusions. Complications include pneumothorax, air embolism, pulmonary edema, hypertension, and bradydysrhythmias.
Open lung per biopsy: At the time of a scheduled biopsy procedure, a sputum sample can be obtained.	The patient is anesthetized. A surgical opening is made, the lung is visualized, and aspiration and lung tissue samples are taken.	Complications include bleeding, pneumothorax, bradydysrhythmias, and respiratory arrest.

sputum (containing pus) commonly results from acute bacterial pneumonia or ruptured pulmonary abscess. *Viscous* (thick, sticky) sputum is common in cystic fibrosis. Watery, muddy sputum with plugs indicates bronchial asthma.

Examination of sputum **color** may also be helpful. *Yellow-green* sputum is associated with pneumococcal pneumonia; *grayish-black* sputum, with smoke inhalation; *pink, frothy* sputum, with congestive heart failure; and *blood-streaked* sputum, with *Klebsiella* and streptococcal pneumonia. Hemoptysis is often an indication of neoplasm, tuberculosis, or trauma.

Evaluation of Findings

Fewer than 25 squamous epithelial cells seen on the slide indicates a sputum sample from the lower respiratory tract. Culture results of the sputum must be interpreted along with the patient's clinical signs and symptoms and therapeutic response to treatment. More than 25 leukocytes seen on the slide indicates an infectious or inflammatory process. Because bacterial growth occurs in 2 to 3 days in a petri dish, whereas growth of viral cultures takes at least 5 days, culture is not a very useful clinical tool. Specific findings for sputum slide smears are given in Table 4-3-2.

 CLINICAL PEARLS

○ Collect 2 to 3 mL of sputum for a culture and at least 4 mL if a microscopic sputum cell count or staining is required.

○ Sputum left to stand for 24 hours will turn green from the enzyme verdoper-oxidase found in neutrophils. Place the sputum specimen on ice for a maximum of 2 hours before sending it to the laboratory for examination.

○ Food or tobacco particles found in a sputum specimen indicate that a poor sputum specimen has been obtained.

○ Induced sputum adequately reflects the findings of direct bronchoscopy, except bronchoscopy shows higher proportions of lymphocytes and macrophages.

○ Antibiotic therapy decreases the percentage of PMNs microscopically seen on the slide; thus, if the patient has taken antibiotics within 10 days before collection, be sure to note this on the laboratory slip.

 Table 4-3-2. Microscopic Findings of Sputum Smear on a Slide

FINDINGS	ASSOCIATED DISEASES
Albumin	Bronchial asthma
Curschmann's spiral structures	Asthma
Eosinophilic cationic protein (ECP)	Positive correlation with severity of bronchial asthma
Eosinophils + bronchial epithelial cells	Asthma, allergic inflammation
Large alveolar macrophages with iron that stains blue	Congestive heart failure, pulmonary edema, pulmonary infarction
Mast cells	Allergic bronchitis
Polymorphonucleocytes (PMNs)	Allergic inflammation, chronic bronchitis

Blood Glucose Specimen Collection and Monitoring

Section 4   Joanne M. Bullard

OVERVIEW

Blood glucose monitoring is essential in the treatment of diabetes. The health care provider is important in the assessment, evaluation, and implementation of interventions to assist the diabetic patient in reaching and then maintaining glycemic control within the prescribed target range. This section covers the basic methods of blood glucose monitoring, interpretation of the results, and interventions for signs of hypoglycemia and hyperglycemia.

PRINCIPLES OF CARE

Blood glucose monitoring is essential to prevent and reduce the complications of hypoglycemia and hyperglycemia.

Hypoglycemia

Hypoglycemia occurs when the blood glucose level falls below 70 mg/dL. Acute hypoglycemia occurs when the blood glucose level falls below 50 mg/dL. This is dangerous, because the central nervous system depends on glucose for energy, and permanent brain damage or death may result if not treated promptly. The signs and symptoms of hypoglycemia and the blood glucose level at which they occur vary among individuals. A patient may be asymptomatic with glucose levels between 60 and 70 mg/dL; however, most patients are symptomatic when the blood glucose level is between 50 and 60 mg/dL. Whenever hypoglycemia is suspected, the blood glucose level should be measured immediately. Hypoglycemia occurs most often in patients receiving insulin, sulfonylurea, or metformin therapy. It may be caused by an incorrect or excessive dose of insulin or oral antidiabetic agent, inadequate food intake due to missed snacks or meals, increased physical exercise, alcohol ingestion, emotional stress, or drug interactions that decrease blood glucose levels. Hypoglycemia may also be caused by disease processes, including liver diseases, liver cancer, and insulin-secreting tumors. See Chapter 18, Section 1 for signs of hypoglycemia and interventions to correct it. It is important to avoid overtreating hypoglycemia, which can cause hyperglycemia.

Hyperglycemia

Hyperglycemia occurs when the blood glucose level exceeds 110 mg/dL. An elevated glucose level is caused by the insufficient production of insulin and/or ineffective utilization of the insulin that is produced. Diabetes mellitus and hyperosmolar nonketotic syndrome (HNKS) are the primary causes of hyperglycemia. HNKS usually occurs in persons with undiagnosed or type 2 diabetes and presents with symptoms of severe hyperglycemia, hyperosmolarity, and dehydration. Diabetic ketoacidosis (DKA) usually occurs in type 1 diabetics as a result of ketosis. DKA is characterized by severe hyperglycemia and metabolic acidosis. Other causes of hyperglycemia include Cushing's syndrome; extreme stress, as occurs with multiple trauma or surgery; excessive growth hormone secretion; total parenteral nutrition; enteral feedings; and pregnancy.

DECISION-MAKING
Blood Glucose Monitoring

Capillary and venous glucose testing provide a means to evaluate the treatment plan and determine whether any changes are needed in the medication, diet therapy, or exercise plan.

Self-Monitoring Blood Glucose

Self-monitoring blood glucose (SMBG) is recommended by the American Diabetes Association (ADA) for patients attempting to maintain near-normal glycemic levels. This includes all type I diabetics, diabetic patients taking insulin or sulfonylurea, and patients not attaining glycemic control through diet, exercise, or medication therapy. The frequency and timing of SMBG are individualized according to each patient's needs and goals. SMBG three to four times a day is recommended for most patients with type I diabetes. For patients being treated with insulin or sulfonylureas, daily SMBG is recommended to monitor glycemic control and detect hypoglycemia.

SMBG is done by finger stick, using a drop of capillary blood placed on a reagent strip. Depending on the method, the result is then determined either visually, making a comparison with a reference color strip, or electronically, using a meter to measure glucose level; see Table 4-4-1.

Table 4-4-1. Finger Stick Capillary Method

Purpose	• To obtain blood glucose level to monitor glycemic control
	• Used in SMBG and bedside monitoring in hospital setting
Procedure	• Using a lancet device, a puncture is made off the center of the finger to obtain a large drop of blood, which is applied to a reagent strip.
	• *Visual reading:* After the specified time period, blot blood off the strip and visually compare the color on the strip to the color chart that comes with the strips.
	• *Meter testing:* According to manufacturer's instructions, after the specified time period, blot the strip and insert it into the meter for reading.
	• *Direct-read meter:* Some meters do not require timing or blotting. With these meters, blood is applied either directly to meter window or to the strip, which is then inserted into meter for reading.
Precautions	• The drop of blood must cover the entire designated area on the reagent strip for accurate results.
	• Timing, if required, must be exact as specified for the meter. Short-timing causes decreased test results. Longer timing causes elevated test results.
	• The meter must be clean, or results will be affected.
	• Do not use reagent strips after the expiration date.
	• Calibrate the meter according to manufacturer's directions with provided control solutions to check for accuracy.
	• Color-blind or visually impaired patients cannot perform visual testing.
Evaluation of Findings	Each patient has an individualized target goal for blood glucose level, usually between 80 and 100 mg/dL
	• If <80 mg/dL, assess for hypoglycemia and treat as needed.
	• Between 80 and 120 mg/dL indicates good glycemic control.
	• If >120 mg/dL, diet, exercise, and/or pharmacologic therapy may need adjustment.
	• A patient performing SMBG may have been given prescribed formula by physician to self-adjust diet, exercise, and/or medication when blood glucose level is elevated.

Fasting Blood Glucose Test

Fasting blood glucose is a laboratory test that measures the amount of glucose in the blood. Fasting is defined as eating or drinking nothing but water for 8 to 12 hours before blood is drawn for the test. Fasting blood glucose is the preferred diagnostic test for diabetes. It is also used to test SMBG accuracy or to assess glycemic control in a patient not taking insulin whose oral hypoglycemic medication is being adjusted (see Table 4-4-2).

Glucose Tolerance Test

The glucose tolerance test (GTT) is a sensitive laboratory test used to diagnose diabetes mellitus in patients whose fasting blood glucose is between 110 and 126 mg/dL. The GTT is also used as a further test to confirm the diagnosis when diabetes is suspected. Specific preparation and procedure guidelines must be followed to ensure an accurate test (see Table 4-4-2).

Glycosylated Hemoglobin Test

The glycosylated hemoglobin (HbA_{1c}) test is a laboratory test used to monitor glycemic control. Glucose glycosylates, or permanently attaches to, hemoglobin molecules in the RBCs, with the amount directly proportional to the glucose concentration in the blood. The average life span of RBCs is 120 days. Thus, this test can accurately reflect blood glucose levels over the previous 2 to 3 months. This test is not affected by food ingestion, stress, exercise, or earlier administration of diabetic medications (see Table 4-4-2).

False Values

Various factors can produce erroneous results from capillary SMBG; for example, application of excessive or insufficient blood to the strip, inaccurate meter calibration, and environmental variations such as moisture and temperature. Causes of false values in the fasting blood glucose, glucose tolerance, and glycosated hemoglobin tests are listed in Table 4-4-3.

Insulin Coverage Formula

A personal sliding scale may be developed by the physician for the patient to use in lowering blood glucose levels and maintaining set glycemic goals. Table 4-4-4 presents a sample sliding scale.

The ADA recommends the following goals: 80 to 100 mg/dL before meals, 100 to 140 mg/dL at bedtime, and below 180 mg/dL 2 hours after meals. An individual patient's goals may vary, depending on the patient's type of diabetes, age, weight, sensitivity to insulin, exercise regimen, and other medical conditions. As the patient's health or lifestyle changes, adjustments need to be made to the sliding scale. To use a sliding scale, the person must be willing to do SMBG frequently, at least before each meal and at bedtime. The dosage of short-acting regular or lispro (Humalog) insulin is adjusted according to the sliding scale. Because of these insulins' quick onset and peak times, the results of the correction will be evident by the next glucose check.

Urine Testing for Ketones

Monitoring the urine for ketones is important, especially for persons with type I diabetes, because ketones in the urine may indicate ketoacidosis. The ADA recommends that a person with diabetes test the urine for the presence
Text continued on page 114

Table 4-4-2. Venous Methods of Blood Glucose Testing

TEST	PURPOSE	PROCEDURE	EVALUATION OF FINDINGS
Fasting blood sugar	Detects problems of glucose metabolism. Used as a diagnostic test for diabetes mellitus*	Blood is drawn by venipuncture after the patient has fasted for 8 to 12 hours. The sample is tested to measure the amount of glucose present in the blood.	70–110 mg/dL: Normal <70 mg/dL: Assess for signs of hypoglycemia 110–126 mg/dL: Impaired glucose tolerance, risk factor for developing diabetes ≥126 mg/dL: Provisional diagnosis of diabetes mellitus*
Glucose tolerance test	Evaluates the rate at which glucose is removed from the bloodstream. Used as a diagnostic test for diabetes mellitus*	• Instruct the patient to: – Eat a balanced diet with at least 150 g of carbohydrate intake for 3 days maintaining normal activity – Fast 8–12 hours before the test. – Avoid alcohol, coffee, or physical activity 8 hours before the test. – Avoid smoking during the test. • Blood is drawn by venipuncture to obtain a fasting sample.* • The patient drinks a beverage containing 75 g or 100 g of glucose (specified by the physician). • Additional blood samples are drawn after 30 minutes, 1 hour, and 2 hours. (The test may continue up to 5 hours in some instances.) * Hold drugs that may influence test results for 3 days before the test.	<140 mg/dL 2 hours postload: Normal glucose tolerance ≥140–<200 mg/dL: Impaired glucose tolerance, risk factor for future diabetes ≥200 mg/dL: Provisional diagnosis of diabetes mellitus*
Glycosylated hemoglobin	Monitors blood glucose levels over the previous 2 to 3 months	Blood is drawn by venipuncture. No fasting is necessary.	<6%: Good diabetic control 6.0–7%: Fair diabetic control >7%: Poor diabetic control

*For a diagnosis of diabetes, results must be confirmed by a second test under similar circumstances on a subsequent day according to ADA criteria.

Table 4-4-3. Causes of False Values in Glucose Testing

TEST	CAUSES OF HIGH VALUES	CAUSES OF LOW VALUES
Fasting blood sugar (FBS)	Drugs: Anabolic steroids, androgens, ascorbic acid, aspirin, baclofen, benzodiazepines, chlorpromazine, chlorthalidone, cimetidine, clonidine, corticosteroids, dextran, dextrothyroxine, diazoxide, disopyramide, phosphate, epinephrine, estrogens, ethacrynic acid, furosemide, glucose infusions, haloperidol, imipramine, isoproterenol, heparin, hydralazine, indomethacin, isoniazid, levodopa, lithium, mercaptopurine, methimazole, methyldopa, nalidixic acid, nicotine, oral contraceptives, oxazepam, phenolphthalein, phenytoin, progestins, promethazine, propranolol, propylthiouracil, reserpine, ritodrine, terbutaline, tetracyclines, thiazides, tolbutamide, triamterene	Drugs: Allopurinol, amphetamines, aspirin, beta-adrenergic blockers, caffeine, chlorpropamide, clofibrate, ethanol, guanethidine sulfate, insulin, isocarboxazid, marijuana, nitrazepam, oral hypoglycemics, phenazopyridine, phenazopyridine hydrochloride
Glucose tolerance test	Strenous exercise Drugs: Same as listed for FBS	Smoking Drugs: Same as listed for FBS
Glycosylated hemoglobin	Hypertriglyceridemia Thalassemia Chronic renal failure Dialysis Splenectomy Elevated hemoglobin F level Alcohol Lead poisoning	Hemolysis Hemolytic anemia Blood loss Abnormal hemoglobins S, C, or D Pregnancy

Table 4-4-4. Sample Sliding-Scale Algorithm

CAPILLARY BLOOD GLUCOSE (mg/dL)	REGULAR INSULIN DOSE (Units)
<60	Notify physician
61–120	No insulin
121–150	1 unit
151–180	2 units
181–240	3 units
241–300	4 units
>300	6 units and notify physician

of ketones during periods of acute illness or stress, or if blood glucose levels are consistently elevated above 300 mg/dL. The ADA also recommends ketone testing whenever any symptom of ketoacidosis (e.g., abdominal pain, nausea, vomiting) is present.

 CLINICAL PEARLS

- Instruct the patient when doing SMBG to hold the hand in a downward position before pricking the finger to promote blood flow to the fingertips.
- To help increase blood flow, try lightly massaging and warming the patient's fingertips.
- For proper blood glucose control, strive to maintain the following blood glucose levels: 80 to 100 mg/dL before meals, 100 to 140 mg/dL at bedtime, and below 180 mg/dL 2 hours after meals.
- To determine the number of units of regular insulin for sliding scale coverage use the following formula

$$(BS - 100) \div 30 = \quad \text{units of reg insulin.}$$

 RESOURCES

- American Association for Respiratory Care: 972-243-2272
- American College of Gastroenterology: www.acg.gi.org
- American Diabetes Association: 800-232-3472 or www.diabetes.org
- American Lung Association: 800-LUNG-USA or www.lungusa.org/diseases/lungchronic.html *or* www.lungusa.org/diseases/lungpneumonia.html
- Journal of the American Medical Association Asthma Information Center: www.ama-assn.org/special/asthma/
- Johns Hopkins Health: www.intelihealth.com/IH/ihtIH
- National Diabetes Education Program: www.cdc.gov/diabetes
- National Diabetes Information Clearinghouse: 301-654-3327 or www.aerie.com
- National Heart, Lung and Blood Institute: www.nhlbi.nih.gov/index.htm
- National Institute of Diabetes and Digestive and Kidney Diseases: 800-GET-LEVEL or www.ndei.org
- www.drhull.com (click under urine specimen)
- www.drkoop.com (click under "U" for urinary)
- www.healthcare.com (click under urine culture)

chapter 5

Decision-Making for Oxygenation Alterations

Assessment of Oxygenation

Section 1

Lorie Arata ■ Lee Farris

OVERVIEW

Alterations in oxygenation affect not only the respiratory system, but also every other body system. The respiratory system is responsible for providing oxygen to the organs, tissues, and cells of all body systems. Therefore, assessment of oxygenation is critical to providing optimal patient care. This section discusses hypoxemia and hyperoxemia, as well as calculation of partial pressure of oxygen, use of pulse oximetry, respiratory failure, and interpretation of arterial blood gas (ABG) values.

PRINCIPLES OF CARE
Oxygen

Oxygen is transported in the blood in two ways: dissolved in plasma (PaO_2) and combined with hemoglobin (SaO_2). PaO_2 and SaO_2 are the most common methods for assessing oxygenation status.

In **PaO_2**, the "P" refers to partial pressure, the "a" means arterial, and, of course, "O_2" is oxygen. PaO_2 is a measure of the partial pressure or tension that oxygen exerts as a gas exerts in plasma. It is simply the amount of oxygen dissolved in plasma. PaO_2 is frequently shortened to PO_2. To measure PaO_2, an arterial blood gas (ABG) sample must be obtained. PaO_2 accounts for only 2% to 3% of the oxygen carried in the blood. Normal PaO_2 is 80 to 100 mm Hg. This value decreases with age after 60 years of age. To estimate a normal PaO_2 for this age group, subtract the number of years over 60 from 80. For instance, in a 70-year-old patient, an acceptable PaO_2 is 70 mm Hg ($80 - 10 = 70$).

In **SaO_2**, the "S" refers to saturation, and the other elements translate as for PaO_2. SaO_2 is defined as the arterial oxygen saturation of hemoglobin, the ratio of the amount of oxygen in the blood that is bound to hemoglobin. SaO_2 may be obtained by ABG analysis or pulse oximetry. SaO_2 accounts for the majority of oxygen (97% to 98%) carried in the blood. Normal SaO_2 is 93% to 99%.

Fraction of Inspired Oxygen

The fraction of inspired oxygen (FIO_2) is the percentage of oxygen being inspired. Only 21% of air is oxygen; the rest consists of nitrogen (78%) and other gases. The clinical term "room air" refers to the patient breathing 21% FIO_2. The PaO_2 of a patient receiving supplemental oxygen is expected to rise. There is no way to calculate how much the PaO_2 will rise given the amount of supplemental oxygen in patients with sick lungs. However, in persons with

115

healthy lungs, the expected PaO_2 can be estimated by multiplying the FIO_2 value by five. For example, a patient with normal lung function receiving 40% FIO_2 will have an expected PaO_2 of at least 200 mm Hg (40 × 5). How far off the patient's value is from this estimation provides information of lung function. To perform these calculations, the O_2 must be in percent (%) concentration as opposed to L/min. Therefore, it is important to know the differences in oxygen concentration by L/min and percentage of oxygen (FIO_2). For an estimation of FIO_2 in comparison to L/min, see Table 5-1-1.

Hypoxemia

Hypoxemia is defined as decreased oxygen level in arterial blood (PaO_2 <80 mm Hg). This differs from hypoxia, which is decreased oxygen at the tissue level. If hypoxemia is left untreated, hypoxia will develop. Table 5-1-2 lists causes of hypoxemia. Signs and symptoms of hypoxemia include pallor, cyanosis, diaphoresis, dyspnea, tachypnea, increased work of breathing, use of accessory muscles, tachycardia, chest pain, anxiety, restlessness, confusion, and fatigue.

A PaO_2 below 60 mm Hg requires immediate intervention unless the patient has a chronic lung disease, such as bronchitis, and has adapted to such low levels of oxygen. A PaO_2 below 40 mm Hg is life-threatening, because at this level oxygen is no longer available to the cells.

Oxygen Toxicity (Hyperoxia)

Excessive oxygen can be just as detrimental as insufficient oxygen. Oxygen toxicity can occur in any adult patient receiving oxygen at concentrations of

Table 5-1-1. Comparison of FIO_2 to L/min

L/MIN	FIO_2
Nasal cannula	
1	24%
2	28%
3	32%
4	36%
5	40%
6	44%
Simple mask	
5	40%
6	50%
8	60%
Venturi mask	
4 (blue)	24%
4 (yellow)	28%
6 (white)	31%
8 (green)	35%
8 (pink)	40%
Partial nonrebreather mask	
6	35%
8	45–50%
10–15	60% +
Nonrebreather mask	
6	60%
8	80%
10–15	80–90%

Table 5-1-2. Causes of Hypoxemia

MECHANISM	COMMON CLINICAL CAUSE
Decrease in inspired oxygen	High altitude
	Low oxygen content of gas mixture
	Enclosed breathing spaces (suffocation)
Hypoventilation	Lack of neurologic stimulation of the respiratory center (oversedation, drug overdose, neurologic damage)
	Trauma, rib fractures, severe pain
	Chronic obstructive pulmonary disease
Alveolocapillary diffusion abnormality	Emphysema
	Fibrosis
	Edema
Ventilation-perfusion mismatch	Asthma
	Chronic bronchitis
	Pneumonia
Shunting	Adult respiratory distress syndrome
	Respiratory distress syndrome
	Atelectasis

From McCance, K. & Huether, S. (1998). *Pathophysiology: The biological basis for disease in adults and children* (3rd ed). St. Louis: CV Mosby.

50% or greater for longer than 24 hours. Administration of such high doses of oxygen produces an abundance of oxygen free radicals. These oxygen free radicals cause a severe inflammatory response that damages the alveolar-capillary membrane, disrupts the production of surfactant, causes interstitial and alveolar edema, and reduces lung compliance. Clinical manifestations of oxygen toxicity include a dry hacking cough, chest discomfort, nausea and/or vomiting, fatigue, restlessness, numbness in the extremities, and dyspnea. These symptoms are very similar to those of respiratory failure.

Over time, the patient with oxygen toxicity develops objective clinical manifestations. Pulmonary function testing reveals decreased vital capacity, decreased compliance, and decreased functional residual capacity. After several days of normal oxygen concentrations, these abnormalities are completely reversed.

DECISION-MAKING

Decision-making for assessment of oxygenation is aimed at maintaining adequate oxygen supply to meet tissue needs and monitoring for and preventing respiratory failure. Assessment methods include physical examination (see Chapter 1, Section 3), pulse oximetry, and ABG analysis.

Respiratory Failure

Respiratory failure occurs when the lungs fail to maintain adequate gas exchange. It results in hypoxemia with or sometimes without hypercarbia or hypercapnia (increased CO_2 levels). Respiratory failure is sometimes defined as a Pao_2 below 60 mm Hg and CO_2 above 50 mm Hg with a pH below 7.30 when the patient is breathing room air. Respiratory failure may be pulmonary related (intrapulmonary) or can be caused by another disorder, producing pulmonary manifestations (extrapulmonary). The hallmark of acute respiratory

Table 5-1-3. Clinical Manifestations of Respiratory Distress

EARLY FINDINGS	LATE FINDINGS
Increased heart rate	Inability to maintain Pao_2 50–60 mm Hg
Increased cardiac output	Respiratory acidosis
Increased respiratory rate	Increased $Paco_2$
Decreased tidal volume	Somnolence
Hypertension	Increased work of breathing
Confusion	Increased accessory muscle use
Decreased mental acuity	Hypotension
Anxiety	Cyanosis
	Bradycardia
	Stupor and coma

failure is hypoxemia. Clinical manifestations are related to hypoxemia and hypercapnia. Table 5-1-3 lists early and late findings of respiratory failure.

Because symptoms of respiratory failure can be so varied, the most reliable diagnostic tool is ABG analysis. In patients with chronic hypercapnia (e.g., those with chronic obstructive pulmonary disease), checking the pH is particularly important. A pH below 7.35 in such patients aids the diagnosis of respiratory failure.

Management goals in respiratory distress/failure are aimed at treating the underlying cause. Other goals include maintaining a patent airway, promoting adequate gas exchange, providing ventilatory support, and promoting clearance of secretions (Table 5-1-4).

Table 5-1-4. Nursing Goals and Interventions for Respiratory Failure

GOAL	NURSING INTERVENTION
Establish a patent airway.	Establish an airway.
	Provide bronchodilator therapy as ordered.
	Administer corticosteroid medication as ordered.
Promote clearance of secretions.	Encourage the patient to cough to clear secretions or remove secretions mechanically via suctioning.
	Provide adequate hydration.
	Provide chest physiotherapy as ordered.
Maintain oxygenation.	Administer oxygen therapy as ordered.
	Institute pulse oximetry.
	Limit activities that consume oxygen.
	Reduce anxiety.
	Perform procedures only when necessary.
	Allow adequate rest time between procedures.
	Control fever.
Provide ventilatory support (prevent hypoventilation, control Pco_2, and normalize pH).	To facilitate deep breathing, raise the head of the bed at least 30 degrees.
	Provide frequent position changes (at least every 2 hours).
	Provide incentive spirometry.

Pulse Oximetry

Although ABG analysis is the standard for measuring arterial oxygen concentration, it is expensive, invasive, and painful and involves a delay between the sampling time and the time when results are available. Pulse oximetry is a simple, noninvasive, and relatively inexpensive way to perform continuous SaO_2 monitoring. It is clinically referred to as pulse oxygen saturation (SpO_2). The pulse oximeter measures the absorption of light in oxygenated hemoglobin in comparison with that of reduced or deoxygenated hemoglobin. A probe with a light sensor can either be clipped on or adhered to a finger, earlobe, or other vascular pulsatile site, such as a toe, the forehead, or the nose. Blood flow to the location of the sensor should be unrestricted.

SpO_2 may be lower in dependent extremities than in nondependent extremities. Nose and forehead probes tend to perform poorly when the SaO_2 is low. If the probe is placed on a finger, nail polish should be removed or the probe should be attached sideways. Acrylic nails without polish do not affect the accuracy of oximetry.

Use of pulse oximeters is recommended for any patient at risk for hypoxemia, as desaturation may be detected much quicker than by clinical assessment. An SaO_2 (or SpO_2) reading of 95% means that 95% of the total hemoglobin is saturated with oxygen molecules. Note that only the percentage of hemoglobin that is carrying oxygen is measured; therefore, pulse oximetry is neither an indicator of overall hemoglobin levels nor an indicator of oxygen delivery to the tissues. Numerous studies have shown excellent correlation between pulse oximetry and arterial oxygen saturation via ABG analysis; this is particularly true of SaO_2 measurements ranging from 70% to 100%.

In general, an oxygen saturation greater than or equal to 95% is considered within normal range. Table 5-1-5 interprets SaO_2 values in comparison with PaO_2 values.

Notice that an SaO_2 of 95% is comparable with a PaO_2 of 80%; however, an SaO_2 of 90% compares with a PaO_2 of only 60%.

Although a useful tool, especially in monitoring trends, the pulse oximeter does have limitations and variables that may affect the accuracy of readings (see Table 5-1-6).

Remember, pulse oximetry measures only oxygenation, not ventilation.

Table 5-1-5.   Comparison of SaO_2 and PaO_2

SaO_2	PROBABLE PaO_2
97	100
95	80
94	70
90	60
85	50
75	40
57	30
32	20
10	10

From Hartshorn, J., Sole, M. L., & Lamborn, M. (1997). *Introduction to critical care nursing* (3rd ed., p. 139). Philadelphia: WB Saunders.

Table 5-1-6. Limitations of Pulse Oximetry

VARIABLES THAT MAY IMPAIR ACCURACY	NURSING CONSIDERATIONS
Motion artifact	The ear is usually least affected by motion.
Parkinson's disease	
Seizures	
Shivering	
Ambient light	Move the sensor or cover it with
Sun	something opaque (e.g., washcloth).
Overhead exam light	
Low perfusion state	Always make certain the pulse rate on the
Weak or absent peripheral pulse	oximeter correlates with the patient's
Hypotension	heart rate.
Hypovolemia	Move the sensor to another site.
Hypothermia	Warm the extremity.
Vasoconstrictive drugs	
Abnormal hemoglobins	The accuracy of pulse oximetry in patients
Carbon monoxide poisoning	with such abnormalities is questionable.
Sickle cell anemia	Could be used as a trend; such patients
Cystic fibrosis	may require ABG analysis.
Severe anemia (hematocrit $<$ 10)	Oximetry will not be accurate.
Fingernail polish	Remove polish.
	Place sensor on toe, ear, or other pulsatile site.
	Can position the fingertip sensor sideways on the finger (may require tape).

Changes in ventilation, such as CO_2 retention and apnea, are not assessed. Pulse oximetry is also not a reliable indicator of hyperoxia, which can lead to oxygen toxicity. As discussed earlier, oxygen toxicity is a serious and detrimental problem associated with oxygen free radicals that damage lung tissue. If you are uncertain of the accuracy of your patient's pulse oximeter or his or her clinical presentation does not correlate with the SaO_2 reading, obtain an ABG analysis for confirmation.

Arterial Blood Gas Analysis
Interpretation

ABG analysis is used to help evaluate a patient's oxygenation status, adequacy of gas exchange in the lungs, and acid-base balance (Table 5-1-7). For the body to maintain homeostasis, it must maintain a balance of acids and bases (alkaline substances.)

Understanding ABG interpretation requires an understanding of the body's buffer systems. A buffer system is a mechanism for neutralizing acids and maintaining homeostasis by combining or separating acids and bases as needed. Three buffer systems exist: the blood, the respiratory system, and the renal system. In the blood, hemoglobin and plasma proteins serve as buffers against CO_2. The respiratory buffer system works through elimination of excess CO_2 by hyperventilation or the retention of CO_2 by hypoventilation. When CO_2 combines with water, it creates carbonic acid, a potent acid. If the blood is too alkalotic, then the respiratory system holds onto CO_2, creating carbonic acid and decreasing the pH. If the blood is acidotic, then the respira-

Table 5-1-7. Arterial Blood Gases

VALUE	FUNCTION	NORMAL	ABNORMAL
pH	Assessment of acid-base balance	7.35–7.45	< 7.35: acidosis > 7.45: alkalosis
Pao_2	Measurement of the partial pressure of oxygen in arterial blood; a reflection of oxygenation and an indicator of how much oxygen the lungs are delivering to the tissue	75–100%	<80 mm Hg is generally considered an indicator of hypoxia.
$Paco_2$	Measurement of the partial pressure of CO_2 dissolved in the arterial blood; a reflection of ventilation and an indicator of how effectively the lungs are eliminating CO_2	35–45 mm Hg	45: acidosis <35: alkalosis
HCO_3	Metabolic component of the body's acid-base balance; reflective of kidney function	22–26 mEq/L	<22: acidosis >26: alkalosis
Sao_2	Measurement of the amount of oxygen bound to hemoglobin	95–100%	

tory system blows off CO_2, reducing the amount of carbonic acid and increasing the pH.

Bicarbonate is the main base in the blood. The renal buffer system excretes or retains bicarbonate when necessary to maintain a normal pH. Nonvolatile acids (those that cannot form a vapor), such as lactic acid and ketoacids, are removed by the kidneys. The respiratory buffer system is activated immediately after an acid-base imbalance is detected; the renal system is much slower and may take up to 2 days to compensate.

The normal pH of arterial blood ranges from 7.35 to 7.45; this is slightly alkaline (Table 5-1-8). The pH value is based on the number of hydrogen ions present; the pH is inversely proportional to the number of hydrogen ions. The fewer the H^+ ions, the higher the pH (alkaline); the more the H^+ ions, the lower the pH (acidic).

Various methods can be used to interpret ABGs. It is important to find a step-by-step method to ensure accuracy; one such method is as follows:

Step 1: Evaluate oxygenation. Look at the Pao_2—is the level indicative of hypoxemia?

Step 2: Evaluate acid-base status. Look at the pH—is it normal (7.35 to 7.45), acidotic (<7.35), or alkalotic (>7.45)?

Table 5-1-8. Quick Reference for Arterial Blood Gas Analysis

	RESPIRATORY ACIDOSIS	RESPIRATORY ALKALOSIS	METABOLIC ACIDOSIS	METABOLIC ALKALOSIS
pH	Decreased	Increased	Decreased	Increased
$Paco_2$	Increased	Decreased	Normal	Normal
HCO_3	Normal	Normal	Decreased	Increased

Step 3: Evaluate respiratory status. Look at the $Paco_2$ level—is it normal (35 to 45), acidotic (>45), or alkalotic (<35)?

Step 4: Evaluate metabolic status. Look at the HCO_3 level—is it normal (22 to 26), acidotic (<22), or alkalotic (>26)?

Now, list the three values that represent acid-base balance: pH, $Paco_2$, and HCO_3. Beside each value, write "A" for acidotic, "B" for basic (alkalotic), or "N" for normal. The pH will indicate whether the patient is acidotic or alkalotic. Next, check which component (respiratory or metabolic) matches the pH. For example: pH 7.20, A; $Paco_2$ 75, A; HCO_3 25, N. The pH indicates acidosis, as does the $Paco_2$, the respiratory component, whereas HCO_3, the metabolic component, is normal. Therefore, these ABG values indicate respiratory acidosis.

Compensation is an attempt by one of the buffer systems to maintain homeostasis. If the value of the unmatched component is normal, then no compensation has occurred. If compensatory mechanisms are seen, but the pH is still abnormal, then compensatory is partial. If the pH is normal and compensatory mechanisms are noted, then compensation is complete. When there is complete compensation, look at the pH to determine the primary imbalance. The primary disorder is what will have caused the pH to shift before compensation. Therefore, whichever side of 7.40 on which the pH falls is considered to be the underlying disorder. For example, pH 7.43, N (leaning toward B); $Paco_2$ 50, A; HCO_3 38, B. Here the pH is normal, indicating that compensation has occurred. But although normal, the pH is leaning toward the alkaline. Therefore, the underlying problem is metabolic alkalosis (as the pH and HCO_3 both indicate alkalosis). This would be interpreted as compensated metabolic acidosis.

Table 5-1-9. Causes of Acid-Base Imbalances

Respiratory acidosis	Metabolic acidosis
Chronic obstructive pulmonary disease	Lactic acidosis
Sedation	Ketoacidosis:
Head trauma	Diabetes
Drug overdose	Starvation
Pneumothorax	Alcoholism
Central nervous system disorders	Diarrhea
Pulmonary edema	Parenteral nutrition
Sleep apnea	
Chest wall trauma	**Metabolic alkalosis**
	Vomiting
Respiratory alkalosis	Nasogastric suction
Pulmonary embolism	Diuretics
Pregnancy	Steroids
Anxiety/fear	Hypokalemia
Hypoxia	Excessive ingestion of antacids
Pain	Administration of HCO_3
Fever	Banked blood transfusions
Sepsis	Cushing's syndrome
Congestive heart failure	
Pulmonary edema	
Asthma	
Acute respiratory distress syndrome	

Table 5-1-10. Manifestations of Acid-Base Imbalances

Respiratory acidosis	Metabolic acidosis
Restlessness	Headache
Dizziness	Drowsiness
Disorientation	Coma
Drowsiness	Seizures
Coma	Hypotension
Headache	Cardiac dysrhythmias
Tremors	Decreased cardiac output
Dyspnea	Nausea/vomiting
Decreased reflex response	Diarrhea
	Hyperkalemia
Respiratory alkalosis	Hyperventilation
Anxiety	
Lightheadedness	**Metabolic alkalosis**
Tinnitus	Numbness and tingling of extremities
Syncope	Agitation
Palpitations	Nervousness
Cardiac dysrhythmias	Confusion
Diaphoresis	Seizures
Nausea/vomiting	Nausea/vomiting
Tightness in chest	Cardiac dysrhythmias
Positive Trousseau's sign	Hypokalemia
Positive Chvostek's sign	Hypoventilation
	Hypocalcemia
	Hypochloremia

Management

The numerous causes of acid-base imbalances (Table 5-1-9) produce varying signs and symptoms (Table 5-1-10). Treatment is always directed to the underlying cause of the imbalance and, therefore, is variable. For example, if the cause of a patient's respiratory alkalosis is hyperventilation related to pain, then the nursing goal would be to decrease the patient's pain, thus decreasing his or her respiratory rate and normalizing acid-base balance. If the cause of a patient's metabolic acidosis is excessive GI output related to diarrhea, then the nurse would administer antidiarrheal agents and fluids as ordered with the goal of preventing excessive elimination of HCO_3 and restoring the acid-base balance.

 CLINICAL PEARLS

○ A patient with a Pao_2 below 60 mm Hg requires immediate intervention; a Pao_2 below 40 mm Hg is life-threatening.
○ Any patient receiving an Fio_2 above 50% for longer than 24 hours should be closely monitored for signs and symptoms of oxygen toxicity.
○ To estimate a patient's expected Pao_2, multiply the percentage of oxygen he or she is receiving (Fio_2) by 5.
○ Pulse oximetry is a noninvasive method of monitoring a patient's oxygen saturation level. In general, an Sao_2 above 92% is considered normal.
○ For patients older than 60 years of age, an acceptable Pao_2 range is from 60 to 80 mm Hg.

Oxygen Delivery Devices

Section 2   Lorie Arata ■ Lee Farris

OVERVIEW

Oxygen therapy is now commonly used in both the hospital and home settings. The implementation, management, assessment, and evaluation of oxygen delivery are important nursing responsibilities. This section covers the basic concepts of oxygen therapy and the various oxygen delivery devices in common use.

PRINCIPLES OF CARE
General

The primary indications for the therapeutic use of oxygen are hypoxemia and tissue hypoxia. (See Section 1 for a detailed discussion of hypoxemia and hypoxia.) Some patient conditions that may necessitate the need for oxygen therapy include, but are not limited to, acute myocardial infarction, chest pain, pulmonary edema, acute or chronic respiratory failure, pulmonary embolism, hypoxemia, severe trauma, acute blood loss, pneumothorax, and carbon monoxide poisoning.

The goal of oxygen therapy is to provide a sufficient concentration of oxygen to ensure adequate tissue oxygenation. Therapeutic use of oxygen can increase alveolar oxygen tension, thus allowing more oxygen to diffuse into the capillaries. Room air contains 21% oxygen; oxygen therapy can deliver 22% to 100% supplemental oxygen.

The choice of a particular oxygen delivery device depends on the severity of the hypoxemia and the underlying cause or disease process. Other factors to be considered include the patient's age, mental status, and overall health, as well as the setting or environment in which the oxygen is to be delivered. In general, the amount of oxygen prescribed should provide a PaO_2 of 60 to 90 mm Hg and an SaO_2 above 90%. It is important to realize that the required PaO_2 and SaO_2 are very individualized and depend on various factors, including patient age, severity of illness, and presence of a chronic disease process.

To evaluate the effectiveness of oxygen therapy, ABG values and SpO_2 may be measured. The nurse should also monitor the patient's respiratory rate and pattern, assess for shortness of breath, decreased work of breathing, improved breath sounds, blood pressure and heart rate within the patient's normal range, and decreased anxiety.

Complications of Oxygen Therapy

Oxygen is considered a medication and as such requires a physician's or advanced practice nurse's prescription. As with all medications, oxygen has both benefits and potential complications. Because high levels of oxygen can cause serious adverse effects, it is important to use the least amount of required oxygen to produce the desired response. Three of the most harmful complications of oxygen therapy are hypoventilation, absorption atelectasis, and oxygen toxicity.

Hypoventilation

In patients with chronic obstructive pulmonary disease (COPD), the drive to breathe is stimulated by hypoxia. Too much oxygen can diminish the drive to breathe, causing hypoventilation and respiratory depression. However, oxygen therapy must be considered if the COPD patient's PaO_2 is below 55 mm Hg. Therapy should start at 2 L/min and can be increased to reach a PaO_2 of about 60 mm Hg or an SaO_2 of 90%. Monitor for signs or symptoms of respiratory compromise, including decreased respiratory rate, decreased PaO_2, decreased SaO_2, headache, and changes in mentation.

Absorption Atelectasis

Atelectasis is defined as the collapse of lung tissue. High concentrations of oxygen can wash nitrogen from the lungs. Room air contains approximately 21% oxygen and 78% nitrogen, as well as small amounts of other gases. Nitrogen, with its high partial pressure, plays an important role in holding the alveoli open. When oxygen concentrations of 90% to 100% are inspired, all nitrogen is washed out of the alveoli. The resulting lack of nitrogen will cause the alveoli to shrink and eventually collapse, producing atelectasis. Manifestations of atelectasis include dyspnea, fever, cough, diminished breath sounds, increased dullness on percussion, and leukocytosis. Prevention includes deep breathing, frequent position changes, and early ambulation, all of which hyperinflate the lungs.

Oxygen Toxicity

High-concentration oxygen therapy causes an increase in oxygen free radicals, which are known to damage the alveolar-capillary membrane. Oxygen toxicity can occur in patients receiving greater than 50% oxygen concentration for longer than 24 hours. It is most frequently seen in patients who are intubated and mechanically ventilated with high concentrations of oxygen for prolonged periods. Section 1 provides an in-depth review of oxygen toxicity.

DECISION-MAKING

There are two types of oxygen delivery systems: low-flow and high-flow. Table 5-2-1 provides information on management of oxygen delivery devices.

Low-Flow Systems

Low-flow oxygen delivery systems supplement oxygen that the patient receives from room air. They provide flow rates that are lower than the patient's inspiratory volume. The balance of inspiratory volume is pulled from room air. Thus, the oxygen from the device and room air mix with each inspiratory effort (tidal volume), so that the actual concentration of oxygen delivered with these devices is not known.

Low-flow devices are indicated for patients who can maintain normal respiratory rates, patterns, and volumes. The nasal cannula, simple face mask, partial rebreather mask, and nonrebreather mask are all low-flow oxygen delivery devices.

High-Flow Systems

High-flow devices provide oxygen flow rates in amounts that are two to three times the patient's inspiratory volume. They are independent of the

Table 5-2-1. Comparison of Oxygen Delivery Devices

DEVICE	L/MIN FLOW TO Fio₂ DELIVERED	ADVANTAGES	DISADVANTAGES	IMPLICATIONS
Nasal cannula Low flow; indicated for patients with spontaneous expirations and oxygen requirements of less than or about 40%.	1 to 24% 2 to 28% 3 to 32% 4 to 36% 5 to 40% 6 to 44%	Generally well tolerated Commonly used Does not interfere with talking or eating Inexpensive	Cannot be used with nasal obstruction Unstable; easily displaced Can cause headache and dry mucous membranes Can cause irritation of nares and skin behind the ears	The patient should have a normal tidal volume. Assess to determine if the patient is a mouth breather. Inspect the nostrils for patency and irritation. Watch for kinks or occlusions in the tubing. Ensure that humidity is always provided. Greater than 6 L/min does not increase oxygenation, but does increase irritation. May need to pad pressure points with gauze.
Simple face mask Low-flow; for patients with higher oxygenation needs than the nasal cannula can provide.	5 to 40% 6 to 50% 8 to 60%	Generally well tolerated Can deliver up to 60% oxygen	Hot Requires tight seal, which may cause patient discomfort Interferes with eating and talking May produce feelings of claustrophobia Aspiration risk	Recommended flow of 8–10 L/min to prevent accumulation of exhaled air in the mask. Has vents to allow exhaled air to escape.
Face tent High-flow; useful for patients with facial trauma. Provides increased patient comfort over the face mask.	10–30 to 55%	High humidity Does not dry out mucous membranes Can be used for patients who cannot tolerate pressure on the nose/face	Not a precise oxygen delivery	Monitor for condensation in the tubing related to high humidity.

Device	Flow rate / Concentration	Characteristics	Nursing considerations	Comments
Partial rebreather mask. Low-flow; useful for patients breathing spontaneously but requiring oxygen concentrations greater than 40%.	6 to 35% 8 to 45–50% 10–15 to 60–80%	Can deliver oxygen concentrations of 35–60%	Same as with all masks	Has a reservoir bag that is always open to the mask. Flow should be sufficient to keep the reservoir bag inflated at end inspiration. Oxygen flows into the mask during inhalation and into the bag during exhalation. Conserves oxygen by having the patient rebreathe some of the exhaled air, which is high in oxygen.
Nonrebreather mask. Low-flow; useful for the treatment of severe hypoxemia in an effort to prevent intubation.	6 to 55–60% 8 to 60–80% 10–15 to 80–90%	Delivers 60–90% oxygen. Does not dry mucous membranes. Delivers highest possible percentage of oxygen of the low flow systems.	Same as with all masks	A one-way valve between the bag and mask prevents air from entering the bag during exhalation; exhaled air leaves the mask via a flap in the face piece. Flow should be sufficient to keep the reservoir bag inflated at end inspiration. Very accurate oxygen delivery. Must fit snugly
Venturi mask. Precise oxygen delivery makes these masks most useful for COPD patients.	Color-coded adapters: Blue 4 to 24% Yellow 4 to 28% White 6 to 31% Green 8 to 35% Pink 8 to 40%	Most reliable control of oxygen delivered. Flow is precisely determined by air entrained, color-coded adapters.	Same as with all masks	
Tracheostomy collar. High-flow	10 to 28–100%	Provides high humidity		Has two ports: an exhalation port that is open at all times and an oxygen attachment port. Monitor for accumulation of water, which can enter the trach. Empty the tubing frequently. Monitor for condensation in the tubing from the high humidity, and empty tubing frequently.
Aerosol face mask. High-flow; useful for patients with thick secretions. Commonly used postextubation and following upper airway surgeries.	10 to 24–100%	Provides high humidity	Same as with all masks	

patient's respiratory pattern. The Venturi mask is an example of a high-flow oxygen delivery device. The primary indications for high-flow devices are for patients who require a consistent oxygen concentrations (FIO_2) related to dependence on the hypoxic drive to breathe, and for patients with abnormal respiratory patterns. If these systems fail to provide adequate oxygenation, then intubation and mechanical ventilation will be necessary.

Regardless of the delivery system chosen, the nurse needs to monitor the patient's skin under the mask, straps, and tubing for signs of irritation or breakdown. Systems should be checked at least once a shift, or per hospital policy, for correct flow rate and patency. Assess for kinks in the tubing and for excess condensation in the system, which will restrict oxygen delivery to the patient.

CLINICAL PEARLS

○ Oxygen should be considered a drug. It is important to remember that although oxygen can be extremely beneficial, it can also cause serious complications.
○ For most patients, the amount of oxygen ordered, if therapeutic, should provide patients with PaO_2 levels of 60 to 90 mm Hg and SaO_2 levels below 90%.
○ For the patient with COPD with a PaO_2 below 55 mm Hg, start oxygen therapy at 2 L/min.
○ A patient who breathes solely through the mouth requires a mask or tent; a nasal cannula will not be effective.

Tracheostomy Care

Section 3   Beverly George-Gay

OVERVIEW

The term "tracheostomy" actually refers to an opening into the trachea through the neck. "Tracheotomy" is the procedure for creating the opening. Clinically, tracheostomy refers to both the opening and the procedure. Tracheostomies have been performed since as far back as 1500 BC. The procedure may be performed *percutaneously* (a relatively new method), which involves a surgical skin incision and needle puncture with stoma dilation of the trachea; or through the *open standard* method, which involves surgical incisions through the skin and through the third and fourth tracheal rings. In both methods, an indwelling tube is inserted to facilitate air passage or evacuation of secretions.

PRINCIPLES OF CARE

A tracheostomy (trach) is necessary to ensure adequate airway management in many patient populations. The procedure was historically performed in the operating room; however, today it is performed more frequently at the bedside in intensive care units (ICUs) in patients who may be too unstable to move. The percutaneous procedure is preferred for the ICU.

A *temporary tracheostomy* involves placement of the tube with an intact

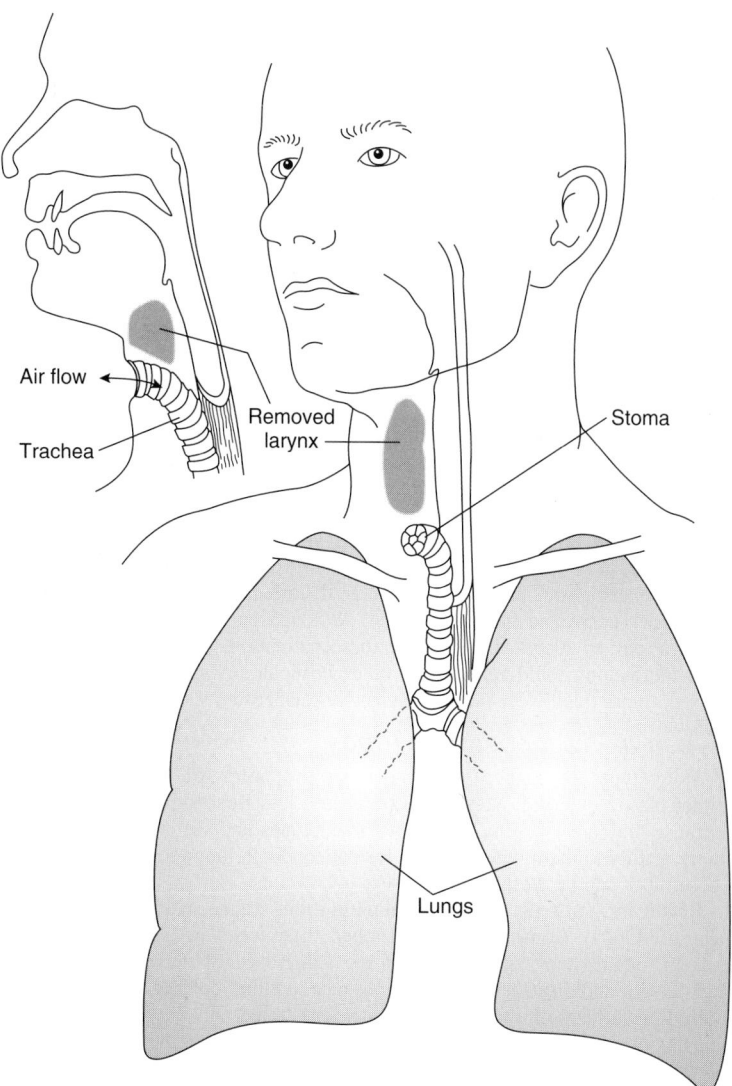

Air flow

Trachea

Removed
larynx

Stoma

Lungs

Figure 5-3-1. Throat after a laryngectomy.

larynx, keeping the trachea in anatomical alignment. The stoma will close once the tube is removed. A *permanent tracheostomy* is usually indicated when the larynx is removed, as in the case of laryngectomy for laryngeal cancer. An incision is made in the neck, and the larynx and part of the upper trachea are removed. The remaining trachea is bent toward the front of the neck, and its edges are sutured to the outside of the neck (Fig. 5-3-1).

In emergency situations outside the hospital and in some emergency departments, a *cricothyroidotomy* may be performed to open the airway until a true tracheostomy can be done. In this procedure, either a 14-gauge needle puncture or a small stab incision is made into the cricothyroid membrane, creating an opening for air flow.

Temporary Tracheostomy
Indications

Tracheostomies are indicated for patients who are in danger of developing respiratory failure due to hypoventilation or ventilation-perfusion mismatch from the following causes.

Airway Obstruction. Obstructions may be caused by soft tissue edema from facial injuries, postoperative swelling after head and neck surgery, inflammation or allergic reactions, tumors, epiglottitis, or foreign bodies. Significant obstructive sleep apnea refractory to conventional therapy may also be an indication.

Secretion Retention. Secretions are easily removed via a tracheostomy tube. This is especially valuable for patients with inadequate cough or those who have lost their gag reflex, which occurs in, for example, patients with a decreased level of consciousness owing to a closed head injury.

Poor Ventilation. Decreases in overall ventilation can occur in many patients because of respiratory center depression from drug overdose, anesthesia, excessive analgesia, and neuromuscular disturbances, leading to ineffective pulmonary nerve and muscle function. Although endotracheal intubation provides a way to adequately ventilate these patients in the acute setting, long-term intubation should be avoided. When artificial airway ventilation is necessary for more than 7 to 14 days, an elective tracheostomy should be performed.

Types of Tracheostomy Tubes

Many types of tracheostomy tubes are available. All types are made of either plastic or metal. **Metal tubes** are used less frequently than other types, because they are irritating to mucous membranes and secretions tend to stick more readily to them. Used mainly for patients with long-term tracheostomies, these tubes can be washed and reused.

Plastic or synthetic polyvinyl chloride tubes are the standard tracheostomy tube used today. Compared to metal tubes, these tubes are less irritating to the mucous membranes and allow for less adherence of secretions. They are lightweight and disposable. These tubes can be either double- or single-lumen, cuffed or cuffless, and fenestrated or nonfenestrated.

The *double-lumen tube,* also called the universal tube, is the most commonly used tracheostomy tube. It has an inner cannula and an outer cannula. The inner cannula fits into the outer cannula, and the outer cannula fits into the stoma. A face plate on the outer cannula with holes on either side allows the cannula to be secured in place with cotton or Velcro ties.

Single-lumen tubes are longer than the universal tube, and are used for patients with exceptionally long or thick necks. These tubes require additional humidification to prevent the buildup of secretions.

The *cuffed tube* is a balloon-type component around the outside of the tube that, when inflated, seals off the surrounding airway. Cuffed tubes are used to prevent aspiration of food and secretions. They are used for patients receiving mechanical ventilation or tube feeding and for patients with excessive secretions. A pilot balloon is attached to the cuff, which indicates the amount of air in the cuff.

The *cuffless tube* has no cuff, enabling aspiration. Adult patients with cuffless tubes are those who are able to protect their airways. Cuffless tubes are used in the pediatric population. Patients with cuffless tubes can speak by covering the opening of the tube on expiration. Air flow on exhalation moves from the bronchus up and around the tube cannula to the vocal cords of the larynx to produce sound.

Fenestrated tubes have a precut opening or fenestration that, when capped, allows air on exhalation to flow from the bronchus up through the vocal cords of the larynx to produce sound, thereby allowing the patient to speak. Both the inner and outer cannulas are fenestrated (Fig. 5-3-2).

Tracheostomy buttons are short, straight tubes that fit into the stoma but do not enter the tracheal lumen. These are frequently used during weaning for decannulation, because they create less airway resistance.

Parts of the Tracheostomy Tube

Outer Cannula. The outer cannula keeps the airway open and should not be removed except for downsizing. It has a swivel-neck face plate that indicates its size and type. For example, "8 DFEN" on the face plate means that the trach tube is a size 8 disposable cannula, fenestrated, cuffed tube. The outer cannula also houses the pilot balloon and the inflatable cuff. The **pilot balloon** is a plastic saclike component connected to the cuff inflation line that acts as

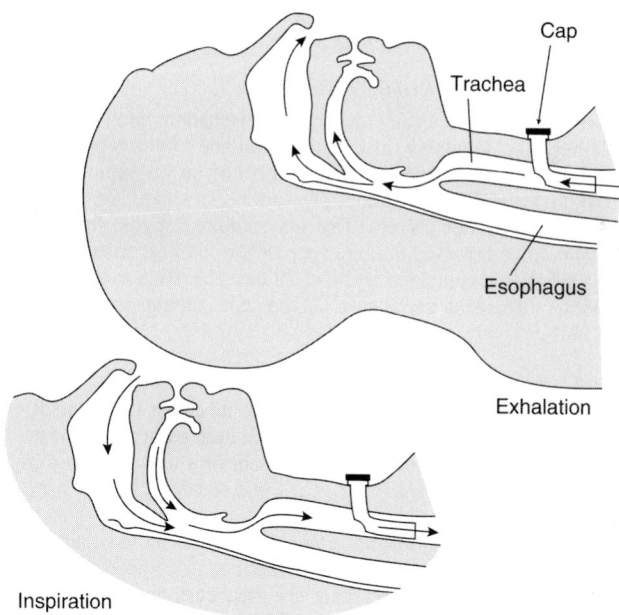

Figure 5-3-2. A fenestrated tracheostomy tube.

an indicator for the amount of air pressure in the cuff. The **cuff** is a balloon component that, when inflated, acts to seal the trachea to prevent air from leaking around the tube and prevent oral or gastric secretions from entering the lungs. When the cuff is inflated, breathing must occur through the tube. Some cuffed tracheostomy tubes have a **pressure-relief valve** that automatically limits the internal pressure of the cuff.

Inner Cannula. The inner cannula fits into the outer cannula and can be removed for cleaning and reuse or disposed of and replaced. The inner cannula can be fenestrated or nonfenestrated.

Obturator. The obturator is a stylet used to direct insertion of a tracheostomy tube. It must be removed immediately after the tracheostomy tube is inserted and kept with the patient in case of accidental decannulation.

DECISION-MAKING
Assessment
Breath Sounds

Breath sounds should be assessed every 1 to 2 hours during the first 24 hours after surgery. This determines how frequently the patient will need suctioning and also helps to assess for pneumothorax. Always keep suction equipment at the bedside.

Oxygenation

SaO_2, measured by pulse oximetry or ABGs, may be monitored in the initial postoperative period. Maintain the SaO_2 above 92%. Observe for signs and symptoms of hypoxemia (i.e., restlessness, agitation, confusion, tachycardia). Section 1 of this chapter provides more details on assessing oxygenation.

Cuff Pressure Measurements

Excessive cuff pressures can cause tracheal ischemia, necrosis, and erosion. Cuff inflation should involve auscultating over the larynx while inflating the cuff in 0.5- to 1-mL increments, until the rush of air on expiration is significantly diminished (for cuffs without pressure-relief valves) or disappears (for cuffs with pressure-relief valves). This may require bagging the patient. Cuff pressures should be assessed during every shift to prevent tissue damage. Cuff pressures should be maintained at 14 to 20 mm Hg. Higher pressures may be needed with mechanical ventilation. In no case should pressure exceed 25 mm Hg.

Air Leak

Air leakage around the cuff can occur if the tube size is too small or if the balloon ruptures. A rush of air will be heard on each expiration despite balloon inflation. An air leak necessitates the placement of a new tracheostomy tube.

Secretions

Assess secretions for consistency, color, and odor as an indication of pulmonary infection or improvement. Provide humidified air to keep secretions loose. Dried secretions can clump and plug the tracheostomy tube. Maintain the patient on 2 to 3 L of fluid/day, which will help keep secretions loose. Trach care with suctioning should be performed every 8 hours or as needed. Teach the patient to take a deep breath and momentarily cover the tracheostomy tube with one finger, then cough while simultaneously removing the finger. This maneuver, called the "glottal stop," helps increase intrathoracic pressure, which aids secretion removal.

Wound Site

Assess the stoma site for signs and symptoms of infection, such as purulent drainage, pain, redness, and swelling. The initial dressing can be reinforced but should not be changed for the first 48 hours after the procedure; this gives the stoma edges time to retract. After the first 48 hours, dressing changes and trach tie changes can be performed daily or as needed.

Decannulation
Accidental Decannulation

If the tracheostomy tube is expelled accidentally within the first 48 hours of placement, the stoma may be held open with a pair of hemostats and reinsertion attempted. This situation is a medical emergency and may require ventilation by ambu bag. A new tube and obturator should be kept at the bedside. A stoma more than 72 hours old will have retracted edges and will maintain an open airway for a short period until the tube can be replaced. A displaced tracheostomy tube occurs more frequently in overweight patients with large necks; therefore, these patients should be monitored more closely.

Planned Decannulation

Once it is determined that the patient can maintain adequate ventilation, the tracheostomy tube may be downsized to size 6 or 4, then capped. If respiratory distress develops, remove the cap and notify the physician. If the patient tolerates the tube being capped for 12 to 24 hours, then the tube may be removed. The stoma edges may be taped shut or covered with an occlusive dressing, and they will heal within 5 to 7 days.

Communication

Provide an alternative method of communication, such as a pad and pencil or a picture chart for a patient who cannot read and write. Carefully watch for nonverbal communication cues. The patient with intact vocal cords will be able to talk by either covering the tube or using a fenestrated tube, a talking trach, or a Passy-Muir valve. When the patient is ready to talk, provide good mouth care and a way for the patient to easily get rid of oral secretions.

Covering the Tube

When the tracheostomy tube is covered with a finger and the cuff is deflated, the flow of air on exhalation will go through the vocal cords, and the patient will be able to make sound. Ensure that the cuff is reinflated for meals.

Fenestrated Tube

Fenestrated tubes allow for better air flow, because they come with an opening in the tube and a cap. The fenestrated tube must also be covered or capped with the cuff deflated for best results. Reinflate the cuff for meals (see Fig. 5-3-2).

Talking Tracheostomy

This type of tube is for long-term trach patients who require mechanical ventilation. An extra channel is incorporated into the tube that can be attached to an air source that provides a continuous flow of air through the vocal cords. This air flow can dry the mucous membranes and thus should be used only when necessary. The cuff remains inflated with this tube.

Speaking Valve (Passy-Muir Valve)

This commonly used speaking tracheostomy device has a one-way valve that is placed over the hub of the tracheostomy tube and opens on inhalation, allowing air to enter the trachea and lungs. The valve closes at the end of inspiration and remains closed throughout exhalation. The air is directed up through the vocal cords on exhalation, enabling the patient to speak. The speaking valve is used most easily with fenestrated trachs, but can be used with other types. If it is being used with a cuffed tracheostomy tube, the cuff must be deflated to allow the upward flow of air. A speaking valve is contraindicated for unconscious patients and patients with thick copious secretions.

Postoperative Complications

Hemorrhage

Mild oozing from the site is common for the first few days postoperatively and can be controlled with gauze packing to the site. If the bleeding is bright red and continuous and the tube is pulsating, the physician should be notified immediately and the patient prepared to return to the operating room. These findings indicate that the tube is resting on the innominate artery, which may perforate and rupture. If rupture occurs, death is imminent. This is a rare occurrence.

Subcutaneous Emphysema

Subcutaneous emphysema may occur as air enters the subcutaneous tissue of the neck and upper chest wall. The crepitus that is produced, although benign, should be reported to the physician, especially if it reaches the face or lower chest. The patient and the family should be told that this is a common complication during the first 24 hours after the procedure and will dissipate after a few days.

Respiratory Distress

Respiratory distress can result from blockage of the tube by a mucus plug, mucosal edema, or increased secretions that the patient is not able to clear.

Pneumothorax/Pneumomediastinum

Pneumothorax may result from damage to the parietal pleura at the apexes of the lungs during the tracheostomy procedure. Pneumomediastinum occurs when air is forced into the mediastinal space from coughing. Pneumomediastinum may also cause pneumothorax. Both are early complications of the procedure and can be treated with chest tube placement.

Long-Term Complications

Infection

Infection at the wound site (tracheitis) or pulmonary infections may develop. It is important to maintain sterile technique when suctioning and caring for the wound, and to maintain aseptic technique for all other care. Monitor for an elevated white blood cell count and for erythema and purulent drainage at the stoma site. Prophylactic antibiotics are not routinely recommended for patients undergoing tracheostomy; however, many patients do receive antibiotics for other reasons.

Tracheal Stenosis

Tracheal stenosis is a narrowing for the tracheal lumen due to scar formation from excessive pressure exerted by the cuff of the tracheostomy tube. Assessing and maintaining desired cuff pressures will help prevent this complication. Tracheal stenosis requires surgical repair.

Tracheoesophageal Fistula

A tracheoesophageal (TE) fistula is an opening created between the trachea and the anterior esophagus. This erosion is caused by excessive cuff pressure on the posterior wall of the trachea; thus, it can be prevented by maintaining proper cuff pressure. A patient with a TE fistula is at high risk for aspiration and its significant sequelae.

Tracheomalacia

Tracheomalacia is the softening, dilation, and potential erosion of the tracheal cartilage from constant pressure exerted by the inflated cuff. This complication is becoming less common because of the pressure-relief valves provided on today's cuffed tubes. Tracheomalacia should be suspected if the patient has a continuous air leak necessitating a larger tube.

 CLINICAL PEARLS

○ Examine the tracheostomy tube's face plate to determine the patient's tube type and size.
○ Air flowing upward to the vocal cords is what allows the patient to speak.
○ Fenestrated tracheostomy tubes allow air to flow upward to the vocal cords, allowing the patient to speak.
○ To inflate the balloon cuff, inject air into the pilot valve in 1-mL increments while auscultating the neck over the cuff until no air leak is heard.
○ Balloon air pressure should not exceed 25 mm Hg.

Chest Drainage Systems

Section 4 Lorie Arata ▪ Lee Farris

OVERVIEW

Chest drainage systems are indicated for patients with conditions that involve a compromise in the negative pressure of the chest cavity. When disease or injury results in the loss of negative pleural pressure, a chest drainage system may be required to reestablish negative pressure. Chest drainage systems are also used to collect blood and other fluids from the thoracic cavity. The nurse assesses, maintains, and troubleshoots chest drainage systems as part of patient care.

PRINCIPLES OF CARE

Chest tubes inserted primarily to remove air are usually placed in the fourth or fifth intercostal space at the midaxillary line. Tubes inserted at this site can also remove fluid. If significant fluid drainage is expected, then a second tube may be placed in the inferior posterior area of the pleural cavity.

In a normal thoracic cavity, the pressure in the pleural space is below atmospheric, or negative, at all times. This negative pressure maintains normal lung inflation. The loss of negative pressure results in collapse of the lung. Chest tubes are inserted into the pleural space between the visceral and parietal pleura to reestablish negative pressure. Chest tubes are indicated in various conditions (Table 5-4-1).

Chest tubes are always connected to a closed system to prevent reentry of air into the pleural space. The closed system usually consists of a three-chambered collection device. Although devices may differ slightly depending on the manufacturer, the functions of the individual chambers remain the same.

- The *underwater seal chamber* allows air and fluid to escape from the pleural space while preventing its reentry and maintaining negative pressure. Water from the water seal chamber cannot flow backward into the pleural space.
- The *drainage collection chamber* allows for the collection and measurement of blood and other fluids.
- The *suction control chamber* allows the proper negative pressure for the patient to be set.

There are two types of suction regulatory chambers. In a *wet suction control* chamber, the amount of negative pressure is increased by increasing the amount of water in the chamber. In a *dry* device, the amount of suction is regulated by adjusting a dial to the necessary specification. Although the suction control chamber regulates the amount of negative pressure applied to the patient, the chest drainage device must be connected to a suction machine to activate the negative pressure. The suction machine should be adjusted so that gentle bubbling is seen in the suction control chamber. Vigorous bubbling hastens the evaporation of water and may contribute to inadvertent changes in the negative pressure setting.

Drainage collection devices have other important features. A rubber diaphragm in the water seal chamber allows the nurse to refill the chamber with a needle and syringe when evaporation occurs. A rubber diaphragm in the drainage chamber allows fluid to be removed for laboratory sampling. Pressure-release valves, either automatic or manual, protect the patient from excessively high positive or negative pressures.

Types of Devices/Systems
Glass Bottles

Although still in use, glass bottle collection systems are not as prevalent as they were before the development of commercially prepared plastic collection units. The bottle systems function essentially the same as the chambers described earlier.

A glass bottle system may have one, two, or three bottles. In a one-bottle setup, the water seal and collection chambers are combined in the one bottle. There is no suction capability; the system works by gravity alone. In a two-

Table 5-4-1. Indications for Chest Tube Placement

Pneumothorax	A pneumothorax occurs when air enters the pleural space, causing the lung on the affected side to completely or partially collapse. A pneumothorax can occur spontaneously or traumatically. A spontaneous pneumothorax occurs when a bleb or bulla ruptures, allowing air to enter the pleural space. A traumatic pneumothorax occurs when the pleura is penetrated by an object such as a broken rib, bullet, or knife, or as a result of a therapeutic medical procedure, such as a central line insertion. A pneumothorax larger than 20% requires chest tube placement for lung reexpansion. Uncomplicated pneumothorax may resolve in 3 to 4 days. Resolution of complicated pneumothorax may take longer, especially if the patient is on positive-pressure ventilation.
Tension pneumothorax	A tension pneumothorax occurs when air enters the pleural space and is not able to escape. The buildup of air in the chest causes increased intrathoracic pressure. This increase in pressure can cause a shift in the structures of the mediastinum from the affected side to the unaffected side. This can result in compression of the heart, lung, and great vessels. Compression of the vena cava results in decreased venous return to the heart. The trachea will deviate toward the unaffected side. This is a life-threatening condition.
Hemothorax	A hemothorax is blood in the pleural space. Like a pneumothorax, a hemothorax can occur spontaneously or as a result of injury. A spontaneous pneumothorax may occur from neoplasms, infection, blood dyscrasias, or rupture of the thoracic aorta. Traumatic hemothorax may occur from a chest injury or an injury that occurs during chest surgery. Hemothorax is classified by the amount of blood in the pleural space. Bleeding of 300 to 500 mL is considered a minimal hemothorax; 500 to 1000 mL, a moderate hemothorax; and more than 1000 mL, a large hemothorax. A moderate or large hemothorax requires chest drainage. Reexpansion of the lung should occur within 7 to 10 days; if it does not, then surgical intervention may be required.
Empyema	An empyema is the collection of pus in the pleural space. It occurs secondary to an infection such as pneumonia. The length of time required for chest drainage varies according to the patient's condition.
Thoracotomy	A thoracotomy is a surgical opening into the thoracic cavity. It is indicated in any surgical procedure that compromises the pleural space, such as lung resection. The chest tube is removed when the condition requiring the thoracotomy is resolved.
Cardiac surgery	Cardiac surgery is an indication for a mediastinal chest tube. This tube is placed in the pericardial space to facilitate drainage of blood from around the heart. This tube uses the same type of chest drainage system, but assessment is different. The nurse observes the drainage collection chamber for bright-red blood that eventually changes to pink or straw-colored drainage. The patient should be observed for signs and symptoms of cardiac tamponade (compression of the heart from expanding fluid in the pericardial sac), including muffled heart tones, decreased blood pressure, increased heart rate, increased central venous pressure, and decreased pulmonary artery pressure. Changes in the color of the drainage back to bright red may indicate new bleeding. These chest tubes are usually removed within the first 24 hours postoperatively.

bottle system, one bottle is the drainage collection chamber and the other is the water seal chamber. This setup also works by gravity alone, with no suction. In a three-bottle system, the first bottle is the collection chamber, the second bottle is the water seal chamber, and the third bottle is the suction control chamber. In a three-bottle system, suction is controlled by the depth at which a manometer is submerged in the water in the bottle, not by the amount of suction applied. Care for patients with glass bottle systems is similar to that for patients with plastic disposable systems.

Commercially Prepared Plastic Units

Various devices are available from several manufacturers. For example, Genzyme Surgical Products produces the Pleurovac dry suction control, the Pleur-evac wet series, and the Thora-Klex waterless (dry) system; Atrium Medical Products manufactures the Oasis dry suction chest drain unit and the Ocean water seal (wet) chest drain. The various models are available within each series. Chest drain autotransfusion products are also available. Specific features of these devices are discussed in Section 2 of this chapter. Features vary slightly depending on the model and manufacturer.

These devices have many benefits that may make them preferable to glass bottle units. They are disposable, small, easy to transport, and convenient. Many safety and diagnostic features are available.

Other Types of Chest Drainage Devices

The Heimlich chest drain valve is a specially designed one-way flutter valve that can be used as an alternative to a three-chamber collection device. The valve is constructed of rubber tubing enclosed in a transparent plastic chamber with tapered ends. The valve allows fluid, air, and clots to escape the chest and drain into a plastic collection container. Backward flow of fluid and air into the chest is prevented by the one-way valve mechanism. The valve can also be connected to regulated suction. The Heimlich valve is indicated for use with any clinical condition in which chest tube drainage is required. The valve must be connected properly so that air can escape from the chest. If the valve is connected incorrectly (backward), air becomes trapped, and a tension pneumothorax may develop.

The pleuro-peritoneal shunt device provides a pathway between the pleural space and the peritoneal cavity. The device is used to treat chronic pleural effusions by removing the fluid from the pleural space to the peritoneal cavity, where it can be absorbed. The pump must be surgically inserted and manually pumped to transfer the fluid.

DECISION-MAKING

Care of the patient with a chest drainage system includes assisting with setup and insertion, providing continuous assessment, troubleshooting, monitoring drainage, monitoring and changing dressings as indicated, assisting with removal, and assessing after removal.

Insertion
Preparing the Patient
Prepare for insertion by teaching the patient about the procedure. Allow time for questions, and obtain informed consent.

Administer a sedative or pain medication if ordered.
Preparing the Equipment
Prepare the necessary equipment and supplies (chest tube, chest drainage system, insertion tray, suction machine, dressing supplies, petrolatum gauze, lidocaine HCl 1%, Betadine solution, and suture material). The most com-

mon chest tube sizes are 28F, 32F, and 36F in adults and 16F, 20F, and 24F in children.

Preparing the System

Prepare the chest drainage system using aseptic technique according to hospital policy and manufacturer's guidelines. In most commercially available systems, the nurse must add sterile water to the water seal chamber. In wet suction control chamber units, sterile water must also be added to the specified level in the suction control chamber. In dry suction control chamber units, the setting is dialed in by the nurse until the indicator reads that the correct setting has been reached. Suction levels may vary from low (-10) to high (-40), with -20 the most common setting. Connect the chest drainage system to the suction machine. Ventilated patients should be disconnected from positive airway pressure before the pleura is entered, to prevent the lung from being pushed against the insertion site and out of the wound. If positive pressure is not discontinued, lung damage may occur. After the tube has been inserted and connected to the chest drainage system, turn on the suction slowly. Verify that the correct amount of suction is being applied by checking the indicator. The type of indicator varies depending on the manufacturer. In a wet device, there should be gentle, not vigorous, bubbling. After the tube has been inserted and the chest drainage device connected to suction, assess the patient according to the guidelines presented in the following section. The patient should be assessed on a regular schedule.

Assessment

Patient Assessment

- Assess vital signs and lung sounds at least every 4 hours. The lung sounds on the affected side may be diminished, depending on the patient's condition.
- Assess the entire chest drainage system. Start with the patient and work toward the closed system.
- Assess the chest tube insertion site. Examine the insertion site for air leaks by listening for whistling or sucking air. Check the end of the chest tube to verify that it has not slipped out of the chest wall. If the chest tube has slipped enough so that the eyelets near the end of the tube are visible, air may be able to enter the chest wall. Notify the physician promptly.
- Assess the dressing; it should be clean and dry.
- Verify that all connections between the patient and the chest drainage system are tight, with no air leaks. The connections may be secured with tape.

Chest Tube Assessment

Water Seal Chamber

Observe the water seal chamber. In a disposable chest drainage system, the water level should be at 2 cm (or 1 inch). In a bottle system, the glass tube that is attached to the patient's chest tube should be submerged to 2 cm (or 1 inch) below the water level. Assess the water in the water seal chamber for *tidaling* or *fluctuation*. In a patient not on a ventilator and not connected to suction, the fluid in the water seal chamber will rise during inspiration (when the pressure is above atmospheric pressure) and fall during expiration (when the pressure is below atmospheric pressure). Tidaling (or fluctuation) will not occur if the patient is connected to suction. Suction may be temporarily discontinued to assess for tidaling. In a patient connected to a mechanical ventilator, the tidaling pattern is reversed; the fluid will rise with expiration and fall with inspiration, because ventilator breaths are delivered with positive pressure. Tidaling will cease if the tube becomes obstructed or kinked or if the lung fully expands.

Air Leaks

Also assess the water seal chamber for air leaks. *Bubbling* in the water seal chamber indicates an air leak. Air may leak from the patient or from the closed drainage system, and it may or may not indicate a problem. A bubbling pattern that corresponds with the patient's respiratory pattern indicates a leak in the patient's lung. A ventilated patient with an air leak receiving positive end-expiratory pressure (PEEP) will demonstrate a pattern of continuous bubbling because of the continuous positive pressure. A nonventilated patient who has continuous bubbling most likely has a leak somewhere in the closed drainage system and should be assessed as follows.

Check the entire system for air leaks by systematically inspecting the chest drainage system for cracks, holes, and disconnections by starting at the patient and working to the collection container. If there is no visible problem, use a rubber-tipped chest tube clamp to clamp the tube where it exits the patient's chest. If the bubbling stops, the air leak is in the patient's lung. If the bubbling continues, it is in the system. Continue to move down the connecting tubing clamping and unclamping the tubing while checking for bubbling in the water seal chamber. If the bubbling stops, the leak is between the clamp and the patient. This indicates a leak in the tubing, and the tubing will have to be replaced. If the bubbling continues when the tubing is clamped at the end where it connects to the collection device, then the leak is in the device, and the device must be replaced. If a new air leak from the patient's lung develops or a previous air leak worsens, notify the physician.

Suction Control and Drainage Collection

Assess the suction control and drainage collection chamber. Verify the appropriate negative pressure setting. In a wet system, evaporation of water can change the desired setting. The suction should be set at a level that allows for gentle bubbling; vigorous bubbling contributes to evaporation. Additional sterile water can by added to achieve the desired level. Evaluate and document the amount and color of drainage in the collection chamber.

Pain Control

Pain control is an important aspect of nursing care. Pain medication may be given through various routes. A highly effective method of pain control in patients who have undergone thoracic surgery is epidural administration of an opioid. This local administration is used during the immediate postoperative period and/or over the following 3 to 4 days. The medication of choice, usually morphine or fentanyl, can be administered via injection at the time of anesthesia as intermittent injections or as a continuous infusion. Closely monitor the patient for side effects associated with narcotic administration.

Removal

Before a chest tube is removed, there should be minimal drainage and the patient should be able to tolerate clamping of the chest tube or placement of the chest tube in a water seal for 12 to 24 hours without air leaks or further accumulation of fluid. The patient is evaluated with a chest tube before the tube is removed.

CLINICAL PEARLS

○ Never clamp a chest tube for more than 1 or 2 minutes. Clamping for longer periods can increase intrapleural pressure, resulting in a tension pneumothorax and/or subcutaneous emphysema.

○ As an alternative to clamping a chest tube in an emergency situation (e.g., a broken collection chamber), you can temporarily reestablish the water seal by placing the exposed end of the tube in a bottle of sterile water.

○ If the patient's suction is discontinued, turn off the wall suction and disconnect the tubing from the suction unit. Leave the connecting tubing open to air. If the system remains closed, air can become trapped, causing a tension pneumothorax and/or subcutaneous emphysema.

○ Milking or stripping of chest tubes is discouraged. This procedure can significantly increase intrapleural negative pressure (-400 cm H_2O) and may have more risks than benefits to patients. An alternative method of removing clots in connector tubing is to gently pinch around the clot to facilitate its movement into the collection chamber.

○ Changes in patient position may facilitate the removal of pooled drainage. Bright red blood or significant increases in drainage not associated with a position change may indicate new bleeding.

○ Chest tubes are discontinued when the chest x-ray indicates lung reexpansion, when there is an absence of air leaks, and when drainage is minimal (<100 to 150 mL/24 hr).

RESOURCES

• American Association for Respiratory Care: www.aarc.org/
• American Lung Association: 800-586-4872 or www.lungusa
• Atrium Medical Corporation: 800-528-7486 or www.atriummed.com
• Genzyme Surgical Products: 800-367-7874
• National Heart, Lung and Blood Institute: www.nhlbi.nih.gov/nhlbi/lung/lung.htm
• Passy-Muir tracheostomy and ventilator speaking valves: www.passy-muir.com
• Veralius Clinical Folios: www.versalius.com/graphics/cf_procedure/trach
• www.cmclungctr.com
• www.dailylung.com
• www.healthgate.com/HealthGate/free/dph.0015.shtml (ABGs)
• www.healthgate.com/HealthGate/free/dph.0200.shtml (Pulse Oximetry)
• www.medicinenet.com (Procedures and Tests-Tracheostomy)
• www.pulmonarydata.com
• www.respcarejournal.com
• www.springnet.com
• www.twood.vinu.edu/students/cpgs/othefcpg.html

chapter 6

Decision-Making for Renal Alterations

Renal Assessment

Section 1   Charlotte Mackey

OVERVIEW

The basic function of the renal system is to eliminate wastes and excess fluid from the body and help maintain homeostatic, electrolyte, and acid-base balance. Renal failure can cause changes affecting all body systems. This section discusses assessment of the patient with suspected or actual renal dysfunction. Laboratory data are discussed in Chapter 11, Section 5.

PRINCIPLES OF CARE

Renal disorders affect millions of Americans and are associated with significant morbidity. At some point during their lifetime, 20% of women in the U.S. will suffer a urinary tract infection. Kidney stones affect at least 1% of the U.S. population. Billions of health care dollars are spent on programs such as dialysis and renal transplants for persons with renal failure. Acute renal failure (ARF) is seen in approximately 5% of hospitalized patients. Historically, a high mortality rate has been associated with chronic renal failure (CRF). However, because of dialysis improvements and renal transplants, the outcome for patients with CRF has greatly improved. Although morbidity rates are high for renal disease, mortality rates are not, at least as compared with heart disease, cancer, and stroke.

DECISION-MAKING
History

Diseases known to be related to renal dysfunction should be identified. Family history of kidney disease is an important factor to assess. Polycystic disease of the kidneys is an inherited disorder that can lead to renal insufficiency and end-stage renal disease (ESRD). In addition to sickle cell disease, autoimmune diseases such as lupus, Goodpasture's syndrome, Berger's disease, and AIDS may also manifest as nephropathy and renal failure.

The most prevalent cause of CRF in the U.S. is diabetic nephropathy. Both type 1 and 2 diabetes mellitus may be associated with nephropathy. Approximately 35% of patients with diabetes develop CRF, and 30% of CRF cases are caused by hypertension. Direct nephron injury is called *hypertensive nephropathy* (HTN). HTN generally is seen in persons older than 50 years of age. Native Americans and African Americans are affected at higher rates, because of the higher incidence of diabetes and hypertension in these groups.

Table 6-1-1.   Common Nephrotoxic Drugs

Antibiotics by class	Aminoglycoside, cephalosporins, sulfa-based drugs, tetracyclines
Individual antibiotics	Amphotericin B, bacitracin, polymyxin B, vancomycin, rifampicin
Radiographics	Contrast agents
Antihypertensives	Angiotensin-converting enzyme inhibitors, thiazides, loop diuretics
Analgesics	Prostaglandin inhibitors, nonsteroidal anti-inflammatory drugs, acetaminophen
Heavy metals	Mercury, lead, gold, copper

Medication History

Certain medications can have a serious effect on the renal system, because the renal system is frequently the primary system responsible for clearance. All medications, both prescribed and over-the-counter, should be assessed for nephrotoxic effects (Table 6-1-1). Other drugs may cause changes in urine color (e.g., rifampin, pyrazinamide).

Clinical Presentation

Patients usually present with dysfunctional voiding, hematuria, or pain. These signs and symptoms are what usually prompt a patient to seek health care.

Dysfunctional Voiding

The patient may experience *urinary frequency*, caused by decreased bladder capacity from infection, inflammation, neurogenic disorders, or the presence of a foreign body. *Nocturia* (increased urination at night) can occur for the same reasons, but it may be a sign that the kidney is losing its ability to concentrate urine. It is a common manifestation of prostate enlargement. *Hesitancy* usually signifies an obstruction of the lower urinary tract. *Dysuria* (burning or discomfort on urination) and *urgency* (a sudden strong desire to void occurring after having voided) are signs of infection and may also point to renal calculi (stones), nonbacterial inflammation, tumors, or prostatitis. Increased volume (*polyuria*) occurs in diabetes mellitus, diabetes insipidus, and at some point during CRF.

Pain

Pain is usually due to distention, inflammation, or the presence of a foreign body within the urinary tract. *Kidney pain* is dull in the flank area or the costovertebral angle (CVA), the area in the back between the 12th rib and the vertebral column. *Renal colic* is a sharp, excruciating pain that radiates to the perineum, groin, scrotum, or labia. It is usually associated with obstruction or the passing of a stone. *Prostatic pain* is a diffuse discomfort in the perineal and rectal areas. It is usually associated with acute prostatitis with obstruction and may be accompanied by back pain.

Hematuria

Hematuria with pyuria indicates infection and should be treated with antibiotics. A single episode of hematuria can be caused by a viral illness, allergy, exercise, or menstruation. Multiple episodes point to a more significant urologic lesion. Hematuria can be described as either gross or microscopic. Gross hematuria is often indicative of a problem in the urine collection system. Common causes include tuberculosis, neoplasm, stones, trauma, and prostatitis. Microscopic hematuria is defined as 2 to 3 red blood cells (RBCs) per high-power field. When accompanied by misshaped RBCs, this is suggestive of glomerular disease.

Systemic Manifestations of Renal Failure

Neurologic

Retained toxins may cause *altered mental status*. The patient may become irritable and exhibit changes in cognitive behavior and, eventually, altered level of consciousness. The cells of the nervous system are especially sensitive, and the patient may report altered peripheral sensation. Altered sensation and increased spontaneous movement of the feet and lower legs is called *restless legs syndrome*. Weakness and decreased deep tendon reflexes may also occur.

Hematopoietic

Erythropoietin is a glycoprotein hormone produced primarily in the kidneys in response to decreased pressure of oxygen in arterial blood. Patients with renal failure are unable to produce erythropoietin, leading to *anemia*. It is not uncommon to see hemoglobin (Hgb) levels of 5 to 7 in patients with CRF. This anemia in turn causes *chronic fatigue*. In ARF, anemia may result from the glomerular filtration of erythrocytes, or bleeding associated with platelet dysfunction. Platelet disorders can lead to prolonged bleeding times and easy bruising.

Integumentary

Because of absorption of urinary chromogens, decreased sweat gland activity, and calcium phosphate deposits in the skin, the skin appears pale and dry with a yellowish discoloration. The hair is brittle and dry. Retained toxins in the skin cause pruritus. A powdery white coating of the skin, called *uremic frost,* occurs due to crystallization of uric acid. The kidneys' inability to regulate sodium and water leads to edema.

Cardiovascular

Cardiac workload is greatly increased in ARF. Accumulated nitrogenous wastes are often irritating to the pericardium, and *pericarditis* commonly develops. Elevated potassium levels may trigger cardiac arrhythmias. Sodium and fluid retention may *increase blood pressure*, which, along with increased renin levels, place an additional burden on the heart and exacerbate edema.

Musculoskeletal

Calcium regulation is directly related to vitamin D and phosphorus levels. The kidneys are responsible for the conversion of vitamin D to its most active form (1, 25-dihydroxycholecalciferol). When active, vitamin D enhances serum calcium levels by increasing reabsorption by the kidney tubules, promoting bone resorption with release of calcium salts, potentiating the effects of parathyroid hormone (PTH), and increasing absorption of calcium ions from the intestine. At the same time, the kidneys are responsible for regulation of phosphate levels via the proximal tubules. Early in the course of CRF, phosphate excretion becomes impaired, and serum phosphorus levels rise. As the glomerular filtration rate (GFR) falls in renal disease, the kidney tubules become resistant to the effects of PTH, which normally raises serum calcium and continues to be produced in response to low calcium levels. Demineralization of the bone, called *renal osteodystrophy*, results from decreased renal activation of vitamin D, retention of phosphate, and increased PTH. *Bone pain and pathologic fractures* commonly occur as a result of this process.

Acid-Base Disturbance

Metabolic acidosis results from decreased secretion of hydrogen by the failing kidneys. Respiratory compensation occurs in response to the metabolic acidosis. The rate and depth of respirations increase as acid levels build up, producing a characteristic respiratory pattern known as *Kussmaul's breathing.*

Respiratory

Pulmonary edema and pleural effusion may develop due to fluid overload, especially if serum albumin levels are decreased.

Gastrointestinal

Mucosal inflammation caused by excessive urea results in *anorexia, nausea and vomiting*, and diarrhea. *Mucosal ulcerations* result from the bacterial breakdown of urea, which produces ammonia. *Uremic fetor* (urinous breath odor), *stomatitis*, and *metallic taste* in the mouth result from urea in the saliva. *Constipation* results from the use of phosphate-binding antacids. *Gastrointestinal bleeding* is common due to clotting abnormalities and increased levels of circulating gastrin.

 CLINICAL PEARLS

○ Monitor the patient with renal failure for drugs that can be potentially nephrotoxic. These drugs include the aminoglycosides (e.g., gentamicin, tobramycin) and tetracyclines.

○ The kidneys normally excrete meperidine, which is converted by the liver to normeperidine. In severe renal failure, this substance accumulates in the body, causing seizures.

○ A side effect of erythropoietin administration is iron deficiency, resulting from the body's need to support RBC production.

Hemodialysis

Section 2   Eden Zabat

OVERVIEW

Once CRF progresses to ESRD, the patient must undergo renal replacement therapy in the form of dialysis or renal transplantation. Dialysis is the most well-known form of ESRD therapy. It is seen as a definitive and life-saving treatment for the acutely or chronically ill renal patient. The current modality of treating ESRD is hemodialysis or peritoneal dialysis (PD) followed by renal transplantation when medically appropriate.

The past decade has brought an increase in the number of patients seeking renal replacement therapy for ESRD, mainly because of advances in dialysis therapies and the support of federal programs. In 1997, more than 304,000 people were being treated for ESRD in the U.S. Medicare and private insurance help pay for much of the cost of renal replacement therapy. Medicare funding for dialysis therapy began in 1973 with enactment of the U.S. Medicare End-Stage Renal Disease program, which extended Medicare coverage to all U.S. citizens with renal disease. This program guarantees dialysis to those needing renal replacement therapy.

The major forms of dialysis used in the clinical settings are hemodialysis and peritoneal dialysis. The clinical picture is expanding for those needing dialysis as newer and more efficient renal devices are developed. Although dialysis therapy has a solid history, significant risks remain.

PRINCIPLES OF CARE
Components of Hemodialysis
Dialyzer

The dialyzer serves as an artificial kidney to remove waste products, toxins, excessive electrolytes, and fluid. Each dialyzer unit has an ultrafiltration (water removal) component that can remove excess intravascular fluid. The dialyzer has a semipermeable membrane between the patient's blood and the dialysate, preventing the patient's blood and dialysate solution from mixing with each other. The semipermeable membrane allows removal of unwanted substances from the blood while adding desirable components.

Dialysate

Dialysate is a fluid and electrolyte solution that flows on one side of the semipermeable membrane. It contains varying amounts of electrolytes and other substances, which control the amount and direction of movement of wastes and unwanted products across the semipermeable membrane. It also contains acid buffers that are absorbed and assist in correcting the metabolic acidosis that occurs with renal failure. Dialysate essentially provides the transport medium to move the waste products, excess electrolytes, excess water, and toxins from the patient's blood across the semipermeable membrane through osmosis, diffusion, and filtration. Other functions of the dialysate include preventing the removal of "essential" electrolytes and preventing excessive water removal during the procedure.

The dialysate solution is composed of water, glucose, and electrolyte ingredients (i.e., sodium, chloride, potassium, magnesium) in varying concentrations. The chemical composition of the dialysate corresponds as closely as possible to normal plasma water and usually includes sodium chloride, sodium bicarbonate or sodium acetate, calcium chloride, potassium chloride, and magnesium chloride. Acetate-based and bicarbonate-based concentrates are the most common dialysate preparations.

Description

Dialysis can be temporary, indicated until the return of kidney function, or permanent, when nephron function falls to 10% to 15% of normal, as in ESRD. Dialysis is a process of cleansing the blood of waste products (urea and creatinine) that have accumulated due to renal dysfunction. Through the physiologic mechanisms of osmosis, diffusion, and ultrafiltration, dialysis can regulate fluid volume and manage electrolyte levels.

A patient needing chronic therapy can receive dialysis in the hospital or in a freestanding dialysis center. An acutely ill patient manifesting hypotension may need dialysis in a critical care environment, which has the capacity for more frequent assessments and hemodynamic monitoring. For the more critically ill patient who may not be able to tolerate hemodialysis, continuous renal replacement therapy (CRRT) modalities are an option. CRRT is similar to hemodialysis and uses an extracorporeal circuit, but the flow through the circuit is relatively slow, thereby limiting the circuit's stability effect. Popular CRRT modalities include continuous arteriovenous hemofiltration (CAVH) and continuous venovenous hemofiltration (CVVH). As a hospital-based therapy, CRRT is performed by a critical care nurse specifically trained in CRRT procedures.

Indications

The indications for dialysis are similar in both ARF and CRF. However, in ARF, hemodialysis is usually initiated after realizing that the patient's hyperkalemia, acidosis, or volume overload cannot be controlled by more conservative measures such as fluid management and medical therapy. In ARF, hemodialysis involves daily treatments; for CRF, hemodialysis is used as maintenance therapy, performed two or three times per week. Hemodialysis is generally indicated for patients with ARF or ESRD who exhibit uremic signs such as an elevated blood urea nitrogen (BUN) and creatinine levels. Typical serum values in hemodialysis patients are:

- Potassium: 4.5 to 6 mEq/L
- BUN: 60 to 90 mg/dL
- Creatinine: 10 to 15 mg/dL

Indications for hemodialysis are severe hyperkalemia, acidosis, and volume overload. Hemodialysis is the therapy of choice for most drug overdoses and chemical poisonings. Tables 6-2-1 and 6-2-2 list additional indications. Patients undergoing hemodialysis are routinely evaluated for associated hemodynamic changes resulting from rapid fluid shifts in the vascular compartments.

Function of Hemodialysis

Hemodialysis removes toxins and excess fluid via extracorporeal circulation of blood through a dialyzer or "artificial kidney." For example, in treating severe hyperkalemia, hemodialysis moves potassium from the blood into the dialysate through the process of diffusion. Establishing adequate dialysis is a priority when managing the hemodialysis patient. The most widely used tool

Table 6-2-1. Indications for Hemodialysis

Acute renal failure
Uremia
End-stage renal disease
Hyperkalemia
Acidosis
Major drug overdoses
Chemical poisonings

Table 6-2-2. Absolute Indications for Hemodialysis in the Patient with End-Stage Renal Disease

Pericarditis
Uremic encephalopathy or neuropathy
Volume overload or pulmonary edema unresponsive to loop diuretics
Bleeding attributed to uremia
Hypertension unresponsive to treatment
Persistent nausea/vomiting
Serum creatinine >12 mg/dL and blood urea nitrogen >100 mg/dL
Seizures

for assessing dialysis adequacy is urea kinetic modeling (UKM). UKM can assess the amount of dialysis delivered by measuring urea clearance and urea generation. It is considered an accurate predictor of hemodialysis outcomes.

Nutritional Considerations

Patients on hemodialysis usually plan their meals with a renal nutritionist because of dietary restrictions as a result of renal dysfunction and the process of hemodialysis. Hemodialysis patients are advised to limit their fluid intake and decrease sodium intake, because fluid can build up quicker in renal disease. The usual daily diet plan for a hemodialysis patient includes 2 g sodium, 2 g potassium, and 1.5 to 2 kg protein. Specific dietary intake of potassium should be controlled. The intake of fruits and vegetables high in potassium, such as tomatoes and oranges, must be closely monitored. Limiting protein restricts the amount of urea and creatinine produced as byproducts, thereby avoiding waste production that can cause further renal impairment. Limiting phosphorous-containing foods (e.g., milk, cheese, soft drinks) is also recommended, because the kidneys no longer have the ability to control phosphorous levels in the body.

DECISION-MAKING
Vascular Access

Access to the bloodstream requires adequate circulation and placement of an invasive vascular device. Vascular access aids the removal of blood and the return of cleansed blood. Monitoring vascular access patency is a priority in the management of a renal patient on dialysis therapy. Proper handwashing is critical before contact with the patient and the vascular access site.

Arteriovenous Fistula

The preferred vascular access device for maintenance hemodialysis in ESRD patients, the arteriovenous (AV) fistula is a surgically created anastomosis of the radial artery to the cephalic vein. Blood is redirected from the artery to the vein, causing the vein to dilate and bulge from the increased pulsatile flow of arterial blood. Patency and quality of blood flow are evaluated by assessing for a bruit (a "whooshing" sound audible over the fistula using the bell of a stethoscope) and a thrill (a vibrating sensation palpable over the fistula). A bruit auscultated over the fistula and a palpated thrill indicates patency of this vascular access.

An AV fistula typically matures within 2 to 6 weeks; using this fistula as access or cannulation during this time is not recommended. The maturation process allows the fistula to dilate and toughen in response to the increased turbulence, changing its appearance. No venipuncture or blood pressure should be performed on the arm with the vascular access. In addition, the nurse must be careful to monitor for any instances where blood flow is restricted in the affected arm. Constriction of the access area can lead to thrombosis problems. Once the fistula is mature, it has an excellent long-term patency rate (Fig. 6-2-1).

Synthetic Grafts

If AV fistula creation is contraindicated, then a synthetic or AV graft is the next choice for access. Contraindications for an AV fistula include inadequate vessels, as usually seen in patients with diabetes or peripheral vascular disease. The AV graft is a surgically created anastomosis of an artery to a vein, but the one difference is the anastomosis is done with a synthetic material, polytetrafluoroethylene (PTFE). The graft is typically placed in the upper arm, forearm, or upper thigh. The graft matures in 2 to 4 weeks, but it has been cannulated as early as 7 to 10 days, when swelling at the graft site dissipates. The PTFE is known to be durable and can withstand multiple thrombectomies and revisions. Assessing graft patency is similar to that described for AV fistulas. Neurovascular assessment of the extremity is a priority intervention. Synthetic grafts are more susceptible to infection and thrombosis than AV fistulas.

Thrombosis of both grafts and fistulas accounts for most of the hospital admissions of this patient population. Clotting of the access device can occur if blood flow through the device is reduced for any reason, such as a drop in blood pressure, an infection somewhere in the body (infection increases serum viscosity), or the application of a tourniquet or blood pressure cuff above the site. This is why avoiding needle sticks, tourniquets and blood pressure cuffs in the extremity with the access device is so important. Treatment for access thrombosis involves surgical declotting.

Central Venous Catheters

Besides AV fistulas and grafts, short- and long-term vascular access catheters are used for hemodialysis. The jugular, subclavian, and femoral veins are the access sites for cannulation using specifically designed semirigid or rigid, single- or double-lumen Teflon catheters. Once placement has been verified by a radiograph, the catheters can be used immediately for hemodialysis. Only the dialysis nurse can instill heparin into these ports. Heparin is usually given after a hemodialysis treatment to maintain catheter patency, and is removed before the next hemodialysis treatment to avoid an inadvertent bolus. The hemodialysis catheters are reserved for dialysis use only and should not be used to obtain blood samples or instill medications. Bleeding at the incision site and clotting of the catheter are common complications of central venous catheters.

Double-Lumen Silastic Catheters with Felt Cuffs

These catheters are usually inserted in the jugular vein for more permanent use or for temporary hemodialysis while the AV fistula or synthetic grafts are

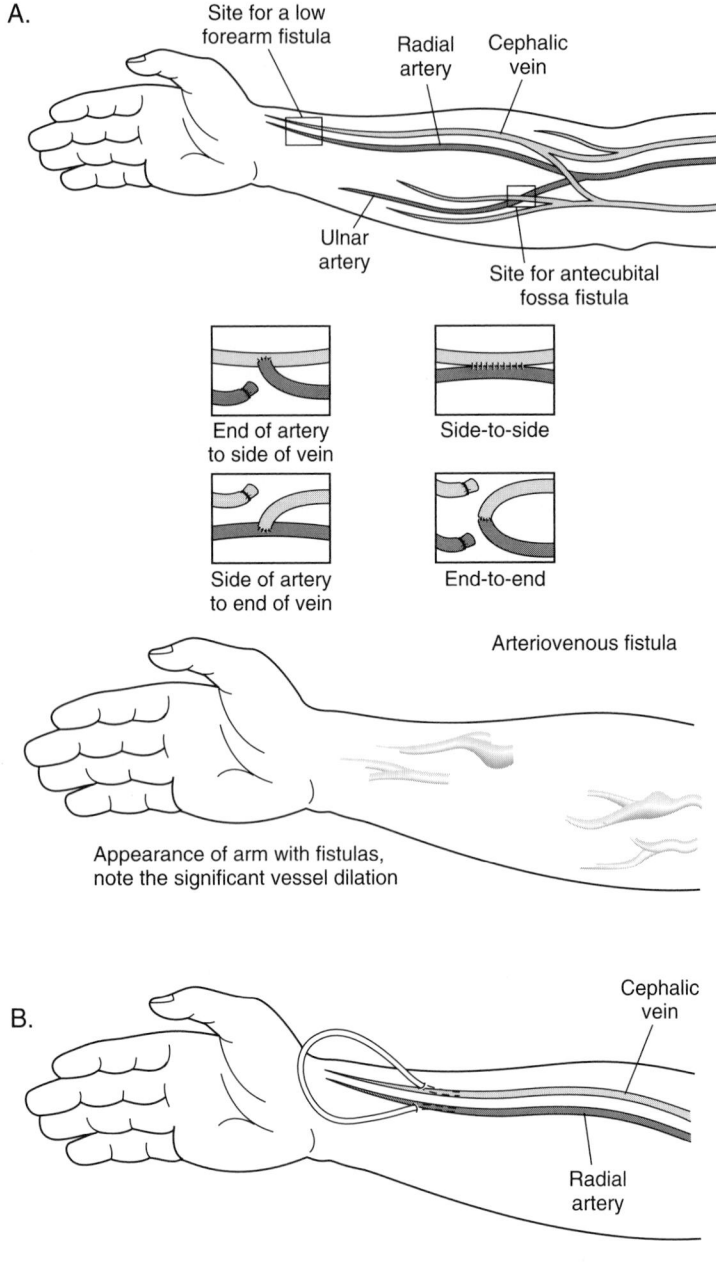

A.

Site for a low
forearm fistula

Radial
artery

Cephalic
vein

Ulnar
artery

Site for antecubital
fossa fistula

End of artery
to side of vein

Side-to-side

Side of artery
to end of vein

End-to-end

Arteriovenous fistula

Appearance of arm with fistulas,
note the significant vessel dilation

B.

Cephalic
vein

Radial
artery

Arteriovenous graft

Figure 6-2-1. An internal arteriovenous fistula and graft.

maturing. They can also be used in patients who have exhausted their vascular access sites and who still need long-term vascular access. Patients who have peripheral vascular disease and those who cannot tolerate the requisite 10% increase in cardiac output associated with AV fistula placement are also candidates for Silastic catheters. However, these double-lumen catheters are more often seen in cases where acute hemodialysis is necessary because the patient's renal function is rapidly deteriorating. Infection, thrombosis, and inadequate blood flow are major complications of this type of vascular access.

Postinsertion Care

Care after insertion of a vascular access device involves thorough assessment of the access device, pain management, and neurovascular checks. The fistula or graft must be assessed for patency. A weak or absent bruit or thrill usually indicates poor blood flow or a clot in the vascular access device. Changes in the quality of the bruit or thrill must be immediately reported to the nephrologist or surgeon. In addition, a complete neurovascular assessment of the affected extremity or the extremity distal to the access must be performed and documented. Blood pressures or venipunctures should not be obtained in the affected extremity, and this restriction should be clearly communicated in the chart as well as in the patient's room. After insertion, the site must be observed for signs and symptoms of infection. The patient's vital signs and lab work must also be carefully assessed for any signs of infection. Dialysis nurses are excellent resources for the care of a hemodialysis patient and should be consulted with any questions regarding vascular access.

Hemodialysis Procedure

Dialysis nurses can cannulate either the AV fistula or graft to begin the hemodialysis procedure. Hemodialysis requires frequent access to the vascular access sites capable of providing rapid extracorporeal blood flow. Dialysis nurses have been known to rotate the specific area of access to improve the likelihood of successful cannulation. Hemodialysis is most commonly scheduled three times per week; each session lasts 3 to 4 hours. It can be done in a hospital-based unit, a free-standing center, or in the patient's home.

Physical Examination

Before hemodialysis therapy, the patient and dialyzer machine are both evaluated. For the acutely ill patient requiring dialysis therapy, a dialysis nurse at the bedside is responsible for monitoring machine parameters. The clinical nurse works collaboratively with the dialysis nurse to critically examine the patient during the entire procedure. The patient is monitored before, during, and after the dialysis procedure. The focus of assessment during dialysis is on monitoring vital signs, weight, fluid intake and output, electrolyte levels, and respiratory assessment to determine tolerance of the dialysis procedure.

Dialyzable Pharmacology

The healthy kidney effectively excretes medications. However, the renal disease process modifies drug excretion for hemodialysis patients who are

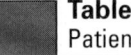

Table 6-2-3. Common Medications for Hemodialysis Patients

DRUG	USE	ADMINISTRATION TIME
Oral calcium-phosphate binder	To counter high phosphate levels in the blood when the kidneys are no longer able to control serum levels	Taken with or immediately after meals. Can be taken with a meal *before* hemodialysis.
Erythropoietin (EPO)	For chronic anemia to stimulate red blood cell production in the bone marrow	Given IV or SQ *during or at end* of hemodialysis treatment. Monitor predialysis hematocrit to determine the amount of erythropoietin
Iron	To produce red blood cells	The parenteral form can be taken with a meal *before* hemodialysis.
Antihypertensive agents	To regulate hypertension	Morning dose is held and *given after* hemodialysis
Sodium heparin	To prevent clotting in the extracorporeal circuit	*Given during* hemodialysis by dialysis nurse

typically receiving medications specific to ESRD. These patients require numerous medications specific to renal disease and/or other chronic disease (Table 6-2-3). Therefore, health care professionals must be able to recognize problems associated with medication use.

Hemodialysis has a known effect on drug clearance. It is not uncommon to hold medications before hemodialysis or to administer supplemental doses for patients receiving hemodialysis. Antihypertensives are usually held before and during dialysis to prevent hypotension. The physician may also order an extra dose before and after dialysis.

Drug dialyzability is determined by two factors: the drug's physicochemical characteristics and the dialysis procedure. Table 6-2-4 lists common dialyzable

Table 6-2-4. Dialyzable Drugs: Drugs that will be Dialyzed Out during Hemodialysis

Acetaminophen (Tylenol)	Cephapirin (Cefadyl)	Methylprednisolone
Acyclovir (Zovirax)	Cephradine (Velosef)	Metoprolol (Lopressor)
Amikacin (Amikin)	Chloral hydrate (Notec)	Nadolol (Corgard)
Amobarbital (Amytal)	Chloramphenicol	Netilmicin (Netromycin)
Atenolol (Tenormin)	(Chloromycetin)	Ofloxicin (Floxin)
Bretylium (Bretylol)	Cimetidine (Tagamet)	Pentazocine (Talwin)
Carbenicillin (Geocillin)	Disopyramide	Phenobarbital (Luminal)
Cefamandole (Mandol)	(Norpace)	Primidone (Mysoline)
Cefazolin (Ancef)	Ethosuximide (Zarotin)	Procainamide (Pronestyl)
Cefoperazone (Cefobid)	Gentamicin	Quinidine
Cefotaxime (Claforan)	(Garamycin)	Ranitidine (Zantac)
Cefoxitin (Mefoxin)	Isoniazid (INH)	Theophylline
Ceftazidime (Fortaz)	Kanamycin (Kantrex)	Ticarcillin (Ticar)
Ceftizoxime (Cefizox)	Meprobamate (Equanil)	Tobramycin (Nebcin)
Cephalexin (Keflex)	Methotrexate (Folex)	Tocainide (Tonocard)
Cephalothin (Keflin)	Methyldopa (Aldomet)	

Table 6-2-5. Drugs Requiring Supplemental Dosing During Hemodialysis

Aspirin	Nadolol
Aztreonam	Phenobarbitol
Captopril	Solu-Medrol
Enalapril	Sotalol
Fluconazole	Theophylline
Imipenem	Tobramycin
Lithium	Vasotec
Lopressor	Zestril

drugs. Drugs with high protein-binding properties are generally not dialyzable. Consulting with a nephrologist or expert will provide vital information for assessing a drug's pharmacologic properties and determining whether modifications in drug or dosage are necessary (Table 6-2-5).

Complications and Interventions

The major cause of death in patients receiving long-term hemodialysis is cardiovascular disease. This is probably related to the inadequate treatment of hypertension and hyperlipidemia in dialysis patients. Other complications that can occur with hemodialysis include hypotension, hypovolemia, bleeding, infection disequilibrium syndrome, muscle cramps, and cardiac dysrhythmias (Table 6-2-6).

 CLINICAL PEARLS

- Rapid reduction of BUN or urea from hemodialysis causes altered levels of consciousness, somnolence, and seizures.
- Application of a tourniquet or blood pressure cuff above the site of a venous access device can cause the device to clot, necessitating surgical declotting.
- The graft site should be evaluated for a thrill and bruit at each patient assessment.
- Withhold routine antihypertensive medications before hemodialysis; may administer them afterward after assessing blood pressure.
- The patient's predialysis nutritional status is a significant predictor of post-dialysis nutritional status.
- Placing a pressure dressing over the puncture site for 10 to 20 minutes can decrease the likelihood of bleeding from a heparin effect at the end of dialysis. Too tight a dressing can compromise the patency of the fistula or graft.
- Hypotension during hemodialysis therapy may indicate a volume deficit.
- To decrease the risk of infection, maintain aseptic technique when accessing the vascular device and to allow antiseptic wiping of the site to dry for more than 3 minutes before puncturing.

Table 6-2-6. Common Complications of Hemodialysis

COMPLICATION	INTERVENTIONS
HYPOTENSION	
Commonly results from rapid ultrafiltration, accidental administration of antihypertensive agents, or increased body temperature from dialysate infusion	Continue blood pressure monitoring. Treat early by elevating the legs or providing replacement IV fluid (normal saline 100–300 mL/hr), or have a dialysis nurse decrease ultrafiltration pressures. Assess for use of antihypertensive agents.
HYPOVOLEMIA	
Results from blood loss in the circuit, accidental tubing separation or membrane rupture, or needle dislodgement	Assess for signs of hypovolemia early and immediately notify the physician, who may order IV normal saline at rapid rate (100–300 mL/hr). Blood transfusions and plasma expanders may need to be given through the dialysis circuit. Continue to monitor intake and output, and note any complaints of dizziness.
BLEEDING	
May occur after needle removal from excess heparin	Monitor for postdialysis bleeding at the vascular access site and puncture sites. Hold pressure for at least 20 minutes and reevaluate. Assess for bleeding from the gastrointestinal and urinary tracts, as well as epistaxis. Instruct the patient about the risk of bleeding.
INFECTION	
Usually related to the vascular access device; may also result from poor handling of dialysis equipment	Assess the vascular access site for erythema, drainage, and unusual warmth or tenderness. Culture and report any drainage. Remember that sterile procedure is indicated when in contact with any vascular access areas. Report any temperature elevations. Strictly monitor susceptible patients, as hemodialysis can increase the risk of infection in those whose immune system is already compromised.
MUSCLE CRAMPS	
Result from rapid water and sodium removal	Have a dialysis nurse decrease the ultrafiltration rate. Hypertonic or isotonic saline may be needed to replace the rapid losses.
DISEQUILIBRIUM SYNDROME (DS)	
Results from the rapid decrease in osmolality of extracellular fluid, which creates a high osmotic gradient in the brain, causing fluid to shift into the brain (cerebral edema). DS involves confusion, clouding of consciousness, and seizures.	Hypertonic or isotonic saline may be needed to replace the rapid losses. Albumin or mannitol may be used to draw fluid back into the vascular space. Reorient the patient as needed. Provide protection against potential seizures.

Peritoneal Dialysis

Section 3   Eden Zabat

OVERVIEW

Peritoneal dialysis (PD) is the other popular form of dialysis for patients with ESRD. An estimated 35% of the ESRD population receives this form of dialysis therapy. PD is also used in the management of ARF, and is the renal replacement therapy of choice for those on "home" dialysis therapy for CRF. PD patients have a greater sense of control with this form of dialysis, because they can actually perform the PD exchanges. This form of dialysis is slower and does not require a specific extracorporeal circuit for the actual dialysis. Therefore, specially trained medical-surgical nurses can be taught this much simpler dialysis procedure. Compared with hemodialysis, peritoneal dialysis has several advantages, including simpler technique, lower cost, increased patient mobility, fewer dietary restrictions, avoidance of heparinization, and better control of hypertension. However, this procedure is not free of significant and serious complications. This section focuses on the specific care management of the patient receiving PD therapy.

PRINCIPLES OF CARE
Description

PD is a dialysis process in which dialysate is infused into the peritoneal cavity through a surgically implanted catheter. The peritoneal membrane serves as the semipermeable membrane between peritoneal capillary blood and the dialysate solution. PD therapy removes accumulated waste products (urea and creatinine) and fluid. PD uses the peritoneal membrane (which lines the abdominal wall) as the surface for dialysis, and the mechanisms of osmosis, diffusion, and ultrafiltration. The dialysate solution is infused during the "fill" time. It remains in the peritoneal cavity for a period of time to "dwell." The dwell is a specific time during which the dialysate sits in the peritoneal cavity, allowing osmosis, diffusion, and filtration to occur. Dwell times vary from several hours in continuous ambulatory PD (CAPD) to 1 hour or less in other forms of PD.

After the fill, waste products, toxins, and fluid leave the body in the dialysate outflow as it is drained during the drain time. Several cycles (exchanges) of fill, dwell, and drain are needed to adequately clear the body of the wastes and excess water. PD is a much slower process than hemodialysis. It takes almost 48 hours for PD to accomplish what hemodialysis can accomplish in 6 to 8 hours.

PD is considered a more conservative form of renal replacement therapy, but electrolyte imbalance problems can still occur. Therefore, careful assessment for electrolyte imbalances—particularly hyperkalemia, hypokalemia, hypocalcemia, and hypernatremia—is required.

Indications

PD is an acknowledged alternative to hemodialysis because of its relative safety. Indications for PD include ARF, CRF, chemical poisoning, acidosis, hypervolemia, and ESRD in patients awaiting renal transplantation. PD may have an advantage over hemodialysis in the cardiovascular patient because of its slower clearance rates. The slower rate reduces the rapid changes in fluids and electrolytes that can occur with hemodialysis.

Because of peritoneal access issues, contraindications to PD include recent abdominal surgery, paralytic ileus, peritonitis, abdominal adhesions, hernia, and abdominal cancer.

Components of Peritoneal Dialysis

Dialysate

The PD dialysate is a sterile solution containing dextrose that is similar in composition to plasma. Dextrose is an important ingredient because it acts as an osmotic gradient between the plasma and dialysate. The dextrose makes the solution hyperosmolar, thereby affecting fluid movement and ultrafiltration. The dialysate carries away the waste products and also prevents the removal of essential electrolytes.

Catheter

The dialysis catheter provides access to the peritoneum for short-term or long-term dialysis. If acute PD is indicated, the catheter may be placed at the bedside. A surgically implanted catheter is indicated for the chronic patient on PD. The PD catheter can be used immediately after insertion. The most familiar PD catheter is the Tenckhoff, an indwelling, Silastic-type catheter. Uses of PD catheters are limited to dialysate instillation and PD exchange.

Nutritional Considerations

Patients on PD therapy have more freedom in their diet than those on hemodialysis. However, malnutrition is a common problem in ESRD and all dialysis patients. These patients commonly experience loss of appetite because of glucose absorption from the dialysate solution. Thus, careful nutritional monitoring is indicated. Referral to a renal nutritionist may be needed, especially for the diabetic or more debilitated patient. In addition, patients with PD require more protein in their diet than hemodialysis patients, because large amounts of protein can be lost in each dialysate exchange.

DECISION-MAKING

Peritoneal Access

Rigid or soft silicone catheters are used in PD. These catheters are placed surgically into the peritoneal cavity during a laparotomy or via a laparoscope. These indwelling catheters are designed to stay in place but may be removed in the event of dialysate leakage, local infection, dislodgement, or peritonitis. These catheters are used for both acute and chronic PD and for neonates and adult patients. Because of healing time requirements, CAPD should be avoided for at least 10 days after catheter placement.

Exit site infections limit the life of PD catheters. Thus, aseptic technique is a priority intervention in maintaining a PD catheter. In addition to the Tenckhoff, other chronic PD catheters include the column disc, Toronto Western, Cruz, Moncrief, and swan neck catheters.

Dialysis Procedure

One PD "exchange" consists of the fill (or inflow), dwell, and drain (or outflow) cycle. Once attached to the peritoneal catheter, a warmed dialysate solution infuses by gravity into the peritoneal cavity. The dialysate is then allowed to dwell in the peritoneal cavity until an adequate time for osmosis, diffusion, and filtration has been achieved. The dialysate usually comes in 2-L bags of 1.5%, 2.5%, or 4.25% dextrose concentration.

Once the dwell is complete, the bag is usually lowered to the floor as the outflow is drained. The outflow drainage is then carefully inspected for bleeding, cloudiness, and fibrin clots. The process is then repeated as needed. In general, PD is indicated for patients who need dialysis but cannot tolerate the hemodynamic changes associated with hemodialysis. Recent advances in laparoscopic techniques have led to fewer catheter complications.

Types of Peritoneal Dialysis

Intermittent Peritoneal Dialysis

Intermittent peritoneal dialysis (IPD) can be continuous or scheduled for sustained periods. IPD can be performed as an acute temporary procedure (for ARF) with continuous hourly exchanges done for 48 to 72 hours, or three to five times per week (for CRF) for 10 to 12 hours each time, for a total of 30 to 60 hours per week depending on the patient's condition. With IPD, the peritoneum is left empty between exchanges. A predetermined amount of dialysate (usually 2 L) is instilled over 20 to 30 minutes. The dialysate is then allowed to drain, and the outflow is inspected.

Continuous Ambulatory Peritoneal Dialysis

Continuous ambulatory peritoneal dialysis (CAPD) is the most common, cost-effective, and viable of the PD treatments. It is popularly known as the "self-care" peritoneal treatment, because it a simpler procedure, is easy to teach, and does not require a programmed machine. The patient attaches a 2-L dialysate bag to the peritoneal catheter for a 10-minute fill time. The patient can then disconnect from the dialysate bag and ambulate freely during the dwell period. The dwell time lasts from 4 to 10 hours. Following the dwell, the patient must connect to a bag for the drain. Three to five exchanges are performed each day. The patient can schedule exchanges around daily activities, for example, before meals and at bedtime.

Continuous Cycling Peritoneal Dialysis

Primarily a home treatment, continuous cycling peritoneal dialysis (CCPD) is a combination of IPD and CAPD. CCPD is becoming more familiar and is now as popular as CAPD for ESRD. This form of PD is unique in the sense that it uses a machine called a cycler. The cycler performs three to five automatic exchanges at night while the patient sleeps. Cyclers can also perform other functions, such as measuring and warming the dialysate before infusion, timing the frequency of exchanges, and measuring ultrafiltration. The cycler significantly reduces the risk of infection because it is a closed system with no breaks between exchanges.

Basic Equipment

PD therapy requires certain equipment and supplies. However, equipment and the actual procedure can vary between institutions.
- Dialysate (the inflow solution)
- Warming device (for dialysate)
- Sterile povidone wash
- Alcohol wipes
- Administration tubing
- Functioning peritoneal catheter
- Sterile mask and gloves

Physical Examination

Before Dialysis. Assess baseline data. Priority data are vital signs, fluid status, electrolytes, and patient weight. Document the exchange start time and record the amount of dialysate on the dialysis flow sheet.

During Dialysis. Continue to assess the patient's temperature, pulse, respirations, and blood pressure throughout each exchange. Carefully assess for fluid overload or underload, and note any signs of peritonitis and other possible complications of PD. Table 6-3-1 lists critical signs and symptoms to monitor during dialysis. Also, keep in mind that as fluid is removed, blood pressure tends to drop. Continue to monitor for acute hemodynamic or circulation changes.

After Dialysis. The priority action during this phase is monitoring for complications. Table 6-3-2 lists potential complications of PD therapy, along with appropriate interventions.

Carefully record all inflow and outflow amounts. Notify the physician if the outflow amount exceeds 500 mL more than the amount instilled. Consider selecting a dialysate of higher or lower tonicity depending on outflow amount and clinical symptoms of volume deficit or overload. For specific criteria and protocol regarding the PD procedure, familiarize yourself with your hospital's policy and procedures manual.

Dialysate Solutions

The dialysate solution comes in bags of 1.5%, 2.5%, or 4.25% dextrose or sorbitol. The more hypertonic the solution, the greater is the ultrafiltration, leading to greater removal of fluid and electrolytes. Several peritoneal dialysis solutions are commercially available. Solutions include Dianeal PD-1, Dianeal PD-2, and Dianeal Low Ca (from Baxter Healthcare), and Delflex (from Fresenius USA).

Dialyzable Pharmacology

PD in itself does not alter pharmacological metabolism. Renal dysfunction generally alters drug metabolism through the accumulation of waste products that can affect drug clearance. Therefore, selecting medications and appropriate dosages for the PD patient is actually similar to selecting medications for the

 Table 6-3-1. Signs and Symptoms to Monitor During Dialysis

FLUID OVERLOAD	FLUID UNDERLOAD	PERITONITIS
Hypertension	Hypotension	Abdominal pain during exchange
Pitting edema of feet, ankles, and hands	Tachycardia	Nausea/vomiting
Crackles in lung fields	Muscle cramps (legs)	Cloudy outflow fluid (effluent)
Shortness of breath		Systemic infection symptoms
Jugular vein distention		
Pulmonary edema		
Fatigue		
Ascites		
Periorbital edema		

Table 6-3-2. Potential Complications of Peritoneal Dialysis

COMPLICATIONS	SIGNS AND SYMPTOMS	INTERVENTIONS
Peritonitis	Hallmark signs include abdominal pain, cloudy outflow drainage, and fever	Maintain meticulous aseptic technique with all bag connections and with collecting samples. Perform exit site care daily. Clean tubing or injection ports with bactericidal solution before adding additives; allow 30 minutes of air drying after cleansing the ports. Once symptoms manifest, report and send a sample of the first outflow for culture and cell count. Discuss initiating empirical antibiotic therapy with the physician.
Pain	Abdominal cramping. Shoulder pain due to diaphragm irritation (Kehr's sign)	Slow the dialysate flow rate, as patient may have sensitivity to the dialysate (common with the first exchanges). Monitor for pain associated with peritonitis.
Exit site infection	Redness, bleeding, drainage, crusting at the exit site; possibly abdominal or intra-abdominal swelling	Maintain strict sterile technique with exit site care. Keep the exit site dry. If blood cultures are negative, application of a topical antibiotic to the exit site may be indicated.
Fibrin formation	White strands or clots in catheter tubing or within outflow drainage	Report to the physician or, if ordered, add heparin to dialysate exchanges.
Positive fluid balance and respiratory problems	Signs of hypervolemia; weight gain, shortness of breath, longer dwell times with less outflow amounts	Decrease fluid intake. Raise the head of the bed to decrease pressure of dialysate inflow on the diaphragm. Decrease dwell time. Increase the hypertonicity of the dialysate.
Dialysate leakage	Clear liquid discharge around the catheter; possibly localized swelling of the genitalia or subcutaneous anterior abdominal wall tissue	Discontinue CAPD and notify the surgeon or nephrologist. Prepare for possible CT scan and probable surgical repair. Temporary hemodialysis may be necessary

CAPD, continuous ambulatory peritoneal dialysis; CT, computed tomography.

ESRD patient. During PD therapy, medications are less likely to be removed, mainly because the dialysate flow rate is slower than with other dialysis methods. As a result, supplemental dosages are not commonly ordered for patients on PD therapy.

Complications/Interventions

Historically, peritonitis is the major complication associated with PD therapy; however, because of technologic advances, such as new delivery systems and connection devices, the incidence of peritonitis is on the decline (see Table 6-3-2).

CLINICAL PEARLS

○ The priority action after PD catheter placement is to check for bowel and bladder perforation within 12 hours of insertion.

○ Correct outflow drainage problems by increasing the distance between the dialysate infusion or collection bag and the peritoneum, or changing the patient's position and having the patient turn from side to side.

○ Peritonitis is a major complication of PD therapy, usually caused by a break in sterile technique during the bag connection procedure.

○ Hallmark signs of peritonitis include fever (temperature >101°F), increased fibrin in dialysate, cloudy outflow, and abdominal pain.

○ Dialysate output should be clear and straw-colored. Note any cloudiness or whitish fibrin clots in the bag. Document and report such findings.

○ Meticulous aseptic technique and accurate recording of each dialysis exchange—including dialysate solution, inflow amount, dwell time, and outflow appearance and amount—are required.

Renal Transplantation

Section 4   Charlotte Mackey

OVERVIEW

Improved surgical technique, immunosuppressive treatment, and more accurate compatibility testing has made renal transplantation a successful therapy for the renal failure patient. One-year survival rates for living and cadaver kidneys ranged between 94% and 97% in 1997. Five-year survival rates for patients receiving living related transplants range from 82% to 93%. Because there is no cure for CRF, the only treatment option available is dialysis, either PD or hemodialysis. Dialysis requires a permanent change in lifestyle and a large time commitment. Many patients need to be dialyzed three times a week and are unable to work. Therefore, kidney transplantation is an option that many patients can explore. However, not all patients with ESRD are candidates for renal transplantation.

PRINCIPLES OF CARE

Indications for renal transplantation include ESRD, glomerulonephritis, insulin-dependent diabetes, nephrosclerosis, polycystic kidney disease, systemic lupus, chronic pyelonephritis, and congenital ureteral valves. Diabetic patients represent 25% of renal transplant patients. Some transplant centers offer a combined kidney-pancreas transplant for insulin-dependent diabetics, which eliminates the need for both insulin and dialysis. In addition, some centers recommend that a diabetic transplant candidate seek a living related kidney donor. Patients who are not candidates for transplant include those with active infection, metastatic disease, morbid obesity, or ongoing substance abuse.

The potential donor–recipient evaluation is extensive. A complete history and physical/psychological examination is performed. Laboratory tests include CBC, BUN, GFR, serum creatinine, creatinine clearance, urinalysis, and urine specific gravity. Evaluative radiography procedures include kidneys-ureters-bladder (KUB), renal ultrasound, renal scan, renal angiography, renal magnetic resonance imaging (MRI), renal biopsy, and cystourethrography. The potential recipient is screened for HIV, cytomegalovirus (CMV), Epstein-Barr virus, and herpes simplex virus. The transplant team evaluates a potential recipient's status individually to determine whether any of these factors exclude the individual from receiving a donated organ. Blood typing, tissue typing, and antibody detection are also completed.

DECISION-MAKING
Procedure

Donor sources for kidneys include cadavers, living related donors, and living unrelated donors. Living related donors can be close family members, including parents, children, brothers, and sisters. Distant family members can also be living related donors. Overall, living related and unrelated kidney donors have the highest success rate, followed by cadaver donors. Related donors have a greater chance of tissue compatibility, and the transplant procedure can be scheduled ahead of time, rather than waiting for a cadaver donor. Kidneys received from a living donor tend to function immediately after transplant, whereas functioning of cadaver organs can take several days or weeks. A living unrelated donor can be someone with close emotional ties to the patient, such as a spouse or close friend. Cadaver organs are donated at the time of death.

The transplant procedure takes 3 to 4 hours. A 2-cm incision is made above the pubis in the iliac fossa. The kidneys normally are located bilaterally in the flank or lumbar areas, behind the abdominal cavity in the small retroperitoneal space. The donor kidney is placed in the iliac fossa and connected to the recipient's renal vein. The donor's renal artery is connected to the recipient's iliac artery, and the donor's ureter is implanted into the recipient's bladder. The recipient's kidneys are not removed unless they are identified as a source of hypertension.

Management

Patient management is similar regardless of the source of the donor kidney. For the first 12 to 24 hours, the patient may be monitored in an ICU. Intake and output are assessed each hour to ensure adequate fluid balance. The patient may need analgesics for pain management. A Jackson-Pratt drain may be placed intraoperatively near the kidney to prevent accumulation of lymph drainage; this is removed when drainage is less than 30 mL for 2 consecutive days. Fluid is usually replaced hourly (based on previous hours' urine output) with 0.45 normal saline IV to avoid renal hypoperfusion. Daily weight must be monitored, as must electrolytes, especially potassium.

Complications/Interventions

Every transplanted organ undergoes some degree of rejection. Immunosuppressive drugs significantly prevent or reduce organ rejection. Rejection of the donated kidney takes various forms and can be mediated by humoral or cellular immunity. Humoral immunity involves the B lymphocytes. They are responsible for producing antibodies known as immunoglobulins. Cell-mediated immunity involves the T lymphocytes and the chemical messengers that T cells produce. These messengers, called lymphokines, perform numerous functions, including recruitment of uncommitted lymphocytes, retaining these cells and phagocytes at the site of inflammation, and activating the retained cells so that they can take part in the inflammatory response.

Acute rejection is manifested by abrupt signs and symptoms of rejection, including inflammation, edema, fever, pain, graft tenderness, malaise, and tachycardia. Blood chemistries reflect organ dysfunction. A definitive diagnosis is made by organ biopsy. This cell-mediated rejection may be resolved with additional antirejection therapy with agents such as OKT_3.

Chronic rejection can occur months or years after the transplant. With chronic rejection, the patient exhibits gradual loss of organ function. The production of antibodies against the transplanted organ eventually leads to a compromised circulatory problem and eventual graft loss. This type of rejection does not respond to any currently available immunosuppressive therapy.

Infection is a complication of posttransplant immunosuppression. Although immune suppression is essential to prevent rejection, pathogens may take advantage of the decreased immune system activity. Opportunistic infections are the leading cause of death in the immunocompromised patient. Three mechanisms are primarily responsible for these opportunistic infections: (1) acquisition of a particularly virulent pathogen, such as meningococcal meningitis or pneumococcal pneumonia; (2) reactivation of an organism that has been latent in the patient's system, such as herpes zoster or tuberculosis; and (3) invasion of bacteria, viruses, fungi, or parasites. Because of this, patients are also started on antifungal and antiviral medication. Bactrim is started prophylactically to prevent *Pneumocystis carinii* pneumonia (PCP).

Skin cancer is a side effect of immunosuppressive therapy. Ultraviolet radiation from the sun damages the skin and makes it susceptible to cancer. Normally, the immune system destroys these damaged cells, but with a suppressed immune system, cancer risk increases. The overall risk is approximately 35% in the U.S. For this reason, transplant patients must do everything possible to protect themselves from sun exposure.

Immunosuppression

Immunosuppression prolongs graft survival but does not replace extensive tissue matching of donor and recipient. The goal of immunosuppression is to suppress the natural immune response to prevent rejection of the transplanted organ.

During the induction phase, a combination of immunosuppressive medications is given in the first few weeks/months after the transplant. The doses of these drugs are gradually reduced. Once the patient stabilizes, a low maintenance dose is maintained, which the patient continues to take for the life of the graft.

Currently, more than 270 medical institutions in the United States operate organ transplant programs. The protocol for immunosuppression varies from center to center. The major immunosuppressive agents used include: immune cell inhibitors (drugs that inhibit B cell and T cell functions); corticosteroids, which produce anti-inflammatory effects (decrease the function of WBCs); and antirejection drugs (Table 6-4-1).

Table 6-4-1. Immunosuppressive Therapy

DRUG	INDICATIONS	NURSING IMPLICATIONS
Azathioprine (Imuran)	Immunosuppression in induction and maintenance protocols. Adjunct for preventing rejection	Assess for leukopenia, thrombocytopenia, macrocytic anemia, and hepatotoxicity. Institute infection-control measures; monitor hemoglobin and hematocrit; assess for infection; assess for jaundice.
Prednisone (Deltasone)	Immunosuppression in induction and treatment of acute rejection. Prevention of rejection	Assess for mood swings, sodium and water retention, muscle wasting, gastrointestinal upset, skin fragility, moon face, and buffalo hump. Avoid adhesive tape; guaiac test stools; assess mood swings; encourage a low-sodium diet; monitor daily weights.
Cyclosporine (Sandimmune)	Immunosuppression in induction and maintenance. Not effective for acute rejection. For prophylaxis of organ rejection. Used with corticosteroids.	Assess for nephrotoxicity tremors, hepatotoxicity, and gingival hyperplasia. Monitor trough levels, serum creatinine and BUN; assess for edema and jaundice; provide meticulous mouth care.
Tacrolimus (FK 506)	Immunosuppression in induction and maintenance. Not used in combination with cyclosporine	Assess for nephrotoxicity, neurotoxicity, gastrointestinal toxicity, and insulin-dependent diabetes. Monitor trough levels, neurologic status, daily weights, intake and output, and blood glucose; consult a dietitian.
OKT₃ (antirejection)	Steroid-resistant acute allograft rejection	May cause flu-like symptoms; administer acetaminophen and treat symptomatically. First dose may cause severe fulminant pulmonary edema, leading to death.
Mycophenolate mofetil (MMF)	Immunosuppression, in combination with cyclosporine. For prophylaxis of organ rejection. Used with corticosteroids	Assess for gastrointestinal toxicity (nausea, vomiting, diarrhea, abdominal cramps, and dyspepsia). Monitor daily weights; assess for edema; auscultate lungs.

Adapted from United Network for Organ Sharing, Donation & Transplantation: Nursing Curriculum. Health Resources & Services Administration, 1996.

Two new monoclonal antibodies approved by the FDA can be given to prevent rejection. These are basiliximab (Simulect) and dacliximab (Zenapax), which work by blocking interleukin-2 receptors on T lymphocytes.

Diet and Lifestyle

Wound Care

Staples are generally left in for 2 to 3 weeks. Patients should avoid tub baths but may shower. Steri-Strips then replace the staples; the Steri-Strips fall off within 2 weeks or can be removed by the patient.

Diet

The patient should maintain a diet low in salt, fat, sugar, and cholesterol. This is individually determined for each patient based on the presence of other medical problems such as diabetes or high blood pressure.

Activity

Immediately following the surgery, the patient should avoid strenuous exercise. The patient should be advised to not lift anything weighing more than 10 pounds and to avoid driving for 2 weeks posttransplant. Exercise such as walking, swimming, or low-impact aerobics should be started slowly and only under the supervision of the transplant team.

Sexual Activity

Because transplant patients are at increased risk for infection, they should avoid having unprotected sex. Pregnancy is not recommended until 1 year after transplant. Female patients should discuss some form of birth control with the transplant team. Papanicolaou smears and mammograms should be done at least once a year, because immunosuppressed patients are at increased risk for cancer.

Medications

The patient should know the name, indication, dosage schedule, and side effects of each prescribed medication. The patient should be encouraged to never miss a dose or run out of a medication, and to promptly report any side effects to the transplant team. The patient should be instructed to avoid over-the-counter medications until first checking with the transplant team.

Infection

The patient should try to avoid people who are sick with a cold or infectious disease. A patient requiring dental work should make the dentist aware of the transplant surgery, because antibiotics may need to be started before the dental procedure.

Rejection Warning Signs

Acute rejection is seen in 40% of transplant patients within the first month after transplant. Thus, the patient, nurse, and family need to be aware of signs and symptoms of rejection (as discussed earlier in the Complications/Interventions section). Rejection can happen weeks, months, or years after the transplant. The patient needs to be instructed to notify the transplant team immediately if any of the following signs and symptoms occur:

- Fever of 100°F or higher
- Pain or tenderness around the surgical site
- Edema of the hands, feet, or eyelids
- Weight gain of more than 2 lb in 1 day
- Decreased urine output or blood in the urine, dysuria, cloudy or foul-smelling urine
- Flu-like symptoms (cough, shortness of breath, sore throat, earache)
- Elevated blood pressure

 CLINICAL PEARLS

○ Transplant patients need to be monitored for signs of rejection every month for the remainder of their lives.
○ Organ rejection can occur years after the transplant surgery.
○ Transplant patients should be encouraged to wear a sunscreen with an SPF factor of at least 29 to protect exposed areas of the skin.
○ Research has shown that monitoring serum creatinine levels in posttransplant patients can help to predict rejection.
○ Medications must be taken on time and as directed. Once a transplant is rejected it is very difficult to find a new kidney that will not also be rejected.

 RESOURCES

- American Association of Kidney Patients (AAKP): 800-749-2257 or e-mail at AAKPnat@aol.com
- American Kidney Foundation: www.afud.org
- American Kidney Fund: 800-638-8299 or www.akhhc.org
- American Nephrology Nurses' Association (ANNA): 888-600-2662 or www.anna.inurse.com
- Colorado HealthNet—Kidney Disease and Kidney Dialysis Research and Information Library: www.coloradohealthnet.org/dialysis/dial_lib.html
- International Society for Peritoneal Dialysis: www.ispd.org
- National Institute of Diabetic and Kidney Disease: www.nidkd.nih.gov
- National Kidney Foundation: 800-622-9010 or www.nephron.com/NKF.html
- National Kidney and Urologic Diseases Information Clearinghouse: e-mail at nkudic@info.nidkd.nih.gov
- Renal Diseases Electronic Journal: www.hdcn.com
- United Network for Organ Sharing (UNOS): www.unos.org

chapter 7

Decision-Making for Neurologic Alterations

Neurologic Assessment

Section 1   Lori Schumacher ■ Michelle Grace

OVERVIEW

Neurologic assessment is a very important aspect of nursing care for any patient regardless of the admitting diagnosis. The foremost goal of a neurologic assessment is to establish the patient's baseline neurologic status so that changes in neurologic function can be detected. Patients may exhibit a wide range of functioning and impairment. A deterioration in neurologic status can be either acute or subtle and may occur over a duration of minutes to months. It is imperative that a thorough neurologic assessment be performed and documented, graphically describes the patient's behavior and reaction to stimuli.

PRINCIPLES OF CARE

Various conditions can cause changes in neurologic status and function, including:
- **Mass lesions**, such as blood clots, tumors, abscesses, edema, and hydrocephalus
- **Disruptions in blood flow**, as caused by an ischemic or hemorrhagic stroke
- **Metabolic disorders**, such as electrolyte imbalances, high ammonia levels, decreased oxygen levels, and chemical imbalances
- **Infectious disorders**, such as a bacterial or viral infection

Variables that provide the most reliable information about the progression and level of neurologic involvement include: level of consciousness; motor function; pupil size, reactivity, and eye movement; cranial nerve assessment; and deep tendon reflexes.

DECISION-MAKING
Level of Consciousness

Consciousness is defined as the state of awareness of the self and environment. Level of consciousness is the most sensitive indicator of changing neurologic status. Consciousness can be considered as existing on a continuum ranging from completely conscious and neurologically normal to comatose and totally unresponsive. Changes in a patient's level of consciousness may be very subtle, making your description of neurologic status crucial. The following is a list of common terms used to describe a patient's level of consciousness:
- **Full consciousness.** The patient is awake, alert, and oriented to person,

place, and time. The patient understands spoken and written commands and is able to express ideas. Behavior is appropriate.

- **Confusion.** The patient is disoriented to person, place, or time with a shortened attention span, memory difficulties, difficulty following commands, altered perception of stimuli, possible hallucinations, agitation, restlessness, and irritability.
- **Lethargy.** The patient is oriented to person, place, and time but very slow with mental processes, speech, and motor activities.
- **Obtundation.** The patient can be readily aroused with stimulation and can follow simple commands appropriately when stimulated; otherwise, the patient may appear very drowsy.
- **Stupor.** The patient lies quietly in bed with minimal spontaneous movement and is generally unresponsive unless vigorous and repetitive stimuli are used. The patient may respond by using incomprehensible sounds or by opening the eyes. The stuporous patient will respond appropriately to painful stimuli.
- **Coma.** The patient will appear to be in a sleep-like state with the eyes closed. The patient will not respond appropriately to stimuli or make any verbal sounds.

Glasgow Coma Scale

The **Glasgow Coma Scale** (GCS) is a standardized neurologic assessment tool that assists in determining a patient's level of consciousness or detecting any changes in level of consciousness in the patient with neurologic deficits. The GCS is designed to decrease the subjectivity associated with the measurement of level of consciousness. The advantages of the GCS are its simplicity and its universal usage. The purpose of the GCS is to assist health care providers in applying the findings of a neurologic assessment.

The GCS has three areas of assessment: eye-opening ability, verbal response, and motor response (Table 7-1-1). These three areas are the most important

Table 7-1-1. Glasgow Coma Scale

Eye Opening	
Spontaneously	4
To command	3
To pain	2
No response	1
Verbal Response	
Oriented to person, place, and time	5
Disoriented	4
Inappropriate words	3
Incomprehensible sounds	2
None	1
Motor Response	
Obeys commands	6
Localizes pain	5
Withdraws from pain	4
Abnormal flexion	3
Extension	2
None	1
Glasgow Score:	

variables reflecting progression and level of neurologic function. Scores in each area are based on the patient's best response in each aspect of that area. The total GCS score ranges from a maximum of 15 to a minimum of 3.

Eye-Opening

The eye-opening response is an easily evaluated indicator of arousal. Always begin with the **mildest stimulus** necessary to obtain a response, then progress to more noxious stimuli.

First, use auditory stimuli, by speaking to the patient. Give the patient a score of 4 (spontaneously) if he or she opens the eyes spontaneously without any type of external stimulation. If the eyes do not open spontaneously, then address the patient by name and/or give a command (e.g., "Mr. Smith, open your eyes for me"). If the patient responds by opening the eyes, then give him or her a score of 3 for eye-opening.

Painful stimuli can be produced by, for example, pinching the inner part of the upper arm or thigh, tapping the sternum, applying firm pressure on the trapezius muscle, or applying pressure to the nail beds. Never use a nipple twist, because this can be extremely traumatizing. If the patient responds to pain, give him or her a score of 2 for eye-opening. If no eye-opening occurs with painful stimuli, give the patient a score of 1. If the eyes are closed by swelling, give a score of 1 with the letter "C" for closed and provide a descriptive comment of the situation.

Verbal Response

The verbal response aspect of the GCS evaluates the appropriateness of the patient's speech. Verbal response is a reflection of language function and orientation to self and environment, which are controlled by the cerebral cortex. The patient receives a score of 1 to 5. To perform this component of the GCS, elicit a conversation with the patient. A patient who is oriented should be able to state his or her name (person), where he or she is (place—location, city, state), and the date (day, month, and year). A patient with expressive aphasia will not be able to answer orientation questions directly, but should be able to answer "yes" or "no" to questions posed in yes-or-no format. Identify the response to the question asked. Give the patient who is oriented to person, place, and time a score of 5 for verbal response.

A patient is considered disoriented when he or she is not oriented to all three components of person, place, and time. When assessing verbal response, it is important to differentiate a patient who is fully oriented from a patient who is confused. A patient may sometimes be oriented to one or possibly two of the components. Even though the patient is partially oriented, consider him or her disoriented and assign a verbal response score of 4.

"Inappropriate words" is defined as random words or phrases that do not make sense, which may include swearing, or words that are an inappropriate response to the stimulus applied. Give a patient with inappropriate words a verbal response score of 3.

A verbal response that consists of moans, groans, and mumbles and unrecognizable words is considered incomprehensible words. A patient using incomprehensible words generally has a depressed level of consciousness and receives a verbal response score of 2.

If the patient does not respond verbally, even in response to pain, assign a verbal response score of 1. A patient who has a tracheostomy or endotracheal tube in place still needs to be assessed for orientation. Even though the patient cannot directly speak because of the breathing tube, he or she can still communicate in various ways (e.g., communication boards, finger signals, shaking/nodding head, eye blinking). If you are unable to assess orientation even when using such nonverbal methods, then give the patient a verbal response score of 1.

Motor Response

The motor response aspect of the GCS provides information on the patient's ability to process stimuli and respond to the stimuli by moving. Motor response also evaluates the function of the brain's cerebral motor strip. Sometimes, it is possible for the patient to have a different motor response on each side. Appropriate response to commands, localization, or an attempt to move away from a painful stimulus demonstrates that the patient's motor strip is functioning at least partially.

Posturing is an inappropriate motor response that is seen in injuries to the corticospinal tract pathways. Posturing can be demonstrated by abnormal flexion, decortication, and abnormal extension decerebration and can indicate extensive damage to the cerebral hemispheres, diencephalon, or brainstem.

To assess motor response, give the patient a simple command to follow. For example, ask him or her to stick out the tongue, squeeze your hand or fingers, or wiggle the toes. A patient may sometimes exhibit an abnormal grasp reflex when you ask him or her to squeeze your hand. To ensure that the patient is following commands and that you did not elicit an abnormal grasp reflex, ask the patient to let go of your hand. If the patient follows any of the commands you have given, making even a weak attempt, then give this response a score of 6.

If the patient cannot follow commands, then observe for localization. Pain localization means that the patient perceives a stimulation as unpleasant and tries to move away from it. For example, the patient responds to a light needle prick on the left hand by moving the left arm away from the needle or by trying to push your hand away with his or her right hand. Give a patient who localizes to painful stimuli a motor response score of 5.

Withdrawal from pain is a reflex response to pain that involves flexion of the arm at the elbow in an attempt to move away from the stimulus. The reflex response is usually seen in the stimulated extremity. This response is not as brisk as the response for localizing to pain. The withdrawal from pain indicates a lower neurologic level of functioning, because it is more of an autonomic reflex. Give the patient who displays withdrawal to pain a score of 4 on the motor response scale.

Abnormal flexion, also known as decortication, is exhibited by flexing the arms at the elbow with internal rotation of the wrists, bringing the arms up toward the chest, and rigidly extending the legs. (An easy way to remember decortication is that the patient's arms are flexed and brought up to the vocal cord area.) A patient who exhibits this response is given a score of 3 on the motor response scale.

Abnormal extension, also known as decerebration, is an indicator of brain stem damage. It involves extension of the arms at the elbows and internal rotation of the shoulders and wrists, along with rigid extension of the legs. A patient displaying abnormal extension receives a motor response score of 2.

A patient displaying no motor response, even to painful stimuli, is given a motor response score of 1. Absence of motor response (assuming that the patient is not taking any medication that prohibits motor movement) is indicative of severe brain stem injury and impending death.

Motor Function

Motor function is controlled by the corticospinal tract. The corticospinal tract begins in the frontal lobe of the brain, crosses in the brainstem, and continues in the spinal cord until it connects with spinal nerves, which ultimately control the skeletal muscles. Because the corticospinal tract crosses sides at the brainstem, injuries above or below the brainstem will result in different motor dysfunctions. If the injury is above the brainstem (or in the brain), then the motor dysfunction will present on the opposite side of the body. For example, an injury on the left side of the brain typically manifests as motor weakness on the right side of the body. If the spinal cord is injured, motor weakness occurs on the same side as the injury.

Assessing Motor Function

Motor function assessment involves comparing muscle strength and tone for symmetry. A patient's motor response is evaluated by using stimuli to obtain a response. As always, begin with the least amount of stimulus possible to evoke a response and progress to more noxious stimuli. Thus, start with auditory stimuli; if the patient does not respond, then attempt tactile stimulation. Reserve painful stimuli for a patient with decreased level of consciousness. To perform a motor function assessment, ask the patient to:

- Move the arms and legs laterally (from side to side).
- Lift the arms and legs against gravity.
- Extend, then retract each arm and leg against your resistance (while you apply slight pressure in the opposite direction of the patient's movement).

When assessing a patient's motor strength, be sure to compare the strength of each extremity bilaterally.

A patient can earn a score of 0 to 5 on the motor strength scale. A patient who exhibits normal movement against gravity and maximum resistance receives a score of 5. A patient who demonstrates movement against mild-to-moderate resistance (i.e., your hand placed on his or her lifted arm or leg) gets a score of 4. A patient who has movement against gravity (i.e., can lift the arm or leg), but not against resistance, receives a score of 3. A patient who can move an extremity but not against gravity (e.g., can roll the leg inward or outward, but cannot lift the leg) receives a score of 2. A patient who is unable to move an extremity but exhibits muscle contraction in an attempt to move gets a score of 1. Finally, a patient who is flaccid with no visible or palpable muscle contraction or movement receives a motor strength score of 0.

Evidence of Drift

For the patient who is able to follow commands, testing for evidence of drift is an important aspect of assessing muscle strength. When, for example, the patient is asked to extend the arms with the palms upward and close the eyes and hold this position, the normal response is to be able to maintain this position without difficulty. A patient who has deficits in proximal muscle strength or altered level of consciousness may exhibit drift, indicated by the arm drifting downward and the palm pronating, suggesting weakness. If the patient is unable to follow commands, this assessment can be done by raising the patient's arms and letting them fall to the bed. The weaker arm will drop faster and outward. The test for drift, when done serially, may indicate extension of weakness or progress toward improvement in muscle strength.

Response to Painful Stimuli

Response to painful stimuli is classified as purposeful, nonpurposeful, or unresponsive. A purposeful motor response is seen when the patient withdraws from the painful stimuli (localization). A patient localizing to pain must make contact with the stimuli that is causing the discomfort—for example, by pushing away your hand when you apply pressure to the nail bed. A nonpurposeful response occurs when the stimulated extremity moves slightly in response to the stimulus and the patient does not attempt to withdraw from the source of pain. An unresponsive response is noted when the patient shows no signs of reacting to a painful stimulus.

Pupillary Signs

Pupillary dysfunction is an early sign of increased intracranial pressure. Pupils are assessed for size, reaction to light, symmetry, and any changes from previous assessment findings. The size and reactivity of pupils are sensitive to numerous influences, including local eye damage, drugs, seizures, and anoxia.

The oculomotor nerve, the third cranial nerve (CN III), is responsible for pupillary constriction. If the oculomotor nerve is damaged or ceases to function (as may occur, for example, when the brain swells and pushes against the nerve or as a result of surgical trauma due to the stretching of the nerve), pupillary dilation occurs.

When assessing pupils: (1) make sure the room is dimly lit, (2) examine each eye and note pupil size in millimeters, and (3) shine a penlight from the outer corner to the inner corner of each eye and note the response.

Normal pupils measure 2 to 7 mm and are equal in size. Be sure to note pupil size before shining a light into the patient's eyes. The normal pupillary reaction is a rapid constriction of the pupil to direct light. To document pupillary assessment, record the pupil size before constriction. Next, record the pupil's reaction to light: brisk, sluggish, or fixed/nonreactive. If the patient's eyes are swollen shut, making pupil assessment impossible, note this in the documentation.

Cranial Nerves

The peripheral nervous system contains 12 pairs of cranial nerves. The cranial nerves emerge from the lower surface of the brain and pass through openings in the skull. The name of each cranial nerve implies that nerve's primary function. Cranial nerves are classified as motor, sensory, and mixed nerves. They are numbered in the order from which they originate from the brain.

The patient's condition and/or procedures that the patient has undergone help identify the nature of cranial nerve involvement. Rather than attempt to assess all 12 cranial nerves, a more effective approach is to identify those nerves most likely to be affected and assess their function serially (Table 7-1-2).

Vital Signs

Patients with neurologic problems commonly exhibit a relationship between vital signs and neurologic function. The brain requires a continuous flow of

Text continued on page 177

Table 7-1-2. Identifying Cranial Nerves

CRANIAL NERVE	FUNCTION	AFFECTED BY	ASSESSMENTS	DEFICITS SEEN
Olfactory (I)	Smell from the nose to the brain. All sensory fragile fibers connect nerve to frontal lobe. Easily disrupted with head injury. Often disrupted with tumors along the nerve path (olfactory meningiomas)	• Closed head injuries • Tumors • Intracranial surgery	To detect dysfunction in sense of smell, must specifically test the sense of smell. Ask the patient to identify a smell such as rubbing alcohol.	• Decrease in the ability to taste • Decrease/absence of sense of smell
Optic (II)	Runs from the retina to the optic chiasm, below the hypothalamus, next to carotid arteries. Provides pathway from visual input from the retina. Represents only one part of visual pathway.	• Posterior communicating artery aneurysm • Lesions, compression of the nerve • Frontal lobe tumors • Optic neuritis • Pituitary tumor	Assess central peripheral vision by testing visual acuity and visual fields • Have patient read off a Snellen chart or whatever is available • Move a pencil or finger from the periphery into the patient's field of vision and ask the patient to indicate when the object is first seen	• Decreased visual acuity • Blind spots in the visual field
Oculomotor (III)	Critical to remember oculomotor functions. Controls motor function of four extraocular muscles (moves the eye up, inward, down, and inward & down).	• Injury to an extraocular muscle • Injury to the oculomotor nerve • Brainstem ischemia • Neoplasm • Trauma • Infection	• Note the patient's ability to look side to side, and up and down • Patient at rest, eye assumes a lateral side position • Pupils are unequal in size	• Compression is represented by pupil dilatation. • Prosis of eyelids • Nerve paralysis prevents the eye from moving inward. • Dilatation of pupil, inability to respond or sluggish response to light stimuli. • Eye drifts outward, unopposed lateral, outward movement

172

Nerve	Function	Conditions/Causes	Assessment	Signs/Symptoms
Trochlear (IV)	Moves the eye down and to a smaller degree inward, crosses midline, innervates contralateral eye, exits the eye dorsally	• Resection of large tumors in the posterior fossa area • Basilar tip aneurysm clippings (involving extensive above and below approaches) • Brain stem ischemia • Neoplasm • Trauma • Infection	• Positioning of the patient's head Midline or assumes tilted side positioning	• Head tilted toward side of weak muscle to compensate for ocular balance
Trigeminal (V)	• *Sensory:* *Ophthalmic* sensory from cornea to forehead *Maxillary* sensory over the maxilla *Mandibular* sensory to lower jaw • *Motor:* Muscles of mastication	• Trigeminal neuralgia (tic douloureux) • Head trauma • Cerebellopontine lesion • Sinus tract tumor/metastatic disease • Compression of trigeminal root by tumor	• Light touch is tested by touching the forehead, cheek, and jaw with a whisp of cotton • Pain perception is tested by the patient's ability to determine between sharp and dull on the forehead, cheek, and jaw • Temperature is tested by the patient's ability to determine between hot and cold on the forehead, cheek, and jaw	• Pain in face • Unable to differentiate touch • Unable to differentiate between sharp and dull • Unable to differentiate between hot and cold
Abducens (VI)	Movement of the eye outward	• Conditions causing increased intracranial pressure • Brainstem ischemia • Neoplasm • Trauma • Infection	• Vision unclear, most pronounced with lateral gaze • Extraocular movements limited upon patient demonstration • Have patient read the time on the clock or describe the number of fingers/object held out in front of the patient	• Blurred or double vision • Unable to move eye outward to any degree • Double vision with extreme lateral gaze

Table continued on following page

173

Table 7-1-2. Identifying Cranial Nerves *Continued*

CRANIAL NERVE	FUNCTION	AFFECTED BY	ASSESSMENTS	DEFICITS SEEN
Facial (VII)	• Motor functions to the face • Sensory	• Bell's palsy • Facial nerve tumor • Intracranial lesion • Herpes zoster	• Ask patient to smile and show his/her teeth • Ask the patient to close his/her eyes tight and purse the lips • Test the corneal reflex	• Facial dysfunction; weakness, paralysis • Hemifacial spasm • Diminished/absent taste
Glossopharyngeal (IX)	*Sensory:* Function includes touch, temperature, and pain from the palate and pharynx *Motor:* Function to the stylopharyngeus muscle involved in swallowing	• Surgeries using a low posterior fossa approach such as posterior fossa meningiomas • Glossopharyngeal neuralgia from neurovascular compression of the IX and X nerves • Trauma • Inflammatory condition • Tumor • Vertebral artery aneurysms	• Note the gag reflex with suctioning • Note the patient's ability to eat and swallow without choking and coughing • Note the patient's holding of secretions/food and drooling • Note the patient's voice as wet or gurgley	• Decreased ability to swallow and control swallowing • Pain at the base of tongue • Loss of gag reflex • Palatal, pharyngeal, and laryngeal paralysis
Vagus (X)	• Motor function to pharynx, larynx, and esophagus • Modulates heart rate and gastrointestinal functions	• Bulbar paralysis (spastic palsy of larynx) • Guillain-Barré syndrome • Carotid endarterectomy • Vagal body tumors • Nerve paralysis from malignancy, surgical trauma	• With procedures and suctioning, note the quality and presence of a gag response • Note the character and quality of voice, with weak or absent innervation of palate, the voice character is affected	• Weak or absent gag reflex • Hoarseness, breathy and/or whispering voice • Uvula, posterior palate will not elevate with stimulation • Nasal quality to voice

Spinal accessory (XI) (bulbar and spinal accessory)	*Bulbar:* swallowing function. Travels with the glossopharyngeal and vagus nerve. Acts upon the pharynx and larynx *Spinal Accessory:* motor function of trapezius and sternocleidomastoid muscles	• Spinal cord disorder • Amyotrophic lateral sclerosis • Trauma • Guillain-Barré syndrome	• Observe patient eating and drinking • Note difficulties with solids, fluids, or both • Note the patient's ability to move and position himself/herself • Ask the patient to shrug the shoulders and turn the head from side to side	• Weak swallowing function • Unable to elevate the shoulders and turn head • Weakness/paralysis of the head rotation, flexion, extension
Hypoglossal (XII)	Motor function to the tongue	• Carotid endarterectomy due to the nerve's close position to the carotid bifurcation • Medullary lesions • Amyotrophic lateral sclerosis • Poliomyelitis • Multiple sclerosis • Trauma	• Ask the patient to stick out the tongue • Note the position of the tongue as mid-line or off-center	• Tongue position is not midline; the tongue sets to either side • Weakness/paralysis of the tongue muscles • Difficulty in talking, chewing, and swallowing

Table 7-1-3. Clinical Manifestations of Neurologic Insults

CLINICAL MANIFESTATION	NEUROLOGIC INSULT
Cheyne–Stokes respirations, characterized by a pattern of increased and then decreased respiratory depth, followed by a period of apnea	Bilateral cerebral infarction Hypertensive encephalopathy Metabolic disease
Central neurogenic hyperventilation, characterized by rapid, regular respiration with a slight increase in depth	Lesions in the front of the fourth ventricle in the lower midbrain to the middle of the pons Infarction Anoxia Ischemia and tumors of the midbrain or pons Hypoglycemia
Apneustic respirations, characterized by a prolonged inspiration with a pause	Injury, infarction, or lesion to the respiratory control center (middle to lower third of the pons)
Cluster breathing, characterized by an irregular respiratory pattern with periods of apnea at irregular intervals	Lesion, injury, or infarction of the lower pons or upper medulla
Ataxic breathing, characterized by totally irregular and unpredictable patterns of breathing	Cerebellar and pontine hemorrhage Medullary compression from supratentorial tumors Severe meningitis
Increased systolic blood pressure	Progression of increased intracranial pressure
Bradycardia	Increased intracranial pressure causing a compensatory bradycardia as the heart attempts to pump blood upward through compressed cerebral vessels Seen only in the decompensatory stages of increased intracranial pressure
Tachycardia	Increased sympathetic outflow associated with ischemia or medullary compression
Dysrhythmias	Spinal shock leading to loss of autonomic innervation
Hypothermia	Metabolic or toxic coma Drug overdose Brainstem or hypothalamic lesions Terminal central nervous system disease
Hyperthermia	Infectious process of the central nervous system and other major systems Subarachnoid hemorrhage Lesions, hemorrhages, or infarctions of the hypothalamus or brainstem Heat stroke Anticholinergic drugs

oxygen-rich blood to supply adequate cerebral tissue perfusion. Alterations in respiratory function, heart rate, blood pressure, and temperature may indicate a neurologic insult (Table 7-1-3).

Cushing's triad is a compensatory mechanism occurring in response to increased intracranial pressure. Its three components—bradycardia, hypertension, and bradypnea—attempt to protect the brain from the damaging affects of inadequate blood flow. This response signifies rapid deterioration and decompensation of protective reflexes. Therefore, skill in interpreting vital signs and neurologic assessment findings is essential in determining the patient's ongoing status.

Rancho Los Amigos Scale

The Rancho Los Amigos cognitive scale is another tool used to classify brain-injured patients. This tool describes the recovery phases that a brain-injured patient must go through. It evaluates cognitive function and aims to evaluate and classify patients according to their behavior.

Deep Tendon Reflexes

Assessing deep tendon reflexes (DTRs) provides important information on central nervous system (CNS) status. Commonly tested DTRs include the brachioradial tendon, triceps tendon, biceps tendon, patellar tendon, and Achilles tendon. DTRs are tested with the muscle relaxed, by tapping the tendon with a reflex hammer. A normal response is a quick movement of the extremity or structure due to the contraction of the muscle that the tendon innervates. Altered DTRs may occur with herniated disks, metabolic changes, or drug toxicities.

DTRs are usually scored on a scale of 4+ to 0:

- 4+: brisk, hyperactive reflex with intermittent or sustained clonus (clonus is the rapid, involuntary contraction and relaxation of skeletal muscle)
- 3+: slightly hyperactive reflex
- 2+: active or normal reflex
- 1+: diminished or hypoactive reflex
- 0: absent reflex

 CLINICAL PEARLS

○ Pupils of unequal size (anisocoria) are found in approximately 15% of the general population.
○ A decreased sense of smell may be attributed to heavy cigarette smoking, chronic rhinitis, or sinusitis.

Increased Intracranial Pressure

Section 2   Michelle Grace ■ Lori Schumacher

OVERVIEW

The ability to recognize increased intracranial pressure (IICP) is a critical assessment skill for nurses. The skull serves as a closed, rigid vault containing brain tissue (84%), blood (4%), and cerebrospinal fluid (CSF) (12%). Each element is compressible—an increase in any one element may result in increasing pressure and fluctuations in intracranial pressure (ICP). Sustained IICP can result in irreversible CNS injury. With sustained IICP, cerebral blood flow (CBF) and cerebral perfusion pressure (CPP) may be seriously diminished, causing brain ischemia and leading to coma and, eventually, death. Table 7-2-1 reviews important concepts associated with IICP.

TABLE 7-2-1. Definitions

Intracranial pressure (ICP)	The pressure of cerebrospinal fluid (CSF) within the skull. Normal ranges of ICP in adults and older children <0–15 mm Hg
Increased intracranial pressure (IICP)	Described as pressures ≥20 mm Hg
Cushing's response	Occurs as a result of IICP. When pressure of the CSF increases close to the cerebral artery pressure, the arteries compress and collapse thus decreasing cerebral perfusion pressure (CPP). Cushing's response causes arterial pressure to rise. As arterial pressure exceeds CSF pressure, CPP is reestablished and blood flow to the tissue is maintained.
Cushing's triad	A clinical presentation in response to intracranial hypertension (IICP). It presents as bradycardia, hypertension, and irregular respirations. The presentation is a result of increasing pressure on the medullary center and signals deterioration and decompensation of vital signs and basic protective reflexes.
Cerebral perfusion pressure (CPP)	The difference between the arterial blood entering the neurovascular system and the return of venous blood exiting the system. This is viewed as a pressure gradient across the brain and the pressure difference and is calculated as the difference between the incoming arterial blood pressure and the opposing intracranial pressure on the arteries, affected of course by the ability of the venous volume to exit. Normal CPP = 60–160 mm Hg.
Autoregulation	A compensatory mechanism to protect the brain when events threaten CPP. This process maintains perfusion over a wide range of blood pressures. Autoregulation is the automatic constriction or dilation of cerebral blood vessels in response to changes in blood pressure. CPP is protected by either the opening (dilation) of vessels in response to decreased systemic blood pressure or constriction of blood vessels in response to an increase in systemic blood pressure. Autoregulation is maintained with a mean arterial pressure of 50–70 mm Hg.
Compliance	The ability of the brain to tolerate increases in intracranial volume without adverse increases in ICP. A response in volume changes with no increase in ICP indicates normal and adequate compliance. Low compliance is indicated when a small increase in volume causes a response of elevated ICP.
Elastance	An effect represented as the tightness or stiffness of the intracranial compartment. It is the brain's ability to tolerate and compensate for an increase in volume. High elastance results in a significant increase in ICP. A tight brain is a poorly compliant brain and has high elastance.
Cerebral edema	The abnormal accumulation of fluid in the intracellular space, extracellular space, or both resulting in increased tissue volume and IICP. In the injured brain, autoregulation is disrupted and the cells leak proteins in the white matter, thus causing an accumulation of fluid (vasogenic edema). Fluid accumulation in the intracellular gray matter is called cytotoxic edema.

PRINCIPLES OF CARE

ICP is a dynamic physiologic process with mild transient elevations and fluctuations occurring in all individuals with such actions as coughing, straining, blood pressure alterations, and sneezing. The normal physiological processes of autoregulation and compliance (see Table 7-2-1) make adjustments to accommodate these fluctuations. Autoregulation causes cerebral blood to shift to extracranial areas through cerebral vasoconstriction, and compliance allows for the displacement of CSF to the spinal column. Together, these compensatory mechanisms prevent significant increases in ICP.

When normal physiologic compensatory responses are impeded, as in the injured brain, autoregulation is lost, compliance is low, and the brain is unable to accommodate any fluctuations. Even small increases in volume (CSF, blood, or tissue) can cause dangerous elevations in ICP, making the brain swollen and tight.

IICP can be caused by increases in any of the three intracranial components:
- *Increased brain volume* from a cerebral mass or lesion (e.g., brain tumor, abscess, hematoma, aneurysm), cerebral edema, or local hemorrhage into brain tissue
- *Increased blood volume* from engorgement of cerebral blood vessels from vasodilation or obstruction of venous outflow
- *Increased CSF* from obstructed circulation or decreased absorption or increased production of CSF, as seen with hydrocephalus

Patients at risk for IICP include those with known head injury, known or suspected space-occupying lesion (e.g., tumor, abscess, hematoma), a GCS score below 8, decorticate and/or decerebrate posturing, hypoxia, hypercarbia, or edema secondary to surgery, trauma, or hemorrhage.

Elevations in ICP produce changes in neurologic assessment findings. These changes may be subtle, occurring over hours to days, or acute, occurring rapidly and progressing quickly to coma and death.

Early signs and symptoms of IICP include:
- Altered level of consciousness (e.g., restlessness, irritability, mild confusion, decreased GCS score, personality changes)
- Pupillary changes (gradual dilation, sluggish reaction)
- Papilledema (edema of the optic nerve from compression), causing diplopia, and decreased visual acuity
- Motor and/or sensory deficits related to the area being compressed
- Changes in speech (slurred, inappropriate, aphasia)
- Headache (early morning, on awakening)
- Vomiting (frequently without nausea) without related gastrointestinal symptoms

Late signs and symptoms of IICP include:
- Further deterioration in level of consciousness, decreased level of arousal, further decreasing GCS score
- Pupillary changes (unilateral or bilateral dilation, nonreaction to light)
- Motor deficits (weakness, abnormal posturing, flaccidity, hemiparesis, hemiplegia, drift)
- Sensory deficits, from decreased reaction to painful stimuli to no response at all
- Changes in speech (slurred, inappropriate, none)
- Changes in respiratory patterns (character, quality irregular rate to apnea)

- Changes in vital signs (Cushing's triad—hypertension, bradycardia, and bradypnea)
- Loss of protective reflexes, cranial nerve dysfunction (cough, gag, corneal reflex)
- Seizure activity
- Hypotension and tachycardia (very late findings)

If untreated, IICP will decrease cerebral blood flow to levels that are incompatible with life or cause compression of the brainstem through herniation.

DECISION-MAKING
Monitoring

ICP monitoring devices include ventricular catheters, subarachnoid screws/bolts, parenchymal implanted devices, and epidural sensors. Each device has certain advantages and disadvantages. The choice of one device over another often depends on the patient's injury or anticipated interventions.

Continuous ICP monitoring of the brain and supratentorial compartment is routine in the evaluation of intracranial disorders. The purposes of monitoring are to detect IICP before it reaches dangerous levels, to guide interventions, and to provide a tool for predicting level of injury and patient outcome. Monitoring ICP requires a sensing device placed in the patient's brain that is connected through cables to the bedside monitor. The pressure signal is conducted through an external transducer or, in some advanced monitoring systems, the transducer is placed in the brain tissue or ventricles. The transducer translates the pressure to a visual picture (waveform) and a numerical value. Insertions of monitoring devices may be done either in the operating room or at the bedside.

Systemic Interventions

Interventions in the treatment of IICP include body positioning (keeping the patient's head in straight alignment), elevating the head of the bed, providing ventilation/airway management, administering medications, and controlling environmental conditions.

Neurologic

Baseline and ongoing evaluations of the patient's level of consciousness, GCS, and ICP and CPP values are critical. The nurse's bedside neurologic assessment is critical in identifying early findings. (See Section 1 for information on neurologic assessment.) Craniotomy may be performed to allow for expansion of brain tissue or for the removal of a space-occupying lesion.

Pulmonary
Prevention of Hypercarbia (Hypercapnia)

Carbon dioxide (CO_2) is a potent vasodilating agent. Vasodilation (engorged vessels) increases ICP. Controlled hyperventilation through mechanical ventilation to maintain a reduced CO_2 level (27 to 35 mm Hg) may be necessary. Keep in mind, however, that significantly low CO_2 levels (<25 mm Hg) can lead to cerebral ischemia from vasoconstriction.

Oxygenation

Monitoring oxygen levels and preventing hypoxia is a critical aspect of care. Oxygenation is monitored with pulse oximetry and arterial blood gas analysis. Prevention of hypoxia is achieved by oxygen, usually through intubation and mechanical ventilation. Maintaining Pao_2 levels above 80 mm Hg during treatments can be accomplished through such actions as positioning and preoxygenation. Positive end-expiratory pressure (PEEP) is used with caution because of its possible affect on decreasing venous drainage/outflow and thus increasing ICP/CPP. Position the patient with the head of the bed elevated 30 degrees and the neck maintained in the midline position. This position not only improves ventilation, but also enhances venous outflow.

Monitoring respiratory patterns is critical. Erratic respiratory patterns are key assessment findings in IICP. Compression of the brainstem causes changes in respiratory patterns, heralding possible herniation.

Cardiovascular Assessment

Monitoring and maintaining blood pressure within desired limits is critical in maintaining ICP/CPP and cerebral blood flow as autoregulation is lost. The physician will determine the mean arterial pressure and systolic blood pressure parameters to be maintained. Desired CPP levels are 60 to 70 mm Hg, and desired mean arterial pressure is greater than 60 mm Hg. Antihypertensive drugs may be needed if CPP exceeds 85 mm Hg or if systolic blood pressure exceeds 160 mm Hg. IICP and compression of the brainstem are likely to result in cardiovascular arrhythmias from CNS or autonomic responses.

Fluid and Electrolyte Management

Monitoring intake and output is a critical aspect of care for patients with neurologic disease or injury. Abnormalities in the sodium potassium pump and irregular levels of antidiuretic hormone (ADH) commonly occur in neurologic illness. Compression of the pituitary gland and hypothalamus can affect electrolyte and hormonal control. Diabetes insipidus (DI) and syndrome of inappropriate antidiuretic hormone (SIADH) commonly occur (Table 7-2-2). Monitoring sodium and potassium levels are critical in preventing changes in level of

Table 7-2-2. Comparison of Diabetes Insipidus and Syndrome of Inappropriate Antidiuretic Hormone Secretion

	DIABETES INSIPIDUS	SYNDROME OF INAPPROPRIATE ANTIDIURETIC HORMONE SECRETION
Description	• Decreased secretion of ADH • Large amounts of urine (polyuria), 4–10 L/day • Dehydration, hypovolemia, polydipsia	• Increased or continual secretion of ADH • Water continually reabsorbed (concentrated urine), urine output 400–500 mL/day • Excessive water retention (weight gain)
Laboratory Findings	• Low urine specific gravity (1.001–1.005) • High serum osmolality • Elevated serum sodium (>145 mEq/L) • Decreased urine osmolality	• Low serum osmolality • Decreased serum sodium (<130 mEq/L) • High urine sodium • High urine osmolality (higher than serum)

ADH, antidiuretic hormone.

consciousness. Glucose-containing intravenous (IV) solutions should be avoided, because these solutions can exacerbate cerebral edema and cause further ischemic damage (see Chapter 2, Section 1).

Pharmacologic Therapy

Certain pharmacologic agents may be given to reduce cerebral edema and ICP. **Osmotic diuretics**, such as mannitol (Osmitrol), may be effective in decreasing ICP because of their rapid action and ability to draw fluid out of the brain tissue into the bloodstream. Another commonly used drug, acetazolamide (Diamox), decreases CSF production. **Corticosteroids**, such as dexamethasone (Decadron), may be given to reduce cerebral edema associated with intracranial tumors, around the area of the mass if the edema is due to an increase in extracellular fluid (vasogenic edema). However, corticosteroids do not decrease ICP. **Anticonvulsants**, such as phenytoin (Dilantin), are given prophylactically to prevent seizures. **Antipyretics** may not be effective in reducing temperature if elevated temperature is caused by hypothalamic dysfunction rather than infection.

Brain Death

If IICP is left untreated or if treatment efforts are ineffective, brain death will ensue from a failure in cerebral circulation or herniation. Cerebral circulation fails when the CPP falls to below 30 mm Hg, so that there is virtually no flow to the brain, leading to ischemia and ultimately necrosis.

Herniation is a displacement of cerebral structures that can progress to brainstem compression and result in brain death. Table 7-2-3 lists the types of herniation syndromes. Signs and symptoms of brain tissue shifts include altered level of consciousness, typically beginning with drowsiness and then progressing to stupor and coma. Regional brain swelling and global IICP produce other manifestations, which may include pupillary abnormalities, decerebrate posturing, and Cushing's triad.

Brain death is absence of clinical brain function that is demonstrably irreversible with a known cause. Brain death is a clinical diagnosis based on such criteria as absence of motor responses to pain in all extremities, absence of brainstem reflexes [oculocephalic (doll's eyes), vestibulo-ocular (caloric

Table 7-2-3. Herniation Syndromes

TYPE	DIRECTION OF DISPLACEMENT
Supratentorial (involves structures located above the tentorium such as the cerebrum)	
Uncal herniation	Lateral and downward
Cingulate herniation	Lateral
Central or transtentorial herniation	Downward
Infratentorial (involves structures located below the tentorium such as the cerebellum)	
Cerebellar tonsillar herniation	Downward into the foramen magnum

test), corneal, cough and gag], and absence of respiratory effort. Confirmatory tests include cerebral angiography showing absent intracerebral circulation, electroencephalography (EEG) revealing no electrical activity, and transcranial Doppler ultrasonography exhibiting absent signals. Most institutions require that the diagnosis of brain death be made by two physicians several hours apart.

CLINICAL PEARLS

- Extremes in sodium levels can cause neurologic symptoms, such as confusion, seizures, and death.
- Avoid IV infusions containing glucose, because glucose will increase cerebral edema and potentiate ICP.
- Elevating the head of bed 30 degrees and maintaining the neck in a neutral position improves ventilation and increases venous outflow.
- Avoid hypotension, which can lead to cerebral ischemia, and hypertension, which can lead to cerebral edema in the patient who has lost autoregulatory functions.

Pathologic Brain Lesions

Section 3   Lori Schumacher ▪ Karen R. Crawford

OVERVIEW

The past decade has brought many advances in the treatment of patients with brain tumors. These advances include new diagnostic tools, surgical equipment, and techniques. The diagnosis of a brain tumor triggers feelings of uncertainty, fear, and hope for the patient and family. Significant loss of neurologic function, treatment options, and quality of life become primary issues. An interdisciplinary approach and a broad knowledge base provide the health professional with the essential skills and information to help provide a positive experience and safe outcome for the patient.

PRINCIPLES OF CARE
Incidence and Etiology

In the U.S., the annual incidence of brain tumors is 17,500 for primary intracranial neoplasms and 17,400 for secondary neoplasms due to metastasis. Neoplasms occur in people of all ages, with peaks in early childhood and in the fifth, sixth, and seventh decades of life. The overall incidence is slightly higher in men than in women, with a higher incidence of neuromas in men and of meningiomas and pituitary adenomas in women.

Classification

Brain tumors can be classified based on a number of distinguishing criteria, including primary or secondary, anatomic location, histologic origin, malignant or benign, and childhood or adult tumors.

Primary brain tumors originate from various cells and structures normally found within the brain. They are described as either malignant or benign (Table 7-3-1).

Table 7-3-1. Benign vs Malignant Tumors

| Benign | Rarely spread; they consist of slow-growing cells with well-defined borders. Life-threatening if located in vital area or if surgically inaccessible, even if the cells are benign. |
| Metastatic | Rapidly growing cells that can spread to other areas of the brain and spinal cord. Always life-threatening. |

In a sense, all brain tumors are potentially malignant, because they may lead to death if not treated. Brain tumors are graded by severity from I to IV. The World Health Organization (WHO) has developed a system that has been fairly widely accepted (although all systems have some limitations). The WHO system identifies the severity of malignancy to assist in developing a treatment plan, as well as to predict outcome (Table 7-3-2).

Secondary brain tumors are metastatic and originate from structures outside the brain, most often from primary tumors of the lungs, breast, and gastrointestinal and genitourinary tracts.

Major Types

Intracerebral Tumors

About 50% of all primary brain tumors and 20% of all primary spinal cord tumors are gliomas, meaning that they grow from glial or neuroglial cells. Glial cells are the cells that support, protect, insulate, and metabolically assist the neurons (Table 7-3-3).

Gliomas usually occur in the cerebral hemispheres but may also strike other areas, especially the optic nerve, the brainstem, and (particularly in children) the cerebellum. The higher the grade, the more malignant the tumor. Gliomas are subclassified by the cell from which they originate as astrocytomas, oligodendrocytomas, or ependymoma (Table 7-3-4). More malignant tumors include anaplastic astrocytomas and glioblastoma multiforme.

Extracerebral Tumors

Meningiomas. Meningiomas constitute about 15% of all intracranial tumors, originate from the dura mater, are encapsulated, and do not invade surrounding tissue. They are considered benign. Signs and symptoms are not manifested until the meningioma reaches a certain size, because of its slow-growing nature. Complete excision is possible with excellent prognosis.

Acoustic Neuromas. These account for 5% to 7% of all intracranial tumors. They arise from the sheath of Schwann cells of the root of CN VIII (acoustic

Table 7-3-2. World Health Organization Tumor Grading System

GRADE	DESCRIPTION
Grade I	Slow-growing; have an excellent prognosis; usually cured with surgery
Grade II	Relatively slow-growing but may spread and can recur at a higher grade
Grade III	More active growth; will spread to adjacent tissue and often recur at a higher grade
Grade IV	Rapid growth, spread widely

Table 7-3-3. Glial Cell Functions

GLIAL CELL TYPE	FUNCTION
Astrocytes	Help form the blood-brain barrier; allow for the transport of nutrients and chemicals for metabolism
Oligodendroglia	Form the myelin sheath
Microglia	Act as phagocytes to remove debris
Ependymal	Line and protect the ventricles

nerve). This slow-growing tumor is considered benign and may involve CN V, VII, IX, X, and the cerebellum. Complete excision is possible with excellent prognosis.

Pituitary Tumors. Between 7% and 10% of all intracranial tumors are located in the pituitary gland, most commonly the anterior pituitary. They are slow-growing and encapsulated. Complete excision is possible followed with hormonal replacement therapy.

Vascular Tumors

Blood vessel tumors, angiomas and hemangioblastomas, account for 3% to 4% of all intracranial tumors. Both are slow-growing in nature. Angiomas arise from malformed arteriovenous connections and occur primarily in the posterior cerebral hemispheres. Hemangioblastomas arise from embryonic vascular tissue and occur primarily in the cerebellum.

Metastatic Tumors

An estimated 25% of individuals with a carcinoma develop metastasis to the brain, most often in the meninges or brain surface. Metastatic brain tumors usually have a poor prognosis, and care typically is palliative, focusing only on relief of symptoms.

Table 7-3-4. Categories of Glial Tumors

GLIAL CELL	TUMOR CELL	PROGNOSIS
Astrocytes	Astrocytoma:	
	• Pilocytic astrocytoma (grade I)	• Usually occurs in children; excellent survival
	• Astrocytoma (grade II)	• 5-year survival with surgery and radiation
	• Anaplastic astrocytoma (grade III)	• Surgery, radiation, and chemotherapy may increase survival
	• Glioblastoma multiforme (grade IV)	• Debulking, chemotherapy, and radiation for palliation; 5- to 18-month survival or less
Oligodendroglia	Oligodendroglioma (grades I to IV)	Complete excision possible; usually benign
Ependymal	Ependymoma (grades I to IV)	Surgical excision possible; usually with grades I and II

DECISION-MAKING

The most common presentation of brain tumors is progressive neurologic deficits, including motor weakness, alterations in cognition or consciousness, seizures, and especially headache. Headache is a common initial sign, but most patients will experience headaches at some point in the course of their illness. Typical brain tumor headaches usually do not throb. They are worse on awakening, sometimes arousing the patient from sleep, and improve by midmorning.

Because of its limited compressibility, the brain has limited compensatory mechanisms for maintaining normal ICP by decreasing the volume of brain tissue, CSF, and cerebral blood volume. Its ability to compensate depends on how rapidly the tumor grows. As a tumor progresses, the patient may become confused, restless, stuporous, and even comatose. Depending on the location of the tumor, abnormalities in pupillary function, as well as deficits in extraocular movement, may occur. Motor deficits (paresis, paralysis, posturing), sensory deficits, and changes in respirations and vital signs may also develop. Table 7-3-5 lists signs and symptoms related to tumor areas. Generalized effects from a neoplasm include IICP (see Section 2 of this chapter) from compression of tissue, obstruction of CSF flow, bleeding around the tumor, or development of cerebral edema.

Diagnostics

The diagnosis of a brain tumor is made from clinical observations, patient history, and a complete neurologic examination. The most common and conclusive test is a computed tomography (CT) or magnetic resonance imaging (MRI) scan to identify the presence of a tumor. Other diagnostic tests may be ordered to evaluate the type of tumor and related conditions and to guide treatment:

- **Cerebral angiography** determines the vascular supply to the tumor and aids in deciding the best surgical approach.
- **Chest films** detect lung lesions that may have metastasized to the brain.
- **Visual field and funduscopic exams** evaluate the visual field and any visual deficits. They also determine the presence of papilledema.
- **Audiometric studies** determine and evaluate hearing loss that may be caused from a tumor such as an acoustic neuroma.
- **Endocrine studies** evaluate hormones controlled by the pituitary gland.
- **Needle biopsy** identifies the specific type of tumor and grade and aids in making appropriate treatment decisions.
- **Positron emission tomography (PET)** is useful in detecting metastatic tumors at distant sites.

Treatment

Brain tumors are treated by medications, surgery, radiation, and/or chemotherapy. When selecting the appropriate treatment, the type, size, and location of the tumor, along with the patient's overall condition and specific signs and symptoms, are considered.

Surgery is done to identify the pathology of the tumor (biopsy), to reduce the size of the tumor (debulking) for palliation, or to remove the tumor completely. Advanced microsurgical techniques, ultrasonic aspiration, stereotaxy, and laser surgery have improved the success of neurosurgical resections.

Table 7-3-5. Signs and Symptoms Related to Tumor Areas

ANATOMIC LOCATION	SIGNS AND SYMPTOMS
Frontal lobe	Behavior changes
	Inattentiveness
	Inability to concentrate
	Emotional lability
	Indifference
	Loss of self-restraint
	Inappropriate social behavior
	Impairment of recent memory
	Difficulty with abstraction
	Flat affect
	Expressive aphasia
	Slowness of movement/generalized response
	Incontinence caused by lack of social control
	Hemiparesis, seizures (particularly focal)
Parietal lobe	Hyperesthesia
	Paresthesia
	Loss of two-point discrimination
	Astereognosis
	Autopanosia
	Disorientation of external environment
	Agraphia
	Construction apraxia
Temporal lobe	Psychomotor seizures (visual, auditory, olfactory hallucinations)
	Mental changes
	Irritability
	Depression
	Poor judgment
	Childish behavior
Occipital lobe	Visual loss in half of each visual field on the side opposite the lesion
	Visual hallucinations
	Possible focalized or generalized seizures

Radiation therapy is based on the fact that tumor cells are more sensitive to radiation than normal cells. Radiation is used for tumors that cannot be excised or can be only partially excised. Depending on the nature of the tumor, radiation therapy can prolong survival.

The use of chemotherapy in treating brain tumors has been limited by the blood-brain barrier (BBB). Today, however, several chemotherapeutic agents can effectively cross the BBB.

 CLINICAL PEARLS

○ Seizures occur in approximately 40% of patients with brain tumors.
○ Some 75% of the headaches experienced by patients with brain tumors are due to IICP. ICP increases when the patient is in a flat position, because of decreased venous return.
○ Typical brain tumor headaches occur on awakening and subside by midmorning.
○ Headaches generally occur over the tumor region.

RESOURCES

- American Association of Neuroscience Nurses: 888-557-2266 or www.aann.org
- American Cancer Society: 800-ACS-2345 or www.cancer.org
- Brain Injury Association Inc.: 703-236-6000 or www.biausa.org
- Brain Trauma Foundation: 212-772-0608 or www.braintrauma.org
- Cancer Information Line: 800-4-CANCER or www.cancercare.org
- National Brain Tumor Foundation: 800-934-2873 or www.braintumor.org
- National Institutes of Health: 800-352-9494 or cancernet.nci.nih.gov

chapter 8

Decision-Making for Cardiovascular Alterations

Cardiac Assessment

Section 1

Becki Hodges

OVERVIEW

Based on statistics from the American Heart Association (AHA), almost 59 million Americans have one or more forms of cardiovascular disease, including high blood pressure, coronary artery disease, stroke, and rheumatic heart disease. Cardiovascular diseases are responsible for approximately 40% of all deaths in the U.S. The scope of the problem makes cardiovascular assessment an essential part of patient assessment. This section covers the basics of cardiovascular assessment.

PRINCIPLES OF CARE

Cardiac assessment requires several different methods of examination. The nurse's role in this assessment includes gathering data for the patient history, measuring vital signs, auscultating heart sounds, and assessing pain. All areas must be closely evaluated to avoid missing subtle changes. A cardinal principle to keep in mind when performing a cardiac assessment is that cardiac function that may be adequate at rest may be inadequate during exertion.

The process can also cause the patient to feel anxious and concerned about potential findings. The nurse should exhibit a relaxed, courteous, confident demeanor during the assessment process to encourage the patient to be as physically relaxed as possible.

DECISION-MAKING

The decision-making process begins while gathering information from the health history, vital signs assessment, pain assessment, and complete physical assessment. Clinical judgment assists the nurse in assimilating the information gathered to help develop a plan of care for appropriate nursing/medical interventions.

Health History

The health history begins with the reason that the patient is seeking care, or the chief complaint. This should include a description of the present illness. The past history includes previous illnesses, injuries, surgeries, and other medical interventions. Risk factors for cardiovascular disease are also assessed.

189

These include family history, sex, age, diet, smoking, sedentary lifestyle, obesity, diabetes, hypertension, and stress.

The patient should be questioned about allergies, current medications (prescription and over-the-counter medications, including herbal remedies), diet, exercise and lifestyle activities, and environmental factors. Specific symptoms to investigate include episodes of chest pain, orthopnea, dyspnea on exertion, paroxysmal nocturnal dyspnea, claudication, peripheral edema, and palpitations.

Vital Signs

Evaluation of vital signs includes heart rate, respiratory rate and rhythm, temperature, and blood pressure. Heart rate is most commonly evaluated by palpating the radial pulse. If the rhythm is not regular during palpation, the irregularity may be further evaluated by monitoring the patient's rhythm by ECG or auscultating of heart sounds.

When evaluating pulse rhythm, note whether the rhythm changes with respiration, is totally irregular, or is basically regular with some beats that occur early.

When evaluating respirations, note the rate and depth of breathing. Also note how hard the patient is working to breathe. Anatomically, the structures of the heart and lungs are in close proximity to each other, and pressure changes in one system often affect the other.

Temperature assessment includes determining whether the patient is hyperthermic or hypothermic. (The normal body temperature range is 98.6°F ± 1 degree.) Elevated temperature points to possible infection or thyroid-related problems. Hypothermia can reflect metabolic abnormalities, such as hypothyroidism, or exposure.

Blood pressure is evaluated with the center of the blood pressure cuff placed over the brachial artery. Make sure the cuff size is appropriate for the patient's size; otherwise, readings may be inaccurate. Once the reading is obtained, whether by a manual cuff, an automated blood pressure device, or an indwelling arterial line, the pressure is evaluated.

Pulse

Evaluation of arterial pulses includes the radial, brachial, carotid, femoral, popliteal, dorsalis pedis, and posterior tibialis pulses. Each pulse should be assessed for pulse amplitude and compared with same pulse on the opposite extremity. (See Section 2 for a pulse amplitude scale.)

Estimation of jugular venous pressure and central venous pressure (right atrial pressure), although usually done by physicians, can provide useful information. This information is obtained by the examination of the jugular veins and jugular pulsations. The patient is positioned with the head of the bed elevated 30 to 45 degrees. The patient's head is turned away from the examiner. The pulsations of the external jugular vein are located and the highest point of pulsation identified. A centimeter ruler is used to measure the distance between this point and the sternal angle. Venous pressures 3 cm or more above the sternal angle are considered elevated.

Pain Assessment

The PQRST method of pain assessment is useful when evaluating chest pain. Question the patient with regard to the following:

- What provokes (P) the pain?
- What is the quality (Q) of the pain? Is it sharp and stabbing, or does it feel like tightness, squeezing, pressure, or indigestion?
- Does the pain radiate (R)? If so, does it radiate to the jaw or down the arm?
- What is the severity (S) of the pain?
- What time (T) did the pain start?

Pain can be rated on a pain scale of 1 to 10, with 1 being almost no pain and 10 being the worst pain that the patient has ever experienced.

Remember that pain is subjective. The pain scale is most effective when used to assess interventions or changes in pain. However, a baseline reference is essential. Types of chest pain are discussed in Table 8-1-1.

Cardiac pain is typically characterized by pressure, tightness, or a feeling of

Table 8-1-1. Differentiating Chest Pain

TYPE OF PAIN	LOCATION AND DESCRIPTION	ASSOCIATED FACTORS
Angina	Substernal or retrosternal pain or discomfort that may radiate to either arm, shoulders or jaw Sudden onset, typically brought on by effort. May feel like indigestion	Pain usually subsides within 10 minutes after rest and administration of sublingual nitroglycerin.
Myocardial infarction	Caused by prolonged myocardial ischemia Sudden onset, crushing, viselike or severe burning pain	The patient may experience shortness of breath, nausea, vomiting, weakness, perspiration, feeling of doom, changes in vital signs. Immediate intervention is essential Evaluation of enzymes, ECG, and patient history are needed.
Pericarditis	Intermittent pain in the precordial area, may radiate; sharp, knifelike, pain	Usually accompanied by a pericardial friction rub. Pain may be relieved when the patient sits up and leans forward. Nonsteroidal anti-inflammatory agents may be used.
Pleural pain	Located in the chest wall, resulting from inflammation of the parietal pleura; sharp, knifelike pain aggravated by coughing	May be associated with a pleural friction rub.
Esophageal pain	Substernal pain, may radiate to back, arms, jaw; burning, possibly squeezing pain	May mimic cardiac pain. Antacids may provide relief. If due to esophageal spasm, sublingual nitroglycerin may relieve the pain (which can confuse the picture).
Chest wall pain	Often begins along costal cartilages as a dull aching, may have increasing intensity over a few days; tenderness is usually localized	Muscle relaxants, analgesics may relieve the pain.

indigestion brought on by exertion and relieved by rest and nitroglycerin. Cardiac pain is *not* typically sharp or stabbing in quality.

Inspection and Palpation

Inspect the chest for any obvious skeletal deformities that might impede internal anatomic structures. Inspection and palpation will help locate the apical pulse, which can reflect the size of the left ventricle. Normally the apical pulse is slightly medial to the left midsternal line at the fifth intercostal space. Palpation may also reveal the presence of a thrill (a palpable murmur).

Auscultation

Using the Stethoscope

A stethoscope with a diaphragm for auscultation of high-pitched sounds and a bell for listening to low-pitched sounds is imperative for cardiac assessment. When using the diaphragm of the stethoscope, be sure to apply firm pressure to the skin during auscultation. Place the bell very lightly on the skin to seal the edge. If too much pressure is applied with the bell, the skin surface will act as a diaphragm and block out low-pitched sounds, letting you hear only high-pitched sounds.

Auscultating Heart Sounds

When auscultating heart sounds, the room should be quiet and comfortably heated. Auscultation should be done systematically. Begin by listening with the diaphragm at the aortic area; then move to the pulmonic area, inch down the sternal border to the tricuspid area, and then move to the mitral area (Table 8-1-2).

Listen specifically at each area for the first heart sound (S1) and then the second heart sound (S2) for intensity, timing, and regularity. Also note any duplication of sound or extra heart sounds during systole or diastole. After auscultating with the diaphragm, repeat the same process with the bell of the stethoscope, starting at the mitral area and moving back to the tricuspid area, then inching up the sternal border to the pulmonic and aortic areas (Table 8-1-3).

Split Heart Sounds

Split S1. Right and left ventricular contraction occur almost simultaneously, but with left ventricular contraction slightly earlier. Splitting of S1 may occur if these events are not timed closely together. A common cause of split S1 is right bundle branch block, which delays the onset of right ventricular systole.

Split S2. Normal physiologic splitting of S2 occurs during inspiration, as pulmonic sounds occur later than aortic sounds. Wide splitting of S2 can result

Table 8-1-2. Auscultation Areas

AUSCULTATION AREA	LOCATION
Aortic area	Second interspace to the right of the sternum
Pulmonic area	Second interspace to the left of the sternum
Right ventricular area (tricuspid area)	Fifth intercostal space at the sternal border
Left ventricular area (mitral area)	Fifth intercostal space, midclavicular line

from late closure of the pulmonic valve in such conditions as right bundle branch block, pulmonic stenosis, and atrial septal defect.

When trying to differentiate a split heart sound from other sounds, remember that normally an S1 or S2 is best heard with the diaphragm of the stethoscope. A split S1 or S2 (or delayed sound) is also best heard with the diaphragm.

Gallop Heart Sounds

A third heart sound (S3) is an extra sound heard after S2. Because S2 indicates the onset of diastole, S3 is considered an early diastolic sound. It is a low-pitched sound best heard at the apex or mitral area using the bell of the stethoscope. S3 is considered a ventricular gallop rhythm that is a normal finding in children and young adults.

The presence of a third heart sound in an older person with heart disease may be one of the earliest indicators of heart failure.

A fourth heart sound (S4, or atrial gallop) is an extra sound heard just before S1. It is considered a late diastolic sound and is best heard with the bell of the stethoscope at the apex or mitral area. S4 results from decreased left ventricular compliance and increased ventricular resistance to filling (stiff ventricles). Causes of S4 include hypertensive cardiac disease, coronary artery disease, and aortic stenosis.

Pericardial Friction Rub

Inflammation of the pericardium (pericarditis) may result in a harsh scraping or grating sound heard along the precordium, usually loudest at the left sternal border. Pericardial friction rub has a systolic and diastolic component. The intensity of the sound may increase when the patient leans forward.)

Murmurs

Murmurs are sounds caused by turbulent blood flow. Pathology may include stenotic valves (narrowed), septal or atrial defects, and incompetent valves (valves that do not seal completely when closed).

When auscultating heart sounds, listen selectively for murmurs. Note whether the sound occurs during systole or diastole. Also note whether the murmur is heard best with the diaphragm (high-pitched) or the bell of the stethoscope (low-pitched). Determine the area in which the sound is loudest; a murmur is usually associated with pathology in that area.

Murmurs are graded on a scale of I to VI (Table 8-1-4).

Classification of Functional Capacity

The severity of functional impairment should be determined in all patients with heart disease. The New York Heart Association (NYHA) has developed a system for classifying the severity of heart failure based on symptoms and exercise capacity. This system, called the NYHA Classification, is helpful in determining disease outcome and monitoring the response to treatment.

- Class I: Asymptomatic. Patients with heart disease with no limitation on physical activity. An example is a patient diagnosed with coronary artery disease who is able to participate in any physical activity without chest pain or shortness of breath.
- Class II: Mild. Patients with heart disease with slight limitation of physical activity (i.e., ordinary activity results in fatigue, palpitation, dyspnea, or angina). An example is a patient who has been diagnosed with coronary artery disease who knows that he can mow half of his yard without

Table 8-1-3. Auscultation of Heart Sounds

HEART SOUND	TIMING	PHYSIOLOGY	AUSCULTATION SITE	INDICATIONS
S1 (Lub) High-pitched sound best heard with the diaphragm	Onset of systole	Closure of mitral and tricuspid valves	Best heard at mitral and tricuspid areas (apex and right lower sternal border)	Normal First heart sound
S2 (Dub) Best heard with the diaphragm	Onset of diastole to the end of systole	Closure of pulmonic and aortic valves	Heard loudest at pulmonic and aortic areas (second interspace just to the left of sternum and second interspace just to right of sternum)	Normal Second heart sound
Split S1 Best heard with the diaphragm	Beginning of systole	Mitral valve closure occurring before tricuspid valve closure	Mitral and tricuspid areas	Often normal May be due to right bundle branch block or pulmonary hypertension
Split S2 Best heard with the diaphragm	End of systole	Delayed closure between the pulmonic and aortic valves	Best heard at pulmonic area of inspiration	Physiologic Normal, if heard on inspiration. Wide splitting may be due to right bundle branch block or pulmonary stenosis.
S3 ventricular gallop rhythm (Sounds like "Ken-tuc-ky") Low-pitched sound best heard with the bell	Early diastole	Early, rapid ventricular filling resulting in vibrations	Best heard at the apex (mitral area) or tricuspid area	One of the earliest indicators of ventricular failure in adults with heart disease. May be a normal finding in children and young adults
S4 atrial gallop (Sounds like "Ten-nes-see") Low-pitched sound-best heard with the bell	Late diastole, just before the next systole	Atria is working harder to fill against a stiff ventricle	Best heard at mitral area	May indicate ventricular hypertrophy, hypertension, aortic stenosis, or coronary artery disease
Pericardial friction rub Harsh grating, scraping sound	Has a systolic and diastolic component	Caused by inflamed pericardial surfaces rubbing together	Usually loudest along the left sternal border	Pericarditis

Table 8-1-4. Grading Murmurs

Grade I: Very faint; may not be heard in all positions
Grade II: Quiet, heard immediately when placing stethoscope on chest
Grade III: Same intensity as normal S1, S2
Grade IV: Loud; may be associated with a thrill
Grade V: Very loud; stethoscope may not be completely on the chest, associated
     with a thrill
Grade VI: May be heard with the stethoscope off the chest, associated with a thrill.
Thrill: A palpable murmur

symptoms, but becomes fatigued and short of breath if exceeding that work effort.

- Class III: Moderate. Patients with heart disease producing marked limitation of physical activity (i.e., fatigue, palpitation, dyspnea, angina with less than ordinary activity). An example is a patient who has been diagnosed with coronary artery disease who experiences chest pain or shortness of breath while climbing one flight of stairs.

- Class IV: Severe. Patients with heart disease that results in the inability to participate in any physical activity without discomfort. Symptoms may be present even at rest. An example is a patient who has been diagnosed with valvular heart disease who cannot arise from a chair and walk to the bathroom or kitchen without shortness of breath and extreme fatigue.

Conclusion

Health history, vital sign measurement, and heart auscultation are important components of the cardiac assessment. When assessing a patient, observe for clues to clinical findings. Integrate the information from the cardiac assessment into other system assessment findings for a complete understanding of the entire physical examination.

 CLINICAL PEARLS

○ Information gathered during the health history can provide clues to use in the decision-making process.

○ Make sure that the environment is warm and quiet when performing physical assessment and auscultating heart sounds.

○ Practice listening to normal heart sounds (lub [S1], dub [S2]) for intensity, timing, and reference to systole and diastole.

○ In a patient with tachycardia in whom it is difficult to differentiate between S1 and S2, remember that S1 just precedes the carotid upstroke.

○ Split sounds are best heard with the diaphragm of the stethoscope.

○ The area of auscultation where a heart sound is heard is one of the most important clues to the possible cause of the sound (e.g., sounds heard over the aortic area usually indicate a problem with the aortic valve).

○ Gather all clues, including the patient's history, and piece the puzzle together.

Vascular Assessment

Section 2   Judy Graham-Garcia ▪ Rebecca Rule

OVERVIEW

Assessment of the vascular system and detection of alterations in blood pressure and blood flow is accomplished through inspection and palpation of the skin and inspection, palpation, and auscultation of the vessels. The postprocedure nursing management of the patient undergoing arteriography and venography requires essential vascular system assessment skills. This section discusses the basic components of vascular assessment.

PRINCIPLES OF CARE

Peripheral vascular disorders may involve the arteries and/or the veins. Atherosclerosis, cardiac disorders, and hypertension are significant contributing factors to the pathogenesis of peripheral vascular disease.

Arterial insufficiency may be acute or chronic. Chronic arterial insufficiency is a progressive debilitating disorder characterized by inadequate blood flow in arteries because of occlusive atherosclerotic plaques or emboli, damaged or diseased vessels, aneurysms, hypercoagulability states, or heavy use of tobacco. Thromboangiitis obliterans is the primary cause of chronic arterial insufficiency, caused by an inflammatory reaction to cigarette smoking, most commonly in men between age 20 and 40 years. Acute arterial insufficiency may result from thrombi originating from cardiac disorders. It is characterized by a sudden decrease in the arterial blood supply to an extremity. Obstruction of any major artery can precipitate symptoms.

Venous insufficiency may be acute or chronic. Venous thrombosis is the most common venous disorder. The triad of stasis, intimal damage, and hypercoagulability is responsible for most venous thrombosis. Venous thrombosis may lead to chronic venous insufficiency, characterized by chronic, noninflammatory edema of the lower legs.

DECISION-MAKING

A thorough vascular examination involves assessing arterial and venous pulses, blood pressure, capillary filling, skin, pain, and ankle-brachial index. Aspects of this assessment include inspection, palpation, auscultation, and vital signs.

Characteristic findings in arterial insufficiency include:
- Bruits
- Coolness
- Cyanosis or mottling
- Decreased or absent peripheral pulses
- Delayed capillary filling
- Exertional limb pain relieved with rest
- Loss of hair on limbs
- Pallor on raising limbs
- Redness (rubor) on lowering limbs
- Sensitivity to cold

- Thin, tight, shiny skin
- Thickened, brittle nails
- Ulceration on an extremity

Arterial System

Three characteristics of the arterial pulse are assessed: rate, rhythm, and amplitude.

Pulse Rate

Normal resting heart rate for an adult is 60 to 100 beats/min. A rate below 60 beats/min likely indicates sinus bradycardia; however, junctional rhythm or heart block must be considered. A rate above 100 beats/min usually indicates sinus tachycardia, which is often associated with episodes of intense emotion or exercise. A rate in an adult above 120 beats/min at rest points to some type of arrhythmia and calls for further investigation.

Pulse Rhythm

The pulse rhythm should be regular or demonstrate sinus arrhythmia. Occasional irregularity of a pulse with an underlying regular rhythm may indicate ectopic beats. An irregularly irregular pulse may indicate atrial fibrillation.

Pulse Amplitude

The amplitude is the fullness or force of the pulse. All pulses except the carotid pulse are palpated simultaneously and compared in terms of amplitude, graded on a scale of 0 to 4:

0 = absent pulse
1 = diminished, easily obliterated
2 = normal
3 = increased
4 = bounding, cannot be obliterated

Important variations in amplitude include pulsus paradoxus and pulsus alternans. In *pulsus paradoxus*, amplitude decreases with inspiration and increases with expiration. It is caused by changes in intrathoracic pressure. A systolic blood pressure decrease of more than 10 mm Hg on inspiration indicates pulsus paradoxus. This change in amplitude may be associated with cardiac tamponade, pneumothorax, pleural effusion, or chronic obstructive pulmonary disease.

Pulsus alternans is characterized by a regular rhythm with alternate pulsations of varying amplitudes. It is often associated with left ventricular failure.

Doppler Assessment

Doppler assessment of pulses is used whenever peripheral pulses cannot be palpated. A water-soluble lubricant is applied to the approximate location of the pulse. The Doppler ultrasound probe placed directly on the lubricated skin sends a beam to the artery. Movement of the red blood cells through the vessel is reflected as a sound indicative of the velocity of blood flow through the artery. An audible signal is heard with each heartbeat.

Blood Pressure

Blood pressure measurement reflects blood volume (cardiac output) and elasticity of the arterial walls (peripheral vascular resistance). The systolic number represents the force against the arterial wall as the ventricle contracts; the diastolic number reflects the force produced during ventricular relaxation and filling.

Blood pressure should be evaluated in both arms, and with the patient lying, sitting, and standing. Differences in positional measurements may indicate orthostatic changes and provide important diagnostic clues to alterations in volume and neurohormonal status. Differences among extremities may indicate significant pathology caused by changes in the vasculature.

Capillary Refill Time

Assessing capillary refill time evaluates peripheral perfusion. Depress the nail bed until it blanches. Remove the pressure and note how quickly the color returns. Color should return in less than 3 seconds.

Elevate the supine patient's legs to 45 degrees. Moderate pallor on elevation indicates that circulation to the extremities is impaired. Lower the patient's legs to a dependent position; color should return within 10 seconds. A delay in color return points to arterial insufficiency. Venous filling should occur after the patient's legs are dependent for 15 to 20 seconds.

Auscultation

Auscultate the carotid arteries for bruits. Bruits are low-pitched blowing sounds best heard with the bell of the stethoscope. Have the patient hold his or her breath while you place the stethoscope over one artery at a time. Bruits occur during systole and result from a narrowing of the vessel secondary to arteriosclerosis.

Skin

Skin assessment includes temperature, color, texture, hair distribution, and the presence of ulcers. With decreased perfusion, skin temperature will be cool. Warmth may indicate inflammation. Pallor is present in compromised superficial circulation, which is especially notable with elevation of the extremities. Cyanosis occurs with inadequate oxygenation or decreased circulation. Rubor (dusky red skin) is seen with tissue ischemia, which again is especially notable on dependency.

Normal skin texture is soft and smooth, with appropriate hair distribution. Arterial insufficiency is marked by tight, shiny, dry, atrophic skin, thick and brittle nails, and hairless feet and toes. Arterial ulcers, typically found in easily traumatized areas, are the result of skin breakdown; they may become gangrenous and necessitate amputation.

Pain

The patient may present with intermittent claudication (exercise-induced pain that is relieved with rest). This can eventually progress to pain at rest.

Ankle-Brachial Index

The ankle-brachial index (ABI) is a noninvasive way to assess arterial perfusion. This assessment involves obtaining blood pressure measurements in both arms (using the higher systolic pressure for the calculation), then obtaining the ankle blood pressure measurement. Divide the systolic ankle pressure by the systolic brachial pressure to get the ABI. An ABI below 0.95 indicates normal perfusion to the extremity.

Venous System

Characteristics of venous insufficiency include:

- Atrophy of skin and soft tissue
- Coldness and pallor of extremities
- Edema of lower extremities
- Gangrenous changes
- Leg pain during menstruation
- Nocturnal cramping
- Swollen, ropelike, or ruptured superficial leg veins

Skin

The venous component of vascular assessment begins with skin assessment. Skin temperature may be warm with chronic venous insufficiency. It is important to note, however, that skin temperature is of limited value, because of extraneous variables such as environmental temperature. Redness along the path of a vein is indicative of phlebitis, whereas light-brown discoloration results from chronic venous insufficiency. In chronic venous insufficiency, ulcers may also be present, usually located on the medial malleolus. These ulcers may be pigmented, and the pain is not usually severe. Pain may indicate necrosis of the ulcer. When the affected limb is placed in a dependent position, the patient may experience an aching-type pain.

Edema

To assess for edema, press the thumb for at least 5 seconds over the dorsum of each foot, behind the medial malleolus, and over the shins. Edema is graded on a four-point scale from slight to very marked. Normally, no pitting edema is seen; pitting edema may be indicative of chronic venous insufficiency, deep vein thrombosis, or congestive heart failure. Nonpitting edema is associated with inflammation.

Superficial Veins

Inspect and palpate for varicosities, dilated or tortuous veins. These are best seen in the standing position, which promotes gravitational flow. With venous insufficiency, the patient will present with palpable, cordlike segments, distended superficial veins, or streaking.

Nursing Management of the Patient Undergoing Angiography and Venography

- Assess blood pressure, pulse, respirations, and pain every 15 minutes for the first 2 hours, and then hourly until stable.
- Assess the pulse, capillary refill, color, temperature, numbness, and tingling of the affected extremity every 15 minutes for the first 2 hours, and then hourly until stable.
- Continue assessing the pulse in the affected extremity every 2 hours for 24 hours.
- Monitor the pressure dressing for signs of bleeding. Assess for areas of redness, swelling, and bleeding around the dressing every 15 minutes for the first 2 hours, and then hourly for the next 4 hours.
- Maintain the patient on bed rest with the affected extremity immobile and a pressure dressing intact for 2 to 4 hours after the procedure.

CLINICAL PEARLS

○ Nurses often assess the arterial pulse by palpating the right radial artery. However, comparison of the apical and radial pulses is important to detect variations that may indicate arterial occlusion.

○ To assess apical pulse rate, if the rhythm is regular, count the number of beats auscultated in 15 seconds and multiply by four. If the rhythm is irregular, double the number of beats counted in 30 seconds. Normal pulse rate in a resting adult is 60 to 100 beats/min.

○ Also assess pulses in the radial, brachial, carotid, femoral, dorsalis pedis, and posterior tibial arteries bilaterally to detect variations suggestive of occlusive disease.

○ Do not palpate the carotid pulses simultaneously—this can trigger bradycardia or syncope.

○ Pulse amplitude and quality are best appreciated in the brachial or carotid arteries.

○ Blood pressure may be up to 10 mm Hg higher in a person's dominant arm than in the nondominant arm.

○ A 4- to 6-second delay in capillary refill may indicate ischemia.

Basic Electrical Conduction

Section 3   Denise Thompson

OVERVIEW

Cardiac muscle is unique in that it is endowed with an electrical conduction system that can generate electrical impulses as well as respond to electrical impulses. The normal electrical conduction pathway is as follows:

Sinoatrial node → internodal and intra-atrial pathways → atrioventricular node → bundle of His → bundle branches → Purkinje's fibers → ventricular muscle (Fig. 8-3-1).

This section covers the basics of the electrical conduction system of the heart.

PRINCIPLES OF CARE
Depolarization and Repolarization

The electrical cells generate and conduct electrical impulses that produce contraction and relaxation of the myocardial cells. Cardiac muscle consists of many single cells that contain negatively charged ions and positively charged ions. In a resting state, these cells normally have negatively charged ions on the inside of the cell and positively charged ions on the outside. Cells in this state are said to be *polarized*, or in the ready state.

When a pacemaker cell generates an electrical impulse, positive ions move rapidly into the cell and negative ions begin to exit, converting the electrical forces inside the cell to a positive charge. This is called a *depolarized* state. As soon as the cardiac cell depolarizes, negative ions reenter the cell and positive ions exit, returning the inside of the cell to its resting negative charge. This process is called *repolarization*, or the recovery phase. Depolarization of the cardiac cell acts as a stimulus on adjacent cells and causes them to depolarize.

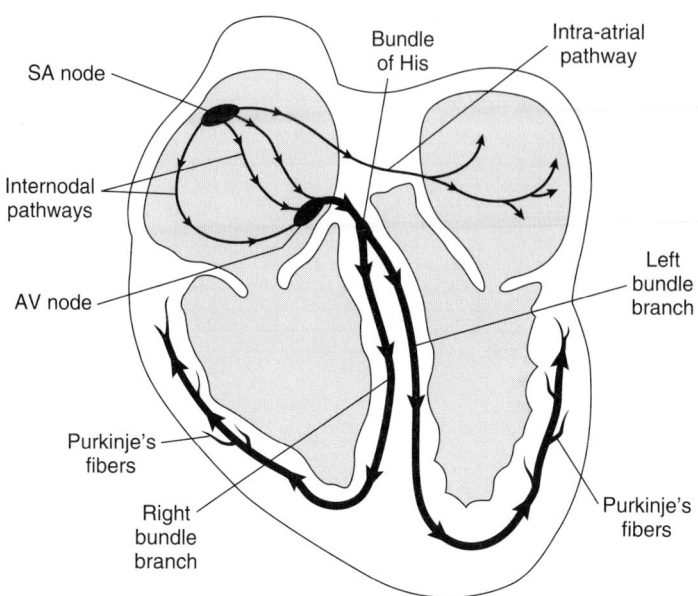

Figure 8-3-1. Normal electrical conduction pathway. AV, atrioventricular; SA, sinoatrial.

Conduction System
Sinoatrial Node

The sinoatrial (SA) node is located in the upper portion of the right atrium near the inlet of the superior vena cava. It is called the master or dominant pacemaker of the heart, generating 60 to 100 beats/min under normal conditions. The electrical impulse travels through the left atria by way of Bachmann's bundle and through the right atria by the internodal tracts. This electrical impulse causes depolarization of the atria.

Atrioventricular Node

Following atrial depolarization, the electrical impulse temporarily stops or is delayed at the atrioventricular (AV) node. The AV node is located in the lower right atrium near the septum. The electrical impulse is delayed here for $\frac{1}{10}$ second, allowing time for atrial emptying and ventricular filling. During this time, 70% to 75% of the blood in the atria flows into the ventricles by gravity. The remaining 25% to 30% is forced into the ventricles with an atrial contraction sometimes referred to as "atrial kick," which normally occurs at the end of atrial depolarization.

If the SA node fails, then the AV node takes over as the pacemaker. The AV node usually generates 40 to 60 beats/min under normal conditions.

Bundle of His

Following ventricular filling, the electrical impulses leave the AV node and travel into the ventricles by way of the bundle of His. The bundle of His,

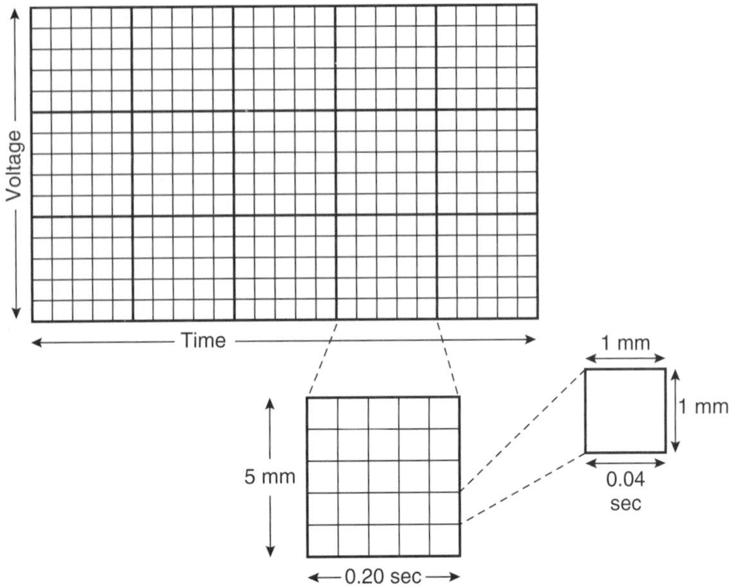

Figure 8-3-2. ECG paper.

located just below the AV node, continues the transmission of electrical impulse to the right and left bundle branches.

Bundle Branches

The bundle of His splits into two branches, the right bundle branch (leading into the right ventricle), and the left bundle branch (leading into the left ventricle). The bundle branches provide for transmission of the electrical impulse to the Purkinje fibers.

Purkinje Fibers

Located deep within the ventricular muscle, the Purkinje fibers conduct electrical impulses from the bundle branches to the cells of the ventricular muscle.

Ventricular Muscle

In response to an electrical stimulus from the Purkinje fibers, the ventricular muscle contracts. If an electrical impulse is not received from the SA node or the AV junction or if they fail as pacemakers, an impulse can be generated from Purkinje fibers or the bundle branches. These impulses are generated at a rate of 20 to 40 beats/min.

Autonomic Nervous System

In addition to the inherent rates, the heart can be influenced by the autonomic nervous system (ANS). The ANS is divided into two parts: the sympathetic nervous system (SNS) and the parasympathetic nervous system (PNS).

The SNS influences both the atria (SA node, intra-atrial and internodal pathways, and the AV junction) and the ventricles. Stimulation of the sympathetic branch by anger, stress, or fright will cause the atria and ventricles to react in several ways: increased rate, increased conduction through the AV node, and increased irritability. The SNS prepares the body to react in times of stress, in what is known as the "fight or flight" response.

The PNS has the opposite effect. The heart slows to normal, and conduction through the AV node is normal. The PNS influences only the atria. This reaction usually occurs after stress subsides.

DECISION-MAKING

Electrical conduction is measured, recorded, and printed on ruled graph paper. The graph paper is divided into 1-mm squares (Fig. 8-3-2). Graph paper measures both time and amplitude. Time is measured on the horizontal line; each square equals 0.04 second. Amplitude, the force of the electrical impulse (voltage), is measured on the vertical line. Each square is equal to 0.1 mV (Fig. 8-3-3).

Each wave recorded on the graph paper represents an electrical impulse in a specific part of the heart.

Waveforms
Baseline

The baseline, or isoelectric line, is the straight line between complexes on the graph paper (Fig. 8-3-4). This represents no electrical activity. A wave

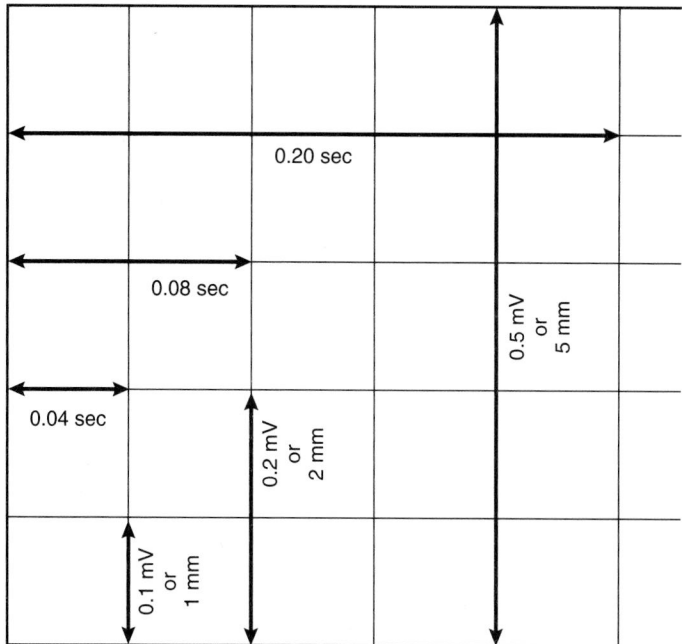

Figure 8-3-3. Relationship between time and voltage.

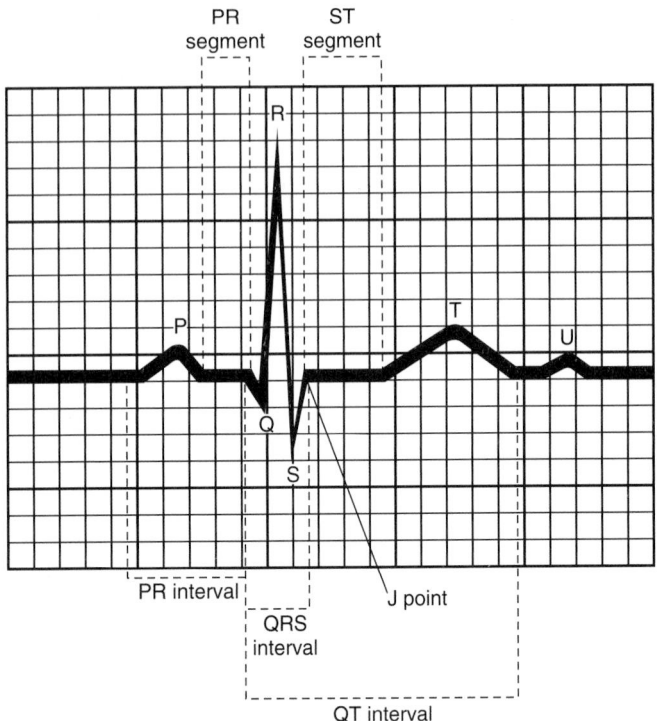

Figure 8-3-4. ECG waveforms.

above the baseline is called a positive deflection; a wave below the baseline, a negative deflection.

P Waves

The first positive deflection, the P wave, represents the depolarization of both the right and left atria. The repolarization of the atria is not seen on ECG because it occurs at approximately the same time as the QRS complex and is buried in the QRS wave.

PR Interval

The PR interval represents the time that it takes an electrical impulse to travel through the atria and AV node to the ventricles or, more specifically, to the bundle of His. The interval is measured from the beginning of the P wave to the beginning of the next deflection. The normal PR interval is 0.12 to 0.20 second.

QRS Complex

The QRS complex represents ventricular depolarization. The complex contains three waves: Q, R, and S. The first negative deflection, the Q wave, should be small (less than one quarter of the size of the R wave) and commonly is not present at all. A larger Q wave is considered pathologic and indicates myocardial infarction (MI). The first positive deflection is called the R wave. The first negative deflection after the R wave is the S wave. The complex is measured from the beginning of the Q wave (or the R wave if the Q is not present) to where the S wave meets the isoelectric line. The normal QRS complex measures less than 0.12 second.

ST Segment

The ST segment extends from the end of the S wave to the beginning of the T wave. The segment should be flat or isoelectric. Elevation or depression of the ST segment may be a sign of myocardial ischemia, injury, or infarction and must be evaluated.

T Wave

The T wave follows the ST segment. This wave indicates the repolarization of the ventricles. An elevated T wave, more than half the height of the QRS, may indicate new ischemia. Also, tall, peaked T waves may be a sign of hyperkalemia. A depressed T wave that follows an upright QRS and looks upside down is frequently an indication of previous cardiac ischemia.

U Wave

The U wave is a small waveform following the T wave. It is frequently a normal finding, but can be related to pathology such as hypokalemia and damage from MI. All U waves should be investigated.

Heart Rate

Heart rate represents the number of electrical impulses conducted through the myocardium in 1 minute. Atrial rate is determined by counting the number of P waves; ventricular rate, by counting QRS complexes. Ventricular rate should be the same as pulse rate; the ventricular rate is preferred for determining heart rate. Rates above 100 beats/min are considered tachycardia, and rates below 60 beats/min are considered bradycardia.

An easy way to calculate heart rate is by the 6-second strip method. The ECG graph paper has hash marks every 3 seconds above the graph. Two of the 3-second intervals equals a 6-second strip. A 6-second strip can be easily multiplied by 10 to evaluate 60 seconds (1 minute) of time. For example, if there are 7 QRS complexes within the 6-second interval, multiply 7 by 10 to arrive at a heart rate of 70 beats/min (Fig. 8-3-5).

Another method is to count the number of R waves in 30 large squares and multiply by 10. This gives an approximate heart rate. A more accurate method is to divide 300 by the number of large squares between R waves (e.g., 300 divided by 4 squares = 75).

 CLINICAL PEARLS

○ To accurately determine heart rate with the 6-second strip method, be sure to count only the complexes in which the entire QRS complex is present within the 6-second markers.

○ Regularity of heart rhythm is determined by measuring the R-R intervals for consistency. If intervals are consistent, then the rhythm is regular.

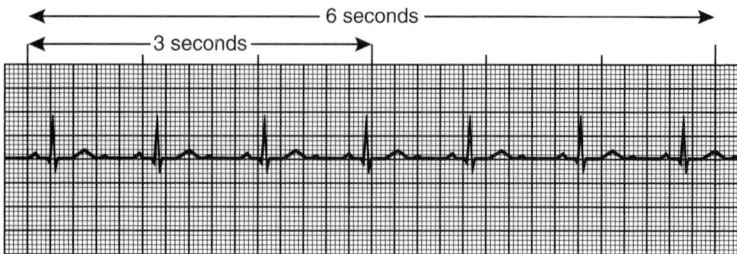

Figure 8-3-5. Six-second ECG strip.

○ A pulse should be felt for every QRS complex seen.

○ The atria rate may differ from the ventricular rate.

○ In a normal sinus rhythm, the P wave should precede the QRS complex, and there should be only one P wave to each QRS.

○ Dysrhythmias are treated only when they cause or are likely to cause symptoms.

Telemetry Monitoring

Section 4   Denise Thompson

OVERVIEW

Cardiac monitoring is no longer done exclusively in the critical care setting. Various ambulatory cardiac monitoring (telemetry) methods are now available. Nurses play a crucial role in teaching and monitoring patients with these devices. This section discusses the basics of ambulatory cardiac monitoring, as well as pacemakers and automatic implantable cardiodefibrillators (AICDs).

PRINCIPLES OF CARE

Ambulatory diagnosis and management of many abnormal cardiac rhythms can be done effectively and safely with the proper use of electrocardiography (ECG) monitoring devices. In ECG monitoring, the heart's electrical activity is picked up by external skin sensors (electrodes), and recorded on graph paper (see Section 3). Some indications for ECG monitoring that may be suited to outpatient evaluation and management include palpitations, syncope, antiarrhythmic drug therapy monitoring, and dysrhythmia surveillance in patients with already documented or potential abnormal heart rhythms.

Holter monitors and transtelephonic ECG monitors are used to diagnose palpitations and syncope and to monitor antiarrhythmic drug therapy. AICDs provide detailed information on the detection of abnormal rhythms and the therapies delivered. Pacemakers are used to treat patients with syncope from bradycardia and patients with documented or potential dysrhythmias.

Lead Placement

The term "leads" can refer to two situations. First, leads are the wires leading from electrodes to a monitor. In this case, the term is not capitalized.

Second, "Leads" with a capital "L" can refer to the different patterns of electrode placement. Electrodes are placed at different parts of the body to allow for different angles of the heart to be viewed on ECG paper. Electrode placement is standardized to avoid confusion in ECG interpretation. Patterns of electrode placement are discussed in Section 5.

Monitoring units are available with three or five electrodes. The five-electrode devices have the advantage of providing two views of the heart simultaneously. Most modern systems use five electrodes. Lead II and Lead MCL (modified chest lead) 1 are the most popular leads in telemetry monitoring.

In **lead II**, electrodes are placed in the right shoulder area under the clavicle (negative electrode), left shoulder area under the clavicle (ground electrode), and the left lower chest (positive electrode).

Chest Wall

| − | + |
| | G |

The electrical impulse normally produced in the heart starts in the SA node, which is approximately located in the right upper chest, and moves toward the left lower chest. Thus, when in Lead II, the electrical impulse is moving *from* the *negative* electrode *toward* the *positive* electrode. This produces positive (upward) wave deflections on the ECG paper. Lead II best depicts atrial activity and is very helpful in determining underlying rhythms.

In a five-electrode system, the additional electrodes are placed on the left lower chest and the fourth interspace, at the right sternal border.

Chest Wall

| − x | + |
| x | G |

In **lead MCL1**, the negative electrode is placed in the left shoulder area under the clavicle, the positive electrode is placed in the fourth intercostal space to the right of the sternum, and the ground can be placed anywhere, usually on the left lower chest.

Chest Wall

| + | − |
| | G |

In this case, the electrical impulse of the heart is now moving *from* the *positive* electrode *toward* the *negative* electrode. Because the electrical impulse is moving away from the positive electrode, negative (downward) wave deflections are recorded on the ECG paper. Lead MCL1 best depicts ventricular activity.

In a five-electrode system, placement is the same as for Lead II. With the five-electrode system, both Leads II and MCL1 can be observed simultaneously without the need to move electrodes around. Other Leads may also be observed simply by turning the dial on the telemetry box.

ECG electrodes have a jelly-filled sponge on one side that serves as a conductive material. Electrodes transmit best when in contact with direct skin. Avoid placing electrodes on bony prominences or hairy areas. If the skin is moist or soiled, clean the area with alcohol or soap and water. Allow the area to dry thoroughly before applying electrodes. Electrodes dry out in about 3 days, so change them at least that often.

DECISION-MAKING
Holter Monitoring

This technique provides continuous recording of the heart's electrical activity during the patient's normal routine. Essentially, the Holter monitor is a portable ECG machine with a memory. The patient wears an ECG recording device, which weighs about 2 lb, connected to electrodes placed on the chest for 24 to 48 hours without interruption. A shoulder strap or a special belt is provided to carry the recorder. The patient keeps a diary of activities, such as walking, eating, urinating, defecation, sexual activities, emotional upsets, and medication use. The patient is also instructed to record any symptoms such as chest pain, shortness of breath, dizziness, or fainting. The patient's diary is compared with the Holter recording to determine any correlation between the patient's symptoms and any underlying cardiac dysrhythmias.

Telemetry

Telemetry units use a small portable transmitter that is usually powered by a standard 9-volt battery and carried in a pouch. Telemetry allows continuous monitoring away from the bedside, while giving the patient freedom to move around and maintain a more regular routine. Lead wires connect the transmitter to standard ECG electrodes. Radio waves then transmit the heart's electrical activity to a central monitoring station. Cellular phones can disrupt this transmission; therefore, they are not permitted in or near telemetry units.

Home Telemetry
Home Monitoring Systems

A home monitoring system is capable of transmitting 12-lead ECG or 3-lead event recording with memory, blood pressure, and pulse oximetry data. The patient wears a monitor while in the home and downloads stored data directly into a base station in the home. The base station transfers the data via telephone line to a central monitoring station.

Transtelephonic Electrocardiographic Monitors

Transtelephonic electrocardiographic monitors (TEMs) transmit recordings by telephone via the conversion of ECG data to audio signals. The audio signals are received at a central station, where they are converted into a conventional ECG recording. TEMs may be worn continuously or applied only at the time of recording. A major strength of these recorders is the extended duration of monitoring that they allow. They may be carried or worn for weeks to months, depending on the indication. These devices also have a high degree of specificity, achieved by requiring the patient to activate the monitor at the time of perceived symptoms.

Pacemakers

Pacemakers are electronic devices that provide an alternative source of electrical power when the heart's own intrinsic pacemaker network fails. A pacemaker is designed to electrically stimulate the heart muscle, but if the heart muscle is irreversibly damaged, it cannot be stimulated. Modern pacemakers are completely programmable in terms of sensitivity, rate of firing, and refractory period.

Pacemakers may be used temporarily or permanently. Temporary pacemakers are used when conditions are thought to be transient and likely to improve. Transvenous, epicardial, and transcutaneous routes are used for temporary pacemaking. All temporary pacemakers have a programmable external pulse generator.

Permanent pacemakers are needed if the problem causes organic changes. With permanent pacemakers, the generator box is implanted either under the skin on the chest wall or abdominal wall, which requires a surgical procedure usually with a local anesthetic. A battery powers the generator. Depending on type, the battery may last for 10 to 40 years before needing to be replaced A pacing lead is threaded into a vein and into the heart, where the tip is placed.

Cardiac pacing can be accomplished in the right atrium, right ventricle, or both. If the atrial method is used, then a pacer "spike" immediately precedes the P wave. If the ventricular method is used, a pacer spike immediately precedes the QRS.

The most popular pacemaker today is a demand pacemaker. This type fires only when the patient's own rate falls below a preset level. A demand pacemaker set at, say, 70 beats/min will remain inactive as long as the patient's heart rate is above 70 and will fire only when the heart rate drops below 70. The patient should not feel the electrical impulse.

The pacemaker committee of the Inter-Society Commissions for Heart Disease Resources has developed a three-letter pacemaker code to describe the operation of the pacemaker.

- The first letter indicates the chamber in which pacing can occur: A, atrial pacing; V, ventricular pacing; or D, both atrial and ventricular pacing.
- The second letter indicates the chamber in which the sensing of intrinsic cardiac activity occurs: again A, atrium; V, ventricle; or D, both.
- The third letter indicates the mode of response to the intrinsic activity: I, inhibited; T, triggered; or D, both inhibited and triggered responses can occur.

An example of this code is "DDI," a mode of dual chamber pacing. The first "D" indicates that both the atrium and the ventricle are to be paced; the second "D" indicates that both the atrium and the ventricle are to be sensed; and the "I" indicates that if intrinsic activity is sensed, then the pacing impulse will be inhibited from discharging. Other common modes include, DDD, VVI, AAI, and VDD.

Automatic Implantable Cardiodefibrillator

An AICD is a fully implantable battery-operated system designed to recognize and terminate ventricular tachyarrhythmias that can cause sudden cardiac death (i.e., ventricular tachycardia and ventricular fibrillation). It consists of a lead system in contact with the myocardium and a pulse generator that delivers electrical shocks. It is inserted in the same fashion as a pacemaker. The battery lasts 5 to 10 years.

All AICDs can recognize and terminate potentially lethal dysrhythmias. However, modern AICDs provide other programmable features, including antitachycardia pacing, low-energy cardioversion, antibradycardia pacing, data storage, and diagnostic algorithms.

Similar to the pacemaker, the AICD also has an identifying code, developed by the North America Society of Pacing and Electrophysiology (NASPE) and the British Pacing and Electrophysiology Group (BPEG). Position one indicates the shock chamber; position two, the antitachycardia pacing chamber; position three, the tachycardia detection chamber; and position four, bradycardia detection chamber. Similar to pacing codes, activity is described by the letters A (atrium), V (ventricle), D (dual), and O (none).

Patients with AICDs should avoid strong magnetic fields, which may cause changes in the device. They should also avoid contact with high-power electricity sources (e.g., large motors, welding currents). Microwaves, hair dryers, shavers, and security detectors in the airport pose no dangers to the device. Cell phones held closer than 6 inches to the pulse generator can interfere with defibrillator operation. Normal function is restored once the telephone is removed.

CLINICAL PEARLS

o Electrodes need to be in contact with direct skin, not bony prominences or hairy areas.
o Electrodes should be changed every 3 days.
o Do not use cell phones in or near telemetry units, because they may interfere with the transmission of telemetry radio waves.
o A patient with an AICD should avoid strong magnetic fields.
o Cell phones may interfere with the operation of AICDs if held within 6 inches of the pulse generator.
o A patient with an AICD commonly feels a mild to strong electrical current when the device fires. Anyone touching the patient during the discharge may also feel a very mild shock.
o A patient with newly placed permanent pacemakers should remain in semisitting position (with the head of the bed at 30 degrees) for at least 12 hours postsurgery.
o A patient wearing a Holter monitor should not allow water from a shower or bath to beat on the electrodes.

12-Lead Electrocardiogram

Section 5   Becki Hodges

OVERVIEW

This section covers use of the 12-lead ECG as a tool to quickly assess for myocardial ischemia, injury, and infarction. It also discusses the expanded ECG with additional right-sided and posterior leads.

PRINCIPLES OF CARE

It is important to remember that the 12-lead or expanded 18-lead ECG is only one tool in the diagnosis of acute MI. The ECG gives helpful information in the assessment of ischemia, injury, and infarction; however, the patient's clinical presentation, assessment findings, and laboratory test data (including cardiac enzymes and troponin I levels) must all be considered.

Indications

The ECG is a graphic display of the electrical activity of the heart. An ECG is indicated for patients with history of heart disease, those with risk factors for heart disease, and those experiencing chest pain. The ECG is also a useful diagnostic tool in differentiating between bundle branch blocks, identifying dysrhythmias, identifying atrial and ventricular hypertrophy, and recognizing and locating ischemia, injury, and infarction. Other diagnostic tools, including echocardiography, stress testing, and nuclear imaging test, can play important roles in the assessment of the cardiac patient. This section addresses use of the ECG in patients who present with acute chest pain.

Lead Placement

Each lead in an ECG represents a different view of the electrical activity of the heart. In analyzing a 12- or 18-lead ECG, there are 12 or 18 different views or perspectives of the electrical activity.

To understand the ECG waveforms that represent one cardiac cycle, it is necessary to understand the physiology of electrical conduction within the heart. The process of depolarization begins in the SA node with the exchanges of electrolytes; the wave of depolarization continues via the intra-atrial pathways to the AV node, the bundle of His, the right and left bundle branches, and the Purkinje fibers to the ventricular cells. This process is an electrical event that can be documented via the ECG. The mechanical event that follows results in cellular contraction contributing to cardiac output (see Fig. 8-3-1).

The process of SA node firing and atrial depolarization is represented on the ECG by the P wave. Delay at the AV node is represented by the PR segment, and ventricular depolarization (the electrical activity from the bundle of His to the ventricular cells) is represented by the QRS complex. Repolarization, the electrical process in which the electrolytes (primarily sodium and potassium) return to the extracellular and intracellular compartments, respectively, is represented on the ECG by the ST segment and the T wave.

Atrial repolarization occurs at approximately the same time as ventricular depolarization and thus is hidden in the QRS waveform.

Analyzing an ECG for ischemia, injury, and infarction requires an understanding of the components of the QRS complex. The Q wave is the first negative waveform of the QRS complex. The R wave is the first positive waveform, and the S wave is the negative waveform that follows the R wave or the second negative waveform.

DECISION-MAKING
ECG Changes: Ischemia

MI is defined as necrosis (death) of myocardial tissue. When an MI occurs, a series of electrical events produce ECG changes. It is recognized that most MIs occur from thrombotic events superimposed on preexisting atherosclerotic plaques in the coronary arteries. As it narrows, the coronary artery is unable to supply the myocardium with sufficient oxygenated blood to meet the work demand of the heart, resulting in ischemia. This is known as angina.

Ischemia is seen on the ECG as an inversion of T waves. Because ischemia is a reversible process (once the work demand is diminished and oxygen supply meets demand), the ECG changes seen with ischemia are also reversible. Therefore, to document changes associated with ischemia, the ECG must be obtained during the angina attack.

ECG Changes: Injury

If a clot occludes the narrowed coronary artery, the myocardial cells that are most distal to the occlusion will first become ischemic. As time lapses and if blood supply to the ischemic area is not reestablished, the cellular changes of injury occur. Injury is also considered a reversible process; however, if there is not immediate intervention and reestablishment of blood supply to the oxygen-deprived myocardium, then infarction (cell death) will occur. An injury current is represented on the ECG by ST segment elevation.

Myocardial injury means urgency! A MI will occur if oxygen supply–demand balance is not restored.

ECG Changes: Myocardial Infarction

Once tissue death involves the entire thickness of myocardium from the endocardial surface to the epicardial surface, a Q wave develops on the ECG. The Q wave is the result of the development of an "electrical window." One of the basic principles of electrocardiography states that electrical waves of depolarization travel toward the positive electrode, producing a positive deflection on the ECG. When electrical waves of depolarization travel away from a positive electrode or toward a negative electrode, a negative deflection occurs on the ECG.

After myocardial tissue becomes necrotic, the cells in the area of damage do not depolarize in a normal fashion. Thus electrical activity travels around the necrotic tissue, but not through it. Therefore, any lead with a positive electrode that overlies the area of damage will interpret that electrical activity as traveling away from the positive electrode, thus forming a negative deflection or Q wave.

Lead Placement
Bipolar Leads

The ECG can be useful in locating the area of myocardial damage. A discussion of lead placement is essential to the understanding of which lead views which area of the heart. In a 12-lead ECG, 12 different views, or leads, provide information about the electrical activity of the heart as well as in a particular surface area of the heart. This section discusses the location of myocardial surface areas.

Leads I, II, and III are bipolar leads (having positive and negative electrodes). In lead I, the positive electrode is placed at the left shoulder with the negative electrode at the right shoulder. Lead I provides information about the left lateral surface of the myocardium. In lead II, the positive electrode is placed at the left foot with the negative electrode at the right shoulder. Lead II provides information about the inferior surface of the myocardium. In lead III, the positive electrode is placed at the left foot and the negative electrode is placed at the left shoulder. Lead III also provides information about the inferior myocardial surface.

Unipolar Leads

Leads aVR, aVL, and aVF are unipolar, with a positive electrode but not a negative electrode. The ECG averages the signal from the other leads for an

Table 8-5-1. Lead Placement

CHEST LEAD POSITION	LEAD PLACEMENT
V1	Fourth intercostal space to the right of the sternum
V2	Fourth intercostal space to the left of the sternum
V3	Midway between V2 and V4
V4	Fifth intercostal space, midclavicular line
V5	Same level as V4 at anterior axillary line
V6	Same level as V4 at midaxillary line

opposite pole. The positive electrode for lead aVR is placed at the right shoulder and, with the exception of a suspected right ventricular MI, this lead is ignored. Lead aVL is placed at the left shoulder and best views the left lateral surface of the heart along with lead I. Lead aVF is placed at the left foot and best views the inferior surface of the myocardium along with leads II and III.

Precordial Chest Leads

The precordial chest leads are also unipolar leads. Their placement is specified in Table 8-5-1. Appropriate placement of the electrode is essential for accurate recording of electrical signals.

Leads V1 through V4 view the anterior surface of the heart, and leads V5 and V6 view the lateral wall. Normal ventricular activation in the precordial chest leads causes a small R wave in V1 with R wave progression (i.e., R waves becoming taller with progression from V1 through V6).

Indicative Changes of Myocardial Damage (Fig. 8-5-1; see also Fig. 8-5-2)

Ischemia

An indicative change is defined as an expected change. T wave inversion represents the indicative change associated with ischemia. T wave inversion alone is a nonspecific diagnostic sign and should be considered with the clinical presentation of the patient. ST depression may be an earlier sign of

	ECG change	Myocardial Damage
A	T wave inversion	Ischemia
B	ST segment elevation	Injury (ST elevation indicates acuteness)
C	Q wave (0.04 sec) wide or ¼ height of the R wave	Infarction

Figure 8-5-1. Significance of ECG changes.

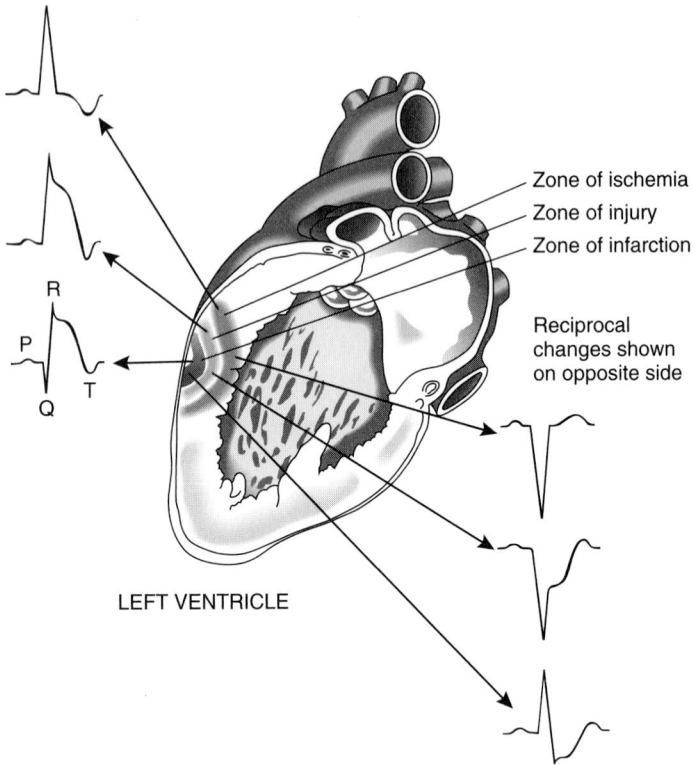

Figure 8-5-2. Zones of ischemia.

ischemia. Other causes of T wave inversion and ST depression include nonspecific changes, digitalis therapy, reciprocal changes, and posterior MIs. It is important to consider the clinical picture along with cardiac enzymes and other diagnostic information (see Figs. 8-5-1A and 8-5-2).

Injury

Injury results from prolonged ischemia with cellular damage. This is the acute phase of an MI. The cells are injured but not dead. Injury can be reversed if treated. The classic ECG sign of injury is ST segment elevation. Normally the ST segment is isoelectric and elevation is measured from the J point (the end of the QRS complex). ST segment elevation greater than 1 mm in the precordial leads can be considered significant.

When an injury current is recognized, medical intervention is essential to preserve myocardial tissue. Therapeutic intervention includes relieving chest pain, decreasing the workload of the heart, improving ventricular performance, and preventing complications. Patients should be assessed for contraindications to thrombolytic therapy and interventional approaches to therapy such as

Table 8-5-2. Interventions for Myocardial Infarction

INCREASE OXYGEN SUPPLY	DECREASE OXYGEN DEMAND
Increase oxygen extraction	• Decrease heart rate
Increase arterial oxygenation	• Decrease preload
Increase coronary blood flow	• Decrease afterload
	• Decrease contractility

angioplasty, stents, atherectomy, or coronary artery bypass grafting (see Figs. 8-5-1*B* and 8-5-2).

Infarction

If oxygenated blood flow is not restored, necrosis will result. Once myocardial necrosis has occurred, cell death (infarction) is irreversible. Early intervention is the key to preventing necrosis or limiting the amount of myocardial damage (Table 8-5-2). The ECG sign of transmural infarction is the development of a Q wave at least 0.04 second wide or one fourth of the height of the R wave (see Figs. 8-5-1C and 8-5-2).

Locating the Infarction

Indicative changes of myocardial ischemia, injury, and infarction (T wave inversion, ST segment elevation, and the development of pathologic Q waves) are evident in the leads that overlie the area of damage (Table 8-5-3). Reciprocal changes are opposite changes in opposite leads (upright T waves, ST segment depression, and tall R waves; see Fig. 8-5-2). When scanning an ECG, look for indicative changes. Consider the clinical clues and laboratory test information.

Expanded Electrocardiogram
True Posterior Myocardial Infarction

No leads in a normal 12-lead ECG directly reflect the posterior surface of the myocardium. Therefore, in a standard 12-lead ECG, if reciprocal changes

Table 8-5-3. Locating the Infarction

LOCATION	INDICATIVE LEADS (LEADS WHERE CHANGES OCCUR)
Inferior MI (usually involves the right coronary artery) (Fig. 8-5-3)	II, III, aVF
Anterior wall MI (usually involves the left anterior descending coronary artery) (Fig. 8-5-4)	V1–V4
Lateral wall MI (usually involves the circumflex branch)	I, aVL, V5, V6
Anterior-lateral MI (usually involves a significant portion of the left coronary artery system)	V1–V6
True posterior MI (may involve the circumflex or distal/posterior portion or RCA)	Tall R waves in V1 and V2 ST segment elevation in leads V7, V8, and V9

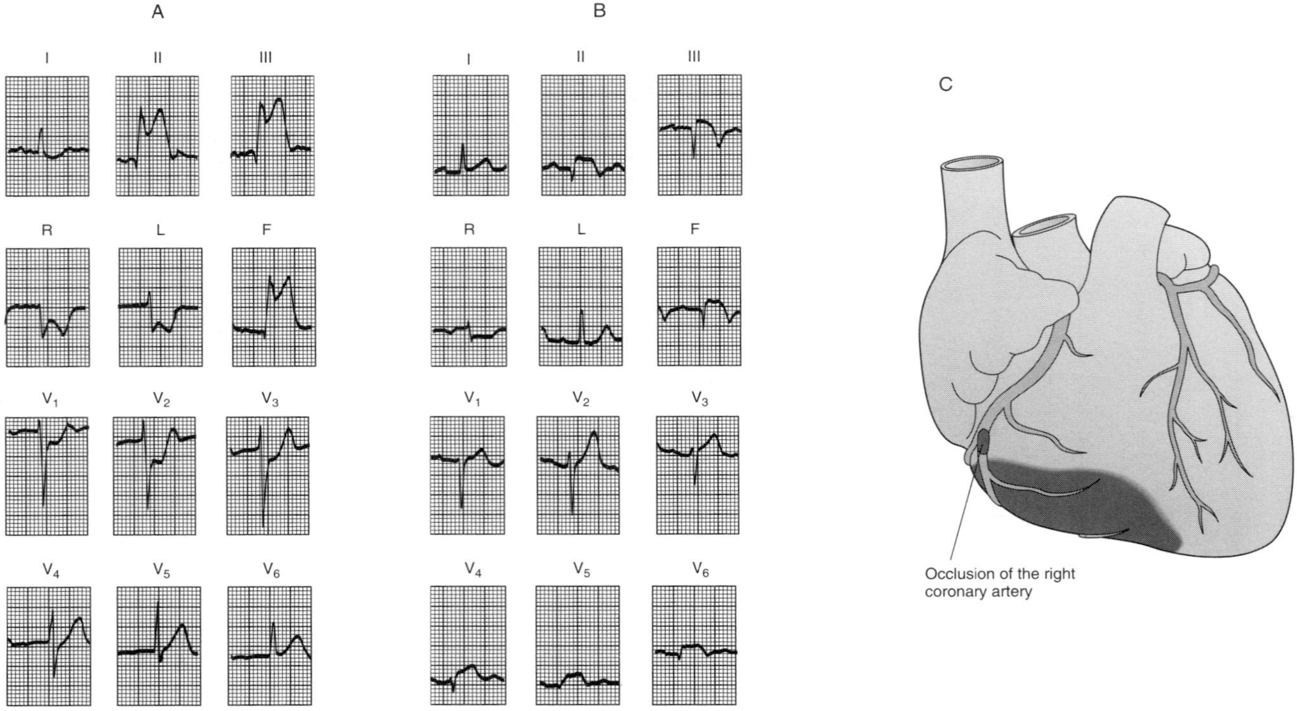

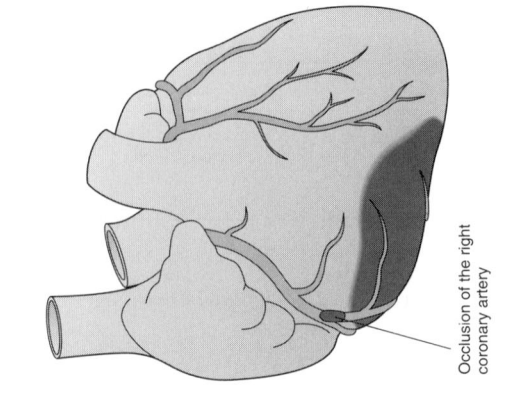

Figure 8-5-3. *A–C.* Inferior wall myocardial infarction. *A.* Acute inferior wall injury reflected in ST segment elevation occurring in leads II, III, and aVF. *B.* Infarction has occurred in the same patient 3 days later with the development of Q waves in the same leads. *C.* With occlusion of the right coronary artery, the inferior or underside of the myocardium is affected.

Occlusion of the right coronary artery

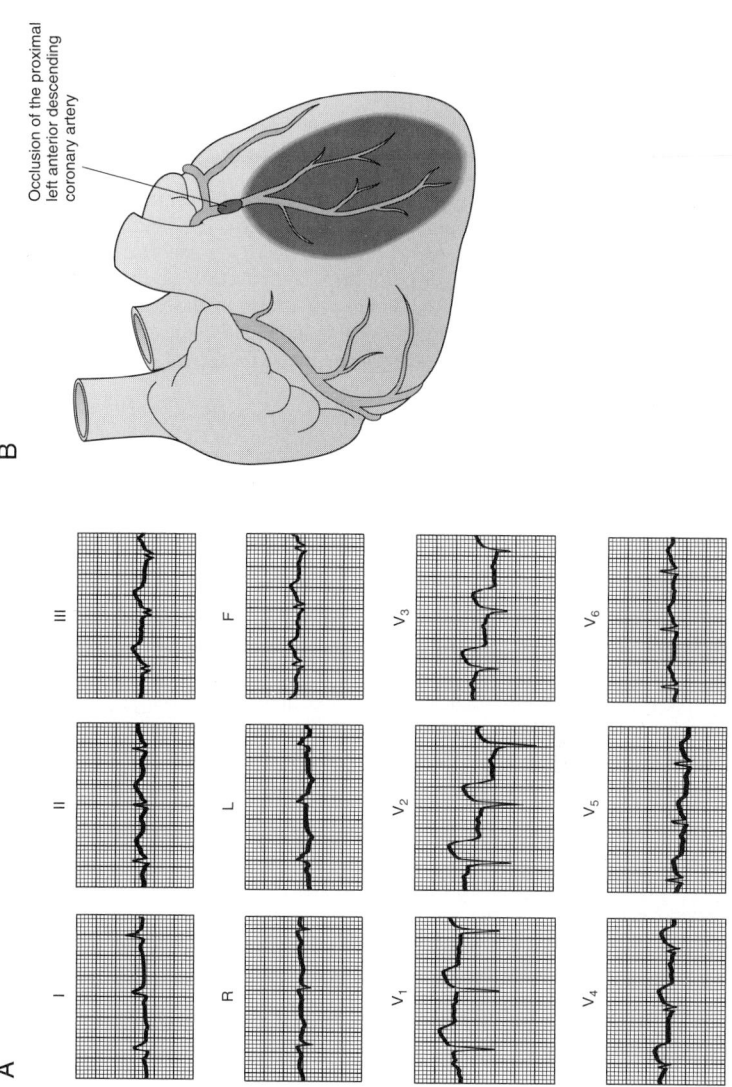

Figure 8-5-4. *A* and *B,* Anterior wall myocardial infarction. *A,* Acute anterior wall injury reflected in ST segment elevation in V_1 to V_4. *B,* With occlusion of the proximal left anterior descending coronary artery, the anterior portion or front side of the myocardium is affected.

217

are noted in the reciprocal leads (opposite changes in opposite leads) of the posterior surface, a true posterior MI should be suspected. The reciprocal leads for the posterior surface are leads V1 and V2. Reciprocal changes include tall R waves, ST segment depression, and upright T waves. Again, reciprocal changes should be considered along with clinical signs and symptoms and cardiac enzyme values.

If a posterior infarction is suspected, then the ECG can be expanded to include V7, V8, and V9 leads. Lead V7 is placed at the same level as V6 in the posterior axillary space. Lead V9 is placed at the fifth intercostal space next to the vertebral column. Lead V8 is placed at the fifth intercostal space between V7 and V9. Attach the cables from leads V4, V5, and V6 to the posterior leads V7, V8, and V9. Label the ECG paper for the changed leads to avoid confusion. These leads would then be reflective of the posterior surface of the heart and considered indicative leads. In the case of a true posterior transmural MI, these leads would show the indicative signs of ischemia, injury, and infarction (T wave inversion, ST segment elevation, and the development of pathologic Q waves).

Right Ventricular Infarction

Right ventricular infarctions should be suspected in patients who have sustained inferior wall MI and whose clinical picture appears worse than the ECG suggests (i.e., signs and symptoms of right ventricular failure without left ventricular failure).

Because no indicative leads in the standard 12-lead ECG look at the entire right ventricle, the ECG can be expanded to include V3R, V4R, V5R, and V6R leads. This is done by leaving the V1 and V2 electrodes in their standard position and moving the standard V4, V5, and V6 electrodes to the same position on the right side of the chest.

If a patient has right ventricular involvement, indicative changes are noted in the right ventricular leads (Table 8-5-4). It is important to obtain the right-sided leads early to guide appropriate clinical intervention. The ECG is also a useful diagnostic tool in assessing wall motion in areas of the heart that may have damage.

Evolutionary Changes in Acute Q Wave Myocardial Infarction (Transmural Infarction)

The first sign of oxygen supply–demand imbalance is the process of ischemia, resulting in inversion of T waves. Injury follows, with ST segment elevation, and necrosis results in the development of pathologic Q waves. As the balance of oxygen is restored to the myocardium, the ST segment returns

Table 8-5-4. Locating a Right Ventricular Infarction

LOCATION	INDICATIVE LEADS
Right ventricular MI (involves the right coronary artery)	ST elevation in V4R; be aware of the possibility of right ventricular infarction. With inferior MI, look for jugular venous distention with clear lung fields.

to baseline first, and eventually the T wave returns to the upright position. In a patient with a transmural MI, the Q wave is a permanent ECG indicator of myocardial damage.

Electrocardiogram Pitfalls

When scanning the ECG for ischemia, injury, and infarction, look for indicative changes in indicative leads. Always look for the acute process first (injury current produces ST segment elevation). There may or may not be pathologic Q waves or T wave inversion indicative of ischemia. Drugs, electrolytes, ventricular aneurysms, hypertrophy, and left bundle branch block patterns can confuse the interpretation.

Conclusion

An ECG can provide useful information in the assessment of a patient presenting with chest pain. Scan the ECG for an acute process. Look for ST elevation indicating an injury current. Look for changes of ischemia represented by T wave inversion. If a transmural MI has occurred, Q waves will develop on the ECG in the leads reflective of the area damaged.

No permanent ECG changes occur in a nontransmural MI.

In addition to the ECG changes, consider the clinical clues, which include patient presentation and laboratory values. Treat the patient and consider the pitfalls. Remember to consider other sources of ST segment elevation. Remember the evolutionary stages of an MI. Q waves persist indefinitely in transmural damage. Q waves may not be apparent early; their development may take hours to days. As the MI evolves, the ST segments return to normal first, then T waves revert to normal. Early intervention is the key to preserving myocardial tissue.

 CLINICAL PEARLS

○ Consider the patient's clinical presentation (e.g., chest pain, diaphoresis, color).
○ Look for indicative changes of acute MI on the ECG (i.e., ST segment elevation) first.
○ Look for ECG changes of ischemia.
○ Consider laboratory values that indicate MI (cardiac enzyme levels and troponin I).
○ Consider other causes of ST segment elevation (e.g., subepicardial injury, pericarditis, ventricular aneurysm); what are the clinical assessment findings?
○ Consider other causes of ST segment depression (e.g., subendocardial injury/ischemia, digitalis therapy, true posterior MI); what are the clinical assessment findings?
○ Look for permanent ECG changes of an old MI.
○ Remember that there are no permanent ECG changes in a non–Q wave infarction; rely on clinical clues, patient presentation, laboratory values, and ST segment elevation.
○ Treat the patient! Consider the drawbacks!

 RESOURCES

• Agency for Healthcare Research and Quality: 800-358-9295 or www.ahrq.-gov

- American Association of Critical Care Nurses: www.aacn.org
- American College of Cardiology: 800-252-4636, ext. 694, or www.acc.org/
- American Heart Association: 800-242-8721 or www.americanheart.org
- American Venous Forum: www.dvt-info.com
- National Heart, Lung, and Blood Institute Information Center: 800-592-8573 or www.nhlbi.nih.gov/
- Society of Vascular Nursing: www.svtnet.org
- Society of Vascular Technology: www.svtnet.org
- Vascular Disease Foundation: www.vdf.org
- Vascular Surgery Society: www.vascsurg.org
- Vascular Web: www.rogers3.com/vascular/

chapter 9

Decision-Making for Nutritional Alterations

Nutritional Assessment

Section 1   Patricia B. Graham

OVERVIEW

Nutritional status affects an individual's health throughout the lifespan. Nutritional needs vary from the premature infant to the elderly adult, and nutritional status is a key factor in any age group. Nutritional assessment involves collecting and interpreting data to identify nutritional risks and poor nutritional status.

PRINCIPLES OF CARE

Malnutrition is considered to be a problem in developing countries, but it also appears in industrialized countries and affects all socioeconomic groups. Malnutrition may be caused by inadequate intake of protein and calories (primary malnutrition) or by altered digestion, absorption, or metabolism (secondary malnutrition). Nutritional status may be affected by other factors, for example, inadequate financial resources, a particular problem in the elderly population. The current emphasis on thinness has caused many women to place themselves on restrictive diets that eliminate not only calories, but also essential nutrients. Eating disorders in adolescents and young women have been on the rise in recent years and are not always easily detected.

The nurse is in a key position to identify adequacies and inadequacies of nutrition through assessment by observation, history taking, and interpretation of laboratory test results. The nurse is then involved with planning care to improve or maintain nutritional status. This is done with the patient, setting short-term and long-term goals while taking into consideration food preferences, ethnic origin, age, and other factors. Planning also involves other members of the patient's health care team. The physician may be writing diet prescriptions, and in institutional settings the patient may meet with the dietitian. Patients who reside at home may need a referral to social services such as "Meals on Wheels." Nursing interventions include teaching, assistance with diet management, and monitoring. Evaluation is accomplished by follow-up on the patient's progress toward meeting goals.

At the same time, an increasing problem, particularly in the United States, is overnutrition. Twice as many children are overweight today when contrasted with children in the early 1970s. This is attributed to a decline in physical activities that burn calories. Research has shown that many Americans fail to meet even the minimum requirements for physical activity. Children today spend more hours watching TV than their parents did. In addition to the

221

passive nature of TV watching, viewers are bombarded with food ads at almost every station break, which often prompts viewers to get up and eat. Internet activities may involve hours of sitting when a child might otherwise be engaged in physical activity.

DECISION-MAKING

Because a significant number of hospitalized patients enter hospitals already malnourished or at risk for malnutrition, the Joint Commission on Accreditation of Health Care Organizations (JCAHO) specifies that every patient receive a nutritional assessment soon after admission. Nutritional assessment involves a considerable amount of data collection. The data are frequently organized using the acronym ABCD, where A is for anthropometrics, B is for biochemical tests, C is for clinical observation, and D is for diet evaluation and history.

Anthropometrics

These are body measurements that can provide a quick and easy means to assess nutritional status.

Direct Measurements

Height and Weight. Height and weight measurement are the most common direct measures and the nurse can consult a height/weight chart or growth chart to see if the patient falls within the norms for height to weight. Measurements should be accurate and standardized. Adults should be weighed on a beam balance scale, because bathroom scales are often inaccurate. Height is measured using a movable headpiece that is lowered until it touches the crown of the head. This headpiece is often attached to a beam balance scale.

Triceps Skinfold. Measurements are made with skinfold calipers at the midpoint between the acromial process and the olecranon of the nondominant arm. The layer of skin and subcutaneous fat, excluding the underlying muscle, is firmly pinched and measured. Three measurements are taken and the results averaged.

Calculated Measurements

Ideal Body Weight. Calculation of ideal body weight (IBW) is simple and requires no special training or tools. The procedure is as follows:

- Females: Allow 100 pounds for the first 5 feet of height; add 5 pounds for each additional inch over 5 feet. Calculations are based on average frame size; subtract 10% for a small frame, and add 10% for a large frame. By this method, a female with a small frame who is 5 feet, 9 inches tall has an IBW of 130.5 pounds.
- Males: Allow 106 pounds for the first 5 feet of height; add 6 pounds for each additional inch over 5 feet. Calculations are based on average frame size; subtract 10% for a small frame, and add 10% for a large frame. By this method, a male with a large frame who is 5 feet, 9 inches tall has an IBW of 176 pounds.

Body Mass Index. Many health professionals now consider body mass index (BMI) the most precise parameter for determining healthy body weight. The BMI is a height-to-weight ratio represented by the following formula:

$$BMI = \frac{weight\ (kg)}{height\ (m^2)}$$

Charts are available for quick reference. A quick method for determining BMI is shown in Figure 9-1-1. General guidelines for evaluating BMI are as follows (Fig. 9-1-2):

- BMI below 18.5: underweight
- BMI 18.5 to 24.9: normal
- BMI 25 to 29.9: overweight
- BMI 30 or above: obese

BMI has been related to mortality in both underweight and overweight persons. Mortality risks are shown in Figure 9-1-3.

Waist-to-Hip Ratio. This is an indicator of fat distribution. To calculate, divide the number of inches around the waistline by the number of inches around the hips. For instance: a woman with a 26-inch waist and 36-inch hips would have a waist to hip ratio of 26/36 or .72. Women with a ratio of 0.80 or higher and men with a ratio of 0.95 or higher are considered to be at greater risk for developing obesity related health problems.

Biochemical Data: Blood Tests
Blood Glucose

This test is performed to detect diabetes, pancreatic tumors, and hypoglycemia and to monitor glucose tolerance in adults. Blood glucose level is very significant in neonates, particularly those that are small for gestational age (SGA) and large for gestational age (LGA).

Serum Proteins

Serum proteins are used in nutritional assessment. They appear to be indicators of mortality and morbidity. Their use is limited, however, because values can shift for reasons other than malnutrition. Degrees of nutritional depletion are identified with albumin, prealbumin, and total lymphocyte count (TLC) as markers in Table 9-1-1.

Albumin. In the clinical setting, albumin has been the serum protein used as a standard for nutritional assessment in ill patients. During illness, albumin is redistributed into the extravascular space as part of the metabolic response to injury or illness. As a result, the serum albumin level decreases. This response can occur in 24 to 48 hours. In contrast, patients with anorexia nervosa, although nutritionally compromised, often maintain normal albumin levels until late in the course of the illness. In patients with chronic protein energy malnutrition (PEM), serum albumin level remains normal despite depletion of body proteins. For these reasons, current recommendations are that albumin be considered a marker of stress rather than overall nutritional status. Repeated

Table 9-1-1. Degrees of Nutritional Depletion

PARAMETER	DEPLETION		
	MILD	**MODERATE**	**SEVERE**
Albumin (g/dL)	3.4–3	3–2.5	<2.5
Prealbumin (mg/dL)	15–10	10–5	<5
Total leukocyte count (mm³)	1500–1200	1200–800	<800

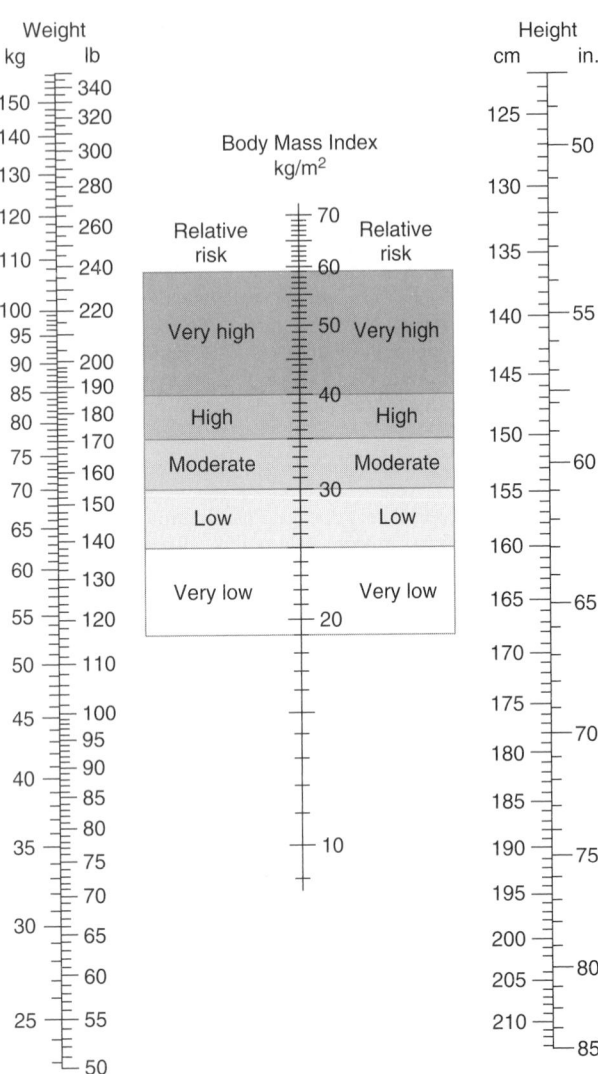

Figure 9-1-1. A nomogram for determining the body mass index (BMI). Lay a straight edge across the nomogram, and connect the patient's weight and height values. The point at which the straight edge crosses the BMI line is the patient's BMI.

studies have shown that low albumin levels correlate with longer hospital stays, medical complications, and increased mortality. Albumin degrades slowly, with a half-life of 20 days. For this reason also, albumin is not an ideal means of measuring day-to-day changes in nutritional status. Normal adult values are 3.5 to 5 g/dL. Cutoff points in albumin levels that distinguish severe malnutri-

Women

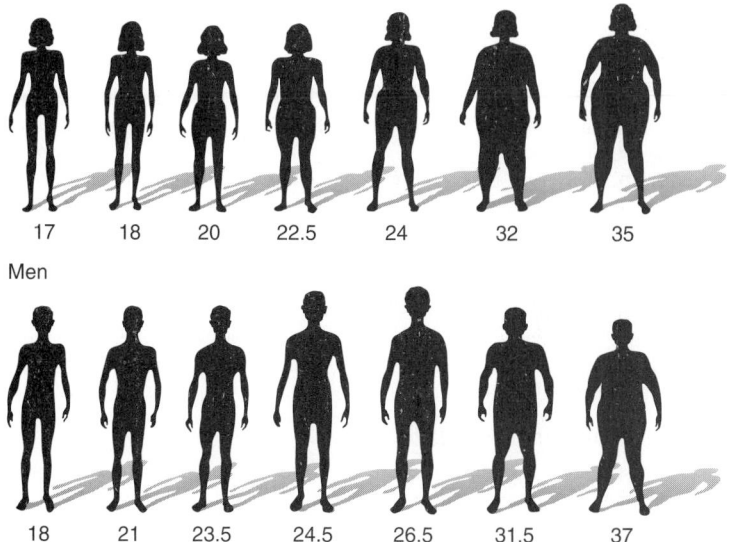

Men

Figure 9-1-2. Examples of various body mass indices in women and men.

Figure 9-1-3. Body mass index (BMI) and mortality. As shown, the optimal BMI lies between 18 and 25.

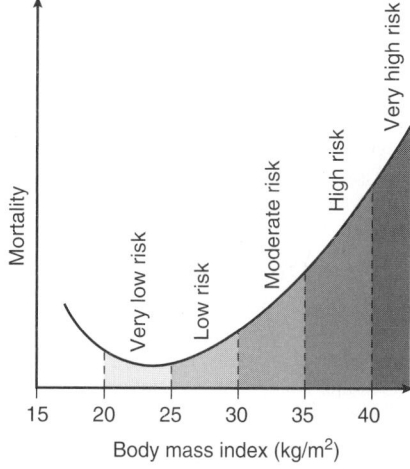

tion from moderate malnutrition can vary somewhat between institutions. Consult an institutional nutrition support person for clarification.

Prealbumin. Measurement of prealbumin is useful as an indicator of nutritional risk as well as a tool for monitoring short-term changes in nutritional status. In contrast to albumin, prealbumin has a half-life of only 1.9 days, which means that response to therapy can be assessed in as early as 2 days. Normal adult values are 17 to 40 mg/dL.

Total Lymphocyte Count. Immune status is also correlated with protein status and malnutrition, and may be useful in nutritional assessments. Lymphocytes are normally 25 to 33% of all white blood cells. Total lymphocyte count (TLC) is 1500 to 4000/mm³.

Transferrin. This is a blood protein that binds with iron and transports it throughout the body. Transferrin is frequently used as a marker of nutritional status. Levels are high when iron stores are low with concurrent normal protein levels, because much transferrin is circulating with no iron for it to bind with. Conversely, in malnutrition where all protein stores are low, transferrin (a protein) is also low. Decreased transferrin may be associated with malnutrition, liver disease, nephrotic syndrome, anemia, or neoplastic disease. Transferrin has a half-life of 7 to 8 days and is usually tested weekly. Normal adult values are 200 to 400 mg/dL.

Hemoglobin and Hematocrit

These test for anemia. Further testing should be done to determine the cause of the anemia. The many possible causes include dietary deficiencies of iron, vitamin B_{12}, or folate.

Cholesterol

This test assesses the risk of heart disease. A total cholesterol level above 200 mg/dL indicates increased risk. However, it is necessary to look at the entire profile, which includes high-density lipoproteins (HDLs) and low-density lipoproteins (LDLs). LDLs, often referred to as "bad cholesterol," carry two-thirds of the body cholesterol to the tissues. Values above 129 mg/dL are considered elevated. HDLs, "good cholesterol," help transport cholesterol from the tissues to the liver for catabolism and elimination. High serum levels of HDLs are considered protective against cardiovascular disease. The normal range is 30 to 65 mg/dL for males and 30 to 85 mg/dL for females.

Triglycerides range from 40 to 150 mg/dL. Levels increase after meals and during stress. Triglycerides have a direct correlation with LDLs and an inverse correlation with HDLs.

Clinical Observation

Clinical observation is usually the first opportunity to assess nutritional status. Does the patient look healthy? Does he or she appear alert and energetic with clear skin, shiny hair, and bright eyes? Many systems are affected by nutritional status, but it is possible to make a quick assessment by looking at the patient, particularly the skin, hair, and eyes (Table 9-1-2). It is sometimes possible to assume that an observation is a result of malnutrition when it is really something else. Dull, dry hair is a sign of protein depletion, but it can also result from overexposure to the sun. Clinical observation does not detect subclinical malnutrition that does not produce physical signs.

Table 9-1-2. Clinical Observations for Nutritional Assessment

BODY AREA	SIGNS OF GOOD NUTRITION	SIGNS OF POOR NUTRITION
General appearance	Alert and responsive	Listless, cachexic, easily fatigued
Weight	Normal for height, age, and build	Overweight or underweight
Hair	Shiny, firm	Dull, dry, brittle
Face	Uniform color	Dark color over cheeks and under eyes, facial edema
Eyes	Bright, clear, moist	Dry (xerophthalmia), pale membranes, dull or scarred corneas
Lips	Pink, moist	Swollen, puffy, stomatitis
Tongue	Red, surface papillae	Smooth, raw, hypertrophy or atrophy of papillae
Teeth	Straight, no caries	Caries, mottled (fluorosis), loose or missing
Gums	Firm, pink	Spongy, bleeding, swollen, inflamed
Glands	No enlargement	Enlarged thyroid (goiter), enlarged parotids
Skin	Smooth, slightly moist	Rough, dry, decreased subcutaneous fat, decreased surface temperature, bruises, petechiae
Nails	Firm, pink	Spoon-shaped, brittle, pale
Skeleton	Good posture	Poor posture
Musculature	Well developed, firm	Flaccid, poor tone
Skeletal	No malformations	Prominent bony structures: scapula, ribs, iliac crest, spinal vertebrae
Abdomen	Flat	Protruding
Nervous system	Normal reflexes	Decreased or absent ankle and knee reflexes, psychomotor changes, depression, sensory loss. Motor weakness, paresthesia
Cardiovascular system	Normal	Cardiomegaly, tachycardia, elevated blood pressure, body edema
Gastrointestinal system	No palpable organs or masses	Hepatosplenomegaly, diarrhea, flatulence
Renal system	Normal blood urea nitrogen and creatinine levels	Negative nitrogen balance, nocturia, decreased urine output

Modified from Christakis, G. (Ed.), Nutritional Assessment in Health Programs. Washington, DC: American Public Health Association.

Dietary History

A major component of nutritional assessment is the dietary history. A complete diet history, including cultural, economic, and medical factors along with food intake patterns, is desirable but not always feasible. Health professionals often face time constraints and need to find a method that is time-efficient and reliable. Because dietary data are usually acquired through self-report and depend on the patient's memory, they may not be accurate or reliable. For example, a patient asked for a 24-hour recall of all the foods eaten during that time period may not be able to recall specifics about intake, quantities, or portion size, particularly when very ill and/or confused. Underreporting or overreporting may occur either by accident or through attempts to make the diet appear more favorable. As a result, the diet over the previous 24 hours may be thought to be typical for this patient when it is not the case.

Another method of assessment is the food record. The food record tracks food intake for a selected period (3 to 7 days) through the use of a food diary and is considered a better means of assessment than the 24-hour recall. A problem with this method is that recordkeeping tends to deteriorate after the first few days.

A food-frequency checklist is another tool to provide additional diet history information. The list can help trigger memory and provide a more complete picture of food intake. The patient must indicate how often a food item is consumed from a list of commonly eaten foods. Portion sizes are not shown. Although this may make the food more acceptable to the patient, the accuracy of the tool is limited.

In essence, dietary data need to be as complete as possible, and the methods described here can improve accuracy when used in conjunction with one another. Use of a food diary in addition to the food frequency checklist can provide more information than either method used alone. Once the data are obtained, they can be evaluated through comparison with the food pyramid or fed into a computer program (see Resources) that analyzes the intake for deficiencies.

CLINICAL PEARLS

○ A quick indication of good nutrition is energy, clear skin, shiny hair, and bright eyes.
○ For detailed nutritional assessment, think ABCD.
○ Maintaining normal weight involves balancing food intake with physical activity.

Daily Requirements

Section 2   Patricia B. Graham

OVERVIEW

To educate the public about nutrition, nutritional information and recommended daily allowances need to be presented to a broad range of individuals in an understandable way. In the early 1940s, a chart of recommended daily allowances (RDAs) was developed to help plan and secure food supplies for national defense during World War II. Since then, RDAs have been revised and updated every 5 years.

Today, however, as new knowledge is acquired about the influence of certain nutrients on chronic diseases, the RDA is under revision to a new standard known as dietary reference intakes (DRIs). The new DRIs include four sets of values: (1) RDAs, (2) adequate intake, (3) tolerable upper intake levels, and (4) estimated average requirements (Table 9-2-1). An example of the current DRIs to date for adults is shown in Table 9-2-2. The remaining RDAs for adults not yet revised are shown in Table 9-2-3.

Although RDAs and DRIs provide basic information needed to meet daily

Table 9-2-1. Four Dietary Reference Intakes and Their Uses

REFERENCE VALUE	DESCRIPTION
Recommended daily allowances (RDAs)	Nutrient intake goals for individuals. RDA values are based on scientific data and aim to prevent deficiencies.
Adequate intakes (AIs)	Suggested nutrient intake targets for individuals. AI values are to be used wherever RDA values are lacking.
Tolerable upper intake values (ULs)	A guide to the risks of higher nutrient intakes.
Estimated average requirements (EARs)	Values used by scientists to evaluate intakes of populations and to generate new RDA values.

Adapted from Food and Nutrition Board, Institute of Medicine, National Academy of Sciences, Dietary Reference Intakes for Calcium, Phosphorus, Magnesium, Vitamin D, and Fluoride. (1997). *Nutrition Today*, **32**, 182–190.

nutritional requirements, the charts are lengthy and not easily interpreted by nonprofessionals. The U.S. Department of Agriculture first published its Food Guide Pyramid in 1992 (Table 9-2-4). Considered the official food guide for the United States, the pyramid is designed to illustrate dietary guidelines for Americans across a broad range of age and educational levels. The pyramid suggests a range of daily servings in four tiers of food groups, from the lowest number of servings to the highest number of servings. It addresses both undernutrition and overnutrition.

In addition to the food pyramid, dietary guidelines published by the U.S. Department of Agriculture specify the following:

Table 9-2-2. 1997–1998 Dietary Reference Intakes (DRIs)

RECOMMENDED DIETARY ALLOWANCES (RDAs)	MEN AGE 19 to >70	WOMEN AGE 19 to >70
Thiamin (mg)	1.2	1.1
Riboflavin (mg)	1.3	1.1
Niacin (mg-NE)	16	14
Vitamin B_6 (mg)	1.3 (age 19–50)	1.3 (age 19–50)
	1.7 (age >50)	1.5 (age >50)
Folate (μg DFE)	400	400
Vitamin B_{12} (μg)	2.4	2.4
Phosphorus (mg)	700	700
Magnesium (mg)	400 (age 19–30)	310 (age 19–30)
	420 (age >30)	320 (age >30)
Adequate intakes (AIs)		
Vitamin D (μg)	5 (age 19–50)	5 (age 19–50)
	10 (age 51–70)	10 (age 51–70)
	15 (age >70)	15 (age >70)
Pantothenic acid (mg)	5.0	5.0
Biotin (μg)	30	30
Choline (mg)	550	425
Calcium (mg)	1000 (age 19–50)	1000 (age 19–50)
	1200 (age >50)	1200 (age >50)
Fluoride (mg)	3.8	3.1

Table 9-2-3. Adult RDAs

AGE (years)	ENERGY (kcal)	PROTEIN (g)	VITAMIN A (µg RE)	VITAMIN E (mg)	VITAMIN K (µg)	VITAMIN C (mg)	IRON (mg)	ZINC (mg)	IODINE (µg)	SELENIUM (µg)
MEN										
19–24	2900	58	1000	10	70	60	10	15	150	70
25–50	2900	63	1000	10	80	60	10	15	150	70
51+	2300	63	1000	10	80	60	10	15	150	70
WOMEN										
19–24	2200	46	800	8	60	60	15	12	150	55
25–50	2200	50	800	8	65	60	15	12	150	55
51+	1900	50	800	8	65	60	10	12	150	55

Table 9-2-4. Groups and Servings of the Food Pyramid

TIER	GROUPS/SERVINGS	
1	Fats, oils, sweets Use sparingly Provides calories and essential fatty acids	
2	Milk, yogurt, and cheese 2 to 3 servings Provides protein, calories, calcium, riboflavin, vitamin B_6	Meat, poultry, fish, dry beans, eggs, and nuts 2 to 3 servings Provides protein, iron, niacin, thiamine, zinc, folic acid
3	Vegetables 3 to 5 servings Provides calories, folic acid, vitamins A and C	Fruits 2 to 4 servings Provides calories, vitamins A and C
4		Bread, cereal, rice, and pasta 6–11 servings Provides protein, calories, iron, niacin, thiamine

- Eat a variety of foods.
- Maintain or improve body weight and balance food intake with physical activity.
- Choose a diet with plenty of grain products, vegetables, and fruits.
- Choose a diet low in fat, saturated fat, and cholesterol.
- Choose a diet moderate in sugars.
- Use salt and sodium in moderation.
- Drink alcoholic beverages sparingly if at all.

To assist a patient in planning his or her daily intake, teach the patient how to read food labels. The Nutrition Labeling and Education Act was fully implemented in 1994, requiring mandatory labeling with few exemptions (coffee, tea, spices, and other foods that have little food value). The "% daily value" found on labels is based on a 2000-calorie/day diet. Food producers voluntarily list the daily value for protein by percentage, which is based on 50 g/day. Nutrition information is provided on a voluntary basis for fresh fruits and vegetables and some meats.

PRINCIPLES OF CARE

Energy is required for all body functions even when an individual is at rest. These functions include respiration, digestion, absorption, maintenance of body temperature, and many others. The sum of all of the internal workings of the body at rest is known as the basal metabolic rate (BMR). Interchangeable terms in general use include resting energy expenditure (REE), basal energy expenditure (BEE), and resting metabolic rate (RMR).

Calories provide the fuel for energy expenditure. Calories from food are supplied by different groups, including proteins, carbohydrates, and lipids or fats. Carbohydrates and fats are the main suppliers of calories. Protein and carbohydrates provide 4 kcal of energy per gram; lipids, 9 kcal/g.

Food Energy

Carbohydrates (sugars and starches) are the major sources of calories (energy) for most people. In the U.S. population, about 50% of the daily caloric intake comes from carbohydrates. In the population of developing countries, this figure is 80% to 90%. Current recommendations for carbohydrate intake include choosing a diet with plenty of vegetables and grain products and using sugars in moderation.

Fats, or lipids, are the most concentrated sources of energy and the second major source of calories for most people. Current recommendations are to limit fats to 30% of the daily caloric intake. They aid the absorption of fat-soluble vitamins and provide insulation, structure, and temperature control. In typical American diets, fats comprise about 37% of total daily calories.

Protein (Nitrogen Balance)

The largest portion of the body (excluding water) is made up of protein, often referred to as the body's "building block." Although protein plays a role in supplying calories for energy, its primary functions are to repair worn out, wasted, or damaged tissues and to build up new tissue. In addition, protein plays a role in water balance, metabolism, and the body's defense system. This nutrient is of particular concern during illness and injury because of its role in repair and in building new tissue.

Proteins found in foods have two classifications: complete and incomplete. Complete proteins contain all nine amino acids. These proteins are of animal origin and are found in meats, poultry, cheeses, and milk. Incomplete proteins are of plant origin and are missing one or more of the nine essential amino acids. Incomplete proteins are found in vegetables, legumes, nuts, grains, fruits, and vegetables. Proteins contain 16% nitrogen; therefore, nitrogen excretion can be used to indicate the adequacy of protein intake. Nitrogen excretion can be evaluated by urine urea nitrogen levels and creatinine clearance.

Zero nitrogen balance occurs when the amount of nitrogen taken in from protein sources is equivalent to the amount of nitrogen excreted. A *positive nitrogen balance* occurs when the amount of nitrogen taken in is greater than the amount excreted. This occurs during periods of rapid growth, in healing after trauma or surgery, or during pregnancy. A *negative nitrogen balance* occurs when the amount of nitrogen consumed is less than what is excreted. This occurs during illness, trauma, fever, major surgery, or burns and results in tissue wasting and weight loss. Negative nitrogen balance occurs in the absence of adequate amounts of calories from carbohydrates. When carbohydrate supplies are inadequate, proteins are converted to carbohydrates and used as fuel (calories) for energy rather than for the repair and maintenance of tissues. Thus if calories are inadequately supplied, protein wasting occurs.

Nutritionally depleted patients, or those under the stress of surgery or illness, should maintain a positive nitrogen balance. Table 9-2-5 lists protein requirements.

DECISION-MAKING
Determining Caloric Requirements

Food energy is measured in heat units, or kilocalories (kcal), commonly called calories. Determining an individual's daily caloric requirements is based on that individual's BMR or REE. A general method for calculating REE is as follows:

- Men: Allow 1 kcal per kilogram of body weight × 24 hours. (Convert

Table 9-2-5. Protein Requirements for Hospitalized Adults

PROTEIN (g/kg)	CLIENT STATUS
0.8–1.0	Healthy, non-stressed
1.2–1.6	Mild to moderate stress
1.7–2.0	Severe stress, burns
2.1–2.5	Severe burns, abnormal protein losses

Adapted from Ogawa, A.M. (1997). Macronutrients. In S.A. Shikova & G.L. Blackburn (Eds.), *Nutrition support: Theory and therapeutics* (pp. 54–65). New York, Chapman and Hall.

weight in pounds to kilograms by dividing by 2.2.) Thus, for a 150-lb (68-kg) man, 68 kg $\times$ 1 kcal $\times$ 24 hr = 1632 kcal/day are required to maintain basic functions.
- Women: Allow 0.9 calories (kcal) per kg of body weight per 24 hours. Thus, for a 150-lb (68-kg) woman, 68 kg $\times$ 0.9 kcal $\times$ 24 hr = 1469 kcal/day are required to maintain basic functions.

The stress of illness places increased physiologic demands on hospitalized patients. The Harris-Benedict equation is the classical method of estimating the REE in these patients. This equation takes into account height and age factors in addition to weight and sex. Stress and illness factors may also be added in. By the Harris-Benedict equation, taller persons have a higher REE and older persons have a lower REE:
- Men: REE = 66.5 + (13.8 $\times$ weight in kg) + (5 $\times$ height in cm) $-$ (6.76 $\times$ age). For a 150-lb (68-kg), 5'10" (178 cm), 35-year-old man:
  66.5 + (13.8 $\times$ 68) + (5 $\times$ 178) $-$ (6.76 $\times$ 35)
  66.5 + 938 + 890 = 1894 $-$ 237 REE = 1657 kcal.
- Women: REE = 655 + (9.56 $\times$ weight in kg) + (1.85 $\times$ height in cm) $-$ (4.68 $\times$ age). For a 150-lb (68-kg), 5'8" (173 cm), 35-year-old woman:
  655 + (9.56 $\times$ 68) + (1.85 $\times$ 173) $-$ (4.68 $\times$ 35)
  655 + 650 + 320 = 1625 $-$ 163.8 REE = 1461 kcal.

A useful guideline for calculating energy requirements in hospitalized patients is given in Table 9-2-6. Many health professionals believe that this simplified formula is preferable to the Harris-Benedict equation, which can be inaccurate in the individual patient.

Table 9-2-6. Energy Requirements for Hospitalized Adults

Kcal/kg OF BODY WEIGHT	INJURY/ILLNESS/CONDITION
25–29	Mild stress, such as uncomplicated surgery, prolonged illness
30–35	Moderate stress, such as sepsis, penetrating trauma, burns on <30% of body surface area
35–40	Severe stress, such as skeletal trauma, burns on >30% of body surface area

Adapted from Ogawa, A.M. (1997). Macronutrients. In S.A. Shikova & G.L. Blackburn (Eds.), *Nutrition support: Theory and therapeutics* (pp. 54–65). New York, Chapman and Hall.

Determining Protein Requirements

Based on the RDA for protein (see Table 9-2-5), a healthy adult weighing 150 lb (68 kg) requires 54 to 68 g/day of protein.

Vegetarians must plan their diet carefully to ensure that they receive adequate amounts of protein. Some vegetarians are allowed dairy products and eggs (lacto-ovo vegetarians). A second group (lacto-vegetarians) includes dairy products from animal sources. The third group (vegans) uses no animal foods. Because their entire diet comes from plant sources, vegans need to select combinations of foods that will provide complete proteins. Rice and beans is an example of an appropriate combination of incomplete proteins.

Determining Fluid Intake

Adults consume 2% to 4% of their total body weight in fluids each day. The average daily intake for a healthy adult is 2600 mL. Recommendations for daily fluid needs are difficult to establish, because they can vary based on other conditions, heat, humidity, exercise levels, and other factors. In general, 2 to 3 L/day (8 to 12 cups) are recommended. Fluid intake should be balanced by fluid loss (urine output). Fluid loss by other means (perspiration, respiration, feces) is approximately balanced by fluid intake through other means (food, oxidation).

A variety of fluids in addition to water may be ingested to meet daily fluid requirements, but persons should be encouraged to drink nutritious fluids such as juices and reduced-fat milk. Coffee and tea are acceptable but have no real food value. Soft drinks should be limited, because they contain "empty" calories (i.e., high sugar content, but no other nutrients).

Other Influences on Nutrition

Planning balanced diets for individuals requires an understanding of ethnic origin, geographical location, religious beliefs, and personal preferences that govern food choices. For example, Orthodox Jews follow specific dietary laws regarding meat and dairy products, Hindus are vegetarians, and Muslims cannot eat pork. First-generation Americans are likely to prefer foods of their ethnic origin; others may serve the ethnic and traditional dishes only on holidays. Food preferences are highly individualistic and may vary widely within the same ethnic group. Orthodox Christians follow specific dietary laws that include periods of fasting.

Finance is another factor that has a major impact on food choices. This is a problem particularly for elder adults living on fixed incomes, who often must make choices between food and medicine. Dietary deficiencies frequently include protein and fiber because of the relatively high cost of meats, fruits, and vegetables. Food selections are likely to include large amounts of soups and other canned foods that have limited nutritive values. When feasible, persons on limited incomes should be encouraged to consult a nutritionist to help them to find ways to get the most value for their food dollar.

 CLINICAL PEARLS

○ Food energy is measured in heat units called kilocalories (kcal), commonly called calories.

○ A positive nitrogen balance should be maintained during periods of stress and illness.

○ Serum protein levels should be assessed when performing a nutritional assessment.

○ Patients needing increased fluids frequently require more than 3 L/day (125 mL/hr).

Diets and Supplements

Section 3   Patricia Graham

OVERVIEW

Eating is a pleasurable human experience across all age groups and cultures. Food is a part of celebration of major life events (e.g., weddings, births, graduations) and of all major American holidays. Many people report a gain of 5 to 10 lb between Thanksgiving and New Year's Day. If this happens each year and there is no effort to take the weight off, an individual can become obese over the years.

Ideally, an individual should eat a basic healthy diet all of the time, allowing for the celebration times by eating less at the next meal or the next day. However, increasing numbers of Americans are becoming obese, and there are major concerns about their health status.

Studies have shown that obese individuals who lose even small amounts of weight are likely to improve their health by reducing the risk of conditions associated with obesity. Weight loss provides greater ease in performing daily activities. Consequently, individuals who lose weight are likely to become more physically active, which further improves health. Although there are multiple approaches to weight loss (e.g., diet, physical activity, behavior modification, drug therapy, and gastric surgery), the most common weight loss method is dieting.

Unfortunately, more than 90% of weight loss programs are unsuccessful. Many individuals lose and gain hundreds of pounds in a series of failed attempts to keep the weight off. Quick weight loss programs and "fad" diets do not produce a change in eating habits, so when the individual stops the diet, he or she is likely to return to previous unhealthy eating habits.

Despite claims that low-carbohydrate, high-fat, low-protein diets are the fastest way to lose weight, the method that has been shown to work best over time is to eat a well-balanced diet while limiting serving size and caloric intake. This approach allows the individual to develop new eating habits that he or she can maintain after reaching the desired weight.

Diets may also be therapeutic. Following a specific dietary regimen may be beneficial in certain conditions. For example, persons with diabetes usually need to follow a diabetic diet, and persons with certain kidney problems may require a renal diet.

PRINCIPLES OF CARE

The 1995 Dietary Guidelines emphasize the importance of eating a variety of foods and balancing food intake with physical activity to maintain or improve weight. Six principles are useful to remember when diet planning, whether the purpose of the diet is to maintain nutrition, to lose weight, or as diet therapy for a physiologic problem or illness. These principles are:

- Adequacy: provides all essential nutrients, fiber, and energy to maintain health and body weight
- Balance: provides foods of various types to ensure distribution of nutrients
- Calorie control: management of food intake
- Nutrient density: a measure of the nutrients that a food provides relative to the energy that it provides
- Moderation: enough, but not too much, of a dietary constituent
- Variety: using different foods to obtain the same nutrients on different occasions

An adult who wishes to follow a healthy diet should first determine his or her daily caloric requirement, then use the food pyramid (see Section 2) and other daily allowance recommendations (see Section 2) to ensure adequate nutrient intake from all food groups.

DECISION-MAKING
Weight-Reduction Diets

Four types of diets are commonly used in weight-reduction plans.

Balanced Energy-Deficit Diets. These diets provide 1200 kcal/day and are nutritionally adequate when the minimum number of servings in the food pyramid are included. Because they normalize food patterns, these diets have the potential for permanently changing food habits. The diets are generally safe and have no adverse effects. Calories may need to be adjusted upward for very active individuals.

Decreased Dietary Fat Diets. In these diets, dietary changes to reduce fat are introduced gradually to prevent a sense of deprivation. This approach can be important in maintaining weight loss.

Low-Calorie Diets. These diets provide 800 to 1200 kcal/day. They may use regular foods or commercial products designed as meal replacements.

Very Low Calorie Diets. These modified fasts are used in hospitals and clinics where patients can be under medical supervision. These programs are usually restricted to persons who are moderately to severely obese and have been unsuccessful with other approaches. Rapid weight loss occurs, but long-term maintenance of the loss is limited.

Fad Diets

The emphasis on weight loss and dieting has caused many persons to turn to fad diets. These diets often promise dramatic weight loss and may limit one or more food groups or place emphasis on a particular food. This discussion of fad diets is not meant to suggest endorsement; the information is provided because health professionals are often asked about these diets and wish to be informed about them.

The *Atkins diet* is a ketogenic diet that restricts carbohydrate consumption while allowing an unlimited quantity of protein. The theory behind the diet is that rather than burning carbohydrates as fuel, the body burns stored fat through ketosis. According to its originator, limiting carbohydrate intake allows this mechanism to work. Once a person achieves his or her weight loss goals, he or she can move on to a carbohydrate intake level of 30 to 90 g/day. This amount is still significantly lower than the American Heart Association's (AHA's) recommendation of 300 g/day. This diet is not endorsed by the American Dietetic Association or the AHA.

Therapeutic Diets

Cardiovascular

Hypertension (high blood pressure) is one of the major health care problems in the United States today. This condition is a major predictor of an individual's risk for circulatory problems such as stroke, heart disease, peripheral vascular disease, and renal insufficiency. Hypertension can be influenced by nutritional factors that reduce the risk of illness.

Obesity, sodium intake, and cholesterol have been shown to be major contributors to hypertension. At the same time, mineral deficiencies (e.g., potassium, calcium, magnesium) have been seen as possible causes of hypertension. There is increasing evidence that omega-3 polyunsaturated fatty acids help to lower blood pressure. The primary source of these fats is cold-water fish.

Patients with hypertension should reduce their intake of sodium chloride from 150 to 100 mEq/day, which is less than 2.3 g of sodium. The average American consumes 4 to 6 g/day. Approximately 75% of this intake comes from processed foods. Reducing sodium intake is usually accomplished by not cooking with salt and avoiding table salt.

Reading food labels can help consumers make wise selections. Products with words like "health," "healthy," or "healthful" on their labels often have reduced calorie, fat, and sodium levels. All of these reductions can be beneficial for persons with hypertension.

Diets that contribute to lowering blood pressure also contribute to preventing atherosclerosis. Atherosclerosis, the formation of plaque within the arterial wall, is the most common cause of arterial obstruction. Serum cholesterol levels are often elevated in patients with atherosclerosis. Table 9-3-1 lists classification of serum cholesterol levels and recommendations for intervention.

Dietary intervention involves fat and cholesterol restriction. The AHA's step 1 diet recommends a total daily fat intake of less than 30%, with less than 10% coming from saturated fats, up to 10% from polyunsaturated fats, and 10% to 15% from monounsaturated fats. Cholesterol is limited to less than 300 mg/day. If the cholesterol level does not drop significantly, the patient may be referred to a dietitian for placement on a step 2 diet. The step 2 diet limits saturated fat to less than 7% of total calories and cholesterol to less than 299 mg/day.

Diabetic Diets

Several goals are involved in planning diets for diabetics. These include:
- Maintenance of near-normal blood sugar levels
- Achievement of optimal serum lipid levels: low-density lipoproteins (LDLs) below 130 and triglyceride level below 200
- Maintenance of blood pressure below 140/90 mm Hg
- Adequate caloric intake based on individual needs

Table 9-3-1. Classification of Serum Cholesterol Levels

SERUM CHOLESTEROL LEVEL (mg/dL)	CLASSIFICATION	INTERVENTION
<200	Optimal level	Provide dietary information. Determine cholesterol levels again within 5 years.
200–239 with no coronary artery disease (CAD) or risks for CAD	Borderline high blood cholesterol	Provide dietary information. Determine cholesterol levels again within 1 year.
200–239 with CAD or risks for CAD; 240 or higher with or without CAD or risks for CAD	High blood cholesterol	Obtain serum low-density lipoprotein (LDL) and high-density lipoprotein (HDL) cholesterol levels. If LDL is 130–159 mg/dL, advise the patient to follow a fat-modified diet, and repeat LDL annually. If LDL is 160 mg/dL or higher, provide dietary therapy and frequent monitoring.

From Ignatavicius, D.D., Workman, M.L., and Mishler, M.A. (1999). *Medical-surgical nursing across the health care continuum* (3rd ed.), Philadelphia, W.B. Saunders.

- Prevention and treatment of chronic complications of diabetes (e.g., renal disease, cardiovascular disease)
- Improvement of overall health through optimal food choices

Although diabetic diets should be individualized and planned by a dietitian, some general principles may be followed. Most diabetic diets use the exchange system. This system is based on three food groups: carbohydrates, protein, and fats. The patient is given a list of the items from each food group that may be eaten at a meal or a snack. For example, in the carbohydrate group, the patient has the choice of 1 slice of bread, half of a bagel, half of a hamburger bun, half cup of corn, or half cup of mashed potatoes. Each of these choices has the same nutrient content and can be substituted for various meals. Studies have shown that diets based on the exchange list produce predictable blood glucose responses.

Recommendations for diabetic diets are as follows:
- 10% to 20% of daily calories from protein
- 45% to 60% of daily calories from carbohydrates
- 30% or less of daily calories from fats

High-Fiber Diets

Current recommendations for daily fiber intake for the general population are 20 to 35 g/day. High-fiber diets help to maintain intestinal health and may aid weight loss and regulation of blood lipids. Persons with constipation and diverticulosis benefit from high-fiber diets. Table 9-3-2 lists foods high in fiber.

Low-Residue Diets

Low-residue diets are used in situations where the intestinal tract is narrowed by inflammation or gastrointestinal (GI) motility is slow. They are often used before and after GI surgery. Persons at risk for small bowel obstruction or those with inflammatory bowel disease may benefit from low-residue/low-fiber

Table 9-3-2. High-Fiber Foods

Whole-grain breads and cereals	Whole wheat, pumpernickel, rye, wheat germ, bran, bulgur, oatmeal, brown or wild rice
Fruits	Apples, berries, figs, papaya, prunes, pears
Vegetables	Artichokes, broccoli, brussels sprouts, raw carrots, chicory, kohlrabi, legumes, shiitake mushrooms, sweet potatoes, rutabagas, turnips, yams
Other	Peanut butter, popcorn

From Cataldo, C.B., DeBryne, L.K., and Whitney, E.N. (1999). *Nutrition and diet therapy: Principles and practice* (5th ed.). Belmont, CA: Wadsworth.

diets. Low residue is the same as low fiber, except that milk and milk products are restricted in low-residue diets. Milk is low in fiber but may contribute to fecal mass and thus is limited in low-residue diets. Long-term use of a low-residue diet necessitates nutritional supplements to supply nutrients normally obtained from fruits and vegetables.

Lactose-Free Diets

Lactose intolerance results from a deficiency of the digestive enzyme lactase, which splits lactose into glucose and galactose in the small intestine. When lactose absorption is blocked in the small intestine, the intestinal osmotic pressure is increased, resulting in cramps, distention, and diarrhea. Lactose-restricted diets are highly individualized, because people vary in their tolerance of this substance. Some persons can tolerate up to 2 cups of milk per day. Cheese is often well tolerated. Milk and milk products treated with lactase are available. Persons with lactose intolerance are at risk for calcium and vitamin D deficiencies and may require supplementation.

Neutropenic Diets

Patients who are immunosuppressed need to be careful with the foods that they eat. These patients need to eat a low-bacteria diet and avoid salads, raw fruits and vegetables, undercooked meat, pepper, and paprika.

Postgastrectomy Diets

Gastrectomy involves partial or total removal of the stomach. Several types of procedures may be done to treat ulcers, cancer, or marked obesity. After gastric surgery, the patient is maintained on nothing-by-mouth (NPO) status with a nasogastric (NG) tube in place until bowel sounds return. Once the tube is removed, the diet begins, starting with small amounts of clear liquids and progressing to larger amounts and then to other liquid and pureed foods. The patient may then be placed on a postgastrectomy diet.

The purpose of this diet is to control the dumping syndrome that may occur when food passes too quickly into the jejunum. At this point, the partially digested food is highly concentrated. As fluids move in to dilute the concentration, the volume of circulating blood diminishes rapidly, creating physical symptoms such as vertigo, tachycardia, syncope, sweating, and diarrhea within 30 minutes after eating. Dietary adjustment in which concentrated sweets are avoided and liquids are limited can help alleviate the symptoms. As time goes on, most persons are able to add some sweets and more liquids.

Renal Diets

Dietary adjustment in renal disease depends on the degree of renal impairment. Chronic renal insufficiency can result from various disorders, including diabetes and cardiovascular disease. Chronic renal failure is a syndrome of progressive and irreversible kidney injury. When renal function declines gradually, 90% to 95% of the nephrons are destroyed before disease becomes evident. Acute renal failure may happen suddenly as a result of disease or injury. When renal deterioration is sudden, failure may occur with the loss of 50% of functioning nephrons.

Clinical symptoms of renal failure can affect almost all body systems. As function diminishes, the ability to maintain vital metabolic balances also diminishes. There is an interference with water and electrolyte balance, particularly sodium and potassium. Nitrogenous wastes (urea and creatinine) are retained. Fewer red blood cells are produced, resulting in anemia. Decreased blood flow to renal tissue results in hypertension, which causes cardiovascular damage that can result in further deterioration of the kidneys. As the disease progresses, anorexia, weight loss, diarrhea, vomiting, and internal bleeding may be seen. Neurologic symptoms include lethargy and, in later stages, coma and convulsions. Renal failure may be treated with hemodialysis, which removes waste products and restores water and electrolyte balance.

Renal failure is managed in part by dietary intervention. The aims of dietary intervention are to:
- Maintain optimal nutritional status
- Correct electrolyte imbalances
- Reduce protein breakdown
- Prevent dehydration
- Postpone the ultimate need for dialysis
- Retard the rate of renal failure

Renal diets are individualized based on the degree of renal insufficiency present. Dietary restrictions vary for patients undergoing dialysis. Close monitoring of electrolytes, blood pressure, and urine output are essential when planning dietary interventions. Dietary protein intake should be just enough to maintain tissues; excessive protein intake can contribute to renal damage.

Research has indicated that a protein-restricted diet prevents some of the symptoms associated with chronic renal failure and may help preserve kidney function. Guidelines for protein limitation are based on the patient's glomerular filtration rate (GFR). A patient with a severely reduced GFR who is not on dialysis is usually allowed 0.55 to 0.60 g of protein per kg of body weight. This is equivalent to 40 g/day of protein for a 150-lb adult. Patients on diets that limit protein to 40 g or less require long-term follow-up by a nutritionist because of the risk of malnutrition. Patients on dialysis require more protein because of losses from the dialysis. These patients are allowed a protein intake of 1 to 1.2 g/kg of body weight. Patients on peritoneal dialysis require 1.2 to 1.4 g/kg because of the loss of protein with each exchange.

Sodium restriction is often necessary, particularly if edema and hypertension are present. Dietary intake of potassium should be limited for patients with advanced renal failure. Patients need to be advised to read food labels, to avoid using salt substitutes, and to check the potassium content of other seasonings. Hyperphosphatemia occurs as the kidneys fail to clear excess phosphorus from the blood. Therefore, phosphorus intake must be limited in patients with renal failure.

Dietary Supplements
Oral Supplements

Oral nutritional supplements are supplied as liquids, powders, and puddings in a variety of flavors. Supplements are intended to add to a diet to provide additional nutrients that are not obtained through normal dietary intake. These supplements may be used in conjunction with a full liquid diet or to meet increased dietary requirements following surgery or stress. One serving may supply 25% to 50% of recommended daily requirements. Supplements are available to provide full nutritional support via tube feedings. See Section 5 for a full discussion on enteral nutrition and tube feeding.

A wide variety of supplements are currently available. Some formulas provide total nutritional support (e.g., Compleat Regular Formula), whereas others provide partial support. The supplements are manufactured by pharmaceutical companies. Consult a current *Physician's Desk Reference* (*PDR*) or the manufacturer's web page for nutritional content of an individual product.

Vitamin, Mineral, and Herbal Supplements

Severe vitamin deficiencies are rare in the United States and other developed countries. However, many persons self-prescribe vitamins believing that their diet may be deficient or that vitamins will give them increased energy, enhanced strength, or increased ability to cope with stress. Supplementary vitamins and/or minerals are indicated in some conditions, including pregnancy and lactation, burns, and multiple injuries. Persons who self-prescribe vitamins should be careful not to exceed recommended daily amounts because of the potential for adverse reactions. Unlike drugs, these dietary supplements are not regulated by the government. Consumers should be advised to read all labels carefully and to consult a health professional (i.e., nurse, nutritionist, pharmacist, or physician) as needed.

In recent years, herbal supplements have received much attention. For example, St John's wort has been recommended as a remedy for depression; gingko biloba is said to improve circulation; and feverfew may help to reduce the pain of migraine headaches. Studies have revealed adverse effects associated with some of these remedies. For example, feverfew and garlic have been shown to increase bleeding time, particularly when taken in conjunction with anticoagulants; St John's wort may potentiate the effects of central nervous system depressants; and ephedra has been linked to numerous adverse events, including deaths. As with other supplements, consumers should be advised to consult a health professional before initiating self-treatment.

CLINICAL PEARLS

- In addition to blood glucose, diabetic diets should achieve optimal serum lipid levels of low-density lipoproteins (LDLs) below 130 and triglyceride level below 200 mL/dL.
- Patients with neutropenia should not eat salads, raw fruits and vegetables, undercooked (rare) meat, pepper, or paprika.
- Patients in end-stage renal failure are generally on a low-protein, low-potassium, low-sodium, and low-phosphate diet.

Parenteral Nutrition

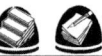

OVERVIEW

Parenteral nutrition (PN), also called total parenteral nutrition (TPN), consists of amino acids, dextrose, electrolytes, minerals, and trace elements. Lipid infusion, although packaged separately, is also considered a component of PN.

PN supplementation is appropriate for patients who are unable to use their GI tract safely. Care of a patient receiving PN requires collaboration from physicians, nurses, dieticians, and pharmacists.

PRINCIPLES OF CARE

Malnutrition is defined as any disorder of nutrition that may result from an unbalanced, insufficient, or impaired absorption, assimilation, or use of foods. PN is indicated in nutritional deficiencies, medical surgical conditions that put the patient at risk for malnutrition, and/or when the GI tract cannot or should not be used.

PN preparations are administered directly into the circulatory system via a peripheral IV or central venous catheter. Preparations for central vein use are hyperosmolar (approximately 1600 milliosmols) and provide high caloric and protein needs for patients with preexisting severe malnutrition or severe catabolic states. These preparations are diluted by blood in a large central vein, such as the superior vena cava. The osmolality of blood is approximately 300 milliosmols. If central PN is administered via peripheral vein, thrombophlebitis will be induced, as the hyperosmolality is damaging to tissues.

Peripheral parenteral nutrition (PPN) is considered a temporary measure to be used for no longer than 2 weeks, because this route cannot meet complete nutritional requirements. PPN is less hyperosmolar (~850 mOsm) than central PN but should still be administered through a large peripheral vein (although phlebitis may still occur). After 2 weeks, if the patient requires continued nutritional support, PN via a central line should be initiated.

Before PN is initiated, a thorough assessment of the patient's nutritional status should be completed (see Section 1 of this chapter).

DECISION-MAKING

The PN solution is prepared commercially or in-house by a qualified pharmacist. Its composition is based on specific patient needs. (See Section 2 for daily requirements.) PN should provide water, protein, and calories in the form of glucose and lipids for energy, electrolytes, minerals, and vitamins. Nutritional components are listed in Table 9-4-1.

- Protein, required for growth, antibody formation, and wound healing, is usually supplied as a mixture of essential and nonessential amino acids. Proteins contain 16% nitrogen; thus nitrogen excretion is used as an indicator of protein intake. The patient is said to be in *nitrogen balance* when the amount of nitrogen taken in via protein sources is equal to the amount of nitrogen excreted. (See Section 2 of this chapter for definition of nitrogen balance.) A major goal of PN is to prevent a negative nitrogen balance. Formulations can be prepared for patients with special protein needs, such as those with renal failure.

- Glucose provides the majority of calories for energy expenditure in the form of a simple carbohydrate, dextrose. A sufficient supply of carbohydrate must be provided simultaneously with protein to prevent the utilization of protein as an energy source.
- Lipids provide the balance of the calories needed for energy requirements. They also act as carriers for fat soluble vitamins and provide linoleic acid, an essential fatty acid. Linoleic acid deficiency can result in dermatitis. *Allergy to eggs is an absolute contraindication for using lipids.*
- Water is necessary for adequate urine production and for the replacement of insensible losses. Insensible losses for each degree of fever (Celsius) equal 200 mL/day; losses from sweat can be up to 2 L/day. The average patient requires an estimated 35 mL/kg/day to maintain adequate renal function.
- Electrolytes are added to provide daily requirements and to replace losses.
- Minerals help maintain osmotic pressure and acid-base balance. Most are provided as trace elements in a mixture or as individual supplements.
- Vitamins are prepared in a multivitamin IV solution that provides all of the daily requirements except vitamin K. The nurse must safely administer and monitor PN infusion.
- The solution's contents should be verified against the physician's order to ensure that the correct solution is being administered to the patient.
- The patient's name and room number and the solution's ingredients, additives, and expiration date should be verified.
- The solution should be checked for discoloration and particulate matter.
- If there are any questions related to the solution, the nurse should not hang the bag and should contact the pharmacist.
- The nurse should administer the PN solution using the type of filter designated by the agency to collect particulate matter. The FDA recommends using 0.22-ng filters and changing them every 24 hours.
- An infusion pump should always be used when administering PN to maintain a constant rate. Strict asepsis is vital to preventing catheter infection. The correct rate of administration should be verified. PN volume ranges from 30 to 40 mL/kg/day; a 200-lb (91-kg) adult would receive between 100 and 150 mL/hr.
- Lipid emulsions, bottled separately from other components of PN, carry a great risk for supporting microbial growth. The Centers for Disease Control and Prevention recommends that all tubing for lipid emulsions be replaced within 24 hours. They further recommend that the infusion of separate lipid emulsions be completed within 12 hours. Lipids are usually infused via a Y-connector into the amino acid and dextrose solution administration tubing.

The patient receiving PN requires frequent monitoring including laboratory values, especially glucose and electrolytes (Table 9-4-2). To monitor therapy for effectiveness, serum proteins are evaluated biweekly or weekly. Prealbumin and transferrin are most commonly used. (See Section 1 of this chapter for descriptions of these tests.) Cholesterol and triglyceride levels may be assessed to prevent the administration of excessive fatty acids. Table 9-4-3 lists common complications associated with PN.

Text continued on page 249

Table 9-4-1. Nutritional Components of Parenteral Nutrition

COMPONENT	FUNCTION	REQUIREMENTS
Protein Parenteral nutrition solution provides amino acid concentrations that vary from 3%–15% solution and contain essential and nonessential amino acids.	Repair of worn body tissue. Synthesis of new tissue growth. Formation of hormones, plasma proteins (albumin, hemoglobin), neurotransmitters, and certain enzymes.	Healthy (nonstressed) individuals should receive the recommended 0.8 g/kg/day. For the stressed patient, current recommendations of 1.2 to 2 g/kg of body weight/day may be excessive. Research suggests providing 1.2 g/kg of preillness body weight/day. If that information is not available, 1.0 g/day/kg of measured body weight is adequate for optimal protein requirements. Also, 10%–20% of dietary calories are derived from protein.
Carbohydrates Dextrose is the commercial preparation of glucose. Concentration varies from 2.5% (25 g/L) to 70% (700 g/L).	Provides energy for the body. Brain, skeletal muscle, red and white blood cells, kidneys, intestines, primary fuel.	50%–60% of daily calories should come from carbohydrates. A minimum of 150 to 200 g (500–700 kcal/day) is necessary to support function of tissues. Infusion of glucose should not exceed the maximum oxidative rate of 4–7 mg/kg/min (5.8–10 g/kg/day).
Fats (lipids) Available in an oil-in-water emulsion made of soybean oil and safflower oil. Do not filter emulsion.	Can be used quickly for energy by all cells except central nervous system cells and erythrocytes. Assist in function and integrity of capillaries and cell membranes.	Provides 9 kcal/g. No more than 30% of calories should come from fat. Essential fatty acids (linoleic and linolenic) are not manufactured by the body; must be obtained in diet. Available in 10% solution, which provides 1.1 kcal/mL; 20% solution, which provides 2 kcal/ml; and 30% solution, which provides 3 kcal/mL.

Fluid	Provides fluid for urine production and the replacement of measurable and insensible losses.	Total fluid: 2.5 L/day. Replacement will vary depending on patient age, weight, and health status. Measurable losses include urine output, drainage tube output, and losses from diarrhea. Insensible losses will be increased in burn patients and those who are febrile, tachypneic, or edematous.
Electrolytes Additive amounts vary based on patient need. Frequent laboratory monitoring is required.	Chemical compounds serve many functions within the body.	Daily: Sodium: 60+ mEq; potassium: 60+ mEq; chloride: as need to maintain acid-base balance; magnesium: 10–20 mEq; calcium: 10–25 mEq; phosphorus: 450+ mmol.
Vitamins Additive amounts vary based on patient need. Frequent laboratory monitoring required.	Assist in the regulation of body functions. Must be obtained from diet, because they are either produced either insufficiently or not at all in the body.	Daily: Vitamin A: 3300 IU; vitamin D: 200 IU; vitamin E: 10 IU; vitamin C: 100 mg; folacin (folic acid): 400 mg; riboflavin: 3.6 mg; thiamin: 3.0 mg; pyridoxine (B_6): 4.0 mg; cyanocobalamin (B_{12}): 5.0 µg; pantothenic acid: 15 mg; biotin: 60 mg.
Minerals Additive amounts vary based on patient need. Frequent laboratory monitoring required.	Inorganic elements on which many body structures and functions depend.	Daily: Calcium: approximately 1000 mg (varies depending on age and sex); phosphorus: 1000–1700 mg; magnesium: 238–321 mg.
Trace elements Adjusted to maintain correct balance.	Found in the body in amounts < 5g; needed in small amounts.	Daily: Iron: 10–15 mg; iodine: 150 µg; zinc: 12–15 mg; selenium: 55–70 µg; copper: 1.5–3.0 mg; manganese: 2.0–5 mg; fluoride: 1.5–4 mg; chromium: 50–200 µg; molybdenum: 75–250 µg.

Table 9-4-2. Laboratory Monitoring Guidelines for Parenteral Nutrition

LAB	FREQUENCY OF TESTING	RATIONALE
Electrolytes (sodium, potassium, chloride, bicarbonate)	Before beginning parenteral nutrition (PN)	To assess for therapeutic levels. Prevent electrolyte imbalances.
Creatinine	Before beginning PN Daily for the first 3 days, then several times/week	To assess the kidney's ability to excrete the increased end products of protein metabolism associated with the amino acid content in PN
Blood urea nitrogen (BUN)	Before beginning PN Daily for the first 3 days, then several times/week	Same as for creatinine
Calcium	Before beginning PN Within 24 hours of initiating therapy Weekly or more frequently depending on patient condition	To assess for therapeutic levels. Prevent electrolyte imbalances. Monitor for refeeding syndrome
Magnesium	Before beginning PN Within 24 hours of initiating therapy Weekly or more frequently depending on patient condition	To assess for therapeutic levels. Prevent electrolyte imbalances. Monitor for refeeding syndrome
Phosphorus	Before beginning PN Weekly	To assess for therapeutic levels. Prevent electrolyte imbalances. Monitor for refeeding syndrome
Aspartate aminotransferase (AST)	Before beginning PN Within 24 hours of initiating therapy	To assess liver for fatty liver syndrome (Liver dysfunction can occur in patients receiving too many calories from carbohydrates.) Weekly or more frequently depending on patient condition

Alkaline phosphatase	Before beginning PN Weekly	To assess liver for fatty liver syndrome (Fatty liver syndrome does not occur in short-term therapy; it takes several weeks or months to evolve.)
Bilirubin	Before beginning PN Weekly	To assess liver for fatty liver syndrome
Cholesterol	Before beginning PN Weekly	To assess toleration of fat emulsion therapy
Triglycerides	Before beginning PN Weekly	To assess tolerance of fat emulsion therapy
Serum proteins (albumin, prealbumin, transferrin)	Before beginning PN Biweekly, then weekly	To assess severity of disease, nutritional status, response to PN. Albumin may be obtained only once, as a baseline.
Complete blood count	Before beginning PN Weekly	To assist in assessing nutritional/fluid status. Hemoglobin is especially used to evaluate dietary deficiency anemia.
Serum glucose	Every 6 hours	To assess for and correct hypoglycemia/hyperglycemia. Regulate insulin dosage.
Urine glucose and ketones	Four to six times a day	To assess for and correct hypoglycemia/hyperglycemia. Regulate insulin dosage.
Creatinine clearance	Before beginning PN; during therapy as necessary	To assess the kidneys' ability to excrete the increased end products of protein metabolism associated with the amino acid content in PN
Urine urea nitrogen (UUN)	Before beginning PN; during therapy as necessary	To assist in determining nitrogen balance

Table 9-4-3. Complications Associated with Parenteral Nutrition

COMPLICATION	CAUSE	NURSING CARE
Refeeding syndrome	Usually occurs within the first 48 hours after initiation of parenteral nutrition (PN). Shift in electrolytes (particularly potassium and phosphorus) from serum into the cells. Results in hypokalemia and hypophosphatemia. Can cause acute congestive heart failure, pulmonary edema, or myocardial infarction.	Closely monitor serum electrolytes. Patients at high risk for refeeding syndrome may have electrolytes checked every 4–6 hours. Be alert for respiratory depression, lethargy, confusion, weakness, and electrocardiogram changes. Introduce PN at a slow rate and increase rate slowly.
Catheter infection	Microorganisms on the skin travel down the tract made by the catheter. Contamination of the fluid or tubing. Contamination from a remote site of infection. The more the system is broken, the greater the risk.	If sepsis is suspected, anticipate catheter removal and catheter tip culture. Blood urine, sputum, and wound cultures may also be ordered.
Air embolism	Air entering the central venous catheter travels through the bloodstream and lodges in a vessel.	Always clamp tubing before disconnecting. Maintain tightness of all connections. If air embolism is suspected, place the patient in the left lateral position with the head down and prepare for oxygen administration while notifying the physician.
Hyperglycemia	High dextrose concentrations and glucose intolerance.	Monitor glucose levels approximately every 6 hours until levels stabilize. The administration rate and/or glucose concentration may need to be reduced.

Note: Other complications related to PN may occur; these are discussed elsewhere in this chapter.

Termination of PN can also lead to complications if not performed correctly. Planned discontinuation must be tapered with the addition of oral carbohydrates if possible. If the PN solution runs out or is abruptly terminated, a 10% dextrose solution should be infused either peripherally or centrally, if possible.

Frequently, medications are added to PN. A histamine-2 antagonist may be added for stress ulcer prophylaxis. Heparin is added to prevent subclavian vein thrombosis and to aid in the conversion of triglycerides to a free fatty acid state. Whether or not to use this additive may depend on institutional and practitioner preference. Insulin is added to control hyperglycemia resulting from infusion of high concentrations of dextrose or underlying diabetes. Only regular insulin should be added. A common recommendation is 0.1 U of insulin for every gram of dextrose in the solution.

 CLINICAL PEARLS

○ A solution containing more than 10% dextrose or more than 5% protein (amino acid) must be administered via a central line, because thrombophlebitis will occur if hyperosmolar solutions are delivered via a peripheral vein.

○ A chest radiograph must be taken after insertion of a central line to verify placement and assess for pneumothorax.

○ A PN solution should not hang longer than 24 hours, to reduce the risk of bacterial and fungal growth.

○ Elevated cholesterol and triglyceride levels may indicate that the patient cannot tolerate the lipid component of PN, requiring discontinuation.

○ Elevated liver function tests may indicate the patient is developing a condition called fatty liver syndrome related to receiving excessive calories from carbohydrates.

○ Elevated serum blood urea nitrogen (BUN) and creatinine levels may indicate renal insufficiency.

○ Blood glucose levels will indicate how well the patient is tolerating the increased amounts of dextrose.

○ Only regular insulin may be added to PN.

○ A common recommendation is to add 0.1 U of insulin for every gram of dextrose in the solution.

Enteral Nutrition

Section 5   Lee Farris ■ Lorie Arata

OVERVIEW

Enteral nutrition, or tube feeding, is defined as the provision of nutrition via the GI tract through a tube. Enteral nutrition is indicated for patients who have a functioning GI tract but for some reason cannot or will not ingest sufficient food. Conditions in which enteral nutrition may be indicated include anorexia, impaired chewing or swallowing, head and neck cancers, and malabsorption syndromes.

Enteral nutrition is preferred over parenteral nutrition for numerous reasons. The GI tract is important in the maintenance of the body's immunologic defenses; such defenses are stimulated by the presence of food in the GI tract.

Table 9-5-1. Types of Enteral Formulas

STANDARD FORMULAS (Polymetric)	HYDROLYZED FORMULAS (Monometric)
• Complex	• Simple
• Require digestion	• "Predigested"; very little digestion is required
• Used for patients with intact digestive and absorptive capabilities	• Used only for patients with impaired digestion or absorption
• Usually contain 1 kcal/mL and are of intermediate osmolality, but may contain up to 2 kcal/mL and be hypertonic	• Usually contain 1 kcal/mL and are hypertonic
• Most contain 10%–15% protein, 50%–60% carbohydrates, and 25%–40% fats; may contain added fiber	• Are low in fat
• Clinical uses include coma, CVA, burns, anorexia. Concentrated formulas may be used for patients with chronic obstructive pulmonary disease, congestive heart failure, and liver disease	• Clinical uses include irritable bowel syndrome
• Products include: Ensure, Isocal, Osmolite, TwoCal (concentrated), and Nutren (concentrated)	• Products include Criticare and Reabilan
• Cost-effective	• High cost

Studies have shown a lower incidence of sepsis in patients who receive enteral feedings than in those who receive total parenteral nutrition (TPN).

PRINCIPLES OF CARE
Nutrition

Enteral feedings can provide all of the required nutrients, or they can be used to supplement an oral diet when given in smaller amounts. There are two major categories of formulas: standard and hydrolyzed (Table 9-5-1). Standard formulas are complex, require digestion, and are used for patients with intact digestive and absorptive capabilities. Hydrolyzed formulas are simple, require little digestion before nutrient absorption, and are used for patients with impaired digestion or absorption.

Various disease-specific formulas provide the appropriate nutritional breakdown and osmolality to ensure adequate nutrition. More than 100 different enteral feeding formulas are available, many of which are interchangeable. Some formulas are specifically designed for the disease process involved. (For information on nutritional assessment, see Sections 1 and 2.) This section provides an overview of the basic nutritional components of formula.

Calories

A calorie is the standard unit for measuring energy. It is the amount of energy required to raise the temperature of 1 mL of water by 1°C. A person's required caloric intake is based on numerous factors, including weight, height, age and energy expenditure. Before enteral feedings are initiated, a complete nutritional assessment should be done (see Section 1) to help determine the patient's daily calorie requirements.

Protein

Protein consists of building blocks known as amino acids. The body requires amino acids to build its own proteins. There are 22 amino acids, 9 of which must be consumed in the diet because the body cannot synthesize them; these are essential amino acids. The amino acids that can be synthesized by the body are nonessential amino acids. See Section 2 of this chapter.

Proteins contain carbon, hydrogen, and oxygen, as do carbohydrates and fats. However, protein is the only dietary component that contains nitrogen. High intake of protein can cause large amounts of urea to be produced; this can overload the kidney, leading to renal problems. As an energy source, proteins provide 4 kcal/g, the same as carbohydrates. However, much more energy is required to metabolize protein than carbohydrates. The recommended daily allowance of protein is 0.75 g/kg. Most enteral formulas provide 14% to 17% of calories as protein. Patients with trauma, sepsis, or burns may need increased protein concentrations.

Fluid and Electrolytes

The average adult requires approximately 1 mL of water/kcal, or 35 mL/kg of normal body weight. Patients receiving enteral feedings may not get enough free water to meet the body's requirements. Standard formulas contain 80% to 85% water; nutrient-dense formulas may contain as little as 60% water.

It is important to remember to measure and record all fluid given to the patient, including water used for tube irrigation, water used to flush and dilute medications, and any IV fluid that the patient may be receiving. Serum sodium, blood urea nitrogen (BUN), hemoglobin, and albumin levels are indicators of fluid status. In general, hemoconcentration indicates underhydration, whereas hemodilution indicates overhydration. The nurse should also assess skin turgor and mucous membranes and check for the presence of edema when monitoring a patient's hydration.

Medications

It is important to know that not all medications can be given via feeding tubes; doing so can alter the therapeutic effect of some medications. Enteric-coated, sustained-release, and sublingual or buccal forms should never be given via a feeding tube. Crushing or releasing the contents of such medications alters the effect and may lead to toxic drug levels. Tablets may be crushed and dissolved in approximately 30 mL of water. Crushing can cause problems, because small particles of the medication can adhere to the tube, altering the dosage and possibly causing tube obstruction. Gel capsules may be opened and the liquid contents diluted with 15 to 30 mL of water.

Liquid medications are the recommended form of administration via feeding tubes. Although liquids seem to cause fewer problems with tube obstruction than crushed medication, liquids can cause complications related to osmolality, sorbitol content, and incompatibility with the formula. Many liquid medications have a high osmolality, which can contribute to diarrhea; dilution of such medication may be helpful.

Sorbitol is used as a sweetener to enhance the taste of certain medications. However, sorbitol can cause cramping, GI distress, and diarrhea. Again, dilution may decrease such side effects.

A medication–formula interaction can cause tube obstruction. Medications that have been found to have such an effect include potassium chloride, iron, paregoric, and phosphasoda.

Two medications with documented significant drug–formula interactions that alter drug absorption are phenytoin (Dilantin) and warfarin (Coumadin). For unknown reasons, enteral feedings lower serum drug concentrations of phenytoin. Tube feeding should be held 1 to 2 hours before and after the phenytoin, and serum phenytoin levels should be monitored closely. The vitamin K content in enteral formulas may cause resistance to warfarin in tube-fed patients, leading to low serum levels. Again, serum drug levels should be closely monitored.

Medications should never be added to tube feeding formulas. Medications also should never be mixed together; rather, each medication should be given separately, with the tube flushed with 5 to 10 mL of water between drugs. It is also important to remember where specific drug absorption occurs. For example, medications that require absorption in the stomach should not be given through an intestinal feeding tube.

DECISION-MAKING
Methods of Feeding

Enteral feedings may be delivered by several methods: bolus, intermittent, continuous, and cyclic. Feedings are administered via a tube inserted directly into the GI tract, usually by a NG or gastrostomy tube.

Bolus feedings consist of 200 to 500 mL of formula every 4 to 6 hours. This type of feeding is administered via a large syringe inserted into the feeding tube. The formula is poured into the syringe, which serves as a funnel device and allows the formula to flow by gravity into the stomach. Formula should not be administered faster than 30 mL/minute; more rapid administration may lead to gastric pooling, thereby increasing the risk of aspiration. An advantage of bolus method is that such feedings are similar to normal meal patterns.

Intermittent feeding consists of 300 to 400 mL of formula delivered over about 30 to 60 minutes using a gravity-drip or infusion pump. This feeding is delivered several times daily. The slower administration of an intermittent feeding may reduce complications associated with bolus feedings, such as nausea, diarrhea, cramps, vomiting, and risk of aspiration.

Continuous-drip feedings provide the necessary calories over a 24-hour period and are usually administered via an infusion pump. The infusion pump allows for more accurate administration of the formula. Continuous-drip feedings may be administered via a NG, gastrostomy, or jejunostomy tube.

Cyclic feedings are similar to continuous feedings except that they deliver the calories required for a 24-hour period in a shorter time. Cyclic feedings may be administered at night to promote appetite during the day and provide freedom from the infusion pump.

Tube Feeding Complications

Various complications are associated with enteral feedings. Many are preventable or manageable with appropriate nursing care. "Dumping syndrome" is a physiologic response to rapid emptying of the gastric contents into the jejunum. This may occur in patients receiving concentrated solutions of high osmolarity. The high osmolarity causes water to move from surrounding tissues into the stomach and intestines. Signs and symptoms of dumping syndrome include dehydration, hypotension, tachycardia, feeling of fullness, nausea, and diarrhea.

Table 9-5-2 lists complications of tube feedings, along with their possible causes and nursing care considerations.

Feeding Tubes
General

Tubes placed nasally are considered short-term access and are used for less than 6 weeks. Tubes placed in the stomach are appropriate for patients with normally functioning GI tracts and patients who are at low risk for aspiration. Patients requiring long-term therapy need surgically placed gastrostomy or jejunostomy tubes. Jejunostomy tubes are preferred for patients with altered GI function and for long-term use in patients at risk for aspiration. Jejunostomy tubes may also be used for short-term nutrition after GI surgery.

Insertion

Assess both nares, and choose the side less likely to have an obstruction. Measure the tube length to be inserted by measuring from the patient's nose to the earlobe to the xiphoid process. Position the patient in high-Fowler's position. Insert the lubricated tube into the desired naris.

Once the tube has passed through to the back of the pharynx, ask the patient to tilt the head forward with the chin toward the chest. If possible, have the patient take sips of water while passing the tube. Do not force the tube.

Monitor closely for excessive coughing, gagging, and difficulty breathing during tube insertion. If these symptoms occur, stop advancing the tube and assess the patient. It may be necessary to withdraw the tube partially or totally and restart the procedure.

Advance the tube to the desired measurement and secure with tape. Check tube placement using the following techniques and an x-ray before beginning an enteral feeding or administering medications.

For insertion of a nasoduodenal tube (e.g., Keofeed II) into the duodenum or jejunum, the same procedure is followed at the bedside. After insertion, the tip of the tube is usually in the stomach. It takes approximately 24 hours for the tip to advance through the stomach and into the intestines. The weighted tip facilitates passage. The patient may be placed on the right side to allow gravity and peristalsis to aid passage of the tube. This type of tube is generally made of a flexible material such as silicon and has a very small diameter. A stylet is used during insertion to prevent kinking. The stylet must be removed after insertion and never reinserted while the tube is in place. An alternative to bedside placement is the use of fluoroscopy.

Placement

Checking placement of an enteral feeding tube is an important nursing responsibility. All enteral tubes used for feeding should be verified with a radiograph before feeding is initiated. Placement of nasally placed tubes should also be checked using the following methods before instilling anything into a feeding tube and every 4 to 6 hours thereafter.

Auscultating the stomach while injecting air into the tube is the first method.

Text continued on page 257

Table 9-5-2. Feeding Tube Complications

COMPLICATION	POSSIBLE CAUSE	NURSING CARE
GASTROINTESTINAL		
Gastric retention, gastroesophageal reflux, aspiration	• Diminished gag reflex	• Assess gastric residuals every 4 hours, if greater than 100 mL (or less in patients receiving smaller feedings), hold the tube feeding for 1 hour and then recheck residual. Resume feeding after residuals are less than 100 mL.
	• Large formula volume or high feeding rate	• Position patient with the head of the bed elevated 30-45 degrees for at least 1 hour after feedings.
	• Tube placement hindering normal function of esophageal sphincter	• Monitor for aspiration by adding tube food coloring to the feeding formula. Check breath sounds every 4 hours.
	• Improper patient positioning	• Verify tube placement before all bolus feedings and every 4 hours with continuous feedings.
	• Delayed gastric emptying	• Add Reglan or a similar medication to enhance gastric emptying.
Nausea and vomiting	• Rapid feeding rate	• Reduce feeding rate and volume.
	• Large feeding volume	• Warm feedings to room temperature.
	• Cold feedings	• Assess for gastric residuals.
	• Delayed gastric emptying	• Consider antiemetics or Reglan to enhance gastric emptying.
	• Improper tube placement	• Verify tube placement.
	• Formula intolerance	• Assess for formula intolerance; if necessary, change to a more tolerable formula.
	• Anxiety	• Keep the head of the bed elevated 30 degrees.
Diarrhea (cause often is multifactorial)	• High formula osmolarity	• Reduce osmolarity by changing formulas or diluting the current formula.
	• Large infusion volume	• Reduce volume, reduce rate, and consider continuous rather than bolus method of feeding.

	Causes	Interventions
	• Rapid infusion volume • Contamination of formula or infusion equipment • Infection with *Clostridium difficile* • Antibiotic use • Lactose intolerance • Impaired gastrointestinal function • Hypoalbuminemia	• Ensure strict hand washing and cleaning of all equipment. • Hang only a 4-hour supply of formula at a time; refrigerate unused, open formula; replace infusion canisters after 24 hours. • Collect stools and examine for *C. difficile*. • Treat with appropriate antidiarrheal medications when not contraindicated. • Use lactose-free formula. • Assess albumin levels; consider parenteral nutrition for patients with significant hypoalbuminemia. • Assess for other malabsorption syndromes that may contribute to diarrhea.
Constipation	• Inadequate fluid intake • Low-residue formula • Medications • Inactivity • Obstruction	• Increase fluid volume. • Increase residue. • Limit use of constipating medications when appropriate. • Provide/promote activity. • If obstruction occurs, stop the feeding. • Administer a laxative if indicated.
MECHANICAL		
Improperly placed tube	• Improper placement • Improper verification of placement • Migration of tube related to coughing, vomiting, or improper taping • Improper taping or security of tube	• Verify tube placement after insertion using radiography. • Reassess tube placement before administering anything via the tube. • Securely tape the tube or use a tube-holding device. • Elevate the head of the bed 30 degrees.
Ear, nose, or throat irritation	• Mechanical irritant to skin and mucous membranes	• Assess for irritation. • Use a smaller-bore tube if possible; consider gastric placement of tube if irritation is severe enough to cause necrosis or infection.

Table continued on following page

Table 9-5-2. Feeding Tube Complications *Continued*

COMPLICATION	POSSIBLE CAUSE	NURSING CARE
Tube clogging	• Viscous formula • Medication administration via the tube • Inadequate flushing • Aspiration of gastric contents into tube	• Always verify tube placement before flushing. • Flush feeding tubes with 15–30 mL of water before and after administering medication. • Administer liquid medications when available; crush tablets thoroughly and dilute in 15 to 100 mL of water before administration. • Stop continuous tube feedings and flush thoroughly before and after administering medications. • Flush tube after checking for residual. • Flush all tubes routinely every 6 to 8 hours. • May use warm water or sodium bicarbonate to clear a clog.
METABOLIC		
Electrolyte and glucose disturbances	• Excessive or inadequate electrolytes in formula • Excessive or inadequate fluid intake • Excessive fluid loss • Preexisting diabetes, stress, high levels of glucose in formula, or use of steroids	• Monitor intake and output carefully. • Use an infusion pump to regulate intake. • Monitor laboratory values closely. • Use an appropriate formula for patients with electrolyte or glucose disturbances.
Drug-nutrient interactions	• Drug availability altered by form and administration technique, amount of medication absorbed, or drug-nutrient interaction	• Do not crush time-release, enterics coated, or capsule forms. • Use liquid medications when available. • Do not add medication to enteral feeding bags. • Hold tube feedings 1–2 hours before and after administration of phenytoin or warfarin. • Monitor drug therapeutic levels closely.
Dehydration	• Infection • Fever • Inadequate intake • Excessive fluid loss	• Closely monitor intake and output. • Monitor daily weights. • Replace fluid losses.
Essential fatty acid deficiency	• Lack of necessary essential fatty acids in formula	• Monitor patient and lab values; this complication is rare.

The nurse should be able to auscultate a gurgle in the stomach. Although this method is frequently used, it is not considered the most reliable method. Aspiration of gastric contents via the tube is another method. Care must be taken to distinguish respiratory secretions from gastric and intestinal secretions.

Evaluating the pH of aspirated fluid is another method for verifying tube placement. The pH of gastric secretions is between 1 and 4; that of intestinal and respiratory secretions is 6 or higher. When placement is questionable using the pH method, a radiograph should be obtained.

It is recommended that patients at risk for aspiration be fed into the small bowel. Residual from a tube placed in the duodenum or jejunum should also be checked regularly. Residual amounts greater than 30 mL indicate that the tube may have migrated into the stomach.

Care of Feeding Tubes

Feeding tubes should be measured or marked so that tube migration can be readily detected. Many tubes are already marked; the nurse should note and record the measurement located at the entrance to the nose or stoma. If the tube is unmarked, then the nurse should mark the tube at the insertion site using either ink or tape or place a sign over the bed specifying the marking.

Nasoenteric tubes should be taped or secured with a tube holder. Tape should be removed and new tape applied, preferably at a different skin site, at least every other day, unless tincture of benzoin is used, in which case the tape should be replaced when it becomes soiled or loose.

The site may be left open to air for 24 hours after the insertion of a gastrostomy or jejunostomy tube. Old crusty drainage may be removed with a half-strength peroxide solution. However, this should not be used to clean the actual stoma site, because it may delay healing. Daily care includes cleaning with soap and water and then rinsing thoroughly.

 CLINICAL PEARLS

- There are two major categories of tube feeding formulas: standard and hydrolyzed. Standard formulas are used for patients with intact digestive and absorptive capabilities, whereas hydrolyzed formulas are used for patients with impaired digestion or absorption.
- Nasally placed tubes are for short-term (<6 weeks) use. Patients who require long-term therapy should have a surgically placed gastrostomy or jejunostomy tube.
- Nasoenterically placed feeding tubes should be verified with an x-ray after initial insertion. Thereafter, placement should be verified before instilling anything into the tube and every 4 to 6 hours thereafter. Methods of placement verification include aspirating gastric contents, instilling an air bolus while auscultating for "gurgle" in stomach, and evaluating the pH of aspirated fluid.
- All feeding tubes should be marked and the placement markings clearly documented so that migration can be readily detected.
- Administration of liquid medications through feeding tubes is recommended. Enteric-coated, sustained-release, and sublingual or buccal forms should never be given through a feeding tube.
- Two drugs with significant drug–formula interactions that alter drug absorp-

tion are phenytoin (Dilantin) and warfarin (Coumadin). The vitamin K content of tube feedings decreases the effects of warfarin.

 RESOURCES

- American Diabetes Association: www.diabetes.org/
- American Dietetics Association: 800-877-1600, ext. 5000, or www.eatright.org/
- American Society for Clinical Nutrition: www.faseb.org
- American Society of Parenteral and Enteral Nutrition: www.clinnitr.org/
- Diet Analysis Web Page: dawp.anet.com
- Food and nutrition Information Center: www.nal.usda.gov
- Herbals: www.altmedicine.com
- Nutrition journal: www.hbz_nrw.de/elsevier/08999007
- www.challengenet.com/g~tube/jlinks.html
- www.is.dal.ca/~pharmwww/druginfo/parent.htm
- www.rossmn.com/ross/clinical/clinical.htm

chapter 10

Decision-Making for Immunologic Alterations

Assessment

Section 1   Phyllis Peterson

OVERVIEW

Advances in medicine and health care have led to increasingly aggressive treatments and therapies, many of which affect immunologic function. Congenital abnormalities, infections, disease states, injuries, and trauma may also have adverse effects on immune function. These changes can be temporary or permanent in nature, but they almost always alter a patient's overall health and well-being.

All patients in acute care settings are at risk for some degree of immunocompromise. Invasive procedures, therapies, and monitoring devices compromise the integrity of skin and mucous membranes, increasing the risk of infection, and thus are particularly hazardous in patients with decreased immunity. The stress of illness, be it physical or psychological, may also have a negative effect on immune response.

PRINCIPLES OF CARE
Immunity and Inflammation as Protective Mechanisms

Intact skin and mucous membranes serve as the first line of defense against foreign organisms and proteins that may cause injury. When these barriers fail or are damaged, inflammatory and nonspecific immune responses form the second line of defense. The third line of defense consists of specific immune responses by antibodies and activated cells directed toward identified foreign organisms or neoplastic cells (Table 10-1-1).

Immunity must be both nonspecific and specific. Nonspecific immunity is present at birth and enables a generalized inflammatory response against foreign cells. Specific immunity is developed as a consequence of exposure to antigens, and allows the body to release cells and chemicals targeted against those specific antigens.

Components of the Immune System

Lymphocytes and other immune system cells form and mature within the bone marrow, liver, and thymus. Specialized tissues, including lymph nodes throughout the body and Peyer's patches in the intestines and spleen, may also have the ability to generate an immune response against antigens. These tissues

Table 10-1-1.　Types of Immunity

RESPONSE	ORIGIN	PROTECTIVE MECHANISM
Innate or natural immunity	Present at birth, tends to be species specific	Offers protection against environmental pathogens
Passive acquired immunity	Obtained by transfer of maternal antibodies or via therapeutic interventions	Conveys temporary protection against pathogenic organisms
Active acquired immunity	Produced by the host after exposure to an antigen or immunization	Conveys sustained protection against pathogens

act as specialized filters able to destroy antigens circulating in the lymph and blood.

B lymphocytes are created in the fetal bone marrow. From there, they move to the fetal liver and lymphatic tissues, where they mature and become functional cells. When exposed to antigens, B cells differentiate into two distinct cell lines, plasma cells and memory cells. Plasma cells secrete immunoglobulins, also called antibodies. These antibodies initiate the chain of events that ideally lead to the ultimate destruction of the antigen. Antibodies offer protection in one of four ways:

- Inactivating bacterial toxins
- Neutralizing viruses
- Destroying bacteria by rendering them susceptible to phagocytosis
- Activating the inflammatory response

T lymphocytes originate in the bone marrow, then move to the thymus to mature. Hormones in the thymus stimulate the T cells to differentiate into suppressor T cells, helper T cells, and cytotoxic T cells. When activated, helper T cells stimulate B cells to produce antibodies and a series of proteins called lymphokines that act directly on other immune system cells. Helper T cells are destroyed or neutralized by the AIDS virus, with catastrophic effects on the immune system.

Cytotoxic T cells bind with and lyse infectious organisms and some cancer cells. Suppressor T cells depress the immune response so that the body does not inadvertently damage its own cells. In the presence of a foreign antigen, macrophages in lymphoid tissue engulf the antigen and then present it to B cells.

Natural killer (NK) cells are lymphocytes that grow and evolve in the bone marrow but are neither T nor B cells. These cells are able to destroy some tumor cells, as well as cells infected with viruses. In addition, they can augment the B cell immune response and promote cell-mediated immunity.

Suppressor T cells are believed to dampen or turn off the functions of both cytotoxic and helper T cells, thereby allowing the immune system to identify the body's own cells. This characteristic is known as "self-tolerance." The body's inability to distinguish its own cells is thought to be one of the causative factors behind autoimmune diseases such as rheumatoid arthritis and systemic lupus erythematosus.

Inflammation
Vascular Phase

In the normal healthy person, inflammation is a reaction of vascular tissue to local injury. Tissue responds to injury with dilation of blood vessels in the injured area and increased permeability of the vessels. Depending on the nature of the injury, this vasodilation may be caused by chemical mediators, such as histamine and serotonin. The vasoactive effects of histamine and serotonin cause rapid constriction of the smooth muscle of large vessel walls and dilation of the postcapillary venules. These effects ultimately increase blood flow into the capillaries.

Vasodilation and increased permeability cause the characteristic warmth, redness, and swelling seen in tissue injury. Increased vascular permeability allows exudates to move out of the blood vessels into the interstitial spaces, often increasing edema. Movement of exudates from the vessels causes a subsequent increase in the concentration of red blood cells in the small blood vessels, producing increased blood viscosity and decreased rates of blood flow. This process minimizes cell damage and death by diluting harmful substances. Because blood flow is more sluggish, clotting occurs at the site of the injury, decreasing the risk of the infection becoming blood-borne. This decreased blood flow heralds the cellular phase of inflammation.

Cellular Phase

Many different types of white blood cells (WBCs) participate in the inflammatory response. Neutrophils are usually the first cells to arrive to a damaged area of the body. They are phagocytic cells, able to engulf and destroy foreign substances and bacteria. Circulating neutrophils have a life span of only 10 to 12 hours after they are released from the bone marrow and must be constantly replaced to provide effective protection against infection and cell damage. In the event of tissue injury or infection, WBC release from the marrow increases in a process called leukocytosis.

Eosinophils are specialized leukocytes that increase during allergic reactions and parasitic infections. Monocytes, another type of phagocytic WBC, have a longer life span than granulocytes and are able to engulf and destroy larger amounts of foreign substances than are neutrophils. Monocytes have the ability to migrate to lymph nodes to provide specific immunity, and can wall off foreign material that cannot be broken down and destroyed. When monocytes move out of the circulation into tissue, they may swell to five times their normal size and become tissue macrophages, which provide an effective defense against disease. Tissue-specific macrophages include the Kuppfer cells of the liver and alveolar macrophages of the lungs.

The effectiveness of WBCs is increased by the presence of antibodies. *Antibodies*, also called immunoglobulins, attach to the surface of bacterial cells and make it easier for the phagocytes to destroy the cells. Interactions between the cells are orchestrated by cell-derived substances called *cytokines*. Cytokines trigger the activities of various cells, helping them to act in a coordinated fashion to defend the body against foreign organisms and pathogens. During the cellular response phase, phagocytic cells destroy harmful agents and foreign proteins, and lay down a fibrin matrix that promotes tissue healing.

Very early in the cellular response phase, lymphokines are cytokines released from T lymphocytes at the site of injury. This causes granulocytes and monocytes to move toward the blood vessel lining and begin to adhere to the endothelial layer, in processes known as pavementing and adhesion. The WBCs then begin to squeeze between the endothelial cells and the basement membrane and eventually move into the extravascular spaces, where they travel to the injured area and begin to attack and destroy foreign organisms.

Complement System

Other factors that regulate inflammatory response include the complement system and arachidonic acid metabolites. The complement system comprises many different proteins that can affect the vascular system, WBC function, and phagocytosis. Complement is responsible for activating neutrophils, monocytes, eosinophils, and basophils and stimulating them to move to the site of tissue injury. These proteins are activated in sequence and help decrease injury and promote healing.

Arachidonic Acid Metabolites

This group of substances includes prostaglandins, thromboxane, and the leukotrienes. Prostaglandins cause fever and enhance the transmission of pain impulses. Leukotrienes cause vasodilation and improve vessel permeability. Thromboxane affects the response of platelets to vessel injury.

To accurately evaluate the patient's resistance to infection, the number of segmented and band neutrophils, or granulocytes, must be determined. Granulocytes are the first cells to arrive at a site of infection or inflammation and constitute the body's first line of defense. In the healthy adult with a normal WBC count (5000 to 10,000 mm^3), the normal granulocyte count is 54% to 62% of the WBC count, or 3800 mm^3 (see Chapter 11, Section 2). Depending on the granulocyte count, a patient's risk for infection may range from insignificant to severe (Table 10-1-2). A patient who experiences prolonged neutropenia or has a total granulocyte count of below 100 mm^3 is at high risk for an overwhelming infection.

Patients suffering defects in cellular immunity are often plagued with chronic or recurrent infections. Genetic disorders, disease processes, malnutrition, alcohol, and certain drugs (e.g., steroids) may adversely affect leukocyte function (see Table 10-1-2).

Table 10-1-2. Autoimmune Disorders

DISORDERS	NATURE OF DEFECT
Systemic lupus erythematosus	Sustained abnormal activation of B lymphocytes
Graves' disease	Excessive stimulation to the thyroid gland from thyroid-stimulating immunoglobulins
Myasthenia gravis	Antibodies developing against acetylcholine receptors at the neuromuscular junction
Type I diabetes	Thought to be the result of a chronic autoimmune process
Rheumatoid arthritis	Thought to be caused by an autoimmune response that damages connective tissue
Goodpasture's syndrome	Deposition of antibodies and complement along the glomerular basement membrane

An exaggerated inflammatory response, as seen with overwhelming infection or major trauma, may lead to life-threatening septic shock. Initially, increased cardiac output and widespread vasodilation occur. Ultimately, capillary leak syndrome develops, with a concomitant drop in blood pressure. Hypoperfusion of vital organs leads to further vasodilation and hypoperfusion and, eventually, multisystem organ failure. Septic shock has a high mortality rate and is a leading cause of death in critical care units.

Types of Immunity

Natural immunity is present at birth and is a product of innate tissue defense mechanisms. Innate immunity in the healthy individual conveys protection from disease and injury by a combination of one or more processes:

- Destruction of bacteria and foreign organisms by white blood cells and cells of the macrophage system
- Destruction of foreign bacteria and organisms by the acid secretions of the digestive tract
- Protective covering provided by intact skin
- Cytotoxic chemical compounds in the blood that destroy foreign organisms

Acquired immunity develops as a result of exposure to foreign antigens that trigger the development of defensive immunity. Immunity may be passively acquired by means of immunization, or may result from contact with other infected people. Short-term or passive immunity may also be obtained from antibodies or T cells developed outside the body and administered as an immunization.

DECISION-MAKING

Comprehensive information must be gathered to appropriately evaluate and manage potential immunologic abnormalities.

History and Physical Examination

Information gathering begins with a thorough review of the patient's medical and social history. Special attention is given to a history of allergy, malignancies, and frequent and opportunistic infections. A patient who has received cytotoxic therapy for malignancies, organ transplants, or prolonged immunosuppressive therapy also requires careful scrutiny.

Lifestyle and social habits may also adversely affect immune status. Because chronic alcohol use can lead to severe myelosuppression, the patient is asked about the amount and duration of alcohol intake. Prolonged inadequate protein calorie intake may also lead to impaired lymphocyte function. A patient who engages in unprotected sex with multiple partners or intravenous drug abuse needs to be screened for HIV disease. For every patient, a complete list of medications (prescription and over-the-counter) should be obtained and evaluated for potential drug–drug interactions and possible immunosuppressive effects.

When performing the physical examination, special attention should be given to sites of recurrent infection, rashes, enlarged lymph nodes, telangiectasis, and hepatosplenomegaly. One or more positive findings in these areas provide further evidence of possible immune defects.

Immunosuppressive Therapies

Various diseases and disorders are treated with immunosuppressive agents and therapies. Patients undergoing treatment for malignancies may experience varying degrees of immunosuppression, depending on the types and doses of cytotoxic agents administered. Radiation therapy may cause profound immunosuppression, particularly if given in conjunction with cytotoxic agents.

Glucocorticoids are administered for their immunosuppressive and anti-inflammatory effects, which are desirable in treating rheumatologic and autoimmune disorders such as lupus and rheumatoid arthritis. Immunosuppressant agents (e.g., cyclosporine, CellCept) are given to prevent the rejection of grafted organs.

Recent developments in recombinant DNA technology have brought the use of various cytokines to treat a wide variety of disease processes. Alpha interferons have been very useful in treating such disorders as hairy cell leukemia, malignant melanoma, and chronic hepatitis. These substances are derived from macrophages and promote T and B cell activity. Colony-stimulating factors (CSFs), such as Neupogen and oprelvekin, have revolutionized the treatment and supportive care of patients with myelosuppressive diseases and those undergoing myelosuppressive therapy by increasing granulocyte counts.

Diagnostic Studies

Serologic and pathologic studies may provide important information about the immunologic status. The most useful and cost-effective serologic test is the complete blood cell count (CBC) with differential (detecting the various types of WBCs). Evaluation of lymphocyte subsets is used to confirm the presence of opportunistic infections and as a part of the diagnostic workup for AIDS. As the number of CD4 cells and T lymphocytes decreases, the risk, severity, and incidence of opportunistic infection increases. Overall lymphocyte counts decrease concurrently with declining immune status.

Besides HIV, possible causes of depressed lymphocyte count include steroids and general anesthesia. Patients with a decreased CD4 and T lymphocyte count are screened for HIV with enzyme-linked immunosorbent assay (ELISA). The HIV antibody must be confirmed via the Western blot test. Anergy panels may be done to evaluate cell-mediated immunity. In these tests, minute amounts of infective organisms (e.g., histoplasmosis, candida) are injected intradermally. The sites are then observed for local erythema and induration, which indicate a normal immune response.

Other diagnostic tests used in the evaluation and treatment of immunodeficient states include erythrocyte sedimentation rate (ESR) and C-reactive protein. ESR tends to be elevated in acute inflammatory processes and in acute and chronic infections. C-reactive protein tends to rise dramatically in the presence of acute inflammation and certain inflammatory and malignant diseases, but tends to return to normal quickly after the inflammatory condition is resolved.

 CLINICAL PEARLS

○ Patients may be at high risk for immunocompromise, depending on age, disease processes, medical history, and medical therapy.

○ Medical therapies contributing to immunocompromise include immunosuppressive drugs, cytotoxic chemotherapeutic agents, and radiation therapy.
○ Immunocompromised patients require careful monitoring and evaluation for the presence of infections, with prompt aggressive treatment.
○ Immunity and inflammation serve as protective mechanisms to safeguard the host from infection, tissue damage, and disease.
○ Adults lose approximately 1% of their immune function every year past age 50.
○ A patient with an ANC count below 500 is considered a severe risk for the development of a potential infection.
○ Bone marrow biopsy is a diagnostic test that predicts changes in the peripheral blood that will occur within the subsequent 2 weeks.

Immunocompromised Host

Section 2   Phyllis Peterson

OVERVIEW

The immunocompromised host may be seen in a wide variety of health care settings, including both acute and outpatient settings. The nurse must be skilled in assessing the immunocompromised patient and in developing and implementing a plan of care to protect the patient from complications associated with immunosuppression and promote rapid recovery if complications do occur. This section covers the basic precautions indicated for an immunocompromised patient.

PRINCIPLES OF CARE

Protective measures and interventions must be planned around each patient's unique requirements. Because stringent protective isolation measures are costly and cause emotional distress to the patient, the need for isolation precautions should be carefully evaluated in light of the patient's risk factors, current immune status, and concurrent disease processes.

Depending on the etiology of the immunocompromised state, protective isolation measures may be a short- or long-term requirement. Patients, caregivers and family members are more likely to comply with isolation restrictions if they receive thorough teaching about the reasons for and protective benefits of isolation.

DECISION-MAKING
Determinants of Isolation Requirements

During the assessment phase, the patient's immune status is carefully determined. A patient with normal cellular and humoral immunity but with an alteration in the protective barrier, such as a surgical wound or burn, may still need protective measures. Conversely, a patient with impaired cellular function may exhibit signs and symptoms of infection and yet have intact skin and mucous membranes. This is why assessment must include not only physical status but also a review of current medications and laboratory tests, particularly CBC with differential.

Many patients fall into a high-risk category because they are debilitated or have a history of previous immunosuppressive therapy or disease. Standard precautions may be sufficient for these patients, provided that they receive ongoing monitoring and evaluation for evidence of declining immune status or infection.

Neutropenic Precautions

The term "neutropenic precautions" refers to a specialized set of precautions instituted for patients with low neutrophil counts. The extent of neutropenic precautions depends on the degree of risk, based on the patient's CBC and differential results (Table 10-2-1).

Neutropenic precautions are directed toward minimizing the risk that an immunocompromised patient may become infected from exogenous or endogenous organisms. Specialized filtered air flow systems offering high-efficiency positive pressure may decrease the incidence of infection in the high-risk patient who is expected to undergo a prolonged period of neutropenia.

Visitors and staff with active infections, recent vaccinations with live vaccines, or recent exposure to contagious illnesses are barred from the patient's

Table 10-2-1. Relative Risk for Infection

NEUTROPHIL COUNT (mm³)	RELATIVE RISK	NURSING IMPLICATIONS
1500–2000	Insignificant	Provide patient education on signs and symptoms of infection, prevention of infections, and when to seek medical and nursing intervention.
1000–1500	Minimal	Help the patient maintain adequate nutrition. Promote integrity of skin and mucosa. Promote good personal hygiene. Provide patient education on signs and symptoms of infection and prevention of infection. Monitor for evidence of infection every 8 hours. The patient should not share a room with those with active infections.
500–1000	Moderate	Assess every 4 to 6 hours for evidence of infection. Inspect invasive devices and tubes for evidence of infection. Obtain daily CBC and cultures as prescribed. Implement neutropenic precautions. Provide patient education regarding prevention of infections.
<500	Severe	Assess every 2–4 hours around the clock for evidence of infection. Implement neutropenic precautions. Provide patient and family education. Collaborate with physician regarding obtaining cultures, antibiotic therapy, and possible use of colony-stimulating factors (e.g., G-CSF).

Adapted from Biebman, M. C., & Camp-Sorrell, D. (1996). *Multimodal therapy in oncology nursing.* St. Louis: Mosby–Year Book.

room. The room is free of carpet, drapes, and cloth-upholstered furniture, because these surfaces are difficult to clean. No live plants or cut flowers are permitted, because of the risk of contamination by soil and water organisms. Standing water and open food containers are avoided because of the risk of bacterial and fungal growth. A humidifier is used only when absolutely necessary, and respiratory equipment must be changed according to institutional policy.

Patients at moderate risk of infection are encouraged to be careful of food safety, and avoid food from open containers that has not been appropriately stored. A patient with severe neutropenia (absolute neutrophil count [ANC] below 500) requires a low-bacteria diet. The patient needs to avoid raw foods, including fresh fruits, vegetables, meats, and shellfish. In some institutions, fresh fruits with thick, intact peels (e.g., bananas, grapefruit, oranges) may be allowed.

Proactive measures are also taken to support and maintain the patient's natural defenses. These include maintaining the integrity of skin and mucous membranes, avoiding invasive procedures whenever possible. Rectal temperatures and rectal manipulation are avoided because of the risk of rectal abscess. Careful attention is given to the patient's hygiene, because many neutropenic patients develop severe infections from their own body flora. The patient is reminded of the importance of hand washing, especially after every toileting. Assistance with bathing and oral care should be provided if the patient is unwilling or unable to do it independently.

All invasive devices (e.g., IV catheters, central lines) must be evaluated daily for evidence of inflammation and erythema. (It is important to note here that because severely neutropenic patients are unable to form purulent drainage at an infected site, caregivers must be alert to other, more subtle signs of infection, such as warmth, pain, and redness.) An invasive device should be evaluated as the possible source of infection should the patient become septic.

Reverse Isolation

Reverse isolation, or protective isolation, is implemented to protect the severely immunocompromised patient from contact with pathogens in the environment. Depending on institutional policy and on previous experience with nosocomial infections in the institution, caregivers and visitors may be required to wear special clean garb (i.e., masks, gown, and hair and foot covers) before entering the patient's room. Caregivers and visitors with contagious illnesses (e.g., colds, flu) are barred from direct contact with the patient. Special disinfection and decontamination measures may also be used to maintain an aseptic environment for the patient.

If a prolonged period of significant immunosuppression is anticipated, the patient may be put in a sterile laminar air flow room. This provides a smooth, even flow of filtered air under positive pressure, which prevents airborne organisms from entering the environment. Special precautions are needed to maintain sterility, including sterilizing the patient's personal items with either chemicals or a gas autoclave and severely restricting contact with most visitors.

Strict protective isolation measures are time-consuming and costly, and they may not improve the outcomes of patients with mild or moderate granulocytopenia, especially neutropenia. Standard protective isolation precautions provide an equal measure of protection for most patients.

Table 10-2-2. Common Pharmacologic Prophylaxis

DRUG	ORGANISM
Fluconazole (Diflucan)	Cryptococcal meningitis, systemic candida
Trimethoprim- sulfamethoxazole (Bactrim)	*Pneumocystis carinii* pneumonitis; shigellosis enteritis
Acyclovir	Herpes simplex virus

Pharmacologic Prophylaxis

Drug therapy plays an important role in decreasing mortality and morbidity in immunocompromised patients. Prompt treatment with broad-spectrum antibiotics has been life-saving for many patients with neutropenic sepsis. For those scheduled to experience prolonged severe neutropenia, prophylactic therapy with antibiotics may be given to protect against gram-negative organisms. Fungal and viral prophylaxis also may be administered to a patient who is at very high risk for sepsis due to neutropenia (Table 10-2-2). Opportunistic organisms may be life-threatening for the immunocompromised patient. Thus, broad-spectrum antibiotic therapy is started immediately at the first indication of infection.

To minimize the duration of immunosuppression associated with cytotoxic chemotherapy, or to support the patient experiencing hematopoietic failure secondary to disease, CSFs may be administered to increase the growth of hematopoietic WBCs. Filgrastim (G-CSF) acts by regulating the production of neutrophils. Sargramostim (GM-CSF) has a somewhat broader range of activity and enhances the growth and effectiveness of neutrophils, monocytes, and macrophages. Both of these drugs have proven effective in regenerating myeloid cell lines after high-dose chemotherapy. In some settings, these drugs are also used to increase the WBC count in patients with AIDS and renal failure.

 CLINICAL PEARLS

○ Consistent meticulous hand washing, along with avoiding direct contact with infected persons, has proven highly effective in preventing the transmission of pathogenic organisms to immunocompromised patients.

○ Immunocompromised patients have varying degrees of risk for infection. A patient's risk may be evaluated by determining the ANC from the WBC differential results.

○ Isolation precautions must be adjusted according to each patient's unique needs. Even patients in stringent protective isolation must be carefully monitored for evidence of infection so that treatment may be initiated promptly.

○ Major causative organisms in sepsis induced by a venous access device are *Staphylococcus aureus*, *Staphylococcus epidermis*, and *Candida*.

○ If blood cultures are positive for *Enterobacter cloacae*, *Enterobacter agglomerans*, or *Pseudomonas cepacia*, avoid administering D5W or higher concentrations of IV fluids, in which these organisms grow rapidly.

○ CSFs take 1 to 2 days to produce changes in laboratory values.

○ Common side effects of CSFs include localized redness and pain at the injection site and excessive leukocytosis.

o An ANC below 500 or a CD4 count below 200 plus a T lymphocyte count or total lymphocyte count below 14 indicates severe risk of infection.
o The patient should be prohibited from contact with contagious individuals and meticulously wash hands often.

Isolation Precautions

Section 3   Phyllis Peterson

OVERVIEW

Isolation precautions should be implemented when a patient harbors pathogenic organisms that may be readily transmitted to others in the environment. Measures to prevent the transmission of organisms are particularly important when caring for immunocompromised patients. Even patients with normal immune systems who have been subjected to many invasive procedures while in the acute care setting may be at risk for serious infections.

Standard precautions should be applied to all patients in the health care setting regardless of their immune status or the presence of possible infections. These precautions involve hand washing and barrier protection (i.e., gowns, gloves, and goggles) to prevent direct contact with all blood and body fluids except sweat. Standard precautions can be highly effective in preventing the transmission of infections via direct contact. They are particularly important in preventing nosocomial infections in immunocompromised patients.

PRINCIPLES OF CARE

Different isolation measures are needed for different patient populations and care settings. Specific isolation precautions are determined based on the patient's immune status, as well as on the immune status of other patients in the unit. Other considerations include the type(s) of infectious organisms either suspected or documented by culture, and their mode of transmission.

Isolation practices must be implemented whenever a patient has a potential or known source of infection. In many regards, hospitals and health care facilities are incubators for infection because they contain so many potential sources and reservoirs for pathogens. Organisms may be brought into the facility by patients, caregivers and visitors. Poor cleaning, decontamination, and sterilization practices regarding the environment, transportation equipment, and medical supplies may further contribute to the spread of infection. Still other infections may arise from the patient's own body flora and can spread to other individuals, particularly if caregivers are negligent about hand washing practices.

Body fluids (urine, feces, mucus, wound drainage, blood) contain potentially infectious organisms that may pose a danger to any patient, regardless of immune status. For this reason, standard precautions are implemented for all patients, regardless of health care setting. These precautions specify the use of hand washing, impermeable protective clothing, waterproof gloves, and splash-resistant face and eye protection to shield the caregiver from direct contact with infectious body secretions. The level of protective garb used is directly influenced by the needs of the patient and the type and amount of body secretions present. When properly used, protective shields and clothing not only protect the caregiver but also help decrease the transmission of pathogenic organisms to other patients.

DECISION-MAKING
Blood and Body Fluids

All body fluids contain potentially infectious organisms; however, not all patients require the same degree of barrier protection. For example, caring for a bedridden patient with multiple bleeding bedsores requires more extensive protective garb than needed when caring for an ambulatory patient with intact skin.

Impermeable masks, goggles, and/or face shields must be worn during procedures and care that may generate splashes or sprays of blood or other body fluids. Because the mucous membranes have a rich supply of blood vessels, infections are readily transmitted via these body surfaces. Surgical masks offer short-term protection only from large droplets from infected individuals who are coughing and sneezing.

Gloves must be worn whenever there is a possibility of contact with any body fluids, or when contact will occur with the mucous membranes or broken skin of any patient. Gloves must be changed after each patient contact, and the hands washed immediately.

Protective garb must be worn to provide protection when contact with body secretions is anticipated. Impermeable gowns are worn to prevent contact of clothing and skin with infectious secretions and to reduce the transmission of organisms to others. Shoe covers and boots may also be required whenever splashes, sprays, or large quantities of infectious material may occur.

Transmission-based precautions may be needed in addition to standard precautions, based on specific characteristics of the suspected or known disease or organism. It cannot be overemphasized that careful hand washing practices must be an integral part of all levels of isolation precautions.

Isolation Precautions

1. Strict isolation precautions may be indicated for a patient with an extremely virulent or contagious infection transmitted through the air or by direct contact. A private room with a closed door is mandatory and medically necessary. Two patients with the same organisms may be cohorted and share the room. Masks, gowns, and gloves are required for all persons entering the room. Items contaminated with body fluids must be bagged and labeled as infectious waste before leaving the room. Meals are provided on disposable plates with disposable utensils.

2. Contact isolation is required for diseases or readily transmissible infections spread by close contact. A private room is medically necessary, except for two patients with the same organism, who can share a room. The door must be closed at all times. Masks are required if caregivers or visitors will be in close quarters with the patient, and gowns should be worn if contact with infectious secretions is likely.

3. Respiratory isolation is designed to prevent the spread of airborne droplets containing infectious organisms. A private room is required, except for two patients with the same organism, who can share a room. The door must

be kept closed at all times. Gowns and gloves are not required unless contact with infectious secretions is possible or anticipated. Masks are required for all persons entering the room. Strict hand washing must be observed. Contaminated items must be bagged and labeled as infectious waste before they may be removed from the room. A patient leaving the room must wear a mask.

4. Airborne precautions, also known as tuberculosis isolation, is indicated for patients with suspected or confirmed pulmonary tuberculosis. These patients require special precautions because of the small size of the droplet nuclei. As the nuclei evaporate, the infectious organisms may remain airborne and be widely dispersed by air currents. The patient must be placed in a private room with negative airflow and an anteroom to prevent the escape of microorganisms into the general environment. Air from the room must be exhausted directly to the outside of the building. If air cannot be vented to the outside, it should be treated with high-efficiency particulate air filters before being circulated to other areas of the building. The room should also have a minimum of 6 to 12 air exchanges per hour. Everyone entering the room must wear a particulate filter facemask. Gowns and gloves are not required unless the possibility exists of contact with contaminated secretions. If the patient must leave the room, he or she must wear a particulate filter mask.

5. Enteric precautions may be initiated to reduce the transmission of infections by direct or indirect contact with feces. In most cases, a private room is unnecessary unless the patient is incontinent, is mobile, or has poor hygiene. Patients with the same organism may share a room. Masks are not required, but gown and gloves are necessary if the possibility exists of contact with infected material. Items contaminated with infectious waste must be bagged and appropriately labeled before they leave the patient's room.

Drug-Resistant Organisms

The widespread use of antibiotics, often in inappropriate circumstances, has led to the development of serious drug-resistant organisms that affect patient care and outcomes in a variety of health care settings. Methicillin-resistant *Staphylococcus aureus* (MRSA) is a major source of nosocomial infections. By definition, MRSA is resistant to all beta-lactam antibiotics, including penicillins and cephalosporins. MRSA is no more infectious or aggressive than ordinary *S. aureus*—it is simply more challenging to treat. This organism is seen in a wide variety of health care settings, including acute care hospitals, long-term-care facilities, prisons, and rehabilitation centers. Health care providers may become colonized with this organism, particularly in the nares, but rarely develop an infection. This is a source of concern, because they may then transmit the organism to patients while providing care.

The incidence of vancomycin-resistant enterococci (VRE) has risen 35-fold since 1989; patients in intensive care settings are particularly susceptible. Enterococci are normally present in the bowel and the genitourinary tract. After exposure to antibiotics, the drug-resistant bacteria may survive and multiply, leading to an overgrowth of the resistant organism in the gut. Patients who are debilitated due to disease processes, immunosuppressant therapy, or numerous surgeries or invasive procedures are at risk for either becoming colonized or developing an active infection with VRE.

Transmission

Research indicates that caregivers' hands are the most frequent mode of transmission of MRSA from patient to patient. The primary reservoir of MRSA is colonized and infected patients. VRE may be spread from patient to patient by direct contact with the hands of personnel or by indirect contact with contaminated environmental surfaces. VRE can survive on hands, gloves, and environmental surfaces for as long as 7 days.

Isolation Precautions for Resistant Organisms

As with other organisms, isolation precautions must be determined based on the status of the organism within the patient. A patient who is colonized with MRSA but has no active infection, draining wound, incontinence, or uncontrolled coughing or sneezing may require only standard precautions. A patient with VRE in the gut who is continent of stool and able to maintain hand washing precautions may also be placed on standard precautions.

Contact isolation is indicated for patients with

- Indwelling catheter–associated MRSA or VRE urinary tract infections or colonization
- Wounds heavily colonized or infected with MRSA or VRE
- Tracheostomy or infected respiratory tract

If a cluster of infections is identified, then all patients with positive cultures should be placed on contact isolation. Personnel need to wear gloves, gowns, and masks in accordance with standard precautions whenever direct patient contact is anticipated. These items need to disposed of safely before leaving the patient's room. Nurses and other caregivers should take care to not touch potentially contaminated surfaces in the patient's environment after removing gloves and washing hands, to prevent transmission of organisms to other patient care areas.

Patient care equipment (e.g., thermometers, glucometers) used by the VRE-positive patient should not be shared with other patients. If the use of shared equipment is unavoidable, then the equipment must be cleaned and disinfected before it is used for another patient.

 CLINICAL PEARLS

○ Always maintain a high index of suspicion for possible infections in patients who are debilitated, malnourished, or immunocompromised.
○ Monitor results of cultures of blood and body fluids carefully. Promptly report positive cultures and determine whether the current therapy is effective for the identified organism(s).
○ Standard precautions involve the use of protective garb to prevent contact with infectious body secretions.
○ Transmission-based precautions must be followed consistently by all caregivers to minimize the risk of nosocomial infections.
○ Isolation precautions may be cumbersome, expensive, and psychologically distressing for the patient. Avoid instituting more precautions than are necessary for safe care.
○ VRE colonization is increased in patients who are in hospitals of more than 300-bed capacity, are on ventilators, are immunocompromised, are neutropenic, have oral mucositis, have diarrhea, or use vancomycin.
○ MRSA has been found on hospital ward curtains. Colonization is increased in patients who are in skilled nursing homes, have received an organ

transplant, have pressure sores, are receiving tube feedings, or have been hospitalized within the preceding year, as well as in persons employed in health care facilities.

 RESOURCES

- American Association of Occupational Health Nurses: www.aaohn.org/
- American Autoimmune Related Diseases Association: www.aarda.org/
- American Journal of Infection Control: www.apic.org/ajic/
- Centers for Disease Control and Prevention, Hospital Infections Program: www.cdc.gov/niddod/hip/DEFAULT.HTM
- The Immune Deficiency Foundation: 708-799-2481 or www.primenet.com/ ~vohnout/immunology.html
- *Journal of Immunology* home page: jimmunol.org/
- Medical Management of Lupus: www.mtio.com/mclfa/lal_3.htm
- National Center for Infectious Diseases: www.cdc.gov/ncidod/index.htm
- National Institute for Occupational Safety and Health: www.cdc.gov/niosh/ homepage.html
- National Institute of Health Web Site on Immunodeficiency Disorders: www.niaid.nih.gov/Publications/pid/contents.htm
- On-Line Review of *Essentials of Immunology*: www.imc.gsm.com/inte-grated/frameset.htm
- Primary Immunodeficiency Association: www.ipopi.org/pia/living/ liv1.html
- U.S. Department of Labor: 202-693-1999
- www.osha.gov/oshpubs/perpro.html (personal protective equipment)
- www.osha-slc.gov/SLTC/bloodbornepathogens/index.html (blood-borne pathogens)

chapter 11

Decision-Making for Common Laboratory Data

Red Blood Cell Counts

Section 1   Kitty Garrett

OVERVIEW

The most frequently ordered laboratory test is the complete blood count (CBC). The CBC is used in physical examinations, preoperative screening, and evaluation of acute disease or symptoms of anemia or infection. Serial values are often used to track the progress of a disease state or a patient's response to treatment. The CBC is a simple method of confirming or ruling out many conditions and determining whether other tests are needed. The CBC assesses the function of all three components of the blood. Red blood cells (RBCs) are assessed for their oxygen-carrying capacity. White blood cells (WBCs) are assessed for their ability to protect the body against foreign matter. Platelet counts are assessed to determine if the numbers are adequate to provide proper clotting. This section discusses RBC count and platelets; the WBC count is discussed in Section 2.

PRINCIPLES OF CARE
Red Blood Cells

RBCs, or erythrocytes, are flexible biconcave disks (like a donut with the hole partially filled) whose primary function is to deliver oxygen from inspired air to the tissues and to carry carbon dioxide back from the tissues to the lungs for elimination. They are derived from the pluripotent stem cells (Fig. 11-1-1) in the bone marrow. RBCs are containers for hemoglobin (Hb); their unique shape allows an increased surface area for Hb to combine with oxygen. Mature RBCs have no nucleus and, therefore, cannot divide. They are constantly being produced and destroyed. The average life span is 120 days. When the body needs more RBCs (e.g., in anemia, tissue hypoxia), a hormone called erythropoietin from the kidneys stimulates the bone marrow to differentiate stem cells into RBCs. This process is called erythropoiesis.

Platelets

Platelets (or thrombocytes) are the smallest cells found in the blood. All of the body's platelets could easily fit into a teaspoon. They play a vital role in hemostasis. Platelets prevent blood loss by adhering together at the site of an injured blood vessel to clump until a more stable clot can form. A platelet plug forms within 3 to 5 minutes of injury.

Cells seen in
bone marrow

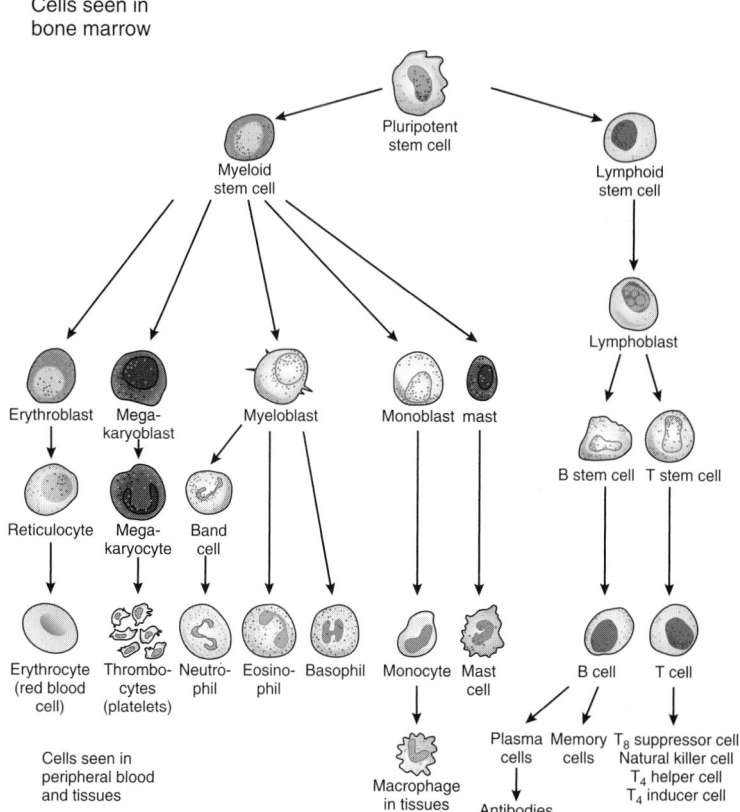

Figure 11-1-1. Origin, development, and structure of thrombocytes, leukocytes, and erythrocytes from pluripotent stem cells.

DECISION-MAKING
Laboratory Tests Related to RBCs
Red Blood Cell Count

The RBC count is measured as the number of erythrocytes in millions per cubic millimeter of blood. The number of RBCs varies according to age, sex, and altitude but averages 5 million/mm³ of blood. Indications for RBC counts are to diagnose blood disorders and to furnish a number for calculating erythrocyte indices that help to define the cause of anemias. *Normal value for males is 4.5 to 6.2 million/mm³; females, 4.0 to 5.5 million/mm³.*

Disorders of Red Blood Cells
Decreased Levels (Anemia)

Anemia is a reduction in the total number of circulating RBCs or a decrease in the quantity or quality of Hb and/or Hct. It is not a disease but rather a clinical syndrome with symptoms of many possible diseases. Conditions that cause anemia include (Table 11-1-1):

-Altered erythropoiesis (as seen in renal failure and with chemotherapeutic agent use, aplastic anemia, leukemia)

-Conditions that cause extreme RBC destruction (as seen in hemolytic or type II hypersensitivity blood transfusion reactions)

-Blood loss

-Nutritional deficiencies including iron deficiency anemia (decreased Hb production), pernicious anemia (decreased RBC production), and folate deficiency anemia (decreased RBC production)

Increased Levels: Erythrocytosis

An elevated level of RBCs is called erythrocytosis (see Table 11-1-1). Polycythemia may also be used to describe an increase in RBC count but actually refers to a specific group of disorders that cause erythrocytosis. Types of polycythemia include primary polycythemia vera, which is caused by a relatively rare myeloproliferative disease of the bone marrow, and secondary polycythemia, which is an increase in RBCs as a physiologic compensatory mechanism for decreases in oxygen delivery. This may be seen in high altitudes or in patients with cardiopulmonary disease such as congestive heart failure (CHF), chronic obstructive pulmonary disease, or cardiovascular malformation.

Reticulocyte Count

Reticulocytes are immature RBCs. They mature into adult RBCs within 24 to 36 hours after their release into the bloodstream from the bone marrow. Therefore, normally there should only be a few in the bloodstream (1% to 2% of total RBC count). Their presence is an indication that the bone marrow is being stimulated to produce RBCs. Reticulocyte counts may be measured to assist in the diagnosis and differentiation of bone marrow depression from other anemias, hemorrhage, hemolysis, or radiation and to evaluate the patient's response to treatment. A raised reticulocyte count (5% to 7%) in a patient who is anemic is a normal expected response and indicates that the bone marrow is able to respond appropriately in attempting to replace sudden RBC loss from destruction or hemorrhage. A normal or low reticulocyte count in an anemic patient indicates bone marrow dysfunction (a production prob-

Table 11-1-1. Red Blood Cell Count: Causes of Abnormal Values

DECREASED RBCs (anemia)	INCREASED RBCs (erythrocytosis)
• Hemodilution	• Polycythemia
• Blood loss	• COPD
• Hemolysis	• High altitude
• Thalassemia	• Dehydration
• Chronic infection	• Gentamicin
• Multiple myeloma	• Methyldopa
• BM depression	• Excessive exercise
• Iron deficiency	• Anxiety, pain
• Renal failure	

BM, bone marrow; COPD, chronic obstructive pulmonary disease; RBC, red blood cell.

Table 11-1-2. Reticulocyte Count: Causes of Abnormal Values

DECREASED RETICULOCYTE COUNT	INCREASED RETICULOCYTE COUNT

• Decreased RBC production (problem with bone marrow) due to:
  • Alcoholism
  • Cirrhosis
  • ↓ Erythropoietin
  • Blood loss
  • Radiation
  • Decreased adrenal function
  • Chronic infection
	• Anemia (normal response)
	• Treatment of iron deficiency anemia
	• Thalassemia
	• Pregnancy
	• High altitude
	• RBC loss (hemorrhage)
	• RBC hemolysis
	• Confirms that problem is NOT in the RBCs or due to Hb production

lem). The number of reticulocytes per thousand erythrocytes is measured and expressed as a percentage (Table 11-1-2). *Normal values are 0.5% to 2.5% in females and 0.5% to 1.5% in males.*

Red Blood Cell Indices

In order to maintain normal oxygen-carrying capacity, RBCs must be adequate in size, shape, and amount of Hb. Alterations in any of these will affect the ability of the RBC to carry oxygen. Erythrocyte indices describe these characteristics and therefore help to identify causes of anemia. They are mean corpuscular volume (MCV), mean corpuscular hemoglobin (MCH), and mean corpuscular hemoglobin concentration (MCHC). RBC indices can also provide an indication of fluid volume status. They are calculated using the results furnished by the RBC, Hb, and Hct.

Mean Corpuscular Volume. The MCV measures the relative *size* or volume in an average RBC. This is important to differentiate, because it helps to identify causes of anemias (Table 11-1-3). Cells that are undersized are called microcytic. Microcytic cells are seen in iron deficiency anemia and thalassemia. Cells that have an average size are called normocytic; examples are hemolytic and hemorrhagic anemias. Cells that are oversized are called macrocytic. Macrocytic cells are seen in pernicious anemia and folate deficiency.

The MCV is also used to diagnose blood disorders and to monitor the course of therapy. The MCV is decreased in dehydration and increased in overhydration. The MCV is calculated by dividing the Hct by the RBC count (MCV = Hct × 10/RBC). *Normal adult values are 82 to 93 μm^3.*

Mean Corpuscular Hemoglobin. MCH measures the average *weight* of Hb in an average RBC. The MCH is of some value in diagnosing severe anemia but is not as useful as the MCHC. It usually goes along with the MCV; that is, if the cell size is smaller, the cells contain less Hb. MCH (like MCV) is increased in macrocytic anemia and decreased in microcytic anemia. It is calculated by dividing the Hb by the RBC count (MCH = Hb × 10/RBC). *Normal adult values are 26 to 34 picograms (pg).*

Mean Corpuscular Hemoglobin Concentration. MCHC measures the average concentration of Hb in an average RBC. MCHC is calculated by dividing the Hb by the Hct (MCHC = Hb × 100/Hct). *The normal value is 31% to 38%.* Cells that are pale because they contain less Hb are said to be

Table 11-1-3. Differentiation of Anemias by Red Blood Cell Indices

MCV*	MCHC*	TYPE OF ANEMIA	SECONDARY TO
Normal 82–93 μm^3	Normal 31–38%	Normocytic, normochromic (normal RBC size and Hb content)	Early iron deficiency, ↓ RBCs due to chronic illness or malnutrition, acute hemorrhage, hemolytic anemia, sickle cell, renal failure, aplastic anemia, leukemia
↓ Level <82	↓ Level <31	Microcytic, hypochromic (small RBC size; decreased Hb content)	Late iron deficiency (most common), chronic infections, thalassemia, lead poisoning
Normal 82–93	↓ Level <31	Normocytic, hypochromic (normal RBC size, decreased Hb content)	Systemic diseases, lead poisoning
↑ Level >93	Normal 31–38	Macrocytic (megaloblastic), normochromic (large RBC size, normal Hb content)	Vitamin deficiency (B_{12}, folic acid), advanced liver disease, alcoholism, pernicious anemia

Hb, hemoglobin; MCV, mean corpuscular volume; MCHC, mean corpuscular hemoglobin count; RBC, red blood cell.

hypochromic, whereas normal-colored cells are said to be normochromic. Hyperchromic cells are rare. MCHC is increased in dehydration and decreased in overhydration.

Red Blood Cell Morphology

In addition to the RBC indices, other characteristics of the RBCs are important. Anisocytosis refers to the abnormal *variation in the size* of the RBCs. There may be combined microcytosis and macrocytosis. Poikilocytosis refers to abnormal *variation in the shape* of the RBCs. These characteristics may be detected when the routine CBC is run, but they must be verified with a slide analysis. Both conditions can affect oxygen-carrying capacity. They usually result from premature release of reticulocytes owing to an accelerated production of erythropoietin. They may also be caused by the use of fertility drugs. Sickle cell anemia causes crescent-shaped RBCs owing to the presence of Hb S. Schistocytes are fragmented RBCs seen in hemolytic anemias and disseminated intravascular coagulopathy.

Hemoglobin

Hb is a complex protein made of heme and globin. It attaches to the RBC to carry oxygen and accounts for approximately 90% of the dry weight of the RBC. It gives blood its red color. Measurement of Hb is performed to identify certain types of anemias, to follow the course of a disease, to monitor therapy, to detect abnormal types, and to provide a number for calculating RBC indices (Table 11-1-4). Hb is measured in grams per 100 mL of whole blood. *Normal Hb is 14 to 18 g/dL in men and 12 to 16 g/dL in women*, although these values vary with altitude.

Hematocrit

The Hct is defined as the total volume of RBCs relative to the total volume of whole blood in cubic millimeters. It is also called packed cell volume (PCV). The word *hematocrit* means "separate blood." Results of Hct are reported as a percentage. The Hct value depends on age, sex, altitude, and RBC size. It should be approximately three times the Hb value and should parallel the RBC when the cells have a normal size and shape. Indications for Hct include the diagnosis of blood disorders, determining the fluid balance, measuring the percentage of RBCs in the circulation, determining the amount of blood loss after surgery/trauma, and providing a number for calculating RBC indices. *Normal Hct values are 40% to 54% for men and 37% to 47%*

Table 11-1-4. Hemoglobin: Causes of Abnormal Values

DECREASED Hb	INCREASED Hb
• Anemia	• Polycythemia
• Blood loss	• COPD
• RBC hemolysis	• High altitude
• ↓ RBC production	• Dehydration
• Fluid retention	• CHF
• Hemodilution	• Smoking
• Pregnancy	

CHF, congestive heart failure; COPD, chronic obstructive pulmonary disease; Hb, hemoglobin; RBC, red blood cell.

Table 11-1-5. Hematocrit: Causes of Abnormal Values

DECREASED Hct	INCREASED Hct
• Anemia	• Polycythemia
• Blood loss	• Late COPD (chronic hypoxemia)
• RBC hemolysis	• Dehydration
• Hemodilution	• Burns
• Iron deficiency	• Acidosis
• Overhydration	• Smoking
• Poor kidney function	
• Multiple myeloma	
• Leukemia	
• Rheumatoid arthritis	

COPD, chronic obstructive pulmonary disease; Hct, hematocrit; RBC, red blood cell.

for women. Elevated sodium and glucose values can also cause the RBC to take in fluid and swell, making RBCs larger and increasing the Hct. Any deficit in plasma volume (dehydration) can cause a falsely increased level of Hct (Table 11-1-5). This increase may require fluid administration to decrease viscosity and to reduce the chance of thrombus formation.

Erythrocyte Sedimentation Rate

The erythrocyte sedimentation rate (ESR) measures how fast RBCs descend in a tube of anticoagulated blood. RBCs in certain states tend to adhere to each other and descend more quickly. A positive test result suggests that an infection or malignancy is present, but it is nonspecific. Many conditions can cause an increase in the ESR. It is used as a supplementary test to aid in the diagnosis of infection or malignancy, inflammation, and some autoimmune diseases (Table 11-1-6). ESR rates tend to increase with age. The ESR can be

Table 11-1-6. Erythrocyte Sedimentation Rate: Causes of Abnormal Values

DECREASED ESR—USUALLY NOT CLINICALLY SIGNIFICANT	INCREASED ESR
• Sickle cell anemia (IS significant)	• Acute or chronic inflammation
• Hypoproteinemia	• Increased plasma protein
• Some anemias	• Severe anemia
• Polycythemia	• Malignancy
• Hyperviscous plasma	• Rheumatoid arthritis
• CHF	• Some anemias
• Mononucleosis	• Multiple myeloma
• Low fibrinogen	• Autoimmune disease
	• All collagen diseases
	• Tissue destruction
	• Acute MI
	• Syphilis
	• Hepatitis
	• Pregnancy (last 2 trimesters)
	• Tuberculosis

CHF, congestive heart failure; MI, myocardial infarction; ESR, erythrocyte sedimentation rate.

determined in several ways. The most common way is the one whose values are applied by the Westergren method. *Normal values for males are 15 to 30 mm/hr and those for females are 20 to 40 mm/hr (Westergren method).*

Laboratory Tests Related to Platelets
Platelet Count

The platelet count measures the number of platelets in 1 mL of blood. It is used to evaluate platelet production and destruction but does not evaluate platelet *function*. Platelet counts are indicated in routine screening and assessment of bleeding disorders and also in the evaluation of the bone marrow in response to chemotherapy or radiation. Platelets circulate for about 10 days and are then replaced. *The normal platelet count is 150,000 to 400,000 mm³/mL.*

Platelet Function

The test that is most indicative of platelet function is the *bleeding time*. It actually measures the time that it takes for a small skin incision to form a platelet plug. Several methods are used for this test; normal results range from 1 to 8 minutes depending on the method.

Disorders of Platelets

Decreased: Thrombocytopenia. The normal platelet count in adults is 150,000 to 400,000 mm³/mL blood. A platelet count of less than 150,000 is called thrombocytopenia; a platelet count greater than 400,000 is called thrombocytosis. The average platelet count is 250,000. Values of less than 20,000 or greater than 1,000,000 are critical and must be reported. Bleeding does not occur until the level drops below 50,000. Counts under 20,000 significantly increase the risk for mortality owing to brain or gastrointestinal hemorrhage. Causes include decreased production in the bone marrow or increased consumption or destruction.

Increased: Thrombocytosis. Transient thrombocytosis is a physiologic response to physical stress, exercise, trauma, infection, and ovulation. An increased level of platelets is not clinically significant unless the patient reaches a level greater than 1,000,000. Increased, inappropriate clotting can then occur. Primary thrombocytosis is a myeloproliferative disorder of the stem cells. See Table 11-1-7 for causes of thrombocytosis and thrombocytopenia.

 CLINICAL PEARLS

○ One unit of packed RBCs increases the Hb by 1 g and the Hct by 3%.
○ Hb/Hct values obtained soon after a hemorrhage may not yet reflect the severity of blood loss; these values may take several hours to drop. Use the heart rate and blood pressure as better indicators of the severity of hemorrhage.
○ Even after a blood transfusion, it takes 12 to 24 hours for the Hb and Hct to increase.
○ The MCHC should be approximately twice the Hb.
○ Dehydration can give a falsely elevated Hct and RBC count.
○ Hemoconcentration can make the blood thicker with an increased risk of thrombi. IV fluid can help to dilute viscous blood and decrease the chance of thromboembolism. Check for CHF.

Table 11-1-7. Causes of Abnormal Platelet Counts

THROMBOCYTOPENIA (<150,000 mm³)	THROMBOCYTOSIS (>400,000 mm³)
• Bone marrow depression/anemia due to medications, chemotherapy, radiation • Leukemia • Infection • Vitamin B₁₂, folic acid deficiency • DIC • Splenomegaly with hyperfunction of the spleen • AIDS • Platelet destruction (either mechanical or autoimmune—idiopathic thrombocytopenia purpura)	• Polycythemia • Malignancies • Inflammatory disease • Rheumatoid arthritis • Infectious disease • Pregnancy • Pulmonary embolus • Trauma/hemorrhage • Fractures • Some anemias • Post splenectomy • Ovulation

AIDS, acquired immunodeficiency syndrome; DIC, disseminated intravascular coagulation.

○ It takes 500 mL blood loss to drop the Hb by 1 g and the Hct by 3%.
○ A transfusion of packed RBCs increases the Hct by 3% and the Hb by 1 g.
○ If no parameters are given and no trends are available with the Hct, in general, the physician should be notified if the Hct is less than 16% or greater than 60%.
○ For every 200 mL blood loss, it takes 20 days to restore Hb to normal without a blood transfusion.
○ The frequency of blood donation is based on the fact that new RBCs are manufactured every 120 days.
○ Thrombi are likely to occur when platelet counts are elevated; bleeding is likely to occur when platelet counts are decreased (<20,000 to 30,000).
○ One 5-grain aspirin can "coat" platelets and prevent blood clotting for the life of the platelet (9 to 12 days).
○ Elective surgery is not usually performed if the Hb is below 10 g.

White Blood Cell Count with Differential

Section 2   Patricia Catalano

OVERVIEW

The WBC count and differential is a commonly ordered laboratory test in the acute care setting. It is an excellent and simple screening test that provides important diagnostic information. Nurses' competency in examining and interpreting laboratory data, specifically the WBC count and differential, can play a significant role in the patient's outcome.

PRINCIPLES OF CARE
Development of Leukocytes (White Blood Cells)

All blood cells develop in the bone marrow from one pluripotent stem cell by a process of cell division and differentiation. This stem cell gives rise to five morphologically and functionally distinct mature WBCs (leukocytes), which are released from the bone marrow into the circulation (see Fig. 11-1-1).

Classification of Leukocytes

Leukocytes are classified according to structure as either *granulocytes* or *agranulocytes* and according to function as either *phagocytes or immunocytes*. The granulocytes, which include neutrophils, basophils, and eosinophils, are all phagocytic cells. Of the agranulocytes, the monocytes and macrophages are phagocytes, whereas the lymphocytes are specific immune cells called immunocytes.

Phagocytes
Granulocytes

Granulocytes get their name from the granules present in their cytoplasm (Fig. 11-2-1). These granules contain mediators that serve inflammatory and immune functions. Granulocytes also contain enzymes in their cytoplasm that are capable of destroying microorganisms and catabolizing debris ingested during phagocytosis. They take about 1 week to develop in the bone marrow. Granulocytes circulate for only about 6 to 12 hours in the bloodstream and 2 to 3 days after entering the tissue. There are three types of granulocytes: *neutrophils, eosinophils,* and *basophils.*

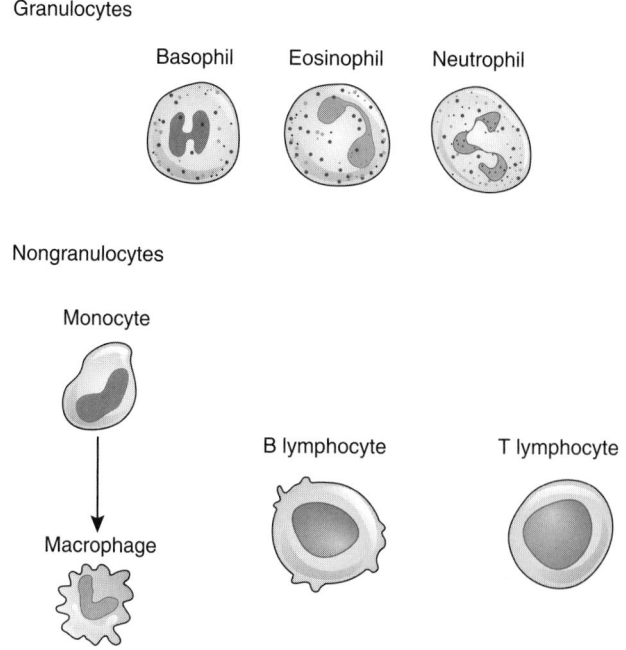

Figure 11-2-1. Human blood smear of granulocytes and nongranulocytes.

Neutrophils

The most populous of the circulating WBCs are neutrophils. Accounting for between 50% and 70% of all circulating WBCs, they are the body's primary line of defense against bacterial infection. Normally, most of the neutrophils circulating in the bloodstream exist in a mature form. Because the nuclei of neutrophils are segmented into three to five lobes connected by thin strands, they are clinically referred to as *segmented neutrophils or "segs."* Another term that is used to refer to these cells is *polymorphonuclear neutrophils (PMNs), or polys*, again because of the shape of the nucleus. These cells, which are highly mobile, are the first to arrive in response to acute inflammation or infection—usually within 90 minutes. They migrate out of the capillaries and into the inflamed site in a process called diapedesis or emigration. They ingest microorganisms and debris, then they die and form purulent exudate that is removed by the lymphatics or through the epithelium.

Bands or stabs are immature neutrophils released from the bone marrow when there is increased demand for neutrophils, usually in response to acute infection. These immature cells have unsegmented nuclei that resemble bands or rods.

Eosinophils

Eosinophils have large, coarse granules and constitute only 1% to 4% of the total leukocyte count. They are often seen at the site of invasive parasitic infestations and allergic (immediate hypersensitivity) responses. Individuals with chronic allergic conditions (e.g., allergic rhinitis or asthma) typically have elevated eosinophil counts. The eosinophils may serve a critical function in mitigating allergic responses, because they can: (1) inactivate the slow reacting substance of anaphylaxis (SRS-A); (2) neutralize histamine; and (3) inhibit mast cell degranulation.

Basophils

Basophils make up less than 1% of all leukocytes. They appear to help the body resist systemic allergic reactions and anaphylactic states. Basophils have cytoplasmic granules that contain vasoactive amines (i.e., histamine, bradykinin, serotonin) that are released to help mediate the inflammatory response. Tissue basophils are called *mast cells*.

Agranulocytes (Nongranulocytes)

Agranulocytes are so called because they do not contain granules in their cytoplasm. There are two types: monocytes and lymphocytes.

Monocyte/Macrophage

Monocytes comprise 2% to 8% of WBCs. They represent the body's second line of defense. Monocytes increase during chronic bacterial infection and viral diseases. They circulate in the blood as monocytes, but once they move into the tissue spaces (usually in response to infection), they mature into larger phagocytic cells called *macrophages*. After maturation the amount of protein-digesting enzymes that they contain increases, thus enhancing their ability to destroy bacteria. Monocyte levels increase as patients recover from the acute phase of infection. These cells arrive on the scene in about 5 hours after an injury and become the predominant WBC in 48 hours.

Table 11-2-1. Tissue Macrophages

MACROPHAGE	TISSUE
Kupffer cells	Liver
Alveolar macrophage	Lung
Histocytes	Connective tissue
Pleural and peritoneal macrophages	Serous cavities
Microglial cells	Nervous system
Osteoclasts	Bones
Mesangial	Kidneys
Langerhans	Skin
Dendritic cells	Lymphoid tissue

Specialized macrophages called *tissue macrophages* reside in certain tissues (i.e., the Kupffer cells in the liver) and can live there for several months (Table 11-2-1). Because macrophages concentrated in these organs sequester and destroy bacteria before they enter the bloodstream, they provide a degree of protection even when a patient is neutropenic.

Steroids slow the proliferation and function of monocytes as well as of neutrophils, thus a patient rendered neutropenic by chemotherapy who is also receiving steroids has lost the secondary protection of the monocytes. Such a patient requires vigilant nursing care and strict enforcement of neutropenic precautions (see Chapter 10, Section 2).

Lymphocytes/Immunocytes

Lymphocytes are also agranulocytes. They are involved in specific immune responses (see Chapter 10, Section 1). There are three classes of lymphocyte—the T lymphocyte (T cell), the B lymphocyte (B cell), and the natural killer cell. These cells have surface molecules on them called cluster of differentiation (CD), which assists in defining their function.

T Cell

The T cell matures in the thymus and is responsible for cell-mediated immunity. It also stimulates B cell activation. The T cell has several subtypes that are produced in response to infection and can be divided into regulator or effector cells.

Regulator Cells

1. Helper T cells are the master switches of the immune system. These cells act as surveyors of the system; they secrete cytokines that influence and stimulate the production of other immune cells. These cells are CD4 T cells.
2. Suppressor T cells suppress this response once the battle is won.

Effector Cells

1. Cytotoxic T cells directly attack and kill invading cells by attaching and releasing enzymes to destroy them. These cells are called CD8 T cells.
2. The memory T cells rapidly respond to a second attack by the same organism. The average survival time for these cells is approximately 5 years.

B Cell

The B cell matures in the bone marrow and is responsible for humoral or antibody-mediated immunity. When activated, B cells produce plasma cells, which release antibodies.

Natural Killer Cell

The natural killer cells remain in circulation to defend against infected host cells and cancer cells.

DECISION-MAKING: ANALYZING THE WHITE BLOOD CELL WITH DIFFERENTIAL

The Sample

The sample is obtained by venipuncture and is collected in a lavender top tube. The sample is viable at room temperature for up to 10 hours. The patient should ideally be at rest for 10 to 15 minutes before the sample is obtained.

Peripheral Smear

The peripheral smear (Fig. 11-2-2) identifies the morphology and amount of cellular elements. The presence of blasts (i.e., immature granulocytes) in the peripheral smear is a finding suggestive of leukemia or a myeloproliferative disorder. Eosinophils stain red; basophils stain dark blue or violet.

Counts

The total WBC count is used to assist in the identification and severity of infection or inflammation. This count is also used to assess the bone marrow's response to radiation therapy and chemotherapy. The WBC differential allows for the critical evaluation of the hematologic status of a patient. One must consider the individual counts of each type of leukocyte (Table 11-2-2).

Elevated Levels

Leukocytosis is the elevation in the total WBC and occurs when the WBC is greater than $11,000/mm^3$. Leukocytosis is usually caused by an increase in one of the five types of WBCs and is given the name of the cell that shows the primary increase. Elevated values may be caused by bacterial infection; tissue necrosis associated with disorders such as acute myocardial infarction, burns, gangrene, inflammation, leukemia, or lymphoma.

Neutrophilia. Neutrophilia is an increased total neutrophil count (including both segs and bands). This increased count is commonly caused by acute infection, inflammation, or tissue destruction. It is also caused by myeloproliferative disorders, such as polycythemia vera and chronic myelocytic leukemia, which increase stem cell proliferation in the bone marrow. This condition may also be referred to as granulocytosis, because neutrophils account for the majority of all granulocytes. If neutrophils are elevated, further evaluation of the bands and segs would be indicated.

Bands. An elevation in bands is referred to as a *shift to the left.* In this situation, an increased number of immature neutrophils are released from the bone marrow and circulate in the blood. This occurs when an overwhelming infection depletes bone marrow reserves of mature neutrophils and resorts to releasing the immature bands.

Segs. A *shift to the right* means that the number of hypermature segmented neutrophils increase. Hypermature segmented neutrophils are those in which nuclear segmentation is impaired and the number of segments increase (greater

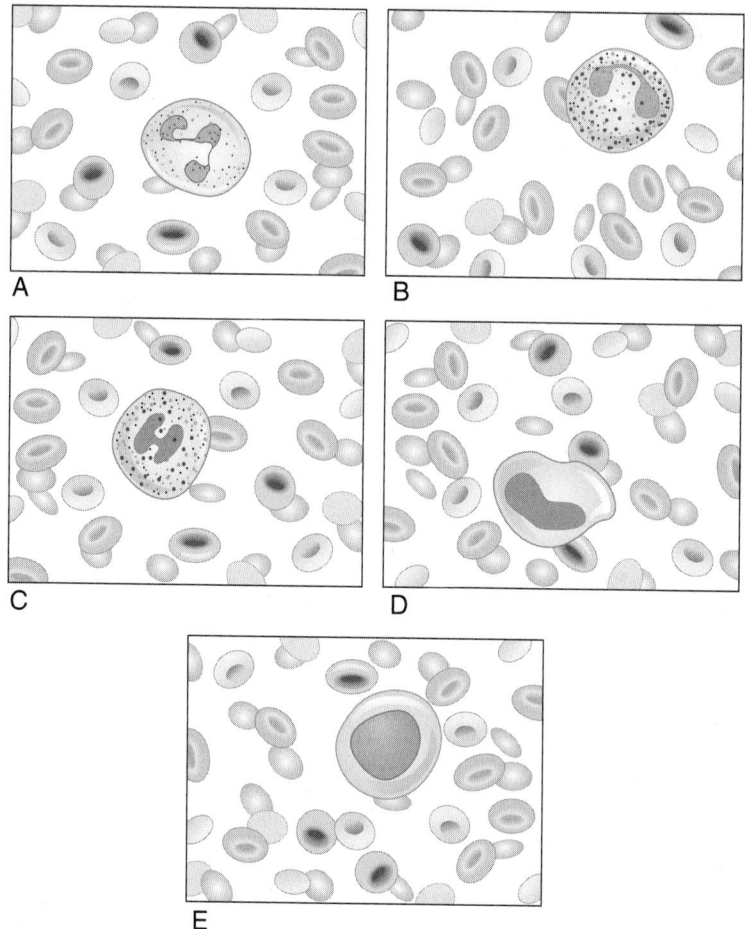

Figure 11-2-2. *A–E,* Granulocytes and nongranulocytes. (*A,* neutrophil; *B,* eosinophil; *C,* basophil; *D,* monocyte; *E,* lymphocyte.)

than five). This shift is seen with liver disease and Down syndrome as well as megaloblastic anemia and pernicious anemia.

Eosinophilia. Increased eosinophils occur with allergic disorders associated with asthma, hay fever, and drug reactions. Eosinophilia is also caused by parasitic diseases and adrenal insufficiency.

Basophilia. Increased basophils are present. Basophilia is rare and is usually related to myeloproliferative disease or basophilic leukemia. Basophilia may be seen with immediate hypersensitivity reactions.

Monocytosis. Increased monocytes are present. Monocytes increase late during the acute phase of infection and during chronic infections such as

Table 11-2-2. Normal White Blood Cell Counts

CELL TYPE	ABSOLUTE (mm³)	DIFFERENTIAL (%)
Total WBCs	4500–11,000	100
Granulocytes		
Neutrophils	3000–7000	60–70
• Segmented	2800–5600	54–68
• Bands	150–600	3–5
Eosinophils	50–400	1–5
Basophils	25–100	0–0.75
Nongranulocytes		
Monocytes	100–800	3–7
Lymphocytes (Immunocytes)	1000–4000	25–33
• T cells	800–3200	80*
• B cells	100–600	10–15*
• NK cells	50–400	5–10*

*Percentage of the total lymphocyte count.
NK, natural killer; WBC, white blood cell.

tuberculosis, subacute bacterial endocarditis (SBE), inflammatory bowel disease, and systemic lupus erythematosus (SLE).

Lymphocytosis. Increased lymphocytes occur in acute viral and chronic infections. Lymphocytosis occurs in mononucleosis, viral hepatitis, cytomegalovirus, measles, mumps, rubella, and early human immunodeficiency virus (HIV) disease.

Decreased Levels

Leukopenia. Leukopenia is a decrease in the total WBC count and is defined as a WBC count below 4500/mm³. Leukopenia is caused by decreased production (as seen in bone marrow depression) or increased destruction (as seen in exhaustive infection) of WBCs. Total WBC counts fall with radiation therapy and chemotherapy. Decreased levels in WBCs result in granulocytopenia and neutropenia.

Granulocytopenia. Granulocytopenia is a decrease in all granulocytes (i.e., neutrophils, eosinophils, and basophils). Most granulocytes are neutrophils. Neutrophils account for more than 96% of all granulocytes. Because of this, in the clinical setting the terms *granulocytopenia* and *neutropenia* are used interchangeably.

Neutropenia. Neutropenia is clinically defined as a neutrophil count of less than 2000/mm³. Although most bacterial infections stimulate an increase in neutrophils, some bacterial infections (e.g., typhoid fever and brucellosis) and many viral diseases, including hepatitis, influenza, rubella, rubeola, and mumps, decrease the neutrophil count. An overwhelming infection can also deplete the bone marrow of neutrophils and produce neutropenia. Patients with a neutrophil count of less than 2000/mm³ are at high risk of developing serious infections. The nurse should carefully monitor the WBC count to watch for downward trends, and neutropenic guidelines should be implemented in the patient's plan of care.

Types of drugs that can produce neutropenia include some antibiotics, the psychoactive drug lithium, phenothiazines, and tricyclic antidepressants. Many antineoplastic drugs that are used to treat cancer produce bone marrow depression and can significantly lower the neutrophil count. WBC production slows dramatically 7 to 15 days after induction of most chemotherapeutic agents, and the bone marrow is generally suppressed for about 3 to 4 weeks after chemotherapy is completed. Severe neutropenia occurs with a neutrophil count of less than 500/mm³. This condition is clinically referred to as *agranulocytosis*, meaning without granulocytes. Immunocompromised patients must have their neutrophil counts closely monitored for this condition. An absolute neutrophil count can be calculated using the following formula:

$$\text{Absolute neutrophil count} = \frac{\underset{\text{(segs and bands)}}{\text{total \% of neutrophils}} \times \text{WBC count}}{100}$$

Therefore, if the patient's WBC count is 3600 and her differential lists 24% segs and 0 bands, her absolute neutrophil count is:

$$\frac{24 + 0 \times 3600}{100} = 864$$

Eosinopenia. Eosinopenia is a decreased number of eosinophils resulting from migration from circulation to areas of inflammation. Eosinopenia is seen in mononucleosis, heart failure, and stress.

Basopenia. Basopenia is a decreased number of basophils. Few normally circulate, thus a periodic lack on the differential is normal. Hyperthyroidism, stress, and prolonged steroid therapy can also cause basopenia.

Monocytopenia. Monocytopenia is a decrease in monocytes. This condition is rare but has been seen with glucocorticoid therapy, hairy cell leukemia, and aplastic anemia.

Lymphocytopenia. Lymphocytopenia is a decrease in lymphocytes; it occurs normally as a person ages, or it may signify an immunodeficiency. This condition is most significant with HIV and acquired immunodeficiency syndrome (AIDS). A CD4 count of less than 200 is one indicator of an individual's conversion from HIV to AIDS. Lymphocytopenia is also seen with SLE.

General Assessment

The WBC count is a part of a big picture. You must also look at the patient and put all information into proper perspective. Trends can help to identify abnormal findings. For example, infection may be indicated if a patient has a total WBC count of 7000 mm³ for 3 days, increasing to 10,000 mm³ on the fourth day. Assess for other signs of infection. Recognize that minor alteration may be a reflection of age. Determine whether the patient has enough neutrophils to combat infection by calculating the absolute neutrophil count.

 CLINICAL PEARLS

○ It is important to consider both the relative and absolute values of various types of WBCs when interpreting a WBC differential.

- Pregnancy results in leukocytosis, primarily owing to an increase in neutrophils.
- A WBC of less than 500 (i.e., severe neutropenia) places the patient at risk for a fatal infection.
- When a patient with severe neutropenia suddenly spikes a temperature, the most appropriate initial nursing action is to notify the physician immediately.
- A WBC over 30,000 indicates massive infection or a serious disease such as leukemia.
- Gerontologic patients have slightly lower total number of WBCs.
- Neutropenic patients should not have intramuscular injections, rectal temperatures, or enemas.
- Leukocytosis as a sign of infection can be masked in a patient taking corticosteroids.
- Neutropenic patients often do not develop an elevated temperature or other signs and symptoms of infection such as redness, swelling, or pus.
- Scrupulous handwashing is the most effective method of preventing a life-threatening infection in a patient with neutropenia.
- An increase in stabs or band cells would indicate *a shift to the left* (i.e., a sign of an overwhelming infection) on a WBC differential.
- A decrease in lymphocytes (lymphopenia) would indicate that a patient is immunodeficient.
- T lymphocytes are the body's master immune cells.
- Fresh fruits and raw vegetables are eliminated from the diet of a patient with severe neutropenia to reduce the chance of infection.
- Signs and symptoms of infection in the neutropenic patient include the following: fatigue, weakness, dehydration, tachypnea, tachycardia, cough, pharyngitis, hypotension, and change in mental status.

Electrolytes

Section 3   Diane Anthony Manghram

OVERVIEW

The examination of serum studies is an important tool used in the diagnosis of numerous diseases and conditions. Disturbances in electrolytes commonly contribute to many illnesses and can be life threatening. Nurses may be challenged to evaluate patients' electrolytes while providing health management for individuals with various health problems in the hospital and community health care settings.

PRINCIPLES OF CARE

Electrolytes are important components essential for cellular homeostasis and function within the human body. Electrolytes are found in all fluid compartments within the human body. They help to regulate water distribution; they govern acid-base balance; and they transmit nerve impulses. Furthermore, they contribute to energy generation and blood clotting.

Electrolytes are solutes that break down into positive or negative ions in solution and generate an electrical charge in solution. Cations are positively charged ions. The anions are negatively charged ions. They are expressed in milliequivalents per liter (mEq/L). Normal serum levels may vary slightly with different laboratories. A healthy diet provides all daily requirements of electrolytes.

Electrolyte imbalances occur secondary to many conditions such as endocrine disturbances, renal dysfunction, and all too frequently, iatrogenically, by inadvertent overadministration. The goal of therapy for all imbalances is early identification and return of the electrolyte to normal serum levels as quickly as possible. *A primary implication of management involves identification and alleviation of the cause in all cases.* Some imbalances require long-term and even lifelong replacement, such as for hypocalcemia following parathyroidectomy. Management also requires knowledge of common clinical findings and assessment of these findings, especially during therapy, to monitor for improvements or deterioration.

DECISION-MAKING
Sodium

Normal serum sodium (Na^+) is 135 to 146 mEq/L. Minimum daily requirements are 2 g/day. The average amount consumed in the United States is 6 g/day.

Sodium is obtained from food intake, a major source being from seasonings (table salt). One teaspoon of salt contains 2 g of sodium. *Sodium is excreted* through the kidneys for the most part with small amounts being excreted through perspiration.

Functions. *Fluid balance maintenance*: Na^+ maintains the osmotic pressure of the extracellular fluid. Thus, it maintains plasma volume and regulates the size of vascular compartments. *Neuromuscular activity*: Na^+ aids in the impulse transmission in nerve and muscle fibers, thus helping to control muscle contractility. *Renal activity*: Na^+ affects the concentration, excretion, and absorption of potassium chloride. Na^+ aids in the maintenance of acid-base balance by combining with bicarbonate and chloride ions.

Regulations. The kidneys regulate sodium levels. When sodium levels are elevated, the kidneys retain water to dilute the elevated level back to normal. When sodium levels are low, aldosterone is secreted by the adrenal glands and results in sodium retention in exchange for potassium by the kidneys.

Hypernatremia

Hypernatremia is a serum sodium level > 145 mEq/L. It is due to a water deficit or to an excess of sodium.

A *water deficit* occurs owing to inadequate water intake. Iatrogenic causes include failure to provide adequate fluid to the NPO or unconscious patient. Diabetes insipidus causes hypernatremia, because the posterior pituitary gland fails to secrete antidiuretic hormone (ADH).

An *excessive sodium intake* is rare. Iatrogenic causes of excessive sodium include administration of sodium bicarbonate and a less severe condition associated with an excess of mineralocorticoid agents. Hypernatremia also occurs in primary aldosteronism owing to increased aldosterone levels, which lead to increased sodium retention by the kidneys. This is frequently of a mild degree and is asymptomatic.

Clinical Findings. These findings relate to cellular dehydration, especially in the brain, and decreased water content in the interstitial fluid. As the brain cells shrink, symptoms of central nervous system (CNS) irritability lead to irritation, lethargy, and confusion and may progress to convulsions and coma. Signs of systemic dehydration include dry oral mucous membranes, tachycardia, hypertension, thirst, and oliguria.

Treatment. Sodium-poor fluids such as dextrose 5% in water (D_5W) is most efficient at correcting hypernatremia. The water moves easily into the interstitium and cells and restores their volume. Serum sodium should not be reduced any faster than 1 to 2 mEq/hr, and levels should be monitored throughout therapy. If corrected too quickly, cerebral edema may occur. Monitor for signs of CNS depression.

Hyponatremia

This problem is the most common electrolyte abnormality and is observed in 2% of all hospitalized patients. It is considered to be a deficiency in sodium in relation to body water and is referred to as diluted body fluids. Severe hyponatremia can result in seizure, coma, and permanent neurologic damage.

Hyponatremia can be caused by an inadequate sodium intake (depletion or deficit hyponatremia) or water excess (dilutional hyponatremia).

Sodium depletion hyponatremia is caused by extrarenal losses from vomiting, diarrhea, and gastrointestinal suctioning or burns, inadequate sodium intake owing to low sodium diets, and the use of diuretics. Sodium depletion can also occur as a result of adrenal insufficiency, where the adrenal glands are unable to secrete aldosterone resulting in the kidneys' failure to retain sodium.

Dilutional hyponatremia occurs when an excess of total body water (TBW) occurs relative to the amount of total body sodium. This can arise when there is a failure of water excretion by the kidneys (e.g., in renal failure), the excessive administration of sodium-free water (e.g., D_5W). Excessive water intake with little or no salt replacement results in a condition called *water intoxication.* A shift of fluid from the intracellular space to the extracellular space, as seen with hyperglycemic osmotic diuresis, can also cause dilutional hyponatremia. *Syndrome of inappropriate antidiuretic hormone (SIADH)* causes hyponatremia because the posterior pituitary gland secretes excessive amounts of ADH, resulting in water retention and inappropriate renal excretion of sodium. SIADH is commonly the result of CNS conditions such as tumors, trauma, infection, medications (e.g., certain antidepressants), chemotherapy, narcotics, pneumonia, tuberculosis, malignancies, and hypothyroidism.

Clinical Findings. CNS irritability results from cerebral edema when brain cells become overhydrated. Findings include anxiety, confusion, delirium, and seizures. Fluid shifts into the interstitial spaces result in hypotension, tachycardia, decreased skin turgor, and decreased urine output (UOP) as well as edematous states.

Treatment. Replace fluid volume with 0.9% normal saline (NS) solution to increase the sodium level. Diuretics may be administered in the case of dilutional hyponatremia to decrease body water. In severe cases, hypertonic solutions may be needed, such as 3% or 5% saline solutions. Assess the patient closely for volume overload (see Chapter 15, Section 5) during therapy.

Potassium

Serum potassium has a normal value of 3.5 to 5.5 mEq/L. The daily dietary intake requirement is approximately 40 mEq. An average dietary intake is 60 to 100 mEq/day.

K^+ is present mainly in muscle (60%), perspiration, gastric and intestinal secretions, and saliva. It is also found in bone.

Function. Potassium is the major cation found in the intracellular fluid (95%). It affects cardiac muscle contraction and electrical conduction. It is vital for the transmission of electrical impulses within the heart. It aids in the neuromuscular transmission of nerve impulses and assists in maintaining the acid-base balance.

Regulation. Maintenance of adequate K^+ level is dependent upon daily ingestion from food and fluids. Many sodium chloride salt substitutes are high in potassium. It is excreted mainly in the kidneys, and a small amount is excreted in perspiration.

Hypokalemia

In hypokalemia, the serum potassium level is less than 3.5 mEq/L. Inadequate intake of potassium or excessive excretion by the kidneys contributes to a deficiency of total body potassium. In certain situations, potassium shifts from the extracellular compartment to the intracellular compartment, thus decreasing the amount of potassium measurable in the blood. Various conditions can cause hypokalemia, such as the use of prolonged diuretic therapy, which increases renal excretion; inadequate dietary intake of potassium; severe loss of gastrointestinal fluids from gastric suctioning or lavage, vomiting, diarrhea, laxative overuse without potassium replacement; and Cushing's syndrome, which causes increased aldosterone secretion, resulting in sodium retention and potassium loss. When any of the three intracellular elements are lost (i.e., magnesium, potassium, phosphorus), deficiencies of the others may follow.

Clinical Findings. Cardiac manifestations include the following electrocardiogram (ECG) changes: decreased amplitude and broadening of T waves and also premature ventricular contractions. The pulse may be weak and irregular. Cardiac arrest occurs from ventricular fibrillation in severe cases. Neuromuscular assessment may reveal skeletal muscle weakness, respiratory muscle weakness (shallow respirations), hyporeflexia, or decreased or absent leg tendon reflexes, and flaccid paralysis may occur in severe cases. Decreased bowel motility results in decreased bowel sounds and possible paralytic ileus, causing anorexia, nausea, and vomiting. Hypokalemia increases the incidence of digitalis toxicity in patients who take digitalis glycoside.

Treatment. Oral replacement by foods high in potassium or potassium supplementation is indicated for mild hypokalemia (3 to 3.4 mEq/L). *Some foods high in $K+$ are avocado, raisins, cantaloupe, banana, beef, pork, veal, spinach, skim milk, tomatoes, and potatoes.* Oral K^+ can be administered up to 100 mEq/day for replacement therapy. Doses of 20 mEq/day are used for prevention. Oral therapy rarely produces hyperkalemia.

Intravenous (IV) potassium is required if the patient cannot take potassium by mouth (PO) and usually if hypokalemia is moderate (2.5 to 2.9 mEq/L) or severe (<2.4 mEq/L). Potassium should never be administered by IV push. It must be diluted and administered at rates no faster than 10 mEq/hr. It may be given at rates of 20 mEq/hr via a central line in monitored situations, such as in an intensive care unit. Central line administration via an infusion pump is preferred because K^+ is irritating to peripheral veins and can cause a chemical phlebitis. Too rapid administration can result in cardiac arrest owing to hyperkalemia. Ensure that no other IV fluids contain K^+. Potassium replacement may be administered in the adult by the following manner:

For $K^+ < 2.4$, give 80 mEq IV over 8 hours, check levels every 1 to 2 hours.

For K^+ 2.5 to 2.9, give 60 mEq IV over 6 hours, check levels at 6 hours and then at 12 or 24 hours.

For K^+ 3.0 to 3.4, give 40 mEq PO or IV over 4 hours; check levels in 12 to 24 hours.

A K^+ of 3.5 to 3.9 may be treated with 20 mEq PO or IV over 2 hours for the seriously ill patient, the patient with cardiac disease, or the patient following surgery. Monitor magnesium and phosphorus levels. If hypomagnesemic, correct the magnesium level prior to potassium.

Hyperkalemia

Hyperkalemia occurs when $K^+ > 5.5$ mEq/L. Conditions associated with hyperkalemia include *renal dysfunction or failure*, because the kidneys are responsible for potassium excretion; *massive tissue damage*, because potassium is released from ruptured cells; *adrenal insufficiency* (hypoaldosteronism), resulting in the retention of K^+ in exchange for Na; and *acidosis*, because H ions move into the cells and K ions move out.

Clinical Findings. Cardiac findings include: ECG changes (approximately half of patients with serum K^+ greater that 6.5 mEq/L do not manifest ECG changes); peaked T waves, of increased amplitude; widening QRS; and biphasic QRS-T complexes. Bradycardia, irregular pulse, or heart block may occur. Cardiac arrest may occur from asystole or ventricular fibrillation. Neuromuscular irritability results in irritability, diarrhea, general muscle weakness, and abdominal cramping.

Treatment. Confirm elevated serum K^+ and withhold any additional administration. Avoid foods high in K^+, and avoid salt substitutes.

Treatment for emergent care consists of the following:

- Insulin and glucose IV: This causes K^+ to shift from plasma into the cells, thus temporarily reducing serum potassium levels.
- Calcium gluconate or calcium chloride IV: Calcium temporarily protects the heart from the cardiotoxic effects of hyperkalemia. Calcium augments the effects of digoxin on the heart. Sodium bicarbonate intravenously in severe hyperkalemia increases blood pH and results in a shift of K^+ into cells. Never mix calcium solutions with sodium bicarbonate, because this results in precipitation.
- Albuterol (a beta-2 agonist), when nebulized, decreases serum potassium in patients on hemodialysis. This modality distributes K^+ into the cells for 2 to 4 hours. Albuterol and insulin are equally effective in lowering potassium in uremic individuals. Both drugs can be given concurrently with glucose without hazard.

Nonemergent Treatment. Loop diuretics are given to increase renal K^+ excretion. Sodium polystyrene sulfonate (Kayexalate), which is a K-binding resin, may be given orally or rectally via an enema. It binds with K^+, which is removed in the stool. Hemodialysis or peritoneal dialysis may be instituted to remove K^+ in the presence of protracted renal insufficiency.

Calcium

Normal total plasma or serum calcium concentration is 9 to 10.3 mg/L. Approximately 45% of serum calcium is bound to protein (albumin) and is thus physiologically inactive. Another 10% is connected to other anions such as citrate, bicarbonate, and phosphate. Free (ionized) calcium makes up the remaining 45% of calcium that is present in plasma. Normal ionized calcium is 4.6 to 5.2 mg/dL.

Function. Calcium assists in bone and teeth formation and provides rigidity and strength along with phosphorus. Calcium has a soothing or sedative type effect on nerve cells and helps to maintain normal transmission of nerve impulses to muscles. Calcium maintains cell membrane structure, function, and permeability and assists in the active process for blood coagulation.

Regulation. Absorption of calcium takes place in the small intestines only in the presence of vitamin D. The parathyroid hormone (PTH) is released in the presence of low serum calcium levels, causing the transfer of calcium from bone to plasma, increased intestinal absorption, and conservation in the renals with resultant excretion of phosphorus. Urinary excretion of calcium is increased by the thyroid hormone calcitonin (decreases renal and intestinal absorption), which is secreted when serum calcium levels are high.

Hypocalcemia

A common cause of hypocalcemia is renal failure. In renal failure, the kidney is unable to produce 1,25-dihydroxycholecalciferol, which is necessary to convert vitamin D to its active form. Without active vitamin D, calcium cannot be absorbed from the gastrointestinal tract and hypocalcemia develops. Hypocalcemia may also be caused by hypoparathyroidism (see Chapter 18, Section 4), parathyroidectomy, or thyroidectomy with inadvertent removal of one or more parathyroid gland resulting in decreased PTH. Hypoalbuminemia is a common cause of low total serum calcium. For each 1 g/dL drop in serum albumin, total calcium drops 0.8 to 1 mg/dL. Citrate present in banked blood may bind calcium and result in hypocalcemia in which large amounts are transfused. Hypomagnesemia may precipitate hypocalcemia.

Clinical Findings. Hypocalcemia increases excitation of nerve impulses to muscle cells as the soothing effect is lost. The neuromuscular and cardiovascular systems are primarily affected.

Neuromuscular irritability produces hyperactive deep tendon reflexes; tingling of fingers, toes, nose, ears, tetany (tonic spasms), and seizures; positive Chvostek's sign (i.e., contraction of the facial muscle in response to tapping the facial nerve anterior to the ear); positive Trousseau's sign (carpal spasm result after occlusion of the brachial artery with a blood pressure cuff for 3 minutes). ECG changes include a prolonged QT interval owing to a lengthened ST segment.

Treatment. For patients with tetany, seizures, or cardiovascular manifestations, calcium gluconate should be administered IV. Calcium should not be administered faster than 0.5 to 1 mL/min. Levels should be monitored every 4 to 6 hours until stable. Magnesium replacement is required when the magnesium level is low, which usually allows for the correction of hypocalcemia. If the level of magnesium is not corrected, correction of calcium is not effective. For chronic hypocalcemia, vitamin D preparations (i.e., dihydrotachysterol, calcitriol) increase calcium absorption from the gastrointestinal tract, and oral calcium preparations are initiated. *Calcium-rich foods should be encouraged such as low-fat yogurt, skim milk, whole milk, cheddar cheese,* *rhubarb, and raw collard greens.* Calcium potentiates the effect of digitalis and should be administered with caution in patients receiving digitalis.

Hypercalcemia

Causes of hypercalcemia include: primary hyperparathyroidism (see Chapter 18, Section 2); metastatic diseases of the bone, which causes excessive calcium to be liberated into the blood as bone is destroyed; and immobilization, which causes calcium to be released from the bone into circulation.

Clinical Findings. Symptoms usually manifest at concentrations > 11 mg/dL. Decreased neuromuscular excitability with hypoactive deep tendon reflexes, lethargy, impaired memory, and slurred speech are noted. Kidney stones and pathologic fractures result from the loss of calcium from the bone into the bloodstream. Shortened ST or QT intervals are common ECG findings.

Treatment. 0.45% Saline or 0.9% saline intravenously by rapid infusion 250 to 500 mL/hr is administered to increase urinary excretion of calcium. Diuretics are usually given at the same time to prevent fluid overload. Calcitonin decreases calcium levels by promoting deposition of calcium in the bone and excretion of calcium in urine, feces, and sweat. Glucocorticoids decrease intestinal absorption of calcium by competing with vitamin D.

Phosphate

The normal range is 2.5 to 4.5 mg/dL. Phosphate consists of phosphorus and oxygen (PO_4). It is the major anion found in intracellular fluid and is stored in bone.

Function. Phosphate provides rigidity and strength to bones and teeth. It is crucial in the formation of substances required for cellular energy (e.g., adenosine triphosphate [ATP]) and the metabolism of fats, carbohydrates, and proteins. Phosphate is considered to be a urinary buffer that actively participates in maintaining acid-base balance.

Regulation. Phosphate intake is dependent upon daily ingestion from foods. Absorption mainly takes place in the small intestines. Excretion is dependent on functioning renals and the influence of PTH.

Hypophosphatemia

Hypophosphatemia occurs with inadequate intake from phosphate; poor hyperalimentation; alcoholism, owing to increased urinary phosphate excretion; chronic use of antacids, which bind to phosphate; and hyperparathyroidism (see Chapter 18, Section 2). Shifts from extracellular fluids into the cell may also produce hypophosphatemia; as in the treatment of hyperkalemia, insulin and bicarbonate cause K^+ to shift into the cell as well as phosphorus. A phosphorus deficiency may cause potassium and magnesium deficiencies within the tissues.

Clinical Findings. The major findings are caused by decreased energy within the cells. Symptoms include irritability, confusion, paresthesia, muscle weakness (including respiratory muscles), seizures, impaired cardiac function, and coma.

Chronic hypophosphatemia produces skeletal and neuromuscular problems such as bone pain, muscle weakness, and pathologic fractures.

Treatment. IV phosphate replacement is required for severe hypophosphatemia or when the gastrointestinal tract is nonfunctional with potassium phosphate or sodium phosphate. Administer phosphate at a rate of 0.2 mM of phosphate/kg/hr. For potassium phosphate, limit the rate to 10 mEq/hr. Too rapid administration results in serious hyperkalemia or hyperphosphatemia. Because this therapy may result in severe hypocalcemia, calcium levels should be monitored, and replacement therapy should be initiated when needed. Monitor magnesium and potassium levels.

Oral therapy is preferred for chronic hypophosphatemia or when symptoms are mild. Also, an increased dietary intake of phosphorus is helpful for mild cases. *Foods that are high in phosphorus include white tuna fish (canned), low-fat yogurt, beef liver, pork, fish, skim milk, whole milk, American cheese, beef, and chicken.*

Hyperphosphatemia

Hyperphosphatemia is seen most commonly with chronic renal failure, resulting in decreased renal excretion and hypoparathyroidism (see Chapter 18, Section 4). Hyperphosphatemia may also occur with the overuse of phosphate-containing laxatives.

Clinical Findings. These findings are the same as for hypocalcemia.

Treatment. Acute conditions may be treated by dialysis. Phosphate-binding antacids (see Chapter 25, Section 3) and dietary restrictions of phosphorus are needed for long-term therapy.

Magnesium

The normal plasma magnesium concentration is 1.5 to 2.5 mEq/L. Of the total magnesium content, approximately 50% is stored in bone; 45% is found in the intracellular space; and the remainder is found in extracellular fluid. Like calcium, approximately one third of magnesium is protein (albumin)-bound (physiologically inactive), and two thirds circulates as free cations.

Function. Magnesium helps to activate several intracellular enzymes that drive the sodium-potassium pump in the cell membrane, DNA synthesis, and carbohydrate and protein metabolism. Magnesium acts directly on the neuromuscular junction by depressing the release of acetylcholine, thus affecting the excitability of cardiac and skeletal muscle.

Regulation. Intake is dependent on dietary ingestion. Absorption occurs primarily in the ileum and jejunum. Magnesium is excreted primarily by the kidneys. When serum magnesium levels are low, PTH stimulates the release of magnesium from bone in much the same manner as it does for calcium.

Hypomagnesemia

The common causes of hypomagnesemia are associated with diminished absorption or intake as seen in malabsorption, malnutrition, and alcoholism, which causes decreased absorption and increased excretion, along with poor dietary intake; renal failure; and hyperalimentation with inadequate magnesium content. Causes associated with increased losses include diuretic therapy resulting in increased renal excretion; chronic diarrhea; overuse of laxatives; and prolonged gastrointestinal suction or vomiting.

Clinical Findings. Neuromuscular manifestations are caused by the loss of acetylcholine depression at the neuromuscular junction. Excessive acetylcholine increases neuromuscular excitability. Common signs and symptoms consist of the following: tremor, confusion, anorexia, tetany, positive Chvostek's sign, positive Trousseau's sign, hyperactive deep tendon reflexes, and seizures. Cardiac dysrhythmias can also occur, as well as tachycardia and hypertension. ECG changes include prolonged QT interval (owing to lengthening of the ST segment).

Decreased activation of the sodium-potassium pump causes hypokalemia by preventing K^+ from moving into the cell and increasing its renal excretion. Because of this, it is necessary to correct the hypomagnesemia before the hypokalemia can be corrected.

Hypomagnesemia may cause hypocalcemia when magnesium levels fall below 1.2 mg/dL. Although mild magnesium deficiency may enhance the release of PTH, severe hypomagnesemia blocks PTH release, impairing the normal calcemic response at the level of the skeleton. Chronic malabsorption may be associated with hypocalcemia, hypokalemia, and hypophosphatemia.

Treatment. Acute management requires IV administration of magnesium sulfate. Administer a 10% solution at least over 1.5 mL/min or 150 mg/min. During administration, monitor for hypotension and respiratory distress. Too rapid administration can lead to severe hypermagnesemia, resulting in respiratory or cardiac arrest. Monitor serum potassium, calcium, and phosphorus levels, because these levels can be affected by hypomagnesemia.

Chronic management requires oral supplementation. *Foods that are high in magnesium include raw spinach, avocado, white tuna fish (canned), and yogurt.* Diarrhea is a side effect that limits the use of oral magnesium preparations. Antidiarrheal agents may be needed.

Hypermagnesemia

Magnesium excess usually results from impaired renal excretion and is most commonly seen in chronic renal failure. Excessive ingestion of magnesium-containing medications (e.g., laxatives, antacids) is another common cause and usually occurs in the elderly. Magnesium excess may also be caused by adrenal insufficiency (i.e., Addison's disease).

Clinical Findings. Hypermagnesemia decreases the release of acetylcholine at the neuromuscular junction, resulting in depressed muscular contraction. Symptoms include muscle weakness, hyporeflexia (deep tendon), hypotension, respiratory depression, mental obtundation, and confusion and bradycardia and can result in cardiac arrest or respiratory arrest.

ECG changes consist of an increased PR interval, broadened QRS complexes, and peaked T waves.

Treatment. Management involves volume expansion with saline and diuresis in a manner similar to that found in hypercalcemia. However, this regimen also increases the excretion of calcium, thus calcium replacement therapy is needed. Calcium also antagonizes the effects of magnesium.

 CLINICAL PEARLS

○ Calcium gluconate contains 4.5 mEq of calcium, and calcium chloride contains 13.6 mEq of calcium. Always clarify which type is to be administered.

○ Hypomagnesemia may cause hypokalemia, hypophosphatemia, and hypocalcemia.

○ Avocado, low-fat yogurt, skim milk, and tuna fish are excellent sources of all electrolytes.

- Oral K^+ can be administered up to 100 mEq/day, but IV K^+ must be administered at rates no faster than 10 mEq/hr. Oral therapy rarely produces hyperkalemia.
- Hypomagnesemia must be corrected before hypokalemia.

Laboratory Data Related to Infection

Section 4   Patricia Preston

OVERVIEW

For many years, improvements in public health combined with the discovery of antibiotics and the development of effective vaccination programs greatly diminished the threat of infectious disease. However, changes in our society and environment have brought about an emergence of new virile pathogens as well as a resurgence of diseases that were once thought to be almost eradicated. Identification of microorganisms has become a cornerstone in surveillance and treatment of infectious disease.

PRINCIPLES OF CARE

Pathogenic bacteria excrete exotoxins and release endotoxins upon their lysis. These toxins damage host cells and tissues. The discovery of antibiotics initially decreased the morbidity and mortality that resulted from bacterial infections. Unfortunately, the widespread and indiscriminate distribution of antibiotics has led to the development of strains of bacteria whose mutations had rendered them resistant to antibiotics.

Viruses must incorporate themselves into the host cell to survive. This incorporation damages the host cell by disrupting its plasma membrane. Viruses are much smaller than bacteria. These characteristics make viruses difficult to isolate and even harder to eliminate.

Fungi are large, immobile organisms with thick cell walls. They must reside on other organisms in order to survive. On humans, they can be found on the skin and mucous membranes. Fungi that cause systemic infection are generally opportunistic and found mainly in persons whose immune system is impaired or suppressed.

Parasites such as tapeworms, roundworms, and protozoans invade the intestinal tract and cause diarrhea, abdominal pain, and poor nutrient absorption. In the developed world, parasitic infection is not encountered as commonly as in the developing world.

Even microorganisms known to cause serious or fatal illness can inhabit specific body sites and *not* cause signs or symptoms of infection. This is called colonization. Colonized bacteria can cause infection if spread from one body site to another or from one person to another. For example, *Escherichia coli* are a necessary component of intestinal normal flora, but if the same bacteria become introduced into the urethra, they can cause infection in the urinary tract.

DECISION-MAKING

Four basic tests are utilized for identification of microorganisms: culture and sensitivity (C&S), Gram stain, acid-fast smear, and serologic testing for antibody-antigen markers.

Culture and Sensitivity

C&S requires the introduction of a specimen into a medium that will foster the growth of microorganisms. This allows for identification of the organism, as well as determination of the organism's sensitivity to different antimicrobial agents. Cultures are considered the "gold standard" method for identifying microbes. Obtaining and securing the specimen with the proper technique is essential to ensure accurate results. For the microorganism to grow in a culture, it must be secured in the proper growth medium. There are three basic types of medium: liquid (broth), solid (agar), and cell culture lines. Bacteria and fungi should be placed in a liquid or solid medium, whereas viruses grow only in cell culture lines because they require a host cell in which they can multiply.

Wound Cultures

The wound should be flushed out and free of exudate before a culture is obtained. Avoid using antimicrobial solutions to clean the wound immediately before a culture, because these cleansers can destroy surface bacteria that would decrease the possibility of yielding the microorganism.

Once the wound is cleaned, the specimen should be obtained from a small area of tissue (1 to 2 cm) as opposed to the entire area of infection. In this way, the microorganism recovered reflects the tissue burden and not the surface contaminants that have no role in the tissue infection.

The nurse should note the characteristics of the wound on the laboratory requisition form. The type, location, and circumstances of the wound should be included to help the laboratory personnel look for the appropriate microbials. For example, a dehisced surgical wound may harbor different bacteria compared with a wound resulting from a human bite.

The result of a wound culture is positive if it shows more than 105 organisms/g of tissue. If the host is immunosuppressed, include that information on the requisition form. Bacterial counts < 105 may also indicate infection for patients whose immune function is compromised. Tissue and fluid biopsies are considered to be the best methods for obtaining accurate cultures.

Blood Cultures

When bacteria overwhelm the immune system, they can move from the tissue into the bloodstream and cause a dangerous systemic infection called septicemia, which has a mortality rate of 40% to 50% and occurs in approximately 200,000 persons each year.

Bacteremia usually precedes septicemia. There are three types of bacteremia: transient, intermittent, and continuous. Transient bacteremia occurs after infected tissue or colonized mucosal surfaces are manipulated. Intermittent bacteremia can occur early in the course of an infection or as a result of bacteria harbored in an abscess. Continuous bacteremia, which leads to septicemia, occurs with an intravascular infection such as infective endocarditis but can occur with any suppurative (pus producing) infection.

Blood cultures are the best diagnostic tool for detecting bacteremia and septicemia.

Because microorganisms can take days or weeks to grow, it is essential that the initial specimen is properly obtained and that time is not wasted on a contaminated sample. The accuracy of blood cultures is highly dependent on the technique used while obtaining the specimen. When drawing blood cultures, skin preparation becomes vitally important. Bacteria that naturally reside in the skin can contaminate the results of the test. Strict sterile technique must be observed.

Preparing the Site. The area chosen for venipuncture should be cleaned first with 70% isopropyl alcohol or ethyl alcohol in concentric circles starting in the center. Cleanse again with 1% to 2% tincture of iodine or 10% povidone-iodine solution using the circular technique described earlier. Let the iodine dry for 1 full minute before starting the venipuncture. If the patient is allergic to iodine, a double application of alcohol should be used. The diaphragm of the collection tubes and the bottles of culture medium need to be cleaned with alcohol and allowed to dry before proceeding with the venipuncture. If you need to touch the site before the venipuncture, the tip of the glove should be cleaned with the same technique as the site. If the first attempt at venipuncture is unsuccessful, a new needle and transfer set should be used. After the blood is drawn, transfer it into two bottles—one that contains a medium suitable for the growth of anaerobic bacteria and the other for aerobic bacteria. After transferring the blood to these bottles, gently mix the contents and deliver the specimen to the laboratory within 30 minutes of drawing the blood.

Choosing the Site. The site of vascular access can also affect the results of a blood culture. The femoral area or any site with dermatologic disease is more likely to yield a higher rate of contaminants. If the patient has an IV, the site chosen for the blood cultures should be below the IV site. Samples obtained through percutaneous venipuncture are much more reliable than those obtained through existing intravascular catheters. Venous blood will have the same bacterial yield as arterial blood. Because of the risk of skin contaminants, blood is drawn from two separate sites for each blood culture.

Amount of the Sample. Many bacteremias are of low magnitude; that is, the bacteria, although potent, are sparsely scattered throughout the blood-stream. There is a direct relationship between volume of blood per culture and bacterial yield. It is recommended that 8 to 10 mL of blood be collected per culture for an adult. Often two to three cultures collected over a 24-hour period are ordered to reduce the possibility of false-positive or false-negative results.

Timing. Blood cultures should be drawn before antibiotics or any antimicrobial medication is administered. If an antibiotic has been started, draw the culture immediately before the next dose. A resin can be added to the culture mediums to bind with the antibiotic and thus diminish its effect on the results. Because of the great stress that bacteremia places on the immune system, it generally produces fever and chills. Therefore, drawing a blood culture when a patient is febrile increases the probability of yielding bacteria in an intermittent bacteremia.

Catheter Tip Cultures

Positive culture results from a vascular access devices such as a dialysis catheter, arterial line, pulmonary artery catheter, central lines, or Hickman

Table 11-4-1. Interpreting Culture Results from Vascular Device–Related Infections

RESULT	INTERPRETATION
Cutaneous Segment/Distal Segment/Blood	
+/+/+	Contaminated line with bacteremia/fungemia from the line
+/+/−	Contaminated line, local infection
+/−/−	Entry site infection
−/+/−	Probable contamination
−/+/+	Tip contaminated from an infection in the bloodstream; consider a remote site of infection
−/−/+	Infection from alternate source
−/−/−	No evidence of culturable infection
+/−/+	Flawed technique; catheter-related infection

catheter are called vascular device–related infections. Assessment of a patient with a vascular access device includes culturing the exit site and taking blood from the catheter and from a peripheral stick. A tip or portion of the catheter should be sent for culture. Table 11-4-1 is an interpretation guide to device-related infections (see also Chapter 2, Section 2 on Venous Access Devices).

Culture Report

Nurses are not only responsible for securing specimens for culture but they must also be able to correctly interpret a C&S report. A C&S report usually contains:

1. Test name and collection information, such as the date and time
2. Type of specimen
3. Type of report: preliminary (within 24 hours) or final (after 48 hours)
4. Colony count: the number of colony-forming units (CFUs)

Colonies are the number of bacteria that arise from a single organism. A diagnosis of infection is based on the number of CFUs, but the criteria for infection differ according to the type of specimen and the mode of retrieval.

Blood, cerebrospinal fluid, and joint fluid are normally sterile; therefore, any microbial growth is significant.

When *urine* is cultured, the collection method determines what CFU count indicates infection. In a voided specimen, 100,000 CFU/mL of one organism strongly suggests the presence of a urinary tract infection (UTI). If the urine is obtained from an in-and-out catheterization, the possibility of contamination decreases and a colony count of 10,000 or greater of one organism is considered significant.

Cultures of sputum frequently grow out "normal flora." As mentioned earlier, bacteria that are not pathogenic can be found on every area of the body. If the bacteria are known to reside in the site that is cultured, the bacteria are considered to be normal flora and are not suspected of causing infection. Organisms in a sputum culture that are not identified as normal flora are quantified as scant, moderate, or numerous. The larger the bacterial load, the more likely is the chance of infection.

Sensitivity

Antimicrobial sensitivity is determined by either disk diffusion or an automated technique. In the *disk diffusion* method, disks impregnated with various antibiotics are placed on the agar of the specimen after culture is completed. If the microorganism is susceptible to the antibiotic, a circle appears around the disk, which indicates that the antibiotic has eliminated the bacteria surrounding it. That circle is labeled the *zone of inhibition*. The larger the zone of inhibition, the more effective the antibiotic will be in treating the microorganism.

The *automated technique* reports sensitivity in terms of minimum inhibitory concentration (MIC). The MIC of a medication is the smallest dose that will effectively inhibit the microorganism. Once this dose has been established, it has to be determined whether that concentration of drug is attainable in a person's bloodstream through an established or normal delivery route without causing toxicity.

The microorganism is reported to be *resistant* to any medications that cannot meet these criteria. If the efficacy of a drug is not clear or cannot be predicted after the testing, then the organism is reported to be in the intermediate range of sensitivity to that drug. The distinction between a toxic dose and a therapeutic dose may sometimes be narrow, or the organism may require a higher than usual dose of a medication for elimination. In these cases, the microorganism is reported to be moderately susceptible to that medication.

Gram Stain

Gram stain is a smear technique that provides a quick way to categorize bacteria into two distinct groups—gram-positive bacteria and gram-negative bacteria. A primary stain (crystal violet) is applied to the smear. Gram-positive bacteria retain the violet color. Gram-negative bacteria do not take up the crystal violet but counterstain red when the second stain (safranin O dye) is applied. An acid-alcohol is applied to decolorize or remove the stain.

Gram staining is very useful when antimicrobial coverage is needed immediately and cannot wait for the full culture report. Effective broad-spectrum coverage can be started with Gram stain results alone. The Gram stain can also be used alone to diagnose some diseases. For example, gram-negative intracellular diplococci in a Gram stain of urethral discharge are diagnostic for gonorrhea.

Acid-Fast Smear

Acid-fast smear is used most commonly to identify *Mycobacterium tuberculosis*, the bacterium that causes tuberculosis (see Chapter 13, Section 5) but does identify all mycobacteria. Mycobacteria are gram-positive bacilli of acid-fast genus. The cell wall of an acid-fast bacillus resists decoloration with acid treatment, thus it retains the violet stain applied to the specimen after the slide has been rinsed with an acid-alcohol solution, where other gram-positive organisms will decolorize, hence the term "acid-fast."

Serology Testing

Serology testing, the study of serum, identifies serum antibodies in an infected host. Although not as accurate as a culture, it is useful for pathogens that cannot be cultured, such as the hepatitis B virus. The organism is identified if the antibody level (titer) for a specific pathogen increases during the acute phase of the disease and falls during the recovery phase. Serology testing can also identify the phase of the infectious process that the host is in. Once a person has been exposed or infected, specific antibodies of the IgM class are produced. They rise during the acute phase of the infectious process and fall at the end of the acute phase. IgG class antibodies rise near the end of the acute phase of the infectious process and remain elevated beyond resolution.

Other

Enzyme-linked immunoassays (ELISAs), indirect fluorescent antibody (IFA), complement fixation, and the Western Blot are tests utilized to detect antigens and antibodies for specific viruses. Sometimes serum specimens must be obtained during the acute and convalescent phases of an illness for a diagnosis to be made. Rapid tests have been developed for the identification of influenza, HIV, and Epstein-Barr virus, which causes mononucleosis.

White Blood Cell Count and Differential

The WBC count with differential provides a great deal of information about the type and course of infection (see Section 2).

 CLINICAL PEARLS

○ When obtaining a wound culture, first clear the wound of exudate and then obtain the specimen from a 1- to 2-cm area of the wound.

○ Strict aseptic technique and proper site selection are required when obtaining blood cultures to decrease the number of false-positive results.

○ A positive blood culture indicates that bacteria (or fungi) are present in the blood. Patients with positive blood cultures are at risk for septic shock and circulatory collapse.

○ The determination of the presence or absence of infection in a cultured specimen is based on the number of CFUs of one type of organism. The number of CFUs that indicate infection varies depending on the type of specimen and the method of specimen retrieval.

○ When a culture is positive for microbial growth, that microbe is tested for its sensitivity to different antibiotics. The C&S report contains a list of antibiotics and an indication if the bacteria were sensitive, intermediate, or resistant to that antibiotic.

Laboratory Data Related to Renal Function

Section 5   Patricia Preston

OVERVIEW

Renal function is assessed frequently in response to drug therapy, dialysis, and renal transplantation and to detect damage from nephrotoxic medications. It is also assessed frequently in the critically and seriously ill patient, because renal dysfunction is a common complication of many disorders.

PRINCIPLES OF CARE

The most important indicator of renal function is the glomerular filtration rate (GFR). The GFR is the amount of filtrate that passes through the glomerulus into the Bowman capsule in 1 minute. The normal rate is approximately 125 mL/hr or 180 L/day. The GFR is dependent on several variables, including cardiac output, the number of functioning nephrons, and capillary pressure in the kidney. If blood flow to the kidney is diminished, less plasma passes through the glomerulus and the GFR decreases. Also, injury or obliteration of a portion of the nephrons limits the amount of plasma that can be filtered and lowers the GFR as well.

DECISION-MAKING
Nitrogenous Waste Products

Nitrogenous wastes are the end products of protein metabolism. Creatinine, ammonia, and uric acid are all nitrogenous waste products that can be measured in the serum.

Blood Urea Nitrogen

Urea is nonprotein nitrogen that is formed in the liver from ammonia (a nitrogenous waste) and is excreted only by the kidneys. Blood urea nitrogen (BUN) levels reflect the balance between the production and excretion of urea. BUN is a calculated value derived by measuring the level of nitrogen in the blood. Because nitrogen accounts for 46.7% of the weight of urea, the amount of nitrogen is multiplied by 2.14 to obtain the BUN. Therefore, anything that increases the production of urea affects the BUN level. Because urea is a protein metabolite, increased protein intake increases urea production. Catabolism, the breakdown of the body's own tissue into protein, also raises urea levels. Physical stressors including starvation, infection, and surgery can place the body in a catabolic state. Dehydration raises the fluid-solute ratio and thus raises the BUN. Certain medications, aspirin, acetaminophen, and some antibiotics, just to name a few, can also increase BUN levels. Therefore, BUN by itself is not a reliable indicator of kidney function. *Normal serum levels for adults are 5 to 20 mg/dL.*

Serum Creatinine

Creatinine, the other nitrogenous waste product, is an important and stable indicator of kidney function. Creatine, the precursor of creatinine, is synthesized in the liver and resides in skeletal muscle tissue where it combines with phosphate to form phosphocreatine (an energy storage compound). When energy is released, this process reverses and produces a small amount of creatinine, which is a waste product of the reaction. Because muscle mass does not change precipitously daily, creatinine production remains at a fairly constant level and is not dependent on levels of activity of the skeletal muscle. Creatinine is excreted exclusively by the kidneys with very little interference from diet, fluid intake, or medications. Furthermore, acute problems that result in transient decreases in GFR do not affect the excretion of creatinine to any significant degree. Thus, serum creatinine is a very sensitive indicator of renal function, because for the most part, only changes in renal function alter this level. Creatinine is cleared only by the kidneys. A rise in creatinine levels in the blood signals a failure of kidney function.

Normal values for men are 0.6 to 1.3 mg/dL. Normal values for women are 0.5 to 1 mg/dL.

Serum creatinine levels increase in any renal disease where 50% of all nephrons are lost and the kidney fails to effectively clear this waste product from the blood. Men and people with greater muscle mass will have slightly higher levels, such as those with gigantism or acromegaly, because more creatinine is produced. Trauma resulting in crush injuries to muscle also increases serum creatinine levels. Decreased levels suggest atrophy of muscle tissue.

Blood Urea Nitrogen–Creatinine Ratio

The ratio of BUN to creatinine helps in distinguishing prerenal acute renal failure (volume depletion renal failure) from other forms of renal failure (see Chapter 25, Section 3). The normal ratio of BUN to creatinine is 10:1. Reduced renal perfusion causes the GFR to diminish. When GFR diminishes, BUN levels increase as a result of concentration; however, creatinine levels remain constant, thus increasing the ratio (e.g. >20:1). Other forms of renal failure result from intrinsic nephron damage or loss of nephrons. When a significant number of nephrons are lost, both BUN and creatinine rise. The BUN increases at the same rate as the creatinine; the 10:1 ratio is maintained, with an elevation of both BUN and creatinine (e.g., 100:10). Conditions that cause an elevation in both BUN and creatinine with a 10:1 ratio include acute tubular necrosis, chronic renal failure, and post renal failure. The ratio is decreased with excessive fluid intake and protein-losing conditions, such as nephritic syndrome, liver disease, and malnutrition.

Uric Acid

The kidneys are responsible for the excretion of uric acid, an end product of the metabolism of purine (components of DNA and RNA molecules). Uric acid has two forms—uric acid and urate salts. Urate salts are highly soluble, but the solubility of uric acid depends on the pH of the urine. The more acidic the urine (pH <5.5), the less soluble uric acid becomes. When the urine maintains a low pH, uric acid can form crystals in the kidney or bladder.

A high intake of purine-rich foods (e.g., meat, fish, poultry, legumes) may contribute to the formation of uric acid stones.

Normal Values of Uric Acid. Normal values for men are 2 to 7.5 mg/dL; normal values for women are 2 to 6.5 mg/dL.

Urine Tests of Renal Function

Creatinine Clearance

The best indicator of GFR is creatinine clearance. This urine test measures the rate at which the kidneys clear creatinine from the blood by comparing the level of creatinine in the serum with the amount excreted in the urine from 2 to 24 hours, although 24 hours is the recommended time period. A decreased creatinine clearance indicates a diminished GFR. The creatinine clearance value is calculated. The test involves collection of all urine for 24 hours (see Chapter 4, Section 2). An abbreviated procedure with 2- or 12-hour collections may also be useful. A serum creatinine sample must be collected during the same time period. Clearance is calculated according to the following formula:

Creatinine clearance =
$$\frac{\text{urine creatinine (mg/mL)} \times \text{volume of urine excreted (mL/min)}}{\text{plasma creatinine level (mg/mL)}}$$

The normal range for men is 85 to 125 mL/min; the normal range for women is 75 to 115 mL/min.

The major cause of reduced creatinine clearance is renal disease. Nonrenal causes include shock, hypovolemia, and nephrotoxic chemical exposure.

Urinalysis

Urinalysis is the gross and microscopic examination of urine to evaluate the pH, specific gravity, and presence of abnormal substances and formed elements (urinary sediment).

Samples may be obtained by random collection, clean catch (midstream), urinary catheter, suprapubic catheter, or straight catheterization (see Chapter 4, Section 2). See Table 11-5-1 for normal findings.

Gross Examination

Color. Urine color normally varies from pale yellow or straw colored to dark amber. These variations are caused more by changes in urine concentration than by changes in urochrome levels, because urochrome is produced at a fairly constant rate. Medication metabolites, certain foods, and several disease processes can also influence the color of urine. See Table 11-5-2 for urine color with its associated conditions.

Clarity. Urine is normally clear. Slight cloudiness may be noted owing to normal precipitates such as phosphates and carbonates (seen in alkaline urine) or urates and calcium oxalate (seen in acidic urine). Cloudy urine is most commonly caused by the presence of WBCs, RBCs, bacteria, and epithelial cells; however, these cells must be confirmed by microscopic examination.

Odor. Urine produces the odor of ammonia if it is left standing owing to the breakdown of urea. Several ingested foods and drugs produce specific odors

Table 11-5-1. Urinalysis

NORMAL FINDINGS

Albumin	Negative
Appearance	Clear to faintly hazy
Bilirubin	Negative
Color	Yellow
Glucose	Negative
Ketones	Negative
Nitrite	Negative
Occult blood	Negative
pH	4.5–8.0
Protein	Negative
Specific gravity	1.003–1.030
Urobilinogen	Negative or 0.1–1 Ehrlich U/dL
Cells	
Erythrocyte	<4 cells/HPF
Leukocytes	<5 cells/HPF
Urinary tract	
Epithelium	<11 cells/HPF
Casts	Moderate clear protein casts
Crystals	Small amount
Bacteria	None or <1000/mL
Parasites	None

HPF, high-power field.

Table 11-5-2. Urine Color and Associated Conditions

URINE COLOR	CONDITION
Blue/green	Amitriptyline, some diuretics, methylene blue color found in medications, nitrofurantoin, *Pseudomonas*
Green	Bacterial infection, some diuretics, propofol (Diprivan), vitamins
Light yellow	Diuresis, diabetes insipidus, glucosuria
Orange	Bile, chlorzoxazone, dehydration, fever, jaundice, laxative use, oral anticoagulants, phenazopyridine hydrochloride (Pyridium), phenothiazines, rifampin, sulfasalazine
Red	Eating beet root/rhubarb/senna, hemoglobin, kidney disease, malaria, menstrual blood, phenolsulfonphthalein, rifampin
Red brown	Hemoglobin, dehydration, liver or gallbladder disease
Smoky red	Intact red blood cells, occult blood
Yellow	Bilirubin

in urine. A fruity odor may indicate ketonuria. An offensive fetid or fishy odor is associated with bacterial infection.

Microscopic Examination

The microscopic examination involves centrifuging approximately 10 mL of urine for 5 minutes to evaluate for the presence of RBCs, WBCs, epithelial cells, bacteria, casts, and crystals.

Red Blood Cells. The presence of RBCs in the urine is indicative of injury to the glomerular membrane or the genitourinary tract, usually from trauma, stones, tumors of the kidney, cystitis, or renal vein thrombosis. Nonrenal disorders may also cause RBCs to appear in the urine, especially those that cause bleeding disorders. Menstrual bleeding may cause false-positive results.

White Blood Cells. Increased amounts may indicate infection or inflammation anywhere in the urinary tract. Glomerulonephritis and lupus nephritis may also cause an increase in WBCs in the urine. The inflammatory process of tumors and renal calculi may produce pyuria (i.e., excessive WBC count in the urine).

Epithelial Cells. Large amounts of epithelial cells are shed in acute tubular necrosis, renal transplant rejection, or any ischemic injury to the kidneys.

Casts. Casts are gel-like substances formed around other particles. For example, there may be WBC casts, RBC casts, bacterial casts, and protein casts. Large amounts of casts indicate disease of the renal tubules.

Crystals. Crystals are formed from the accumulation of salts. Increased amounts indicated that the sample was allowed to stand for longer than 2 hours. The presence of certain crystals may indicate disease; for example, uric acid crystals may indicate gout.

Bacteria. Bacterial counts greater than 10^5 indicate the presence of a UTI. The bacterial count increases if the sample is allowed to stand at room temperature. Urine tests positive for nitrites in the presence of bacteria. Nitrates are normally present in urine but are converted to nitrites in the presence of bacteria.

Specific Gravity. Specific gravity measures the density of urine relative to that of water (1.000). Values can range from 1.001 to 1.030. Lower values (dilute urine) occur with increased fluid intake, diabetes insipidus, and distal renal tubular disease. Increased values (concentrated urine) occur with insufficient fluid intake, decreased renal perfusion, dehydration, or in the presence of antidiuretic hormone.

pH. Normally urinary pH averages 5 to 6, with an acceptable range of 4.5 to 8. A high dietary intake of meats and certain fruits such as cranberries will cause urine to be acidic. Acidic urine may be helpful in the presence of UTIs, because some organisms do not multiply as rapidly in an acidic environment. High dietary intake of citrus fruits and vegetables produces alkaline urine. Alkaline urine is useful in the treatment of salicylate poisoning, with sulfonamide therapy in the treatment of UTIs, and in the prevention of kidney stones other than ammonium magnesium kidney stones.

See Chapter 4, Section 2 for urine analysis by reagent strip.

Urine Protein

As discussed, filtration of the plasma through the glomerulus removes all but scant amounts of protein. Normal amounts are considered less than 150 mg/24 hr or 10 mg/100 mL of protein. The presence of larger amounts of protein in the urine is considered proteinuria. If the level is > 3.5 g/24 hr, proteinuria is severe, indicating nephrotic syndrome. A macroscopic urinalysis can detect protein in the urine and also provide a gross estimate of the amount.

A trace positive result is approximately equivalent to 150 mg/24 hr.

1+ = 200–500 mg/24 hr
2+ = 0.5–1 g/24 hr
3+ = 2–5 g/24 hr
4+ = 7 g/24 hr

Urinary Sediment and Sodium

An increase in urinary sediment indicates the decreased ability of the glomerulus to filter the urine. Another urinary finding associated with acute renal failure is a low fraction of excreted sodium (<1%).

Radiologic Procedures

Blockage of a ureter can result in retrograde flow of urine. When the urine accumulates in the renal collecting system (i.e., hydronephrosis), pressure increases in the proximal tubules and thus decreases the GFR. Complete obstruction can cause the GFR to drop to zero, which results in renal failure. Obstruction can be caused by renal calculi, tumors, impingement on the ureters from external organs, or neurologic damage to the bladder. Laboratory and diagnostic tests used to determine if an obstruction exists and elucidate the cause include: kidneys, ureters, and bladder (KUB), intravenous pyelogram (IVP), and cystoscopy.

Kidneys, Ureters, and Bladder

A KUB is a radiograph of the kidneys, ureters, and bladder. This radiograph is used to estimate renal size and to identify and locate stones or calculi in the urinary tract. With the exception of uric acid stones, most renal calculi can be visualized on a radiograph.

In order to assess the bladder with a KUB, a patient must have a full bladder when the radiograph is taken.

Intravenous Pyelogram

An IVP is a radiograph in which visualization of the urinary tract system is augmented through the use of a contrast medium. This technique allows for

Table 11-5-3. Effect of Renal Failure on Electrolytes

BLOOD TEST	EXPECTED CHANGE IN RENAL FAILURE	RATIONALE
Sodium	Increased or decreased	Decreased renal elimination of sodium Water overload and dilution of sodium
Potassium	Increased	Decreased renal elimination of K^+ due to inability to excrete
Calcium	Decreased	Vitamin D is not converted to its active form in renal failure. Without vitamin D, calcium cannot be absorbed from the gut
Phosphorus	Increased	Decreased renal elimination of phosphorus due to inability to excrete
Magnesium	Increased	Decreased renal elimination of magnesium due to inability to excrete

more detailed examination of the organs and can be used to check for filling defects caused by obstruction in the urinary tract. After the dye is injected, a series of radiographs are taken over a 30-minute period to track the passage of the dye through the kidneys, ureters, and bladder. An IVP also shows the size and location of any radiopaque stones.

The dye used in an IVP contains iodine and may cause anaphylactic reactions in persons allergic to iodine. Every patient should be questioned about sensitivity to shellfish, iodine, or IV dye before undergoing an IVP.

The patient is generally given a laxative or enema to use at home the night before an IVP. This helps to ensure visualization of the urinary tract. Fluid restriction may be instituted on the morning of the test so that the dye does not pass through the urinary tract more rapidly than expected.

Cystoscopy

If direct visualization is needed, a small flexible fiberoptic scope can be inserted into the urethra and passed into the bladder. This is done to check for the presence of small or radiolucent stones, diverticuli of the urethra, and lesions such as cancer. In men, this test can determine the size of the prostate and the level of intrusion into the bladder wall. The ureters and kidney cannot be visualized by cystoscopy.

Serum Electrolytes

Serum tests commonly affected in renal dysfunction are: calcium, phosphorus, sodium, potassium, and magnesium (Table 11-5-3).

 CLINICAL PEARLS

○ The BUN can be affected by many factors and alone is not a reliable indicator of kidney function. (About 60% kidney dysfunction is needed before a change in BUN is seen.)

○ The production of creatinine is stable, and it is not reabsorbed in the renal tubules. Therefore, creatinine does provide a reliable indicator of kidney function.

○ The BUN-creatinine ratio helps to distinguish prerenal acute renal failure from other forms of renal failure. If the ratio exceeds 10:1, there is a decrease in the GFR, which is associated with volume depletion. If both the creatinine and the BUN are elevated, and the ratio remains 10:1, it usually signals intrinsic nephron damages as seen in acute tubular necrosis or chronic renal failure.

○ Creatinine clearance test evaluates the GFR by estimating the time that it takes the kidneys to excrete creatinine.

○ Obstruction in the urinary tract can cause renal failure by increasing the pressure within the proximal tubules and decreasing the GFR.

RESOURCES

- American Kidney Fund: 800-638-8299
- American Sickle Cell Association: 216-229-8600
- Cooley's Anemia Foundation: www.thalassemia.org
- Epogen: 800-272-9376 (reimbursement); 800-272-6436 (clinical information)
- http://www.laboratorynetwork.com
- http://www.med.virginia.edu/medicine/clinical/pathology/.labtests
- http://www.renalnet.org/renalnet/renalnet.cfm
- Joint Center for Sickle Cell and Thalassemic Disorders: 617-732-8490
- National Institute of Allergy and Infectious Diseases: http://www.niaid.nih.gov
- National Kidney Foundation: http://www.kidney.org

chapter 12

Decision-Making for Pharmacology

Analgesia

Section 1   Christine Stackhouse

 OVERVIEW

Pain is an unpleasant sensory and emotional experience associated with actual or potential tissue damage. However, the definition that guides nursing practice regarding pain management and analgesia is that pain is whatever the patient says it is, existing whenever the patient says it does. This definition acknowledges the subjective nature of pain and guides how to approach its management or relief.

PRINCIPLES OF CARE
Physiology of Pain

Nociception is the term used to describe the physiologic mechanisms involved in the pain phenomenon. Pain begins when free nerve endings called nociceptors found in the skin, muscle, connective tissue, and organs are stimulated by direct damage or from chemical mediators released at the site of injury, transmitting impulses to the central nervous system (CNS). The impulse travels by means of specialized sensory pain fibers, A-delta myelinated (fast) fibers and C nonmyelinated (slow) fibers. Most fibers enter the spinal cord at the dorsal root, and the impulse is transmitted to the thalamus, and then to the cerebral cortex, basal ganglia, and limbic system.

Types of Pain
Acute Pain

Acute pain is caused by any tissue-damaging event and is usually self-limiting. Healing of the injury or control of the disorder causing the pain is expected to end the pain experience.

Chronic Pain

Chronic nonmalignant pain may be both nociceptive and neuropathic (i.e., stimuli abnormally processed by the nervous system). The pain lasts longer than 6 months. Chronic pain is associated with prolonged tissue pathology or continuation of pain after healing has occurred. Possible injury to the peripheral nervous system or the CNS that results in persistent pain after healing is the perceived cause. Malignant pain can be recurrent, acute, persistent, or a combination with a progressive malignant process. The goal of treatment is to improve quality of life (as defined by the patient) and maintain a pain-free state.

Pain Assessment

Intensity

Intensity is a subjective term usually quantified using a pain scale. A wide variety of pain scales exist aimed at specific patient populations. A scale of 0 to 10 is commonly used, with 0 representing no pain and 10 indicating the worst pain that the patient could possibly have.

Location and Quality

Specific questions about the location and whether the pain radiates to other areas can identify the tissues and nerves affected. Having the patient identify the quality of the pain (i.e., sharp, dull, constant, intermittent, burning, aching, rebound, or pulsating, stabbing, cramping, shooting, splitting, tender, tiring) can assist in determining the cause of the pain.

Pattern

The pattern of pain identifies the onset, frequency, and duration of pain. Onset can help identify the cause of pain. For example, gastric pain that occurs at bedtime suggests peptic ulcer disease or gastric reflux into the esophagus; calf pain that occurs only when walking can indicate intermittent claudication of the calf muscles. Noting the frequency and duration of the pain can also help identify the cause.

Aggravating and Alleviating Factors

Aggravating and alleviating factors identify what increases or decreases the pain. Such factors may include positioning, movement of the affected area, coughing, application of pressure, and analgesic administration.

Objective Behaviors

Behaviors such as splinting of the affected area, distorted posture, agonized facial expression, clenched teeth, impaired mobility, insomnia, anxiety, attention seeking, and depression are important to identify and manage. Some cultures view tolerance of pain as signifying strength and endurance, and thus persons of these cultural backgrounds will be more stoic in their response and desired treatment of pain.

History

Past medical, surgical, medication, allergy, and family history should be collected. All medications, including prescribed, over-the-counter, and herbal substances, should be investigated. All diagnostic tests and procedures should be reviewed. Assessment of sleep patterns and nutritional status of the patient are important to assess stress.

Psychosocial

The psychological and social aspects of pain should be addressed, especially in patients with chronic or malignant pain. The patient's past experiences with pain and its management can also influence pain levels. Common contributing factors (e.g., depression, fear, anxiety, grief, feelings of loss of control, feelings about work, support systems, and isolation) should be investigated. If possible, the patient's significant others should be involved in the care and management plan. Use of alcohol, nicotine, or recreational drugs should be identified. A patient may turn to other substances as a result of inadequate pain control.

DECISION-MAKING
Opioids

Opioids are used in the treatment and management of moderate to severe pain because of their effectiveness, ease of titration, and favorable risk–benefit ratio. It is believed that opioids (endogenous or exogenous) bind to receptor sites at the nerve endings in the dorsal root of the spinal cord, which blocks pain transmission to the brain or alters perception and interpretation of pain by the brain. Opioids act on two main types of opioid receptors, kappa (κ) and mu (μ), both of which provide analgesia. In addition to analgesia, stimulation of μ receptors causes respiratory depression, constipation, urinary retention, and euphoria; stimulation of κ receptors causes sedation (without respiratory depression). Another receptor that may be activated is the sigma receptor. Stimulation of sigma (σ) receptors causes vasomotor stimulation and psychomimetic effects (hallucinations and paranoia).

Various drugs bind to the opioid receptors tightly (pure) or partially and act as agonists to turn on activity or antagonists to turn off (block) activity. *Agonist* drugs activate both the mu and kappa receptors. *Agonist-antagonist* drugs activate kappa receptors (agonist) and block or have minimal effects on the mu receptors (antagonist), or vice versa. Pure agonists block all opioid effects.

Opioid Classification
Pure Agonists. Morphine, codeine, fentanyl, hydromorphone (Dilaudid), and meperidine (Demerol) bind with the mu sites and do not antagonize activity at the kappa and sigma sites. Morphine is the standard by which all other opioids are measured and is particularly suitable for severe continuous pain of either visceral or soft-tissue origin.

Opioid Agonists-Antagonists. Butorphanol (Stadol), dezocine (Dalgan), nalbuphine (Nubain), and pentazocine (Talwin) bind with the kappa sites for pain relief and block the effects of pure agonists at the mu sites. These drugs produce less analgesia than pure opioids, have a low potential for abuse, and produce less respiratory depression. Buprenorphine (Buprenex) is a partial μ agonist and a κ antagonist. If an agonist is given in combination with an agonist-antagonist, the analgesic effect of the agonist may be diminished.

Pure Antagonists. Naloxone (Narcan), naltrexone (Trexan), and nalmefene (Revex) are used for reversal or overdose of opioids. They block the opioid effects of analgesia and relieve the related complications of respiratory depression and sedation.

Dealing with Opioid Side Effects
Most side effects occur as a result of blocking simulation of opioid. Table 12-1-1 lists common side effects and their treatment.

Selection of Route
The proper route of administration depends on patient condition and needs.
Oral Route. This is the most convenient, cost-effective, and least invasive method of administration for all degrees of pain.

Table 12-1-1. Opioid Side Effects

SIDE EFFECT	TREATMENT
Constipation	• Laxatives; bisacodyl (Dulcolax); hyperosmotic (lactulose); adequate hydration, fiber, physical activity
Nausea and vomiting	• Antiemetics; switching to another opioid
Neurologic side effects	• Supportive and safety measures for sedation and dizziness
Respiratory depression	• Naloxone (Narcan)
Xerostomia and diaphoresis	• Xerostomia (dry mouth): oral hygiene; humidified air; providing ice cubes, gum, or candy Diaphoresis: dosage titration
Pruritus	• Antihistamines (diphenhydramine [Benadryl] and cimetidine [Tagamet]); skin care; dosage changes
Hyperalgesia/allodynia	• Decreased or eliminated if another opioid is selected (e.g., fentanyl, methadone)
Urinary retention	• Urinary catheterization; discontinuing the adjuvant drug; changing to another opioid or route
Miosis	• Maintaining a brightly lit room

Intravenous Route. The intravenous (IV) route provides immediate relief when the oral route is contraindicated. IV administration includes bolus dosing, continuous infusion, and patient-controlled analgesia (PCA).

Continuous Infusion. Continuous infusion provides consistent absorption for the highest level of analgesia with the smallest amount of opioid.

Patient-Controlled Analgesia. PCA delivery devices can be programmed to administer basal (continuous infusion) rates of medications and patient-controlled bolus doses for breakthrough pain. PCA use is not appropriate for sedated or confused patients.

Intramuscular Route. If the IV route is not possible, the IM route can be used for acute pain.

Transdermal Route. This route is appropriate for individuals already on opioid therapy, who have constant pain, and who have infrequent episodes of breakthrough pain; it is also recommended for unconscious individuals with end stage disease.

Mucous Membranes. Use of nasal, sublingual, and buccal routes is increasing, as absorption into the bloodstream is relatively quick. Fentanyl lollipops or lozenges (Actiq and Oralet) and buccal morphine tablets are now available.

Epidural Analgesia. This route is of benefit to patients who have thoracic, orthopedic, and abdominal pain. Pain relief occurs from the direct drug effect on spinal cord opioid receptors. Close monitoring is required for movement of the opioid above or across motor pathways causing unwanted complications such as respiratory depression.

Opioid Administration

See Table 12-1-2 for recommended starting dosages for adults. Consult a drug handbook for methods of IV administration. Table 12-1-2 also provides guidelines for switching from one analgesic to another, providing the same pain relief in comparison. This is called "equianalgesia." Thirty mg of morphine by mouth, for example, produces the same amount of analgesia as 130 mg of codeine by mouth; or, 30 mg of morphine by mouth produces the same analgesia as 10 mg of morphine by IV.

Table 12-1-2. Opioid Analgesic Dosages for Adults Weighing Greater than 50 Kg

DRUG	RECOMMENDED STARTING DOSAGES (ORAL)	RECOMMENDED STARTING DOSE (PARENTERAL)	APPROXIMATE EQUIANALGESIC ORAL DOSE TO MORPHINE	APPROXIMATE EQUIANALGESIC PARENTERAL DOSE TO MORPHINE
Morphine	30 mg q 3–4 hr	10 mg q 3–4 hr	30 mg q 3–4 hr; around-the-clock dosing	10 mg q 3–4 hr
Codeine	60 mg q 3–4 hr	60 mg q 2 hr IM or SC	130 mg q 3–4 hr; doses over 65 mg not recommended	75 mg q 3–4 hr; doses over 65 mg not recommended
Hydromorphone	6 mg q 3–4 hr	1.5 mg q 3–4 hr	7.5 mg q 3–4 hr	1.5 mg q 3–4 hr
Hydrocodone	Not available	10 mg q 3–4 hr	30 mg q 3–4 hr	Not available
Levorphanol	4 mg q 6–8 hr	2 mg q 6–8 hr	4 mg q 6–8 hr	2 mg q 6–8 hr
Meperidine	Not recommended	100 mg q 3 hr	300 mg q 2–3 hr	100 mg q 3 hr
Methadone	20 mg q 6–8 hr	10 mg q 6–8 hr	20 mg q 6–8 hr	10 mg q 6–8 hr
Oxycodone	10 mg q 3–4 hr	Not available	30 mg q 3–4 hr	Not available
Oxymorphone	Not available	1 mg q 3–4 hr	Not available	1 mg q 3–4 hr

Note: Published tables vary in suggested doses that are equianalgesic to morphine. Clinical response is the criterion that must be applied for each patient; titration to patient response is necessary. Because there is not complete cross-tolerance among these drugs, it is usually necessary to use a lower-than-equianalgesic dose when changing drugs and to retitrate to response. Recommended doses do not apply to a patient with renal or hepatic disease or other conditions affecting drug metabolism and distribution. Adapted from U.S. Department of Health and Human Services Clinical Practice Guideline for Acute Pain Management.

Opioid Reversal

If stimulation is ineffective in arousing and increasing respiration, then the use of an antagonist, such as naloxone (Narcan), is needed. Naloxone should be administered slowly; several doses may be required. After mixing 0.4 mg of naloxone with 10 mL of normal saline in a syringe, approximately 0.5 mL is administered over 2 minutes. The patient's response is assessed and the dose titrated to effect every 2 minutes. When the patient's respiratory rate and depth increase or the patient becomes responsive, IV administration is stopped. If no increase in respirations and/or depth occurs, dosage titration is continued every 2 to 3 minutes (up to a total of 0.8 mg). The patient is monitored for the next few hours, because the duration of naloxone may be shorter than that of the opioid, and repeated dosing may be needed until the opioid is metabolized and excreted. Naloxone should be titrated in doses that improve respiratory function but not reverse analgesia. If IV access is not available, naloxone is administered 0.4 mg via subcutaneous (SC) or intramuscular (IM) injection. The patient should respond within 5 minutes. If the patient remains unresponsive, SC/IM dosing is repeated every 5 minutes up to 2 mg total.

Drug Tolerance and Dependence

There is a difference between opioid physical dependence and psychological addiction. Physical dependence is the body's adaptation to the opioid, and abrupt termination of the opioid will cause signs of physical withdrawal in all patients who have used opioid for long periods. Addiction is the sociologic term used to describe the psychological compulsion to use drugs for the psychic effects despite harm and does not improve the person's quality of life. Patients with chronic pain using continuous opioid therapy will probably become physically dependent, but only 1% have the potential for addiction. Reports of uncontrolled pain by a patient should first be considered a failure of treatment or physical tolerance, not psychological addiction.

Nonopioid Analgesics

Nonsteroidal anti-inflammatory drugs (NSAIDs) and acetaminophen are often used to control mild to moderate pain alone or as adjunctive therapy with opiates.

Nonsteroidal Anti-Inflammatory Drugs

Also used to treat fevers and to suppress inflammatory disorders such as rheumatoid arthritis. An additional action is the reduction of thrombus formation by suppression of platelet aggregation. NSAIDs work by blocking the synthesis of prostaglandins and other mediators of the inflammatory response at the site of tissue injury, preventing stimulation of pain receptors. NSAIDs cause a potentiating effect when used with opioids, resulting in opioid sparing. Table 12-1-3 presents dosage information and information on general management.

Adverse Effects

- Mild GI upset to severe GI ulceration and bleeding may occur. Nonopioid therapy is responsible for 20% of all hospitalizations for GI bleeding. To minimize these effects, these drugs should always be administered with food or milk.

Table 12-1-3. Nonsteroidal Anti-inflammatory Drug Dosages for Adults

NSAID	USUAL ORAL ADULT DOSE	COMMENTS
Acetylsalicylic acid (aspirin, ASA, many brands)	650–975 mg q 4 hr	The standard against which other NSAIDs are compared. Inhibits platelet aggregation and may cause postoperative bleeding
Choline magnesium trisalicylate (Trilisate)	1000–1500 mg bid	May have minimal antiplatelet activity; also available as oral liquid
Diflunisal (Dolobid)	1000 mg initial dose followed by 500 mg q 12 hr	
Etodolac (Lodine)	200–400 mg q 6–8 hr	
Fenprofen calcium (Nalfon)	200 mg q 4–6 hr	Available in several brand names and generic forms. Also
Ibuprofen (Advil, Motrin)	400 mg q 4–6 hr	available in oral suspension
Ketoprofen (Actron, Orudis)	25–75 mg q 6–8 hr	
Ketorolac (Toradol)	Generally begin with a 30 or 60 mg IM initial dose, followed by 15 or 30 mg q 6 hr; oral dose following IM dosage: 10 mg q 6 hr	Available in oral and parenteral preparations. IM dose not to exceed 5 days
Magnesium salicylate (Doan's)	650 mg q 4 hr	Many brands and generic forms are available
Meclofenamate sodium (Meclomen)	50 mg q 4–6 hr	
Mefenamic acid (Ponstel)	250 mg q 6 hr	
Naproxen (Naprosyn)	500 mg initial dose followed by 250 mg q 6–8 hr	An oral liquid is also available
Naproxen sodium (Anaprox, Aleve)	550 mg initial dose followed by 275 mg q 6–8 hr	
Salsalate (Disalcid)	500 mg q 4 hr	May have minimal antiplatelet activity
Sodium salicylate (Urasel-5)	325–650 mg q 3–4 hr	Available in generic form from several different companies

Adapted from U. S. Department of Health and Human Services Clinical Practice Guideline for Acute Pain Management.
IM, intramuscular; NSAID, nonsteroidal anti-inflammatory drug.

- Bleeding is a potential risk because of the suppression of platelet aggregation.
- Renal impairment is most common in elderly patients, cardiac patients, and those with preexisting renal disease.
- Salicylism occurs with elevated aspirin levels. Signs include sweating, headache, tinnitus, and dizziness. The drug should be discontinued if this occurs.

Acetaminophen

Acetaminophen prevents the synthesis of prostaglandins but only in the CNS. It has little or no direct effect at the site of injury and thus lacks the peripheral anti-inflammatory activity of NSAIDs. The usual oral adult dose is 650 to 975 mg every 4 hours.

Adverse Effects

- Toxic levels can cause hepatic failure. Avoid exceeding 4 g in 24 hours. Alcohol intake increases the risk of hepatic injury. Also monitor over-the-counter medications, as many contain significant amounts of acetaminophen.
- Toxicity may be treated with acetylcysteine.

World Health Organization Analgesic Ladder

The World Health Organization (WHO) has developed a three-step analgesic ladder for control of pain. The WHO ladder is widely regarded as being the most appropriate approach to the management of pain, whether it is acute, chronic nonmalignant, or chronic malignant pain. The ladder begins with interventions using nonopioids and progresses through weak opioids to strong opioids, according to the severity of pain.

Step 1: Nonopioid With or Without Adjuvant Therapy

The first step in this approach is the use of acetaminophen, aspirin, ibuprofen, naproxen, or another NSAID for mild pain. Adjuvant analgesic therapies can also be initiated, including corticosteroids, anticonvulsants, antidepressants, and antihistamines.

Nonpharmacologic adjuvant therapies (e.g., application of heat or cold packs, massage, transcutaneous electrical nerve stimulation [TENS], distraction, relaxation, imagery, biofeedback, prayer, aroma therapy, music, and acupuncture) can often provide additional pain relief. Unfortunately, these techniques are frequently underused. If pain persists or increases, move to step 2.

Step 2: Opioid for Mild to Moderate Pain, Plus a Nonopioid, With or Without Adjuvant Therapy

When pain persists or increases, an opioid such as codeine, hydrocodone, oxycodone, hydromorphone, meperidine, or morphine should be added to (not substituted for) the NSAID. Opioids for this step are readily available in fixed prepared oral dose combinations with acetaminophen (e.g., Darvocet-N, Lortab, Percocet, Tylenol No. 3) or aspirin (e.g., Darvon-N, Percodan), because the combination of NSAIDs and opioids provides additive analgesia.

Step 3: Opioids for Moderate to Severe Pain, With or Without a Nonopioid, With or Without Adjuvant Therapy

At this step, separate dosage forms of the opioid and NSAID should be used to avoid exceeding maximally recommended doses of NSAIDs. Pain that is persistent, or moderate to severe at the outset, should be treated beginning at step 3 and titrated upward, increasing opioid potency or using higher dosages. Drugs such as codeine or hydrocodone are replaced with more potent opioids (usually morphine, hydromorphone, methadone, fentanyl, or levorphanol). Medications for persistent pain should be administered on an around-the-clock basis, with additional as-needed doses for breakthrough pain.

Geriatric Concerns

Many persons feel that pain is a natural part of growing old; this attitude can lead to inadequate pain treatment. Pain contributes to deconditioning, gait disturbances, falls, cognitive dysfunction, and malnutrition in older patients. Renal and hepatic functions are generally decreased, allowing for drug accumulation. Increases in the proportion of body fat and decreases in serum proteins affect the percentage of bound and free circulating drug levels. Age-related changes may necessitate slightly lower doses and/or lengthened frequency of doses in elderly patients. Cognitive impairments (delirium or dementia) present serious barriers to pain assessment and treatment; in patients with cognitive deficits, behavior changes (e.g., agitation, restlessness) may provide the best clues to pain.

 CLINICAL PEARLS

○ Opioid use during the acute phase of an illness should not be an issue when caring for patients with addiction problems. In fact, these patients will typically require larger doses of opioids because of their physical tolerance to them.

○ Drug-seeking behavior should be considered a failure of treatment and/or physical tolerance rather than a psychological addiction to narcotics. Patients in pain will attempt to find measures to relieve the pain whether provided by health care professionals or other sources.

Anticoagulants

Section 2   Christine Stackhouse

OVERVIEW

Coagulation, simply stated, is the formation of a thrombus or blood clot to maintain hemostasis. It is a complex process that involves a chemical chain reaction of substances or factors within the blood. When normal hemostasis becomes pathological, leading to the inappropriate production of thrombi (stationary blood clots within a blood vessel or the heart) and emboli (a broken-off piece of a thrombus circulating through the blood), pharmacologic manipulation of the coagulation process is initiated.

The use of anticoagulation therapy has been shown to prevent and reduce the morbidity and mortality of several conditions, including deep vein thrombosis (DVT), pulmonary embolism (PE), unstable angina, myocardial infarction (MI), and cerebrovascular accident (CVA). Other conditions such as immobility, surgery, trauma, large bone fractures, and atrial fibrillation, which can lead to DVT, PE, or CVA, are also treated prophylactically with anticoagulants.

PRINCIPLES OF CARE
Phases of Hemostasis

The normal process of coagulation is best described in five sequential phases.

Vascular Phase

Known as vasospasm or vessel spasm, this is the immediate constriction of the injured vessel that serves to decrease further blood loss.

Platelet (Thrombocyte) Phase

This phase involves the formation of an unstable platelet plug. As platelets strike the rough edges of a damaged vessel, they become activated and change shape, and also become sticky. They then line up on exposed subendothelial tissue with the help of von Willebrand's factor (a plasma protein that helps bind the platelet to exposed collagen). This process, called *platelet adherence*, is followed by *platelet aggregation*, in which the platelets stick to each other, forming layers. Substances released by the platelets themselves (e.g., adenosine diphosphate [ADP], thrombin, and thromboxane A_2) induce the aggregation process. Platelets achieve hemostasis by forming a platelet plug within 3 to 5 minutes.

Coagulation Phase

The coagulation phase is extremely complex involving a stepwise series of reactions known as the clotting (or coagulation) cascade, which results in formation of a firm fibrin clot. The clotting cascade can be considered to be three pathways in one (Fig. 12-2-1):
- The *intrinsic pathway* is triggered from internal vessel damage, exposing underlying layers of the vessel wall, or from plaque formation.
- The *extrinsic pathway* is triggered from external damage such as trauma, and involves tissue thromboplastin. Tissue thromboplastin (factor III) is a lipoprotein released from injured cells outside the blood vessel. The extrinsic pathway is a more rapid system with fewer steps.
- Both pathways converge into the *common pathway.* In the common pathway, the prothrombin activator catalyzes the conversion of prothrombin (factor II) into thrombin. Thrombin then acts as an enzyme to convert fibrinogen (factor I) into fibrin threads that enmesh the platelets. Fibrin threads transform the temporary platelet plug into an insoluble fibrin clot.

Without the coagulation phase, the platelet plug is swept away within 7 to 10 days, and bleeding occurs. If even one factor is deficient, the entire process may fail. Table 12-2-1 lists conditions that can result in coagulation problems.

Calcium (factor IV) is required in almost all steps; adequate levels must be

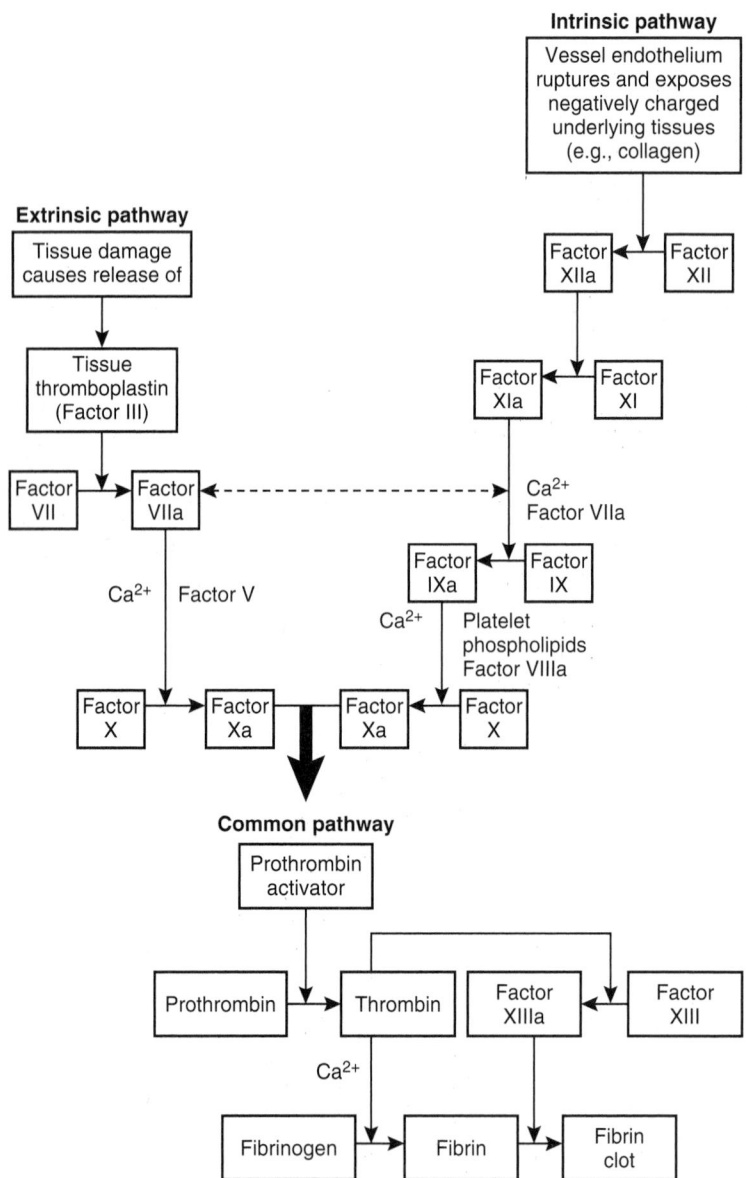

Figure 12-2-1. Extrinsic and intrinsic pathways. (With permission from Hansen, M. [1998]. *Pathophysiology: Foundations of disease and clinical intervention.* Philadelphia: WB Saunders.)

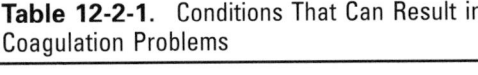

Table 12-2-1. Conditions That Can Result in
Coagulation Problems

CONDITION	DIMINISHED FACTORS
Autoimmune disease	VIII
Congenital deficiency	I, II, V, VII, VIII, IX, X, XI, XII
Disseminated intravascular coagulation	I, V, VIII
Fibrinolysis	I, V, VIII
Heparin administration	II
Liver disease	I, II, V, VII, IX, X, XI
Vitamin K deficiency	II, VII, IX, X, XI
Warfarin (Coumadin) administration	II, VII, IX, X, XI

maintained. There must be adequacy of both platelets and clotting factors to form a firm fibrin clot. Excessive or inappropriate clotting is prevented by an intact endothelium and by antithrombin III (AT III) as well as a number of other circulating anticoagulant factors. AT III is a factor synthesized by the liver and endothelial cells that binds to and inactivates any activated thrombin outside of the clot.

Clot Retraction

This is the final stage of the "stasis" part of hemostasis. The fibrin strands contract or shorten, becoming stronger and denser. This contraction approximates (brings together) the edges of the injured vessel and seals the site of injury. Contraction also causes expression of the serum from the cells within the fibrin meshwork, producing serous drainage.

Clot Destruction (Fibrinolysis)

Plasminogen is an anticlotting protein that continuously circulates in its inactive form. As the clot is being formed, the circulating plasminogen is deposited into it. Once retracted, vascular endothelial and liver cells release two naturally occurring plasminogen activators, *tissue plasminogen activator* (t-PA), and *urokinase plasminogen activator.* These activate the plasminogen trapped in the clot, to form plasmin. *Plasmin*, a proteolytic enzyme, breaks down fibrin and any fibrinogen in the area. Fibrin is broken down (fibrinolysis) into fibrin fragments called *fibrin split (degradation) products*, including a cross-linked D-dimer fragment. Measurements of the D-dimer are used clinically to determine the rate of clot lysis. Fibrinogen is broken down (fibrinogenolysis) to *fibrinogen degradation products.* These products serve as anticoagulants by binding to any free, broken strands of fibrin, preventing further clot formation.

DECISION-MAKING
Coagulation Testing

Although the coagulation process involves many factors and pathways, only a few of the factors are manipulated to produce anticoagulation for various therapeutic treatments. Several tests are performed to monitor therapeutic drug actions and to determine dosing requirements. Coagulation testing is also important in monitoring bleeding disorders (Table 12-2-2).

Table 12-2-2. Laboratory Values in Coagulation Testing

TEST	NORMAL VALUE	CRITICAL VALUE
Activated partial thromboplastin time (APTT)	30–40 sec	70 sec
Partial thromboplastin time (PTT)	60–80 sec	100 sec
Prothrombin time (PT)	11.2–13.2 sec	20 sec or International Normalization Ratio (INR) >4.5
Platelets	150,000–400,000/mm³	<20,000 >1 million

Prothrombin Time

Prothrombin time (PT) is used to screen the extrinsic pathway. PT can detect deficiencies in factors II, V, VII, and fibrinogen. It is commonly used to regulate warfarin (Coumadin) therapy. Prolonged PT can also indicate vitamin K deficiency, liver disease, disseminated intravascular coagulation (DIC), and the presence of fibrin split products. *Blood samples* are collected in blue-top tubes. These tubes contain sodium citrate, which binds with the calcium in the blood to prevent clot formation until the test can be performed. In this test, a reagent, tissue thromboplastin, and calcium are added to the plasma sample. These directly activate the extrinsic pathway, and the time it takes for the sample to clot is measured. *Normal values* range from 11.2 to 13.2 seconds, depending on the reagent used.

PT can vary significantly, depending on the type of *tissue thromboplastin* reagent used. Each commercially prepared tissue thromboplastin reagent has a different sensitivity, as they are prepared from rabbit brain and/or lung or human tissue factor. This results in varying values with each test. This situation led to the development of the *international normalization ratio* (INR) by the World Health Organization (WHO) in 1983. The INR is a method of standardizing the thromboplastin reagents used in PT testing. The INR takes into account the International Sensitivity Index (ISI) and the mean normal range of the reagent. The ISI designates the sensitivity of a particular thromboplastin to an international reference plasma. The mean of the normal range is used as the control. Both the ISI and the mean are found on the reagent's package insert. The INR is the patient's PT in seconds, divided by the mean of the normal range of the reagent, squared to the ISI:

$$INR = \left[\frac{\text{Patient PT in seconds}}{\text{Mean of the normal range of the reagent}} \right]^{ISI}$$

If the patient's PT is 16.1, look on the PT reagent's package insert for the mean normal range and the ISI. Then:

$$\left[\frac{16.1}{11.6} \right]^{2.77} = 2.5$$

The use of the INR significantly decreases the differences seen between laboratories and reagents used, which provides more consistent and meaningful results for patients on warfarin. The INR is preferred for oral anticoagulation monitoring; however, a PT must still be obtained to calculate the INR.

Activated Partial Thromboplastin Time or Partial Thromboplastin Time

These tests are used to screen for coagulation disorders in the intrinsic system, including hemophilia (type A: deficiency in factor VIII; type B: factor IX) and DIC, and for monitoring heparin therapy. Partial thromboplastin time (PTT) is a precursor to activated partial thromboplastin time (APTT). The APTT is more widely used today, because it is faster and more reliable than the PTT. It measures the time that it takes for a firm fibrin clot to form after a reagent is added to the sample. The sample is collected in the same manner as for PT. Again, testing values may vary from one laboratory to another, and each laboratory determines the normal ranges for the specific reagent used. Normal APTT generally falls between 22.1 and 34.1 seconds.

Fibrinogen Assay

Normal fibrinogen concentration is 175 to 400 mg/dL. Deficiencies suggest liver disease, thrombolytic therapy, or DIC.

Fibrin Degradation Products

The normal value is below 2.5 μg/mL. An elevated value suggests DIC.

D-dimer

The D-dimer tests for the cross-linked D region of degraded or split fibrin strands. This test is more specific for split products from fibrinolysis, thus distinguishing fibrinolysis from fibrinogenolysis. It thereby confirms the presence of DIC. The normal range is negative to below 0.5 μg/mL.

Bleeding Time

Normal bleeding time is 2 to 9 minutes. This test is commonly used for assessing the effectiveness of platelets, but not the platelet count. A drug that alters platelet function is aspirin. While aspirin does not alter the number of platelets within the circulation, it does alter the platelets' ability to aggregate or stick together. Altered platelet functioning is referred to as *thrombocytopathia*. Bleeding time is also useful for screening for von Willebrand's disease.

Platelet Count

Platelets are produced by bone marrow, and then released to circulate within the blood (see Chapter 11, Section 1). Normal platelet count is between 150,000 and 400,000/mm^3. Platelet plugs are important for closing the minute ruptures in very small blood vessels that occur hundreds of times daily. A platelet count below 150,000/mm^3 indicates thrombocytopenia; a count above 400,000/mm^3 indicates thrombocytosis.

Drug Therapy
Heparin

Heparin inactivates prothrombin (factor II), thus preventing the formation of thrombin. Heparin is not thrombolytic, but it inhibits clot formation. IV

▮ **Table 12-2-3.** Heparin Sliding Scale Example

HEPARIN STANDING ORDERS

Client's weight: _____

Initiate heparin therapy with bolus (80 U/kg) = _____ U IV

Begin IV heparin (18 U/kg/hr) = _____ U/hr standard mix: 20,000 U heparin in 500 mL of
    D5W = 40 U/mL

Warfarin _____ mg PO, q day to start on day 2 of anticoagulation therapy

Laboratory: APTT, PT, CBC, urinalysis, and hemocult stool now
    CBC and platelet count q 3 days
    STAT APTT 6 hr after heparin bolus
    Daily PT starting on day 1 of heparin therapy

Adjust heparin infusion according to sliding scale below:

APTT <35 give 80 U/kg bolus = _____ units IV and increase drip by 4 U/kg/hr = _____ U/hr

APTT 35 to 45 give 40 U/kg bolus = _____ units IV and increase drip by 2 U/kg/hr = _____ U/hr

APTT 46 to 70 No changes

APTT 71 to 90 decrease drip by 2 U/kg/hr = _____ U/hr

APTT >90 hold heparin drip for 1 hr and reduce drip by 3 U/kg/hr = _____ U/hr

APTT 6 hr after each dosage change for nontherapeutic results, after 2 consecutive therapeutic
    APTT results change APTT to every morning.

Date/signature: _____ of ordering physician

APTT, activated partial thromboplastin time; CBC, complete blood cell count; PO, by mouth; PT, prothrombin time.

heparin is used for the initial treatment of DVT, CVA, acute MI, and PE, because of its immediate onset of action and short half-life (1.5 hours).

Dosage. The use of fixed-dose heparin has been replaced with weight-based nomograms and sliding scale standing orders (Table 12-2-3). A heparin bolus of 80 U/kg is initially given, followed by an IV infusion of 18U/kg/hr. Continuous IV heparin infusion is always administered with an infusion pump.

Laboratory Monitoring. Initial testing includes baseline APTT, PT, platelet count, hemoglobin and hematocrit, urinalysis, and stool for occult blood. This is done to identify any current bleeding problems and is used as a comparison during anticoagulation therapy.

APTT should be monitored at 6-hour intervals for the first 24 hours after the start of the infusion, with dosages adjusted accordingly. After two consecutive therapeutic APTTs are obtained, daily monitoring is usually sufficient. If at any time the APTT results are not considered therapeutic, the heparin dose is titrated and every-6-hour APTT monitoring is initiated again until therapeutic levels are reached. *Therapeutic APTT results should be between 1.5 and 2.5 times the control values (45 to 70 seconds).* Note that APTT testing exhibits a *diurnal variation* (as much as 50%) during continuous heparin infusion. APTT is generally highest around midnight and lowest around 7 AM. Elevated late evening levels can result in decreased heparin infusion, causing a subtherapeutic APTT the next morning because of the diurnal variations.

Adverse Reactions. Mild adverse reactions to heparin include fever, chills, rash, and a burning sensation at the injection site. More serious side effects include prolonged bleeding, hemorrhage, thrombocytopenia, and heparin-induced thrombocytopenia and thrombosis, or white clot syndrome (WCS). For mild reactions and mild bleeding, heparin should be gradually switched to another anticoagulant. For severe bleeding, IV protamine sulfate, 10 to 50 mg over 1 to 3 minutes (not to exceed 20 mg/min or 50 mg in 10 minutes), is given to reverse the action of heparin. Blood and blood product administration may be needed.

WCS can occur 2 or more days after the initiation of therapy in patients who have had heparin in the past, or 10 to 15 days later in those never previously exposed to heparin. WCS is characterized by severe thrombocytopenia, increasing resistance to heparin dosing, and thromboembolism. Thromboembolism associated with WCS can result in limb amputation, PE, or CVA. WCS can be diagnosed with a platelet count below 100,000/mm^3 or platelets that decreased 50% before heparin therapy. If WCS is suspected or diagnosed, heparin should be stopped immediately and protamine sulfate administered or plasmapheresis performed (removes IgG factor). Alternative drugs to provide anticoagulation should then be used.

Warfarin (Coumadin)

Warfarin blocks vitamin K–dependent coagulation factors (II, VII, IX, and X), leading to production of nonfunctional clotting factors. Warfarin therapy is the drug of choice for long-term anticoagulation as it can be taken orally, requires less monitoring, and has a longer half-life (36 to 44 hours) than heparin. The duration of warfarin therapy for DVT and PE without known cause should last 6 months. For recurrent DVT, CVA, or other conditions that significantly increase the risk of thrombosis or emboli, such as atrial fibrillation, long-term warfarin therapy is warranted. Warfarin therapy reduces the risk of CVA in patients with atrial fibrillation by about 70%. *Patients on long-term warfarin therapy should wear a Medic-Alert bracelet.*

Dosage. Warfarin therapy can begin on the second day of heparin therapy. The usual first dose of warfarin for adults is 5 mg/day. If the INR is not between 2.0 and 3.0 after two dosages, then the daily dosage can be increased. (But elderly or postoperative patients should not receive more than 5 mg/day.) It is common to stop heparin therapy on the same day that the INR becomes therapeutic (2 to 3 days). However, overlapping heparin and warfarin therapy for 5 days is recommended.

Laboratory Monitoring. Monitoring of warfarin therapy is becoming safer and more convenient with the development of nurse-led clinics. Target INR for the treatment of arterial and venous thrombosis and the prevention of systemic embolism is 2.0 to 3.0. For therapy with mechanical heart valves, the target INR is 2.5 to 3.5.

Adverse Reactions. INR values below 2.0 call for immediate treatment. The risk of bleeding does not significantly increase until INR rises above 4.5. Current guidelines for elevated PT/INR values without hemorrhage are as follows:

- INR above therapeutic level and below 6: Hold the next one or two scheduled doses of warfarin and start at lower doses when INR returns to therapeutic levels.
- INR above 6 and below 10: Hold warfarin and give 1 to 2 mg vitamin K via SC injection. Generally, the INR will return to more therapeutic levels in 8 hours.
- INR between 10 and 20 without bleeding: Hold warfarin; administer 3 mg of vitamin K via SC or IM injection, and check PT and INR at 6-hour intervals.
- INR over 20: Hold warfarin; give 10 mg vitamin K IM, and check PT at 6-hour intervals.

If hemorrhage occurs with an elevated PT/INR, administer vitamin K, fresh frozen plasma, whole blood, or plasma concentrate of vitamin K–dependent clotting factors, and hold warfarin. It may take several weeks for vitamin K to be eliminated.

Drug Interactions. Warfarin can interact with various drugs. *Drugs that interact with warfarin and elevate PT values include* acetaminophen, amiodarone, cephalosporins, chloramphenicol, ciprofloxacin, clofibrate, diflunisal, thyroid drugs, heparin, anabolic steroids, cimetidine, disulfiram, glucagon, methimazole, metronidazole, propylthiouracil, sulindac, sulfinpyrazone, sulfonamides, and vitamin E.

Drugs that decrease responsiveness to warfarin and decrease PT values include barbiturates, griseofulvin, ethchlorvynol, carbamazepine, paraldehyde, phenytoin, and rifampin.

Drugs that increase ulcer incidence and increase PT values include indomethacin, mefenamic acid, oxyphenbutazone, phenylbutazone, and salicylates. These drugs should not be used in combination with warfarin.

Oral hypoglycemic agents, such as sulfonylureas, increase the hypoglycemic response when used with warfarin. Blood glucose levels should be closely monitored.

Low Molecular Weight Heparin

Low molecular weight heparin (LMWH) has been found to be as effective as, or more effective than, standard heparin, and minimal to no monitoring is necessary. Outpatient use of LMWH, given SC, is increasing rapidly. Patients can be taught to self-administer the medication SC and can be discharged from the hospital sooner, with home health follow-up.

LMWHs disrupt the coagulation cascade by blocking the conversion of factor X to its activated form. Because they have no effect on thrombin (as does standard heparin), the risk of bleeding is greatly reduced. Also, standard (unfractionated) heparin binds extensively to plasma proteins, which causes unstable levels. LMWHs bind much less, which produces a longer half-life (two to four times longer than heparin) and makes plasma levels predictable, alleviating the need for APTT monitoring.

LMWHs are approved for prevention of DVT in patients who are immobilized, have undergone surgery, have sustained hip fracture, or are being treated for unstable angina, non–Q wave MI, or acute DVT.

Dosage: Therapy is started immediately after diagnosis (Table 12-2-4). Warfarin, 5 mg/day, is started 1 to 2 days later.

Laboratory Monitoring. Other than baseline CBC, platelet count, PT, and APTT, no laboratory monitoring of LMWHs is recommended. Most patients receiving LMWH for DVT can be treated on an outpatient basis.

Patient Education

Patient education is extremely important as anticoagulation therapy alters many aspects of the patient's life. Lifestyle changes include avoiding contact sports, to decrease the incidence of trauma, and avoiding certain prescription and nonprescription drugs. Dietary changes may be needed to maintain a constant, stable vitamin K intake. Vitamin K intake does not have to be low, as long as there are no fluctuations that will alter the effects of LMWH. Patients need frequent follow-up assessment and laboratory testing to avoid hypercoagulation and hypoanticoagulation states and complications.

Table 12-2-4. Low Molecular Weight Heparin Dosing

DRUG	RECOMMENDED USES	DOSAGE
Ardeparin (Normiflo)	Deep vein thrombosis (DVT) prophylaxis following knee replacement	50 U/kg SC q 12 hr; begin the evening of the day of surgery or the morning and continue for 14 days or until ambulatory
Dalteparin (Fragmin)	DVT prophylaxis following hip and abdominal surgery	2500–5000 IU SC daily, begin just before surgery and continue for 5–10 days
	Treatment of unstable and non–Q wave myocardial infarction (MI)	120 IU/kg SC q 12 hr combined with aspirin 75–165 mg PO daily until stable
Danaparoid (Orgaran)	DVT prophylaxis following hip surgery	No more than 10,000 IU SC q 12 hr 750 units SC bid; begin 1–4 hours preoperatively and continue no sooner than 2 hours postoperatively for 7–14 days
Enoxaparin (Lovenox)	DVT prophylaxis following hip, knee, and abdominal surgery	30 mg SC q 12 hr; begin 12 hr following surgery for 7–10 days or 40 mg SC daily
	Unstable angina and non–Q wave MI	1 mg/kg q 12 hr combined with aspirin 100–325 mg PO daily for 2–8 days
	Acute DVT	1 mg/kg q 12 hr for 5–7 days until therapeutic warfarin levels are reached

Antiplatelet Drugs

Platelets are involved in the intrinsic pathway of the clotting cascade and begin the clotting process. Antiplatelet drugs alter the platelets' ability to adhere to damaged vessels and one another. The drugs do not necessarily decrease the number of platelets. However, thrombocytopenia can be a side effect. Antiplatelet drugs are used to prevent arterial thrombosis. They are indicated for prophylaxis against MI, both primary and recurrent (see Chapter 14, Section 5), and in stroke prevention (see Chapter 19, Section 2).

Aspirin remains the most commonly used antiplatelet drug. The common dosage range is 81 to 325 mg/day. Some patients can benefit from dosages as low as 40 mg/day. (Lower doses reduce the risk of GI ulceration and upset and may increase compliance.) Dipyridamole has been shown to be more effective in decreasing the risk of stroke in combination with aspirin than either drug alone. Ticlopidine is slightly more effective than aspirin in preventing CVA in patients with TIA, but is much more expensive with more side effects. It is also more effective when combined with aspirin to prevent thrombosis of coronary stenting. Clopidogrel is as effective as ticlopidine, but again more expensive than aspirin. Clopidogrel is used when aspirin is ineffective or not tolerated. Abciximab is used in coronary balloon angioplasty and may also have a role in stent implantation, as an adjunctive therapy to thrombolysis in acute MI, and in unstable angina and non–Q wave MI. Table 12-2-5 lists the uses and dosages of antiplatelet drugs.

 CLINICAL PEARLS

- Asymptomatic patients with atrial fibrillation do not require urgent warfarin therapy. They can be started on a less aggressive outpatient basis. The goal is to achieve an INR of 2 to 3 over a 1- to 2-week period.

- Elderly patients require smaller dosages of anticoagulants because they metabolize the drugs more slowly. Patients age 75 and older can begin on warfarin 2.5 mg/day.

- When beginning warfarin as an outpatient, check the INR at least three times the first week, twice the second week, and monthly thereafter if PT levels are stable.

- To reduce the incidence of bleeding with patients on LMWH following the removal of catheters (epidural, arterial, or central venous), wait 6 hours after injection of dose.

- Collection of blood for tests to evaluate APTT levels should not be drawn from central venous catheters. Studies show that results are unreliably high, even after a blood waste of 12 mL before collection. One study noted accurate APTT levels with the use of an 18-gauge peripheral saline lock placed distal to the heparin infusion. The first 0.5 mL should be withdrawn before the sample is collected.

- Warfarin is teratogenic (causing permanent damage to developing fetus) and should not be given to women attempting pregnancy or already pregnant. Heparin or LMWH is a better choice because neither is associated with malformations; however, both can increase the risk of pregnancy loss and premature delivery.

- Patients taking warfarin need to maintain a constant intake of vitamin K, not necessarily a low vitamin K intake. The idea is to avoid fluctuations in

Table 12-2-5. Antiplatelet Drugs

DRUG	USES	DOSE	COMMON ADVERSE EFFECTS
Aspirin	Angina, myocardial infarction (MI), prosthetic heart valves, postcoronary bypass surgery	81–325 mg PO daily	Indigestion, gastrointestinal (GI) upset, GI ulcers, tinnitus, rash, bruising, bleeding
Abciximab (ReoPro)	Unstable angina and percutaneous transcoronary angiography (PTCA) intervention used in combination with aspirin and heparin	IV bolus 0.25 mg/kg followed by a 12-hour infusion at 10 μg/min for up to 12 hours, and concluding 1 hr after PTCA	Nausea, vomiting, hypotension, bradycardia, bleeding
Clopidogrel (Plavix)	Atherosclerotic diseases; prevention of MI, cerebrovascular accident (CVA), peripheral vascular disease	75 mg PO daily	Indigestion, GI ulceration, neutropenia, rash, thrombocytopenia, bleeding
Dipyridamole (Persantine)	Used in combination with warfarin for prosthetic heart valves, peripheral vascular disease	75–100 mg PO qid	Headache, dizziness, hypotension, syncope, nausea, vomiting, bleeding
Ticlopidine (Ticlid)	Angina, MI, post-PTCA and stent placement, transient ischemic attack (TIA), CVA	250 mg PO bid with food	Anemia, pancytopenia, thrombocytopenia, hypotension, nausea, vomiting, GI upset, rash, hepatic dysfunction, bleeding

331

vitamin K intake, which will cause fluctuation in PT levels when the patient is taking a constant dose of warfarin.
○ Optimal time to test INR is 16 hours after the administration of warfarin.

Antidepressants

Section 3   Robert Mead

OVERVIEW

Depressive disorders are among the most common health problems in the United States. Major depressive disorders are associated with a high degree of functional disability, resulting in an increased use of medical services. The exact prevalence of depressive disorders is not known. Depression is two to three times as frequent in females as in males and can occur at any age, although it is most prevalent in adults age 25 to 44. However, trends indicate that the gender difference is decreasing, the typical age of onset is dropping, and the overall rate is increasing. Depressed mood or loss of interest and pleasure in usual activities are the major characteristics of depressive disorders (Table 12-3-1).

The cause of depressive disorders is not known. Various coexisting factors likely precipitate depression. Reduced functional activity of one or more of the brain neurotransmitters (i.e., NE and serotonin) appears to cause many of the symptoms of depression. What causes these changes is unknown. Stressful events, concomitant medical illnesses, other medications, and genetics can play roles in the development of major depressive disorder.

Table 12-3-1.   Types of Depressive Disorders

TYPE	CHARACTERISTICS
Atypical	Anxiety, hypersomnia, increased appetite, weight gain
Catatonic	Bizarre posturing, motor immobility, stupor
Melancholic	Decreased appetite, depressed mood, disordered sleep, guilt, loss of interest or pleasure, mood unreactivity, psychomotor retardation, weight loss
Mixed-anxiety disorder	Persistent anxiety, depressive symptoms
Postpartum	Severe depression within 1 month of childbirth, may involve psychotic symptoms
Premenstrual dysphoric disorder	"PMS"; severe depression, anxiety mood lability, headache, fatigue, sleep and appetite changes; remits after onset of menses
Psychotic	Delusions, hallucinations, depressed mood, loss of interest or pleasure; high incidence of suicide; family history
Recurrent brief depression	Severe depression for 2–4 days with functional impairment; recurs routinely or randomly
Seasonal	Regular occurrence of symptoms following a seasonal pattern (fall/winter), with full remission in other seasons (spring/summer)
Subsyndromal symptomatic depression	Less severe depressive symptoms and less functional impairment

Table 12-3-2. Individual Antidepressant Medications

TYPE AND GENERIC NAME	BRAND NAME	USUAL DAILY DOSAGE RANGE
Tricyclic Antidepressants (TCAs), Tertiary Amines		
Amitriptyline	Elavil	25–300 mg
Clomipramine	Anafranil	25–250 mg
Doxepin	Sinequan	25–300 mg
Imipramine	Tofranil	30–300 mg
Trimipramine	Surmontil	50–300 mg
Tricyclic Antidepressants (TCAs), Secondary Amines		
Amoxapine	Asendin	50–600 mg
Desipramine	Norpramin	25–300 mg

PRINCIPLES OF CARE

The underlying treatment of depressive disorder is psychological counseling and support. This must occur routinely and involve all family members. Pharmacologic treatment should start soon after counseling begins. A medical workup must be completed before antidepressant therapy is initiated, to rule out secondary causes of depression, such as other disease states (e.g., thyroid disorders, adrenal disorders, infections, malignancies, neurologic disorders, metabolic disorders) and/or medications, including nonprescription, prescription, herbal remedies, food supplements, alcohol, and other drugs of abuse.

It is not known how the antidepressant agents work. All but the monoamine oxidase inhibitors (MAOIs) block the reuptake of NE and/or serotonin to various degrees. The differences in the amount of reuptake blockade are reflected in the various side effects associated with each group of antidepressant agents. MAOIs inhibit the enzyme system that metabolizes dopamine, epinephrine, NE, and serotonin. This results in increased levels of these neurotransmitters. Current theory is that long-term use of an antidepressant agent causes a reregulation of an abnormal receptor-neurotransmitter relationship. This hastens the natural recovery process from depression by returning neurotransmission to normal.

Once an antidepressant medication (Table 12-3-2) is started, the patient (and family members) must be counseled that improvement in symptoms will not be seen until 2 to 4 weeks or longer. Improvement will be gradual; adequate time (4 to 6 weeks) should be allowed to determine the effectiveness (and the most effective dose) of an antidepressant medication.

Antidepressant therapy should be continued for 6 to 12 months after the first depressive episode, 5 years after the second episode, and indefinitely for three or more episodes. When discontinuing antidepressant therapy, the dose should be slowly tapered over at least 1 to 2 months.

Antidepressants can be taken with or without food. Agents that can cause sedation should be taken at bedtime.

Antidepressant medications have varying side effects (Table 12-3-3) and potential drug-drug interactions. (Consult a drug handbook for potential interactions.) Patients must be monitored for these effects, and should be taught what to watch for and what to do if untoward effects occur.

▮▮▮▮ **Table 12-3-3.** Adverse Effects

ANTIDEPRESSANT CLASS	COMMON ADVERSE EFFECTS
Monoamine oxidase inhibitors	Sedation, orthostatic hypotension, anxiety, seizures, sexual dysfunction, weight gain, hepatocellular damage
Tetracyclic antidepressants	
Maprotiline	Seizures, sedation, anticholinergic effects,* cardiac conduction abnormalities
Mirtazapine	Sedation, anticholinergic effects,* increased appetite, weight gain
Other antidepressants:	
Nefazodone, trazodone	Sedation, orthostatic hypotension, seizures
Bupropion	Anxiety, seizures, nausea, headache
Selective serotonin reuptake inhibitors	Anxiety, sexual dysfunction, nausea, headache, extrapyramidal effects†
Tricyclic antidepressants	Anticholinergic effects,* sedation, orthostatic hypotension, weight gain, seizures, cardiac conduction abnormalities
Serotonin/norepinephrine reuptake inhibitors	
Venlafaxine	Anxiety, seizures, sexual dysfunction

*Anticholinergic effects include dry mouth, constipation, blurred vision, dry eyes, tachycardia, and urinary hesitancy or retention.

†Extrapyramidal effects include akathesia, acute dystonic reactions, and parkinsonian symptoms.

DECISION-MAKING

The treatment goals for a patient with a depressive disorder are to decrease the symptoms of depression and to return the patient's level of function to where it was before the episode began. Depressed patients should be hospitalized in cases of perceived increased suicide risk, poor health, absent social support system, and symptoms of psychotic or catatonic depression. Severely depressed patients should be placed on suicide precautions during initial antidepressant therapy, to decrease the risk of suicide by overdose.

Various pharmacologic and nonpharmacologic treatments are used for depressive disorders. The initial choice of pharmacologic therapy is made empirically, because which specific treatment will be the most effective cannot be predicted. Overall, up to 85% of patients treated with an adequate dose of an appropriate agent will show improvement.

The choice of antidepressant agent may be influenced by differences in the types and incidence of adverse effects (see Table 12-3-3). Antidepressant medications are involved in a number of potentially significant drug-drug and drug-food interactions. Table 12-3-4 lists potential MAOI food interactions. All concomitant medications must be considered when monitoring the safety and effectiveness of any antidepressant medication.

Nonpharmacologic treatments include:

- Electroconvulsive therapy (ECT), most useful in severe, resistant depression, or when medications must be avoided
- Phototherapy, useful in treating seasonal depression in patients who do not respond well to medications. Daily light exposure is provided for 30 minutes to 2 hours.
- Transcranial magnetic stimulation (TMS). Useful for research and diagnostic purposes, it is finding clinical application in treating depressive disor-

Table 12-3-4. Potential Monoamine Oxidase Inhibitor Food Interactions Resulting in Hypertensive Crisis and/or Death

Cheese (American, Blue, Boursault, Brie, Camembert, Cheddar, Emmenthaler, Gruyere, Mozzarella, Parmesan, Romano, Roquefort, Stilton, Swiss)

Dairy products (sour cream, yogurt)

Meat/fish (anchovies, beef or chicken liver, other meats, fish [unrefrigerated, dried, fermented, spoiled, smoked, pickled], caviar, bologna, salami, pepperoni, summer sausage, dry sausage, game meat, meat extracts, meat prepared with tenderizer, shrimp paste)

Alcoholic beverages (beer, red wine, sherry, distilled spirits, liquors)

Fruits and vegetables (avocados, bananas, bean curd, broad [fava] beans, dried fruits such as raisins and prunes, figs, miso soup, raspberries, sauerkraut, soy sauce, yeast extracts), caffeine (coffee, tea, colas), chocolate, ginseng

ders. An electromagnet is placed on the scalp, causing depolarization of cortical neurons. Treatment for 1 to 2 weeks has been found to be effective in patients who have not responded to medication.

 CLINICAL PEARLS

○ Antidepressant medications work slowly, and several weeks may be required to achieve the maximal effect of an appropriate dose of the agent.

○ All of the antidepressant agents are metabolized in the liver. They have a long elimination half-life. Doses can be held for 1 to 2 days without causing a clinically significant decrease in the efficacy of the medication.

○ Antidepressant medications have many adverse effects and potential drug-drug interactions. Care must be taken to give the correct dose of the antidepressant medication to avoid untoward effects.

○ Overdose of many of these agents produces rapid multisystem complications and can result in negative outcomes for the patient. Suicide attempts using these agents result in a long period of potential danger, especially involving the cardiovascular system. Patients who receive an overdose (intentional or unintentional) require immediate care and intense monitoring, even if they appear to be normal.

○ Elderly patients are more prone to adverse effects of antidepressant agents, as well as to long-term sequelae from these adverse effects (e.g., nursing home placement after suffering a hip fracture from a fall secondary to an adverse drug effect). To prevent these adverse effects, therapy is usually started with the lowest dose of an agent. Dosage increases are small and are done over a longer period. Elderly patients also are more likely to experience drug-drug interactions, because they tend to take more concomitant medications. Again, care must be taken to avoid potential drug-drug interactions.

○ Special consideration must be given to pregnant or nursing women. The risk of potentially exposing a fetus or newborn to these antidepressant agents must be weighed against the risk of exposing the fetus or newborn to an untreated depressed mother.

Antihypertensives

Section 4   Linda McCuiston

OVERVIEW

Antihypertensive drugs are increasingly common in hospital and community settings. Nurses play a crucial role in patient education about these medications. Patient compliance with a prescribed regimen depends in large part on the patient's awareness and knowledge imparted by the nurse. This section covers basic pharmacologic aspects of antihypertensive medications.

PRINCIPLES OF CARE

Blood pressure (BP) is determined by the amount of cardiac output (CO) and peripheral vascular resistance (PVR), and can be reduced by pharmacologic action on either or both of these factors. Pharmacologic agents may decrease CO by either inhibiting myocardial contractility or decreasing ventricular filling pressure. Reduced ventricular filling pressure may be achieved by decreasing venous tone or blood volume through renal system control. Pharmacologic agents can decrease PVR by acting on vascular smooth muscle to cause vessel relaxation and resultant vasodilatation. PVR can also be reduced by interference with the sympathetic nervous system and vessel constriction, resulting in vasodilatation.

The 1997 sixth report of the Joint National Committee on Prevention, Detection, Evaluation and Treatment of High Blood Pressure (JNC-VI) established new guidelines to help physicians and advanced practice nurses improve the standard of care for hypertension. A classification scheme for determining the severity of hypertension was created by this group (see Chapter 15, Section 4). *The JNC-V recommends beta-adrenergic blockers as initial treatment for stage 1 and 2 hypertension.*

DECISION-MAKING
Drug Classification

Antihypertensive therapy includes drugs that are classified as angiotensin-converting enzyme (ACE) inhibitors, angiotensin receptor antagonists, calcium channel blockers, alpha-adrenergic blockers, beta-adrenergic blockers, alpha-beta-blockers, central alpha-adrenergic blockers, peripheral adrenergic neuron antagonists, direct vasodilators, and diuretics.

Angiotensin-Converting Enzyme Inhibitors

Action. Angiotensin-converting enzyme (ACE) inhibitors reduce blood pressure by interfering with the renin-angiotensin-aldosterone system (RAAS). In the RAAS, renin is released because of decreased blood flow to the kidneys. ACE inhibitors block ACE, which prevents the conversion of angiotensin I to angiotensin II. Angiotensin II is a potent vasoconstrictor and stimulator of aldosterone. Aldosterone is a stimulator of sodium and water reabsorption. Blockage of ACE produces a decrease in sodium and water reabsorption, fluid volume, PVR, and vasoconstriction, leading to a drop in blood pressure.

The major contribution of ACE inhibitors is vasodilatation. Because ACE inhibitors affect both the arterial and venous systems, both preload and afterload are reduced. The vasodilatation of renal arteries improves renal flow. However, ACE inhibitors can precipitate acute renal failure in severe cases of renal artery stenosis, congestive heart failure, and severe sodium or water depletion. On initiation of ACE therapy, a progressive decline in blood pressure occurs, reaching maximum effectiveness in approximately 1 week.

Use. ACE inhibitors are well tolerated in all age groups but have been found to be more effective in younger and middle-aged white patients with normal renal function. Age-related structural and functional changes include decreased number of renal glomeruli and glomerular surface area, renal blood flow, renin and aldosterone secretion, and glomerular filtration rate. Therefore, the elderly (especially African American elderly) are more resistant to ACE monotherapy. ACE inhibitors appear to be more effective in African American patients when combined with a low-dose thiazide diuretic.

Because of their efficacy and tolerability, ACE inhibitors are often used as a first-line drug option in treating hypertension. Because of their cardioprotective effects, ACE inhibitors are used to treat patients with stable post-MI, bronchospastic problems, congestive heart failure, as well as older patients with low CO and high PVR. Because ACE inhibitors slow the development of diabetic glomerulopathy and nephropathy, they are useful for patients with peripheral vascular disease and diabetes mellitus. In addition, ACE inhibitors improve insulin sensitivity and do not increase lipid levels. They are also suggested when beta-blockers and diuretics are contraindicated, but are most effective when used concurrently with a diuretic.

Common Adverse Effects. Some adverse effects common or uniquely related to ACE inhibitors include headache, dizziness, postural hypotension, rash, and nonproductive cough.

Angiotensin Receptor Blockers

Action. Angiotensin receptor blockers (ARBs), also called angiotensin II inhibitors or antagonists, act by selectively blocking the binding of angiotensin II to specific receptors (AT_1 receptors) found in vascular smooth muscle and adrenal gland sites. Whereas ACE inhibitors block the conversion of angiotensin I to angiotensin II, other enzymes that are not blocked by ACE inhibitors can form angiotensin II. By blocking the renin-angiotensin system and aldosterone release, ARBs inhibit vasoconstrictive and aldosterone effects. ARBs relax smooth muscle, promoting vasodilatation, and increase renal sodium and water excretion, thereby decreasing plasma volume. With decreased vasoconstriction and blood volume, CO and PVR are reduced and blood pressure drops. Because other enzymes in the body that are not blocked by ACE inhibitors also produce angiotensin II, ARBs were formulated to further assist in the interference of the RAAS in blood pressure reduction. Finally, like ACE inhibitors, ARBs improve insulin sensitivity.

Use. ARBs are effective in all age groups, but less effective in African Americans if used as monotherapy. Losartan (Cozaar) is especially successful in decreasing blood pressure in patients with renal insufficiency without worsening creatinine clearance and renal function. ARBs are beneficial in patients who are unable to tolerate ACE inhibitors. Maximum reduction of blood pressure from ARBs is not typically observed until 3 to 6 weeks after initiation of therapy. If blood pressure is not controlled adequately, a low-dose diuretic combination may be given for greater efficacy.

Common Adverse Effects. The most common adverse effects of ARBs include headache, dizziness, nasal congestion, cough, insomnia, and fatigue.

Calcium Channel Blockers

Action. Calcium channel blockers (CCBs) inhibit calcium influx into muscle cells through slow calcium channels during membrane depolarization. Calcium is blocked in pertinent intracellular sites, including vascular smooth muscle, the myocardium, and the cardiac conduction system. Inhibition of transmembrane movement of calcium and the resultant decrease in total amount of calcium reaching intracellular sites results in relaxation of the smooth muscle of small arteries and decreased PVR. The normal adrenergic response to CCBs is a reflexive vasoconstriction, which acts to attenuate the hypotensive drug effect. In the elderly with diminished reflexes, this protective vasoconstriction is decreased and can lead to excessive hypotension. Three types of CCBs are available: dihydropyridines (e.g., nifedipine [Procardia]), diphenylalkylamines (e.g., verapamil [Calan]), and benzothiazepines (e.g., diltiazem [Cardizem]).

Use. CCBs are beneficial and safe in African American patients and patients with chronic obstructive pulmonary diseases, dysrhythmias, variant angina, hyperlipidemia, diabetes mellitus, and renal dysfunction. They are also effective in older patients with low CO, decreased blood volume, high PVR, and high catecholamine or low plasma renin levels.

This drug category should be used cautiously in patients with a history of bradycardia and never be used in those with atrioventricular (AV) heart block and any other conduction disturbances, or heart failure patients, as CCBs have a profound vasodilatation effect and, therefore, an ability to compromise cardiac performance. Diphenylalkylamines and benzothiazepines have less vasodilating action with negative inotropic (or force of cardiac muscular contractility) and chronotropic (or rate of rhythmic heart rate) properties than dihydropyridines. Therefore, they should be used with caution when given concurrently with a beta-adrenergic blocker to patients with AV block, bradycardia, and heart failure. All CCBs are equally effective in monotherapy for mild to moderate hypertension. There is greater efficacy of CCB monotherapy than other classifications of antihypertensive agents in elderly and African American patients, in whom renin levels are usually low. If the CCB does not adequately reduce the blood pressure, the efficacy may be increased with a beta-adrenergic antagonist or diuretic.

Common Adverse Effects. The common adverse effects of CCBs include dizziness, headache, flushing, weakness, and dysrhythmias.

Alpha-Adrenergic Blockers

Action. An alpha-adrenergic blocker selectively blocks postsynaptic stimulation of alpha-1 receptors that regulate vasomotor tone and reduces PVR by dilating vessels with resultant reduced blood pressure. This blockage reduces arteriolar resistance, inhibits NE reuptake, and causes a sympathetically mediated reflex increase in the heart rate and plasma renin activity. Vasodilatation persists during long-term therapy of this class, but CO, heart rate, and plasma renin activity return to normal. Renal blood flow is generally unchanged during therapy. Retention of sodium and water occurs in many patients during continued administration, and this attenuates the typical postural hypotension.

Use. Alpha-adrenergic blockers are effectively used in mild to moderate hypertension with monotherapy or in combination therapy with a diuretic and beta-blocker. Alpha-adrenergic blockers are beneficial in hypertensive patients with increased sympathetic nervous system activity, such as pheochromocytoma crises, hypertension owing to clonidine (Catapres) withdrawal, or with the use of MAOIs. Generally, alpha-adrenergic blockers are contraindicated in severe hypertension, cardiovascular disease, renal disease, and peripheral vascular disease.

Common Adverse Effects. The most common adverse effects associated with alpha-adrenergic blockers include first-dose phenomenon and orthostatic hypotension.

Beta-Adrenergic Blockers

Action. These blockers are also known as beta-blockers. They are beta or cardio-selective, with a greater effect on beta-1 (adrenergic receptors of myocardium) than on beta-2 (adrenergic receptors in the smooth muscle of the bronchi and blood vessels). By blocking beta-adrenergic receptors of the sympathetic nervous system, cardiac response to sympathetic nerve stimulation is inhibited. Blocking sympathetic stimulation and impeding catecholamine activity reduce the release of renin and aldosterone. This action reduces angiotensin II–mediated vasoconstriction and fluid volume. Beta-1 adrenergic blockers reduce CO, cardiac contractility, heart rate, impulse conduction, vasoconstriction, and PVR, resulting in lowered blood pressure.

Use. Beta-adrenergic blockers have been found to reduce morbidity and mortality associated with hypertension. This category of antihypertensives is effective in young hypertensive patients with high CO, normal PVR, normal blood volume, and high plasma renin levels, and is recommended in post-acute MI. Nonselective beta-blockers that block beta-1 and beta-2 improve exercise tolerance. African Americans do not respond well to beta-blockers except when the beta-blockers are combined with diuretics. Elderly patients and smokers seem to have a decreased antihypertensive response to beta-blockers. Beta-adrenergic blockers should be avoided in people with chronic obstructive airway disorders, depression, bradycardia, heart block, PVD, and heart failure caused by systolic dysfunction. Beta-adrenergic blockers should be used with caution in diabetes mellitus and severe liver disease.

Common Adverse Effects. The most common adverse effects or uniquely associated effects of beta-blockers include bradycardia, postural hypotension, dizziness, headache, fatigue, and bronchospasm.

Alpha-Beta Blockers
(Mixed Adrenergic Antagonists)

Action. Alpha-beta antagonists block the alpha and beta receptors with the effect being stronger on the alpha receptors. By blocking stimulation of vasomotor tone (alpha receptors), vasodilatation is achieved. By inhibiting cardiac response to sympathetic nerve stimulation (beta-receptors), reduction of blood pressure, heart rate, and cardiac contractility is achieved. However, AV conduction time, refractory period, CO, and renal function are essentially unaffected by alpha-beta blockers.

Use. Alpha-beta blockers are used in stage 1 or 2 of hypertension. They may be used alone or with a thiazide diuretic. Labetalol, when given IV, can decrease blood pressure rapidly and is used in the treatment of hypertensive emergencies.

Common Adverse Effects. The most common or uniquely associated adverse effects of alpha-beta blockers include headache, dizziness, drowsiness, palpitations, tachycardia, nasal congestion, nausea, and the first-dose phenomenon. The first-dose phenomenon or orthostatic hypotension can be severe with the first drug dose.

Central Alpha-Adrenergic Agonists (Sympatholytics)

Action. Central alpha-adrenergic agonists work by depressing sympathetic nervous system outflow from the brain stem to the heart, kidneys, and peripheral vessels with resultant suppression of vasomotor and cardiac centers causing a decrease in systemic vascular resistance. Decreased vascular resistance allows systolic and diastolic blood pressure reduction, while lowering the heart rate only slightly. Rebound hypertension may occur with abrupt discontinuation of sympatholytics, except for methyldopa.

Use. This category of antihypertensives can be used for treating mild to moderate hypertension. Methyldopa is usually preferred for hypertension during pregnancy. Generally, central alpha-adrenergic agonists are not used as a first-line drug option for hypertension.

Common Adverse Effects. The most common or uniquely associated adverse effects following sympatholytics include drowsiness, dizziness, weakness, hypotension, dry mouth, nasal congestion, constipation, decreased libido, impotence, and weight gain from sodium and water retention.

Peripheral Adrenergic Neuron Antagonists

Action. The action of this classification focuses on the CNS and sympathetic nerve stimulation reduction. Vasoconstriction is decreased by the accumulation of these drugs in adrenergic neurons because they disrupt the release of NE. These drugs concentrate in the neurosecretory vesicles, where they replace NE. By depleting the normal transmitter catecholamine supply of NE in peripheral sympathetic postganglionic fibers, peripheral adrenergic neuron antagonists can be released by stimuli that normally release NE. By inhibiting vasoconstriction, vasodilatation is allowed, whereas preload, PVR, CO, heart rate, and blood pressure are reduced.

Use. Peripheral adrenergic neuron antagonists are usually administered concurrently with other medications for efficacy. They are primarily used for moderate to severe hypertension. They are contraindicated in depression, pheochromocytoma, and heart failure. Give with caution in patients with diabetes mellitus, impaired renal or hepatic function, a recent MI, PVD, asthma, and patients taking MAOIs.

Common Adverse Effects. The most common adverse effects associated with this drug category include headache, dizziness, drowsiness, fatigue, orthostatic hypotension, impaired ejaculation, diarrhea, and shortness of breath.

Direct Vasodilators

Action. Direct vasodilators reduce blood pressure through vasodilatation by the relaxation of smooth muscles in the arterioles and decreased PVR. Some direct vasodilators affect both the arterial and venous systems reducing both preload and afterload. Blood pressure reduction in this manner can consequently stimulate the baroreceptors to increase heart rate, CO, cardiac contractility, and lead to increased cardiac workload. This increase in cardiac workload is attenuated by the concurrent administration of beta-adrenergic blocking agents.

Use. This category is used for moderate to severe hypertension, or hypertension unresponsive to other medications. This category is also the drug of choice for hypertensive crisis. Direct vasodilators are used with caution in the elderly and those patients with coronary artery disease. Because direct vasodilators are generally not used in monotherapy, they are commonly administered concurrently with a diuretic.

Direct vasodilators are beneficial in hypertension associated with end-organ damage and hypertension resistant to other treatment methods. Because of their baroreceptor-stimulating effects, direct vasodilators should be avoided in patients with ischemic heart disease. Concurrent administration with beta-adrenergic blockers or centrally acting drugs compensates for the baroreceptor stimulation. Loop diuretics are usually administered with direct vasodilators to avoid sodium and water retention. When vasodilators are used in conjunction with beta-blockers, centrally acting drugs, or diuretics, the combination can be administered in smaller doses. Smaller doses help to offset the adverse effects.

Direct vasodilators may be used in pregnancy but should be used cautiously in early pregnancy, diabetes mellitus, impaired cerebral or cardiac circulation, and impaired renal function. They are contraindicated in patients with coarctation of the aorta and arteriovenous shunts.

Common Adverse Effects. The most common associated adverse effects of direct vasodilators include headache, palpitations, and tachycardia.

Diuretics

According to the JNC-VI, a diuretic is one of the first-line drugs used in hypertension management. Diuretics may be initiated in monotherapy or efficacy may be enhanced by the addition of virtually all other antihypertensive agents. Thiazide, loop, and potassium-sparing diuretics are helpful in reducing sodium and water retention, which reduces fluid volume and lowers blood pressure. Loop diuretics are not routinely used for hypertension because of the drastic fluid loss. The basic pharmacologic aspects of diuretics are discussed in Section 8.

Choice of Drug

Antihypertensive drug choice is based on laboratory and physical findings, history, and comorbidity. Even when medications are deliberately selected to fit individual needs, the patient's responses may vary. If the first medication selected is not tolerated or is ineffective, then a medication from another category is be added or substituted. Initial therapy usually begins with a diuretic or beta-blocker. African Americans do not respond as well as whites to beta-blockers, but do well with sustained-release verapamil, calcium channel blockers, labetalol, and diuretics. Younger patients with good renal function may be started on ACE inhibitors or calcium channel blockers. If more than one drug is necessary, and a diuretic was not used initially, most physicians or advanced practice nurses would add a diuretic. The elderly are more responsive to calcium channel blockers and diuretics.

- The initial antihypertensive drug of choice for patients with diabetes mellitus is an ACE inhibitor.
- The initial antihypertensive drugs of choice for patients with heart failure are ACE inhibitors and diuretics.
- The initial antihypertensive drugs of choice for patients with MI are ACE inhibitors and beta-blockers.

Administration

Assess baseline blood pressure, pulse, and laboratory values of renal and liver function tests and CBC before initiating antihypertensive therapy. Later, monitor blood pressure, pulse, and laboratory values for effectiveness and adverse effects. Before administration of each dose, the blood pressure should be monitored. If the blood pressure is outside the parameters outlined by the physician, the medication should be held. The blood pressure should be checked again in 1 to 2 hours and the medication may be administered if the BP is within the given parameters. If there are no parameters and the systolic blood pressure is below 100 mm Hg, hold the dose for 1 hour and check the blood pressure again. If it remains low, notify the physician.

Furthermore, as a general rule, antihypertensive medication should be withheld if the heart rate is less than 50. Antihypertensive drugs should generally be tapered off over 1 to 2 weeks. Abrupt discontinuation may result in rebound hypertension or in a withdrawal syndrome characterized by palpitations, headache, trembling, and sweating. Table 12-4-1 gives dosing, drug interactions, nursing implications, and adverse effects.

Patient Teaching

- To avoid lightheadedness, dizziness, and hypotension during antihypertensive therapy, change positions slowly and in stages. On awakening, sit up in bed 1 minute, dangle on the edge of bed for 1 minute, and then stand for 1 minute before walking. Also, avoid hot baths, steam rooms, saunas, hot tubs, excessive exercise, and alcohol, which may cause excessive vasodilatation. Avoid caffeine and nicotine, which cause excessive vasoconstriction.
- Avoid driving or operating potentially hazardous equipment until your reaction to the medication is known.
- Take antihypertensive medication at mealtime to prevent gastrointestinal distress.
- Avoid discontinuing antihypertensive drugs abruptly, because rebound hypertension may occur.

 CLINICAL PEARLS

○ Withhold antihypertensive medication if the patient's heart rate is below 50 beats/min.
○ Palpitations, headache, trembling, and sweating may be signs of abrupt antihypertensive medication withdrawal.
○ Teach the patient to avoid driving or operating potentially hazardous equipment until his or her individualized reaction to the medication is known.
○ Instruct the patient to take antihypertensive medication at mealtimes to avoid gastrointestinal distress.

Text continued on page 348.

Table 12-4-1. Antihypertensive Pharmacology

ANTIHYPERTENSIVE CLASSIFICATION	DAILY DOSE	DRUG INTERACTION	ADVERSE EFFECTS	NURSING IMPLICATIONS
Angiotensin-Converting Enzyme (ACE) Inhibitors Captopril (Capoten) Benazepril (Lotensin) Enalapril (Vasotec) Fosinopril (Monopril) Lisinopril (Prinivil, Zestril) Moexipril (Univasc) Quinapril (Accupril) Ramipril (Altace) Trandolapril (Mavik)	12.5–150 mg 10–40 mg 2.5–40 mg 10–40 mg 5–40 mg 7.5–30 mg 5–80 mg 1.25–20 mg 1–4 mg	The interaction of alcohol, diuretics and other antihypertensives with ACE inhibitors leads to hypotension. NSAIDs decrease ACE inhibitor effects. Tetracycline and quinapril concurrently decrease absorption of tetracycline; antacids decrease ACE inhibitor absorption. Cyclosporin and vitamin K supplements increase the risk of hyperkalemia, lithium increases lithium toxicity, digoxin increases digoxin toxicity. Probenecid increases level of captopril. Rifampin decreases effectiveness of enalapril. Allopurinol increases the risk of hypersensitivity reactions.	Dry hacking cough (an "ACE-cough") is the most common side effect, which usually subsides several days after discontinuation. First-dose phenomenon or severe hypotension is a potential problem in patients who are hypovolemic or are receiving high doses of diuretics. Headache, dizziness, weakness, anorexia, nausea, vomiting, diarrhea, rashes, itching, insomnia, tachycardia are very common. Hyperkalemia may be seen with renal insufficiency. Infrequent but serious and potentially fatal allergic reactions, such as anaphylaxis or angioedema of the lips, tongue, glottis, larynx, face, and extremities may occur. Increased fetal mortality in the second and third trimesters. May precipitate acute renal failure.	Obtain baseline renal and liver function tests before and throughout treatment. Monitor potassium, blood urea nitrogen (BUN), and serum creatinine level increases, decreased sodium level, proteinuria, and liver enzymes. Check complete blood count (CBC) every 2 weeks for 3 months and then periodically for decreased hemoglobin and hematocrit and neutrophils. Monitor blood pressure, especially after the first dose, for detection of first-dose phenomenon, which is often prevented by volume expansion. Caution the patient against excess sweating and dehydration, which may lead to excess blood pressure reduction. Instruct the patient to discontinue taking the drug at the first sign of allergic reaction, angioedema, or pregnancy. *Table continued on following page*

343

Table 12-4-1. Antihypertensive Pharmacology *Continued*

ANTIHYPERTENSIVE CLASSIFICATION	DAILY DOSE	DRUG INTERACTION	ADVERSE EFFECTS	NURSING IMPLICATIONS
Angiotensin Receptor Antagonists (mg)				
Losartan (Cozaar)	50–100 q day	Phenobarbital decreases the effectiveness of irbesartan and losartan. Cimetidine increases blood levels and effects of losartan. Potassium supplements and potassium-sparing diuretics increase the risk of hyperkalemia.	Headache, hypotension, dizziness, nasal congestion, sinusitis, fatigue, dyspepsia, diarrhea, hyperkalemia. muscle cramps, myalgia, back and leg pain, insomnia, renal and hepatic dysfunction may occur. Less coughing and angioedema are reported than with ACE inhibitors.	Instruct the patient to report hypotension. Monitor electrolytes. Monitor renal and liver function tests. The drug should not be taken in the second or third trimester of pregnancy. Monitor for first-dose phenomenon, especially in volume-depleted patients.
Valsartan (Diovan)	80–320 q day			
Irbesartan (Avapro)	150–300 q day			
Candesartan cilexetil (Atacand)	8–32 qd–bid			
Telmisartan (Micardis)	40–80 mg			
Calcium Channel Blockers (mg)				
Benzothiazepines	60–120 qd	Quinidine may cause excessive hypotension. Beta-blockers increase the risk of bradycardia when used with diltiazem and mibefradil. Both verapamil and diltiazem may precipitate heart failure.	Dizziness, headache, weakness, ankle edema, constipation, initial reflex tachycardia, flushing, palpitations, dysrhythmias such as severe bradycardia, peripheral edema, gastroesophageal reflux, hyperglycemia, and sinus arrest. Decreased incidence of drug-induced orthostatic hypotension. May increase digoxin levels.	Assess baseline electrocardiogram (ECG), liver and renal function tests. Monitor hyperglycemia. Take before meals. Change position slowly. Monitor heart rate before administration; hold the drug if heart rate is 50 beats/min.
Diltiazem (Cardizem SR, Cardizem CD, Dilacor XR, Diltia XT, Tiamate, Tiazac)				
Diphenylalkylamines	120–300 qd			
Verapamil (Calan, Calan SR, Isoptin, Verelan, Covera-HS)				
Dihydropyridines	120–240 qd			
Nifedipine (Adalat CC, Procardia XL)	120–360 qd			
Nicardipine (Cardene, Cardene SR)	40–120 tid			
Amlodipine (Norvasc)	40–120 qd or bid			
Felodipine (Plendil)	120–360 qd			
Isradipine (DynaCirc, DynaCirc CR)	120–240 HS			
Nisoldipine (Sular)	10–30 tid			
	30–90 qd			

344

Alpha-Adrenergic Blockers

Drug	Dose	Drug Interactions	Side Effects	Comments
Prazosin (Minipress)	2–20 mg	Antihypertensive effect of phenoxybenzamine is blocked by monoamine oxidase (MAO) inhibitors. Blood pressure is increased with alcohol and tricyclic antidepressant use.	Orthostatic hypotension, headache, nasal congestion, dizziness, palpitations, arrhythmias, weakness, drowsiness, abdominal pain, dry mouth, nausea, vomiting, diarrhea, fluid retention, priapism, impotence. Less tachycardia than with direct vasodilators. First-dose phenomenon within 90 min of the initial dose or when dosage is increased rapidly especially if on a diuretic or beta-blocker.	Use cautiously in patients with chronic renal failure, cerebral thrombosis, and males with sickle cell trait. Monitor for first-dose phenomenon 30–90 minutes after first dose. Give the first dose at bedtime. Syncope may be preceded by tachycardia.
Doxazosin (Cardura)	1–16 mg			
Terazosin (Hytrin)	1–20 mg			
Tamsulosin (Flomax)	0.4–0.8 mg prn			
Phenoxybenzamine (Dibenzyline)	5–60 mg			
Phentolamine mesylate (Regitine)	2–5 mg prn			
Tolazoline (Priscoline)	10–50 mg			

Beta-Adrenergic Blockers

Drug	Dose	Drug Interactions	Side Effects	Comments
Propranolol (Inderal)	25–100 mg	Nonsteroidal anti-inflammatory drugs (NSAIDs) decrease action. Cardiac glycosides, amphetamines, epinephrine, cocaine, and selective beta-blockers with MAO inhibitors can produce severe hypertension and bradycardia. Insulin and oral hypoglycemics alter the effectiveness, and thyroid preparations decrease the effectiveness of beta-blockers. Alcohol and nitrates may cause additive hypotension.	Bizarre dreams, insomnia, dizziness, headache, postural hypotension, fatigue, depression, impotence, peripheral vasoconstriction, bradycardia, and bronchospasm.	May mask symptoms of hypoglycemia. Sudden discontinuance can produce withdrawal syndrome (sympathetic hyperactivity) or rebound hypertension. Should be tapered off over 10–14 days. Avoid with asthmatics. Monitor increased renal and liver function tests, potassium, blood glucose, and triglycerides. If the heart rate is <50 beats/min before administration, hold the drug.
Atenolol (Tenormin)	40–240 mg			
Metoprolol (Lopressor)	50–200 mg			
Timolol (Bicadren)	10–40 mg			
Nadolol (Corgard)	20–240 mg			
Betaxolol (Kerlone)	5–40 mg			
Bisoprolol (Zebeta)	5–20 mg			

Table continued on following page

Table 12-4-1. Antihypertensive Pharmacology *Continued*

ANTIHYPERTENSIVE CLASSIFICATION	DAILY DOSE	DRUG INTERACTION	ADVERSE EFFECTS	NURSING IMPLICATIONS
Alpha-Beta Blockers				
Labetalol (Normodyne, Trandate)	200–1200 mg	Cimetidine may increase the toxicity of labetalol.	Headache, dizziness, drowsiness, palpitations, tachycardia, nausea, nasal congestion, peripheral vascular insufficiency, orthostatic hypotension, bronchospasm, and hepatotoxicity.	May mask hypoglycemia. Discontinuation should be gradual over 1–2 weeks.
Carvedilol (Coreg)	12.5–50 mg			
Central Alpha-Adrenergic Blockers				
Methyldopa (Aldomet)	250 mg–2 g		Nasal congestion, dry mouth, anorexia, vomiting, constipation, abdominal pain, sodium retention with weight gain, impotence, decreased libido, rash, dizziness, drowsiness, weakness, bradycardia, orthostatic hypotension, restlessness, nervousness, forgetfulness, vivid dreams, hallucinations, depression, dyspnea, and rebound hypertension with abrupt discontinuation	Take at bedtime to avoid drowsiness or interference with driving or operating heavy equipment. Avoid hot showers and baths. Avoid drinking more than 4 cups of caffeinated coffee, tea, or cola per day. Withdraw drug over 2–4 days to avoid rebound hypertension.
Clonidine (Catapres)	0.1–0.6 mg			
Guanabenz (Wytensin)	4–64 mg			
Guanfacine (Tenex)	1–3 mg			

Peripheral Adrenergic Neuron Antagonists

Guanethidine (Ismelin)	10–50 mg	Alcohol increases the effects of low-dose central alpha-adrenergic blockers.	May take 3 weeks to achieve full effects. Increased orthostatic hypotension with hot environment, standing, and exercise. Discontinue at first sign of depression.
Reserpine (Serpasil, Serpalan)	0.05–1 mg		
Guanadrel (Hylorel)	10–75 mg		

Nasal congestion, fatigue, headache, drowsiness, visual disturbances, dizziness, weakness, gastric distress, diarrhea, peripheral edema, leg cramps, seizures, decreased libido, impaired ejaculation, hypothermia, profound orthostatic hypotension, bradycardia, nightmares with high doses, tardive dyskinesia, severe suicidal depression, shortness of breath, bronchospasm, respiratory depression, and heart failure; inability to perform complex tasks; exacerbation of peptic ulcer disease.

Direct Vasodilators

Hydralazine (Apresoline)	40–200 mg po	Hydralazine effects are increased with alcohol, other antihypertensives, MAO inhibitors, nitrates, and general anesthetics. Diazoxide with diuretics potentiates hyperuricemia, and hypotension. NSAIDs decrease effects. Beta-blockers decrease tachycardia caused by hydralazine. Hyperglycemia is increased with corticosteroids, estrogen, progesterone, and phenytoin.	Monitor intake and output, decreased urine output, and daily weight, auscultate lungs, and monitor blood glucose frequently. Stay recumbent at least 1 hour after injection. Monitor decreased hemoglobin and hematocrit red blood cell count, blood glucose, renal and liver function tests. Nipride is light sensitive and should be covered with a foil wrapper. Freshly prepare every 24 hours and use with IV infusion pumps and microdrip regulator. Monitor IV site for extravasation. Monitor for cyanide toxicity after 1–2 days, especially in patients with liver disease.
Minoxidil (Loniten)	5–40 mg IM/IV		
Diazoxide (Hyperstat)	2.5–40 mg		
Nitroprusside (Nipride)	0.5–10 µg/kg/min		

Nasal congestion, excess lacrimation, dizziness, throbbing headaches, anxiety, drowsiness, syncope, weakness, lethargy, restlessness, gastric distress, constipation, tremors, euphoria, sodium and water retention, peripheral edema, impotence, palpitations, reflex tachycardia, atrial and ventricular dysrhythmias, blood dyscrasias, leukopenia, agranulocytosis, temporary hearing loss, hyperglycemia, hematuria, nocturia, proteinuria, azotemia, severe rebound hypertension, pulmonary edema, and heart failure. Rarely causes orthostatic hypotension. Minoxidil usually causes hirsutism and can cause severe fluid retention.

347

○ The JNC VI hypertensive treatment algorithm recommends beta-blockers and diuretics as initial therapy for uncomplicated hypertension.
○ The first-dose phenomenon, or orthostatic hypotension, is common when initiating an antihypertensive medication, especially in volume-depleted patients. Avoid this by maintaining adequate hydration and discontinuing diuretics 2 to 3 days before administration. On administration of the initial dose, instruct the patient to lie down for 3 to 4 hours.

Anti-Infectives

Section 5   Brenda K. Shelton ■ Christopher R. Friese

OVERVIEW
Many patients present with conditions that alter immune system function or undergo therapies that predispose them to infection. Various microbes have the capability of causing infection when they breach the body's immune defenses. Specific levels of microbial invasion and their associated clinical responses may influence the decision of whether to treat with anti-infective therapy, as well as the specific agent and dosage. This section focuses on the clinical applications of three major categories of anti-infective medications: antibacterials (antibiotics), antifungals, and antiviral agents.

PRINCIPLES OF CARE
Choosing the Agent
Identify the infecting organism by culture and sensitivity (C&S) testing (see Chapter 11, Section 4). These samples should be obtained before starting anti-infective therapy. C&S preliminary data (Gram staining) are reported within 24 hours, with a complete description of the pathogen and antibiotics that should effectively destroy it available within 3 days. Gram staining rapidly identifies bacteria as gram-positive or gram-negative. Therapy is started before receipt of the full C&S report, based on experience and knowledge of the host and infectious source. This is called *empiric therapy*. Empiric therapy is also used to guide prophylactic therapy. *Host factors,* such as age, immune status, genetic factors, and allergy history, will affect the choice of drug.

Choosing the Route
The most effective and reliable method of delivering antibiotics is via the IV route, although agents such as sulfonamides may actually have a greater bioavailability when given orally. IV therapy is preferred for seriously ill patients; the oral route can be equally effective in otherwise healthy patients. Anti-infective agents may be directly instilled into internal body spaces, such as the bladder, pleural space, peritoneum, and intrathecal space. The direct injection technique is used when there is concern that systemic routes may not achieve the necessary drug levels at the site of infection.

Choosing the Dose
Anti-infective agents must be maintained at therapeutic levels in the blood to be effective and prevent the regrowth of the infecting pathogen. To maintain

Table 12-5-1. Peak and Trough Levels for Selected Antibiotics

DRUG	PEAK	TROUGH
Gentamicin	4–10 μg/mL	<2 μg/mL
Tobramycin	4–10 μg/mL	<2 μg/mL
Amikacin	20–32 μg/mL	4–8 μg/mL
Vancomycin	20–35 μg/mL	5–10 μg/mL

Note: Peak and trough levels vary according to institutional policy. Consult your toxicology laboratory for assistance.

therapeutic drug levels, *peak level* and *trough level* are monitored for certain drugs (Table 12-5-1). Peak level is monitored approximately 1 hour after drug infusion. This shows that the level of the drug is effective, yet not toxic. Trough level is drawn immediately before a dose, to verify that the level of drug remains therapeutic between doses.

Some agents are given in one defined dose for bacteriostatic activity, and a higher dose when bactericidal effects are desired. *Bacteriostatic* agents inhibit protein synthesis of microorganisms so they cannot grow or replicate; these agents are used prophylactically to prevent infection in at-risk persons and to treat infections in patients with relatively normal immune systems. *Bactericidal* agents, which kill the microorganism, are necessary for infected patients with poor immune function or for those who have underlying conditions (e.g., diabetes mellitus) that restrict their ability to minimize the spread of infection.

Determining Adverse Effects of Antimicrobial Therapy

Most anti-infective agents are naturally occurring substances that have the potential for hypersensitivity or anaphylactic reaction. Patients without a previous history of allergic response to a specific antibiotic may experience a reaction because of slowly accumulated antibodies that respond more vigorously with each exposure. Rashes alone may be treated supportively if the drug in use is effectively treating the infection. It is important to recognize antimicrobial agents of similar structure, where cross-reactivity or hypersensitivity across classifications may occur. It is well established that patients with penicillin allergies are more likely to also experience allergic reactions to cephalosporins and carbapenems. Severe hypersensitivity reactions are most common after the first and second doses of IV medications, or during the first 48 hours of oral therapy, although late hypersensitivity has also been reported.

Superinfection is a new infection that appears during the course of treatment for a primary infection. It occurs when the majority of normal flora are destroyed by a broad-spectrum antibiotic, resulting in the overgrowth of a resistant microbe. This resistant microbe no longer needs to compete with other microbes for nourishment and can overgrow to the point of being pathologic, thus producing a second infection. A common superinfection is caused by *Clostridium difficile*. The destruction of normal gut flora by broad-spectrum antibiotics allows the overgrowth of *C. difficile*, which produces an inflammatory process in the colon that causes significant diarrhea. This effect is called *antibiotic-associated pseudomembranous colitis*. Treatment includes discontinuing the offending antibiotic agent, when feasible, and administering oral metronidazole or vancomycin. Superinfection with candida, a fungus, is also common.

Monitoring

Antimicrobial therapy must be monitored to evaluate continued efficacy and detect toxicity. Most antimicrobials will cause defervescence within 72 hours. A new microbe may be the cause of a new fever after the initial 72-hour period. Continued fevers beyond 72 hours after initiation of therapy is an indication for reculturing suspected sites of infection. Patients who are afebrile on antibiotics and have received a full course of antimicrobial therapy do not need reculturing. Patients at generally higher risk for sepsis may be recultured at the conclusion of antimicrobial therapy, or when they are converted to an oral formulation.

Assessment for local and systemic signs and symptoms of infection is also important to evaluate the success of therapy. Significant clinical responses to antibiotics may take 1 to 3 days. Local symptoms include erythema, tenderness, swelling, purulent drainage, skin breakdown, or wound separation. Systemic symptoms include fever, leukocytosis, fatigue, myalgias, and local lymphadenopathy. Early signs of sepsis include hypotension, tachycardia, mental status changes, and decreased urine output. Laboratory monitoring includes tests for renal and hepatic function, because most anti-infectives are cleared renally or hepatically.

Microbial Resistance

Microbial resistance to anti-infective therapy is an escalating problem associated with years of indiscriminate and inconsistent antimicrobial administration practices. As living organisms, microbes have the capacity to change and compensate to survive, which they have done in the face of antimicrobial agents over the past three decades. Three mechanisms have been identified in the development of resistant microbes:

- Point mutations in the genetic sequence of the organism may alter the target site of an anti-infective agent.
- Bacterial chromosomes may experience rearrangements of DNA in large amounts, making them less susceptible to the usual anti-infective agents.
- Foreign DNA can be acquired by the organism, allowing the microbe to adapt to and survive with the anti-infective agent.

Resistant organisms are most likely to develop in patients with immunosuppression, earlier repeated use of broad-spectrum antibiotics, multiple anti-infective treatment regimens, or poor compliance with anti-infective therapy. Anti-infective therapy is timed so that pathogenic organisms are not allowed to grow between doses. Administering a dose late or missing a dose allows the microorganisms that have been suppressed to regrow in an adapted (resistant) fashion, thus creating resistance.

DECISION-MAKING
Antibacterials
Penicillins

Narrow-spectrum (NS): penicillin G, penicillin V; gram-positive coverage

Broad-spectrum (aminopenicillins): ampicillin, amoxicillin, bacampicillin; gram-positive and gram-negative coverage

Penicillinase (betalactamase)-resistant NS: methicillin, nafcillin, oxacillin, dicloxacillin; antistaphylococcal

Extended-spectrum: carbenicillin, piperacillin, ticarcillin; antipseudomonal

Penicillin combined with penicillinase inhibitor: Timentin (ticarcillin/clavulanate), Unasyn (ampicillin/sulbactam), Augmentin (amoxicillin/clavulanate), Zosyn (piperacillin/tazobactam)

Penicillins are natural or synthetic beta-lactam structured antimicrobials that weaken bacterial cell walls, causing cell lysis. They may be bacteriostatic or bactericidal, dependent on the agent or the dose. Penicillinase (betalactamase) is an enzyme produced by resistant bacteria that breaks the beta-lactam structure of penicillins, thus destroying the drug.

1. Administer with food and avoid caffeine to reduce drug-induced nausea. Antidiarrheal therapy may be needed to manage increased bowel motility or gastrointestinal superinfection.

2. Most penicillins enhance renal excretion of potassium. Monitor serum potassium levels and provide supplements as needed. Idiosyncratic glomerulonephritis from glomerular basement membrane damage can occur during renal clearance.

3. Administer an antihistamine or a steroid cream as needed for rash (especially with ampicillin and amoxicillin). Persistent, unexplained fever may be a sign of hypersensitivity. Antipyretics are only partially helpful. Some hypersensitivity reactions are anaphylactoid and require emergency support. Reaction does not involve IgE antibody and thus is not of predictable incidence or severity.

4. Penicillins alter platelet function and coagulation (especially ticarcillin and carbenicillin).

Carbapenems

Imipenem/cilastatin sodium
Meropenem

Carbapenems interfere with bacterial cell wall synthesis and cause cell lysis (bactericidal). Cilastatin inhibits imipenem breakdown in the renal system, making this agent useful in urinary tract infections. These agents provide broad coverage against gram-positive, gram-negative, and anaerobic organisms.

1. Patients with penicillin allergies are also considered allergic to drugs in this class.

2. Administer the drug via central venous access whenever possible and in a large volume of fluid to decrease the risk of phlebitis. Nausea, vomiting, sweating, dizziness, and hypotension may occur idiosyncratically during infusion, and may or may not resolve when the infusion rate is slowed.

3. Neuromuscular twitching may occur (especially with imipenem), and the seizure threshold may be lowered in patients with preexisting conditions. Assess for resting tremors and institute seizure precautions if necessary.

Monobactams

Aztreonam

This synthetic monocyclic antimicrobial disrupts the bacterial cell wall (similar to penicillins) and thus has bactericidal properties. It is used against aerobic gram-negative organisms including *Escherichia coli*, *Klebsiella pneumoniae*, *Proteus*, *Enterobacter*, and *Pseudomonas*.

1. Aztreonam is not used to treat suspected line or skin infections.
2. Dosage adjustment is required with renal insufficiency.
3. Aztreonam has little cross-sensitivity with penicillins and cephalosporins. It may be used as an alternate drug when those drugs are indicated, but there is a history of hypersensitivity reactions.

Cephalosporins

Generations expand the spectrum of antimicrobial coverage:

First generation: cephalothin, cefazolin; gram-positive coverage

Second generation: cefamandole, cefotetan, cefoxitin; gram-positive and gram-negative coverage

Third generation: ceftazidime, moxalactam, ceftriaxone; gram-positive, gram-negative, and CNS coverage

Fourth generation: cefepime; highest gram-positive, gram-negative, and CNS coverage.

Cephalosporins inhibit cell wall synthesis similar to penicillins. First- and second-generation agents are bacteriostatic; the others are bactericidal.

1. Administer the drug via central venous access whenever possible. If central venous access is not possible, then infuse the drug slowly through a large peripheral vessel, to reduce the risk of phlebitis. Give an antidiarrheal agent as needed.
2. Hypersensitivity reactions, including macular, itchy rash, may occur. Apply antihistamine or steroid creams as needed. Persistent, unexplained fever may be a sign of hypersensitivity. Antipyretics are only partially helpful. An anaphylactic hypersensitivity reaction necessitates emergency respiratory support, including epinephrine.
3. Monitor for antibiotic-associated pseudomembranous colitis (AAPC).
4. Rarely, cephalosporins alter platelet function and coagulation, resulting in bleeding.

Tetracyclines

Tetracycline
Demeclocycline
Doxycycline
Minocycline

These drugs inhibit protein synthesis, leading to bacteriostatic effects. They are most active against gram-positive organisms, although resistance is common. Aerobic gram-negative coverage is poor. Common specific indications include rickettsiae (e.g., tick fever), chlamydiae, and *Helicobacter pylori*.

1. Taking a tetracycline with food will reduce drug-related nausea but will interfere with absorption. Because the drug binds to calcium, reducing absorption, avoid calcium-containing foods (e.g., milk and milk products) and antacids. If such foods or antacids are ingested, hold the oral drug for at least 2 hours. Avoid caffeine, which can cause gastrointestinal upset. Administer oral preparations through a straw to prevent tooth staining.
2. Implement safety precautions for potential vertigo from vestibular toxicity.
3. Superinfection of the bowel (AAPC) and vagina can occur. Assess for diarrhea and vaginal itching. Higher doses or IV administration increases the risk of hepatic toxicity. Monitor hepatic enzymes for elevations, indicating organ toxicity. Avoid bright lights because of drug-related

photosensitivity. Long-term therapy requires renal (i.e., blood urea nitrogen, creatinine) and hematologic (to detect leukopenia and thrombocytopenia) monitoring.

4. Tetracyclines have good subcutaneous absorption because of their high lipid solubility.

5. Tetracyclines decrease absorption of oral contraceptives; as appropriate, advise the patient to use another contraceptive method.

Macrolides

Erythromycin
Azithromycin

Macrolides inhibit bacterial replication by inhibiting protein synthesis. These agents are bacteriostatic or bactericidal, depending on the infecting microorganism and the drug dosage. They are effective against gram-positive organisms, and some gram-negative organisms, including *Chlamydia, Legionella*, and *Mycoplasma pneumoniae*.

1. Administer macrolides via central venous access whenever possible. Dextrose 5% in water is the preferred solution. If central venous access is not possible, then administer the drug slowly through a large peripheral vessel and with large volume dilution, to reduce the risk of phlebitis. IV formulations can cause reversible tinnitus, vertigo, and transient hearing loss. Diarrhea is dose-related; administer antidiarrheals as needed.

2. Maintain good oral hygiene to reduce the risk of severe stomatitis. If stomatitis occurs, perform oral rinses with saline or bicarbonate solution four times a day, and use an oral anesthetic agent (e.g., viscous lidocaine, Ulcerease) to reduce discomfort.

3. Monitor bilirubin levels and hepatic enzymes for elevations indicating cholestasis and hepatotoxicity.

4. Apply an antihistamine or a steroid cream if a macular, itchy rash occurs.

5. Macrolides potentiate the effects of theophylline and steroids.

Clindamycin

Clindamycin inhibits bacterial protein synthesis with both bacteriostatic and bactericidal effects. It is effective against serious gram-positive and anaerobic gram-negative organisms.

1. Take clindamycin with food to reduce drug-related nausea; avoid caffeine, which can cause gastrointestinal upset. Administer the IV form in a large volume of fluid and through a large peripheral or central vein to reduce the risk of phlebitis.

2. Assess for superinfection with AAPC, which can be severe.

3. Apply an antihistamine or a steroid cream if a macular, itchy rash occurs.

4. Because clindamycin and its metabolites are cleared through the liver, monitor for hepatic toxicity.

Fluoroquinolones

Norfloxacin
Ciprofloxacin
Levofloxacin
Ofloxacin
Trovafloxacin

Fluoroquinolones are bactericidal; they interfere with DNA gyrase, which is needed for DNA strand development of bacteria. These agents are highly effective against urinary pathogens and also against enteritis-causing pathogens including salmonella, shigella, *Campylobacter jejuni, Yersinia,* and resistant *Enterobacter.*

1. Administer fluoroquinolones with food and avoid caffeine to reduce drug-induced nausea.
2. Fluoroquinolones enhance the physical effects of theophylline, warfarin, and caffeine. Avoid concomitant NSAIDs, which enhance bleeding tendency. Administer acetaminophen as needed for headache.
3. Drug-induced fatigue and malaise may occur. Provide a sleep-conducive environment and facilitate frequent rest periods. Assess for signs and symptoms of depression. Implement safety precautions for potential dizziness or visual disturbances (i.e., blurriness, diplopia).
4. Monitor hepatic enzyme levels for elevations indicating toxicity.

Aminoglycosides

Amikacin
Gentamicin
Tobramycin
Neomycin

Aminoglycosides cross the cell membrane of bacteria and interrupt protein synthesis. These agents are bacteriostatic at lower doses, but are bactericidal at usual doses. They are effective against most aerobic gram-negative bacteria, including enterobacter (e.g., *Serratia, Proteus, Klebsiella, Escherichia coli*), and *Pseudomonas aeruginosa.* Anaerobic bacteria are resistant to aminoglycosides.

1. Aminoglycoside dosage should be reduced in patients with renal failure. Excess drug levels are nephrotoxic.
2. Because aminoglycosides are poorly absorbed orally, they are usually given IM or IV.
3. Peak and trough blood levels are monitored for efficacy.
4. Long-term use causes partially reversible vestibular and auditory damage. Slower administration may reduce incidence. Instruct the patient to report signs of ototoxicity. Assist in hearing evaluation after completion of therapy.
5. A slower administration rate may reduce toxicity and will not alter drug effects.
6. Apply an antihistamine or a steroid cream if needed for rash.
7. Aminoglycosides alter platelet function and may enhance bleeding tendency. Avoid other anticoagulant or antiplatelet medications.
8. Aminoglycosides may prolong or enhance neuromuscular blockade in patients receiving neuromuscular blocking agents (e.g., pancuronium, anesthetic agents), or those with neuromuscular diseases (e.g., myasthenia gravis, multiple sclerosis).

Sulfonamides

Short-acting (e.g., sulfisoxazole)
Medium-acting (e.g., sulfamethoxazole)
Ultra long-acting (e.g., sulfadoxine)
Combination therapy (e.g., trimethoprim-sulfamethoxazole)

Sulfonamides inhibit bacterial cell DNA synthesis, resulting in cell death. These agents are bacteriostatic. Significant bacterial resistance exists with the sulfonamides. The combination of trimethoprim and sulfamethoxazole is particularly effective against aerobic gram-negative bacteria (e.g., *E. coli*, Enterobacteriaceae). It provides activity against common gram-positive organisms like *Staphylococcus* and *Streptococcus*, but is noted for its efficacy against more stubborn organisms such as *Listeria monocytogenes*, *Nocardia*, *Xanthomonas multiphilia*, and protozoal organisms such as *Pneumocystis carinii*.

1. Hypersensitivity skin reactions are common. This may be a macular, itchy rash, but a more severe form called Stevens-Johnson syndrome, or toxic epidermal necrolysis (TEN), may occur. Apply an antihistamine or a steroid cream for mild reactions. Persistent, unexplained fever and serum sickness (fatigue, malaise, myalgias, arthralgias) may indicate hypersensitivity. Antipyretics are only partially helpful. AIDS patients are at increased risk for hypersensitivity reaction.
2. Increase oral fluid intake to more than 1000 mL/day to reduce the risk of crystalluria. Take with food to reduce drug-related nausea, avoid concomitant caffeine to reduce GI upset.
3. Teach the patient to avoid bright light and to use sunscreen when outdoors because of drug-related photosensitivity.
4. Significant symptomatic hemolytic anemia may occur in patients with glucose-6-phosphate dehydrogenase (G6PD) deficiency.
5. Long-term or high-dose use may cause leukopenia and thrombocytopenia. Monitor CBC every 3 months during therapy.
6. Rare diffuse hepatic necrosis may occur 1 to 3 weeks into therapy; monitor hepatic enzyme levels.
7. Sulfonamides may prolong INR and enhance the effects of coumadin and phenytoin.

Miscellaneous Agents

Vancomycin

Vancomycin inhibits cell wall synthesis at different points than penicillin and cephalosporins. It also inhibits bacterial RNA synthesis. Vancomycin has dose-related bacteriostatic and bactericidal properties. It is effective against all gram-positive organisms and is used to treat infections with staphylococcus, *Clostridium difficile*, and *Corynebacterium diphtheriae*. Oral vancomycin is used to treat AAPC.

1. Persistent, unexplained fever may occur; this may be partially relieved with antipyretics.
2. Administer vancomycin over at least 2 hours, because too-rapid infusion may cause warmth, flushing, tachycardia, hypertension, or hypotension ("Redman syndrome"). Reaction usually occurs within 10 minutes of starting infusion, and may be alleviated by slowing the infusion rate. Administer vancomycin via central venous access whenever possible. Administer slowly and with large volume diluent through a large peripheral vessel to reduce the risk of phlebitis.
3. Apply an antihistamine or a steroid cream as needed for rash.
4. Periodically monitor CBC for leukopenia.
5. Increased blood vancomycin levels lead to hearing loss.

6. When given with other nephrotoxic agents, vancomycin can have additive renal toxic effects.

Metronidazole

Metronidazole reduces to metabolites that react with bacterial and protozoal DNA, causing limited bacterial transcription and replication, with bacteriostatic properties. It is used to treat infection with anaerobic GI organisms such as *Bacteroides* and *Clostridium difficile*, and difficult-to-treat infections with *Trichomonas* and *Giardia*.

1. Administer metronidazole with food. Sweet, hard candies may best relieve dry mouth or metallic taste. Administer via central venous access whenever possible. Administer slowly and with a large volume of fluid through a large peripheral vessel to reduce the risk of phlebitis.
2. Administer acetaminophen as needed for headache.
3. Assess peripheral sensation; if neuropathies occur, the drug may be changed.
4. Avoid concomitant alcohol-based preparations, which can cause an Antabuse (disulfiram)–like reaction.
5. Rash is common; administer antihistamines as needed for pruritus.
6. Reversible neutropenia may occur with long-term use. Monitor CBC.
7. The patient may report dark, tea-colored urine. Advise the patient that this is not a sign of toxicity.

Antifungals
Imidazole Agents

Ketoconazole
Itraconazole
Fluconazole

Imidazoles impair ergosterol biosynthesis of fungi and may affect oxidative and perioxidative fungal enzyme systems. They are effective against widely spread, localized fungal infections and oral/mucocutaneous candida.

1. Take the drug with food to reduce drug-related nausea, and avoid caffeine.
2. Monitor hepatic enzymes for elevations indicating drug toxicity.
3. Prepare the patient and family for altered body image (e.g., gynecomastia), changes in secondary sex characteristics (e.g., dysmenorrhea, decreased testicular size), and decreased libido from decreased testosterone levels.

Amphotericin B

This drug binds to ergosterol in the fungal cell membrane, causing pores to open and the intracellular contents to leak out. It is used to treat disseminated fungal infections (e.g., candidal, aspergillar, cryptococcal).

1. Severe, high-spiking fever may occur 30 to 45 minutes into the infusion. Premedication with antipyretics is only partially helpful. Some patients require steroids or antihistamines to relieve fever and chills.
2. Rigors accompanying fever may be relieved by covering the patient with a warm blanket or by administering IV morphine, meperidine (via slow IV push), or a benzodiazepine.
3. Administer potassium supplements, because amphotericin B enhances renal excretion of potassium.

4. Hydration with high sodium fluid before and after administration is thought to reduce renal toxicity.
5. The dosage should be reduced in patients with renal failure.
6. Lipid-based preparations are less nephrotoxic and are indicated for patients with serum creatinine level below 2.5. Lipid-based preparations are considerably more expensive.
7. Periodically monitor CBC for anemia.
8. Administer via central venous access whenever possible, or give slowly through a large peripheral vessel to reduce the risk of phlebitis. The drug is compatible only in D5W solution.
9. Test doses may be ordered to ensure that the patient can tolerate therapy. Infuse 1 mg over 20 to 30 minutes and observe for reaction. The patient may tolerate faster infusions over time if renal function is not compromised.
10. Tachycardia with hypertension or hypotension may occur. Monitor vital signs frequently during administration.
11. Wear gloves if applying amphotericin B topically.

Antivirals
Acyclovir and Valacyclovir (Oral Form); Famciclovir

These virustatic agents act by inhibiting viral DNA synthesis. They are effective against herpes simplex virus (types I and II), varicella zoster (especially famciclovir), and herpes zoster.

1. Administer through central venous access if possible to prevent irritation at the infusion site.
2. These agents are usually given IV over 1 hour. The dose is reduced in patients with renal failure. A slower infusion rate decreases nephrotoxicity.
3. Monitor hepatic enzymes for elevations indicating drug toxicity. Monitor ammonia level, serum chemistry values, and glucose level if the patient exhibits mental status changes. Drug-related metabolic encephalopathy must be differentiated from clinical causes.
4. Apply an antihistamine or a steroid cream as needed for a macular, itchy rash.
5. Periodically monitor CBC for leukopenia and thrombocytopenia. The drug may be discontinued if these effects occur.

Ganciclovir

Ganciclovir blocks viral DNA synthesis. It is equally active as acyclovir against herpes viruses, but more active against Epstein-Barr virus (EBV) and cytomegalovirus (CMV).

1. Ganciclovir is poorly absorbed orally; it is usually given IV for treatment and orally for prophylaxis.
2. Periodically monitor CBC for leukopenia and thrombocytopenia, the most common dose-limiting toxicity of ganciclovir.
3. Monitor hepatic enzymes for elevations indicating drug toxicity.
4. Apply an antihistamine or a steroid cream if needed for a macular, itchy rash.
5. Administer acetaminophen as needed for headache. Antipyretics may be helpful in managing persistent, unexplained fever.

6. Perform frequent mental status assessment. Monitor ammonia level, serum chemistry values, and glucose levels if mental status changes occur. Drug-related metabolic encephalopathy must be differentiated from clinical causes. Myopathy occurs idiosyncratically or with long-term use. Assess muscle strength and motor activity. Implement physical therapy to maintain muscle tone.

 CLINICAL PEARLS

○ Immunocompromised patients, such as those undergoing chemotherapy, may not exhibit normal signs of infection (i.e., fever, pus formation, erythema). Identification of pathogens is especially difficult in this population. Fever and pain are the two most-reported symptoms of infection in neutropenic patients. As such, they are often treated with prophylactic antibiotics.

○ IV infusion of certain antibiotics is more prone to cause phlebitis. When possible, central venous access is recommended. Bactrim, erythromycin, azithromycin, and vancomycin are especially irritating to tissues; extravasation is possible. When infusing these drugs via a peripheral IV, slow the infusion rate and use D5W as a background fluid to minimize difficulty. Antimicrobial agents causing phlebitis are usually more diluted (150 to 250 mL/dose) and infused no faster than 100 to 150 mL/hr. Consult a drug handbook or pharmacist for information on compatibility with other drugs and solutions.

○ Some antibiotic and antifungal agents alter renal excretion of electrolytes. Depletion of sodium, potassium, and magnesium is most common.

○ Some antimicrobial categories—aminoglycosides, carbapenems, and antivirals—lower the seizure threshold. Although they may not actually cause seizures, they do increase the risk in susceptible individuals.

○ Broad-spectrum antimicrobial therapy destroys the body's normal flora and predisposes individuals to superinfection (secondary infection) with less-common microbes usually controlled by the normal flora. This complication occurs with a peak incidence 5 to 7 days after initiation of therapy. The most common sites of superinfection are the oral, GI, and genitourinary systems.

Antiseizure Medications

Section 6

Mia Smitt ▪ Judy Kaye

OVERVIEW

Antiseizure, or anticonvulsant, medications act on the CNS in various ways. These drugs are used to treat epilepsy and other seizure disorders. Some are used for other purposes, including sedation, neurologic pain control, and with other medications to treat certain psychiatric illnesses.

Seizures are a sudden disorderly discharge of activity in the cerebral neurons characterized by sudden transient alteration in brain function. (For more information on seizures, see Chapter 19, Section 8.) The nurse must know the factors that can precipitate seizure activity in patients with seizure disorders, be able to recognize the different types of seizure presentation, and understand appropriate medications and doses. The nurse also must be able to teach patients and their caregivers about the illness, self-care, and treatments.

PRINCIPLES OF CARE

Pharmacologic therapy is frequently based on the specific type of seizure (Table 12-6-1). The goal of therapy with antiseizure medication is to suppress the abnormal discharge and spread of neural activity within the seizure focus. Mechanisms of action of antiseizure medications include stabilization of neuronal membranes, depression of nerve transmission in the motor cortex, modulation of the sodium channels of the neurons, and enhancement of the sodium-potassium-adenosine triphosphatase activity in neuron and glial cells. Many commonly used medications have modes of action that are unknown or not yet clearly defined. The choice of medication is based not only on the type of seizure, but also on such other factors as potential for compliance, age and sex, cost, and even diet.

DECISION-MAKING
Precipitating Factors or Events

Factors that can provoke seizures in adult and pediatric populations include fatigue, physical or emotional stress, hypoglycemia, fever, water intoxication, constipation, alcohol withdrawal, stimulants, hyperventilation with resultant respiratory alkalosis, and some drugs (e.g., tramadol, certain anticonvulsants). Local anesthesia, pregnancy-related hypertension, and systemic lupus erythematosis can also provoke seizures. Some women have increased seizure activity immediately before or during menses. Environmental stimuli (e.g., loud noises, strong odors, certain music, blinking lights) can precipitate a seizure in susceptible individuals. (Controversy and questions continue regarding any adverse effects of prolonged exposure to video games.)

Medication Use

Drug therapy begins with monotherapy, with the initial agent titrated to maximum benefit with minimal side effects. An effective dose may require 3 to 4 weeks of tapering; periodic blood concentrations are helpful, but clinical response should be carefully monitored.

Frequently, two or more drugs are needed for optimal control when seizure activity continues despite maximum doses of a single agent; the drugs in the combination usually will have different modes of action and side effects. Having the patient maintain a log of seizure activity can be helpful in choosing the correct medication or making dosage adjustments.

Nursing management of antiseizure drugs involves proper administration, monitoring, and patient teaching (Table 12-6-2).

Appropriate laboratory follow-up is necessary for optimum efficacy and positive outcomes.

Drug Interactions

A significant number of drug interactions occur with antiseizure medications. These can decrease or intensify the effect of several commonly taken medications, including antihistamines, warfarin, and oral contraceptives, as well as the effect of the antiseizure drug itself.

Text continued on page 364.

Table 12-6-1. Pharmacologic Treatment of Seizures

DISORDER	DRUG GENERIC NAME	BRAND NAME	USUAL DAILY DOSE ADULTS (A) AND CHILDREN (C)	USUAL THERAPEUTIC BLOOD LEVELS	COMMON SIDE EFFECTS
Absence (Petit Mal)					
Drugs of choice	Ethosuximide or	Zarontin	(A) 750–1250 mg (C) 20–40 mg/kg	40–100 μg/mL	Mild drowsiness, nausea
	Valproic acid	Depakote	(C) 15–60 mg/kg	50–120 μg/mL	Drowsiness, hair loss, increased appetite, weight gain
Alternatives	Clonazepam	Klonopin	(A) 1.5–20 mg (C) 0.05–0.2 mg/kg	20–80 ng/mL	Drowsiness
	Lamotrigine	Lamictal	(A) 300–500 mg (C) Not approved	Not established	Drowsiness, visual blurring, clumsiness, changes in balance
Partial, Including Secondarily Generalized					
Drugs of choice	Carbamazepine or	Tegretol	(A) 800–1600 mg (C) 10–30 mg/kg	6–12 μg/mL	Drowsiness, visual blurring, clumsiness, changes in balance, nausea
	Phenytoin or	Dilantin	(A) 300–400 mg (C) 4–8 mg/kg	10–20 μg/mL	Drowsiness, visual blurring, clumsiness, changes in balance, nausea
	Valproic acid or	Depakote	(A) 1000–3000 mg (C) 15–60 mg/kg	50–120 μg/mL	Drowsiness, hair loss, increased appetite, weight gain
	Primidone or	Mysoline	(A) 750–1250 mg (C) 10–25 mg/kg	5–12 μg/mL	Mild to severe drowsiness
	Oxarbazepine or	Trileptal	(A) 1200–2400 mg		Somnolence, dizziness, diplopia, ataxia, nausea, rash
	Levetiracetam	Keppra	(A) 3000 mg		Somnolence, asthenia, and psychiatric symptoms (agitation, anxiety, depression, psychosis)
Alternatives	Phenobarbital	Luminal	(A) 90–150 mg (C) 2–5 mg/kg	5–35 μg/mL	Mild to severe drowsiness, depression, decreased memory
	Lamotrigine	Lamictal	(A) 300–500 mg (C) Not approved	Not established	Drowsiness, visual blurring, clumsiness, changes in balance
As adjunct	Gabapentin	Neurontin	(A) 900–2400 mg (C) Not approved	Not established	Drowsiness, clumsiness, changes in balance
As adjunct	Topiramate	Topamax	(A) 200–400 mg (C) Not approved	Not established	Clumsiness, changes in balance, decreased memory, fever, chills, sore throat

Primary Generalized Tonic-Clonic

Drugs of choice	Valproic acid or	Depakote	(A) 1000–3000 mg (C) 15–60 mg/kg	15–20 µg/mL	Drowsiness, hair loss, increased appetite, weight gain
	Carbamazepine or	Tegretol	(A) 800–1600 mg (C) 10–30 mg/kg	6–12 µg/mL	Drowsiness, visual blurring, clumsiness, changes in balance, nausea
	Phenytoin	Dilantin	(A) 300–400 mg (C) 4–8 mg/kg	10–20 µg/mL	Drowsiness, visual blurring, clumsiness, changes in balance, nausea
Alternatives	Lamotrigine	Lamictal	(A) 300–500 mg (C) Not approved	Not established	Drowsiness, visual blurring, clumsiness, changes in balance
	Primidone	Mysoline	(A) 750–1250 mg (C) 10–25 mg/kg	5–12 µg/mL	Mild to severe drowsiness
	Phenobarbital	Luminal	(A) 90–150 mg (C) 2–5 mg/kg	15–35 µg/mL	Mild to severe drowsiness, depression, decreased memory
	Topiramate	Topamax	(A) 200–400 mg (C) Not approved	Not established	Clumsiness, changes in balance, decreased memory, fever, chills, sore throat

Atypical Absence, Myoclonic, Atonic

Drug of choice	Valproic acid	Depakote	(A) 1000–3000 mg (C) 15–60 mg/kg	50–120 µg/mL	Drowsiness, hair loss, increased appetite, weight gain
Alternative	Clonazepam	Klonopin	(A) 1.5–20 mg (C) 0.05–0.2 mg/kg	20–80 ng/mL	Drowsiness
As adjunct	Felbamate	Felbatol	(A) 2400–3600 mg (C) 15–60 mg/kg	Not established	Anorexia, vomiting, insomnia

Status Epilepticus

Drugs of choice	Lorazepam or	Ativan	(A) 1–2 mg/min (maximum 10 mg) (C) 0.05–0.1 mg/kg IV		
	Diazepam and	Valium	(A) <2 mg/min (maximum 4 mg (C) 4–8 mg/h IV drip 0.05–1 mg/kg rectal		
	Fosphenytoin (hydantoin)	Cerebyx	(A) 15–20 mg phenytoin equivalents (PE)/kg IV at <150 mgPE/min (C) Safety not established; phenytoin 20 mg/kg load at <1 mg/kg/min; may repeat 5 mg/kg q 30 min to a total of 30 mg/kg		

Table 12-6-2. Nursing Management for Common Antiseizure Medications

MEDICATION	NURSING MANAGEMENT
Phenytoin Used for all types of seizures except absence.	Oral administration: • The tablet may be crushed and the immediate release capsule may be opened. Both should be mixed with food (e.g., applesauce). The suspension should be shaken thoroughly to ensure proper mixing. Because it is a strong alkaline preparation, have the patient drink a fluid before administration; this protects the esophagus from irritation. Administer with food to reduce gastric upset. If food is not used, follow with a full glass of water or milk. • Do not interchange prescriptions; drug amounts may be different. For example, a 100-mg tablet contains 95 mg of drug and cannot be substituted with two 50-mg tablets. IV administration: • Administer at a rate of 50 mg/min or slower. Drop the rate to 25 mg/min in elderly patients, severely ill patients, or patients with liver damage. Flush the IV line with normal saline solution following the drug at the same rate. Rapid administration results in possibly severe hypotension and central nervous system depression. • Do not mix with other IV solutions, especially dextrose; precipitation will occur. Do not use a solution if it is not clear. • Phenytoin also may be administered IM. Monitoring and patient teaching: • Gingival hyperplasia occurs in 20% of patients. Effects are minimized with good oral hygiene. • If a measles-like skin rash occurs, withhold the drug; this may progress to exfoliative dermatitis. • Hirsutism may occur; if it is too disturbing for the patient, usually in women, carbamazepine should be considered. • Alcohol intake may increase serum levels, leading to toxicity, and must be avoided.
Carbamazepine Used for all types of seizures except absence. Preferred for women, to avoid the hirsutism and coarsening of facial features that can occur with phenytoin.	Oral administration: • Take with meals to enhance absorption. Monitoring and patient teaching: • Light-headedness, ataxia, gastric upset, and drowsiness frequently occurs during initial therapy but should subside within a few days. If not, notify the physician. • May cause breakthrough bleeding when taken with oral contraceptives; may also decrease the reliability of the oral contraceptive. Blood counts should be monitored closely (see Table 12–6–1), because carbamazepine may cause significant to fatal bone marrow suppression. • If a measles-like skin rash occurs, withhold the drug; this may progress to exfoliative dermatitis.

Phenobarbital Used to treat partial and tonic/clonic seizures.	Oral administration: • The tablet may be crushed and mixed with fluid or food. IV administration: • Reconstitute with at least 10 mL of sterile water for injection and further dilute with another 10 mL of sterile water. Administer at a rate of 60 mg/min or slower. If administered too rapidly, severe CNS depression (respiratory depression) will result. • Do not use if discolored; do not mix with other medications. • Extravasation may cause significant necrosis. Monitoring and patient teaching: • Overdose can result in death from severe respiratory depression. Avoid alcohol and other central nervous system depressants. • May cause birth defects
Valproic acid Used in the treatment of absence and mixed seizures.	Oral administration: • The tablet should not be crushed or chewed. Free drug particles will irritate oral and pharyngeal membranes. • Take with meals to reduce gastric upset. Monitoring and patient teaching: • Hepatotoxicity, although rare, may be life-threatening. Instruct the patient to monitor for signs of liver injury: anorexia, jaundice, nausea, vomiting, light-colored stools, and diarrhea. • May cause birth defects.
Ethosuximide Used mainly for absence seizures.	Oral administration: • Take with food if gastric upset occurs. • Mild without severe adverse effects.
Primidone Used for all types of seizures except absence.	Oral administration: • The tablet may be crushed and mixed with fluid or food. • Therapeutic effects may not be evident for several weeks. • Usually taken in combination with another drug.
Gabapentin Used for adjunctive therapy of partial seizures.	• Do not mix with antacids. Separate antacid from drug by 2 hours. • Mild without severe adverse effects

Patient and Caregiver Education

When patients are aware and in control of their condition, quality of life is improved. Almost all antiseizure medications cause some degree of CNS depression. The patient is advised to take the medication close to bedtime if possible, and to avoid driving or any hazardous activity during the initial phase of therapy. This effect does wane with continued use.

Monitor the use of over-the-counter (OTC) medications, some of which have CNS depressant effects that intensify the depressant effects of antiseizure drugs. Advise the patient to discuss all OTC medications with a health care provider before using.

The patient must understand the importance of never abruptly discontinuing the drug, as status epilepticus may ensue. All patients with seizure disorders should wear some form of identification, such as a Medic-Alert bracelet.

Most treatment failure results from noncompliance, and most noncompliance results from inadequate knowledge and sense of control.

 CLINICAL PEARLS

○ When considering treatment after a first seizure, consider whether precipitating or provoking factors can be avoided or corrected. If so, then antiseizure medication may be unnecessary. Consider the consequences of recurrence, the benefits of drug therapy, and the possible adverse effects.

○ Match the drug to the type of seizure: simple and complex, partial: carbamazepine, phenytoin, and phenobarbital (with gabapentin used as adjunctive therapy in refractory simple and complex partial seizures); absence: valproic acid, ethosuximide; tonic-clonic: valproic acid, carbamazepine; myoclonic and atonic: clonazepam.

○ Myoclonic and atonic seizures are more difficult to treat than other seizure types.

○ Emotional difficulties related to chronic stress, social stigma, and the unpredictability of seizure activity often arise in patients and families. These difficulties need to be addressed.

○ Patients need to be aware of the adverse effects of antiseizure medications. These medications may reduce the effectiveness of oral contraceptives. They are teratogenic. There are numerous interactions between these and other prescription and OTC drugs.

○ The IV infusion rate of phenytoin should not exceed 50 mg/min. Phenytoin must be used with extreme caution because of serious cardiovascular side effects and the potential for soft-tissue or vascular injury at the injection site. Fosphenytoin sodium IV produces less reported tissue injury at injection sites, but recommended infusion rates cannot be exceeded, because cardiovascular collapse can also occur with this drug. Both drugs cause interactions with many other drugs, and a pharmacologic assessment should be completed before administration.

Digestive Tract Medications

Section 7   Mary Jo Gerlach

OVERVIEW

Drugs used to treat disorders of the gastrointestinal (GI) system encompass a wide array of agents. This section discusses the drugs used to treat common conditions affecting the GI tract: heartburn, constipation, diarrhea, nausea, and vomiting. Drugs used to treat inflammatory bowel disease, Crohn's disease and ulcerative colitis are also discussed. Medications used to treat peptic ulcer disease are covered in Chapter 17, Section 4.

PRINCIPLES OF CARE

Gastroesophageal reflux disease (GERD), heartburn, and dyspepsia result from the regurgitation of acid and pepsin into the lower esophagus because of an incompetent lower esophageal sphincter (LES). *Constipation* is determined by consistency of stool (hard and dry versus soft and hydrated) and, to a lesser extent, frequency of bowel movements. *Diarrhea* refers to an increase in the frequency of stools, as well as an increase in the bulk and the fluid content of stools. Various conditions can predispose a person to diarrhea, including infection, inflammatory conditions of the bowel, faulty digestion, and functional disorders (e.g., short bowel syndrome, irritable bowel syndrome).

Nausea is an unpleasant subjective symptom that may precede vomiting. It can be attributed to a number of factors, including pain, medication side effects, or an early sign of a physiologic disorder, such as kidney disease or hepatitis. In nausea, gastric tone is decreased, and gastric peristalsis may be absent. Irritation to the stomach (ulcers, cancer) or ingestion of toxins (including contaminated foods/beverages or poisons) triggers the *vomiting* center via the chemoreceptor trigger zone (CTZ). Pregnancy, motion sickness, and biliary or renal colic can directly trigger the vomiting center. The cerebral cortex may also be responsible for initiating nausea and vomiting through such factors as psychological stress, pain, and stimuli from any of the five senses (Fig. 12-7-1).

Inflammatory bowel disease (IBD) encompasses ulcerative colitis (UC) and Crohn's disease (CD) (see Chapter 16, Section 5). Rectal bleeding may be associated with UC, and both UC and CD may present with abdominal cramps and diarrhea.

DECISION-MAKING
Agents Used to Treat Heartburn
Antacids

Magnesium-, aluminum-, and calcium-based antacid compounds increase esophageal and gastric pH to reduce symptoms associated with hyperacidity. They deactivate pepsin and increase lower esophageal pressure.

Adverse Effects and Drug Interactions. Magnesium-based antacids may cause diarrhea; they must be used cautiously in patients with renal disease. Aluminum- and calcium-based products may lead to constipation. Calcium-based products may cause acid rebound, as the pH of the stomach decreases in response to neutralization with the antacid.

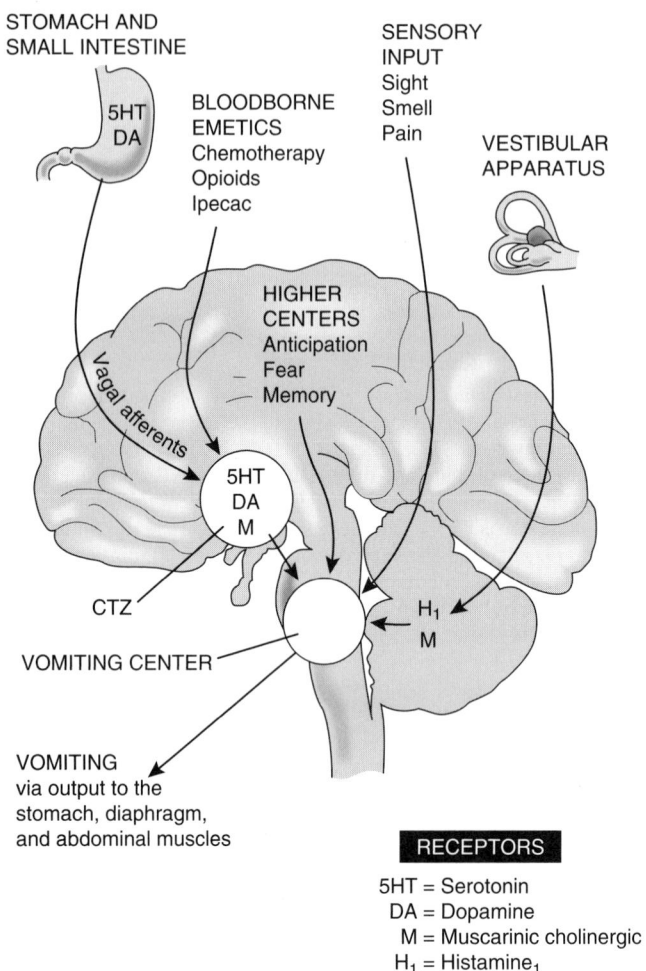

Figure 12-7-1. The emetic response. (From Lehne, R. [2001]. *Pharmacology for nursing care* [4th ed.] Philadelphia: WB Saunders.)

Drug interactions with antacids include decreased absorption of digoxin, INH, phenytoin, iron, tetracycline, and fluoroquinolone antibiotics.

Contraindications. Magnesium-based antacids are contraindicated in patients with renal failure, because the magnesium ions are not excreted.

Histamine-2 Receptor Antagonists

The following drugs are histamine-2 (H₂) receptor antagonists: cimetidine (Tagamet), famotidine (Pepcid), nizatidine (Axid), and ranitidine (Zantac).

H$_2$ receptor antagonists reduce the amount of gastric acid by blocking the H$_2$ receptors on the parietal cells to reduce irritation of gastric mucosa.

Adverse Effects and Drug Interactions

Cimetidine: Confusion, lethargy, agitation, disorientation, especially in elderly patients. Possible drug interactions include increased metabolism of phenytoin, theophylline, and warfarin; monitor serum drug levels. Antacids interfere with drug absorption.

Famotidine: Constipation, headache, elevated BUN and creatinine levels. There are no significant drug interactions.

Nizatidine: Sleepiness, dysrhythmias, increased perspiration. Serum salicylate levels may increase when higher doses of aspirin are taken. Avoid concomitant use of tomato-based juices, which can decrease drug potency.

Ranitidine: Headache, constipation, diarrhea, darkening of stool and tongue. Drug interactions include increased hypoglycemic effect when taking glipizide. Warfarin metabolism may be increased; monitor the PT and INR and adjust dosage as necessary.

Contraindications. H$_2$ receptor antagonists are contraindicated in persons who manifest hypersensitivity to the drug(s).

Proton Pump Inhibitors

Omeprazole (Prilosec) and lansoprazole (Prevacid)

Proton pump inhibitors suppress the secretion of gastric acid by inhibiting the enzyme H$^+$, K$^+$-ATPase, which actually produces gastric acid.

Adverse Effects. There are no significant adverse effects for short-term therapy; headache, nausea, vomiting, and diarrhea may occur. Long-term effects of omeprazole may lead to increased risk of cancer.

Interactions. Proton pump inhibitors affect absorption of drugs that require low gastric acid for absorption: ampicillin, digoxin, iron preparations, and ketoconazole. Sucralfate may delay the absorption of lansoprazole. Concomitant use of omeprazole and diazepam, phenytoin, and warfarin may lead to increased serum drug levels; monitor serum drug levels.

Contraindications. Proton pump inhibitors are contraindicated in persons who may be hypersensitive to the drugs.

Prokinetic Agents

Metoclopramide (Reglan)

This drug enhances the response to acetylcholine at nerve endings in the GI tract, increasing upper GI motility.

Interactions. Drug interactions with metoclopramide include hypertensive crisis with MAOIs. Opiates and anticholinergics antagonize the GI motility effects of the drug. Additive sedation may occur with CNS depressants such as alcohol; avoid concomitant use.

Contraindications. Metoclopramide is contraindicated in patients with Parkinson's disease, pheochromocytoma, GI hemorrhage, perforation, or obstruction, as well as in those taking MAOIs.

Agents Used to Treat Constipation

Laxatives

Peristalsis Stimulants That Increase Bulk

Methylcellulose (Critucel)
Psyllium (Metamucil, Fiberall)

These agents act by increasing the contents of the bowel, which exerts pressure on the colon wall to stimulate peristalsis. They act on the small and large intestines. They are used in the temporary treatment of constipation (acute or chronic), and in therapy for diverticulosis and irritable bowel syndrome. Production of soft stool may take 1 to 3 days.

Adverse Effects. These agents may cause esophageal obstruction if not swallowed with sufficient fluid (a full glass of water or juice) or may be regurgitated (especially by elderly patients).

Interactions. Administration with anti-infective agents, digoxin, oral anticoagulants, or salicylates can decrease absorption of these drugs.

Contraindications. These agents should not be given to patients with fecal impaction or intestinal stricture, in whom they may cause intestinal obstruction. They should not be administered to patients who cannot swallow or who report abdominal pain, nausea and vomiting, or other signs of appendicitis.

Peristalsis Stimulants That Increase Fluid

These agents act on the intestinal walls to increase water/electrolyte secretion. This increases the water content of stool and enhances peristalsis.

Saline Agents

Magnesium sulfate (Epsom salts)
Magnesium phosphate
Magnesium citrate (Citrate of magnesia)

Saline agents are used in preparation for diagnostic and surgical procedures, treatment of constipation, and removal of anthelminthics (deworming agents).

Adverse Effects. Significant water/electrolyte loss can occur, necessitating replacement therapy.

Interactions. Orally administered drugs should be taken 2 hours after these agents to prevent impaired absorption.

Contraindications. Magnesium and potassium toxicity may occur in persons with renal failure. Saline agents should be used with caution in patients with hypertension, congestive heart failure, and edema because of the high sodium content. They should not be administered to patients with abdominal pain, nausea and vomiting, other symptoms of appendicitis or acute surgical abdomen, fecal impaction, and intestinal obstruction or perforation.

Stimulant Agents

Bisacodyl (Dulcolax)
Senna (Senokot, Fletcher's Castoria)

Stimulant agents are used to treat acute constipation and in preparation for surgery or diagnostic procedures. Short-term use is suggested for acute constipation. The preparation should produce stool within 6 to 12 hours.

Adverse Effects. This agent carries a significant water/electrolyte loss potential. Senna may produce a harmless discoloration of urine (pink or yellow-brown) when the drug is excreted in acidic urine.

Interactions. Enteric-coated preparations should not be chewed or crushed. These preparations should not be taken within 1 hour of ingesting milk or milk products or antacid preparations.

Contraindications. These are the same as for saline agents.

Hyperosmotic Agents

Lactulose (Cephulac, Chronulac)
Polyethylene glycol (PEG) (Colyte, GoLYTELY)
Glycerin (Fleet Babylax) (also in suppository form)

These agents act on the large intestine to increase stool mass while incurring no significant loss of fluid and electrolytes. They are commonly used in preparation for diagnostic and surgical procedures. PEG is safe in persons who are dehydrated and those with renal or cardiovascular disease. It may be given via a nasogastric tube. PEG typically begins working 30 to 60 minutes after administration. Glycerin suppositories must be retained for at least 15 minutes; action should occur within 1 hour.

Adverse Effects. Common adverse effects include nausea, bloating, and cramps (lactulose gaseous distention). Lactulose may cause an increase in serum glucose level; monitor serum glucose levels in diabetic patients. If lactulose is administered as an enema and is not retained for 30 minutes, be prepared to repeat the dose to achieve the desired results. With PEG, nausea and abdominal bloating are potential problems for some persons because of the large quantity of fluid ingested (4 L; 240 mL/10 min). Rectal excoriation is possible from the increased number of stools. In addition, glycerin may cause hyperemia of rectal mucosa.

Interactions. Orally administered drugs, transit time is decreased, administer at other times

Contraindications. These are the same as for saline agents.

Stool Softeners

Docusate sodium, docusate calcium, and docusate potassium act in the large intestines. They alter the surface tension of feces, enhancing absorption of water and fats into feces and softening the stool. These agents are especially helpful in patients who have undergone anorectal surgery and in patients with hemorrhoids. They are also given to patients recovering from MI to help prevent straining on defecation.

Adverse Effects. Possible adverse effects include a bitter taste in the mouth, mild abdominal cramping, and diarrhea. Be alert to formulations with sodium, potassium, calcium; note any electrolyte restrictions.

Interactions. Stool softeners should not be given with mineral oil. This could cause toxicity from increased absorption of mineral oil.

Contraindications. These are the same as for saline agents.

Lubricant/Emollient Agents

Mineral oil lubricates the colon, prevents water from leaving the stool, and softens the stool mass. It is helpful in preventing constipation and following anorectal surgery or for a person with hemorrhoids.

Adverse Effects. Lipid pneumonia can occur, especially in the elderly, if the drug is aspirated. Long-term use can result in seepage of mineral oil from the rectum.

Interactions. Repeated doses may result in decreased absorption of fat-soluble vitamins (A, D, E, and K); monitor for deficiencies. Docusate salts may increase absorption of mineral oil.

Contraindications. These are the same as for saline agents.

Agents Used to Treat Nausea and Vomiting

Anticholinergic Agents

Scopolamine (Transderm Scop)

Anticholinergic agents suppress the receptors that connect the vestibular apparatus in the inner ear with the vomiting center in the brain. These agents are most effective in preventing motion sickness.

Adverse Effects. Dry mouth, blurred vision, drowsiness, and constipation are among the most common adverse effects. Others include skin rash, difficult urination, and disorientation.

Interactions. Use with antihistamines, phenothiazines, and tricyclic antidepressants may increase CNS adverse reactions. Scopolamine should be used cautiously with digoxin, with careful monitoring for increased levels to prevent toxicity. Use with alcohol will increase CNS depression.

Contraindications. Use is contraindicated in patients with glaucoma, GI obstruction and paralytic ileus, asthma and other chronic pulmonary diseases, myasthenia gravis, and prostatic hypertrophy.

Antihistamines

Dimenhydrinate (Dramamine)
Meclizine (Antivert, Bonine)

Antihistamines prevent acetylcholine from binding with the receptors in the inner ear by blocking histamine-1 receptors, as opposed to the H_2 blocking agents that suppress gastric acid.

Adverse Effects. Sedation is the primary adverse effect. Other adverse effects are similar to those for anticholinergic agents.

Interactions. Antihistamines should not be used with other CNS depressants, including alcohol.

Contraindications. Antihistamines are contraindicated in persons who manifest a hypersensitivity reaction.

Cannabinoids

Dronabinol (Marinol)

The mechanism of action of dronabinol is complex. By altering the person's perception of the environment, it may inhibit nausea and vomiting. This agent has been found to be helpful in patients undergoing cancer chemotherapy.

Adverse Effects. Adverse effects of cannabinoids include dizziness, sedation, euphoria, hallucinations, dry mouth, and diarrhea.

Interactions. Dronabinol should not be used concurrently with CNS depressants, including alcohol and sedatives, and psychoactive agents.

Contraindications. This agent is contraindicated in persons who are allergic to sesame seed, and should be used cautiously in those with cardiovascular disease because of the potential for tachycardia and hypotension.

Dopamine Antagonists

Prochlorperazine (Compazine)

Prochlorperazine works by blocking dopamine receptors in the chemoreceptor trigger zone (CTZ) in the brain. Larger doses may suppress the vomiting center. This agent may be used to suppress emesis caused by such factors as preoperative nausea, postoperative vomiting, toxins, and cancer chemotherapy.

Adverse Effects. Adverse effects include extrapyramidal reactions, hypotension, blurred vision, sedation, and adverse effects associated with anticholinergic agents.

Interactions. Avoid taking prochlorperazine with antacids, which will inhibit absorption. Use the drug cautiously with anticholinergic and antiparkinsonism agents (increase anticholinergic and parkinsonian symptoms). Increased CNS depression may occur when administered with antihistamines, barbiturates, and benzodiazepines.

Contraindications. Prochlorperazine should be avoided in persons with CNS depression (coma), those receiving spinal or epidural anesthesia, and those ingesting alcohol.

Glucocorticoids

Dexamethasone (Decadron)

The mechanism of action of dexamethasone is unknown. It has proved useful in controlling emesis associated with cancer chemotherapy.

Adverse Effects. No significant side effects are associated with dexamethasone. Single doses are given infrequently.

Interactions. No significant interactions are anticipated, because of the infrequent dosing intervals.

Contraindications. Dexamethasone is contraindicated for persons with systemic fungal infections.

Prokinetics

Metoclopramide (Reglan)

Nausea is relieved by increasing the tone of the lower esophageal sphincter and by blocking the dopamine receptors in the chemoreceptor trigger zone (CTZ) in the brain (see Agents Used to Treat Heartburn).

Serotonin Blockers

Ondansetron (Zofran)

This drug blocks serotonin receptors in the CTZ and on the neurons of the vagus in the GI tract. It is effective when given alone but has a synergistic effect when given with dexamethasone.

Adverse Effects. Headache, fatigue, dizziness, diarrhea, and constipation are the most common adverse effects.

Interactions. Drug interactions may occur with phenobarbital or cimetidine. Absorption of ondansetron may be affected; however, dosage adjustment is usually not necessary.

Contraindications. Ondansetron is contraindicated for persons with hypersensitive response to the agent.

Agents Used to Treat Diarrhea

Local-Acting

Adsorbents

Bismuth subsalicylate (Pepto-Bismol)
Attapulgite (Kaopectate)
Kaolin with pectin
Methylcellulose products
Metamucil
Other bulk-forming laxatives

These agents bind with the diarrhea-causing microorganisms (bacteria and viruses) and allow them to be passed with the stool. They also help reduce water loss. Methylcellulose products provide bulk to diarrhea-like stool by absorbing excess fluid.

Adverse Effects. Adsorbents may predispose to constipation. Bismuth subsalicylate may cause darkening of the tongue and the stool.

Interactions. Simultaneous administration with oral medications may impair their absorption; allow a 2-hour interval between other drugs. Because bismuth is a salicylate, it should not be administered with other salicylates, anticoagulant agents (bruising, increased bleeding time), or antidiabetic agents (increased hypoglycemic effects). Bismuth is radiopaque; its presence may interfere with x-ray examinations of the GI tract.

Contraindications. Bismuth is contraindicated in persons with hypersensitivity to salicylates.

Intestinal Flora Modifiers

Lactobacillus acidophilus (Bacid, Intestinex, Lactinex)

These agents change the bacterial levels in the intestine and reestablish the normal flora. They are particularly effective in replenishing normal flora destroyed by antibiotic therapy.

No significant adverse effects, interactions, or contraindications are associated with the use of these agents.

Systemic Action

Anticholinergics

Atropine
Hyoscine
Hyoscyamine

Anticholinergics are rarely used alone; they are generally used in combination with adsorbents and diphenoxylate. In these combinations, they help relieve the cramping associated with diarrhea. (See Agents Used to Treat Nausea and Vomiting: Anticholinergics)

Opiates (Natural and Synthetic)

Opium tincture
Camphorated (paregoric)
Diphenoxylate (Lomotil) (combined with atropine)
Loperamide (Imodium)

Opiates decrease intestinal motility and encourage increased fluid and electrolyte absorption in the intestine. In addition, less fluid enters the large intestine because of stimulation of opioid receptors in the small intestine.

Adverse Effects. Opiates produce CNS effects, such as dizziness and lightheadedness. They may also cause nausea and vomiting. Because camphorated opium tincture contains dilute morphine, physical dependence is possible with long-term use. Diphenoxylate has no significant CNS effects unless taken in large doses. Atropine has been added to the formulation to discourage high dosing; dry mouth, tachycardia, blurred vision, and urinary retention may occur. The side effect profile for loperamide is similar to that for diphenoxylate.

Interactions. Interactions may occur with use of barbiturates and alcohol. Patients taking diphenoxylate should be closely monitored for CNS depression. MAO inhibitors may precipitate hypertensive crisis.

Contraindications. Use of these agents is contraindicated in persons who have ingested toxic agents and in those with diarrhea that results from infectious diarrhea or pseudomembranous colitis. Diphenoxylate is contraindicated in persons who may be hypersensitive and in those with glaucoma or severe liver disease.

Anti-infective Agents

Anti-infective therapy is indicated for the following types of diarrhea: amebiasis, giardiasis, cholera, *Clostridium difficile*, shigellosis, sexually transmitted (gonorrhea, syphilis, chlamydiosis, and herpes simplex), and "traveler's" diarrhea. The agent should be matched to the infective microorganism. Indiscriminate use of anti-infective agents is cautioned against; resistant strains of microorganisms may develop. Concomitant use of antidiarrheal agents should be avoided.

Agents Used to Treat Irritable Bowel Disease

Symptomatic Relief

Antidiarrheal Agents

Antidiarrheals used to treat Crohn's disease (CD) include loperamide, diphenoxylate with atropine, and tincture of opium. Methylcellulose is used to treat ulcerative colitis (UC) in early stages. (For control of chronic diarrhea, see Agents Used to Treat Diarrhea.) Avoid the use of opiates and anticholinergics in UC, to prevent toxic megacolon.

Antispasmodic Agents

Propantheline bromide (Pro-Banthine), hyoscyamine (Cystospaz, Gastrosed) are antispasmodic agents. These drugs are used in CD to reduce abdominal cramping.

Adverse Effects. Adverse effects include dizziness, headache, confusion or excitement (in elderly patients), palpitations, blurred vision, dry mouth, and urinary retention. Drugs should be discontinued at the first sign of intestinal obstruction.

Interactions. Drugs that may interact with antispasmodics include antihistamines, antiparkinsonism drugs, meperidine, phenothiazines, quinidine, and tricyclic antidepressants.

Contraindications. These agents are contraindicated for persons with glaucoma, GI obstruction, or severe ulcerative colitis, and in persons who are hypersensitive to the drugs.

Specific Therapy

5-Aminosalicylic Acid Agents

Sulfasalazine (Azulfidine)

Mesalamine (Asacol, Pentasa) (slow-release form)

These agents reduce clinical signs of disease (local inflammation) and probably suppress prostaglandin synthesis. They are most useful in treating early-stage disease. Mesalamine may be given locally by retention enema or suppository.

Adverse Effects. Adverse effects of sulfasalazine include nausea, fever, rash, and arthralgias, and hematologic disorders; obtain a baseline CBC and monitor periodically. Side effects of mesalamine include headache and GI upset (e.g., cramps, abdominal pain, flatulence, nausea and vomiting, diarrhea or constipation).

Interactions. Many drugs can interact with sulfasalazine, including antibiotics, digoxin, folic acid and iron, oral anticoagulants, oral antidiabetic agents, and oral contraceptives. Drugs that may interact with mesalamine include lactulose and omeprazole.

Contraindications. These agents are contraindicated for persons who are hypersensitive to salicylates and those with GI or urinary obstruction.

Corticosteroids

Prednisone and budesonide are corticosteroids. The anti-inflammatory action of corticosteroids helps to reduce symptoms but does not alter the course of the disease. Budesonide is a topically active corticosteroid with little systemic action.

Adverse Effects. Avoid prolonged use of corticosteroids to prevent serious adverse effects, including adrenal suppression, peptic ulcer, osteoporosis, cataracts, diabetes, hypertension, and masking of infectious processes.

Interactions. Drugs that may interact with corticosteroids include aspirin and other NSAIDs, barbiturates, phenytoin, rifampin, oral anticoagulants, potassium-depleting diuretics, and salicylates.

Contraindications. Use is contraindicated in persons with hypersensitive reactions to the drugs or those with fungal infections.

Immunomodulating Drugs

Azathioprine (Imuran)
Mercaptopurine (Purinethol)

These immunosuppressant agents are used for patients who need long-term disease management but have been unresponsive to other treatment modalities. The effects of immunomodulating drug therapy may be delayed for up to 6 months, and so these agents are used simultaneously with other treatment modalities.

Adverse Effects. Adverse effects include nausea and vomiting, leukopenia, thrombocytopenia, pancreatitis, and hepatotoxicity.

Interactions. Drugs that may interact with immunomodulating drugs include ACE inhibitors, allopurinol, and warfarin.

Contraindications. Contraindicated in persons who are hypersensitive to any components of the drug.

Nicotine Transdermal System (Nicotrol)

The nicotine transdermal system helps to control mild to moderately active UC.

Adverse Effects. Adverse effects include contact dermatitis, nausea and vomiting, dizziness, headache, and sleep disturbances.

Interactions. Interactions may occur with concurrent use of acetaminophen and caffeine. Concurrent use with insulin may decrease hepatic enzymes that aid in drug metabolism.

Contraindications. Use of this system is contraindicated for persons who are hypersensitive to nicotine, have had a recent MI, life-threatening dysrhythmia, or increased angina pectoris.

 CLINICAL PEARLS

- To prolong antacid action up to 4 to 5 hours, administer antacids 1 hour after meals rather than on an empty stomach.
- Discontinue use of antidiarrheal agents if diarrhea worsens despite treatment, because these drugs may mask symptoms of more serious pathology.
- Be aware that therapy with immunosuppressants may take from 4 to 6 months to be effective.
- During immunosuppressant therapy, monitor WBC and hemoglobin levels

weekly for 1 month, then twice monthly during therapy. These agents depress rapidly regenerating cells and may precipitate a lack of immune response. If the counts drop suddenly or become dangerously low, temporarily discontinue the drug and institute appropriate restorative therapy.

○ Keep the patient's head elevated at least 30 to 45 degrees after administration of bulk-forming laxatives such as Metamucil to prevent regurgitation into the esophagus and potential esophageal obstruction (especially in the elderly).

○ Never administer laxative preparations to persons complaining of abdominal pain, because these agents stimulate peristalsis and may precipitate rupture of the intestine.

○ Ginger is effective in preventing motion sickness. The antiemetic effects result from ginger's local action on the gastric mucosa. Ginger ale or powdered ginger capsules may be effective for some patients.

Diuretics

Section 8   Jan Addy

OVERVIEW

Diuretics are capable of producing increased urine volume by promoting the loss of water and sodium from the body. This is accomplished by various mechanisms.

Body fluid retention depends largely on the retention of sodium. Therefore, the effectiveness of a diuretic is primarily related to its ability to increase sodium excretion. Caring for the patient receiving diuretic therapy requires close monitoring of fluid and electrolyte status and the recognition of acute fluid and electrolyte imbalances.

PRINCIPLES OF CARE
Diuretic Actions in the Nephron

Normally, solutes such as electrolytes, amino acids, and glucose are reabsorbed in the kidney's tubules, and wastes are removed. Approximately 99% of the water, electrolytes, and nutrients that are filtered at the glomeruli undergo reabsorption. Most diuretics act by decreasing the rate of reabsorption of these substances at different points in the kidney's tubules.

Categories of Diuretics

Diuretics are classified according to where they act in the tubules of the kidney, their chemical structure, and their potency. Currently, there are five classes of diuretics:

• Carbonic anhydrase inhibitors
• Thiazide and thiazide-like diuretics
• Loop diuretics
• Osmotic diuretics
• Potassium-sparing diuretics

Table 12-8-1 summarizes classes of diuretics, major sites of action, time course of effects, and types of electrolyte imbalances.

Table 12-8-1. Diuretic Actions, Uses, and Significant Side Effects

DIURETIC	PRIMARY ACTION	USES	SIGNIFICANT SIDE EFFECTS
Carbonic anhydrase inhibitors	Inhibit production of carbonic anhydrase, which blocks the reabsorption of sodium and water in the convoluted tubule	Glaucoma Edema Epilepsy High-altitude sickness	GI: Anorexia, nausea and vomiting GU: Hematuria, impotence, glycosuria CNS: Seizures, paresthesias, drowsiness Hematologic: bone marrow depression, hemolytic anemia Dermatologic: urticaria, Stevens-Johnson syndrome, toxic epidermal necrolysis Metabolic: acidosis
Loop diuretics	Inhibit sodium and water reabsorption in the distal tubule	Hypertension Edema with congestive heart failure Hepatic edema Renal disease Hypercalcemia	CNS: dizziness, headache, tinnitus, blurred vision GI: nausea and vomiting, diarrhea Hematologic: agranulocytosis, thrombocytopenia, neutropenia EENT: ototoxicity Metabolic: hypovolemia, hypokalemia, hypocalcemia, hypomagnesemia CV: circulatory collapse

Thiazide diuretics	Inhibit tubular reabsorption of sodium and chloride in ascending loop of Henle	Hypertension, edema, diabetes insipidus, adjunct with loop diuretics, idiopathic hypercalciuria	CNS: dizziness, headache, blurred vision, paresthesias, decreased libido GI: anorexia, nausea and vomiting, diarrhea, pancreatitis, cholecystitis Hematologic: jaundice, leukopenia, purpura, agranulocytosis, aplastic anemia, thrombocytopenia Dermatologic: urticaria, photosensitivity Metabolic: hypokalemia, glycosuria, hyperglycemia, hyperuricemia, hypochloremic alkalosis GU: impotence
Osmotic diuretics	Inhibit tubular reabsorption of water and solutes by increasing the osmotic pressure of the glomerular filtrate	Early oliguric phase of acute renal failure Increased intracranial pressure/cerebral edema	CNS: seizures, headaches, fever CV: chest pain, tachycardia Lung: pulmonary congestion EENT: blurred vision Hematologic: thrombophlebitis
Potassium-sparing diuretics	Exchange potassium and hydrogen ions for sodium in the distal tubule	Hyperaldosteronism Hypertension Congestive heart failure	CNS: dizziness, headache, weakness GI: cramps, nausea and vomiting, diarrhea GU: urinary frequency

CNS, central nervous system; CV, cardiovascular; EENT, eyes, ears, nose, and throat; GI, gastrointestinal; GU, genitourinary.

377

Carbonic Anhydrase Inhibitors

Carbonic anhydrase inhibitors (CAIs), such as acetazolamide (Diamox), inhibit the production of the enzyme carbonic anhydrase. This enzyme, found in the proximal tubules of the kidney and the eyes, catalyzes the union of water and carbon dioxide to form carbonic acid.

Almost two thirds of all sodium and water is reabsorbed back into the blood in the proximal tubules. CAIs act specifically to inhibit this reabsorption. It does this through a specialized transport system that exchanges sodium for hydrogen ions. Thus, CAIs increase sodium excretion by decreasing sodium–hydrogen exchange throughout the renal tubules.

The diuretic potency of CAIs is weak; therefore, they are usually not effective in acute fluid overload states. CAIs are primarily used in the treatment of chronic open-angle glaucoma, because the drug decreases the secretion of aqueous humor in the eye, which ultimately decreases intraocular pressure.

Other uses include treatment of congestive heart failure that has become resistant to other diuretics, treatment of high-altitude sickness, and as an adjunct in the treatment of epilepsy.

Loop Diuretics (High-Ceiling Diuretics)

Loop diuretics act to inhibit the resorption of sodium and chloride in the ascending loop of Henle. These very potent diuretics can produce significant fluid and electrolyte imbalances. Agents in this category have renal effects as well as cardiovascular and metabolic effects, including reduction of blood pressure, pulmonary vascular resistance, systemic vascular resistance, central venous pressure, and left ventricular end-diastolic pressure. Loop diuretics are used in the treatment of congestive heart failure, edema, hepatic and renal disease, hypercalcemia, and hypertension.

Loop diuretics include furosemide (Lasix), ethacrynic acid (Edecrin), bumetanide (Bumex), and torsemide (Demadex). Furosemide is the most commonly prescribed loop diuretic. These agents share the same side effects and drug interactions. Their onset and duration of action times are also similar except for bumetanide, which has a shorter duration of action (4 to 6 hours). Ethacrynic acid and bumetanide are not approved for the treatment of hypertension.

Osmotic Diuretics

The most commonly prescribed osmotic diuretic is mannitol (Osmitrol). Urea (Ureaphil), glycerin (Osmoglyn), and isosorbide (Ismotic) are also classified as osmotic diuretics. Osmotic diuretics act mainly by increasing the osmotic pressure of the glomerular filtrate, which inhibits the tubular resorption of water and other solutes. Sodium excretion is not significantly increased, because these drugs only excrete an osmotically equivalent amount of water from the body.

These drugs are used mainly to draw fluid from the tissue spaces, such as in the brain and eye. For this reason, they are used to treat increased intracranial pressure and increased intraocular pressure. Osmotic diuretics are rarely used for routine diuretic therapy.

Mannitol and urea are given only IV. Glycerin and isosorbide are administered orally.

GENERIC NAME	TRADE NAME
Chlorothiazide	Diuril, Diurigen
Hydrochlorothiazide	Esidrex, Oretic, Hydrodiuril, others
Bendroflumethiazide	Naturetin
Benzthiazide	Exna
Hydroflumethiazide	Diucardin, Saluron
Methyclothiazide	Aquatensen, Enduron
Polytiazide	Renese
Trichlormethiazide	Metahydrin, Naqua, Diurese

Thiazide and Thiazide-Like Diuretics

Thiazide diuretics act in the distal convoluted tubule and the ascending loop of Henle to inhibit the resorption of sodium and chloride. Through their actions, sodium, chloride, water, and (to a lesser extent) potassium are excreted. Thiazides are commonly used as adjuncts in the management of congestive heart failure, cirrhosis, hypertension, and edematous states. Thiazides produce a lower diuretic effect than the loop diuretics. Of the many thiazide diuretics available, the most widely recognized agent is hydrochlorothiazide (Hydro-DIURIL). All of these agents are administered orally, except for chlorothiazide, which can be administered orally and IV.

Potassium-Sparing Diuretics (Aldosterone-Inhibiting Diuretics)

Potassium-sparing diuretics work in the collecting ducts and the distal convoluted tubules by interfering with the sodium-potassium exchange system, causing a decrease in potassium excretion. They also bind competitively to aldosterone receptors, thus blocking the resorption of sodium and water. Commonly prescribed potassium-sparing diuretics include spironolactone (Aldactone), triamterene (Dyrenium), and amiloride (Midamor). Triamterene combined with the thiazide diuretic hydrochlorothiazide in a single pill yields the benefits of a thiazide while also limiting potassium loss.

DECISION-MAKING

Diuretic therapy poses many challenges for nurses. Understanding the actions, uses, types, side effects, contraindications, patient teaching, drug interactions, and nursing considerations will assist in providing optimal care. Table 12-8-1 summarizes the actions, uses, and significant side effects of the five categories of diuretics. Dosage ranges of the prototype drug are included. Nursing considerations, drug interactions, and significant contraindications are listed in Table 12-8-2. Important information needed in caring for the patient taking diuretics is identified in Tables 12-8-3 and 12-8-4.

 CLINICAL PEARLS

○ Pretherapy baseline data—serum electrolytes, CBC, electrocardiogram, signs with orthostatic vitals, and weight—should be assessed for all patients.
○ Monitor electrolytes, fluid status, weight, and vital signs throughout therapy.

Table 12-8-2. Significant Contraindications, Drug Interactions, and Nursing Considerations of Common Diuretics

DRUG	SIGNIFICANT CONTRAINDICATIONS	DRUG INTERACTIONS	NURSING CONSIDERATIONS
Carbonic anhydrase inhibitors Acetazolamide (Diamox)	Low serum sodium and potassium, renal and hepatic dysfunction, hyperchloremic acidosis, adrenal insufficiency, hypersensitivity to thiazide diuretics	Increased amphetamine effect Increased cyclosporine levels Increased ephedrine effect Increased salicylate level in brain Decreased methotrexate effect Decreased primidone effect Increased quinidine effect	1. Tolerance after prolonged use may necessitate dosage increase. 2. IM administration is painful because of the alkalinity of the solution. 3. Reconstitute each 500 mg with at least 5 mL of sterile water. 4. Administer IV over 1 minute.
Loop diuretics Furosemide (Lasix)	Hypersensitivity to sulfonylureas, severe electrolyte depletion, hepatic coma, lactating mothers, pregnancy	Increased ototoxicity with aminoglycosides Increased anticoagulant activity Increased lithium levels Decreased effect with nonsteroidal anti-inflammatory drugs (NSAIDs) Decreased glucose tolerance Additive effect with thiazides Increased risk of dysrhythmias with digitalis Additive ototoxicity with cisplatin	1. Similar to thiazide diuretics 2. Administer orally with food or milk if GI upset occurs. 3. Ensure ready access to bathroom facilities. 4. Administer IV push dose at a rate of 20 mg/min. For patients with renal impairment, administer at 4 mg/min.

Drug	Contraindications	Drug Interactions	Nursing Considerations
Thiazide diuretics Hydrochlorothiazide (HCTZ)	Anuria, renal decompensation, advanced hepatic cirrhosis, edema from toxemia of pregnancy	Increased risk of hypokalemia with corticosteroids Increased risk of hyperkalemia with diazoxide Increased therapeutic effects of oral hypoglycemic agents Increased risk of toxicity with lithium May prolong induced leukopenia with antineoplastic agents Decreased effect of anticoagulants Enhanced loss of electrolytes with amphotericin B	1. Geriatric patients may manifest an increased risk of hypotension and changes in electrolyte levels. 2. Administer with food or milk to prevent a GI upset. 3. Administer early in the day so that increased urination does not disturb sleep. 4. Ensure that the drug is discontinued for several days before parathyroid function tests.
Osmotic diuretics Mannitol	Anuria, pulmonary edema, severe dehydration, active intracranial bleeding except during craniotomy, progressive heart failure, progressive renal damage after mannitol therapy	No significant drug interactions	1. Use a filter with concentrated mannitol (15%, 20%, 25%). 2. Concentrations greater than 15% may crystallize. To redissolve, warm the bottle in hot water; cool to body temperature before administering. 3. Do not add to other IV solutions or mix with medications. 4. If blood is administered concurrently, add 20 mEq of sodium chloride to each liter of mannitol to prevent pseudoagglutination.
Potassium-sparing diuretics Spironolactone	Acute renal insufficiency, hyperkalemia, anuria	Increased risk of hyperkalemia with acetylcholine (ACE) inhibitors Additive hypotension with general anesthetics Increased risk of hyperkalemia with captopril Increased half-life of digitalis Increased risk of lithium toxicity Increased risk of hyperkalemia with triamterene combination	1. Tablets may be crushed. 2. Food may increase drug absorption. 3. Protect the drug from light.

Table 12-8-3. Key Assessments, Monitoring, and Teaching Points for Patients Receiving Diuretic Therapy

Pretherapy Assessment

1. Assess and record baseline data necessary for monitoring the effects of diuretic therapy. This includes a thorough health history and physical examination, specifically, baseline fluid and electrolyte status, baseline laboratory data, and a baseline weight.
2. Review medical history and documents for existing or past conditions that require cautious use or contraindications for the use of diuretic therapy.

During Therapy Assessments and Interventions

1. Measure and record intake and output. Note the amount and color of initial output after diuretic administration.
2. Assess skin, mucous membranes, level of consciousness, and vital signs for any changes indicating dehydration or electrolyte loss.
3. Assess laboratory values for changes in sodium, potassium, chloride, calcium, magnesium, blood urea nitrogen, creatinine, and uric acid levels.
4. Assess arterial blood gases (if indicated) for signs of acidosis or alkalosis.
5. Assess for the presence of orthostatic hypotension.
6. Assess adequacy of glucose control with diuretic therapy in patients with diabetes.
7. Assess for hypersensitivity drug interactions, and drug-nutrient reactions.
8. Ensure that bathroom facilities are readily accessible to the patient.
9. Assess the adequacy of the patient's diet to replace lost electrolytes.

Surveillance and Evaluation

1. Evaluate the effectiveness of diuretic therapy by noting the absence of side effects.
2. Evaluate the resolution or reduction of edema, fluid volume overload, congestive heart failure, hypertension, increased intracranial pressure, or a return to normal intraocular pressure.

○ Encourage the patient taking loop or thiazide-like diuretics to add potassium-rich foods to the diet.
○ Patients taking osmotic diuretics should be monitored for pulmonary congestion.
○ For diuretics to work effectively, the patient must have a functioning renal system.

PATIENT TEACHING

1. Maintain proper nutritional and fluid volume status by eating potassium-rich foods such as bananas, oranges, dates, raisins, plums, fresh vegetables, potatoes, meat, and fish (not necessary only for patients on potassium-sparing diuretics).
2. If taking digitalis with a diuretic, monitor pulse rate and signs of digitalis toxicity (anorexia, nausea, vomiting, and bradycardia).
3. Monitor glucose level closely because of the hyperglycemic effects of diuretics.
4. Change positions slowly after sitting or lying to prevent dizziness.
5. Keep scheduled follow-up visits with the physician.
6. Monitor daily weight by keeping a log or journal.
7. Recognize and report clinical manifestations of dehydration and hypokalemia.
8. Report any weight gain of 2 lb (1 kg) or more in 1 day or 5 lb (2.25 kg) in 1 week.

Table 12-8-4. Classes of Diuretics, Major Sites of Action, Time Course of Effects, and Types of Potential Electrolyte Imbalances

DIURETIC CLASS	MAJOR SITES OF ACTION	TIME COURSE OF EFFECTS		ELECTROLYTE IMBALANCES
		ONSET	DURATION	
Carbonic anhydrase inhibitor (Acetazolamide)	Proximal tubule and (?) distal tubule	Oral: 1 hr	8–12 hr	Hyponatremic acidosis Hypokalemia Hypochloremic acidosis
Loop diuretics (Furosemide)	Thick portion of the ascending loop of Henle and proximal tubule	Oral: <60 min	6–8 hr	Hypokalemia Hypochloremic acidosis Hyponatremia (excessive diuresis) Hypocalcemia
Osmotic diuretics (Mannitol)	Proximal tubule, descending loop of Henle, and collecting tubule	IV: <5 min IV: 30–60 min	2 hr 6–8 hr	Minimal electrolyte imbalances
Potassium-sparing diuretics (Spironolactone)	Collecting tubules	Oral: 1–3 days	2–3 days	Hyperkalemia
Thiazide and thiazide-like diuretics (Hydrochlorothiazide)	Distal convoluted tubule	Oral: 2 hr	6–12 hr	Hypokalemia Hypochloremic alkalosis Hyponatremia Hypercalcemia

383

- Report any clinical manifestations related to dehydration and electrolyte imbalances.
- Diuretics should be taken early in the day to prevent nocturia.
- Because elderly patients are prone to developing orthostatic hypotension, encourage an elderly patient to change positions slowly.
- Bathroom facilities must be accessible to all patients taking diuretics.
- Documentation of the effectiveness of diuretic therapy should be noted in the patient's medical record.
- IV lasix should be administered at a rate of 20 mg (or fraction of)/minute for low doses. For high doses, the rate is 4 mg/min. This reduces the risk of ototoxicity.

Insulins

Section 9   Joanne M. Bullard

OVERVIEW

Insulin and oral hypoglycemic agents, as well as diet, exercise, and stress management, are important in the management of diabetes mellitus. This section discusses the pharmacologic agents used in the management of type 1 and type 2 diabetes mellitus, as well as the different insulin regimens.

PRINCIPLES OF CARE

The primary goal of pharmacologic treatment of diabetes mellitus is the achievement of normal or near-normal blood glucose levels. The treatment choices are either oral hypoglycemic agents or insulin.

Oral hypoglycemics are used in the treatment of type 2 diabetes mellitus. In this form of diabetes, the beta cells of the pancreas are able to produce insulin. The amount produced may be decreased, normal, or increased; however, a defect prevents the available insulin from binding with cell receptor sites, thus preventing glucose transport into the cell. Insulin resistance—the inability of the target tissues to effectively use the insulin produced—also occurs. Oral hypoglycemic agents are used when normal blood glucose levels cannot be maintained with diet, exercise, and stress management. If oral hypoglycemics are ineffective in controlling blood glucose levels in type 2 diabetics, then insulin may be required.

Insulin is a hormone that lowers blood glucose levels and regulates the metabolism and storage of carbohydrates, fats, and proteins. It is required for the treatment of type 1 diabetes mellitus and also may be required for some patients with type 2 diabetes mellitus. In type 1 diabetes, an absence of insulin production from a marked decrease of beta cells in the pancreas leads to elevation of blood glucose concentrations. Exogenous insulin is required to control blood glucose levels.

DECISION-MAKING
Oral Hypoglycemic Agents

There are five types of oral hypoglycemic agents: sulfonylureas, alpha-glucosidase inhibitors, biguanides, thiazolidinediones, and meglitinides (Table

Table 12-9-1. Oral Antidiabetic Agents

CLASSIFICATION	ADULT DOSAGE	ADMINISTRATION CONSIDERATIONS
Sulfonylureas		
First Generation		
Acetohexamide (Dymelor)	250 mg q day before breakfast Maximum: 1.5 g/day	Doses >1 g/day should be given before breakfast and dinner.
Chlorpropamide (Diabinese)	100–250 mg q day with breakfast Maximum: 750 mg/day	Generally prescribed as a single morning dose; may be divided in two or three doses with meals to decrease gastrointestinal effects.
Tolazamide (Tolinase)	100 mg–1 g q day Maximum: 1 g/day	Doses > 500 mg/day should be given 30 minutes before breakfast and dinner.
Tolbutamide (Airiness)	250 mg–3 g q day in one dose or two divided doses	
Second Generation		
Glipizide (Glucotrol)	2.5–5 mg q day 30 min at breakfast Maximum: 40 mg/day Sustained-release: 5–10 mg q day	Doses > 15 mg/day should be given 30 minutes before breakfast and dinner.
Glyburide (Diabeta, micronase)	1.25–5 mg q day with breakfast Maximum: 20 mg/day	Doses > 15 mg/day should be given in divided doses with breakfast and dinner.
Glimepiride (Amaryl)	1–2 mg q day with breakfast Maintenance dose: 1–4 mg/day Maximum: 8 mg/day	
Alpha-glucosidase inhibitors		
Acarbose (Precose)	25 mg q day to tid with first bite of each main meal Maximum: ≤60 kg: 150 mg/day >60 kg: 300 mg/day	
Miglitol (Glyset)	Initial: 25 mg with meals Maintenance: 50 mg tid Maximum: 100 mg tid	
Biguanides		
Metformin hydrochloride (Glucophage)	500 mg bid Maximum: 3 g/day	Should be taken with morning and evening meals.
Thiazolidinediones		
Pioglitazone (Actos)	15–30 mg q day Maximum: 45 mg/day	May be taken without regard to meals.
Rosiglitazone (Avandia)	4–8 mg q day	May be taken with or without food; either in the morning or in two divided doses.
Meglitinides		
Repaglinide (Prandin)	0.5–4 mg 15–30 min before meals in two to four doses q day Maximum: 16 mg/day	

12-9-1). These agents may be used alone, in combination, or adjunctively with insulin therapy in the treatment of type 2 diabetes mellitus.

Sulfonylureas

Action. Sulfonylureas act to decrease high levels of blood glucose in several ways. They directly stimulate the functioning beta cells of the pancreas to secrete insulin, thus lowering the blood glucose concentration. They also decrease hepatic glucose release by decreasing gluconeogenesis (formation of glycogen in the liver) and glycogenolysis (formation of glucose from glycogen). In addition, sulfonylureas increase sensitivity of the peripheral insulin receptors, which in turn results in increased insulin binding in peripheral tissues.

Use. Sulfonylureas are used in the management of mild to moderately severe stable type 2 diabetes mellitus as an adjunct to diet and exercise. They may also be used as an adjunct to insulin therapy. They are not used in the treatment of type 1 diabetes mellitus, because patients with this form of diabetes do not produce any endogenous insulin.

Test Interferences. Sulfonylureas may produce increased blood urea nitrogen (BUN) and creatinine values, abnormal thyroid function test results, and reduced radioactive iodine uptake (RAI) test results.

Adverse Effects. Hypoglycemia is the primary adverse effect, especially in the elderly and in patients with renal or liver impairment. Other adverse effects include nausea, vomiting, anorexia, diarrhea, cholestatic jaundice, leukopenia, thrombocytopenia, agranulocytosis, hemolytic anemia, aplastic anemia, rash, pruritus, and diuretic effects. Chlorpropamide is an exception, producing an antidiuretic effect. It also has the greatest risk for severe hypoglycemia and may produce a disulfiram-type reaction (facial flushing, sweating, tachycardia, headache, dyspnea), which may last up to 24 hours after administration.

Biguanides

Action. Biguanides decrease blood glucose concentrations by inhibiting hepatic glucose production, reducing glucose absorption in the intestines, and increasing insulin sensitivity in the peripheral tissues. They do not affect insulin secretion.

Use. Biguanides are used to treat patients with type 2 diabetes mellitus who are unable to maintain blood glucose control through diet alone or through combined diet and sulfonylurea therapy. The only biguanide approved for use in the United States is metformin. This agent may be used alone or in combination with a sulfonylurea.

Test Interferences. Metformin may decrease serum potassium levels. It also may decrease vitamin B_{12} levels.

Adverse Effects. The most common adverse effects of biguanides are nausea, vomiting, diarrhea, abdominal pain, abdominal bloating, and a bitter or metallic taste. Another adverse effect may be asymptomatic low vitamin B_{12} levels. The most serious adverse effect is lactic acidosis.

Metformin should be held for 48 hours after the administration of IV iodinated contrast media, to prevent accumulation resulting in lactic acidosis in the presence of renal impairment. Ensure that renal function is normal before administering.

Alpha-Glucosidase Inhibitors

Action. The alpha-glucosidase inhibitors act to reduce blood sugar concentrations by binding to the alpha-glucosidase enzymes in the small intestines. Postprandial hyperglycemia is reduced as a result of the delayed digestion of carbohydrates and glucose absorption in the GI tract.

Use. Alpha-glucosidase inhibitors are used in the management of type 2 diabetes mellitus as an adjunct to diet therapy. They may also be used in combination with sulfonylurea drugs.

Adverse Effects. Abdominal discomfort, flatulence, and diarrhea are the most common adverse effects of the alpha-glucosidase inhibitors. Hypoglycemia is usually seen only when used in combination with sulfonylureas, because alpha-glucosidase inhibitors have no effect on insulin production or on insulin resistance.

Thiazolidinediones

Action. Thiazolidinediones decrease blood glucose concentrations by enhancing the effects of circulating insulin. They improve target cell response to insulin by decreasing insulin resistance, which increases the uptake of glucose by the skeletal muscles and adipose tissue. They also inhibit gluconeogenesis, thus decreasing production of glucose by the liver. Thiazolidinediones are active only in the presence of insulin; they do not stimulate the production of insulin.

Use. Thiazolidinediones are used in the management of type 2 diabetes mellitus. They may be used as an adjunct to diet and exercise to lower blood glucose, or in combination with sulfonylurea, insulin, or metformin to improve glycemic control.

Adverse Effects. Adverse effects include nausea, diarrhea, headache, hepatotoxicity, and decreased hemoglobin, hematocrit, and white blood cell counts. Other adverse effects may include rhinitis, pharyngitis, infection, pain, back pain, asthenia, and urinary tract infection. Hypoglycemia may be a risk for patients who are receiving a thiazolidinedione in combination with sulfonylurea or insulin. Women with insulin resistance who are premenopausal and anovulatory may be at risk for conception, because ovulation may resume with thiazolidinedione therapy. Thiazolidinediones may increase edema in the edematous patient.

Meglitinides

Action. The meglitinides act to reduce blood glucose concentrations by stimulating the pancreatic beta cells to release insulin. This drug requires functioning beta cells for this action to occur.

Use. Meglitinides are used in the management of type 2 diabetes mellitus as an adjunct to diet and exercise to control blood glucose levels. These agents may also be used in combination with the biguanide agent metformin.

Adverse Reactions. The most common adverse effect is hypoglycemia. Meglitinides significantly lower postprandial blood glucose levels. Other possible adverse effects include nausea, vomiting, diarrhea, rhinitis, bronchitis, headache, chest pain, arthralgias, back pain, and paresthesias.

Insulin

Insulin is required for the treatment of type 1 diabetes mellitus and may be needed to treat type 2 diabetes mellitus when diet, exercise, and/or oral hypoglycemic agents are not successful in controlling blood glucose levels. Table 12-9-2 lists specific agents. Regular insulin is used to lower blood glucose levels in emergency treatment of diabetic ketoacidosis or hyperosmotic nonketotic coma, in acute episodes of severe infections or illnesses, in major surgery, and in severe hyperkalemia (promotes intracellular shift of potassium);

Table 12-9-2. Insulins

CLASSIFICATION	DOSE/PHARMACOKINETICS
Rapid-acting Insulin	
Insulin Lispro	5–10 U SC 0–15 min before meals
Humalog	Onset: <15 min
	Peak: 0.5–1 hr
	Duration: 3–4 hr
Short-acting Insulin	
Insulin injection (regular insulin)	5–10 units SC 15–30 min before meals and bedtime
Humulin R, Novulin R,	Onset: 30–60 min
Pork Regular Ilentin II,	Peak: 2–3 hr
Regular Purified Pork Insulin,	Duration: 5–7 hr
Velosulin, Velosulin BR,	
Velosulin human	
Insulin zinc suspension prompt	Onset: 0.5–1 hr
(Semilente)	Peak: 4–7 hr
Semilente Insulin,	Duration: 12–16 hr
Semilente Purified Pork Insulin	
Intermediate-acting insulin	
Isophane insulin suspension	Onset: 1–2.5 hr
(NPH)	Peak: 7–15 hr
Humulin N, Ilente II (pork),	Duration: 22 hr
Insulatard NPH, Mixtard,	
Novolin 70/30, Novolin N	
Insulin zinc suspension (Lente)	Onset: 1–2 hr
Humulin L, Lente Ilentin II	Peak: 8–12 hr
(pork),	Duration: 18–24 hr
Lente Purified Pork Insulin,	
Novolin	
Long-acting Insulin	
Insulin protamine zinc (IPZ)	Onset: 4–8 hr
Ilentin II	Peak: 14–24 hr
	Duration: 36 hr
Insulin zinc suspension extended	Onset: 4–8 hr
(UltraLente)	Peak: 16–18 hr
Humulin U, UltraLente,	Duration: 36 hr
UltraLente insulin	

as stimulating test for growth hormone secretion; and in psychiatry for induction of hypoglycemic shock as therapy. Insulin binds with receptor sites on the cell membranes, facilitating the transport of glucose into the cells to be used for energy. Insulin-specific receptor sites are located on most body cells, primarily the cells of cardiac and skeletal muscle, adipose tissue, and the liver.

Insulin preparations vary by origin (beef, pork, mixture of beef and pork, human, and an analog of human insulin), action times (i.e., onset, peak, duration), and concentration (U-100 and U-500). *Onset* refers to when the insulin begins to work; *peak*, to when the maximum effect of the insulin occurs; and *duration*, to the amount of time that the insulin is active in the body. *U-100 insulin* (the most commonly used preparation) contains 100 units in 1 mL; *U-500* (used only in special cases) contains 500 units in 1 mL.

Insulin can be accurately measured only using a specifically calibrated syringe. The variety of available preparations allows the health care provider to select the insulin that best suits the individual patient's needs and lifestyle.

Human insulin is produced in the laboratory. Biosynthetic human insulin is now most commonly used because of its decreased incidence of allergic reactions and other adverse effects.

Insulin is also available in a subcutaneous infusion pump. This method is suitable only for a highly motivated, disciplined patient, however, as severe hypoglycemia is a significant complication of noncompliance.

Test Interferences

Use of insulin may cause altered thyroid function, decreased serum calcium, and decreased serum potassium.

Administration

To prevent tissue fibrosis, injection sites should be systematically rotated within one anatomic area (e.g., abdomen, thighs, buttocks, lower back, upper arms), with all available sites within that area used before moving to the next area. Insulin is injected with the needle at a 90-degree angle to prevent local reactions. After injection, gentle pressure is applied; vigorous massage may alter the rate of absorption.

An insulin vial should be discarded, unused, if any clumping, solid deposit, or granular appearance is noted. The physician should be consulted for dosages when breakfast is delayed for laboratory testing. At the beginning of insulin therapy, blurred vision may occur; this usually subsides in 6 to 8 weeks. The patient should be given instructions for dosages to be used on "sick days." Added stress due to sickness can cause the blood glucose levels to rise.

Mixing Insulins

In some patients, a mixture of short- and intermediate-acting insulins can achieve a more normal glycemic control than can be achieved by the use of a single type of insulin. The patient's response to a mixture of insulins may differ from his or her response to insulins given separately, because of chemical changes in the mixture, which may occur immediately or over time. Some specific guidelines for the mixing of insulins are as follows:

- Insulin products should not be mixed with other medication or diluent without the prescribing practitioner's approval.
- NPH insulin should not be mixed with Lente insulins. Precipitation and changes in onset or duration may occur.
- NPH insulin and short-acting insulin may be mixed and used immediately or stored for later use.
- When mixing short-acting with intermediate- or long-acting insulin, always draw the short-acting insulin into the syringe first, to prevent possible contamination of the short-acting insulin with the intermediate- or long-acting insulin.
- Animal and human insulins should not be mixed.
- Regular insulin may be mixed with all other types of insulin.

Table 12-9-3 details the procedure of mixing insulins.

Insulin Coverage

In nondiabetic persons, the pancreas continuously secretes a basal amount of insulin and also produces additional insulin after meals to maintain normal

Table 12-9-3. Mixing Insulins

1. Roll the insulin bottle in your hands to mix intermediate- or long-acting insulins (cloudy). Do not shake.
2. When mixing short-acting and delayed-action insulin:
   a. Draw air into syringe, the same amount as the amount of delayed-action insulin prescribed, and inject air into the delayed-action bottle.
   b. Withdraw the empty syringe.
   c. Draw air into the syringe, the same amount as the amount of short-acting insulin prescribed, and inject into the short-acting insulin bottle.
   d. Invert the vial of short-acting insulin and withdraw the prescribed amount. Clear any air bubbles and remove the syringe from the bottle.
   e. With the delayed-action bottle inverted, carefully insert the same syringe and withdraw the prescribed amount of delayed-action insulin. Avoid injecting short-acting insulin injected into vial. The total dosage of short- and delayed-action insulin is now in the one syringe.
3. After insulin is mixed in the syringe, administer within 15 minutes.

blood glucose levels. In diabetic persons, insulin regimens are used in an attempt to parallel the normal secretory pattern of insulin by the pancreas. Insulin dosages are individualized, with adjustments based on blood glucose monitoring. Most insulin regimes use NPH insulin (intermediate-acting) for basal insulin coverage and regular (short-acting) insulin.

Single-Injection Regimen. This regimen involves one injection of either intermediate-acting or a combination of intermediate-acting and short-acting insulin in the morning before breakfast. This coverage may not match the patient's food intake, resulting in afternoon hypoglycemia, or may not be adequate to control the patient's fasting blood glucose level.

Two-Dose Regimen. In this regimen, considered conventional therapy, an intermediate-acting or a combination of intermediate- and short-acting insulin is given twice a day. The initial total dose of insulin is 0.5 to 1.0 units/kg/day. The total dose is divided and given as two-thirds before breakfast and one-third before supper. The total breakfast dose is then divided by type of insulin, two-thirds intermediate-acting and one-third short-acting. The evening dose is also divided as one-half intermediate-acting and one-half short-acting. Table 12-9-4 gives an example. Adjustments are determined by blood glucose monitoring. Disadvantages are that the patient's meal schedule needs to be regular, and hypoglycemia may occur at night.

Table 12-9-4. Two-Dose Insulin Regimen

For a 70-kg person, the dosage is calculated as follows:
70 kg $\times$ 0.5 = 35 U/day (total insulin dose)
Breakfast dose: Two thirds of the total dose (0.66 $\times$ 35 U) = 23.1 U (administer 23 U of intermediate-acting insulin)
If using an intermediate- and short-acting combination, further calculate:
Intermediate-acting: 0.66 $\times$ 23.1 U = 15.2 U (administer 15 U)
Short-acting: 0.33 $\times$ 23.1 U = 7.6 U (administer 8 U)
Evening dose: One-third the total dose (0.33 $\times$ 35 U) = 11.5 U (administer 12 U of intermediate-acting insulin)
If using an intermediate- and short-acting combination, further calculate:
Intermediate-acting: 0.50 $\times$ 11.5 U = 5.75 U (administer 6 U)
Short-acting: 0.50 $\times$ 11.5 U = 5.75 U (administer 6 U)

Three-Dose Regimen. In this regimen, an intermediate-acting insulin or a combination of intermediate- and short-acting insulin is given before breakfast, a dose of a short-acting insulin is given before dinner, and a dose of an intermediate-acting is given at bedtime. This regimen may prevent nighttime hypoglycemia but may not provide adequate noontime coverage.

Four-Dose Regimen. In this regimen, considered to be intensified therapy, a short-acting insulin is given 30 minutes before each meal, and an intermediate-acting insulin is given at bedtime. This regimen allows better flexibility with the timing of meals. The dosage of the short-acting insulin is determined before each meal by blood glucose monitoring.

Snacks

Because the goal of treatment is to maintain normal or near-normal blood glucose levels, timing of food intake and insulin peak times must be considered. Meals should be scheduled to correspond with the peak times of the insulin being administered. Food needs to be taken at these times to prevent hypoglycemia. Snacks may be needed between meals and at bedtime to prevent episodes of hypoglycemia. This need varies among individuals and with the insulin regimen used. Individualized meal planning is needed to identify appropriate food choices for meals and snacks according to the patient's prescribed diet. Additional rapidly absorbable carbohydrate snacks (e.g., fruit, fruit juice, bread products, whole milk) may be needed before and during exercise to prevent hypoglycemia.

Complications of Insulin Therapy

Hypoglycemia is a common problem in patients with type 1 diabetes mellitus. Hypoglycemia resulting from an excess of exogenous insulin is referred to clinically as an *insulin reaction*. It is usually caused by a missed meal or unexpected exercise, but there may be no known precipitating event. Daytime episodes are easily recognized and quickly treated; nighttime episodes may produce night sweats and early-morning headaches. See Chapter 18, Section 1 for further discussion of hypoglycemia.

Hyperglycemia manifests as one of two phenomena. The *dawn phenomenon* is an early morning rise in plasma glucose believed to be due to a nocturnal surge of growth hormone. It may be prevented with a late evening dose of intermediate-acting insulin. The *Somogyi phenomenon* is a rebound morning hyperglycemia following a nighttime episode of hypoglycemia. It is prevented by providing an adequate late evening snack. Somogyi occurs rarely in adults. See Chapter 18, Section 1 for further discussion of hyperglycemia.

Hypersensitivity reaction may occur. Localized reactions include itching and erythema at the injection site. Systemic effects include rash, dyspnea, tachycardia, angioedema, and anaphylaxis. Lipodystrophy is marked by atrophy and dimpling and hypertrophy at the injection site.

Drug Interactions

Use of beta-blockers, salicylates, anabolic steroids, alcohol, MAO inhibitors, clofibrate, tetracyclines, guanethidine, and oxytetracycline may increase the effects of insulin. Corticosteroids, dextrothyroxine, diltiazem, dobutamine, epinephrine, and estrogens may decrease the effects of insulin. Thiazide diuretics, furosemide, phenytoin, and thyroid preparations increase glucose levels. Beta-blockers and propranolol mask signs and symptoms of hypoglycemia.

 CLINICAL PEARLS

- Insulin absorption may be increased with the occurrence of hypoglycemia from massages, saunas, and warmth from baths and the environment.
- Store insulin vials in current use at room temperature. Administer insulin at room temperature.
- Cough syrups and liquid cold medications that contain sugar may raise blood glucose levels.
- Regular exercise improves glycemic control by promoting weight loss, decreasing insulin resistance, and improving glucose utilization.
- For patients with gout, the sulfonylurea of choice is acetohexamide (Dymelor), which has uricosuric properties.
- Insulin cannot be given orally. It is destroyed by proteolytic enzymes in the GI tract. Insulin is given only parenterally, either subcutaneously or IV.
- Regular insulin is the insulin of choice for acute situations, such as diabetic ketoacidosis. It is the only rapid-acting preparation that can be given IV.
- An extra vial of insulin should always be kept in the refrigerator, and a vial of regular (short-acting) insulin should be kept on hand for emergencies.
- Insulin preparations are stable at room temperature for months if temperature extremes are avoided.

Respiratory Drugs

Section 10   Joanne M. Bullard

OVERVIEW

Many pharmacologic agents are used in the management of respiratory disorders. An ongoing nursing responsibility is to ensure the safe and effective administration of these medications. This section covers the basics of respiratory drug categories, as well as the proper use of metered-dose inhalers (MDIs).

PRINCIPLES OF CARE

Respiratory pharmacology can be divided into two categories: drugs used to relieve bronchial obstruction, as occurs in asthma, chronic obstructive pulmonary disease (COPD), and cystic fibrosis; and drugs used to relieve rhinitis, cough, and colds. Drugs used to relieve bronchial obstruction include bronchodilators and inhaled agents (i.e., anti-inflammatory agents and bronchodilators). Drugs used in the treatment of rhinitis, cough, and colds include antihistamines, antitussives, decongestants, expectorants, and mucolytics.

DECISION-MAKING
Pharmacology for Bronchial Obstruction
Bronchodilators

Bronchodilators are agents used to treat and prevent bronchoconstriction caused by asthma, acute and chronic bronchitis, and emphysema. They are also used in the treatment of allergic reactions and exercise-induced broncho-constriction. There are two major groups of bronchodilators: beta-2 adrenergic agonists and methylxanthines (also called xanthines).

Beta-2 agonists stimulate beta receptors to relax the smooth muscles in the bronchioles of the lungs. These agents are usually given by inhalation for acute and chronic bronchoconstriction.

Xanthines promote relaxation of bronchial smooth muscle cells by blocking the inactivation of cyclic adenosine monophosphate (cAMP, the body's natural bronchodilator) and by blocking prostaglandin and adenosine (the body's natural bronchoconstrictors) at the receptor sites. Xanthines are now considered second-line bronchodilators and are used less frequently than before. Xanthines are available in oral and IV forms. The oral xanthine theophylline is normally used for long-term treatment of chronic respiratory disorders, whereas ami-nophylline, a theophylline salt, is administered IV to treat acute bronchocon-striction. Table 12-10-1 gives dosages and information about selected bron-chodilators.

Inhalant Medications

These medications include bronchodilators (adrenergic and anticholinergic) and anti-inflammatory agents (corticosteroids and mast cell stabilizers).

Inhaled Adrenergic Bronchodilators (Sympathomimetics)

Inhaled adrenergic bronchodilators are used primarily for the treatment and prevention of bronchospasm. These sympathomimetics mimic the effects of the sympathetic nervous system (SNS), specifically stimulating the beta-2 receptors of the smooth muscles of the bronchi, causing relaxation. Relaxation of the smooth muscles results in bronchodilation of the bronchial tree, thus reducing airway resistance and increasing the lungs' vital capacity. Stimulation of the SNS also results in tachycardia, palpitations, and increased blood pressure, common side effects to monitor for during the administration of these drugs.

Anticholinergic Bronchodilators

The only anticholinergic recommended for bronchodilation is ipratropium bromide (Atrovent). This drug is used in the maintenance treatment of COPD as a single agent or in combination with an adrenergic bronchodilator, because the two drugs have different mechanisms of action. Ipratropium produces bronchodilation by blocking the acetylcholine receptors of the parasympathetic nervous system (PNS), which cause bronchoconstriction, thus allowing for relaxation of the smooth muscles of the bronchial tree. Adverse effects are usually mild and related to PNS blockade, such as dry mouth.

Inhaled Corticosteroids

Inhaled steroids are used in the management of chronic asthma and for symptom management of rhinitis. Inhaled steroids are administered on a fixed schedule. They inhibit inflammatory responses in the airways and decrease mucus production. They are not useful in acute bronchospasm.

Mast Cell Stabilizers

Mast cell stabilizers are anti-inflammatory medications that prevent reactions to allergens by blocking the release of chemical mediators of the epithelial and eosinophil cells, thus suppressing an allergic response. Mast cell stabilizers block inflammation, whereas steroids suppress inflammation. These medica-

Table 12-10-1. Selected Bronchodilators

CLASSIFICATION	USUAL DOSE/DAY MAXIMUM/DAY	DRUG INTERACTIONS	ADVERSE EFFECTS	NURSING IMPLICATIONS
Beta-2 Agonists		Use of other sympathomimetic bronchodilators may cause possible additive effects that could lead to hypertensive crisis.	CNS: Tremor, anxiety, nervousness, restlessness, convulsions, weakness, dizziness, vertigo, headache, hallucinations	For epinephrine:
Albuterol (Proventil)	2–4 mg PO q 6–8 hr Sustained-release (SR): 4–8 mg PO bid			• Administration of SC injection solution by the IV route may cause fatal hypertension or cerebral hemorrhage.
Ephedrine sulfate	25–50 mg PO q 3–4 hr Maximum: 150 mg/24 hr		Cardiovascular: Palpitations, hypertension, hypotension, bradycardia, reflex tachycardia	• Use of a tuberculin syringe provides greater accuracy in measurement of SC dosages.
Epinephrine (Adrenalin, Bronkaid)	Aqueous solution (epinephrine 1:1000): 0.2–0.5 mL SC; may repeat after 20 min if necessary	Use of monoamine oxidase inhibitors or tricyclic antidepressants may potentiate action on the vascular system.	Eye: Blurred vision, dilated pupils GI: Nausea, vomiting Other: Muscle cramps, hoarseness, hypersensitivity reaction	• Rotate injection sites to prevent tissue necrosis. • Epinephrine may cause elevate blood glucose levels.
Susphrine	Aqueous solution (epinephrine 1:200): 0.1–0.3 mL SC; may repeat after 4 h if necessary	Concurrent use of beta-blockers may negate the therapeutic effects of the adrenergic agonist.		Instruct the patient: • To use caution if driving or performing tasks requiring mental alertness
Metaproterenol (Alupent, Metaprel)	10–20 mg q 6–8 hr			• That tremor is the most common adverse effect associated with oral administration
Terbutaline sulfate (Brethine)	2.5–5 mg PO q 6–8 hr Maximum: 15 mg/day 0.25 mg SC, may repeat after 15–30 min if necessary q 4–6 hr			• Not to use over-the-counter drugs without a physician's approval

Methylxanthines				
Theophylline (Slo-Phyllin, SloBid, Theo-Dur, Theolair-SR, Somaphyllin) Aminophylline (approximately 80% theophylline content)	Note: All dosages are based on ideal body weight. Oral: Acute symptoms Initial dose: 5–6 mg/kg Maintenance: 3–4 mg/kg/day in three or four divided doses (q 6–8 hr) Maximum: 400 mg/day Chronic therapy Initial dose: 6–8 mg/kg Maximum: 400 mg/day in 3–4 divided doses (q 6–8 hr) Then may be increased 25% q 2–3 days to a maximum of 13 mg/kg/day or 900 mg, whichever is less	Cigarette smoking may lower theophylline plasma concentration significantly. Beta-blockers, cimetidine, tacrine, zileuton, ciprofloxacin, erythromycin, oral contraceptives, and caffeine may increase theophylline plasma levels. Theophylline may lower lithium levels.	Nausea, vomiting, anorexia, headache, flushing, insomnia, nervousness, irritability, palpitations, tachycardia, blood pressure changes Reactions associated with plasma theophylline levels: <20 µg/mL: Few side effects 20–25 µg/mL: Nausea, vomiting, diarrhea, headache, insomnia, restlessness >30 µg/mL: Severe dysrhythmias, convulsions, death	Monitor drug levels for evidence of toxicity (>20 µg/mL). The therapeutic theophylline plasma level is 10–20 µg/mL. Instruct the patient to: • Take with milk or food to decrease gastric upset. • Avoid caffeine, colas, chocolate, and coffee to decrease side effects of drug • Avoid charbroiled foods (may reduce the half-life to 50%). • Avoid smoking. • Take the drug only as prescribed, do not exceed the prescribed dose. • Avoid use of over-the-counter drugs without a physician's approval. • Avoid chewing or crushing any SR formulations • Take the drug at the same time every day.

▉ **Table 12-10-2.** Using a Metered-Dose Inhaler

INSTRUCTIONS	RATIONALE
1. Remove the cap from the inhaler and shake the inhaler vigorously for 3–5 seconds.	Shaking mixes the medication.
2. If the MDI was not used recently or is new, release a dose into the air.	Releasing a dose before using tests the spraying ability of the canister.
3. In a standing or sitting position, slightly tilt the head back.	This position and tilting the head back open the airways, allowing the medication to enter the lungs rather than the mouth.
4. Exhale through the mouth until no more air can be expelled.	Exhalation empties the lungs.
5. Hold the canister upright, place the mouthpiece in your mouth and seal with your lips. Alternative position: Open your mouth and hold the mouthpiece 1 to 2 inches in front of your mouth.	
6. Start to inhale slowly through your mouth, pressing down on the inhaler as you begin to breathe in.	This releases the medication directly into airways.
7. Continue inhaling for 3–5 seconds, then try to hold your breath for 10 seconds (or as long as possible).	Taking a full breath and holding 10 seconds allows the medication to be absorbed.
8. Release the canister and exhale.	
9. If prescribed, repeat the dose after waiting 1 minute.	Waiting may allow the second dose to enter the lungs further.

MDI, metered dose inhaler.

tions are used only in prophylaxis of allergic rhinitis and bronchial asthma, because they have no bronchodilating actions.

Administration of Inhalants/Metered-Dose Inhalers

An MDI is a hand-held canister designed to release a measured dose of an inhalant medication. When the pressurized canister is pushed against a dispensing valve, a specific dose is released in the form of a fine powder, mist, or aerosol spray for inhalation. Table 12-10-2 provides details on the use of MDIs.

Patient Teaching

- Administer bronchodilator inhalers at least 5 minutes before steroid inhalers. This facilitates opening of the airways and enhances penetration of the medication into the lungs.
- After using a corticosteroid MDI, rinse the mouth with water. This reduces or prevents the occurrence of oropharyngeal candidiasis, hoarseness, or dry cough.
- Rinse the mouthpiece and cap of the MDI daily with warm, running water. Clean them weekly with mild soap and warm water. Allow to air dry. Cleaning maintains patency and minimizes bacterial exposure.
- To determine whether the canister is full or empty, float the canister in a bowl of water. A full canister will sink to the bottom; an empty canister will float.
- Discard the MDI after 3 months, even if not empty. This ensures that active medication is available for use.

Pharmacology for Rhinitis, Cough, and Colds

Antihistamines

Histamine$_1$ (H_1) is a chemical mediator released during cell injury that produces vasodilatation, increased capillary permeability, and hyperemia, which account for the signs and symptoms of inflammation. Antihistamines reverse vasodilatation and decrease capillary permeability at inflammatory sites. They are used primarily to relieve the symptoms of irritated, swollen mucus membranes and mucosal edema associated with allergic responses, especially allergic rhinitis.

Antihistamines are H_1 receptor antagonists that block the action of histamine by competing for H_1 receptor sites on effector cells. They do not prevent or decrease the amount of histamine released. Histamine acts as a neurotransmitter in the CNS. Some antihistamines produce sedative and antiemetic effects by blocking the effects of the neurotransmitter. Antihistamines also block the muscarinic receptors of the parasympathetic nervous system, causing anticholinergic adverse effects such as dizziness, blurred vision, dry mouth, nausea, vomiting, and urinary retention.

There are two generations of antihistamines; both have similar actions. The first-generation antihistamines have six subclasses. The degree of sedative, antiemetic, anticholinergic, and gastrointestinal (GI) adverse effects vary within the subclasses. Second-generation H_1 antagonist (blocker) drugs produce less CNS adverse effects, such as sedation, because they do not cross the blood-brain barrier. Table 12-10-3 gives dosages and information about selected antihistamines.

Antitussives

Antitussives are used to suppress ineffective or dry, persistent cough that interferes with sleep. They may be either opioid or nonopioid agents and may act either centrally or locally. Centrally acting antitussives suppress the cough reflex by acting on the cough center in the medulla, inhibiting the cough response receptors, whereas locally acting antitussives act directly at the site of irritation. Locally acting agents may be in the form of lozenges, syrups, and gargles. Table 12-10-4 gives dosages and information for antitussives.

Decongestants

Decongestants are used for the symptomatic relief of congestion caused by allergies, coryza, rhinitis, and sinusitis. Decongestants stimulate the alpha-adrenergic receptors of the smooth muscle of the blood vessels to release NE, which causes vasoconstriction. This results in reduced blood flow, reduced fluid exudation, and shrinkage of the mucus membranes, decreasing nasal congestion. Decongestants are available in oral preparations and nasal drops or sprays. Table 12-10-5 provides dosages and drug information.

Expectorants

Expectorants are agents that make the cough more productive. They stimulate mucus glands to increase production of respiratory tract secretions, which decreases the viscosity of the secretions. The increased production and decreased viscosity of the secretions make them easier to expectorate. Table 12-10-6 gives dosages and drug information.

Text continued on page 403.

Table 12-10-3. Selected Antihistamines

CLASSIFICATION	USUAL AND MAXIMUM DAILY DOSES	DRUG INTERACTIONS	ACTIONS AND COMMON SIDE EFFECTS	NURSING IMPLICATIONS
First-Generation			Alkylamines:	Assess for possible contraindications to antihistamines, including hypersensitivity, acute asthma, narrow-angle glaucoma, impaired gastrointestinal (GI) motility or obstruction, prostatic hypertrophy, bladder neck obstruction, or heart disease.
Brompheniramine	4–8 mg PO qid Sustained-release (SR): 8–12 mg PO bid Maximum: 40 mg/day	Central nervous system depressants (intensity and antipsychotic agents, barbiturates, procarbazine, phenothiazides, sedative-hypnotics, alcohol) increase sedative effects	• Minimal sedative effects • Moderate anticholinergic effects • No antiemetic effects Common side effects include drowsiness, dry mouth, and urinary retention Paradoxical excitation may occur.	
Chlorpheniramine (Chlortrimeton)	2–4 mg PO q 6–8 hr (SR): 8–12 mg PO q day Maximum: 24 mg/day			Administer oral antihistamines (except astemizole) with meals or milk to decrease GI side effects. Administer astemizole 1 hour before or 2 hours after meals. Absorption decreases 60% when taken with food.
Dexchlorpheniramine (Polaramine)	2 mg PO q 4–6 hr SR: 4–6 mg PO bid	Monoamine oxidase inhibitors and tricyclic antidepressants increase anticholinergic effects		
Ethanolamines			Ethanolamines:	Instruct the patient to avoid alcohol when taking oral antihistamines.
Clemastine fumarate (Tavist)	1.34 mg PO bid Maximum: 8.04 g/day	Antihistamines decrease the effects of anticoagulants	• Moderate to high sedative effects • Significant anticholinergic effects • Significant antiemetic effects • Low incidence of GI side effects	Encourage fluid intake of 2000–3000 mL/day. Increased fluid intake helps thin respiratory secretions.
Diphenhydramine (Benadryl)	25–50 mg PO q 6–8 hr IM/IV: 10–50 mg to a single dose of 100 mg Maximum: 400 mg/day		Common side effects include drowsiness, dry mouth, and tachycardia.	Instruct the patient not to drive or perform tasks requiring mental alertness when taking antihistamines with sedative effects.
Ethylenediamines			Ethylenediamines:	Tell the patient that gum or hard candy may help relieve dry mouth.
Tripelennamine (P8Z)	25–50 mg PO q 4–6 hr SR: 100 mg PO q 12 hr Maximum: 600 mg/day		• Moderate sedative effects • High incidence of GI distress • Minimal anticholinergic effects • Minimal antiemetic effects	Instruct the patient to discontinue antihistamines at least 4 days before skin testing to avoid false-negative results.

Common side effects include dry mouth, nose, and throat, drowsiness, epigastric distress, anorexia, nausea and vomiting, and constipation.

Instruct the patient not to chew or crush any SR formulations.

Phenothiazines

Promethazine (Phenergan) — 12.5 mg PO q day or 25 mg PO at bedtime

Phenothiazines:
- Marked antihistamine activity
- Potent sedative, antiemetic, and anticholinergic effects

Common side effects include sedation, drowsiness, blurred vision, and dry mouth.

Piperazines

Cetirizine (Zyrtec) (second generation) — 5–10 mg PO q day

Piperazines:
- Low to no sedative effects
- Low to no anticholinergic effects
- No antiemetic effects

Common side effects include drowsiness, sedation, and headache.

Piperidines

Azatadine maleate (Optimine) (second generation) — 1–2 mg PO bid

Cyproheptadine (Periactin) — 4 mg PO tid
Maximum: 0.5 mg/kg/day

Piperidines:
- Moderate antihistamine activity
- Low to moderate sedative effects
- Moderate anticholinergic effects
- No antiemetic effects

Common side effects include drowsiness and dry mouth.

Second-Generation

Astemizole (Hismanal) — 10 mg PO q day

Azatadine maleate (Optimine) — 1–2 mg PO bid

Cetirizine (Zyrtec) — 5–10 mg q day

Fexofenadine (Allegra) — 60 mg PO bid

Loratadine (Claritin) — 10 mg PO q day

Second Generation:
- Moderate to high antihistamine activity
- Low to no sedative effects
- Low to no anticholinergic effects
- No antiemetic effects

Common side effects include drowsiness, sedation, and headache.

Table 12-10-4. Antitussives

CLASSIFICATION	USUAL AND MAXIMUM DAILY DOSES	DRUG INTERACTIONS	ADVERSE EFFECTS	NURSING IMPLICATIONS
Opioid (Sedating)				
Codeine	10–20 mg PO q 4–6 hr Maximum: 120 mg/day	Opioids potentiate the effects of monoamine oxidase (MAO) inhibitors, alcohol, and other central nervous system (CNS) depressants	At low doses, the risks of dependency and adverse effects are reduced.	Instruct the patient to notify the physician of any cough lasting longer than 1 week.
Hydrocodone bitartrate (Hycodan)	5–10 mg PO q 4–6 hr Maximum: 15 mg/day		Antitussives may cause dizziness or drowsiness, CNS depression with very large doses, gastrointestinal (GI) upset, nausea, constipation, and abdominal discomfort.	Instruct the patient to take codeine with milk or food to decrease GI upset. Instruct the patient not to drive or perform tasks that require mental alertness.
Nonopioid (Nonsedating)				
Benzonatate (Tessalon Perles)	100 mg PO tid Maximum: 600 mg/day	Dextromethorphan given with MAO inhibitors can cause excitation and hyperpyrexia.	Benzonatate may cause choking and anesthetic effect if contents of the perle (soft capsules) dissolve in the mouth.	Instruct the patient to swallow the perle whole, not to chew it.
Dextromethorphan (Benylin DM)	10–20 mg PO q 4 hr or 30 mg PO q 8 hr Sustained-release: 60 mg PO bid Maximum: 120 mg/day			Dextromethorphan is the drug of choice. It is the only antitussive with research-proven efficacy, and is comparable to codeine but without codeine's addictive or respiratory depressive effects.
Other				
Diphenhydramine (Benadryl)	See Table 12–10–3.			Although an antihistamine in the treatment of coughs associated with the common cold or irritants, diphenhydramine also has proven efficacy as an antitussive.

400

Table 12-10-5. Decongestants

CLASSIFICATION	USUAL DOSE	DRUG INTERACTIONS	ADVERSE EFFECTS	NURSING IMPLICATIONS
Ephedrine sulfate (nasal drops) (Ephedsol, Vantronol)	Maximum: 2–4 drops qid for 3–4 consecutive days	Monoamine oxidase (MAO) inhibitors, furazolidone, and methyldopa increase vasopressor effects.	Decongestants may cause mild central nervous system stimulation: restlessness,	Instruct the patient not to use nasal sprays for longer than 3–5 days to decrease the likelihood of rebound
Ipratropium bromide (nasal spray) (Atrovent)	2 sprays (0.03% solution) in each nostril bid–tid	Phenothiazides and guanethidine decrease vasopressor effects.	tremors, nervousness, headache, blurred vision, insomnia; with	congestion. Instruct the patient to gently blow the
Naphazoline (nasal spray/drops) (Privine)	1–2 drops or sprays (0.025%) q 3–6 hr for no more than 3–5 days	Theophylline increases the risk of arrhythmias.	higher doses: tachycardia, palpitations, lightheadedness,	nose before using nose drops or sprays to ensure open passages.
Oxymetazoline (nasal spray/drops) (Afrin, Allerest)	2–4 drops or 2–3 sprays in each nostril in morning and at bedtime	Tricyclic antidepressants increase cardiovascular effects.	nausea, and vomiting, especially if the patient is hypersensitive to adrenergic drugs.	For the instillation of nose drops: Instruct the patient to position the head in a lateral, low position to keep
Phenylephrine HCl (nasal drops) (Neo-Synephrine, Sinex)	2–3 drops (0.25–0.5%) in each nostril q 3–4 hr	Urine acidifiers decrease decongestant effects.	Adverse effects are less likely with topical use.	medication from entering the throat. For inhalation of nasal sprays:
Phenylpropanolamine HCl (Contac, Triaminic)	25 mg PO q 4 hr or sustained-release (SR): 75 mg q 12 hr	Urine alkalinizers increase decongestant effects.	Prolonged use (more than 3–5 days) may cause rebound nasal congestion to occur, chronic	Instruct the patient to bend the head slightly forward with the spray nozzle inserted in the nostril (do not occlude
Pseudoephedrine (Sudafed, Sudafed SA, Drixoral)	Maximum: 150 mg/day 60 mg PO q 4–6 hr SR: 120 mg bid		rhinitis, and possible ulceration of nasal mucosa. Rebound congestion is not seen	the nostril) and to sniff briskly. After use, rinse the dropper or spray tip with hot water to prevent
Tetrahydrozoline (nasal spray/drops) (Tyzine)	2–4 drops/spray (0.05% solution) each nostril no more than q 3 hr		with pseudoephedrine. Nasal drops or sprays may cause stinging, burning, or excessive	contamination of the solution. Instruct the patient not to chew or crush SR medications.
Xylometazolin (nasal spray/drops) (Otrivin)	2–3 drops/spray (0.1%) q 8–10 hr Maximum: 3 doses/day		drying of the nasal mucosa and hypersensitivity.	Because of their short duration and rapid effect, decongestants may become habit forming.

401

Table 12-10-6. Expectorants and Mucolytics

CLASSIFICATION	USUAL AND MAXIMUM DAILY DOSES	DRUG INTERACTIONS	ADVERSE EFFECTS	NURSING IMPLICATIONS
Expectorants Guaifenesin (Glycerol guaiacolate, Robitussin)	200 mg (2 tsp) q 4 hr Maximum: 2.4 g/day	Concurrent use of heparin may increase the risk of hemorrhage from inhibition of platelet adhesiveness by guaifenesin.	Low incidence of gastric upset, nausea, vomiting, drowsiness, urticaria, and rash. Concurrent use of caffeine may cause increased nervousness, tremors, or insomnia.	Instruct the patient to: • Follow each dose with a full glass of water • Increase fluid intake to 2–3 L/day to increase mucus viscosity • Notify a health care provider if cough lasts for longer than 1 week or is accompanied by a rash, fever, or persistent headache • Avoid milk and milk products to minimize production of secretions
Mucolytics Acetylcysteine (Mucomyst)	Nebulization: 1–10 mL of 20% solution or 2–20 mL of 10% solution q 4–6 hr Instillation: 1–2 mL of 10–20% solution q 1–4 hr in tracheostomy	Incompatible with antibiotics; must be administered separately.	Nausea, vomiting, rhinorrhea, rash, fever, drowsiness, chest tightness, bronchoconstriction, increased bronchospasm with asthma, respiratory tract irritation, increased bronchial secretions	Have suction equipment available for removal of increased secretions if the patient is unable to expectorate. May cause stickiness on face (with face mask or nebulizer use). Wash the face with water to remove. Medication has a disagreeable, "rotten egg" odor that soon disappears.

Mucolytics

Mucolytics are used to liquefy thick, tenacious secretions in the respiratory tract. The mucolytics act by disrupting the chemical bonds between mucoprotein molecules, causing the secretions to liquefy. Only two agents are recommended for use as mucolytics: hypertonic saline and acetylcysteine (Mucomyst). Both are given via inhalation or direct instillation into the airway. See Table 12–10–6 for dosages and drug information.

Combination Therapy

Many respiratory tract medications are available in combination forms without a prescription. Combination medications should be used only when multiple symptoms exist. If relief of only one symptom is desired, the preferred drug is a single-entity formulation, because the dosage may be individualized. Most combination respiratory medications commonly contain an analgesic (acetaminophen), an antihistamine (chlorpheniramine or diphenhydramine hydrochloride), and a nasal decongestant (phenylpropanolamine or pseudoephedrine). Some may also contain an antitussive (dextromethorphan) or an expectorant (guaifenesin). Various combinations of ingredients are available to provide the best possible symptom relief.

 CLINICAL PEARLS

○ Antihistamines are effective in reducing hay fever symptoms in 75% to 95% of patients with seasonal allergic rhinitis.

○ A productive cough is a protective measure that removes excessive secretions or foreign bodies from the respiratory tract and generally should not be suppressed.

○ Milk and milk products increase mucus production and should be avoided to minimize secretions.

○ Use of caffeine with decongestants may cause increased nervousness, tremors, or insomnia. Caffeine is present in cola drinks, coffee, tea, and chocolate. Decaffeinated colas, coffee, and teas are recommended.

○ Sustained-release forms of oral medications should not be chewed or crushed. If scored, they may be broken in half, but not chewed or crushed. Chewing or crushing interferes with the release mechanism.

Sedatives

Section 11   Robert Mead

OVERVIEW

The pharmacologic actions of sedatives depress the CNS. They are often referred to as antianxiety or anxiolytic drugs. Sleep-inducing drugs in this category are known as hypnotics. Sedatives are commonly prescribed to treat anxiety disorders, sleep disorders, and substance withdrawal and when acting-out or aggressive behavior occurs, such as in acutely ill patients with infections, electrolyte imbalances, or chronic disease states.

The etiology of anxiety disorders is unknown. Abnormalities in multiple neurochemical pathways, including cholecystokinin, dopamine, gamma-amino-butyric acid, norepinephrine (NE), and serotonin (5-HT), play a role in the development of the various anxiety disorders. The drugs most commonly prescribed to treat anxiety are benzodiazepines, followed by barbiturates and nonbenzodiazepines/nonbarbiturates.

PRINCIPLES OF CARE

The prompt treatment of anxiety is necessary to assist in the improvement of a patient's other concomitant disease states. Recognizing the symptoms of an anxiety disorder is the first step toward effective treatment. After secondary causes of anxiety (i.e., other disease states or medications) are ruled out or corrected or modified, an antianxiety agent is selected. Usually oral therapy is appropriate, but parenteral therapy may be needed in those patients who cannot take anything by mouth or who need a rapid onset of action.

Proper rest is essential for the patient's condition to improve. An oral sedative/hypnotic agent can be useful in helping the patient get to sleep and remain asleep. A parenteral sedative agent can also be used to stop or decrease aggressive or combative behavior. This will help the patient to recover, improve the surroundings for other patients, and decrease the risk of staff injuries.

After sedative administration, the patient must be monitored for signs and symptoms of overdose (e.g., decreased respiration rate, altered heart rate, level of consciousness) and for the effectiveness of the medication. Proper documentation in the nurse's notes and the patient's medication administration record will prevent the unintended administration of extra doses before the next scheduled dose is due or the next "as needed" dose can be given.

DECISION-MAKING

Many sedative agents are used to treat anxiety. Table 12-11-1 reviews the available agents.

Ensuring adequate rest while hospitalized is a key component to recovery. The patient may need a medication to help him or her fall asleep and/or

Table 12-11-1. Medications Used to Treat Anxiety

TYPE AND GENERIC NAME	TRADE NAME	USUAL DAILY DOSAGE (mg/day)
Benzodiazepines		
Alprazolam	Xanax	0.75–4
Chlordiazepoxide	Librium	10–200
Clorazepate	Tranxene	3.75–90
Diazepam	Valium	2–40
Halazepam	Paxipam	20–160
Lorazepam	Ativan	0.5–10
Oxazepam	Serax	10–120
Prazepam	Centrax	20–60
Nonbenzodiazepines		
Buspirone	BuSpar	15–60
Diphenhydramine	Benadryl	25–200
Hydroxyzine	Vistaril	50–400
Propranolol	Inderal	80–160

Table 12-11-2. Medications Used to Treat Sleep Disorders

TYPE AND GENERIC NAME	TRADE NAME	USUAL BEDTIME DOSAGE (mg)
Barbiturates		
Pentobarbital	Nembutal	50–100
Secobarbital	Seconal	100
Pentobarbital 50 mg + secobarbital 50 mg	Tuinal	1 capsule
Benzodiazepines		
Estazolam	ProSom	1–2
Flurazepam	Dalmane	15–30
Quazepam	Doral	7.5–15
Temazepam	Restoril	15–30
Triazolam	Halcion	0.125–0.25
Other Agents		
Chloral hydrate	Noctec	500–2000
Doxylamine	Unisom	25–100
Trazodone	Desyrel	50–100
Zaleplon	Sonata	5–10
Zolpidem	Ambien	5–10

remain asleep (Table 12-11-2). Aggressive or combative behavior places the patient and staff at increased risk of harm and does not help the healing process. Table 12-11-3 provides information on medications that can be helpful in controlling this behavior. Table 12-11-4 lists medications used as sedatives for diagnostic procedures.

All of these agents have various adverse effects. The most common adverse effects are oversedation, ataxia, and confusion, especially in debilitated elderly patients. The antihistamine agents (e.g., diphenhydramine, doxylamine, hydroxyzine) can also cause anticholinergic adverse effects, which include dry

Table 12-11-3. Medications Used to Treat Aggressive/Combative Behavior

TYPE AND GENERIC NAME	TRADE NAME	USUAL DOSAGE
Benzodiazepines		
Chlordiazepoxide	Librium	IM: 25–100 mg; may repeat every 6 h (to a maximum of 300 mg/day)
Diazepam	Valium	IM/IV*: 2–10 mg; may repeat every 1–4 hr
Lorazepam	Ativan	IM/IV*: 1–2 mg
Antipsychotic Agents		
Chlorpromazine	Thorazine	IM: 25–50 mg; may repeat in 1 h
Haloperidol	Haldol	IM/IV*: 2–5 mg; may repeat hourly
Trifluoperazine	Stelazine	IM/IV*: 1–2 mg; may repeat every 4–6 h (to a maximum of 10 mg/day)
Other Agents		
Diphenhydramine	Benadryl	IM/IV*: 25–50 mg; may repeat every 6–8 h
Hydroxyzine	Vistaril	IM: 25–100 mg; may repeat every 6 h
Propofol	Diprivan	IV infusion for ICU sedation, 5–50 µg/kg/min

*For IV administration, give slowly over 1–3 minutes. (Long-acting injectable formulations cannot be given IV; they must be given only by deep IM.)

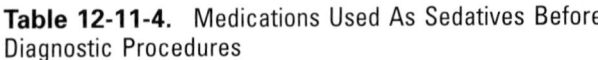

Table 12-11-4. Medications Used As Sedatives Before Diagnostic Procedures

GENERIC NAME	TRADE NAME	USUAL DOSAGE
Benzodiazepines		
Chlordiazepoxide	Librium	Adults: 50–100 mg IM/IV
Diazepam	Valium	Adults: 2–10 mg IM/IV
Lorazepam	Ativan	Adults: 1–2 mg IM/IV
Midazolam	Versed	Adults: 1–5 mg IV
		Children: 0.025–0.1 mg/kg IV
Other Agents		
Droperiderol	Inapsine	Adults: 1.25–2.5 mg IM/IV
Fentanyl	Sublimaze	Adults: 1–2 μg/kg IV
Propofol	Diprivan	Adults Initiation:
		100–150 μg/kg/min IV
		Maintenance: 25–50 μg/kg/min IV

mouth, constipation, urinary hesitancy, tachycardia, and confusion. The antipsychotic agents can cause extrapyramidal side effects (e.g., dystonic reaction, akathisia) after even a single dose, though this is not common. Prolonged use of benzodiazepines or barbiturates can lead to dependence.

Symptoms of withdrawal can occur after 4 to 6 weeks of therapy. These are more likely if the medication is short-acting (e.g., alprazolam, oxazepam), taken regularly for more than 3 months, and discontinued abruptly. Onset can be within 1 to 10 days. Symptoms include increased anxiety, sensory disturbances (e.g., photophobia, hypersomnia), difficulty concentrating, dizziness, vomiting, confusion, delirium, seizures, and even death. A large overdose of a benzodiazepine can cause ataxia, hypotonia, coma, and, rarely, death. The effects of a benzodiazepine overdose can be reversed by giving flumazenil (Romazicon) 0.5 to 1 mg IV every few minutes for a total of 5 mg. In the event of resedation, repeated doses can be given every 20 minutes. If no response is noted within 5 minutes of giving the cumulative dose of 5 mg, then the major cause of the sedation is not likely a benzodiazepine, and giving more flumazenil will not be effective. No reversal agents are available to treat the symptoms of barbiturate overdose.

Drug-drug interactions can occur with any of the sedative agents (Table 12-11-5). Sedative agents given on an "as needed" basis or as a one-time dose have a low potential for drug-drug interactions.

Sedative agents used to treat sleep disorders should have a fast onset of action and a short elimination half-life. Agents with long elimination half-lives (e.g., chlordiazepoxide, diazepam, flurazepam, temazepam) should not be used to treat sleep disorders, to avoid the possibility of the patient waking up in the morning still sedated and feeling "hung over."

Antipsychotic agents used as single doses or on an "as needed" basis would have a low potential for drug-drug interactions, although administering them with other CNS depressants could cause an increase in CNS depression.

 CLINICAL PEARLS

○ Many adverse effects and potential drug-drug interactions are with sedative agents. Care must be taken to ensure that the correct dose of the sedative is

Table 12-11-5. Potential Drug-Drug Interactions

SEDATIVE AGENT	CAN POTENTIALLY INTERACT WITH THE FOLLOWING DRUG(S)	WHICH CAN RESULT IN
Barbiturates	Alcohol Benzodiazepines Monoamine oxidase inhibitors Narcotic analgesics	Increased central nervous system (CNS) depression (sedation, coma, respiratory depression, death)
Barbiturates	Rifampin (Rifamycin)	Decreased serum barbiturate levels
Barbiturates	Beta-blockers Carbamazepine (Tegretol) Clonazepam (Klonopin) Felodipine (Plendil) Corticosteroids	Decreased serum levels of these agents, resulting in decreased pharmacologic effects
Barbiturates	Doxorubicin (Adriamycin) Doxycycline (Vibramycin) Fenoprofen (Nalfon) Griseofulvin (Grisactin) Oral contraceptives Quinidine (Quinidex) Theophylline (Slo-Bid) Verapamil (Calan, Isoptin) Warfarin (Coumadin)	Decreased serum levels of these agents, resulting in decreased pharmacologic effects
Benzodiazepines	Cimetidine (Tagamet) Disulfiram (Antabuse) Fluoxetine (Prozac) Isoniazid (INH) Ketoconazole (Nizoral) Metoprolol (Lopressor) Oral contraceptives Propoxyphene (Darvocet) Propranolol (Inderal) Valproic acid (Depakene)	Increased serum benzodiazepine levels, which can increase the pharmacologic and toxic effects of benzodiazepines
Benzodiazepines	Alcohol Barbiturates Narcotic analgesics	Increased CNS depression (sedation, coma, respiratory depression, death)
Benzodiazepines	Digoxin (Lanoxin) Phenytoin (Dilantin)	Increased serum digoxin or phenytoin levels
Benzodiazepines	Levodopa (Sinemet)	Decreased antiparkinsonian effect of levodopa

given, to avoid the untoward effects of the medication. Abrupt discontinuation of chronic barbiturate or benzodiazepine therapy can cause a withdrawal syndrome with potentially severe symptoms, including confusion, delirium, seizures, and possibly death.

○ Overdosage of many of these agents can result in negative outcomes. Suicide attempts with these agents result in a long period of potential danger, especially involving the central nervous and respiratory systems. Patients who receive an intentional or unintentional overdose require immediate care and intense monitoring.

○ Elderly patients are more prone to the adverse effects from the sedative agents because of age-related declines in liver and kidney function and protein binding. Starting with the lowest dose available should help prevent adverse effects. The elderly are also more likely to experience drug-drug interactions because of the larger number of concomitant medications that many use. Again, care must be taken to avoid potential drug-drug interactions.

○ Most of the sedative agents pose serious risks to pregnant or nursing women. These agents should not be used in these patients.

Adrenocorticosteroids

Section 12   Jan Addy

OVERVIEW

The use of adrenocortical steroids has steadily increased over the last 2 decades, making them one of the most prescribed medications today. Commonly called *corticosteroids*, these medications act both physiologically and pharmacologically. The nurse's responsibility is to correctly administer, monitor the effects of, and evaluate the intended outcome of these medications.

Adrenocorticosteroid agents should not be confused with the term "anabolic steroids" currently sold on the street. Anabolic steroids are androgenic hormones that are used illegally to increase strength, muscle mass, and ultimately athletic performance.

PRINCIPLES OF CARE
Physiology

The adrenal cortex produces three classes of steroid hormones: glucocorticoids (which affect carbohydrate metabolism and other processes), mineralocorticoids (which modulate salt and water balance), and androgens (which contribute to the expression of sexual characteristics). The term "corticosteroid" is limited to glucocorticoids and mineralocorticoids; androgens are not discussed here.

Categories of Corticosteroids
Mineralocorticoids—Regulators of Mineral Salts

Mineralocorticoids naturally occur in the body in the form of aldosterone, which helps maintain water and electrolyte balance. Secreted from the adrenal gland, aldosterone acts primarily in the renin-angiotensin system of the kidney to facilitate the reabsorption of sodium and water from the distal tubule of the nephron. Aldosterone functions in the control of blood pressure, blood pH, and serum potassium level.

Mineralocorticoids exert a primarily physiologic effect by influencing the renal processing of sodium, potassium, and hydrogen through the release of aldosterone from the adrenal cortex. The pharmacologic use of mineralocorticoids is for replacement therapy in adrenal insufficiency.

Fludrocortisone (Florinef Acetate) is the oral replacement mineralocorticoid used to treat adrenal insufficiency and salt-losing androgenital syndrome. This potent mineralocorticoid also exerts a weak glucocorticoid action. The drug is given only orally and is available in 0.1-mg tablets.

Glucocorticoids—Regulators of Carbohydrate, Protein, and Fat Metabolism

Glucocorticoids influence how the body regulates carbohydrate, protein, and fat metabolism. Physiologic effects can occur naturally from the release of glucocorticoids from the healthy adrenal gland or from the administration of exogenous glucocorticoids in low doses to treat adrenal hormone deficiency seen in adrenal disorders. Pharmacologic effects of glucocorticoids are produced when high levels of these agents are administered to treat certain disorders unrelated to problems associated with adrenocortical functioning (e.g., allergic reaction, asthma, or inflammatory states). Tables 12-12-1 and 12-12-2 summarize the physiologic and pharmacologic effects and clinical manifestations of glucocorticoids.

The body's synthesis and release of glucocorticoids are regulated through a negative feedback loop. In times of demand or stress, the hypothalamus secretes corticotrophin-releasing factor (CRF), which acts on the anterior pituitary to cause the release of adrenocorticotrophin hormone (ACTH). ACTH stimulates the adrenal cortex to release cortisol (the pharmaceutical equivalent to hydrocortisone) and other glucocorticoids needed by the body for energy. Once cortisol quantities are sufficient, the hypothalamus and pituitary gland stop further release of CRF and ACTH. Hence, elevated cortisol levels halt further glucocorticoid synthesis, thereby keeping plasma levels of glucocorticoids within an appropriate range. Stimulators of ACTH include stress (surgery, illness, infection, trauma, anxiety, and hypoglycemia) and basal stimulation. Basal stimulation follows a circadian rhythm, which peaks in the early morning and reaches its lowest point late in the evening. When glucocorticoid levels are low (as can occur normally in the evening hours), the hypothalamus is stimulated to begin the process again to replace these vital hormones. Subsequently, when levels are high, the body reacts by suppressing the release of CRF from the hypothalamus, thereby stopping the release of glucocorticoids.

Glucocorticoids are used primarily in three important therapeutic actions: anti-inflammatory, antiallergic, and antistress. In addition, glucocorticoids affect carbohydrate metabolism by stimulating gluconeogenesis (formation of glucose from noncarbohydrate sources such as protein or fat), decreasing glucose utilization by body cells, and promoting glucose storage as glycogen. Increased glucose production results in the breakdown of protein (catabolism) and leads to poor wound healing, muscle wasting, and limited hair growth.

Fat (lipid) metabolism is also affected through the breakdown of triglycerides, increased lipolysis (fat breakdown), and increased fat storage in the adipose tissue. These mechanisms increase glucose levels in the body.

Glucocorticoids are used in the treatment of rheumatic disorders (e.g., rheumatic arthritis), collagen disorders (e.g., systemic lupus erythematosus), allergic disorders (e.g., dermatitis, drug hypersensitivity, allergic asthma, serum sickness), dermatologic disorders (e.g., Stevens-Johnson syndrome, severe psoriasis, poison oak/ivy/sumac, urticaria), ophthalmic disorders (e.g., optic neuritis, uveitis), gastrointestinal disorders (e.g., ulcerative colitis), hematologic disorders (e.g., autoimmune hemolytic anemia, thrombocytopenic purpura), and other disorders including nephrotic syndrome, gout, hypercalcemia, multiple sclerosis, anaphylactic shock, adrenal insufficiency, cerebral edema, and acute spinal cord injuries.

Text continued on page 413.

Table 12-12-1. Physiologic Effects of Glucocorticoids and Their Clinical Manifestations

PHYSIOLOGIC EFFECTS OF GLUCOCORTICOIDS (OCCUR AT LOW DOSES)	CLINICAL MANIFESTATIONS
Metabolic	
Carbohydrate: Glucose availability is increased by forming glucose from noncarbohydrate sources, reducing the use of glucose from peripheral cells and storing glucose in the form of glycogen in the liver.	Elevated serum glucose levels (80–120 mg/dL) (usually seen only in long-term treatment, patients with diabetes mellitus, and patients with beginning stages of insulin resistance)
Protein: Breakdown of protein in the form of amino acids helps produce more glucose in the body.	Muscle wasting, thinning of the skin, negative nitrogen balance, decreased bone matrix (osteoporosis), development of skin changes (purple striae, ecchymosis, acne) (occurs in long-term therapy)
Fat: Breakdown of fat occurs.	Redistribution of fat; "moon face," "buffalo hump," central obesity (potbelly)
Cardiovascular	
Depressed levels cause capillaries to become more permeable and decrease the ability of vessels to constrict.	Falling blood pressure, increased circulating red blood cells, and decreased polymorphonuclear leukocytes, eosinophils, basophiles, and monocytes
Fluids and Electrolytes	
Limited mineralocorticoid activity may occur, causing aldosterone to act on the collecting ducts of the kidney to promote sodium and water reabsorption and potassium and hydrogen excretion.	Mild edema Decreasing potassium levels, leading to hypokalemia (may occur in long-term therapy)
Central Nervous System (CNS)	
CNS excitability increases.	Insufficiency: Mood changes, depression, lethargy, and irritability Excess: "Steroid psychosis" (rare), generalized excitation, euphoria
Stress Response	
Increased amount of glucocorticoids, along with epinephrine, is released during stress. The higher the stress, the more pronounced the clinical manifestations.	Hypotension Hypoglycemia Circulatory collapse; death

Table 12-12-2. Pharmacologic Effects of Glucocorticoids and Their Clinical Manifestations

PHARMACOLOGIC EFFECTS OF GLUCOCORTICOIDS (OCCUR AT HIGH DOSES)	CLINICAL MANIFESTATIONS
Metabolic	
Carbohydrate: Glucose availability is significantly increased.	Hyperglycemia, polyuria, polyphagia, polydipsia
Protein: Accelerated rate of protein breakdown helps increase serum glucose more rapidly.	Increased muscle wasting and skin thinning; increased destruction of bone matrix, making the patient prone to fracture development; more pronounced negative nitrogen balance
Fat: Accelerated rate of fat breakdown and redistribution occurs.	More prominent "buffalo hump," "moon face," appearance changes, and development of Cushing's syndrome
Anti-inflammatory/Immunosuppressant	
Suppression of the immune system by depressing the proliferation of lymphocytes, which decrease the normal immune component of the inflammatory process. The inflammatory response is interrupted by inhibiting chemical mediators needed for a normal response. The infiltration of phagocytes is depressed.	Increased susceptibility to infection; inflammatory response is altered; possibly sepsis without high fever
Fluids and Electrolytes	
Sodium and water are retained; potassium is excreted, producing a limited mineralocorticoid response.	Hypernatremia Hypokalemia and acidosis Peripheral edema Increased blood pressure Manifestations of fluid volume excess

411

Table 12-12-3. Pretherapy Nursing Assessment and Teaching for Patients Taking Corticosteroid Medications

PRETHERAPY ASSESSMENT	PRETHERAPY PATIENT TEACHING
1. Record general baseline data: vital signs, weight, skin color and temperature, orientation, reflexes, muscle tone, pulses, skin pigmentation, bowel sounds, liver palpation, and usual intake and output 2. Review laboratory data: complete blood count (CBC), serum electrolytes, serum cholesterol and triglyceride counts, and urinalysis. 3. Review medical history for previous use of corticosteroids and conditions for which the medication was ordered. Check to be sure the patient does not have a condition that would contraindicate the use of corticosteroids. 4. Review medical and family history for actual and potential conditions that might cause specific side effects of drug therapy (e.g., diabetes mellitus).	1. Explain the actions, dosages, side effects, and rationale for taking corticosteroids. Be sure that the patient has a good understanding of these medications. 2. Explain why the medication is given cautiously to certain patients (e.g., pregnant and lactating patients, patients with diabetes and peptic ulcers). 3. Explain importance of taking medication regularly/daily and not skipping doses. 4. Explain that corticosteroid medications should be weaned and not abruptly stopped for any reason. 5. Explain side effects of drug and that the degree of side effects is influenced by the dosage and duration of drug therapy. Patients on long-term therapy are more likely to experience more severe side effects.

Table 12-12-4. Teaching Points for Patients Taking Corticosteroid Medications

CORTICOSTEROID	PATIENT TEACHING
Mineralocorticoids	1. Stress the importance of adhering to the prescribed dosage. 2. Stress the danger of sudden withdrawal of medication. 3. Explain clinical manifestations of adrenal insufficiency (e.g., nausea, dyspnea, fever, hypotension, myalgia, hypoglycemia). 4. Instruct the patient to monitor weight daily. 5. Urge the patient to monitor blood pressure frequently. 6. Include teaching points for the glucocorticoids.
Glucocorticoids	1. Instruct the patient to take the oral daily dose before 9 AM with food or milk. 2. Stress the importance of adhering to the prescribed dosage and weaning schedule. 3. Emphasize the importance of avoiding infections and notifying a physician immediately if infection is suspected. 4. Instruct the patient on long-term therapy to obtain periodic ophthalmic examinations. 5. Urge the patient to contact a physician when experiencing severe and/or consistent gastric distress. 6. Instruct a patient known to be at risk for diabetes mellitus to monitor blood glucose level. 7. Encourage the patient to use a firm mattress and bedboard and to report persistent backache or chest pain. 8. Inform female patients that menstrual irregularities may occur, especially with long-term therapy. 9. Instruct the patient to carry information describing the condition being treated, the drug, and the dosage at all times. 10. Instruct the patient to limit salt intake and to eat potassium-rich foods. 11. Instruct the patient not to abruptly withdraw medications. 12. Instruct the patient to report a weight gain of 5 lb. (2.25 kg) in 1 week. 13. Explain that mood swings or changes commonly occur during high-dose, long-term therapy.

Among the many glucocorticoids available, the most commonly used include hydrocortisone, prednisone, dexamethasone, and beclomethasone. Glucocorticoids can be administered orally, IV, IM, intranasally, rectally, topically, and by inhalation.

DECISION-MAKING

As nurses' responsibility for the management of patient care increases, so must their knowledge of pharmacology. Pretherapy assessment and teaching are essential to increase compliance and reduce morbidity (Tables 12-12-3 and 12-12-4). Table 12-12-5 presents information on nursing interventions and monitoring for patients taking corticosteroids. The nurse also needs to be familiar with side effects and drug interactions, to help prevent serious prob-

Table 12-12-5. Nursing Interventions and Monitoring for Patients Taking Corticosteroid Medications

NURSING INTERVENTIONS	PATIENT MONITORING
1. Dosages ordered for once a day should be given before 9 AM to mimic normal diurnal corticosteroid levels and minimize hypothalamic-pituitary-adrenal (HPA) suppression.	1. Be alert for possible hypersensitivity reactions with parenteral use.
2. Administer antacids between meals to minimize the risk of peptic ulcer.	2. Assess mental status for any changes in mood and affect.
3. Give oral doses with food or milk to reduce gastrointestinal symptoms.	3. Monitor vital signs for hypertension.
4. Give divided doses 6–12 hr apart.	4. Monitor intake and output for fluid retention.
5. Administer corticosteroid inhalers only as prescribed. Too frequent use may cause rebound laryngeal spasms. Keep inhalers clean with mouthwash to prevent possible fungal infections.	5. Monitor weight. A weight gain of 5 lb. (2.25 kg) in 1 week should be reported immediately.
6. Topical corticosteroids should be administered only as prescribed. Be sure the skin is clean and dry before application. Sterile technique should be used if the skin is not intact. Use caution with occlusive dressings, because these can enhance systemic availability of the drug. Avoid contact with the eyes and mucous membranes.	6. Monitor serum sodium, calcium, and potassium levels for any changes from the mineralocorticoid action of some of these drugs.
7. Nasal passages should be cleared before intranasal administration.	7. Monitor serum glucose level for hyperglycemia from increased glucose availability.
8. Mix all liquid and parenteral doses thoroughly and prepare according to the manufacturer's instructions.	8. Monitor pediatric patients closely; long-term corticosteroid therapy may suppress normal growth pattern.
9. Administer the IM form in a large muscle (gluteal). Prevent tissue trauma by rotating sites.	9. Monitor for possible drug interactions.
10. Arrange to taper doses when discontinuing high-dose or long-term therapy. Do not abruptly withdraw these medications.	10. Closely monitor for clinical manifestations of infection. Patients on corticosteroid therapy may not be febrile because of a suppressed anti-inflammatory response.
11. The lowest possible dosage should be prescribed to reduce side effects.	

Table 12-12-6. Common Side Effects of Mineralocorticoids and Glucocorticoids

DRUG CLASSIFICATION	PRIMARY ACTIONS	MAJOR SIDE EFFECTS
Mineralocorticoids (Fludrocortisone acetate)	Sodium and water resorption Blood pressure regulation Regulation of blood pH Regulation of potassium levels	Fluid retention, hypokalemia (muscle weakness, paresthesias, fatigue), flushing, sweating, headache, hypertension, circulatory collapse, thrombophlebitis, and embolism (also see side effects of glucocorticoids)
Glucocorticoids (Prednisone, hydrocortisone, dexamethasone)	Anti-inflammatory and antiallergic effects Blood pressure regulation Carbohydrate metabolism Protein metabolism Fat metabolism Antistress effects	Central nervous system: Headache, vertigo, mood swings, convulsions, "steroid psychosis" Cardiovascular: Congestive heart failure, hypertension, edema (from electrolyte imbalances) Endocrine: Growth suppression in children, Cushing's syndrome, menstrual suppression/irregularities, hyperglycemia, carbohydrate intolerance, thrombophlebitis, arrhythmias Gastrointestinal: Peptic ulcers, pancreatitis, ulcerative esophagitis, abdominal distention Skin: Petechiae, ecchymoses, poor wound healing, hirsutism, urticaria, fatty redistribution in subcutaneous layers, striae, abnormal pigmentation Musculoskeletal: Loss of muscle mass and weakness, osteoporosis, avascular necrosis of joints, vertebral compression, spontaneous fractures Ocular: Increased intraocular pressure, glaucoma, exophthalmos, cataracts Other: Fluid retention, weight gain, increased appetite, hypokalemia, hypocalemia, alkalosis, negative nitrogen balance, renal stones, leukocytosis, masked signs of infection, fat embolism

Note: The incidence of adverse reactions and side effects increases with higher dosages and increased duration of therapy.

414

Table 12-12-7. Drug Interactions of Corticosteroids

1. The dosage requirements for antidiabetic agents, isoniazid, salicylates, and oral anticoagulants may need to be increased.
2. The risk for gastric ulceration increases when corticosteroids are used with nonsteroidal anti-inflammatory drugs (NSAIDs).
3. Concomitant use of corticosteroids and non–potassium-sparing diuretics and/or amphotericin B can lead to severe hypokalemia.
4. Digitalis toxicity can occur with the use of corticosteroids as a result of potassium loss.

lems associated with the administration of adrenocorticosteroids (Tables 12-12-6 and 12-12-7).

 CLINICAL PEARLS

○ A patient who is on long-term oral corticosteroid therapy (greater than 2 weeks) and is NPO (for any reason) must be given their daily dosage of corticosteroids by another route (i.e., IV, IM injection).
○ Because steroids mask the clinical manifestations of infection, be sure to assess the patient thoroughly for potential infection or infectious states.
○ Immediately report any clinical manifestations of Cushing's syndrome (i.e., hyperglycemia, protein wasting and muscle loss, scanty hair growth, poor wound healing, redistribution of body fat, obesity of torso, "moon face," ecchymoses, cervical dorsal fat pad, sodium retention, potassium loss, edema, mood swings, psychoses/depression, hypertension).
○ Do not skip doses of corticosteroids. If a dose is missed, do not double the next scheduled dose.
○ Encourage the patient to increase the intake of potassium-rich foods and to limit salt intake.
○ Parenteral forms should be diluted according to the manufacturer's guidelines.
○ Weigh the patient daily, and closely monitor intake and output.
○ Closely monitor glucose levels in patients with diabetes.

 RESOURCES

Agency for Health Care Policy and Research (AHCPR): 800-358-9295 or www.ahcpr.gov
American Academy of Allergy, Asthma, and Immunology: www.aaaai.org
American Academy of Neurology: 612-623-8115 or www.aan.com
American Diabetes Association: www.diabetes.org
American Dietetic Association: www.eatright.org
American Epilepsy Society: 860-586-7505 or e-mail aesmain@aol.com
American Gastroenterological Association: www.gastro.org/
American Heart Association: Anticoagulants: www.americanheart.org/Heart_and_Stroke_A_Z_Guide/antico.html
American Lung Association: 800-LUNG-USA (800-586-4872) or www.lungusa.org
American Pain Society (APS): 847-375-4715 or www.ampainsoc.org
American Society of Pain Management Nurses (ASPMN): 800-34-ASPMN or www.aspmn.org

Anticoagulation Forum: www.acforum.org/
Anxiety Disorders Association of America: 301-231-9350 or www.adaa.org
Association for Professionals in Infection Control and Epidemiology (APIC): www.apic.org
Centers for Disease Control and Prevention: www.cdc.gov
Crohn's & Colitis Foundation of America (CCFA): 800-932-2423 or www.ccfa.org
Crohn's & Colitis Foundation of Canada (CCFC): 800-920-5035 or www.ccfc.org
Epilepsy Centers at Washington University: www.wustl.edu.epilepsy/pediatric
Epilepsy Foundation of America: 301-459-3700 or www.efa.org
Epilepsy International: E-mail: Info@epi
Lennox Gastaut Syndrome Support Group: E-mail: wssg@foden.net
National Alliance for the Mentally Ill: (800) 950-6264 or www.nami.org
National Alliance for Research on Schizophrenia & Depression: 516-829-0091 or www.mhsource.com/advocacy/narsad/
National Cancer Institute's International Cancer Care Information Center: www.icic.nci.nih.gov
National Depressive & Manic-Depressive Association: 800-826-3632 or www.ndmda.org
National Institute of Diabetes and Digestive and Kidney Disease: www.niddk.nih.gov
National Institute of Neurological Disorders and Stroke, National Institutes of Health: ninds.nih.gov
National Jewish Center for Immunology and Respiratory Medicine: www.njc.org
National Mental Health Association: 703-684-7722 or www.nmha.org
Oncology Nursing Society (ONS): 412-921-7373 or www.ons.org
Resource Center for State Cancer Pain Initiatives: 608-265-4013
Society of Gastroenterology Nurses & Associates: 800-245-7462 or www.sgna.org
www.AmericasDoctor.com
www.anxiety.mentalhealth.net
www.anxietynetwork.com
www.cdc.gov
www.depression.com
www.helix.com
www.intelihealth.com
www.nursepdr.com
www.onhealth.com

III

Applied Decision-Making

chapter 13

Respiratory

Asthma

Section 1   Judy Kaye ■ Mia Smitt

 OVERVIEW

Asthma is chronic inflammatory disease of the airways with episodic symptomatic exacerbations. It is frequently referred to as reactive airway disease. Approximately 5.4% of the U.S. population (16 million) has asthma. Prevalence is higher in African Americans and Hispanics than in caucasians. The prevalence of asthma increased by 75% from 1980 to 1994 in the United States, with corresponding increases in mortality. Annual associated health care costs are estimated to be more than 6 billion dollars. Asthma morbidity and mortality continue to rise despite medical treatment.

 PATHOPHYSIOLOGY

Asthma is a disease of the airways characterized by hyperresponsiveness of the airways to a multiplicity of stimuli, resulting in widespread bronchoconstriction that reverses either spontaneously of as a result of therapy. Stimuli (e.g., infectious agents, environmental allergens) cause the exaggerated inflammatory response that leads to bronchospasm.

There are two broad classifications of asthma, extrinsic and intrinsic. In clinical practice, these distinctions are not easily made and there may be some overlap in most patients. *Extrinsic*, or allergic, asthma is the most common form. It is triggered by such environmental allergens as air pollution, tobacco smoke, animal dander, dust, insect excrement, pollens, molds, chemicals, foods, and drugs. Initial exposure causes the plasma cells to produce antigen-specific IgE antibodies that bind with the mast cells in the airways. Subsequent exposures then cause mast cell degranulation and the release of inflammatory mediators. Inflammation and bronchoconstriction develop within minutes of the exposure and usually resolve within minutes to hours. There is a personal or family history of allergies.

Intrinsic, or nonatopic, asthma has no known allergic cause. The patient has no personal or family history of allergies and no elevation of serum IgE levels. Respiratory infections, emotional stress, cold dry air, and environmental irritants are known to trigger episodes. Bronchoconstriction may develop several days following the exposure and can last for days to months.

Other subtypes include drug-induced asthma and exercise-induced asthma. Common drug offenders include aspirin, beta agonists, and nonsteroidal anti-inflammatory agents. *Exercise-induced* asthma is more common in young adults. Episodes resolve about 30 minutes after cessation of activity.

Status asthmaticus is a severe episode of asthma lasting for days to weeks without improvement.

The major pathologic feature of all types of asthma is a hyperresponsiveness of the airways in response to inflammation. Inflammatory mediators are released that cause bronchial smooth muscle constriction, vascular congestion, increased vascular permeability and edema, the production of thick mucus, and impaired ciliary function, resulting in airway obstruction. The thick mucus produces plugs that cause air trapping with resultant airway hyperinflation distal to the plug, which increases the work of breathing. Hyperventilation and respiratory alkalosis follow. Without intervention, ventilation is further compromised, with the development of hypoxia and respiratory acidosis. Respiratory failure and death may occur.

Several theories explaining airway hyperirritability have been postulated, but the basic mechanism remains unknown.

 ## SIGNS AND SYMPTOMS

In asthma, the airways are sensitive and often swollen or inflamed to some degree, even when no symptoms are evident. During an episode, the patient complains of decreased activity tolerance and shortness of breath with a tightness or pain across the chest. There may be a nonproductive cough, sometimes with a sensation of anxiety and suffocation. The patient will report a history of allergies, exposure to certain environmental conditions, stress, recent illness, or medication use.

Physical examination usually reveals the patient in an upright position or leaning forward to maximize air space. There may or may not be a change in level of consciousness. Cyanosis of the nail beds or circumoral area may be noted. Other manifestations may include diaphoresis, distended neck veins, hypotension, and hypoxemia (measured by pulse oximetry). A nonproductive cough and tachycardia are common. Chest auscultation usually reveals a short inspiratory period with prolonged expiratory wheezes in more than one lung field. There may be fine or coarse rales and/or rhonchi and decreased breath sounds and movement. Use of accessory muscles of respiration muscles may be seen.

Based on the stepwise approach to diagnosing and managing the illness, asthma is classified as mild intermittent, mild persistent, moderate persistent, or severe persistent.

Mild intermittent asthma symptoms occur less than two times a week. Peak expiratory flow (PEF) is normal between exacerbations. Exacerbations are brief (lasting from a few hours to a few days), and the intensity may vary. Nighttime symptoms occur less that three times a month. PEF is greater than or equal to 80% predictability, with variability below 20%.

Mild persistent symptoms occur more than two times a week but less than 1 time a day. The exacerbations may affect activity and nighttime symptoms occur greater than two times a month. PEF is greater than or equal to 80% of predicted, with variability of 20% to 30%.

Moderate persistent symptoms occur daily despite the daily use of beta-agonist inhalers. Exacerbations may last for days and occur two or more times a week, affecting activity. Nighttime symptoms occur more than once a week. PEF is 60% to 80% of predicted, with variability greater than 30%.

Severe persistent asthma involves continual symptoms with frequent severe exacerbations and limited physical activity. Nighttime symptoms occur frequently. The PEF is less than 60% of predicted, with variability greater than 30%.

DIAGNOSTIC CRITERIA

Chest x-rays may show hyperinflation during an acute episode but will be normal between exacerbations. Pulmonary function tests may show decreased forced expiratory volume (FEV) and flow rates. These usually improve with immediate acting bronchodilators. During the asthma episode, arterial blood gases may show a mild decrease in oxygen saturation (PaO_2) and carbon dioxide saturation ($PaCO_2$), but this is transient. Increased $PaCO_2$ may indicate severe obstruction; acidosis may indicate impending respiratory failure. The white blood cell count with differential likely reveals increased eosinophils and serum IgE related to the allergic component of the disease.

INTERVENTIONS

The stepwise approach to controlling asthma is frequently used when prescribing medications (Table 13-1-1). (See also Chapter 12, Section 10.)

For *mild intermittent asthma*, short-acting beta-2 agonists are used only as needed to control symptoms. If these drugs are needed more than twice a week, the patient may need reassessment and reclassification. Ipratropium may be used for patients who cannot tolerate beta-2 agonists. A short course of oral steroids may be needed occasionally.

Mild persistent asthma is treated with a low-dose inhaled steroid (to inhibit the inflammatory response) or with cromolyn or nedocromil. A leukotriene modifier or sustained-release theophylline may be considered.

In *moderate persistent asthma*, symptoms may be controlled with a medium-dose inhaled steroid and/or a long-acting inhaled beta-2 agonist. An oral beta-2 agonist may be helpful in controlling nighttime symptoms. Sustained-release theophylline may be considered.

Severe persistent asthma is treated with a high-dose steroid and a long-acting inhaled beta-2 agonist or a long-acting oral beta-2 agonist or sustained-release theophylline. An oral steroid is considered when symptoms remain uncontrolled or exacerbations are severe.

Heliox, a helium and oxygen mixture, was first used to treat acute asthma symptoms in 1935, but was discontinued with the use of epinephrine and then the beta-2 agonist drugs. Its use resumed in 1989 when published studies indicated that it improves ventilation, lowers airway pressure and resistance, and decreases dyspnea in patients with severe asthma who are refractory to the initial use of inhaled beta-2 agonists. Studies continue to measure the effectiveness of heliox as a short-term treatment strategy.

Some studies have shown improved asthma control with the use of montelukast (Singulair), a leukotriene modifier, and loratadine (Claritin), a histamine receptor agonist. Leukotriene modifiers are not indicated for acute exacerbations, but studies suggest that they may be beneficial in controlling acute symptoms.

Oxygen therapy may be used during an acute exacerbation at 2 to 4 L/min via nasal cannula. Endotracheal intubation and mechanical ventilation may be needed in severe cases.

Primary nonpharmacologic interventions include patient and caregiver edu-

Table 13-1-1. Medications Used to Treat Asthma

Short-acting Inhaled Beta-2 Agonist Bronchodilators
Albuterol (Proventil, Ventolin) (MDI)
Pirbuterol (Maxair) (MDI)
Terbutaline (Brethaire) (MDI)
Bitolterol (Tornalate) (MDI or nebulizer)
Possible side effects: Tachycardia, skeletal muscle tremor

Long-acting Beta-2 Agonist Bronchodilators
Salmeterol (Serevent) (MDI)
Albuterol (Volmax) (oral)
Metaproterenol (Alupent) (MDI or oral)
Possible side effects: Tachycardia, skeletal muscle tremor, hypokalemia, hyperglycemia

Inhaled Steroids
Beclomethasone (Beclovent, Vanceril, Vanceril DS) (MDI)
Fluticasone (Flovent, Flovent Rotodisc) (dry powder inhaler)
Flunisolide (AeroBid) (MDI)
Triamcinolone (Azmacort) (MDI)
Budesonide (Pulmicort) (dry powder inhaler)
Possible side effects: Cough, oral candidiasis, dysphonia, systemic adverse effects with high doses

Systemic Steroids
Prednisone, prednisolone, methylprednisolone
Possible side effects: Muscle weakness, cataracts, osteoporosis, weight gain, gastrointestinal
  irritation, hypertension, Cushing's syndrome

Inhaled Anticholinergics
Ipratropium bromide (Frequently given in combination with beta-2 agonists. Also used in beta-
  blocker–induced bronchospasm and for patients intolerant of beta-2 agonists.)
Possible side effects: Dry mouth, thickened respiratory secretions, cough, bronchospasm, blurred
  vision

Nonsteroidal Anti-inflammatory Inhalers
Cromolyn (mast cell stabilizer) (MDI)
Possible side effects: Bad taste in mouth, throat irritation
Nedocromil (anti-inflammatory) (MDI)
Possible side effects: Bad taste in mouth, bronchospasm, cough

Leukotriene Modifiers
Montelukast (Singulair) (oral)
Zafirlukast (Accolate) (oral)
Zileuton (Zyflo) (oral)
Possible side effects: Liver toxicity with zileuton, drug-drug interactions with zafirlucast

Methylxanthines
Theophylline (Uniphyl, Uni-Dur, Theo-24) (oral tablets, sustained-release)
Possible side effects: Restlessness, dizziness, seizures, tachycardia, drug-drug interactions,
  gastrointestinal upset, insomnia, hyperglycemia, hypokalemia

MDI, metered-dose inhaler.

cation regarding those triggers to which the patient is susceptible. Awareness and avoidance of such triggers will help prevent an asthma exacerbation. Teaching about the proper use of medications and adherence to the prescribed schedule also encourages the patient to take ownership of the illness and control symptoms and exacerbations.

If a *metered-dose inhaler* (MDI) is prescribed, teach the patient how to use it correctly (see Chapter 12, Section 10). The spacer (if one is used) is attached to the MDI, and the open end of the MDI is put into the patient's mouth. The medication is sprayed once into the spacer. The patient takes a deep breath, holds it for 10 seconds, and then breathes out into the spacer. The patient then takes a second deep breath without spraying and follows the same directions as for the first breath. The process is repeated if the dose is for two puffs. The canister and spacer should be cleaned with warm running water at least once daily.

Breathing exercises and the use of a peak flow meter (PFM) should be taught. Deep diaphragmatic breathing can produce a significant reduction in the intensity of asthma symptoms and in medication use. Peak flow meters are available at low cost and sometimes can be obtained free from some pharmaceutical companies. The patient and the caregiver determine the target zones and monitor the peak expiratory flow several times a day. Results should be reviewed with the primary care provider on a regular basis.

To use a peak flow meter correctly, the pointer is set to zero. While standing (or sitting tall in a straight-backed chair) and holding the PFM horizontally, the patient takes a slow, deep breath and puts the unit in the mouth with the lips held tightly around the mouthpiece. The patient then blows out as hard and as fast as possible. The reading is recorded. After 15 to 30 seconds, these steps are repeated twice more. The patient will establish his personal best when symptoms are controlled (i.e., no bronchoconstriction, inflammation, or excess mucus) and compare future scores with this.

Anxiety can be a major component in an asthma exacerbation. Emotional support given to the patient and caregiver can relieve anxiety, increase relaxation, and promote acceptance of teaching. Guided imagery, music, and art therapy and other relaxation strategies can help to control an exacerbation and prevent an occurrence.

 COMMUNITY CARE

The patient's home should be assessed for triggers and environmental hygiene implemented. Air pollution also can trigger attacks, thus awareness of current air quality should be emphasized.

Diet is important, with an emphasis on balanced meals and adequate hydration. Excessive weight increases dyspnea and exercise intolerance.

Patient and caregiver teaching with return demonstrations (use of PFM, MDI, and spacers) at follow-up visits can enhance the quality of life for patients with asthma.

An individualized "action plan" should be developed. This should be written with the patient and caregiver and include specific actions to take when certain signs and symptoms occur. Breathing exercises, medications, and alternative interventions are listed. Telephone numbers of the patient's primary health care provider, home health nurse, emergency room, ambulance service, and appropriate family members or friends should be included.

The patient should be referred to social service agencies as needed to ensure access to adequate medications, equipment, and follow-up health care services.

 PROGNOSIS

Most patients have mild intermittent to mild persistent asthma. The symptoms will be well controlled, especially if the onset occurred during childhood or early adolescence. Adult-onset asthma tends to be more persistent and more severe, but the exacerbations become milder over time. Fewer than 5% of patients have life-threatening disease, and death usually results from a sudden and very severe exacerbation.

 CLINICAL PEARLS

○ Bubble-blowing (i.e., soap bubbles with a wand) can be an effective technique to slow respiratory rate, ease effort, and reduce anxiety. Instruct the patient and caregiver to inhale deeply and, with pursed lips, to slowly and deliberately exhale, blowing through the bubble wand.

○ Breath-activated inhalation powder delivery systems are available as an alternative to traditional MDIs.

○ To determine the fullness of the MDI canister, float the canister in a bowl of water. If the canister is more than 70% full, it will lie on its side below the surface of the water. If it is 30% to 70% full, it will float vertically just under the surface. If it is 15% to 30% full, it will float at an approximate 30-degree angle with half of the canister above the surface of the water and the valve end submerged. If it is less than 15% full, most of the canister will float above the surface at a 30-degree angle with a corner of the valve exposed.

○ A used MDI should be discarded as soon as the number of doses specified on the container is used.

NURSING PROBLEM/ DIAGNOSIS	NURSING INTERVENTIONS CLASSIFICATION (NIC)
Risk for bronchospasm/Risk for impaired gas exchange	Medication Management Respiratory Monitoring Oxygen Therapy
Deficient knowledge regarding disease process and the use of medications	Teaching: Disease Process Teaching: Prescribed Medication

Bronchitis

Section 2   Judy Kaye ▪ Mia Smitt

 OVERVIEW

Bronchitis is an inflammation of the tracheobronchial tree with excessive mucus production. It is classified as acute or chronic. *Acute bronchitis* (AB) is a common problem produced by various organisms, most often viruses. The incidence is higher in smokers, the very young, and the very old and rises during the winter months. A productive cough is the most common symptom. Treatment is aimed at relieving the symptoms. Codeine-containing cough suppressants and bronchodilators may be necessary. Antibiotics are helpful only if the source is bacterial.

Chronic bronchitis (CB), along with emphysema, fall into the category of *chronic obstructive pulmonary disease* (COPD), a condition that produces chronic obstruction to air flow. CB affects habitual smokers and those with exposure to air pollution, fumes, dust, and frequent bacterial or viral infections. The incidence increases in adults over age 40. Incidence is higher in men than in women.

CB is defined clinically as excessive bronchial secretions and productive cough for at least 3 months in 2 consecutive years. CB can be further subclassified by severity as *simple* CB (productive cough with no evidence of airflow obstruction), *chronic asthmatic bronchitis* (hyperreactive airways with intermittent bronchospasm), and *obstructive* CB (the development of chronic airflow obstruction).

 PATHOPHYSIOLOGY

AB in otherwise healthy adults (without underlying respiratory disease) is an inflammatory process causing hypersecretion of mucus. It usually results from a viral infection, such as influenza, parainfluenza, or adenovirus. Varying degrees of bronchospasm may occur with subsequent hypoxemia.

In CB, permanent inflammatory changes occur in the lower respiratory tract related to chronic irritation by inhaled substances or frequent infections. The bronchial wall thickens and the mucous glands hypertrophy and dilate, leading to increased mucus in the airways. As the disease progresses, normal defenses become impaired, and bronchial scarring of small bronchi causes airway obstruction and weakening of the bronchial walls. Alveolar gas exchange becomes impaired, leading to hypoxemia (causing cyanosis) and an increase in carbon dioxide retention. Hypoxemia causes pulmonary vasoconstriction, resulting in pulmonary hypertension. The pulmonary hypertension strains the right ventricle, as it must work harder to eject blood into the constricted pulmonary vessels. The right ventricle eventually fails, leading to right-sided heart failure, called *cor pulmonale*.

AB can occur as an acute exacerbation of CB known as *acute bacterial exacerbations of chronic bronchitis* (AECB). Unlike AB, these exacerbations are most commonly caused by bacterial pathogens and increase in severity as the disease progresses.

 SIGNS AND SYMPTOMS
Acute Bronchitis

Patients with acute viral bronchitis present with cold symptoms including an occasional low-grade fever ($<101°F$), rhinorrhea, sore throat, a burning sensation in the chest, fatigue, and persistent, usually nonproductive, cough. There may be an increase in sputum production, especially in patients who smoke. Occasionally, a patient may complain of generalized myalgias secondary to coughing. Signs and symptoms of acute bacterial bronchitis include a more productive cough with the aforementioned symptoms, fever, and retrosternal pain aggravated by protracted coughing. Wheezes and rhonchi are found on physical examination, and the pharynx is often erythematous.

The acute symptoms usually last from 3 to 7 days, but the cough may persist for up to 6 weeks in patients with any underlying lung disease.

Chronic Bronchitis

Cough and sputum production is a key symptom. Patients with CB have a high number of leukocytes in their sputum even when not suffering an exacer-

Table 13-2-1. Chronic Bronchitis and Emphysema

SIGNS AND SYMPTOMS	CHRONIC BRONCHITIS	EMPHYSEMA
Body size	Overweight—corpulent and/or edematous	Thin
Age at diagnosis	40–65	50–75
Smoking history	Usually long	Usually long
Cough	Common	Little
Sputum	Much—mucoid and mucopurulent	Little
Breath sounds	Wheezing, rhonchi	Decreased
Respiratory infections	Frequent	Infrequent
Chest radiograph	Normal inflation, rounded diaphragm, increased heart size, increased bronchovascular markings	Hyperinflation, flattened diaphragm, normal heart size, decreased bronchovascular markings
Carbon dioxide retention	Frequent early in disease	Usually later in disease
Hypoxia	Common early in disease	Possible with exertion early in disease and at rest later in disease

bation. *Edema* resulting from right-sided heart failure is noted in the lower extremities and as jugular vein distention. *Cyanosis* caused by hypoxia is noted as the disease progresses. The edema and cyanosis produce the characteristic presentation of CB known as the "blue bloater." Chest auscultation usually reveals inspiratory and expiratory rales, rhonchi, and wheezing with a prolonged expiratory phase. Shortness of breath on exertion is common. Oxygen saturation, measured by pulse oximetry, is less than 92%.

Most patients show clinical findings that suggest a combination of CB and emphysema, because they are usually concurrent (and co-morbid) conditions. The differences in clinical findings between the two are listed in Table 13-2-1. Patients with advanced disease may present with a "barrel chest" appearance.

The patient with AECB presents with wheezing, increasing dyspnea, and increased sputum production with a change in the viscosity and color of the sputum. Fever is not generally a presenting symptom. The white blood cell (WBC) count may be elevated with or without a left shift (Chapter 11, Section 2). Leukocytes and pathogens are seen in the sputum.

 DIAGNOSTIC CRITERIA

Pulmonary function testing reveals decreased FEV and forced vital capacity (FVC) and increased residual volume (RV) and functional residual capacity (FRC). Sputum assessment usually reveals either increased polymorphonuclear granulocytes (indicative of continual bronchial irritation) and/or increased eosinophils (suggestive of an allergic component of the irritation). Chest x-rays often show increased bronchovascular markings in the lower lung fields and increased cardiac size (silhouette) when right-sided failure is present. Hemoglobin and hematocrit are elevated because of increased erythropoiesis from the hypoxic state. Arterial blood gas evaluation reveals hypoxemia, marked by Pao$_2$ below 60 mm Hg, and hypercapnia, marked by Paco$_2$ of 50 to 60 mm Hg, because of decreased alveolar ventilation.

INTERVENTIONS

The treatment of AB is symptomatic and supportive. Acetaminophen, ibuprofen, and aspirin are effective in relieving the discomfort of mild fever. (Remember that aspirin should not be given to children with fever because of the risk of Reye's syndrome.) *Cough* is usually relieved with over-the-counter suppressants, but more severe coughing, especially a cough that interrupts sleep, may be treated with codeine preparations. *Wheezing* can be relieved with a bronchodilator delivered by an MDI for short-term use. Routine use of *antibiotics* is not recommended because most cases of bronchitis are caused by viral pathogens. The patient should be instructed to drink at least 3 L of fluids daily to maintain adequate *hydration* and to thin respiratory secretions. The use of a humidifier or vaporizer also may help to ease congestion.

Patients with CB are treated with *bronchodilators*. As-needed use of bronchodilators may be more effective than regular use early in the disease. Regular use of bronchodilators, postural drainage, deep breathing, and expectorants as the illness progresses will improve gas exchange and improve the removal of secretions. Teaching the patient the technique of *pursed-lip breathing* helps to relieve dyspnea.

Air humidification to help liquefy secretions, and supportive supplemental low-dose *oxygen* (1 to 3 L/min) is given when the patient's Pao$_2$ is below 55 mm Hg. *Chest physiotherapy* is beneficial in mobilizing secretions.

Oral or *parenteral steroids* will reduce inflammation, but studies continue to assess the efficacy of inhaled steroids in reducing the frequency of acute exacerbations. *Prophylactic antibiotics* may be beneficial in patients with severe lung disease, especially during the winter.

The patient should be given *nutrition and exercise counseling* to improve muscle strength, decrease fatigue, and lessen breathlessness. The patient also should be taught to recognize the *early signs of infection* (e.g., increased coughing, darkening of sputum with an increase in thickness and amount, increased dyspnea, and fatigue).

When applicable, *smoking cessation* programs and counseling should be made available to patients and their caregivers.

For acute bacterial exacerbations of CB, antibiotics are appropriate in addition to supportive and symptom management. The choice of agent depends on the bacterial pathogen isolated from the patient's sputum. Short-term steroid use is usually beneficial.

COMMUNITY CARE

A primary disease prevention strategy is the reduction of smoking. Various cessation programs are available through public health departments, private health care provider offices and clinics, schools, and the American Cancer Society, American Lung Association, and other organizations. A number of cessation modalities are available, including pharmacotherapy, psychotherapy, peer support groups, workplace incentive programs, and community programs aimed at smokers of different age groups.

The nurse can encourage community awareness of a common link between influenza and AB during the winter months. Teaching about the importance of frequent hand washing, adequate ventilation, and early management of symptoms may help decrease the frequency and duration of illness. An annual influenza vaccine and appropriate pneumonia vaccine should be encouraged, especially for elderly persons and those with chronic illnesses.

A patient with CB needs to be monitored carefully during winter months, when exacerbations are more likely. A complete environmental and occupational history should be obtained to ascertain exposure to noxious gases, fumes, pollutants, and tobacco smoke. Patient and caregiver education about triggers, prevention, pulmonary hygiene, and wellness promotion will help retard acute bacterial exacerbations and their sequelae. Home care may be advised if certain criteria (e.g., home-bound status) are met. Teaching should be reinforced at every visit.

 PROGNOSIS

AB is a self-limiting illness that usually resolves within several days in previously healthy adults to a few weeks in persons with any underlying respiratory difficulties. Younger and healthier persons who contract AB usually recover with no sequelae or long-term illness. Older persons, smokers, and persons with existing respiratory compromise (e.g., asthma, allergies, emphysema, cystic fibrosis) are at greater risk for long-term illness and potentially serious sequelae. Acute bacterial bronchitis may progress to pneumonia in elderly and debilitated persons.

CB is an irreversible, progressive illness. Rigorous attention to pulmonary hygiene and reduced exposure to respiratory irritants, especially smoking cessation, may slow disease progression. Without lifestyle changes, airway obstruction worsens. If CB is unchecked, pulmonary hypertension ensues, which can lead to cor pulmonale and death.

 CLINICAL PEARLS

○ Hand washing is one of the most effective ways of reducing the spread of infection. The nurse must set an example in this behavior and teach this concept repeatedly to patients and staff.
○ Smoking cessation is vitally important in the reduction of both AB and CB. Second-hand smoke is also an irritant that can cause reactive airway and bronchitis symptoms.
○ AB is a disease of exclusion. Chest radiographs, blood counts, and sputum cultures are not necessary unless symptoms are very severe and the diagnosis is questionable.
○ Antibiotics are sometimes indicated for smokers with AB and CB, because their lungs are often colonized with pathogenic bacteria. Amoxicillin, amoxicillin-clavulanate, macrolides, and trimethoprim-sulfamethoxazole (TMP-SMX) are common agents of choice.
○ Influenza and pneumococcal vaccines should be encouraged for all persons at increased risk for infection.
○ Patients with CB must be taught to recognize the symptoms of early infection and the need for prompt intervention by a health care provider to reduce the risks of complications.

○ Usually healthy adults who present with AB should be taught that antibiotic use is not likely to alter the course of the illness, may destroy normal flora and defenses, and contribute to the growing number of antibiotic-resistant bacteria.

○ Teach the "flotation test" to determine the fullness of MDI canisters (see Section 1, Clinical Pearls).

NURSING PROBLEM/ DIAGNOSIS	NURSING INTERVENTIONS CLASSIFICATION (NIC)
Ineffective airway clearance	Respiratory Monitoring Airway Management Oxygen Therapy Teaching: Prescribed Medication Teaching: Disease Process Smoking Cessation Assistance
Poor nutrition/Unbalanced nutrition: less than body requirements	Nutrition Management
Lack of exercise	Energy Management Exercise Promotion

Emphysema

Section 3   Mia Smitt ▪ Judy Kaye

 OVERVIEW

Emphysema is one of two major airway diseases composing chronic obstructive pulmonary disease (COPD). Emphysema is also known as type A COPD, with chronic bronchitis known as type B. Many persons with emphysema also have CB as the symptoms of each often overlap.

COPD is a major public health issue in the United States and is the second-ranking cause (after heart disease) of permanent disability. According to the American Lung Association, of the 14 million Americans with COPD, approximately 12 million have bronchitis and 2 million have emphysema.

 PATHOPHYSIOLOGY

Emphysema is a chronic lung disease marked by irreversible, abnormal enlargement of the alveolar spaces distal to the terminal bronchioles, with destruction of their walls. Elastic recoil of the alveoli is impaired as elastic fibers that normally hold airways open during expiration are also lost, causing air to become trapped in the distal air spaces, where it is difficult to exhale. Air-trapping leads to the formation of thin-walled, dilated alveoli called emphysematous blebs (smaller than 1 cm in diameter) and bullae (>1 cm in diameter).

Airway enlargement and alveolar wall loss diminishes the pulmonary/capillary network surface area essential for adequate gas exchange, thus ventilation and perfusion decline. The respiratory centers of these patients are more responsive to hypoxia despite the dyspnea. They are less susceptible to cor pulmonale (see Section 2) until late in disease progression and also less prone to polycythemia than those with CB. Principal causes include cigarette smoking, environmental pollution, occupational exposure to asbestos, and mill and mine work.

Primary emphysema is rare, accounting for less than 2% of all cases of emphysema. This type has been linked to a deficiency of the enzyme alpha 1 antitrypsin, which inhibits the actions of those substances that break down proteins, including elastin and other structural proteins in the lungs. Persons with this deficiency are more likely to develop emphysema, because breakdown of the proteins in the lung tissues is not inhibited. Smokers with this autosomal recessive trait are even more susceptible to developing emphysema.

Secondary emphysema is also caused by an inability to inhibit the breakdown of structural proteins in the lung. *The primary cause of secondary emphysema is smoking.* Smoking causes excessive accumulation of neutrophils and macrophages in the lung tissue (parenchyma), leading to the release of large amounts of proteolytic enzymes. These enzymes break down needed lung proteins, resulting in parenchymal destruction. Other irritants and allergens may also set up this pattern of continuous destruction, but the degree of injury has not been seen to equal that associated with tobacco smoke.

Emphysema is classified according to the location of the pathology. Two major classifications are centrilobular and panlobular. *Centrilobular*, or centriacinar, emphysema accounts for 95% of all cases. This type involves the respiratory bronchioles and alveolar ducts, usually in the upper lobes. The alveolar sac (distal to the respiratory bronchioles) remains intact. Centrilobular disease occurs mostly in smokers with chronic bronchitis. *Panlobular*, or panacinar, emphysema involves enlargement of all air spaces distal to the terminal bronchioles, mostly in the lower lobes. This occurs mainly in those with the alpha 1 antitrypsin deficiency and in older adults.

 ## SIGNS AND SYMPTOMS

The patient typically presents with a complaint of *dyspnea on exertion*. This progresses to include dyspnea at rest. Acute exacerbations are typically triggered by respiratory tract infection and exposure to pollen, dust, and other allergens. *Cough* with sputum production usually indicates the presence of chronic bronchitis. The cough is more prominent in the morning because of buildup of secretions during the night.

Physical examination reveals a flushed appearance and visible tachypnea, hence the characteristic term "pink puffer." The patient usually presents with pursed-lip breathing and may sit in a characteristic posture with the chest forward and hands resting on the knees in an attempt to conserve energy for breathing. The use of accessory muscles of the chest and neck is often visible. Breath sounds are diminished with few wheezes and rhonchi. Chest percussion is hyperresonant. Anteroposterior chest diameter is increased (barrel chest). The patient is usually thin (due to anorexia and lack of energy to eat) and male in his 5th decade.

 ## DIAGNOSTIC CRITERIA

Pulmonary function testing shows obstructed air flow during expiration. Airway collapse and air-trapping in the distal portions of the lung lead to decreased FVC and FEV and increased FRC, RV, and total lung capacity (TLC). TLC may be twice normal. Although the diffusing capacity may be greatly reduced because of collapse of the capillary–alveolar exchange, the ventilation and perfusion deficits remain relatively balanced.

A chest radiograph may show a flattened diaphragm that moves less than 3 cm between inspiration and expiration, hyperinflation of the lungs, a small or normal cardiac silhouette (size), a narrow mediastinum, and increased retrosternal air space indicative of extensive air-trapping.

Arterial blood gas analysis reveals mild to moderate hypoxemia (Pao_2 of 55 to 80 mm Hg) and normal $Paco_2$. Hypercapnia usually occurs only in acute exacerbations or in end-stage disease.

INTERVENTIONS

Smoking cessation is the most important factor in slowing the progression of emphysema.

Medications

Inhaled bronchodilating medications are used as first-line therapy, with ipratropium the common drug of choice. In patients who continue to display symptoms after bronchodilator therapy, *corticosteroids* may offer relief. Inhaled steroids are replacing the use of systemic steroids, and fewer adverse effects are noted.

Nutritional Support

Weight loss is associated with a poor prognosis. Dyspnea may cause both an increase in caloric needs and fatigue. Teach patients to weigh themselves regularly, and encourage small frequent meals with favorite foods high in protein and complex carbohydrates, nutritional supplements as tolerated, and adequate rest before meals. Constipation can be prevented with fiber-rich foods, adequate hydration, and stool softeners as needed.

Infection Prevention

Persons with chronic respiratory illness are more susceptible to pulmonary infections from ineffective airway clearance. Teach patients and caregivers to notice changes in secretions such as color, odor, or consistency. Changes in activity tolerance, fever, chills, night sweats, sore throat, and an increase in oxygen use can signal infection. Bronchodilators, increased fluids, incentive breathing, and turning and coughing every 2 hours may help prevent infection. Appropriate antibiotics should be started as soon as an infectious process is identified, to reduce potential complications of the infection.

Oxygen

Impaired gas exchange can compromise blood gas values. Cyanosis, changes in vital signs, and decreased level of consciousness are indicative of worsening hypoxemia. Administering low-flow oxygen, repositioning with the head of the bed at 60 degrees or upright in a chair, and decreasing activity to maximize energy promote patient comfort. The primary health care provider must be notified. Blood gases, complete blood count with differential, and metabolic profiles may be evaluated to further assess the patient's status. *Continuous* *supplemental oxygen is indicated when PaO$_2$ drops below 55 mm Hg.* Nasal cannula is the method of choice for oxygen delivery.

Breathing Techniques

Several breathing techniques can help the patient improve gas exchange.

Pursed-Lip Breathing. Teach the patient the following technique: With the mouth closed, inhale through the nose for approximately 2 seconds. Exhale through the mouth with the lips pursed, as if whistling, for twice as long as the inhalations, approximately 4 seconds. This keeps the airways open longer during exhalation. It also helps reduce anxiety. A novel technique is to teach the patient to blow bubbles with a bubble wand. The expirations are slower, longer, and more forceful. This also relieves anxiety and muscle tension.

Diaphragmatic Breathing. This technique saves energy by reducing the effort of the accessory muscles. Instruct the patient to place one hand on the chest and the other on the abdomen. During inhalation, push the abdominal hand outward while the chest hand remains still. During the slow exhalation, the abdominal hand will fall inward. This technique should be taught while the patient is calm and receptive to teaching. It should be used as much as possible and definitely during episodes of shortness of breath.

Surgery

Surgical bullectomy may provide symptomatic relief in patients with large bullae who have stopped smoking.

Anxiety Reduction

Anxiety is common in patients with chronic pulmonary disease because of dyspnea and feelings of suffocation. Anxiety may also be linked to lack of knowledge and feelings of helplessness. Support groups may be beneficial. Adequate rest periods will conserve energy and may help reduce episodes of dyspnea. Relaxation measures, such as the use of music, guided imagery, and journaling, may help to reduce stress and anxiety. Anxiolytic medications may be helpful.

 COMMUNITY CARE

Smoking cessation programs, as well as community awareness and actions to reduce air pollution, benefit all people and help to reduce the numbers and severity of pulmonary diseases (see Section 2).

Patient teaching points should include the following:

- Keep the home free of allergens, dust, molds, and mildew that will exacerbate symptoms. Pet dander can be an irritant, thus pets should be kept outdoors as much as possible and never allowed to sleep in the patient's bedroom. The use of aerosol sprays may be irritating and, therefore, should be avoided. Wood-burning fireplaces and heating units should be avoided whenever possible. Air filters and humidifiers must be cleaned or replaced regularly.
- The use and actions of prescribed medications, breathing exercises, the correct use of supplemental oxygen, and care of the oxygen unit.

Nutrition and energy conservation counseling should be given to maximize health. *Adequate hydration* should be ensured.

Home health services are very valuable to the patient and caregiver as the patient makes the transition from hospital to home and also in the maintenance of illness stability. *Social services* may be beneficial in helping the patient find available community resources, potential financial assistance, and counseling.

Immunization against influenza should be given annually; immunization against pneumonia should be given every 5 years.

 PROGNOSIS

Emphysema is usually a very prolonged illness with the disability of increasing dyspnea and occasional infections. Activity tolerance declines, with increasing dependence on assistance with activities of daily living. As ventilation worsens, dependence on supplemental oxygen increases. The dyspnea may seriously compromise quality of life and should be addressed with appropriate medication. Appetite decreases, and nutritional status becomes compromised, with progressive weight loss and cachexia. Mental acuity declines, and increasing somnolence is seen. The patient will most likely die of right-sided heart failure, hypoxia, or infection. Lung cancer occurs more frequently in patients with emphysema and chronic bronchitis.

 CLINICAL PEARLS

○ An oxygen facemask may cause anxiety in some patients.
○ Smoking cessation programs are numerous and varied in style and design. It has been shown that multiple modalities and consistent advice with the sincere concern of the patient's health care provider are effective in long-term smoking cessation programs.
○ Respiratory irritants must be avoided as much as possible. Cold temperatures can be mediated by wearing a facemask or muffler.

NURSING PROBLEM/ DIAGNOSIS	NURSING INTERVENTIONS CLASSIFICATION (NIC)
Ineffective breathing pattern	Respiratory Monitoring Airway Management Oxygen Therapy Teaching: Prescribed Medication Teaching: Disease Process Smoking Cessation Assistance
Poor nutrition/Unbalanced nutrition: less than body requirements	Nutrition Management
Lack of exercise	Energy Management Exercise Promotion

Pneumonia

Section 4   Mia Smitt ■ Judy Kaye

 OVERVIEW

Pneumonia is the most common respiratory infection in adults, with an annual incidence of 1200 per 100,000 population for community-acquired

infection and 800 per 100,000 population for nosocomial infection. In the United States, pneumonia is the sixth leading cause of death overall and the leading cause of death from infectious disease. Pneumonia affects males more often than females. The elderly and those with chronic illness or disability are at greater risk (Table 13-4-1).

PATHOPHYSIOLOGY

Disease-causing microorganisms can reach the lungs in several ways. When an infected person coughs, sneezes, or even talks, pathogens are expelled into the air, where they can be inhaled by others. Aerosolized medicines can harbor infectious organisms in contaminated respiratory therapy equipment. The aspiration of oropharyngeal flora can become pathogenic during illness or with poor dental/oral hygiene. Gram-positive bacteria (e.g., *Staphylococcus*) can be spread from the circulatory system from sepsis, systemic infection, or a contaminated needle.

The disease-causing pathogen generally overwhelms a person who becomes ill, and the body's defenses cannot stop the proliferation of the organism. The immune reaction and the endotoxins released by the pathogenic organism can damage the bronchial mucous membranes and result in necrosis of the lung parenchyma. Ensuing edema may cause the terminal bronchioles to fill with infectious exudates, leading to ventilation-perfusion mismatch.

Bacterial Pneumonia

Bacterial pneumonia is associated with the production of copious amounts of exudates that consolidate (solidify) in the alveolar spaces, causing significant ventilation-perfusion mismatch. The distribution of the consolidation may be patchy, as seen in bronchopneumonia, or it may affect an entire lobe (or a portion of a lobe), as in lobar pneumonia. The most common bacterium causing community-acquired pneumonia is *Streptococcus pneumoniae* (accounting for 45% of all cases), followed by *Haemophilus influenzae*, gram-negative bacilli, and *Staphylococcus aureus*. Many of the organisms responsible for hospital-acquired (nosocomial) pneumonia have developed resistance and are more difficult to treat. Hospital-acquired pneumonia has a higher mortality rate than community-acquired pneumonia.

Community-Acquired "Atypical" Pneumonia

The term "atypical" refers to the fact that these pneumonias do not produce alveolar exudates. A more accurate term is *interstitial pneumonitis*. Organisms responsible for atypical pneumonias are viruses (most commonly, influenza virus type A), and *Mycoplasma pneumoniae*. Chlamydia and *Legionella* species may also be implicated. Atypical pneumonia is usually mild and self-limiting. It can be a primary infection, such as influenza pneumonia, or secondary to another illness, such as measles.

Aspiration Pneumonia

This type of pneumonia can occur acutely for the aspiration of volumes greater than 50 mL with a pH below 2.4, or chronically from the aspiration of small volumes on a recurrent basis. *Nosocomial aspiration pneumonias* are

Table 13-4-1. Common Organisms Found in Pneumonia

ORGANISM	HIGH-RISK PATIENTS	SPUTUM	CHEST RADIOGRAPH
Gram Positive			
Streptococcus pneumoniae	Cardiopulmonary disease, viral respiratory infections, immunosuppression	Blood-streaked or rust-colored	Patchy infiltrates
Staphylococcus aureus	Severe diabetes mellitus (DM), immunocompromised status, dialysis, drug abuse, respiratory infections	Yellow, purulent	Consolidation
Gram-Negative			
Haemophilus influenzae	Chronic obstructive pulmonary disease (COPD), alcoholism	Purulent	Consolidation Lower lobes
Klebsiella pneumoniae	Alcoholism, DM, hospitalized patients	Hemoptysis in 30%	Consolidation
Pseudomonas aeruginosa	COPD, cystic fibrosis, tracheostomy, mechanical ventilation	Copious, greenish, foul-smelling	Bilateral patchy infiltrates
Community-Acquired Atypical			
Virus	May be previously healthy	Nonproductive cough	Patchy infiltrates
Legionella	COPD, smoking, cancer, DM, immunosuppression, chronic heart and kidney disease	Dry cough	Consolidation
Mycoplasma pneumoniae	Closed populations (e.g., military bases, college campuses)	Dry cough	Patchy infiltrates

caused by *Escherichia coli, S. aureus, Klebsiella pneumoniae*, and *Pseudomonas aeruginosa* and result from acute aspiration. *Community-acquired aspiration pneumonias* are caused by anaerobes and result from chronic aspiration.

Pneumocystis carinii Pneumonia

Pneumocystis carinii pneumonia (PCP) is acute interstitial plasma cell pneumonia caused by the protozoan *P. carinii*. It is one of the most common opportunistic infections occurring in patients with human immunodeficiency virus (HIV) infections and is the AIDS indicator disease in 43% of patients.

 ## SIGNS AND SYMPTOMS

Most affected patients report an upper respiratory infection followed by fever, chills, cough, pleural pain, dyspnea, and sometimes hemoptysis. Symptoms may start suddenly or gradually. With increasing ventilation-perfusion mismatch, the patient may complain of restlessness and anxiety. Some patients will report associated rhinorrhea, nausea, myalgias, and diarrhea.

Bacterial pneumonia usually begins abruptly. Typical presentation includes shaking chills associated with high fever, pain on inspiration, and dyspnea. Respiratory signs of consolidation include rales, rhonchi, localized and diminished breath sounds, friction rub, egophony, bronchophony, and whispered pectoriloquy. There will likely be dullness to percussion and tactile fremitus. Signs of respiratory distress include tachypnea, tachycardia, and cyanosis. The patient may exhibit nasal flaring, the use of accessory muscles, and intercostal retractions. A productive cough with dark, thick, or rust-colored purulent sputum is often seen. Mentation changes, such as anxiety, restlessness, confusion, and somnolence, may indicate compromised ventilation and perfusion.

Atypical pneumonia has a slower, more insidious onset. The cough is more often nonproductive, and fevers are lower than the fevers associated with bacterial pneumonia. The patient will complain of generalized myalgias, headache, fatigue, and sore throat. The respiratory signs of consolidation may be similar to those of bacterial pneumonia but to a lesser degree.

 ## DIAGNOSTIC CRITERIA

In bacterial pneumonia, laboratory findings show leukocytosis (WBC count of 10,000 to 30,000/mm³ with a left shift on the WBC differential) (see Chapter 11, Sections 2 and 4). In viral pneumonia, the WBC count is often below 5000/mm³.

Sputum for gram staining is helpful in identifying whether the organism is gram-negative, gram-positive, or viral. Acid-fast staining rules out tuberculosis.

Arterial blood gas analysis may or may not reveal hypoxemia. Sometimes there will be an initial hypocapnia followed by hypercapnia. *Blood cultures* will be positive in 10% to 20% of patients with both community-acquired pneumonia and nosocomial pneumonia. *Chest radiographs* may reveal lobar or segmental consolidation, interstitial infiltrates, bronchopneumonia, or pleural effusion.

In a hospitalized patient, a gram-negative organism should be suspected. If the patient is living in the community and was previously healthy, the etiology may be viral, mycoplasmal, or, most likely, a gram-positive organism.

 INTERVENTIONS

Treatment strategies for the patient with pneumonia depend on many factors. Risk factors for a complication or mortality should be carefully reviewed.

Hospitalization should be considered for persons older than 65 years of age, those with comorbid conditions or an impaired immune system, and those who present with altered mental status, hypotension, hypoxemia, or severe symptoms of illness.

Appropriate antibiotics should be instituted immediately when bacterial pneumonia is suspected. Empiric therapy with the following antibiotics is useful until culture and sensitivity results become available. Macrolides, such as azithromycin (5-day therapy), clarithromycin, and erythromycin, are often the first-line empiric therapies for community-acquired pneumonia. For community-acquired pneumonia in patients over age 60, fluoroquinolones with enhanced action against *S. pneumoniae* (e.g., trovafloxacin, levofloxacin, grepafloxacin) or a second-generation cephalosporin plus a macrolide are recommended. Streptococcal pneumonia still is often treated with penicillin V orally.

For hospital-acquired pneumonia, a third-generation cephalosporin plus an aminoglycoside or a fluoroquinolone plus an aminoglycoside are the usual first-line therapies. For antipseudomonal action, piperacilln-tazobactam (Zosyn) or metronidazole (Flagyl) is recommended. Clindamycin can be added for suspected aspiration. Vancomycin is recommended for suspected *S. aureus* in patients from nursing homes or for suspected resistant *S. pneumoniae*.

Viral pneumonia is treated with supportive care, symptom control measures, and antiviral medications such as zanamivir, amantadine, or rimantadine if the pneumonia is secondary to an influenza infection. *Pneumocystis carinii pneumonia* is usually treated with TMP-SMX. An IV macrolide or oral fluoroquinolone is usually the drug of choice for *Legionella*.

Oxygen support should be given for cyanosis, dyspnea, mentation changes, and hypoxia. Oxygenation saturation is monitored by pulse oximetry. Oxygen typically is started at 2 L/min and is increased to maintain PaO_2 above 92%. Mechanical ventilation is warranted for respiratory failure.

Appropriate nutrition (soft foods) and hydration (with electrolyte correction if indicated) should be addressed. IV fluid therapy may be necessary to replace insensible losses and to keep secretions loose. Dairy products should be avoided, because they increase mucus production. Multivitamins, vitamin C, and vitamin E may be useful. All patients receiving enteral nutrition should be maintained on aspiration precautions.

Analgesics should be given for relief of painful coughing. Cough suppressants may be necessary to promote rest. The patient should be on restricted activity to conserve energy.

Percussion, postural drainage, expectorants, and mucolytics can help to relieve airway congestion.

 COMMUNITY CARE

Prevention of both the disease and any complications is the hallmark of community care. Vaccines for the prevention of pneumococcal pneumonia have been available for many years and should be offered to persons at risk, notably those older than 65 years of age and those with chronic illness or immunosuppression. The vaccine is usually effective for 5 years or longer.

Optimizing the health of all patients should be a goal of both nursing and medicine. Smoking cessation, adequate nutrition, good hygiene, sanitation, and ventilation are health promotion measures that may decrease the incidence and prevalence of community-acquired pneumonia. Nosocomial infections can be curbed by meticulous attention to infection control measures, pulmonary hygiene, and staff awareness of nosocomial infection risks. Health departments promote community awareness of the potential for acquiring Legionnaires' pneumonia. This organism can thrive in the standing water of air-conditioning units, humidifiers, water faucets, and water storage systems.

Community education regarding the risks, prevention, symptoms, and treatment of pneumonia will lessen the severity of illness and potential sequelae. Adequate follow-up, including home nursing care services, medication, and supplemental oxygen, helps promote a positive outcome for ill patients. Too many patients do not adhere to their antibiotic regimens (which contributes to the rise in antibiotic resistance worldwide) because they are not aware of the consequences of nonadherence.

 PROGNOSIS

Most otherwise healthy adults recover from acute pneumonia within a week. Improvement in symptoms and the reduction of fever can be expected within 1 to 3 days after the institution of appropriate antibiotic therapy. The overall mortality rate of community-acquired pneumonia is approximately 15% in hospitalized patients and less than 1% in patients cared for outside the hospital. Between 30% and 50% of patients with nosocomial pneumonia will die of pneumonia as a complication of their comorbidities.

The poorest prognoses can be expected for persons of advanced age and those with positive blood cultures, low WBC count, immunosuppression, respiratory failure, inappropriate antibiotic therapy, and delayed treatment.

 CLINICAL PEARLS

- Common associated factors in patients with pneumonia include tobacco smoking, upper respiratory infection, and alcoholism.
- Patients with COPD, asthma, or other chronic respiratory illness are more susceptible to pneumonia infection and should be vaccinated every 5 years.
- Typical bacterial pneumonia is more common in persons 45 years of age and older. Atypical pneumonia is more common in persons younger than 45 years of age.
- Pneumonia is more common during the winter.
- *Streptococcus pneumoniae* is included in the broad category of pneumococcal pneumonia.
- Streptococcal pneumonia can trigger a sudden onset of herpes simplex.
- If a patient has both pneumonia symptoms and diarrhea, consider *Legionella* infection.
- Patients who smoke and those older than 40 years of age should have disease resolution confirmed with a repeat chest radiograph.

○ Bronchogenic carcinoma can present with the same symptoms as those of pneumonia.

NURSING PROBLEM/ DIAGNOSIS	NURSING INTERVENTIONS CLASSIFICATION (NIC)
Ventilation/perfusion mismatch/ Impaired gas exchange	Respiratory Monitoring Airway Management Oxygen Therapy
Airway congestion/Ineffective airway clearance	Airway Suctioning Chest Physiotherapy Cough Enhancement Positioning Fluid Management
Increased fluid and nutritional requirements	Nutritional Therapy Fluid/Electrolyte Management
Risk for aspiration	Aspiration Precautions

Tuberculosis

Section 5   Beverly George-Gay ■ Cynthia Chernecky

 OVERVIEW

Tuberculosis (TB) causes more deaths worldwide than any other infectious disease. A resurgence of TB occurred in the United States from 1985 to 1992 from outbreaks of resistant strains, human immunodeficiency virus (HIV), as well as decreased immunity in persons older than 65 years of age. Movement of infected individuals from high-prevalence areas, transmission in crowded institutional settings, homeless shelters, substance abuse, and lack of access to health care also contributed to the increased incidence.

Since 1993, the number of reported cases has declined; however, TB continues to be reported in every state, and cases in foreign-born persons have increased by 4%. An estimated 10 to 15 million people in the United States are infected with *Mycobacterium tuberculosis*.

 PATHOPHYSIOLOGY

Tuberculosis is a bacterial infection caused by the *Mycobacterium tuberculosis* bacilli (MTB), a nonmotile, aerobic, gram-positive rod of acid-fast genus. The organism is transmitted by microscopic droplets from an infectious person. The organism enters the host's nasal or oral passages and lodges in the alveolar spaces. Once in the lungs, most of the MTB is ingested by alveolar macrophages. A small amount is released when the macrophages die. These surviving bacilli can spread through the lymphatic channels and the bloodstream to areas of high oxygen tension, including the apex of the lungs, kidneys, brain, and bone, and can multiply, forming colonies.

Once again the immune system is activated against these remaining bacilli, and it responds by sending macrophages to the area. The macrophages surround and encapsulate the colonies. The surrounded colonies become necrotic and caseous, forming a tubercle. Scar tissue grows around the tubercle, forming a granuloma. At the same time, macrophages present the MTB antigenic markers to circulating T lymphocytes, activating a cell-mediated immune response that results in the production of killer T cells, memory T cells, and eventually suppressor T cells (see Chapter 10, Section 1).

It may take 2 to 10 weeks for this cell-mediated response to kill most of the bacilli, preventing further multiplication. At this stage, the person has TB infection, which can be detected with a tuberculin skin test. However, he or she is not contagious.

A person with *latent TB infection* (LTBI) is infected but exhibits no signs of disease. The organism is contained. The MTB usually remains dormant within the granuloma for life in most healthy individuals.

Active TB, or TB disease, develops if encapsulation fails and the bacilli overcome the defenses of the immune system, resulting in disease progression and tissue destruction. Infectious disease develops in the lungs (pulmonary TB). Extrapulmonary TB is rarely infectious.

Reactivated TB occurs in patients with LTBI whose immune defenses have weakened, allowing the active process to develop. Immunodeficiency can result from diabetes mellitus, renal failure, and immunosuppressive diseases or drug therapy; however, reactivated TB occurs most commonly in persons with HIV or AIDS. Most reactivated cases occur within the lungs. In the United States, approximately 10% of individuals with normal immune systems who acquire LTBI without treatment will develop active TB at some point in life.

 ## SIGNS AND SYMPTOMS

In LTBI, the patient is infected with MTB but is asymptomatic. Signs and symptoms of pulmonary TB range from mild persistent cough to chronic, productive cough and hemoptysis. Extrapulmonary symptoms depend on the site affected. Systemic symptoms include low-grade fever associated with chills in about 44% of patients; night sweats are seen in 60% of patients. Other nonspecific symptoms can include weight loss, anorexia, fatigue, and pleuritic pain. Although night sweats, hemoptysis, and weight loss are considered the classic findings in active TB, they are not always present.

 ## DIAGNOSTIC CRITERIA
Tuberculin Skin Test

The Mantoux skin test is the gold standard for diagnosing LTBI. It involves an intradermal injection of 5 units (0.1 mL) of purified protein derivative (PPD) containing TB antigenic properties. Hence, the test is commonly called the PPD skin test. In the immunocompetent patient with LTBI, sensitized immune cells recognize this derivative from the initial infection and react, causing local inflammation and producing an area of induration.

The intradermal injection must result in a bleb. A false-negative result may occur if the PPD is injected subcutaneously rather than intradermally, in which case no bleb occurs. The test is usually administered on the left forearm. The test results are read 48 to 72 hours after injection. Only induration or vesiculation is significant; erythema is not. Table 13-5-1 provides details on how to determine a positive reaction by the size of the induration.

False-negative results may occur if cellular immunity wanes over several years. In the elderly, if there is a questionable negative PPD result, a second PPD may be administered 2 weeks later. If the second PPD is positive, then the patient is truly positive. The first PPD stimulated the waning immune response, acting as a booster.

False-negative results also may occur in patients who are immunocompromised and are incapable of mounting an immune response (anergy). Anergy is detected by administering skin-test antigens (i.e., tetanus toxoid, mumps, and candida), to which most people have been exposed at least once. A positive reaction to the panel indicates that the patient can mount an immune response; thus a negative PPD is negative. A negative anergy panel strongly suggests an impaired immune system, increasing the possibility of a false negative, which merits further investigation. Anergy testing is no longer recommended for HIV-positive persons in the United States.

False-negative results may also be seen if the patient is tested too soon after infection, before the activation of immune cells (memory T cells). In this case, the patient should be retested in 1 month.

False-positive results can result from the presence of nontuberculous mycobacterium organisms or because of vaccination with bacille Calmette-Guérin (BCG).

Sputum Testing

Sputum studies are the standard for diagnosing *active TB*. Samples should be collected on three consecutive days, early in the morning after the patient has been on nothing-by-mouth status (NPO) for about 8 hours.

A smear is obtained for staining, and cultures are plated. Positive cultures confirm the diagnosis. With recently developed liquid medium systems, MTB growth can be detected in 4 to 14 days. Because of the length of time needed to grow a culture, smear staining is relied on to some extent for early recognition of MTB.

MTB is an acid-fast bacillus (AFB), which means that it resists decolorization by acid-alcohol during the gram-staining process (hence the term "acid-fast"). Sputum stain results can be obtained within 24 hours of specimen collection. If the smear is positive for AFB, then isolation and drug therapy

Table 13-5-1. Interpretation of Tuberculin Skin Test as Defined in Millimeters of Induration

5 mm	Considered positive in patients who are HIV-positive, those who have had close contact with someone who has active TB, those with fibrotic changes on chest radiograph, or immunosuppressed patients
10 mm	Considered positive in relatively high-risk populations, such as IV drug users who are HIV-seronegative, recent arrivals from high-prevalence countries, residents or employees of congregate settings (e.g., prisons, nursing homes, homeless shelters), and medically underserved and low-income populations (e.g., migrant farm workers)
15 mm	Considered positive for patients who are without risk factors

should be initiated immediately because this is strongly suggestive of MTB. Unfortunately, only 50% of patients with active TB show a positive AFB stain. All samples must be cultured even if the smear is negative for AFB.

If diagnosis of active TB remains questionable after sputum testing, then bronchoscopy for bronchoalveolar lavage, brushing, or biopsy are considered. These techniques have a high diagnostic yield.

Sample Collection

Have the patient rinse the mouth with water to remove debris and normal flora. Then tell the patient to take three deep breaths, then a deep cough, to produce at least 5 to 10 mL (1 to 2 teaspoons) of sputum. Saliva and nasopharyngeal secretions are useless. Ensure that all personnel in contact with the patient are wearing a particulate respirator (HEPA respirator) mask, not a surgical mask. (Only the particulate respirator mask can filter out droplet nuclei.)

If the patient is unable to expectorate sputum spontaneously, then induction by nebulized saline may be performed. This procedure produces an aerosol mist; thus the patient must be in a negative-pressure isolation room or sputum induction booth, and particulate respirators must be worn by all persons. Room access should be limited for at least 1 hour after the completion of sample collection. Nasotracheal suctioning may be used if the patient is unconscious.

Cultures

Active TB may occur outside the pulmonary system. Therefore, specimens of urine, cerebrospinal fluid, or pleural fluid may be needed.

Chest Radiograph

Active TB may yield various radiographic abnormalities, ranging from small shadows to large infiltrates or cavities. Thus, TB cannot be diagnosed by chest radiograph alone; a sputum culture is necessary to confirm the diagnosis.

A patient with LTBI often has completely normal chest radiographs. Occasionally, calcified granulomas known as Ghon's lesions may be seen in the lung periphery.

 INTERVENTIONS

Screening

The Mantoux, or PPD, skin test is the standard for TB screening in the United States. Other tests, including the tine and Heaf tests, have proven unreliable. There are no universal standards for the frequency of PPD testing. Most health care facilities require the test either annually or biannually for employees. Persons in high-risk areas, such as homeless shelters and prisons, may need to be tested two to four times a year.

Isolation

Isolation precautions should be initiated when active TB is suspected even before the AFB smear report is obtained. Strict respiratory isolation precautions include a room with negative air pressure (NAP), in which exhaust air is vented directly outside (where MTB is destroyed by ultraviolet light) and is not vented into another part of the building. A gown, gloves, and a particulate respirator must be worn by every person who enters the patient's room. A patient leaving the NAP isolation room must wear a particulate respirator.

Respiratory isolation can be discontinued when follow-up sputum smears show a definite reduction or clearance of AFB. This generally takes at least 2 weeks of effective antituberculin medication, after which time the patient is no longer considered contagious.

Antituberculin Medication

Drug therapy for LTBI as diagnosed by positive PPD (see Table 13-5-1) consists of 6 to 9 months of preventative isoniazid (INH) therapy. Rifampin may be used in patients with history of exposure to isoniazid-resistant strains of TB. For HIV-positive patients, rifampin and pyrazinamide (PZA) daily for 2 months is recommended.

Therapy for active TB involves multiple drugs, each of which helps prevent the emergence of resistant organisms. Solo drug therapy may lead to resistance. Therapy is usually prescribed for 6 months, with daily doses of INH, rifampin, PZA, and ethambutol or streptomycin for the first 2 months and biweekly doses of INH and rifampin for the remaining 4 months. Lengthier courses with more extensive drug combinations may be necessary if resistance occurs. Persons with HIV should undergo 9 to 12 months of treatment. Table 13-5-2 lists nursing implications for first-line drug therapy; Table 13-5-3 lists nursing implications for second-line drug therapy.

Pulmonary Status Assessment

For a patient with active TB, breath sounds, cough, and sputum are assessed every 4 hours for improvement or deterioration. Symptoms should improve within 2 to 3 weeks of antibiotic therapy.

Table 13-5-2. Nursing Implications for First-Line Antituberculin Drug Therapy

Isoniazid (INH)	Hepatotoxic and may induce hepatitis. Obtain baseline liver functions tests (LFTs). Instruct the patient to report signs of weakness, nausea, vomiting, dark urine, pale stool, or jaundice. Alcohol should be avoided. INH may induce peripheral neuropathy; the patient should be started on pyridoxine (vitamin B_6) to prevent this. INH supresses phenytoin, metabolism, causing levels to rise, potentially to toxic levels.
Rifampin	Causes a red-orange discoloration to urine, feces, sputum, sweat, and tears; also discolors contact lenses. Inform the patient of this occurrence and explain that it is harmless. This drug should be taken 1 hour before meals or 2 hours after meals. Rifampin decreases the effectiveness of oral contraceptives; the patient should consider other forms of contraception. Rifampin may also reduce the effectiveness of corticosteroids, warfarin, methadone, digoxin, and some hypoglycemic agents. Aspirin may interfere with the absorption of rifampin and should be avoided. Rifampin is hepatotoxic (see implications for INH).
Pyrazinamide (PZA)	May cause gastric irritation. Instruct the patient to monitor for and report skin rashes. Hepatotoxic (see implications for INH).
Ethambutol	May induce optic neuritis, decreased visual acuity, and impaired red-green color discrimination. The patient should have periodic eye examinations.
Streptomycin	An aminoglycoside; can be ototoxic and nephrotoxic and may cause hypokalemia. Hearing should be periodically evaluated. Renal function and potassium levels should be monitored.

Table 13-5-3. Nursing Implications for Second-Line Antituberculin Drug Therapy

Para-aminosalicylic acid	May cause gastric disturbance. It is sodium loading and hepatotoxic
Ethionamide	May cause gastric disturbance. It is also hepatotoxic and leaves a metallic taste
Cycloserine	May cause neurologic effects such as psychosis, personality changes, impaired coordination, and seizures; may also cause rash
Capreomycin	Ototoxic and nephrotoxic and may cause hypokalemia
Kanamycin	Ototoxic and nephrotoxic and may cause hypokalemia

Nutritional Support

High-calorie and high-protein diets with nutritional supplements should be encouraged. Dietary consultation may be necessary depending on the degree of weight loss or anorexia. Weight should be monitored biweekly. A fluid intake of 2 to 3 L/day should be maintained.

Bacille Calmette-Guérin Vaccine

BCG vaccines are derived from a live strain of *Mycobacterium bovis*. The Tice strain of this vaccine is currently available in the United States but is rarely indicated, because its effectiveness in preventing active TB has not been clearly shown, it interferes with the diagnosis of a newly acquired infection, and it may cause serious complications in immunocompromised persons because it is a live vaccine. The BCG vaccine may be recommended on an individual basis in specific settings.

 COMMUNITY CARE

Assessment

Obtain a health history and assess risk factors. These include drinking unpasteurized milk (which may contain bovine tuberculosis) and being a member of one or more of the following groups: foreign born, migrant worker, racial or ethnic minority, poor, and homeless. Outbreaks of multidrug-resistant strains have occurred in hospitals, prisons, and community health clinics.

Assess for signs and symptoms of active and advanced TB. Assess factors associated with disease progression: advanced age, history of gastrectomy, substance abuse, diabetes mellitus, chronic renal failure, leukemia, lymphoma, silicosis or sarcoidosis, and HIV infection.

Assess the patient's compliance with medications by taking a pill count. Dipstick the urine to detect isoniazid in urine 24 to 48 hours after the drug is ingested. Ask the patient on rifampin therapy about his or her urine color; it should be orange several hours after medication ingestion.

Determine whether directly observed therapy (DOT) is necessary. DOT includes administering prescribed medications and actually watching the patient ingest them. This may be necessary to ensure compliance. Consider DOT for all patients.

Monitoring

Administer a TB skin test to persons who come in close contact with the patient, including all visitors, children, and spouse.

Assess for pulmonary and extrapulmonary complications of TB:

- Pulmonary: respiratory failure, bronchopleural fistula, atelectasis, empyema, pneumothorax
- Reproductive: In females, pelvic inflammatory disease, impaired fertility, ectopic pregnancy; in males, epididymitis, prostatitis, scrotal pain
- Musculoskeletal: joint arthritis, vertebral collapse, kyphosis
- Hematologic: anemia, leukocytosis, thrombocytopenia
- Cardiac: pericarditis
- Gastrointestinal: peritonitis, malnutrition
- Genitourinary: urinary stricture, urinary tract infection, flank pain from renal involvement
- Neurologic: meningitis, spinal cord compression

Teach the patient to report any of the following: chest pain; hemoptysis; shortness of breath; nausea or vomiting; anorexia; jaundiced skin or eyes; sudden weight gain; swollen feet, ankles, legs, or hands; hearing loss; tinnitus; vertigo; or vision changes.

Notify the Public Health Department of all active cases of TB.

Prevention

Reinforce teaching about the importance of covering the nose and mouth when coughing or sneezing and of properly disposing of tissues. Inanimate objects are not significant means of spreading TB, thus no special precautions are needed for eating utensils, clothing, or books.

 PROGNOSIS

In patients with untreated active TB, 50% die within 5 years, 32% experience spontaneous resolution of disease, and 18% experience relapse. Approximately 85% of persons with LTBI will never develop active TB. The prognosis is excellent unless the person develops a concomitant chronic illness. In patients who are treated and are compliant with the prescribed treatment regimen, the cure rate is 95% with a relapse rate of 5%.

 CLINICAL PEARLS

- A sputum culture, not a smear, is the definitive test for diagnosing active TB. This test is 98% sensitive.
- Persons with LTBI are neither contagious nor harmful. A person with suspected active TB is placed in isolation until active TB is ruled out.
- A patient with suspected TB who has a sputum test identified as AFB positive should be placed in respiratory isolation. A positive AFB is strongly suggestive of MTB.
- Poor compliance with medication therapy for TB has been a major factor in the rise in TB in recent years. DOT is a way to ensure medication compliance.

NURSING PROBLEM/ DIAGNOSIS	NURSING INTERVENTIONS CLASSIFICATION (NIC)
Prevention/screening	Health Education
	Health Screening
Latent infection	Medication Administration: Oral
	Teaching: Disease Process
	Self-Modification Assistance
Active infection	Infection Control
	Medication Administration
	Respiratory Monitoring
	Nutrition Therapy

chapter 14

Cardiac

Angina

Section 1   Judy Graham Garcia ▪ Rebecca Rule

 OVERVIEW

Angina is the presenting symptom of coronary artery disease (CAD) in 38% of men and 61% of women. It is seen most commonly in middle-aged and older men and in postmenopausal women. The likelihood of underlying CAD is enhanced by a history of hypertension, diabetes mellitus, hyperlipidemia, or smoking or a family history of premature ischemic heart disease in first-degree relatives (younger than 55 years).

 PATHOPHYSIOLOGY

Angina, which means "to choke," is caused by a decrease in myocardial oxygen supply. It usually occurs when the coronary artery is more than 75% occluded. The occlusion is due to a thrombus or embolus that blocks the coronary artery, which in turn prevents effective delivery of oxygen to the myocardial cells. This deprivation of oxygen produces ischemia, which causes chest pain. The pain most often occurs during physical activity, when the oxygen supply cannot meet the requirements of the myocardial cells. Emotional distress may also cause angina pectoris.

Causes of angina include atherosclerosis of the coronary arteries, coronary artery spasm, thrombosis, aortic stenosis, hypertrophic cardiomyopathy, primary pulmonary hypertension, severe hypertension, and aortic insufficiency.

 SIGNS AND SYMPTOMS

Stable Angina (Exertional, Classic, or Chronic Angina)

Pressure or heaviness, radiating to the back, neck, or arms, is brought on by exercise, emotional stress, meals, cold air, or smoking and is relieved by rest or nitroglycerin. It lasts several minutes but no longer than 30 minutes. The discomfort may radiate to the neck, lower jaw, teeth, shoulders, inner aspects of the arms, or back. Discomfort may be described as a "clenched fist over the sternum" (Levine's sign). Dyspnea on exertion may be the only symptom in some cases. The electrocardiogram (ECG) is usually normal.

Unstable Angina. Progressive, rest, or postinfarction angina or chest pain is new or has changed in character to become more frequent, more severe, or both. It may precede myocardial infarction (MI) in some patients. Transient ST-segment depression, T wave inversion, or ventricular arrhythmias may be observed.

Printzmetal's Angina (Variant Angina). Chest pain occurs at rest or in an atypical pattern, such as after exercise or nocturnally. Pain is the result of coronary artery spasms, and electrocardiographic changes (usually ST-segment elevation) are noted during symptoms.

Anginal Equivalent. Exertional dyspnea or fatigue results from myocardial ischemia and is relieved with rest or nitroglycerin.

 DIAGNOSTIC CRITERIA

12-Lead Electrocardiogram. The ECG may show evidence of previous MI. During angina, the ECG often shows ST-segment depression, T wave inversion, or both. The changes resolve after the episode ends. Other findings are nonspecific, and traces are usually normal. Bundle-branch block, Wolff-Parkinson-White syndrome, or intraventricular conduction delay may make the ECG unreliable.

Exercise Stress Test: Positive. An exercise stress test is conducted to determine how the heart reacts when it is forced to work under the stress of exercise. It usually involves the patient walking on a treadmill or riding a stationary bike for 30 to 60 minutes, during which an ECG is performed.

Radioisotopes. The use of an intravenously administered radionuclide with a noninvasive cardiac scanner allows for the identification of poor or lack of perfusion of the coronary arteries.

Stress Echocardiography. The myocardium is stressed by the administration of dobutamine, an inotropic agent. Myocardial wall motion is observed on continuous echocardiography.

Stress Thallium Test: Positive. Thallium is taken up by normal cardiac cells to reveal poorly perused areas, which are called "cold spots."

Rapid Sequence Magnetic Resonance Imaging. Magnetic resonance imaging may reveal coronary artery calcification but does not identify obstructive coronary artery lesions.

Cardiac Catheterization with Coronary Angiography

This is an invasive diagnostic test performed to quantify the patency of the coronary arteries. This procedure is capable of measuring cardiac filling pressures and left ventricular function through a ventriculogram.

 INTERVENTIONS

Comprehensive Management of Chronic, Stable Angina

- Identification and treatment of associated diseases, which can precipitate or worsen angina
- Reduction in coronary risk factors (see Section 4)
- General and nonpharmacologic methods, with particular attention toward adjustments of lifestyle
- Pharmacologic management
- Revascularization through percutaneous coronary interventions (PCIs) or coronary artery bypass graft (CABG) surgery

Pharmacologic Management

Only two medical therapies (aspirin and effective lipid-lowering agents) have been convincingly shown to reduce mortality and morbidity rates in patients with chronic stable angina.

- Aspirin, 160 to 325 mg/day PO, is indicated for all patients with coronary disease in whom this medication is not contraindicated (e.g., those with an allergy to aspirin or those on warfarin therapy). It is cost-effective antiplatelet therapy.

- **Hydroxymethyl glutaryl coenzyme A (HMG-CoA) reductase inhibitors** should be started for hypercholesterolemia. These drugs not only have a positive affect on the lipid profile but also decrease the incidence of symptomatic CAD and of MI and death from MI.

Other therapies, such as nitrates and calcium channel blockers, have been shown to improve symptomatology and exercise performance, but their effect, if any, on survival has not been demonstrated.

- **Beta-blockers** are effective in decreasing the heart rate, which reduces myocardial oxygen demand and thus reduces angina. The treatment goal is to maintain the resting heart rate at 50 to 60 beats/min. Side effects are common and include fatigue, exacerbation of peripheral vascular and chronic obstructive pulmonary disease, depression, and erectile dysfunction. Geriatric patients may be very sensitive to these side effects. Beta-blockers must also be used with caution in patients with diabetes because they may mask the signs and symptoms of hypoglycemia.
- **Calcium channel blockers** (calcium antagonists), in the long-acting form, are indicated for the treatment of angina in patients without compromised ventricular function (left ventricular [LV] ejection fraction of more than 40%). The various agents have different side effect profiles. The short-acting calcium channel blockers, such as nifedipine, are contraindicated because they increase the risk of myocardial ischemia.
- **Long-acting nitrates** act through preload reduction and coronary vasodilatation. A daily nitrate-free interval of 10 to 14 hours is necessary to prevent tolerance. A calcium channel blocker or beta-blocker should be used along with the nitrates during the drug-free interval. Tachyphylaxis occurs rapidly. Side effects include headache and hypotension and tend to decrease with continued use.
- **Sublingual nitroglycerin**, 0.4 mg, is the most effective therapy for the treatment of acute anginal episodes. It is available in both tablet and spray form. The dose may be repeated every 5 minutes up to three times, at which time the patient should seek emergency medical care if symptoms are not relieved.
- **Combination therapy,** especially nitrates in conjunction with calcium channel blockers, is common. Triple therapy with the addition of a beta-blocker may be necessary. Beta-blockers and calcium channel blockers may combine to produce symptomatic heart block. Care must be taken when prescribing combination therapy in patients with even moderately impaired LV function.

Treatment goals in the management of unstable angina include symptomatic relief, reperfusion, and prevention of MI. In the acute phase, this is accomplished through the administration of antithrombotic agents and agents such as beta-blockers that decrease the workload of the heart. The goal of long-term management includes repair of the vessel and prevention of recurrence, with treatment strategies that focus on antithrombosis, risk factor modification, and surgical intervention if indicated.

- **Aspirin** is the most common antiplatelet agent prescribed for the treatment of coronary heart disease. After the rupture of an atherosclerotic plaque, aspirin decreases platelet activation by preventing the production and release of thromboxane A_2, a potent platelet activator, from platelets.

- **Heparin** is the most commonly used agent for acute anticoagulation. Current recommendations for anticoagulation in unstable angina include the administration of aspirin, 160 to 325 mg/day PO, as soon as possible, followed by unfractionated heparin (UH) at 80 units/kg IV bolus with maintenance initially at 18 U/kg/hr. Target activated partial thromboplastin time (aPTT) should be maintained at 1.5 to 2 times the control for at least 48 hours or until resolution of the event.
- The current trend is to substitute the **low-molecular-weight heparin** (LMWH) enoxaparin or dalteparin for UH. Efficacy has proved to be similar among the two classes of heparin. The increasing popularity of the LMWHs has evolved from the limitations of UH, which include varying aPTT; frequent monitoring; bleeding; thrombocytopenia; osteoporosis; intravenous administration, which increases inpatient costs; and rebound ischemic events associated with cessation. It is important to note that with the use of combination therapy (i.e., LMWH, aspirin, and glycoprotein [GP] IIb/IIIa platelet inhibitors), there is a much greater propensity for bleeding.
- Management options that are continually evolving include administration of the **GP IIb/IIIa platelet inhibitors**, affecting platelet aggregation through the inhibition of clot-bound thrombin, the final common pathway before platelet aggregation and clot formation after plaque rupture. The GP IIb/IIIa inhibitors can be administered as complementary therapy with UH or the LMWHs. GP IIb/IIIa inhibitors bind to GP IIb/IIIa receptors, preventing the binding of fibrinogen to the platelet. Therefore, the formation or progression of platelet activation is inhibited. When used in combination with UH, inactivation of thrombin results, thus preventing the conversion of fibrinogen to fibrin.

Percutaneous Coronary Interventions

PCIs include angioplasty–repeat dilatation, stent implantation, and directional and rotational coronary atherectomy. Effective antiplatelet therapy is crucial with PCIs because of platelet-mediated restenosis. As a result of this platelet stimulation associated with PCIs, the GP IIb/IIIa inhibitors may be used as adjunctive therapy with PCIs. The GP IIb/IIIa inhibitors are administered intravenously, and the patient must be closely monitored for bleeding.

Aortocoronary Bypass (Coronary Artery Bypass Graft Surgery, Open Heart Surgery)

CABG is a surgical procedure that circumvents obstructive coronary lesions through the process of myocardial revascularization. This results in unobstructed blood flow that oxygenates previously ischemic myocardium. The most commonly used autogenous blood vessels to bridge the occluded areas are the internal mammary arteries and the saphenous veins. CABG is indicated with severe three-vessel disease or diffuse disease in a single vessel.

COMMUNITY CARE

Risk factors must be identified, and reduction strategy must be implemented.

Assessment

1. Take a history, and assess the following risk factors.
   - Family history of premature coronary disease

- Hypercholesterolemia
- Hypertension
- Tobacco use
- Diabetes mellitus
- Male gender
- Advanced age
- Postmenopausal women

2. Assess ability to adapt, dietary patterns, learning and coping abilities and interest, and family participation and support in the medical regimen.
3. Assess knowledge of the disease process, risk factors, required lifestyle adaptations, follow-up care, and knowledge of and compliance with medication and diet.
4. Assess cardiovascular status, and instruct patient to assess pain and characteristics, and precipitating and alleviating factors, with an emphasis on early recognition of onset.
5. Assess lifestyle, participation in activities of daily living, and effects of activity on angina. Identify activities that increase oxygen consumption and cause pain.

Monitoring

1. The frequency and severity of the complaints guide monitoring.
2. Monitor pain for type, location, intensity, and duration to establish individual anginal pattern, and instruct the patient to report any change in established pattern.
3. Hospitalization for the initiation of intravenous heparin therapy is indicated for patients diagnosed with unstable angina.

Prevention

Advise the patient to
1. Discontinue tobacco use.
2. Adhere to a low-fat, low-cholesterol diet.
3. Engage in a regular aerobic exercise program.
4. Take antilipidemic drugs.
5. Minimize emotional stress.

PROGNOSIS

1. The prognosis varies and depends on the extent of CAD as well as on LV function.
2. The annual overall mortality rate is 3% to 4%.

CLINICAL PEARLS

○ The treatment goal with all types of angina is to reduce myocardial oxygen demand or to increase myocardial oxygen supply.
○ Diabetics and women often have silent ischemia.
○ The primary concern when caring for patients who have received heparin, a GP IIb/IIIa platelet inhibitor, or both is potential bleeding complications that can affect the patient's safety. It is essential to monitor patients carefully and be alert for thrombocytopenia as an indicator of a potential problem.

○ When UH is administered, the nurse is responsible for follow-up and reporting of aPTT values to the appropriate provider.

○ Comprehensive patient education and risk factor reduction are important secondary prevention efforts in patients with angina.

○ For patients who receive antiplatelet agents, education before discharge home is of utmost importance. Patients should understand bleeding risks associated with antiplatelet therapy. They should be instructed to take proper precautions to prevent bleeding, which include the use of a soft toothbrush and the avoidance of aspirin-containing products such as Alka-Seltzer, Norgesic, and Goodies and BC Headache Powders. Encourage the patient to comply with the follow-up schedule and to report any bleeding complications.

○ Success in the treatment of a patient who presents with angina requires a well-informed patient who understands the side-effect profile of the agents administered as well as the importance of follow-up.

NURSING PROBLEM/ DIAGNOSIS	NURSING INTERVENTIONS CLASSIFICATION (NIC)
Ischemia/acute pain (chest)	Cardiac care: Acute Pain management Energy management
Effective therapeutic regimen management	Teaching: Disease process Teaching: Prescribed medication Cardiac precautions

Cardiogenic Shock

Section 2   Judy Graham Garcia ■ Rebecca Rule

 OVERVIEW

Shock is a syndrome in which the oxygen delivery system is unable to meet the metabolic demands of the body, therefore compromising organ functions. If untreated, shock may progress to circulatory collapse, impaired cellular metabolism, and, eventually, death.

The hallmark of cardiogenic shock is the inability of the impaired ventricle to adequately perfuse and oxygenate the tissues of the body. The causes of cardiogenic shock include acute MI (AMI), heart failure (HF) (left ventricular [LV] and right ventricular [RV]), cardiomyopathy, severe valvular defects, pulmonary embolism, cardiac tamponade, tachyarrhythmias and bradyarrhythmias, and cardiopulmonary bypass.

Successful nursing care of the patient in cardiogenic shock requires prompt problem identification and rapid intervention. Depending on the degree of altered hemodynamics and the cause of inadequate circulation, patients who present with cardiogenic shock may undergo multiple therapies to promote adequate myocardial and cerebral perfusion.

 PATHOPHYSIOLOGY

Cardiogenic shock results from inadequate tissue perfusion due to inability of the left ventricle to pump sufficient blood to meet the metabolic demands

and oxygen requirements of the body. Cardiogenic shock is most commonly caused by massive MI that damages 40% or more of the left ventricle. The ventricle is unable to meet the demands of the body due to decreased cardiac output, maldistribution of blood flow, or both.

Impaired function of the left ventricle leads to decreased stroke volume and inadequate systolic emptying. The decreased stroke volume results in decreased cardiac output, causing hypotension and decreased tissue perfusion. Inadequate systolic emptying causes blood to build up in the left ventricle and then back up into the pulmonary circulation, which can progress to cause congestion in the right ventricle and systemic circulation. This leads to an increase in LV filling pressure, left atrial pressure, pulmonary venous pressure, and pulmonary capillary pressure, all of which lead to pulmonary interstitial and intra-alveolar edema. The vicious cycle continues.

 ## SIGNS AND SYMPTOMS

The cardinal signs of cardiogenic shock are hypotension, with systolic blood pressures of less than 90 mm Hg, and inadequate peripheral perfusion and eventual end-organ hypoperfusion. Initial compensatory mechanisms in response to the decreased blood pressure cause catecholamine (epinephrine and norepinephrine) release, which results in increased myocardial contractility and heart rate and elevated temperature. Catecholamine release also causes peripheral vasoconstriction in an attempt to shunt blood from the periphery to the major organs. This results in decreased capillary refill time, absent or weak thready peripheral pulses, and decreased pulse pressure. Pulmonary congestion results in dyspnea and crackles. Right-sided heart congestion results in jugular vein distention and peripheral edema.

As shock continues, compensatory mechanisms fail. Inadequate organ perfusion manifests according to the system that is affected (see Chapter 14, Section 3) (Table 14-2-1).

 ## DIAGNOSTIC CRITERIA

Cardiogenic shock can be differentiated from other forms of shock on the basis of specific diagnostic criteria. Typically in cardiogenic shock, blood pressure is low, heart rate is elevated, pulses are diminished, lungs are congested, skin is cool, and jugular neck veins are distended.

Hemodynamic Monitoring via Pulmonary Artery Catheter
Electrocardiography
This is helpful when distinguishing from other forms of shock (see Table 14-2-2). The ECG provides important clues to the cause of cardiogenic shock by assessing for evidence of myocardial ischemia or injury.

Echocardiography
Echocardiography should reveal the following findings if the cause of cardiogenic shock is:
- Bradycardia: normal-sized ventricular chambers with vigorous systolic contraction with a slow rate
- LV failure: dilated left ventricle with reduced systolic performance; regional wall motion abnormalities may indicate old or new myocardial ischemia or infarction
- RV failure: dilated right atrium and right ventricle with reduced RV systolic

Table 14-2-1. Symptoms and Etiology of Cardiogenic Shock

MANIFESTATION	CAUSE
Anxiety	Decreased cerebral perfusion
Restlessness	
Confusion and disorientation	
Lethargy	
Coma	
Presence of S3 or S4 heart sounds	Decreased myocardial perfusion
Cool, moist, clammy, pale skin with marked facial pallor, bluish or mottled extremities, and severe cyanosis of the lips and nailbeds	Increased myocardial demands for oxygen and nutrients
Chest pain	
Increased respiratory rate, later becoming Cheyne-Stokes or apneic	Decreased pulmonary perfusion
Diffuse rales	
Nausea	Decreased gastrointestinal perfusion
Hypoactive bowel sounds	
Decreased urinary output	Decreased renal perfusion
Muscle aches	Decreased perfusion to the musculoskeletal system
Diminished deep tendon reflexes	

contraction; tricuspid regurgitation is usually present; contractility of the left ventricle varies
- Cardiac tamponade: small cardiac chambers with diastolic collapse of the right atrium and right ventricle. Systolic contraction of the right atrium and right ventricle is usually normal unless dysfunction was present previously or coexistent LV or RV failure has occurred.

Pulse Oximetry
This is used to evaluate arterial oxygen saturation; normal adult value is more than 92% without oxygen therapy.

Chest Radiography
The degree of cardiac enlargement and pulmonary vascular congestion is evaluated.

Cardiac Angiography
Obstructed coronary arteries, leading to myocardial ischemia and injury, are identified.

Table 14-2-2. Expected Findings in Cardiogenic Shock

PARAMETER	EXPECTED CHANGE	NORMAL VALUE
Right atrial pressure or central venous pressure	Normal or increased	2–6 mm Hg
Pulmonary capillary wedge pressure or pulmonary occlusion wedge pressure	Increased	6–12 mm Hg
Systemic vascular resistance	Increased	800–1200 dynes/sec/cm^{-5}
Cardiac output	Decreased	4–8 L/min
Cardiac index	Decreased	2.5–4 L/min/M^2

Laboratory Tests

Arterial blood gas, serum lactate, serum chemistry, and cardiac enzyme tests provide indications to the degree of shock, fluid and electrolyte status, oxygenation, and myocardial damage.

INTERVENTIONS

Thrombolysis, Percutaneous Coronary Interventions, and Coronary Artery Bypass Graft Surgery

Only early revascularization seems to reduce the mortality rate associated with cardiogenic shock. Patients who are referred for coronary arteriography should receive interim circulatory support with appropriate pharmacologic agents and intra-aortic balloon pump (IABP) counterpulsation. Ventricular function can be improved by relief of the ischemia that occurs as a result of occluded as well as severely obstructed nonoccluded coronary arteries.

Pharmacologic Management

1. If the cause is *LV failure*, treat the patient with vasopressors and vasodilators. The goal is to correct hypotension, increase forward LV output, and return LV and RV filling pressures to the normal range. Agents to be used may include the following:
   - **Calcium chloride** increases myocardial contractility, but the effect may be modest and short lived.
   - **Dopamine** increases systemic arterial pressure and cardiac output.
   - **Dobutamine** or **milrinone** augments cardiac output and is the agent of choice if ventricular filling pressure reduction is necessary.
   - **Milrinone** reduces preload and afterload through direct arterial vasodilation and has a positive inotropic effect.
   - **Nitroprusside** or **nitroglycerin** may be administered if the systolic arterial pressure is more than 90 mm Hg to increase forward cardiac output and decrease the pulmonary capillary wedge pressure.
   - **Norepinephrine** may be necessary in patients with profound hypotension or systolic arterial pressure of less than 70 mm Hg, to prevent coronary hypoperfusion.
   - **Diuretics** may also be cautiously used to reduce the systemic congestion.
   - **Fluids** and **electrolytes** maintain adequate intravascular volume and support cardiac function.
2. If the cause is *RV failure*, treat the patient with pulmonary vasodilators such as isoproterenol, prostaglandin E_1, or intravenous nitroglycerin and inotropes such as dobutamine. For refractory hypotension that does not respond to these measures, a pulmonary vasodilator may be infused directly into the pulmonary artery via a Swan-Ganz (pulmonary artery) catheter or via inhalation of nitric oxide.
3. If the cause is *cardiac tamponade*, supportive measures are used that include volume expansion intravenous fluids such as plasma protein fraction (Plasmanate) or whole blood and inotropes such as dobutamine.

Intra-aortic Balloon Pump Counterpulsation

Effective for both LV and RV failure, mechanical circulatory support with IABP may be used in conjunction with pharmacologic agents. This can prevent a continuous upward titration of sympathomimetic inotropes and vasoconstrictors that can result in decreased perfusion of the renal, mesenteric, and coronary vasculature. Another advantage of IABP counterpulsation is that it does not increase myocardial oxygen demand.

Left Ventricular Assist Device

LV assist devices may be used if the combination of IABP counterpulsation and pharmacotherapy fails. These devices serve as temporary supports or "bridges" to heart transplantation.

Cardiac Pacing

Pacing is effective for cardiogenic shock secondary to bradyarrhythmias.

Surgical Reexploration

Emergency sternotomy or subxiphoid drainage is necessary for cardiac tamponade after cardiac surgery.

Pericardiocentesis

Pericardiocentesis is effective only for nonsurgical cardiac tamponade.

Heart Transplantation

Heart transplantation has been used successfully to treat cardiogenic shock in appropriately selected patients.

Oxygen Therapy

Oxygen therapy is necessary to support pulmonary congestion and fatigue. Close monitoring of hemodynamic status is essential. Responses to all medications and fluid therapies must be evaluated with efforts to maintain a mean arterial pressure of more than 80 mm Hg, urine output of more than 0.5 mL/kg/hr, and electrolytes within normal limits. Oxygenation status is monitored to maintain oxygen saturation at more than 92% and PaO_2 at more than 80 on blood gas analysis. Breath sounds should also clear with therapy, and respiratory effort should be reduced. Electrolyte and acid-base status is closely monitored and corrected as needed.

 COMMUNITY CARE

Take a history and assess risk factors for CAD, MI, and HF. Take preventative steps as identified for patients with CAD (see Chapter 14, Section 4), MI (see Chapter 14, Section 5), and HF (see Chapter 14, Section 3).

 PROGNOSIS

A diagnosis of cardiogenic shock carries a poor prognosis, with a fatality rate of about 70%.

 CLINICAL PEARLS

o Prompt recognition by the bedside nurse of the signs and symptoms of impending cardiogenic shock can lead to immediate treatment and circulatory support, preventing the downward spiral of the deleterious low output syndrome that can ensue.

○ Clarify the patient's desires regarding end-of-life and resuscitation issues.
○ Involve the family in decision-making, and keep them informed of the disease process, treatment, and prognosis.
○ Identify important nursing diagnoses and implement necessary interventions: fluid volume deficit, altered peripheral tissue perfusion, decreased cardiac output, anxiety and fear, ineffective family coping, knowledge deficit, and altered nutrition, less than body requirements.

NURSING PROBLEM/ DIAGNOSIS	NURSING INTERVENTIONS CLASSIFICATION (NIC)
Pump failure/decreased cardiac output	Hemodynamic regulation
	Shock management: Cardiac
Pulmonary congestion/impaired gas exchange	Oxygen therapy
	Airway management
	Respiratory monitoring

Heart Failure

Section 3   Kitty Garrett

OVERVIEW

HF is a leading cause of death in the United States. It affects 4.8 million persons, accounting for more than 200,000 deaths annually. It is the only cardiovascular disease that continues to increase in incidence, more than doubling each decade from age 45 to 75. As more cardiac patients live longer, the chance of HF developing increases. HF is associated with significant morbidity leading to a high incidence of physician office visits and hospitalizations and a high prevalence of early readmissions. Fifty percent of HF patients die within 5 years after diagnosis. There is a high incidence of sudden death secondary to ventricular dysrhythmias. Despite new research findings regarding the pathophysiology and treatment of HF, it continues to be a chronic, debilitating syndrome and a major public health concern.

The simplest explanation of HF is that the heart is unable to pump sufficient blood to meet the metabolic needs of the tissues due to a reduction in the contractile force of the ventricles. The term *heart failure* is preferred over the commonly used *congestive heart failure* because many patients with HF do not manifest pulmonary or systemic congestion.

Many patients have combined systolic and diastolic components. Even though the symptoms may be similar for both, it is important to make the distinction because the treatment is different for each. Systolic HF is more common, occurring in 70% of cases; diastolic HF is seen less frequently (30%).

PATHOPHYSIOLOGY

The cause of the decrease in ventricular contractility in HF may be secondary to the initial insult (MI, hypertension, cardiomyopathy) or secondary to compensatory mechanisms that become maladaptive. It was discovered that chronic advanced HF is the result of the prolonged action of several factors: ventricular remodeling and hypertrophy, neurohormonal activation of the sympathetic nervous system, the Frank-Starling and renin-angiotensin-aldosterone (RAA) mechanisms, and the secretion of other vasoactive substances.

The increase in muscle mass that occurs in chronic HF with LV hypertrophy initially increases the force of ventricular contraction. However, over time, changes in the structural, functional, and gene expressions of myocardial cells begin to develop. These cellular changes cause the ventricle to assume a more spherical shape; this is called *ventricular remodeling*. The cell growth is abnormal and disorganized, and instead of enhancing contractility, the myocardium becomes stiff and noncompliant with a decrease in contractility. Eventually, the size of the muscle outgrows the blood supply, and ischemia develops. The more decompensated the patient, the more ventricular remodeling occurs. This perpetuates a cycle that exacerbates the HF and can increase the risk of sudden death from ventricular ischemia and dysrhythmias. It is recognized that if ventricular remodeling can be minimized, the progression of HF may be delayed.

The decrease in cardiac output initiates a chain of physiologic events in an attempt to compensate for the decreased blood supply. Compensatory mechanisms such as activation of the sympathetic nervous system, the Frank-Starling mechanism, and the RAA mechanism are initially adaptive and serve to restore cardiac output but eventually become maladaptive.

Catecholamines (epinephrine and norepinephrine) are released in response to the decreased cardiac output; they exert their adrenergic effects on the heart and blood vessels.

Heart

Acute activation of the sympathetic nervous system causes an increase in heart rate and force of contraction that is an attempt to pump out more blood to increase cardiac output. Initially, the increase in heart rate is effective. However, the faster the heart rate, less time for ventricular filling, resulting in decreased rather than increased cardiac output, leading to ischemia and angina if CAD is present.

Blood Vessels

When arterial pressure falls, the baroreceptor reflex responds by constricting peripheral arteries and veins to redistribute blood to the vital organs (brain and heart). The vasoconstriction is again very effective initially, but if prolonged, it may cause increased resistance to flow (afterload) and ultimately also can decrease rather than increase cardiac output. The left ventricle, after months of chronic overworking against this resistance, begins to hypertrophy, and the vicious cycle of ventricular remodeling is perpetuated.

The Frank-Starling mechanism describes the attempt by the heart to increase stroke volume by stretching the LV fibers to elicit a stronger contraction. The greater the volume, the greater the stretch, and the more forceful is the contraction. This occurs only up to a physiologic point where, if overstretched, the force of the contraction decreases, much like an overstretched rubber band. This ultimately results in cardiac dilatation, which is characteristic of HF. The inner chamber of the left ventricle enlarges to accommodate the expanding volume. During this compensated stage (before overstretching), the patient has no symptoms. However, once overstretching and true cardiac dilatation occur, the contraction becomes weaker and less blood is ejected.

The RAA mechanism is the attempt by the body to increase preload by gaining intravascular volume. This is more likely to occur in chronic HF than during an acute episode. When cardiac output is decreased, renal blood flow is also decreased, stimulating the release of renin, which triggers the RAA mechanism. Renin activates the conversion of angiotensinogen to angiotensin 1, which is inert. The presence of angiotensinogen 1 is sensed by an enzyme called angiotensin-converting enzyme (ACE), which facilitates the conversion of angiotensin I to angiotensin II, a potent vasoconstrictor. Once the circulating angiotensin II is detected, there is a release of aldosterone from the adrenal cortex, which promotes the reabsorption of sodium and water by the distal renal tubules. This increases intravascular volume and decreases urinary output, subsequently increasing cardiac output. The increased intravascular volume gained from the actions of the RAA mechanism can eventually cause problems with LV preload (pulmonary edema) and RV preload (peripheral edema). The increased volume also increases blood pressure, which further aggravates the problem of peripheral resistance (afterload). The myocardial fibers become overstretched, leading to decreased contractility and compensatory hypertrophy. This leads to ventricular remodeling, which perpetuates the cycle.

Other substances, such as vasopressin and endothelin, also contribute to the peripheral vasoconstriction, which increases the systemic vascular resistance.

 SIGNS AND SYMPTOMS

HF is characterized by symptoms of **inadequate tissue perfusion, volume overload,** or both. Inadequate tissue perfusion results in reduced exercise tolerance, fatigue, and shortness of breath. Decreased cerebral perfusion may cause cognitive impairment. Decreased coronary perfusion may cause angina. Ventricular dysrhythmias are common. Weight gain results from excess fluid retention. Increased ventricular filling and decreased systolic ejection result in cardiomegaly (increased heart size). Pulmonary edema results from failure of the left ventricle, and peripheral edema results from failure of the right ventricle. Although most patients with left-sided HF eventually develop pulmonary and systemic congestion, it is helpful in understanding the origins by separating congestive symptoms into left-sided (pulmonary) and right-sided (systemic) components.

The **congestive** symptoms of left-sided HF are caused by the inability of the left ventricle to keep up with the amount of blood presented to it, which causes a backup of fluid into the lungs. Because of the increased demands placed on it to pump blood throughout the body to meet metabolic needs, the left ventricle usually fails first, causing pulmonary congestion. Early symptoms may include fatigue, insomnia, irritability, and exertional dyspnea. Physical assessment signs that may occur before symptoms appear include a tachycardia, the presence of diffuse bilateral crackles that do not clear with coughing, and the presence of a third heart sound. Heart size may be enlarged clinically and radiographically. Later signs, which are highly suggestive of the diagnosis, include dyspnea at rest, orthopnea, and paroxysmal nocturnal dyspnea. Acute pulmonary edema may occur when the pressure in the pulmonary vessels becomes so great that fluid floods the alveoli and decreases the availability for

Table 14-3-1. New York Heart Association Functional Classification of Heart Failure

CLASS	DESCRIPTION
I	No limitations of physical activity; ordinary activity produces no symptoms.
II	Slight limitations; patients are generally comfortable at rest, but ordinary physical activity produces symptoms.
III	Marked limitations; patients are usually comfortable at rest, but less than ordinary physical activity produces symptoms.
IV	Severe limitations; inability to engage in any physical activity without discomfort; patients may have symptoms of cardiac insufficiency or anginal syndrome even at rest; symptoms are generally refractory to treatment; considered end-stage disease.

Symptoms = fatigue, dyspnea, palpitations, angina.
From Diseases of the Heart and Blood Vessels—Nomenclature and Criteria for Diagnosis (6th ed.) (1964). Boston: Little Brown.

air exchange. The fluid can accumulate so rapidly that compensatory mechanisms do not have time to develop and the patient experiences air hunger, frothy sputum, and acute respiratory distress.

Elevated pulmonary pressures from LV failure cause resistance to RV pumping. When the right ventricle has to pump against high pulmonary resistance, it eventually weakens and fails, and fluid backs up into the systemic circulation. Right-sided HF is usually the result of left-sided HF. (Pure right-sided failure due to other causes such as pulmonary hypertension is called cor pulmonale.) Symptoms of right-sided failure are peripheral pitting edema, weight gain, liver engorgement and discomfort, abdominal bloating, and nocturia. There may be ascites due to liver congestion. Intra-abdominal pressure may cause anorexia and nausea. Physical assessment signs of right-sided failure are also peripheral in nature: jugular venous distention, engorged liver, and peripheral edema.

Patients in chronic HF may exhibit a range of symptom severity based on the disease progression. **Exercise tolerance** is related to morbidity and mortality. The New York Heart Association (NYHA) functional classification is a universally accepted system of classifying the severity of HF on the basis of physical limitations (Table 14-3-1).

 DIAGNOSTIC CRITERIA

Laboratory Testing

Routine diagnostic tests include complete blood count, urinalysis, electrolytes, blood urea nitrogen, creatinine, serum albumin, and thyroid function studies. These tests may rule out or confirm other treatable causes of symptoms.

Electrocardiography

There are no specific findings of HF on the ECG.

Chest Radiography

Cardiomegaly is highly suggestive of HF.

Physical Examination

Physical examination is not highly sensitive for the detection of HF, especially in the absence of congestive symptoms.

Echocardiography

The most conclusive test for the diagnosis of HF is the transthoracic Doppler two-dimensional echocardiogram. This can be used to rule out valvular disease, assess ventricular size, and determine whether the LV dysfunction is systolic or diastolic.

Exercise Stress Testing

Pharmacologic induction of "ischemia" with agents such as dobutamine, dipyridamole, or adenosine may be used in patients who cannot exercise for other medical reasons. A stress echocardiogram (using exercise or dobutamine) may also detect ischemia and viable myocardium.

Coronary Angiography

Angiography may be performed to evaluate the patient for CAD. It is important to identify HF accompanied by angina because this group of patients stands to gain the greatest benefit from revascularization with CABG to improve symptoms and prognosis. The presence of chest pain suggests that there some viable myocardium remains to salvage.

INTERVENTIONS

The treatment of chronic HF has changed remarkably since the 1990s. HF is no longer considered simply an edematous state in which patients are treated symptomatically with diuretics. Research demonstrating new findings in the pathophysiology of the disease has shifted the emphasis from symptomatic treatment to the prevention of disease progression.

Acute Exacerbations

During hospitalization for acute exacerbations of chronic HF, the following are required for patients.

- Supplemental oxygen, cardiac monitoring, and short periods of bed rest may help decrease myocardial oxygen consumption ($M\dot{V}O_2$) and promote diuresis. To reduce venous return and permit greater lung expansion, a semi- or high Fowler's position is used.
- Deep breathing exercises and repositioning are encouraged at least every 2 hours to prevent atelectasis.
- Intake and output, patient weight, and electrolyte levels are monitored daily.
- Vital signs and mental status are assessed at least every 2 to 4 hours, with any significant changes reported immediately.
- Assess for deep venous thromboses. Elastic stockings or compression devices are used in nonambulatory patients to enhance circulation. Early ambulation is encouraged.

Unless otherwise directed, notify the physician of the following situations:

- Systolic blood pressure of less than 90 mm Hg, heart rate of less than 50 beats/min (suspend use of beta-blockers and digoxin)
- Oxygen saturation less than 92% on oxygen therapy
- Excessive intake compared with output (positive fluid balance of 1000 mL in 24 hours), weight gain of more than 2 lb/day, 24-hour urine output of

less than 30 mL/hr, blood urea nitrogen and creatinine more than baseline, or creatinine of more than 3.0
- Potassium of more than 5.5 mEq/L or less than 3.5 mEq/L

CABG should be attempted in patients with coronary disease and ischemia. Surgical procedures such as cardiomyoplasty are still considered experimental. Heart transplantation may be used as a last resort in patients with end-stage HF.

Chronic Heart Failure

The goal for a patient with chronic HF is improvement in quality of life (i.e., improvement in functional capacity), increase in survival time, and management of the compensatory mechanisms that cause symptoms of pulmonary and peripheral congestion.

Any treatable underlying cause (e.g., hypertension, dysrhythmias, aortic stenosis, mitral regurgitation) should be corrected if possible.

Nonpharmacologic Management

Have the patient limit sodium and fluid intake, lose weight if necessary, and avoid alcohol, because it can decrease contractility. Mild to moderate activity as tolerated is recommended to avoid atrophy of skeletal muscles, improve aerobic conditioning, and improve psychosocial status. Isometric exercises such as pushups and weightlifting should be avoided because they put too much stress on the left ventricle.

Pharmacologic Management

Traditionally, medical treatment was aimed at symptom relief and consisted of administering diuretics, digitalis, and vasodilators. These drugs decrease the workload of the heart by decreasing preload (volume) and afterload (resistance) and by increasing contractility. These drugs are still prescribed, but the focus is on suppression of compensatory mechanisms and prevention of disease progression. ACE inhibitors, aldosterone blockers, and beta-blockers fall into this category (Table 14-3-2).

Angiotensin-converting Enzyme Inhibitors

ACE inhibitors are used in all patients with LV dysfunction, even in those with NYHA functional class I HF, to prevent symptoms. If ACE inhibitors cannot be administered due to allergy, bilateral renal artery stenosis, pregnancy, angioneurotic edema, hyperkalemia, elevated creatinine, cough, hypotension, or other problems, an alpha-2 adrenergic receptor blocker such as losartan or a combination of hydralazine and isosorbide dinitrate may be used. Two commonly used ACE inhibitors are captopril (Capoten) and enalapril (Vasotec).

Hypotension is common with the first dose, especially in patients who are sodium or volume depleted, such as those treated vigorously with diuretics. Doses should be started low and titrated up. The concurrent use of aspirin or nonsteroidal anti-inflammatory drugs may cause sodium retention, decreased renal function, or worsening of HF.

Diuretics

Daily weights and intake and output should be monitored. Daily weight fluctuations are secondary to fluid gains and losses, not to body fat. A weight gain of 2 to 3 lb overnight is considered a significant weight gain. Diuretics should be used only when the patient has signs of volume overload. Patients

Table 14-3-2. Recommended Medications in Chronic Systolic Heart Failure (<40%) Left Ventricular Ejection Fraction

NYHA CLASS	I	II	III	IV
ACE inhibitors (captopril)*	Prevents conversion of angiotensin I to angiotensin II; decreases fluid; retention; ↓ afterload by vasodilatation; improves survival and clinical symptoms; prevents "remodeling"			
Diuretics		↓ Preload; used only with symptoms of volume overload; rapid effect; must be individualized		
Digitalis		↑ Contractility; used to improve symptoms or slow ventricular rate in atrial fibrillation		
Beta-blockers (carvediolol)†		Blocks sympathetic response—prevents excessive increase in heart rate and blood pressure; vasodilates to improve symptoms and clinical status; prevents "remodeling" (effects take 2–3 months)		
Aldosterone blockers (spironolactone)			Blocks renin-angiotensin-aldosterone response; decreases myocardial fibrosis (cardioprotective)	
IV inotropes (dobutamine, milrinone)†			Controversial; palliative; ↑ contractility and ↓ symptoms in patients refractory to maximal medical treatment	

Note: With the exception of IV inotropes and diuretics, these drugs are not used in acute exacerbations.
*In patients who cannot tolerate angiotensin-converting enzyme (ACE) inhibitors, substitute an α_1-adrenergic receptor blocker such as losartan or a combination of hydralazine and isosorbide dinitrate.
†Do not combine beta-blockers with intravenous inotropes; otherwise any combination of the above drugs may be given.

462

with mild HF can usually be managed adequately on thiazides. However, with severe volume overload or when the glomerular filtration rate is low secondary to decreased cardiac output, thiazides are ineffective, and loop diuretics (furosemide, bumetanide, metolazone [Zaroxolyn]) must be used. Loop diuretics are administered intravenously when oral doses do not provide the desired response.

Blood pressure and potassium and magnesium levels should be monitored closely because diuretics can cause hypotension, hypokalemia, and hypomagnesemia. Alkalosis may also be present.

Digitalis

Digoxin has been used for years to treat HF. It is inexpensive and well tolerated and improves quality of life by alleviating symptoms. However, digoxin has not been shown to have an effect on survival or disease progression. It therefore is not recommended for patients with NYHA functional class I but rather for patients with mild to moderate symptoms of HF (class II/III).

The serum digoxin level should be monitored initially until a therapeutic level is obtained and at any point where digitalis toxicity is suspected, renal function deteriorates, or symptoms worsen. The therapeutic level of digoxin is 0.5 to 2 ng/mL; greater than 2.0 is considered toxic. There is a fine line between therapeutic dose and toxicity, especially in patients with impaired renal function. The risk of toxicity is potentiated by hypokalemia, which may occur with the concurrent use of diuretics. Symptoms of toxicity include fatigue, visual disturbances such as green halos, nausea and anorexia, and cardiac dysrhythmias. As long as the patient has normal renal function, any excess digoxin is eliminated through the kidneys. Several drugs, including amiodarone, quinidine, beta-blockers, diuretics, and verapamil, potentiate the effect of digoxin.

Beta-Blockers

The use of beta-blockers has historically been contraindicated in HF due to their negative inotropic effect on the myocardium. Because the focus of the treatment of HF is on the prevention of ventricular remodeling and neurohormonal activation (the causes) rather than on the decreased contractility (the effect), the use of beta-blockers is being reconsidered for patients with NYHA functional class II/III HF.

Carvedilol (Coreg) is the only beta-blocker approved by the Food and Drug Administration for the treatment of HF. Carvedilol is a combination of a beta-blocker and alpha-1 adrenergic blocker, which means that it prevents tachycardia and increased force of contraction and prevents vasoconstriction. It has been shown to reduce the risk of disease progression, and it may improve LV function and increase exercise tolerance.

Beta-blockers should not be used in acute episodes of HF; they are indicated for the long-term management of chronic HF. Treatment is initiated at low doses and gradually increased. Patients are monitored carefully for dizziness, hypotension, bradycardia, and fluid retention during this period. They may feel more fatigue and have worsening HF symptoms initially, but LV ejection fraction improves after 2 to 3 months of therapy. To prevent hypotension, the administration of beta-blockers should be spaced throughout the day so that they are not given at the same time as diuretics and ACE inhibitors. Abrupt withdrawal could result in severe deterioration. The use of beta-blockers should be discontinued if intravenous inotropic therapy (milrinone, dobutamine) is required. Beta-blockers can cause bronchospasm and are contraindicated in patients with bronchial asthma.

Vasodilators

Vasodilators are first-line drugs in HF; they may dilate arterioles or venules to decrease the workload of the heart. ACE inhibitors are the most effective vasodilators. However, if they are contraindicated, a combination of hydralazine (Apresoline) and isosorbide dinitrate (Isordil) may be used. Hydralazine is an arteriolar vasodilator, and isosorbide dinitrate is a venous vasodilator.

Significant side effects of nitrates include orthostatic hypotension and reflex tachycardia. If fluid retention is present, vasodilators should not be administered without diuretics to prevent pulmonary and peripheral edema.

Sympathomimetics (Dobutamine) and Phosphodiesterase Inhibitors (Milrinone)

The intravenous infusion of positive inotropic agents such as dobutamine (Dobutrex) or milrinone (Primacor) may be used in patients with advanced HF (NYHA functional class III/IV) who are refractory to maximum doses of ACE inhibitors, digoxin, and diuretics. Dobutamine and milrinone are considered palliative in helping to relieve symptoms in patients with end-stage HF. Patients may receive infusions as inpatients or outpatients or even in the home setting. Administration through a central venous line and cardiac monitoring during administration are recommended.

Even though there have been many anecdotal reports of improvement in quality of life, several studies have shown that mortality rate, dysrhythmias, and myocardial oxygen consumption demands are increased with positive inotropic drugs.

Aldosterone Blockers (Spironolactone)

Aldosterone blockers are indicated in patients with NYHA functional class III/IV HF. Aldosterone blockers should be administered with ACE inhibitors. Standard doses of ACE inhibitors only transiently suppress the release of aldosterone, whereas aldosterone blockers contribute to a more sustained effect.

The main side effects are hypotension and hyperkalemia.

Anticoagulant Agents

Anticoagulants (warfarin) are indicated in patients with atrial fibrillation to prevent systemic embolization. International normalized ratio (INR) levels should be maintained between 2 and 3. Patients with right-sided HF and liver abnormalities should be monitored carefully for bleeding tendencies.

Antidysrhythmia Agents

Supraventricular dysrhythmias such as atrial fibrillation and atrial flutter are common in the dilated heart. Nearly all HF patients have ventricular dysrhythmias. Unless syncope or severe hemodynamic compromise occurs, these should not be treated. Many antidysrhythmia drugs can decrease contractility of the heart. If treatment is necessary, the patient should be monitored or hospitalized. Amiodarone (Cordarone) is approved for the treatment of refractory ventricular dysrhythmias, but its toxicity limits its long-term use. It is also under investigation for use in atrial dysrhythmias. The patient may be evaluated for insertion of an automated implantable cardioverter-defibrillator if there is a risk of sudden death from ventricular dysrhythmias.

Diastolic Heart Failure

The goal of drug therapy in patients with diastolic dysfunction is to control symptoms by reducing ventricular filling pressure without reducing cardiac output. Diuretics and nitrates are the drugs of choice. Calcium channel blockers, beta-blockers, and ACE inhibitors may be of benefit. Agents with positive inotropic effects (digoxin) are not indicated if systolic function is normal.

 COMMUNITY CARE
Economic Impact

Because of the chronic nature of this serious disease and the high prevalence of readmissions, HF is also a very expensive disease. The medical cost for management of the 4.5 million admissions annually is estimated to be $20 to $40 billion. Because only about half of this amount is being reimbursed to hospitals and physicians, hospitals are investigating new creative approaches to cutting costs and decreasing readmissions.

Disease Management

Studies have shown that most "revolving door" readmissions are due to exacerbations of HF that are preventable and related to noncompliance and patients' lack of knowledge and understanding of their disease. "Disease management" programs are being established in response to the realization that it costs less to keep people well. The emphasis is on tertiary promotion of wellness and prevention of complications in persons with specific diseases such as HF. Depending on available resources, disease management programs may include clinic facilities, telephone follow-up, and home visits. Some insurance companies or disease management companies even provide ongoing monitoring over the telephone. Clinic settings may offer physical assessments, weight evaluation, laboratory tests, patient education, monitored low-level exercise and group support, and intravenous infusions of inotropic agents. Most are designed to use a multidisciplinary approach and follow some type of standardized protocols.

Consistent reinforcement of patient education is one of the most important aspects of the program. Education focuses on signs and symptoms of HF, the rationale for daily weighing and sodium restriction, the importance of medication compliance, the encouragement of physical activity, and instructions on when to call the physician. Overall, it teaches the patient to accept responsibility for his or her own health and to make a concerted effort toward lifestyle changes to improve his or her functional status. The psychosocial support and personalized attention enhance motivation, which increases compliance. This simple yet crucial element has been shown to affect patient outcomes as demonstrated by decreases in readmission rates, emergency department visits, and improvement in quality of life.

Emphasize the following aspects of patient education on discharge:

- Increase activity gradually, as much as tolerated without return of symptoms; avoid isometrics.
- Carefully follow dietary restrictions regarding sodium, fluid, and potassium (if on diuretic therapy, may be on 2 to 3 g sodium restriction).
- Read labels, and be especially aware of foods with hidden sodium content.
- Check with the physician before using salt substitutes that contain potassium if taking ACE inhibitors or aldosterone blockers.
- Weigh daily (without clothes, on same scales, and before breakfast). Report a weight gain of more than 2 lb in 1 day or 5 lb in 1 week.

- Report any shortness of breath, palpitations, swelling, persistent dry cough, decrease in urine output, leg cramps, or confusion.
- Understand the purpose of each medication as well as side effects and the importance of taking medications as prescribed.
- Notify the health care provider if problems arise with social support system or with psychological or emotional status.
- Do not drink more than one alcoholic drink per day, and do not smoke.

Prevention

HF remains a chronic, disabling, and lethal condition that can be controlled but not cured. Primary prevention includes the control of hypertension and the reduction in other risk factors for MI. Secondary prevention includes prompt treatment of MI with thrombolytic therapy, percutaneous transluminal coronary angioplasty, CABG, or a combination. Tertiary treatment involves early identification and aggressive treatment, especially of treatable causes. ACE inhibitors should be initiated even before symptoms occur (NYHA functional class I) to prevent further progression.

 PROGNOSIS

Even with aggressive treatment, the 6-year mortality rate is 80% for men and 65% for women. Functional capacity is a predictor of mortality: as symptoms increase, the prognosis worsens. Patients gradually decompensate as they move from NYHA functional class I to class IV. Patients in class IV HF may be evaluated for eligibility for a heart transplant, but donor hearts are scarce. It is recommended that prognosis be discussed with the patient; advanced directives are encouraged.

The greatest improvement in mortality rates occurs for CABG performed in patients with angina and decreased LV ejection fraction. The second greatest difference occurs is with the use of ACE inhibitors, which have been shown to increase survival.

 CLINICAL PEARLS

○ Diuretics are not automatically prescribed for oliguria. Oliguria is the body's way of conserving water when it is scarce (RAA mechanism). Assess the clinical volume status and blood pressure. Diuretics may cause life-threatening hypotension if administered indiscriminately.
○ If twice-a-day diuretic dosing is required, the first dose should be taken in the morning and the second in mid-afternoon (not after 4 PM) to prevent nocturia.
○ Patients should be weighed daily before breakfast with the same clothes and on the same scales. Report a weight gain of 2 to 3 lb in 1 day. (It takes approximately 10 lb of extra fluid in the intravascular space before interstitial edema develops.)
○ Patients should be encouraged to maintain their own intake and output and daily weight records even while in the hospital.
○ Nonsteroidal anti-inflammatory drugs should be avoided. They can increase sodium retention and swelling and increase serum potassium levels.
○ Patients taking nitrates need a minimum 10-hour nitrate-free period (preferably during the night) to avoid tolerance. For example, a three-times-daily dose of isosorbide dinitrate may be given at 7 AM, 1 PM, and 7 PM.

○ Stagger doses of diuretics, ACE inhibitors, and beta-blockers by intervals of at least 1 hour to prevent hypotension.

○ Avoid calcium channel blockers in patients with systolic HF (they may be used in patients with diastolic failure).

NURSING PROBLEM/ DIAGNOSIS	NURSING INTERVENTIONS CLASSIFICATION (NIC)
Decreased cardiac output	Hemodynamic regulation Cardiac precautions Oxygen therapy
Risk for pulmonary/peripheral congestion/excess fluid volume	Fluid/electrolyte management Respiratory monitoring
Fatigue	Energy management

Coronary Artery Disease

Section 4   Rebecca Rule ■ Judy Graham Garcia

 OVERVIEW

CAD is the leading cause of death in the United States. It is estimated that 13.5 million individuals in the United States have CAD. Approximately 490,000 Americans die annually from CAD–related events, such as stroke, MI, HF, and others. Of every 4.6 deaths in the United States, 1 death is the result of CAD. In addition, there are many individuals living with CAD–related morbidities, including myocardial ischemia, LV dysfunction, and arrhythmias.

Numerous opportunities exist for nurses to intervene in the prevention of CAD at all levels. It is important for nurses to educate their patients and the public about risk factors (modifiable and nonmodifiable), lifestyle changes, and signs and symptoms of CAD. Collaboration with other health care providers is essential in providing optimal patient care and education. An interdisciplinary team consisting of physicians, nurses, pharmacists, dieticians, and exercise therapists, combined with a strong patient commitment, is essential in the effective management and prevention of CAD.

 PATHOPHYSIOLOGY

Atherosclerosis begins when plaques form in the arteries, occluding blood vessels, which in turn decreases the oxygen and nutritional supply to the myocardium. It is an insidious process, and the clinical manifestations may not be observed for 20 to 40 years.

Atherosclerotic lesions are characterized by the accumulation of lipids, both extracellular and intracellular; the proliferation of smooth muscle cells; and the formation of scar tissue and proteins. The lesions begin as an elevated thickening of the intima of the vessel, which is covered with connective tissue and smooth muscle. As the lesions increase in size, the buildup of plaque, fibrin, platelets, and debris eventually decreases the blood flow through the lumen of the artery and predisposes the individual to thrombus formation. In

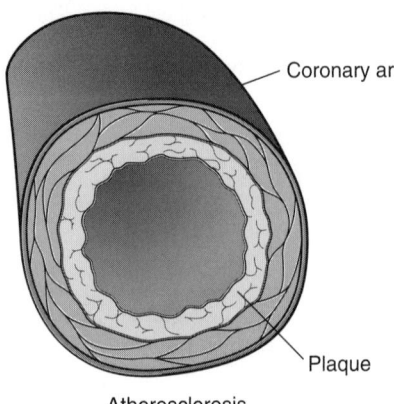

Coronary artery

Figure 14-4-1. Atherosclerosis.

Plaque

Atherosclerosis

the later stage of formation, the lesions may hemorrhage, ulcerate, or develop scar tissue.

As the disease progresses, the severity of reduction in blood flow increases, leading to an imbalance in myocardial oxygen supply and demand. When the demand exceeds the supply, myocardial ischemia develops. Approximately 10 seconds after the coronary occlusion, ischemia develops. This in turn leads to inability of the heart cells to contract, decreasing pump function and depriving the myocardium of glucose and oxygen. If myocardial ischemia persists for more than about 20 minutes, MI occurs (Fig. 14-4-1) (see Chapter 14, Section 5).

Risk Factors

Modifiable. Factors include hypertension, elevated low-density lipoprotein (LDL >160 mg/dL), decreased high-density lipoprotein (HDL <35 mg/dL), elevated triglycerides, diabetes mellitus, cigarette smoking, stress, obesity, sedentary lifestyle, and type A personality.

Nonmodifiable. Factors include age (men older than 45 years, women older than 55 years), gender, postmenopausal women, and heredity or family history of premature CAD (MI in male parent or sibling before the age of 55, or female parent or sibling before the age of 65).

SIGNS AND SYMPTOMS

Angina pectoris (chest pain) occurs when the coronary artery lumen is occluded to the point that there is an inadequate blood supply to the heart muscle. This discomfort usually lasts from 3 to 5 minutes and disappears if blood flow to the area is restored. The pain may be described as ranging as a heavy sensation to severe pain. Individuals often present with discomfort in the chest, which may radiate to the neck, jaw, and left shoulder or arm and down the back. There are three types of angina: stable, unstable, and Prinzmetal.

In stable angina, the lumen is narrow and hard, which does not allow vessels to dilate in response to demand by the myocardium. Rest and nitroglycerin often relieve the pain. If the pain is not relieved by the aforementioned measures, then an infarction may be developing.

Unstable angina is characterized by its unpredictability. The onset and course differ with each attack. It often occurs at rest, and with time, the attacks increase in frequency and duration. It may be a result of impending infarction.

Prinzmetal's angina also occurs without predictability and almost always at rest. This pain is due to the vasospasm of a coronary artery with or without atherosclerosis. It usually occurs during sleep and may have a cyclic pattern.

 DIAGNOSTIC CRITERIA

Evaluation of chest pain should be thorough and complete and include a patient history and physical examination. However, it is important to note that many diseases produce chest pain that may mimic the chest pain associated with myocardial ischemia:

Gastrointestinal: peptic ulcer disease, esophageal reflux, esophageal spasm, cholelithiasis, cholecystitis, pancreatitis

Musculoskeletal: costochondritis

Pulmonary: pulmonary embolism, pleurisy, pneumothorax, pneumonia, pleuritis, pulmonary hypertension

Infectious: herpes zoster

Psychiatric: anxiety

Other cardiac disorders: MI, pericarditis, dissecting aortic aneurysm

Laboratory

Lipoproteins are considered to be accurate predictors of CAD. The purpose of lipoproteins is to transport cholesterol, triglycerides, and other insoluble fats.

LDL is cholesterol rich. LDL is also known as "bad cholesterol." As cholesterol carried by LDL is deposited in the peripheral tissues, increased LDL levels are associated with an increased risk of arteriosclerotic heart disease.

HDL is a carrier of cholesterol that is produced in the liver. It is thought that the role of HDL is to remove the cholesterol from the peripheral tissues for transport to the liver for excretion. HDL, also known as "good cholesterol," may also have a protective effect by preventing the cellular uptake of cholesterol and lipids.

Triglycerides are fatty acids that are located in the bloodstream and transported via LDL. Using glycol and other fatty acids, they are produced in the liver and act as a storage source for energy.

Cholesterol is the primary lipid associated with arteriosclerotic heart disease, and is used to identify those at risk for arteriosclerotic heart disease. The primary source of cholesterol is food. Cholesterol is metabolized by the liver to its free form and is transported in the bloodstream by lipoproteins. About 75% of cholesterol is bound to LDL and about 25% is bound to HDL.

Desired Range

LDL: less than 160 mg/dL for persons with CAD, less than 180 mg/dL for persons without CAD

HDL: more than 45 mg/dL for men, more than 55 mg/dL for women
Triglycerides: from 40 to 160 mg/dL for men, from 35 to 135 mg/dL for women
Total cholesterol: less than 200 mg/dL

Special Tests

Electrocardiography. Check for ST-segment depression and inverted T waves.

Stress Electrocardiography. Assess for symptoms and electrocardiographic changes during exercise.

Imaging

Stress Thallium or Intravenous Dipyridamole Thallium Stress Test. Assess for symptoms and electrocardiographic changes during physiologic or pharmacologic stress.

Echocardiography. This noninvasive stress test assesses for cardiac chamber size and function and valvular structure and function.

Coronary Angiography. This invasive test identifies narrow and occluded coronary arteries. It is the gold standard for diagnosing CAD.

 INTERVENTION

Pharmacologic and nonpharmacologic interventions are delineated in Tables 14-4-1 and 14-4-2.

Special Procedures

Percutaneous Transluminal Coronary Angioplasty. A balloon-tipped catheter is placed in the stenotic portion of the artery. The balloon is inflated, compressing the plaque against the wall of the artery, which in turn dilates the vessel.

Coronary Artery Bypass Graft Surgery. A blood vessel is harvested, usually from the saphenous vein or the internal mammary artery, and is anastomosed to the occluded artery, thus bypassing the occlusion.

Laser Angioplasty. The laser catheter is placed in the stenotic area, is activated, and vaporizes the plaque.

Vascular Stent. A permanent tube is placed in the artery after angioplasty to prevent closure and restenosis.

 Table 14-4-1. Pharmacologic Management to Mediate the Effects of Hypertension and Elevated Cholesterol Levels

CLINICAL MANAGEMENT	RATIONALE
Nitrates	Dilate coronary arteries; decrease preload and afterload
Calcium channel blockers	Dilate coronary arteries and reduce vasospasm
Cholesterol-lowering drugs	Reduce development of atherosclerotic plaques
Elimination of oral contraceptives	Use can cause increased blood pressure and cholesterol levels

From Luckman J. (1997). *Saunders manual of nursing care* (p. 1036). Philadelphia, WB Saunders.

Table 14-4-2. Nonpharmacologic Interventions to Reduce the Impact of Risk Factors

RISK FACTOR	NONPHARMACOLOGIC INTERVENTION
Smoking	Physician emphasis; stop-smoking programs; group support; hypnosis
Hypertension	Weight reduction; dietary salt restriction; exercise; stress reduction techniques; alcohol restriction
Cholesterol	Diet: <30% total calories from fat; <200 mg cholesterol/day; exercise
Diabetes mellitus	Diet, weight control
Stress	Biofeedback; medication; stress management education; exercise; behavioral programs; counseling; relaxation techniques
Physical inactivity	Exercise prescription and instruction
Obesity	Diet counseling and restriction; surgery; gastric bypass (controversial)

From Luckman J. (1997). *Saunders manual of nursing care* (p. 1035). Philadelphia, WB Saunders.

 COMMUNITY CARE

Assessment. Take a complete personal and family health history, and assess for risk factors.

Monitoring. Lipid panel, weight loss, smoking cessation, and adherence to other risk factor modification recommendations are monitored.

Prevention. Promote healthy lifestyle in early childhood and prevention of initial disease as well as further disease progression.

 PROGNOSIS

The prognosis depends on the complications and severity of the disease.

 CLINICAL PEARLS

○ Prevention is the single most important factor in the management of CAD.
○ CAD is most prevalent in older men.
○ CAD risk is most effectively modified through smoking cessation, moderate levels of exercise, weight control, and control of hypertension, diabetes, and lipid abnormalities.
○ Diabetes is a primary risk factor for CAD in Hispanics.
○ Type A personalities have a high correlation with cardiovascular disorders, including hypertension.

NURSING PROBLEM/ DIAGNOSIS	NURSING INTERVENTIONS CLASSIFICATION (NIC)
Risk for ineffective tissue perfusion/effective therapeutic regimen management Lifestyle modifications	Risk identification Teaching: Disease process Surveillance Cardiac precautions Nutrition counseling Smoking cessation assistance

Myocardial Infarction

Section 5　　　　　　　　　　　　　　Judy Graham Garcia ■ Rebecca Rule

 OVERVIEW

Acute coronary syndromes lead to significant morbidity and mortality rates. According to 1999 American Heart Association data, every 29 seconds, an American has a coronary event, and every minute, an American dies from a coronary event. Coronary heart disease, specifically, resulted in 476,124 deaths, or 1 of every 4.9 deaths, in the United States in 1999, earning the position of the No. 1 killer of Americans. More than 4 million patients present to hospitals annually with a diagnosis of unstable angina or AMI. Each year, 250,000 persons die of coronary heart disease within 1 hour of symptom onset.

Annually, more than 1.5 million new and repeat MIs occur. Forty-two percent of women and 24% of men die within 1 year after an AMI. The incidence in the United States is 600 per 100,000 population. AMIs occur predominantly in persons older than 40 years. In the age range of 40 to 70 years, men experience more AMIs than do women, but in those 70 years old or older, women experience more AMIs than do men.

 PATHOPHYSIOLOGY

MI occurs when the blood flow to the myocardium is suddenly interrupted, resulting in deprivation of oxygen and nutrients to the myocardium. Initiating the cascade of potential events is a rupture of atherosclerotic plaque resulting in local thrombus formation. This atherosclerotic plaque is an advanced fibrolipid plaque that consists of an extracellular lipid core, smooth muscle cells, foam cells, and a thin fibrous cap. The stability of the plaque is determined by the physical integrity of this fibrous cap. Plaques prone to rupture are not flow limiting. Without flow restriction, these plaques do not cause classic angina. The plaques most prone to rupture have a lipid-rich core that makes them soft. Stable plaque has less lipids and a stable cap that makes them more resistant to fissuring and formation of thrombi.

After rupture of the vulnerable plaque, several events ensue. Plaque rupture damages the epithelium and activates the clotting cascade via the intrinsic and extrinsic pathways; see Chapter 12, Section 2. The ruptured atherosclerotic plaque becomes a stimulus for platelet aggregation.

Platelets play an important role in the pathophysiology of acute coronary syndromes. First, platelets adhere to the vessel wall in the area of the unstable plaque, resulting in increased production of thrombin. Next, activation occurs of the GP IIb/IIIa platelet receptors, or the final common element in the clotting pathway. This results in the binding of fibrinogen to these receptors on many platelets. Fibrinogen then forms bridges between the platelets and holds them tightly together. Finally, platelet aggregation occurs. At the site of rupture, the plaque lodges locally and, through the attraction of platelets and thrombin, results in the development of a platelet-rich mural thrombus that generates thrombin.

As the end result of the clotting cascade, thrombin converts fibrinogen to fibrin, which ultimately converts the loose aggregation of platelets of a potential thrombus into a tightly woven clot. The thrombus leads to an acute coronary syndrome that may occur in varying degrees: no change in the degree of stenosis, a higher-grade stenosis, or an occluding thrombus that may either be resolved or become chronic. When thrombus occlusion occurs, it may be intermittent, leading to unstable angina, or completely occlusive, leading to AMI. Whether AMI is transmural or subendocardial depends on the degree and the duration of the occlusion and the presence or absence of collateral circulation. Thus, the end result is unstable angina, non–Q wave MI, or Q wave MI. After total occlusion, myocardial necrosis is complete in 4 to 6 hours. Flow to ischemic areas must remain above 40% of preocclusion levels for that area to survive.

 SIGNS AND SYMPTOMS

- Pain in the chest, arm, back, jaw, epigastrium, or neck; may occur exclusively in these areas or radiate from the chest to any of these areas
- Nausea and vomiting
- Diaphoresis
- Dyspnea, rales
- Anxiety, restlessness, fatigue, sense of impending doom
- Lightheadedness, pallor, weakness, syncope
- S3 or S4 heart sound
- Arrhythmias
- Hypertension, hypotension
- Jugular venous distention

Typical Presentation
- Chest pain
- Shortness of breath
- Diaphoresis
- Nausea and vomiting

Atypical Presentation
- Weakness, dyspnea, syncope, confusion, and HF are common atypical presentations in the elderly and diabetics. "Silent" infarcts, which may be unrecognized by both the physician and the patient, occur in up to 20% of infarcts.
- A peripheral neuropathy, or altered sensorium, may mask the pain sensation in the elderly, diabetic, or hypertensive patient who may present with shortness of breath and no chest pain.
- Weakness, fatigue, or back pain may be described by women, who present with more atypical symptoms than do men and describe pain more vaguely than do men. Compared with men, women have more neck, shoulder, back, jaw, and upper abdominal pain; more nausea, dyspnea, and fatigue; and less diaphoresis.

 DIAGNOSTIC CRITERIA
History
1. Take a brief and relevant history, and assess risk factors.

Risk Factors
- Hyperlipidemia-increased LDL; decreased HDL; hypertriglyceridemia
- Premature (<55 years old) familial onset of coronary disease

- Cigarette smoking
- Diabetes mellitus
- Hypertension
- Sedentary lifestyle
- Aging
- Hostile, frustrated personality
- Prior MI

2. Assess the chest pain for consistency with AMI. Follow the mnemonic *NOPQRSTUV:*

N = Normal: What is the patient's baseline function?

O = Onset: Is the pain new, recurrent, sudden, or gradual?

P = Provocation and palliation: What are the aggravating factors (i.e., foods; cold; activity; anxiety, emotions, or stress; inspiration; body position)? What makes the pain feel better or go away (i.e., rest, nitroglycerin, eating, positioning, antacids, heat)?

Q = Quality and quantity: Describe the pain (e.g., sharp, dull, stabbing, pressure, burning, fullness). Rate the pain on a scale from 1 to 10, with 1 being the mildest pain you have ever experienced to 10 being the most severe and disabling pain you have ever experienced.

R = Region and radiation: Where does the pain occur (e.g., epigastric, retrosternal, substernal, precordial, localized, diffuse)? Does the pain spread to any other areas (back, jaw, arms, abdomen, neck)?

S = Symptoms: What symptoms are associated with the pain (e.g., nausea, vomiting, diaphoresis, shortness of breath, dizziness, weakness, headache, heartburn, cough, fever)?

Laboratory

Creatine Kinase. The creatine kinase (CK) level rises after an MI, beginning in 4 to 8 hours; peaks in 18 to 24 hours; and subsides over 3 to 4 days.

Creatine Kinase Isozymes: MM (Skeletal Muscle), BB (Brain and Kidney), and MB (Cardiac). Serum CK-MB elevation is diagnostic for MI. The CK-MB level is elevated within 3 to 6 hours, peaks at 12 to 24 hours, and returns to normal within 12 to 48 hours after an MI.

Troponin I. This inhibitory protein in muscle fibers is the most specific and sensitive indicator for myocardial necrosis. The level rises 6 to 8 hours after the onset of ischemia.

Lactate Dehydrogenase. Levels rises above normal values within 24 hours of AMI, peak within 3 to 6 days, and return to baseline within 8 to 12 days. It is used to date a recent MI well past the acute episode.

Erythrocyte Sedimentation Rate. The rate rises above normal levels within 3 days and may remain elevated for several weeks.

Leukocytes. The level rises within several hours, peaks in 2 to 4 days, and returns to normal within 1 week.

12-Lead Electrocardiogram

Interpret the 12-lead ECG to determine whether an AMI occurred; this is central to the diagnosis of AMI.

- Subendocardial ischemia is indicated by ST-segment depression and T wave inversion.
- Injury, or *acute transmural ischemia*, is indicated by ST-segment elevation

in a regional pattern. This occurs when ischemia is prolonged for more than a few minutes.

- Infarction, or *transmural myocardial necrosis*, is indicated by the development of Q waves, which appear within 24 to 48 hours. This indicates infarcted tissue that extends at least halfway through the myocardial wall. Q wave presence does not indicate when the infarct occurred.
- Changes in leads II, III, and aVF indicate a problem in the inferior wall of the myocardium. Arrhythmias associated with inferior infarction include bradycardia and first-, second-, and third-degree atrioventricular block (Chapter 8, Section 5).
- Changes in leads V_2 to V_5 indicate a problem in the anterior wall.
- Changes in leads V_1, V_6, I, and aVL indicate a problem in the lateral wall.
- Diagnostic clues to acute RV infarction are not provided by the standard 12-lead ECG.

Echocardiography (Ultrasonography of the Heart)

- Echocardiography is useful in evaluating wall motion abnormalities in MI and overall LV function. Regional wall motion abnormalities are associated with MI in 90% to 100% of patients with transmural MI.
- Echocardiography is useful in delineating and assessing mechanical complications (ventricular septal defect, papillary muscle rupture, or pericardial tamponade).

Imaging

- Chest radiography: Findings dependent on severity of MI
- *Radionuclide (Isotope) Studies:* (1) Thallium scanning—accumulates in viable myocardium and (2) technetium-99m–gated blood pool scanning—a noninvasive means of measuring ventricular function; accumulates in recently infarcted myocardium

Hemodynamic Monitoring

- Hemodynamic monitoring with a pulmonary artery catheter is not indicated in patients with uncomplicated AMI.
- Knowledge of pulmonary artery pressure and pulmonary artery wedge ressure (is important for prescribing treatment for patients with complicated MI).
- Indications for placement of a pulmonary artery catheter include the following:
  1. Severe or progressive congestive HF or pulmonary edema
  2. Progressive hypotension or cardiogenic shock
  3. Suspected mechanical complications such as valvular disorders
  4. Wedge pressure, central venous pressure, and cardiac output: Guide treatment decisions by differentiating the RV infarct patient with low filling pressures in need of volume from the LV infarct patient with high filling pressures in need of diuresis, inotropes, and afterload reduction

Cardiac Catheterization with Coronary Angiography

- Cardiac catheterization is indicated for patients with AMI
  1. Within 6 hours of symptom onset in patients who are candidates for PCIs and in patients whom thrombolysis is contraindicated

2. After 6 hours of symptom onset but before hospital discharge in patients with recurrent chest pain, suspected mitral regurgitation, or ruptured interventricular septum causing HF or shock or suspected subacute cardiac rupture

- Cardiac catheterization localizes obstructive coronary artery lesions.
- Cardiac catheterization guides PCIs for the reestablishment of perfusion.
- Right-sided catheterization may be used to obtain right-sided pressures, to evaluate the pulmonic and tricuspid valves, to sample blood oxygen content of right-sided chambers for detection of left-to-right shunt, to determine cardiac output, and to evaluate mitral valve stenosis or mitral valve insufficiency via the transseptal approach.
- Left-sided catheterization is used to obtain pressure measurements to evaluate mitral and aortic valve and LV function, to use angiography to evaluate mitral and aortic valve disease, and to perform left ventriculography.

 INTERVENTIONS

Three Phases of Acute Myocardial Infarction Management (National Heart Attack Alert Program)

Phase I: The patient component of treatment delay. Failure to seek care promptly is the most common reason for treatment delay.

Phase II: Prehospital action, such as emergency medical services.

Phase III: The hospital action component of treatment delay.

Delays to Treatment

In general, denial of symptoms may lead to postponement of care, because patients may delay seeking treatment urgently or emergently. Women delay seeking AMI care longer than men. In-hospital delays are also longer for women receiving thrombolytic therapy.

Admission to Inpatient Coronary Care Unit

Analgesia, prevention, and treatment of electrical and mechanical complications, limitation of infarct size, and salvage of myocardium are the goals. These are accomplished through increasing myocardial blood and oxygen supply and decreasing myocardial oxygen demand.

Arrhythmias

Ventricular Tachycardia. If the patient is unstable or pulseless, use direct current countershock and cardiopulmonary resuscitation, lidocaine, or procainamide.

Ventricular Fibrillation. Use direct current countershock and cardiopulmonary resuscitation.

Atrial Flutter and Fibrillation. Use digitalis or intravenous diltiazem or verapamil. If the patient is hemodynamically compromised, use direct current cardioversion or rapid atrial pacing.

Sinus Bradycardia. If this is accompanied by hypotension or if the patient is hemodynamically compromised, treat with atropine. If this is ineffective, use electrical pacing.

Atrioventricular Block. In inferior infarction, transvenous pacing is required if the patient is hemodynamically compromised. In anterior infarction, pacing is usually required because escape rhythm is unstable, with ventricular asystole occurring quite suddenly.

Aspirin

Aspirin, 160 to 325 mg chewed and swallowed, should be administered as soon as possible followed by enteric-coated aspirin, 160 to 325 mg PO QD. Aspirin is an important adjunct to thrombolytic therapy because it enhances the effects of thrombolytic agents. Platelet activity is increased in the setting of AMI, and aspirin inhibits platelet aggregation and platelet activity and permanently damages platelets.

Heparin

Heparin is an antithrombin that prevents coagulation by interfering with the formation of thrombin from prothrombin, thus preventing thrombin from allowing the conversion of fibrinogen to fibrin. The goal of heparin therapy is to prevent the extension of thrombus. The therapeutic aPTT threshold (1.5 to 2.5 times the control value) should be reached within 24 hours of initiating therapy.

The LMWHs enoxaparin and dalteparin have been replacing the traditional UH. Limitations of UH that have resulted in this substitution include varying aPTT, frequent monitoring, bleeding, thrombocytopenia, osteoporosis, intravenous administration that increases inpatient costs, and rebound ischemic events associated with cessation.

Morphine Sulfate

Pain relief is very important, and morphine should be administered to relieve chest pain quickly. Pain can result in autonomic disturbances, causing dangerous arrhythmias, hypotension, and increased area of infarct. The initial adult dose of morphine is 4 mg IV, administered at a rate of 1 mg/min. Morphine may be repeated at a dosage of 2 to 4 mg at 5- to 15-minute intervals until the patient is pain free.

Beta-Blockers

Beta-blockers are used after MI because of their ability to inhibit the chronotropic (increased cardiac rate) and inotropic (increased cardiac contraction) responses to catecholamines. Beta-blockade is indicated in *all* patients *except* for those with the following contraindications:

- Asthma
- Severe congestive HF
- Hypotension (systolic blood pressure <100 mm Hg)
- Absolute bradycardia (heart rate <60 beats/min)
- Beta-blockers are administered via the oral or intravenous route. They decrease the incidence of myocardial rupture, decrease the size of the infarct, and improve survival if administered within 4 hours of symptom onset.

Nitrates

Nitrates are effective in treating ischemic chest pain and hypertension and in reducing pulmonary congestion. They decrease preload via peripheral vasodilatation, resulting in decreased venous return, reduced filling pressures, and reduced intracardiac volumes. Specific to the coronary circulation, nitrates increase coronary vasodilation, reverse coronary vasoconstriction, and result in dilation of collateral vessels. Nitroglycerin is first administered sublingually every 5 minutes until chest pain is relieved for a maximum of 3 doses. It is recommended for the first 24 to 48 hours for patients with AMI and HF, persistent ischemia, or hypertension (usually intravenous) and beyond 48 hours for patients with recurrent angina or persistent pulmonary congestion (transdermal or oral).

Thrombolytic Therapy

Thrombolytic agents are effective in decreasing mortality rates if administered within 6 hours of onset of chest pain or other symptoms to patients in whom no contraindications exist. The standard of care for an AMI is to administer the agent within 20 minutes of emergency department presentation. Optimal thrombolytic candidates include those with ST-segment elevation or bundle-branch block on the ECG in the setting of an appropriate clinical history. The cornerstone of therapy for AMI is urgent revascularization with direct angioplasty or thrombolytic therapy. Thrombolytic agents include streptokinase, recombinant tissue plasminogen activator (rtPA [alteplase]), and recombinant plasminogen activator (rPA [reteplase]). Through the conversion of plasminogen to plasmin, these agents result in a breakdown of the fibrin strands that bind together a clot. This usually results in dissolution of the thrombus and therefore reestablishes reperfusion to the myocardium.

New Antiplatelet Agents

Management options that are continually evolving include administration of the GP IIb/IIIa platelet inhibitors, affecting platelet aggregation through the inhibition of clot-bound thrombin, or the final common pathway before platelet aggregation and clot formation after plaque rupture. The effectiveness of these intravenous agents has been proved in multiple large-scale clinical trials (Integrelin to Manage Platelet Aggregation to Prevent Coronary Thrombosis [IMPACT II], Platelet IIb/IIIa Underpinning the Receptor for Suppression of Unstable Ischemia Trial [PURSUIT], Platelet IIb/IIIa Antagonist for the Reduction of Acute Coronary Syndrome Events in a Global Organization Network [PARAGON], Platelet Receptor Inhibition for Ischemic Syndrome Management Study [PRISM], Chimeric 7E3 Antiplatelet in Unstable Angina Refractory to Standard Treatment [CAPTURE], Evaluation of IIb/IIIa Platelet Receptor Antagonist 7E3 in Preventing Ischemic Complications [EPIC], Global Utilization of Streptokinase and TPA for Occluded Arteries IV [GUSTO-IV], and Recombinant Plasminogen Activator Angiographic Phase II International Dose Finding Study [RAPID]).

The GP IIb/IIIa inhibitors can be administered as complementary therapies with UH or the LMWHs. GP IIb/IIIa inhibitors bind to GP IIb/IIIa receptors, preventing the binding of fibrinogen to the platelet. Therefore, formation or progression of platelet activation is inhibited. When used in combination with UH, the UH results in inactivation of thrombin, thus preventing the conversion of fibrinogen to fibrin.

The goal of combination therapy with an antithrombotic and a GP IIb/IIIa platelet inhibitor is the synergistic effect that is obtained when one agent blocks fibrin and the other blocks platelets. This results in the prevention of thrombus growth in a platelet-rich arterial clot. Combination therapy also allows for the administration of lower doses of thrombolytic agents, decreasing the bleeding risk.

Percutaneous Coronary Interventions

Angioplasty has been associated with a lower early mortality rate and better long-term outcome compared with thrombolytic agents. PCIs include angioplasty–repeat dilatation, stent implantation, and directional and rotational coronary atherectomy. They represent a treatment alternative to thrombolytic therapy in AMI. However, PCIs are not as readily available in all clinical settings as are the thrombolytic agents. Effective antiplatelet therapy is crucial with PCIs because of platelet-mediated restenosis. As a result of this platelet stimulation associated with PCIs, the GP IIb/IIIa inhibitors and thrombolytic agents may be used as adjunctive therapy with PCIs. The thrombolytic agents are generally administered via the intracoronary route, and the GP IIb/IIIa inhibitors are generally administered via the intravenous route.

With PCIs, GP IIb/IIIa inhibitors are often used as adjunctive therapy, such as a stent plus abciximab. The GP IIb/IIIa inhibitor abciximab produces its antithrombotic effect by directly inhibiting the binding of natural ligands like fibrinogen to GP IIb/IIIa receptors. The result is a dose-dependent inhibition of platelet aggregation.

Surgical Management

Surgical intervention is a mainstay of the treatment of heart disease. Surgical interventions for acquired heart disease include CABG, minimally invasive cardiac surgery, transmyocardial revascularization, cardiomyoplasty, aortic surgery, and heart transplantation.

COMMUNITY CARE

Assessment

1. Instruct the public to call on the emergency medical services system if pain and associated symptoms occur that indicate a heart attack.
2. Nurses must be aware that the field of prehospital management of AMI patients has expanded rapidly. Prehospital management is considered to be the first link in early access to care.
3. Prehospital thrombolysis has shown to improve outcomes in patients with AMI.
4. Prehospital electrocardiography also improves outcomes in patients with AMI.
5. For patients who previously had an AMI, assess their response to medications.

Monitoring

1. Monitor effectiveness of the community-based emergency cardiac care system.
2. Be aware of special considerations regarding women and cardiovascular disease.
   - Women have a higher rate of stroke, major bleeding, and recurrent MIs regardless of whether they receive thrombolytic therapy.

- Treatment with aspirin, heparin, or beta-blockers is less frequent in women.
- Cardiac catheterization, thrombolytic therapy, PCIs, and CABG rates are lower in women than in men.
- Female gender is an important predictor of poor outcome.
- Women have a higher in-hospital mortality rate.
- According to the Framingham Heart Study, 33% of women and 21% of men experience a repeat MI.
- Despite better systolic ventricular function in women, 30% of women and 21% of men are disabled due to HF after an AMI.

Prevention

1. High blood pressure and high blood cholesterol are two of the main risk factors that can be controlled. Because these conditions have no symptoms in the early stages, regular medical check-ups can help to identify the presence of these risk factors.
2. Lifestyle changes can decrease the risk of heart disease by reducing the presence of risk factors. The public should be counseled to
   - Quit smoking
   - Lose weight and maintain ideal body weight
   - Follow a low-saturated fat, low-cholesterol diet
   - Exercise regularly
   - Minimize stress
   - Control alcohol intake
3. Education efforts must be directed to the general public. Special emphasis should be placed on patients with stable CAD and on persons with or at risk for CAD.

 PROGNOSIS

1. The outcome is dependent on the size and location of the infarction and the rapidity with which blood flow can be reestablished through pharmacologic or mechanical modalities.
2. The overall mortality rate is 10% during the hospital phase, with an additional 10% mortality rate during the next year. More than 60% of the deaths occur within 1 hour of the onset of the event.
3. Total occlusion of the left main coronary artery, which usually supplies 70% of the LV mass, is catastrophic and results in death within minutes.
4. Killip classification is as follows:
   Class I: No congestive HF, mortality rate less than 5% (clear lungs)
   Class II: Mild to moderate congestive HF (bibasilar rales, S3 gallop, or both), mortality rate of 10%
   Class III: Severe congestive HF (rales >50% of lung fields, S3 gallop, pulmonary edema), mortality rate of 30%
   Class IV: Cardiogenic shock, blood pressure of less than 90 mm Hg with hypoperfusion (oliguria, confusion, clammy skin), mortality rate of more than 80%

 CLINICAL PEARLS

- A significant percentage of patients have nonspecific findings on presentation, such as peaked T waves and ST-segment elevation of less than 0.2 mV.

- A small percentage of patients, with transmural infarction, present with a normal ECG.
- The combination of a fibrinolytic agent with a GP IIb/IIIa platelet inhibitor has been shown to result in more frequent and more rapid reperfusion.
- Facilitated PCI with fibrinolytic and antiplatelet therapy is emerging as a promising technique for achieving early reperfusion and shows potential for improvement in patency rates.
- The nursing care of patients after cardiac catheterization is directed toward the prevention and detection of complications, which, although infrequent, may be life threatening. The many nursing responsibilities related to cardiac catheterization are outlined in the Guidelines for Cardiac Catheterization and Cardiac Catheterization Laboratories of the American College of Cardiology/American Heart Association Ad Hoc Task Force on Cardiac Catheterization.
- UH can induce thrombocytopenia, thus patients should be monitored closely for signs and symptoms and the platelet count should be followed closely. Patients should be assessed frequently for hemorrhage.
- UH should not be abruptly discontinued because an MI can develop quickly as a result.
- The use of beta-blockers in MI has been shown to improve postinfarction survival rates.
- When beta-blockade is initiated, the target heart rate is 50 to 60 beats/min. Beta-blockers should not be initiated if the heart rate is less than 60 beats/min and should be avoided if the PR interval is more than 0.24 second or if second- or third-degree atrioventricular block is present. Patients should also be monitored for hypotension, because a major effect of beta-blockers is a decrease in systolic blood pressure, and therapy should not be initiated if systolic blood pressure is less than 90 mm Hg.
- Nitroglycerin may result in hypotension, causing a decrease in coronary perfusion pressure with a resultant increase in myocardial ischemia. The nurse should closely monitor the patient's heart rate and blood pressure.
- In comparison with men, women who present with AMI are older, have more comorbidities (hypertension, diabetes, congestive HF), have higher rates of "silent AMI," and have smaller cardiac enzyme elevations.

NURSING PROBLEM/ DIAGNOSIS	NURSING INTERVENTIONS CLASSIFICATION (NIC)
Infarction/acute pain (chest)	Cardiac care: Acute Pain management
Decreased cardiac output	Hemodynamic regulation Fluid/electrolyte management Cardiac care: Rehabilitative

Rheumatic Heart Disease

Section 6   Rebecca Rule ■ Judy Graham Garcia

 OVERVIEW

   Rheumatic heart disease (RHD) develops as a sequela of rheumatic fever (RF). The incidence RF is about 0.6 per 1000 population in the United States

but affects an estimated 15 to 20 million persons worldwide. The lower incidence in the United States is related to multiple factors. Antimicrobial agents for the treatment of RF have played an important role in this decline. Other factors include higher economic standards, improved living conditions (better housing and decreased crowding in homes and schools), and increased health care access.

The incidence of RF is equal among males and females. Populations with increased incidence of RF include military recruits, persons residing in crowded housing conditions, and those in close contact with school-aged children. In the past, RF was considered a disease of temperate climates but now is seen more in warm tropical climates of developing countries. The incidence of RF follows a seasonal pattern that parallels the course of streptococcal pharyngitis and is most common in the United States in the spring. RHD develops in 50% to 75% of children with RF after a long latent period and approximately 35% of adults with RF.

 PATHOPHYSIOLOGY

Strong evidence exists that supports the role of group A beta-hemolytic *Streptococcus* (GABHS) as the causal agent of initial and recurrent episodes of RF. The precipitating event for RF is an untreated GABHS tonsillopharyngitis. The risk of RF is virtually eliminated with antimicrobial eradication of the bacteria. However, important to note is the fact that RF follows a mild, almost asymptomatic pharyngitis in about one third of cases. This is very concerning, because the prevention of RF depends on the clinical diagnosis and antimicrobial treatment of streptococcal pharyngitis.

The pathology of RF is related to both the host and infecting microorganism. The magnitude of the immune response to the antecedent streptococcal infection and the persistence of the infection during recovery are the most important factors. The attack rate is also influenced by variations in the rheumatogenicity of GABHS strains. Evidence exists that RF is associated with infections caused by virulent encapsulated (mucoid) strains that can induce strong type-specific immune responses to M protein and other streptococcal antigens. Although only about 3% of persons with untreated streptococcal pharyngitis develop RF, the incidence of RF among those who have experienced a previous episode of RF is about 50%.

Several studies suggest a familial predisposition to or genetic basis for RF. Almost all patients with RF have a specific B-cell alloantigen, and susceptibility has been linked with human leukocyte antigen (HLA)-DR1, -DR2, -DR3, and -DR4 haplotypes in different ethnic groups.

Exudative and inflammatory reactions of connective or collagen tissue characterize the acute phase of RF, primarily affecting the heart, joints, brain, and cutaneous and subcutaneous tissues, even though the disease process is considered to be diffuse. A generalized vasculitis of small blood vessels also occurs, but thrombotic lesions are not seen, as with some of the other connective tissue disorders.

Within collagen, fibrinoid degeneration occurs. Interstitial connective tissue becomes edematous and eosinophilic. As a result, collagen fibers fray, fragment, and disintegrate. Mononuclear cells, including large modified fibrohistiocytic cells or Aschoff cells, infiltrate and form Aschoff giant cells. The

Aschoff nodule can be identified in rheumatic carditis but are not observed in other affected organs.

RHD develops as the inflammatory process affects the heart. Carditis is the most specific manifestation of RF. Rheumatic carditis is a pancarditis that affects the endocardium, myocardium, and pericardium to varying degrees; it is almost always associated with a murmur of valvulitis (endocarditis). Inflammation of the valvular tissue is responsible for the most commonly recognized manifestations of rheumatic carditis. In endocarditis, edema and cellular infiltration of valvular tissue and chordae tendineae occur. Then, hyaline degeneration of the affected valve leads to the development of verrucae at the valve edge, preventing accurate approximation of the valve leaflets. If inflammation continues, the valve becomes fibrotic and calcified, eventually leading to stenosis. The most characteristic component of valvulitis involves the mitral and aortic valves and the chordae of the mitral valve. The hallmark of rheumatic carditis is mitral insufficiency. Less common, and usually associated with mitral insufficiency, is aortic insufficiency. Involvement of the tricuspid and pulmonic valves rarely occurs.

The severity of carditis spans a wide range, from death secondary to HF from residual valvular damage requiring surgical intervention, at one extreme, to a less intense scarring of the heart valves at the other. Evidence may be subtle, and auscultatory signs of valvular involvement may be easily missed.

In the absence of valvulitis, or endocarditis, myocarditis or pericarditis rarely occurs. In patients with myocarditis, tachycardia and transient arrhythmias may occur. Cardiac failure may result from severe myocarditis or valvular insufficiency. When severe hemodynamic changes occur as a result of valvular, myocardial, or pericardial disease, cardiac enlargement occurs. Pericarditis and the accumulation of pericardial fluid may occur secondary to inflammation of the visceral and parietal surfaces of the pericardium.

 SIGNS AND SYMPTOMS

- Murmur of valvulitis
- Any signs and symptoms of cardiac failure: dyspnea, jugular venous distention, weight gain, edema, hepatosplenomegaly, rales, cough, abdominal bloating, weakness, fatigue
- Sore throat
- Fever
- Arthralgia

 DIAGNOSTIC CRITERIA

Evidence of Antecedent Untreated GABHS Tonsillopharyngitis. Supporting evidence includes a positive throat culture or rapid streptococcal antigen test or elevated or rising streptococcal antibody titer.

Electrocardiography. In acute RF, a common electrocardiographic finding is a prolonged PR interval for age and rate. This finding alone is not diagnostic for carditis and is not associated with the ultimate development of RHD. Other electrocardiographic findings may include tachycardia, atrioventricular block, and QRS-T changes suggestive of myocarditis.

Echocardiography. An echocardiography is a useful tool in detecting endocardial, myocardial, and pericardial involvement. It is important to note that there is a risk of overdiagnosing valvular incompetence, and overreliance on echocardiography for the diagnosis of RHD should be avoided.

Chest Roentgenography. A chest radiograph is a useful tool for the assessment of pericarditis, pulmonary edema, increased pulmonary vasculature, and cardiac size; however, a normal-size cardiac silhouette does not exclude RHD.

Anemia of Chronic Inflammation. This may be mild or moderate and normocytic normochromatic.

Acute Phase of Rheumatic Fever. Fever and arthralgia may occur in conjunction with carditis. Acute-phase reactants, such as the erythrocyte sedimentation rate and C-reactive protein level, are usually elevated in the acute phase when carditis occurs. It is important to note that the erythrocyte sedimentation rate may be suppressed to normal levels in patients with congestive HF.

 INTERVENTIONS
General Intervention

- Admit the patient to the hospital for close observation and appropriate work-up.
- Bed rest is required in the acute phase with ambulation after fever subsides and acute-phase reactants return to normal.
- The patient should avoid strenuous physical activity.
- Penicillin therapy is prescribed for 10 days (erythromycin if penicillin allergy is present).
- If HF occurs, treat with diuretics, oxygen, digitalis, and sodium-restricted diet.

Antirheumatic Therapy

- Supportive therapy is provided to reduce constitutional symptoms, control toxic manifestations, and improve cardiac function.
- For mild carditis, salicylates are particularly effective. Aspirin at dosages of about 100 mg/kg/day, given in divided doses, usually achieves a therapeutic serum salicylate level, for approximately 1 month or until clinical and laboratory evidence support inflammatory inactivity.
- For significant carditis, including pericarditis and congestive HF, corticosteroids may be life saving (e.g., prednisone at 1 to 2 mg/kg/day, for 2 to 3 months, with tapering over 2 weeks).
- No evidence supports that salicylate or corticosteroid therapy affects the course of carditis or reduces the incidence of residual RHD.
- "Rebound" rheumatic activity is possible. If mild symptoms of acute-phase reactants reappear within 2 weeks of the discontinuation of anti-inflammatory agents, they usually subside without any treatment. If more severe symptoms occur, treatment with salicylates may be necessary. It is also acceptable to administer salicylates like aspirin at a dosage of 75 mg/kg/day while tapering corticosteroids.

Surgical Intervention

Surgical intervention consists of replacement of the affected valve, requiring open heart surgery.

 COMMUNITY CARE:
Assessment

1. Promptly recognize and eradicate GABHS from the throat.
2. Assess community for high-risk populations, such as those residing in

crowded living conditions, those working with school-aged children, and military recruits.

3. Assess cardiac involvement in patients diagnosed with RF.
4. Assess for higher risk of recurrences in economically disadvantaged populations.

Monitoring

1. Monitor the response to antimicrobial therapy.
2. Patients with RF who show no clear evidence of carditis on the initial examination should be monitored closely over a few weeks to assess for cardiac involvement.
3. Monitor for focal outbreaks in particular geographic areas.
4. Monitor patients with a history of RF with increased exposure to streptococcal infections, such as children and adolescents, parents of young children, teachers, physicians, nurses, and allied health care personnel in contact with children, military recruits, and others in crowded housing conditions.

Prevention

Primary: Prevention of Primary Attacks of Rheumatic Fever

1. Prompt recognition and proper treatment of GABHS tonsillopharyngitis result in eradication of GABHS from the throat.
2. Penicillin is the antimicrobial agent of choice for the treatment of GABHS and prevention of RHD. Other options include erythromycin, azithromycin, and narrow-spectrum cephalosporins.

Secondary: Prevention of Recurrent Attacks of Rheumatic Fever

A patient with a history of RF is at high risk for recurrent attacks. Asymptomatic GABHS infections may trigger an attack. Even when a symptomatic infection is treated, RF may still recur. Therefore, secondary prevention may require continuous antimicrobial prophylaxis rather than simply treatment of acute episodes of GABHS infection.

Continuous Antimicrobial Prophylaxis. This is recommended for all patients with a well-documented history of RF and for all patients with definite evidence of RHD, initiated at the time of recognition of either acute RF or RHD. Even if throat cultures are negative at the time of diagnosis of acute RF, a full therapeutic course of penicillin should be administered to eradicate any residual GABHS. Family members of rheumatic patients should always be treated promptly for streptococcal infections.

Continuous antimicrobial prophylaxis is the most effective prevention of a recurrence of RF. Patients with a history of RHD are at high risk for recurrences of carditis, with each subsequent case resulting in increasingly severe episodes of cardiac involvement. Therefore, long-term antibiotic prophylaxis, possibly for life, is necessary, with the duration depending on the degree of residual valvular disease. In a patient with a history of RF with carditis but no residual valvular disease, prophylaxis should continue for 10 years or well into adulthood, whichever is longer. If residual valvular disease has occurred, prophylaxis is maintained for at least 10 years after the last episode and at least until age 40, and sometimes for life.

The recommended treatment regimen for secondary prevention is an injection of long-acting penicillin (benzathine penicillin G) every 3 to 4 weeks, usually every 3 weeks with residual rheumatic carditis. Oral agents are appropriate in patients with a low risk of recurrence; however, nonadherence may become an issue. The preferred agent for oral prophylaxis is penicillin V.

Bacterial Endocarditis Prophylaxis. Additional short-term antibiotic prophylaxis before certain dental and surgical procedures is required for patients with RHD. Those at particularly high risk include patients with prosthetic valves or previous endocarditis. Penicillin should be avoided as the agent of choice for bacterial endocarditis prophylaxis because the streptococci may have developed resistance to oral penicillin used for secondary prevention. Current recommendations of the American Heart Association should be followed.

 PROGNOSIS

The prognosis is dependent on the degree of cardiac involvement from previous attacks of RF. The risk of recurrence of RF increases with multiple previous attacks and decreases as the length of time since the last attack increases. Therefore, the frequency of attacks and adherence to antibiotic prophylaxis also affect the prognosis.

 CLINICAL PEARLS

○ Mitral insufficiency is the common murmur associated with RHD.
○ Any patient with a history of RHD should be placed on bacterial endocarditis prophylaxis before dental and surgical procedures per current recommendations of the American Heart Association.
○ Antibiotic regimens used for secondary prevention are ineffective for the prevention of bacterial endocarditis.

NURSING PROBLEM/ DIAGNOSIS	NURSING INTERVENTIONS CLASSIFICATION (NIC)
Infection (cardiac valvular tissue)	Fever treatment Medication administration Teaching: Disease process
Risk for heart failure	See Chapter 14, Section 3

chapter 15

Vascular

Aortic Aneurysm

Section 1   Vallire D. Hooper

 OVERVIEW

Abdominal aortic aneurysms (AAAs) most commonly occur in persons older than 50 years and are twice as prevalent in men as in women. Most aneurysms are asymptomatic until the patient presents to the emergency department with a rupture, thrombosis, or embolization. Symptoms before the rupture are often vague and nonspecific, with the most common complaints being vague and diffuse abdominal or back pain, or both. The aneurysms that are discovered before rupture are generally discovered incidentally as a part of a routine physical examination or a medical work-up for another problem or complaint.

 PATHOPHYSIOLOGY

An *aneurysm* is a localized dilatation or ballooning of a vessel wall. Aneurysms are classified according to their anatomic location and their shape. An aneurysm may occur in any vessel but most commonly occurs in the aorta and iliac arteries. Aortic aneurysms are commonly labeled as *abdominal aortic* or *thoracic* (ascending or descending) *aortic* depending on the anatomic location. Other areas that are commonly associated with aneurysm formation include the popliteal, femoral, and carotid vessels.

Aneurysms are also classified according to their shape.

Fusiform. A diffuse dilatation or ballooning out that affects the entire circumference of a length of vessel.

Saccular. A distinct and localized outpouching of an area of artery wall; may also be called a "berry aneurysm."

Dissecting aneurysms result from a tear in the intimal layer of the vessel that allows blood to accumulate between the vessel walls. A false aneurysm is a complete tear of all vascular layers, usually resulting from a trauma, needle puncture, or suture failure. A pseudoaneurysm is a dilated or tortuous vessel segment without interruption of the vessel layers.

Aneurysm formation is a slow, gradual process; the natural course is gradual enlargement at an average rate of 10% of the current diameter per year followed by rupture.

The exact cause of AAA formation is unknown. The aorta is particularly prone to aneurysm development due to the absence of a penetrating vasa vasorum in the adventitial layer (the purpose of which is to give the vessel strength and support) and the constant stress and tension on the vessel wall. AAA formation is most commonly thought to be a degenerative process that results from atherosclerosis. As atherosclerotic plaque formation and deposit

487

erode the vessel wall, elastin layers in the vessel are fragmented, resulting in a weakened, thin tunica media and eventual aortic dilatation.

Uncontrolled hypertension (HTN) is also thought to greatly contribute to aneurysm formation. Prolonged high pressures destroy the tunica media, weakening the abdominal aortic wall. This constant bombardment of high pressure and expanding blood flow results in eventual aneurysm formation and rupture.

Other risk factors include the following:

- Increased age (decreases the "give and take" of the vessel)
- Sex (greater prevalence in males)
- Congenital syndromes (e.g., Marfan's syndrome, Ehlers-Danlos syndrome, Turner's syndrome, aortic coarctation)
- Blunt or sharp trauma (including surgical)
- Infection and inflammatory conditions
- Family history of aneurysms
- History of smoking
- Peripheral vascular and coronary artery disease
- Chronic obstructive pulmonary disease
- Presence of other aneurysms
- Pregnancy (particularly the third trimester)

 SIGNS AND SYMPTOMS
Asymptomatic/Prerupture Patient

Most patients present without signs and symptoms. As many as one third of all AAAs are detected on routine physical examination as a prominent pulsation at or above the umbilicus. The patient may report an awareness of this pulsation when lying down or resting quietly, and tenderness over the site may be present (particularly with enlarging aneurysms). A bruit may also be auscultated over the aneurysm. The patient may present with very benign symptoms such as constipation, impaired or painful orgasms, testicular pain or edema, scrotal ecchymosis, weight loss, early satiety, or nausea and vomiting. These symptoms are caused by encroachment of the aneurysm on other organs but are very hard to differentiate from other disease processes. The most common sign and symptom of an AAA is vague abdominal or lower back pain, or both. This pain may be described as throbbing or constant and may be indicative of impending rupture.

Symptomatic/Dissecting/Rupture Patient

A ruptured AAA is a medical and surgical emergency. It presents with severe, sharp, sudden, and continuous abdominal pain radiating to the back, hips, scrotum, and pelvis. This is accompanied by vital sign changes associated with hypovolemia, shock, mental alteration, and syncope.

 DIAGNOSTIC CRITERIA
Asymptomatic/Prerupture Patient
Routine Physical Examination

A palpable abdominal mass may be revealed on examination.

Laboratory Values

No routine laboratory values are indicated for the patient with an asymptomatic/preruptured AAA. Any decision to draw blood for laboratory work should be made on an individual basis.

Abdominal Ultrasonography

This in an inexpensive, noninvasive technique frequently used for the initial confirmation of an AAA and for routine follow-up care of smaller aneurysms that require frequent monitoring for potential enlargement. Ultrasonography provides information on both the size and location of the aneurysm, although it is most accurate in the anteroposterior rather than lateral dimension.

Computed Tomography

A computed tomography (CT) scan also is a noninvasive diagnostic tool. It involves radiation exposure and is more expensive than ultrasonography but allows for a more accurate visualization of the arterial wall of the aorta and the surrounding tissues and organs, thus allowing for a more accurate determination of the size and location of an aneurysm. Serial CT scans may also be used to follow small aneurysms that require frequent monitoring and to evaluate postoperative complications such as graft occlusion, hemorrhage, and abscess formation.

Magnetic Resonance Imaging

Magnetic resonance imaging (MRI) may be used in the diagnosis and monitoring of AAAs, but it provides results comparable with those obtained with CT scanning; it is more expensive; and sometimes it is difficult to obtain because the technology is not available in all hospitals.

Transthoracic and Transesophageal Echocardiography

Neither transthoracic nor transesophageal echocardiography requires the use of contrast agents; both are available in most hospitals and can be performed at the bedside. Transesophageal echocardiography is particularly useful in identifying the size and extent of the aneurysm as well as any peripheral vessel involvement. It is also helpful in visualizing true and false lumens and intimal flaps.

Arteriography

Arteriography is an invasive procedure that was once considered the gold standard for AAA diagnosis. It is still used by many surgeons to determine the plan for surgical repair, because the extent of aortic dissection and branch vessel involvement can be easily determined. However, the evaluation obtained from this procedure may be inaccurate if the aneurysm contains a thrombus, because the size of the thrombus may diminish the size of the lumen that is visible with the contrast agent.

Symptomatic/Dissecting/Rupture Patient

When a dissecting or ruptured aneurysm is suspected, patient mortality rates increase in direct proportion to the time to treatment. Diagnosis may be made on patient presentation alone. If confirmation is required, the most readily available, accurate, and safest diagnostic mode should be used. The most common choices include transthoracic echocardiography, transesophageal echocardiography, or CT scanning because they are noninvasive and readily available and allow for continuous patient monitoring. Ultrasonography should not be used for a suspected dissection or rupture because this could enhance the rupture and further deteriorate the patient's condition. Routine preoperative blood work, electrocardiography, and a blood sample for a type and cross should also be obtained.

INTERVENTIONS
Prehospital Monitoring

For the asymptomatic patient with an AAA that is 5 cm in diameter or less:
- Refer all AAAs to a vascular surgeon for assessment and monitoring.
- Assess peripheral pulses and blood pressure (BP), comparing both sides. Pressure differences of 20 mm Hg or greater in the upper extremities may indicate dissection or occlusion of the subclavian, innominate, brachial, or axillary artery.
- Modify risk factors where possible to slow disease progression.
- Maintain BP in a normotensive range.
- Establish appointments for routine follow-up and monitoring every 6 months.

Patient Teaching

Discuss the nature, onset, and course of the disease to include risk factors that should be modified and risk for rupture.
- Emphasize the importance of routine follow-up every 6 months.
- Include pharmacologic and nonpharmacologic measures to control BP when indicated.
- Medication instruction should include purpose, dosage, frequency, side effects, and signs of toxicity.
- Inform the patient and his or her family to seek immediate medical attention if any of the following occurs:
  Onset of diffuse back or abdominal aching
  Onset of severe back or abdominal pain
  Soreness over the umbilicus
  Sudden onset of extremity ischemia
  Persistent elevated BP

Surgical Management

Conventional repair of an AAA involves an open surgical repair in which the abdomen is opened and the aneurysm is exposed for repair. This surgery is a complex procedure that requires general anesthesia. The aortic and iliac arteries are clamped and a prosthetic graft is placed. Mortality rates for an elective procedure are as low as 5%; mortality rates for emergency repairs run as high as 50%. These rates increase in relation to a patient's decreasing health status. Patients with comorbidities such as cardiopulmonary disease who are undergoing elective repairs have an increased mortality rate of up to 40%. Many of these patients require lengthy intensive care unit stays after surgery and often remain ventilated for several days. Large volumes of blood may be lost, and many organ systems are stressed. The patient is at high risk for myocardial ischemia or infarction, stroke, renal ischemia, and hypovolemic shock both during and after the procedure. Pain control is also difficult as the mid-line abdominal incision extends from the below the sternal notch to the pubic area.

Preoperative Care

Preoperative preparation depends on the patient presentation and symptoms. Care for the patient undergoing an emergency procedure for a dissecting or ruptured aneurysm focuses solely on patient survival—on maintaining sufficient circulating volume to get the patient to the operating room for repair. All other preoperative care should be implemented on an "as-needed" basis. An elective procedure allows for adequate and more routine preoperative preparation to include the following:

Routine preoperative diagnostic tests for this patient include a complete blood cell count and a complete electrolyte assay. A urinalysis and clotting studies may also be ordered. A chest radiograph and 12-lead electrocardiograph should be obtained. The patient should also have recently had ultrasonography, CT scanning, MRI, or arteriography to determine the size and location of the aneurysm.

A complete preoperative assessment should be conducted to include height, weight, vital signs, and a complete history and physical examination.

Postoperative Care

Postoperative care is focused on maintaining hemodynamic and ventilatory stability as well as on providing adequate pain control. The patient is transferred from the surgical suite to an intensive care unit after surgery for the first 24 to 48 hours. He or she may also remain ventilated immediately postoperatively and will have a nasogastric tube for intermittent suction for the first 24 to 72 hours.

Vital signs and other hemodynamic parameters should be monitored at least hourly while the patient is in the intensive care unit. Vital signs are generally monitored every 4 hours once the patient is transferred to the general ward. The patient should be watched closely for signs and symptoms of hypovolemic shock, postoperative hemorrhage, or both. An effort should also be made to keep the systolic BP below 120 mm Hg to prevent a strain on the operative sutures. The electrocardiogram should be monitored for dysrhythmias and signs and symptoms of myocardial ischemia or infarction.

The respiratory status should be monitored carefully during ventilation. Once the patient is extubated, good pulmonary toileting should be encouraged, including deep breathing and coughing, and incentive spirometry.

Peripheral circulation should be closely monitored to include neurologic status, presence of pulses, temperature, color, and capillary refill. Extremities should also be monitored for any sensory or motor deficits.

Other organ systems, including the gastrointestinal and renal systems, should be monitored for signs and symptoms of ischemia to include the absence of bowel sounds after 48 to 72 hours, abdominal distention, decreased urinary output, and elevated blood urea nitrogen or creatine.

Serial laboratory work, including complete blood cell count, electrolytes, and arterial blood gases, should be monitored for abnormalities.

Early ambulation should be encouraged to prevent deep venous thrombosis. The patient should be turned at least every 2 hours while bedridden and intubated and should be up in a chair or ambulating within 24 to 48 hours after surgery.

The patient should be monitored for signs and symptoms of infection to include elevated temperature, elevations in the white blood cell count, and changes in the appearance of the surgical incision.

Pain control should be aggressive and may include epidural analgesia as well as intravenous narcotics to include as-needed (PRN) and patient-controlled analgesia (PCA) dosing. Nonpharmacologic pain management techniques such as relaxation and distraction should be included.

Endovascular Repair

Endovascular repair was first pioneered as a surgical alternative to AAA repair in the early 1990s. The technique involves inserting and deploying a graft through the femoral artery to the location of the AAA. The graft is released and secured in place by the normal diameter of the aorta and several metal hooks. Once deployed, the graft creates a circumferential seal that excludes the actual aneurysm from circulation, resulting in the thrombosis and resolution of the aneurysm sac. This procedure, although still in its infancy, is thought to have many advantages over the conventional repair, particularly for the compromised, high-risk patient. The long-term durability and effectiveness of these grafts and this procedure, however, are still being explored.

Preoperative preparation for this elective procedure should include all of the diagnostics, assessment, and teaching recommended for a conventional open repair. In addition to this, some specific issues must be addressed.

Preoperative instruction, while emphasizing the importance of early ambulation and an early return to normal activities, must also address the possibility of conversion to an open procedure if the endovascular graph cannot be placed successfully.

Accurate and current measurements of the aneurysm, the aorta, and the iliac arteries using angiography and contrast-enhanced CT with three-dimensional reconstruction are also crucial to a successful outcome. The following issues must be measured or addressed before surgery:

- The diameter of the common and external iliac arteries must be greater than the diameter of the introducer for the graft system.
- Angiography must also determine that the inferior mesenteric artery is not essential for intestinal perfusion, because the artery may be obliterated during the procedure.
- The normal vessel diameter both above and below the aneurysm must be measured.
- The length and size of the aneurysm must be measured in relation to the proximal and distal arteries.

The patient is usually extubated before leaving the operating room after an endovascular AAA repair. Postoperative care is similar to that for the conventional repair patient and should address the following:

The stability of vital signs and hemodynamic parameters should be monitored, and peripheral perfusion should be assessed.

The patient should be monitored closely for any signs of abdominal or back pain, indicating possible bleeding or rupture of the aneurysm.

Pain is very easily controlled with an intravenous narcotic in the immediate postoperative period. The patient can usually be switched to oral medication within 2 to 4 hours of the procedure.

Most patients can be transferred from the postanesthesia care unit to a monitored telemetry bed within 2 hours of the end of the procedure, eliminating the need for an intensive care unit stay.

Patients are ambulated within 4 to 6 hours of the procedure.

A postoperative chest radiography, arteriogram, and spiral CT scan are obtained 2 to 5 days after surgery to evaluate the graft placement and to ensure that there is no continued filling of the aneurysm.

Most patients are discharged within 2 to 5 days of the procedure.

COMMUNITY CARE

Assessment

Assessment for abdominal masses and pulsations should be part of any routine physical examination. Particular care should be taken to closely assess patients with high-risk factors or a familial history of aneurysms. Some studies advocate routine abdominal ultrasound for men older than 65 years of age, but this has not been widely implemented.

Monitoring

Once an aneurysm is discovered via routine assessment, it is crucial that the patient obtain continuous follow-up and evaluation at a minimal of every 6 months. Postoperative follow-up after both conventional and endovascular repairs should occur at least every 3 months for the first year and every 6 months thereafter.

Prevention

Modification of risk factors associated with coronary artery disease is the most effective method of preventing the development of AAA. Control of HTN is also crucial to prevent aneurysm formation.

PROGNOSIS

The overall mortality rate for AAAs after rupture is 90%; however, this may be reduced to 50% if the patient reaches the hospital alive. Early detection and repair yield the best outcomes, with an overall mortality rate of 5%. Emergency repair after dissection or rupture yields a mortality rate of 50% or higher, with a 30-day postoperative mortality rate also around 50%.

CLINICAL PEARLS

○ Vague abdominal or back pain should be closely evaluated in men older than 55 years of age.

○ The patient who presents with chest pain in whom myocardial ischemia and infarction have been ruled out should be closely evaluated for the presence of an AAA or a thoracic aortic aneurysm.

○ The patient who presents with severe abdominal or back pain with hypotension should be considered a surgical emergency. Multiple intravenous lines should be started, and volume expanders should be administered. The presence or absence of an AAA should be established immediately, and the operating room should be placed on standby for an emergency aneurysm repair.

○ The patient should be closely monitored after AAA repair for hypovolemia, hemorrhage, hypotension, myocardial ischemia, decreased urine output, and peripheral vessel occlusion.

NURSING PROBLEM/ DIAGNOSIS	NURSING INTERVENTIONS CLASSIFICATION (NIC)
Prerupture care/Risk for deficient fluid volume	Teaching: disease process Circulatory precautions Teaching: prescribed medication
Rupture management/Deficient fluid volume	Hemodynamic regulation Cardiac care: acute Fluid/electrolyte management Circulatory care

Buerger's Disease

Section 2   Linda McCuistion

 OVERVIEW

In Buerger's disease, an inflammatory response in vessels intermittently reoccurs. The exact cause of the vascular inflammatory response is unknown but is believed to be a genetic or an autoimmune disorder. Buerger's disease usually affects men between the ages of 20 and 40 years. The prevalence of Buerger's disease in females had been 10%, but due to the increase in female cigarette smokers, the prevalence is 20%, which parallels the percentage of female smokers. Although Buerger's disease occurs worldwide, it is more prevalent in eastern European, Asian, Indian, and Jewish cultures.

 PATHOPHYSIOLOGY

Buerger's disease is a vascular disorder that involves segments of small and medium-sized arteries, veins, and capillaries. The onset is usually gradual and occurs more commonly in arteries than in veins and capillaries. Distal vessels of the extremities initially are affected before proceeding proximally.

The exact cause of Buerger's disease is idiopathic, but it may be caused by an insult of a vessel resulting in recurrent inflammation. Vessel insult may result from direct injury, an autoimmune response, or infectious agents, or it may be secondary to other conditions, such as systemic lupus erythematosus, physical agents, frostbite or exposure to extremely cold temperatures, irradiation or sunburn, mechanical injury, or toxins. The strongest association of a precipitating factor with Buerger's disease is cigarette smoking. A possible theory of the association of cigarette smoking with Buerger's disease is a hypersensitivity to tobacco antigens. In addition, nicotine affects blood vessels by stimulating the sympathetic nervous system to release epinephrine and norepinephrine. These released hormones contribute to potent peripheral vasoconstriction. Carbon monoxide emitted from cigarettes also acts as a chemical irritant that injures the endothelium or inner lining of blood vessels and triggers the inflammatory response, causing edema that narrows the vessel's lumen.

Vessel injury may also be caused by an autoimmune response that causes recurrent inflammatory injury, which involves the endothelial cells and smooth muscle cells of the arterial wall. Despite the cause of the inflammation, the pathophysiologic responses are the same.

Recurrent inflammation can result in thrombosis and permanent tissue damage. The exudate leads to an excessive amount of necrosis and fibrosis, which leaves permanent vascular scarring. Fibrosis leads to vascular thrombosis, occlusion, and ischemia. Often, the entire disease process eventually results in the necrosis of vessels, which leads to ulcerative skin lesions and gangrene of the involved extremities. Necrotic skin lesions may be seen on the affected distal extremity, such as tips of the fingers or toes. Also, larger arteries, such as the brachial and femoral, may be involved.

 ## SIGNS AND SYMPTOMS

The signs and symptoms of Buerger's disease are primarily related to arterial ischemia. When circulation is inadequate due to vessel narrowing from repeated inflammation, the patient experiences pallor and enhanced sensitivity to cold, pain, and paresthesia, such as numbness, tingling, or a burning sensation.

The predominant symptom of Buerger's disease is pain. In this disease, pain is usually characterized as intermittent claudication in the involved extremities. *Intermittent claudication* is pain that is usually felt in the calf of the leg or arch of the foot after walking or exercising and generally relieved in 1 to 2 minutes by resting. This pain is measured in blocks (e.g., one- or two-block intermittent claudication). *Rest pain* is a later characteristic of Buerger's disease; it is an increased sensation of burning, sensitivity to cold, or unexplained pain in an affected extremity at rest. In some patients, pain at rest may be present continuously. As the ischemic disease progresses to later stages, rest pain becomes more persistent and devastating. Owing to the stimulation from severe pain, the sympathetic nervous system overactivity may lead to further coldness of the skin and excessive sweating of the feet.

Severe ischemia develops in many areas of the body. Distal pulses are usually diminished or absent due to the decrease in blood flow of the affected extremities. Decreased blood flow reduces the ability of capillaries to exchange oxygen, nutrition, and other metabolic products. This impaired capacity of metabolic interchange leads to a high oxygen concentration in capillaries, malnutrition, and atonic capillaries. As oxygen accumulates in dilated capillaries, dependent rubor or a reddened skin color is seen. As poor circulation progresses, edema and a cyanotic or purple discoloration of the affected extremity are noted. In addition, trophic skin changes result from a lack of adequate circulation and nutrition to body cells. The skin of the affected extremity may be thin and shiny with decreased hair growth, whereas the nails become thick and malformed.

In later stages, the complications of ulcerations and gangrene usually appear. Ulcerations owing to peripheral arterial diseases result from an inadequate exchange of oxygen and nutrients. The ulceration or excavation of skin surface is caused by inadequacy in cellular metabolism leading to necrosis or cell death. In general, ulcerations due to arterial insufficiency are small, circular, deep lesions on the tips of the toes or between the toes with demarcated edges.

Arterial ulcerations are also characterized by severe pain. Gangrene, which is a considerable mass of necrotic tissue, frequently necessitates amputation.

 DIAGNOSTIC CRITERIA

The physical examination usually reveals diminished or absent pulses in the affected extremity, such as the radial, ulnar, or tibial sites. Pulse oximetry is used to assess cutaneous oxygen delivery to the tissues. Doppler ultrasonography is used to quantify the degree of ischemia by measuring the ankle-brachial index (ABI). The ABI is obtained by measuring BPs with the typical four-cuff technique. By applying four pneumatic cuffs, one each to the upper thigh, the lower thigh, the upper calf, and immediately above the ankle, as well as the upper arm to measure the brachial BP, segmental pressures recorded with the Doppler device can be contrasted. The ABI is calculated by dividing the ankle pressure by the brachial pressure. The normal ABI is less than or equal to 1.0. Asymmetry in brachial pressure of more than 10 mm Hg or an ABI of less than 1.0 is suspected in arterial disease. Plethysmographic studies, which record variations in blood volume of extremities by detecting the amount of blood flow, can also be used to measure blood flow adequacy. This helps to evaluate blood flow and determines the degree of impaired peripheral circulation in diagnosis of the early stages of Buerger's disease. Also, CT scanning and MRI may be used for diagnosis. MRI allows indirect visualization of cross-sectional images, thus it evaluates vascular integrity and disorders with the use of a contrast agent. Arteriograms can determine the location and degree of arterial occlusion in Buerger's disease. They can show the characteristic, smooth, tapering segmental lesions in the affected vessels and collateral vessels at the sites of vascular occlusion.

 INTERVENTIONS

The goals of management for Buerger's disease include improvement in circulation, prevention of disease progression, and protection of the affected extremities from trauma, injury, and infection. The following interventions promote vasodilatation, which meet the management goals of Buerger's disease.

Prevent Vasoconstriction

The patient should be taught methods to prevent vasoconstriction, which include the avoidance of nicotine, caffeine, exposure to cold, constrictive clothing, crossing the legs, and emotional stress. The strong correlation with Buerger's disease and smoking necessitates the complete cessation of cigarette smoking and use of all forms of tobacco. When a patient completely quits cigarette smoking, the signs and symptoms generally improve greatly. Avoidance of caffeine in coffee or tea and prolonged exposure to cold temperatures can also help to prevent vasoconstriction. Emotional stress must be decreased as much as possible. Stress management and relaxation techniques may be taught to minimize vasoconstriction from the stress response.

Promote Vasodilatation

Measures to promote vasodilatation and to improve circulation include appropriate positioning and exercise. Proper positioning uses gravity to promote blood flow, therefore arterial circulation is improved when a body part is positioned below heart level. Buerger-Allen exercises may be prescribed for the arterial insufficiency of Buerger's disease; extremities are placed in elevation, dependent, and horizontal positions in the Buerger-Allen exercises (Fig. 15-2-1). Blood flow is improved by filling and emptying of arteries, with prescribed position changes in a prescribed time frame. If pain and dramatic color changes occur, the patient should discontinue the Buerger-Allen exercises and rest.

Walking Exercises

A program of walking exercises improves blood flow and is a key treatment for peripheral vascular diseases (PVDs). After determination of the severity of intermittent claudication on a treadmill exercise test, patients are instructed to walk until feeling moderate pain and to then rest. Walking exercise sessions should be carried out three or four times a week for approximately 30 to 40 minutes. Studies have shown a significant improvement in exercise tolerance and quality of life by approximately 180%. Walking exercises, however, are contingent on the state of the disease. They are appropriate only when no pain at rest, ulceration, or gangrene is present. If these symptoms are present, then complete bed rest is indicated until resolution.

Medications

Medications may also promote vasodilatation. Examples of antiplatelet agents are acetylsalicylic acid (aspirin), ticlopidine (Ticlid), and dipyridamole (Persantine), which inhibit platelet aggregation and thus prevent thrombus formation and eventual occlusion. Newer medications include pentoxifylline (Trental) and clopidogrel bisulfate (Plavix). These drugs increase the flexibility of red blood cells, decrease blood viscosity by inhibiting platelet aggregation, and decrease fibrinogen, thus increasing blood flow and oxygenated blood to the affected extremities. Calcium antagonists and thromboxane inhibitors are used for their vasodilatation effects. Strict vasodilators are rarely prescribed, because they tend to vasodilate only healthy vessels and may even divert blood flow away from partially occluded vessels. Therefore, vasodilators tend to worsen the ischemic situation in Buerger's disease.

Surgery

Surgical procedures may promote vasodilatation and promote circulation. By blocking or severing a sympathetic nerve that causes constriction of blood vessels, vasodilatation is produced and blood flow is improved. Arterial bypass surgery may also improve blood flow. If ulcerations are present, débridement of ulcers may be necessary to promote healing. If gangrene is present, amputation is the only option to preserve the remaining healthy tissue.

Protection

Safety measures that protect affected extremities from trauma, injury, and infection should be taught to the patient. Teaching proper foot care includes cleanliness of skin by washing the feet daily with a mild soap and lukewarm water. The bath water should be tested for an appropriate temperature before the patient enters the water. Care should be taken to wash between the toes and to rinse thoroughly. Drying should be complete, using a patting method to

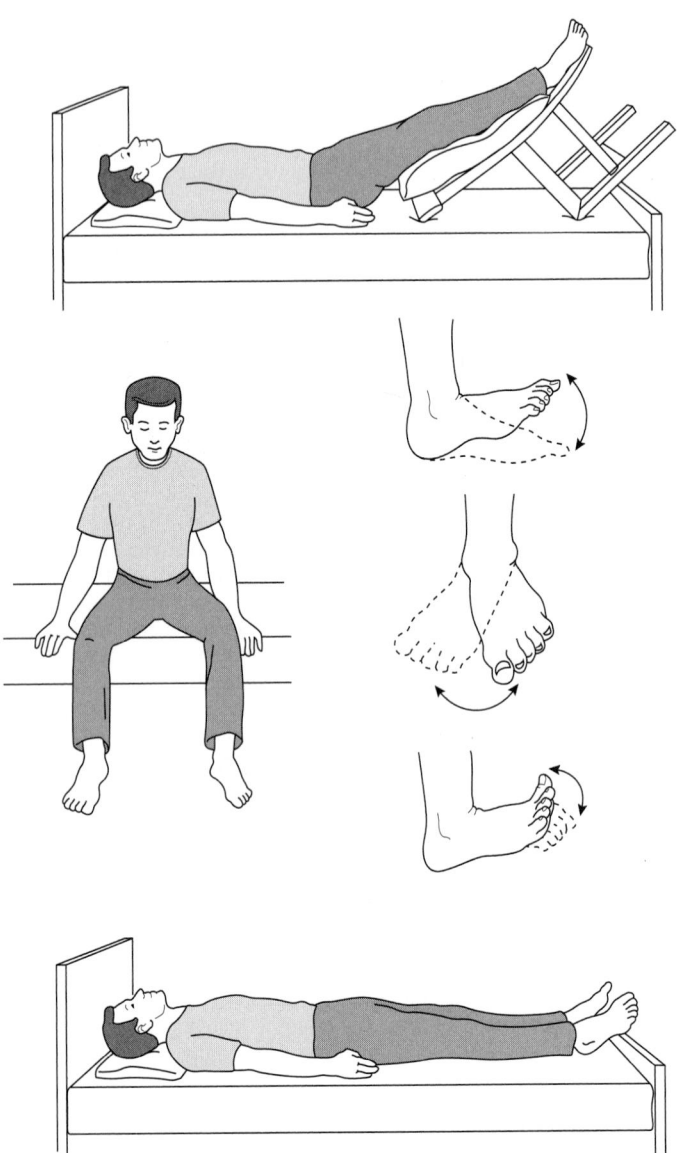

Figure 15-2-1. Buerger's exercises.

dry rather than rubbing. For safety, the feet should be inspected daily for redness, dryness, blisters, or cuts in the skin. For dry skin, a cream with lanolin may be applied, but it should never be applied between the toes. Toenails should be cut straight across when soft after bathing, or a podiatrist may be consulted to cut the nails.

Warmth and safety can be maintained by wearing mittens, cotton socks (cotton absorbs moisture accumulated from sweating), and sturdy shoes or slippers. The patient should be instructed to avoid trauma, extremely cold temperatures, and heating pads because the patient with Buerger's disease has decreased sensitivity to touch, thus a burn or other damage is more likely to occur. Patients should be taught to avoid hindering circulation by crossing the legs or ankles, wearing tight-fitting clothing, or standing for prolonged periods in one position.

 COMMUNITY CARE

Assessment

1. Take a history and assess predisposing factors that are present: cigarette smoking, age, and family disease history.
2. Assess for signs and symptoms of Buerger's disease: intermittent claudication, sensitivity to cold, pallor, excessive sweating of feet, dependent rubor, slow capillary refill, and paresthesia (e.g., numbness, tingling, and burning sensation).
3. Assess for signs and symptoms of advanced disease: cyanosis or purple discoloration, severe pain, rest pain, diminished or absent pulse, edema, and trophic skin changes (e.g., thin shiny skin, decreased hair growth, and thick malformed nails).

Monitoring

1. Monitor patient compliance with prescribed therapeutic treatment regimen.
2. Monitor for signs of healing or infection if ulcerations are present: evidence of healing by secondary intention, fever, edema, and drainage with foul odor.
3. Monitor for hydration and nutritional status: dry scaly skin, poor skin turgor, and tenting of skin.
4. Monitor need for pain medication: intermittent claudication, rest pain, and before dressing changes for anticipated pain.
5. Monitor for ischemic complications of Buerger's disease, such as ulcerations and gangrene.

Prevention

1. Instruct patient regarding measures to reduce vasoconstriction factors: cessation of smoking, avoidance of caffeine, reduction in exposure to cold temperatures or heating pads, and stress reduction.
2. Instruct patient regarding measures to improve circulation: change position every 1 to 2 hours, discourage crossing the legs or placement of pillows under the knees, maintain a comfortable room temperature, provide adequate clothing and blankets, avoid constrictive clothing, refrain from obesity, and avoid sitting or standing for prolonged periods.
3. Instruct the patient regarding prescribed medication regimen.

PROGNOSIS

- Ulceration and gangrene eventually occur in most patients. If gangrene is present, amputations are very likely to follow. When Buerger's disease has progressed to the point of amputation, a toe or even a transmetatarsal amputation is not sufficient. Usually, a below- or above-the-knee amputation is necessary. Amputation is imminent if the patient complains of severe rest pain, if overwhelming infection is present, or if gangrene worsens.
- In patients who stop smoking, only approximately 5% require that a digit or extremity be amputated, whereas in patients who do not stop smoking, approximately 40% require amputation of some type.
- The morbidity and mortality rates are uncertain for Buerger's disease, because patients usually have concurrent more life-threatening conditions, such as coronary artery disease and cerebrovascular disease.

 CLINICAL PEARLS

- Vasodilators make Buerger's disease worse.
- Cigarette smoking has an extremely strong association with Buerger's disease, and if the patient can completely stop smoking, the signs and symptoms improve greatly.
- Buerger-Allen exercises use gravity to fill and empty arteries through properly timed position changes.
- Extreme elevation of lower extremities should be avoided, because this position slows arterial blood flow.
- Instruct the patient with Buerger's disease to never use a heating pad on the lower extremities to avoid burns on vulnerable tissue.
- A program of walking exercises can improve exercise tolerance and quality of life by 180%.

NURSING PROBLEM/ DIAGNOSIS	NURSING INTERVENTIONS CLASSIFICATION (NIC)
Decreased perfusion/Ineffective tissue perfusion	Circulatory care Peripheral sensation management Positioning Exercise therapy
Prevention of vasoconstriction/ Therapeutic regimen management	Environmental management Skin surveillance Smoking cessation assistance

Deep Vein Thrombosis

Section 3   Beverly George-Gay

 OVERVIEW

Deep vein thrombosis (DVT) is a frequent and potentially fatal complication that mainly affects hospitalized patients. Two million Americans experience

DVT each year. It is responsible for approximately 200,000 hospitalizations annually. More than 60,000 patients in the United States die of acute pulmonary embolism (PE) as a consequence of DVT. Only 50% of people with DVT are symptomatic; the other 50% go without treatment, increasing their risk for a significant event.

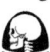 **PATHOPHYSIOLOGY**

A *thrombus* is a stationary blood clot formed within the cardiovascular system (see Chapter 15, Section 8). There are three predisposing factors that stimulate thrombus formation, as described by Virchow in 1856: (1) vessel wall (endothelial) injury or abnormality, (2) stasis, and (3) hypercoagulability.

Vessel Wall Injury or Abnormality

Vessel wall injury or abnormality can occur due to direct injury to the vein, as seen with venipuncture, surgery, or cannulation, or to pressure from surrounding tissue. Patients undergoing lower extremity orthopedic surgery are at the highest risk for the development of DVT due to vessel manipulation during the procedure. Without prophylaxis, the risk of DVT after joint arthroplasty ranges from 45% to 70%. A significant PE will occur in as many as 16% of these patients. Chemical agents introduced into the vascular system such as chemotherapeutic agents, some vasopressor agents (e.g., dopamine), contrast medium, and high-dose antibiotics can cause endothelium damage. Other causes include burns and fractures that cause damage to the vessel (e.g., burns and fractures of the pelvis, femur, tibia, and fibula).

Stasis

Venous stasis occurs when the venous valves are dysfunctional and muscles are inactive. The loss of muscular pumping action and maintenance of unidirection flow result in venous pooling. Pooling allows coagulation factors to accumulate, increasing the chance of platelet aggregation and clot formation (see Chapter 12, Section 2). Risk factors for stasis include: (1) immobilization due to postoperative convalescence, major illness (e.g., stroke), and spinal cord injury; (2) decreased blood flow states, which occur with myocardial infarction, heart failure, and shock; (3) prolonged sitting on a airplane or in an automobile; (4) atrial fibrillation (the loss of atrial contraction allows a small amount of blood to pool in the atria, encouraging clot formation); (5) obesity; (6) diabetes mellitus; and (7) sickle cell anemia.

Hypercoagulability

Accelerated coagulation mechanisms occur with several hematologic disorders such as polycythemia, certain malignancies, and antithrombin III deficiencies. Hypercoagulability also can occur as a protective or reparative mechanism after surgery or trauma, especially with soft tissue injuries. In 10% to 40% of patients undergoing thoracic or abdominal surgery, DVT will develop. Pregnancy results in hypercoagulability; in fact, PE is a leading cause of maternal death secondary to DVT. Other risk factors include estrogen use, systemic infection, autoimmune diseases such as systemic lupus, ulcerative colitis, smoking, and acquired immunodeficiency syndrome.

Additional risk factors include idiopathic thrombophlebitis and previous DVT.

The thrombus can reduce flow and increase turbulence, which enhances the formation of more thrombi or may completely occlude the vessel. DVT can be occlusive or nonocclusive, affecting the deep veins of the pelvis and lower extremities. The thrombus may cause increased venous pressure below the clot, because forward flow is blocked. Increased pressure results in venous dilatation and may eventually cause leakage of intravascular fluid into the interstitial spaces (*edema*). In some patients, deoxygenated hemoglobin within the stagnant blood imparts a cyanotic discoloration to the extremity, a condition called *phlegmasia cerulea dolens* (i.e., a swollen, blue, painful leg). In cases in which edema is excessive, interstitial pressure exceeds capillary pressure, resulting in pallor, a condition called *phlegmasia alba dolens* ("swollen, pale, painful leg"). However, in most cases, patients are asymptomatic.

COMPLICATIONS
Pulmonary Embolism

A life-threatening complication of DVT is a PE. Venous thrombi tend to extend in the direction of blood flow, toward the heart, frequently producing a "tail." The tail, or a part of the thrombus, may dislodge, forming a *thromboembolus* (sometimes called an *embolus* ["a traveling clot"]). The thromboembolus travels through the venous circulation and into the inferior vena cava, the right atrium, and ventricle and enters the pulmonary artery. Up to 80% of PEs are small and clinically silent, because pulmonary circulation has multiple sources of collateral flow. Pulmonary infarction occurs in 10% to 15% of cases, usually in patients with cardiopulmonary disease. Approximately 1% of pulmonary emboli are fatal. Death results when 50% to 60% of the pulmonary vasculature is occluded by a large embolus, causing acute right heart failure and resulting in cardiac arrest in 75% of cases. Death in the other 25% of cases is associated with hypotension. Although most cases of PE are caused by a DVT, PEs may also be caused by fat, tumor, air, amniotic fluid, or bacterial emboli.

Chronic Venous Insufficiency

A common complication of recurrent DVT is chronic venous insufficiency. When chronic venous insufficiency occurs secondary to a thrombus, the condition is called *post-thrombotic syndrome*. After venous thrombosis, valvular closure is prevented as high venous pressures distend the vein and separate the valvular leaflets. Valves also become thickened and contracted, preventing closure. The increased pressure causes plasma proteins and red blood cells, in addition to fluid, to leak into the tissue spaces, causing pigmentation and altering circulation. Secondary varicosities may develop. Stasis ulcerations (see Chapter 3, Section 1) result from the rupture of small skin veins. Skin becomes dry and scaly; subcutaneous tissues fibrose and atrophy; and cellulitis may develop. Findings of venous insufficiency do not usually manifest for years after DVT.

 ## SIGNS AND SYMPTOMS

Venous thrombosis and thrombophlebitis are frequently referred to as the same disorder, but in most cases, DVT does not occur in response to inflammation (phlebitis) and no signs of inflammation are present. If the thrombus is extensive and causes occlusion, the patient will be symptomatic. If, however, the thrombus is small and nonocclusive, no inflammation will be present and the patient will be asymptomatic.

The signs and symptoms of symptomatic patients are discussed.

Signs. On the physical examination, signs reveal the affected extremity to be 3 cm greater in circumference than the unaffected leg, unilateral pitting edema, and dilated, collateral superficial veins (nonvaricose). Homan's sign (calf pain on dorsiflexion of the foot with the knee in about 30 degrees of flexion) is present in only a few patients (10% to 20%) and should not be assessed if DVT is suspected, because it may cause embolization.

Symptoms. Pain caused by pressure on adjacent nerves may be noted in the affected limb and made worse with standing or walking and better with elevation. Swelling of the affected extremity is a sensitive indicator and may be associated with varicosities, edema, cyanosis, or pallor.

The first indication of DVT for some patients is presentation with the signs and symptoms of PE.

Signs and Symptoms of Pulmonary Embolism. Dyspnea, usually with a sudden onset, is the most common symptom of PE, occurring in about 60% of patients. It can vary from mild to severe and from intermittent to progressive. Chest pain worsening with deep breathing is commonly reported. Common findings on examination include tachypnea (respiratory rate >24/min), tachycardia, and fever.

 DIAGNOSTIC CRITERIA

The diagnosis of DVT cannot be made on clinical information alone, because most patients are asymptomatic. Objective diagnostic testing is essential. A scoring system (Table 15-3-1) has been developed that is based on risk factors, signs, and symptoms and allows for the identification of subgroups of patients who are highly likely or unlikely to have DVT. This score provides a pretest probability that helps the clinician to better interpret the test results. This strategy is used to help ensure that patients with DVT receive appropriate therapy and those who do not have DVT are not exposed to the risks of anticoagulation.

Table 15-3-1. Scoring System

CLINICAL PARAMETER	SCORE
Active cancer (treatment or palliation within previous 6 months)	1
Paralysis, paresis, or recent (4 weeks) plaster immobilization of the lower extremities	1
Recently bedridden for more than 3 days or major surgery within 4 weeks	1
Localized tenderness along the distribution of the deep venous system	1
Entire leg swelling (thigh and calf)	1
Calf swelling by >3 cm compared with the asymptomatic leg	1
Pitting edema; symptomatic leg only	1
Dilated superficial veins (nonvaricose) in symptomatic leg only	1
An alternative diagnosis is more likely or greater than that of DVT	− 2

There is a high probability for deep vein thrombosis (DVT) if the score is ≥3, moderate probability if the score is 1 to 2, and low probability if the score is ≤0.

Adapted from Elliott, G. C. (2000). The diagnostic approach to deep venous thrombosis. *Semin Resp Crit Care Med, 21,* 511–519.

Venography

Venography (see Chapter 15, Section 8) is the reference standard for the diagnosis of DVT, but it is expensive and invasive and carries significant side effects, so it is not the first choice for diagnostic tool. Rather, it is used when diagnosis remains unclear after clinical evaluation and initial testing (ultrasonography). Side effects of venography include hypersensitivity to contrast medium, including urticaria, angioedema, bronchospasm, or cardiovascular collapse; pain or discomfort at the injection site; and thrombosis secondary to contrast medium. Contrast medium may also cause renal damage and is contraindicated for patients with serum creatinine levels higher than 2 mg/dL.

Ultrasonography
Duplex Venous Ultrasonography

The method used most often to identify DVT is duplex venous ultrasonography. It is the initial test of choice, but it is less accurate than venography. Its advantages are that it is low cost and noninvasive and lacks associated side effects. This method uses both scanning and compression, thus allowing for the detection of thrombus via either direct visualization or inference when the vein does not collapse on gentle compression. Morbid obesity, severe edema, casts, and immobilization devices can limit the examination. This method is highly sensitive and specific for the diagnosis of symptomatic DVT. It is, however, limited for the detection of proximal and calf DVT for the asymptomatic high-risk postoperative patient.

Impedance Plethysmography

This ultrasound study detects changes in blood volume that can occur with obstruction. A cuff is wrapped around the thigh and inflated to a pressure that exceeds venous pressure but not arterial diastolic pressure (e.g., 50 mm Hg). When the cuff is deflated, rapid venous outflow should occur. If a thrombus is present, venous emptying is significantly slower. False-positive results can occur in patients with pelvic tumors or conditions with elevated venous pressure. This also is limited in the detection of DVT in the asymptomatic patient.

Magnetic Resonance Imaging

MRI may be an alternative to venography. It is particularly useful for the detection of thrombi in the pelvic vein.

D-Dimer

This blood assay detects clot fragments produced by clot lysis. It may be used in addition to other tests to rule out the diagnosis of DVT.

Pulmonary Arteriography (Angiography)

This is the definitive test for PE. A radiopaque dye is injected into the pulmonary vasculature through a catheter inserted into the right side of the heart. Vascular filling defects then can be visualized on radiographs.

Lung Scan

A lung scan (ventilation/perfusion) is used to diagnose PE. Radiopaque agents are inhaled (xenon) and injected peripherally to delineate areas of ventilation and areas of perfusion in the lung. Frequently, the results are inconclusive, especially when the pretest probability for DVT is low.

Computed Tomography

Spiral CT and CT angiography have been found to be helpful in the diagnosis of both PE and DVT.

INTERVENTIONS

Prophylaxis (Thromboprophylaxis)

Prophylaxis is a primary intervention for patients at risk. The goals of prophylaxis is to prevent the onset of either symptomatic or asymptomatic DVT and to prevent pulmonary embolism.

Exercises

Active or passive lower extremity exercises produce muscular contraction that facilitates venous return to the heart. Teach plantar flexion and dorsiflexion of the feet, called "heel pumping," and circumduction of the feet, called "ankle circles." These should be performed every 1 to 2 hours while awake for 10 to 12 repetitions. Deep breathing exercises produce increased negative pressure in the thorax, which allows the large veins to easily empty into the right atrium. These should be done every 1 to 2 hours while the patient is awake.

Mobilization

Early mobilization, especially ambulation, is necessary to stimulate the contraction of leg muscles, which enhances venous return. This can be done hours after surgery or on the first postoperative day, depending on the procedure. Adequate pain control must be provided to facilitate mobilization.

Leg elevation above the level of the heart promotes venous return; elevation should not exceed 45 degrees. Crossing the legs, placement of pillows behind the knees, and elevation of the knee gatch are activities that produce pressure on the popliteal space, which may impede venous flow, and should be avoided. Massaging of the legs is contraindicated, because it may cause thrombi to break off, thus producing emboli.

Mechanical Measures

Intermittent external pneumatic compression provides: (1) increased velocity of venous return, reducing stasis; (2) stimulation of regional fibrinolytic activity, reducing hypercoagulability; and (3) the reduction in venodilatation, reducing endothelial damage.

Sequential Compression Devices

Sequential compression devices are multichamber devices that are applied to the lower extremity to provide sequential compression to milk venous blood forward. They are to be worn with elastic stockings (i.e., thromboembolic disease stockings [TEDS]). Elastic stockings must be applied evenly to prevent wrinkles. Noncompliance may be a problem with this system because patients complain that the sequential compression devices are "too hot" or that the accompanying stockings were bothersome. Some complications that may occur include a venous tourniquet effect when thigh-high stockings roll down and peroneal nerve palsy from constant long-term pressure on the nerve. For intermittent plantar compression, a foot pump is applied around the foot only, providing pulsatile compression of the plantar venous plexus and peripheral veins of the foot. Foot pumps are used without elastic stockings. They are more compatible with other devices such as bulky leg dressings and continuous passive motion devices.

Both sequential compression devices and foot pumps have been found to be effective, but the efficacy depends on patient compliance. Patient education regarding DVT prophylaxis is a priority and has been shown to improve patient compliance. Sympathy in allowing the patient to keep these devices off can be detrimental. Ensure that the devices are sized and applied correctly. Remove devices and elastic stockings at least twice daily for 15 minutes (or as recommended by the manufacturer) for skin inspection and care and then reapply.

Pharmacologic Prophylaxis

Standard (unfractionated) heparin at low dose (low-dose heparin), 5000 units every 8 to 12 hours subcutaneously, is useful for DVT prophylaxis but may predispose the patient to the risk of bleeding. This is used mainly in the postoperative general abdominal surgery patient. Low molecular weight heparins (LMWHs), such as enoxaparin at low doses subcutaneously (see Table 12-2-4), are effective with minimal incidence of bleeding. They are preferred in the postoperative orthopedic patients. LMWHs are also being used on an outpatient bases with close follow-up. Warfarin is one of the most commonly used prophylactic agents in the United States. It is administered the evening after the procedure and takes 36 hours or longer to become therapeutic. PT and INR monitoring are required (see Chapter 12, Section 2). Warfarin may be started at lower doses than for the actual treatment of DVT (e.g., DVT treatment is started at 5 mg and prophylaxis treatment may be started at 2 mg).

Standard weight-based intravenous heparin may be used for patients with previous DVT, followed by warfarin. Anticoagulation for prophylaxis may be recommended for 2 to 6 weeks or up to 3 months for patients at high risk. Monitor for and teach the patient to report signs of bleeding, including ecchymosis, hematomas, nosebleeds, hematemesis, hematuria, and black tarry stools (melena). Faintness, weakness, dizziness, or severe headache may be a sign of cerebral hemorrhage, and abdominal pain may be sign of gastrointestinal hemorrhage; both must be reported (see Chapter 12, Section 2 for administration, antidotes, and care of patients receiving anticoagulant agents).

Surveillance

It is important to identify patients at risk. Monitor for and teach the patient to be alert of the signs of both DVT and PE as previously identified.

Management of Acute Deep Vein Thrombosis and Acute Pulmonary Embolism

Anticoagulation

Anticoagulation prevents further clot formation while allowing the body's clot lysis systems to operate. Standard weight-based intravenous heparin to achieve an activated partial thromboplastin time of 1.5 to 2.5 times mean for approximately 5 days followed by oral anticoagulants is the mainstay of therapy (see Chapter 12, Section 2). Oral anticoagulant therapy with warfarin is started 1 to 2 days after the onset of symptoms to achieve anticoagulation with an INR of 2.0 to 3.0. Subcutaneous use of weight-based dose LMWHs (see Table 12-2-4) is effective for the initial treatment of acute thrombosis for 5 days, followed by oral anticoagulation. Outpatient treatment with weight-based LMWH for 5 to 10 days followed by warfarin has been found to more cost effective and may be a promising alternative for patients with acute DVT. These patients are closely monitored at an anticoagulation clinic; this usually requires 1 day of hospitalization to initiate and teach LMWH administration and to arrange home care. Patients with extensive thrombosis in the iliofemoral veins, massive PE, or concomitant medical illness, as well as those at an increased risk for bleeding, should be treated on an inpatient basis. For patients with DVT and PE, anticoagulation is maintained for 3 to 6 months with warfarin. Signs of bleeding (as identified earlier) must be taught and reported.

Pain Management

Pain may be reduced with mild analgesics; acetaminophen therapy is helpful. Warm compresses may be used for comfort and to increase circulation to the affected area. Leg elevation above the level of the heart reduces venous congestion and pain.

Mobilization and Exercise

Bed rest is usually used for the first 5 to 7 days, with leg elevation, and then as described for prophylaxis. Elastic stockings may be needed for 3 to 6 months to support vein walls and valves and to decrease swelling. Mechanical measures may be used as prophylaxis in the unaffected leg.

Thrombolytic Therapy

Thrombolysis may be used to dissolve current clots in patients with PE, and although it is not commonly recommended for DVT, it may be used in patients with extensive obstruction of venous outflow. Drugs used for thrombolytic therapy act by assisting plasminogen to become plasmin, initiating fibrinolysis. Streptokinase, urokinases, and recombinant tissue plasminogen activator (rtPA) are approved thrombolytic agents. The following adult regimens include: rtPA at 100 mg intravenously over 2 hours; streptokinase at 250,000 IU bolus in normal saline or 5% dextrose in water over 30 minutes, followed by 100,000 IU/hr for 24 hours; and urokinase at 4400 IU/kg intravenous loading dose in 5 mL of solution over 10 minutes, followed by 4400 IU/kg/hr infused for 12 hours. If bleeding occurs, discontinue the agent and administer fresh frozen plasma (contains clotting factors; see Chapter 2, Section 3).

Contraindications to thrombolytic therapy include current active internal bleeding, cerebrovascular accident within the past 2 months, intracranial or intraspinal surgery in the past 2 weeks, and hypersensitivity to the agent. Relative contraindications include trauma or surgery within the past 15 days of PE, diastolic HTN of higher than 100 mm Hg, recent cardiac arrest resuscitation, during pregnancy, and within 2 weeks of delivery.

Oxygen

Supplemental oxygen via nasal cannula may be used to maintain a PaO_2 of higher than 80 mm Hg.

Surgical Management

The primary indication for surgery is to prevent PE in patients at high risk who cannot take anticoagulant agents or for whom anticoagulation was ineffective. Inferior vena cava or caval interruption involves the placement of an umbrella-type filter into the inferior vena cava to prevent thrombi from the lower extremities from passing into pulmonary circulation. The filter is inserted percutaneously through superficial femoral veins. Thrombectomy or embolectomy (rare) may be performed in extreme cases.

 COMMUNITY CARE

During anticoagulation therapy, the patient should be taught to avoid any contact sports that can lead to serious injury. Use a soft toothbrush for oral care, and if there is a need to shave, use an electric shaver. Keep all follow-up appointments and wear a MedicAlert bracelet. If on warfarin, maintain a diet consistent in the amount of vitamin K. Foods high in vitamin K include liver, tea (green), cauliflower, chickpeas, and green leafy vegetables (e.g., broccoli, Brussels sprouts, kale, spinach, turnip greens). Although in the green leafy vegetable family, cabbage, lettuce, asparagus, and green beans are not high in vitamin K. Warfarin should be taken at the same time every day.

Review the disease process with the patient, and evaluate for the signs of bleeding, DVT, and PE.

Teach the patient to avoid sitting and standing for long periods. The patient should ambulate a few minutes every hour while awake. Encourage a gradual walking program for the patient, and review leg exercises. Review the application of elastic stockings, and assess for compliance.

Teach the patient to avoid over-the-counter medications without consulting the health care team. Drugs such as aspirin and ibuprofen are platelet aggregation inhibitors and can cause prolonged bleeding episodes when used in conjunction with anticoagulant agents.

Teach and observe for the signs of venous stasis ulcers, which may not appear for years.

 PROGNOSIS

DVT itself is not fatal; death may result from the development of PE. PE is the third most common cardiovascular cause of death, which may result in up to 55,000 deaths per year. In massive PE, most deaths occur within the first hour.

 CLINICAL PEARLS

○ Heel pumping and ankle circles exercises should be performed every 1 to 2 hours while awake for 10 to 12 repetitions.
○ Leg elevation should not exceed 45 degrees.
○ Avoid popliteal pressure, which is produced by crossing the legs, placing pillows behind the knees, and elevation of the knee gatch.
○ Sequential compression devices should be used with elastic stockings, and foot pumps are used without elastic stockings.
○ Low-dose heparin is standard (unfractionated heparin administered subcutaneously at 5000 U every 8 or 12 hours).

○ Foods high in vitamin K include liver, tea (green), cauliflower, chickpeas, and green leafy vegetables.
○ Do not massage the legs of patients with DVT.
○ Do not repeat Homan's test once DVT is diagnosed or test result is positive.

NURSING PROBLEM/ DIAGNOSIS	NURSING INTERVENTIONS CLASSIFICATION (NIC)
Ineffective tissue perfusion	Circulatory care Embolus care: peripheral Embolism care: pulmonary Respiratory monitoring Surveillance
Anticoagulation	Bleeding precautions Circulatory precautions
Acute pain	Heat/cold application Pain management

Hypertension

Section 4 Diane Anthony Manghram ■ Beverly George-Gay

 ## OVERVIEW

Hypertension is defined as excessive tension that is exerted by blood on arterial walls, which results in an intermittent or sustained elevation in systolic BP (>140 mm Hg) and diastolic BP (>90 mm Hg) in an adult. It is the most common of all cardiovascular disorders and affects persons in all geographic areas and of all socioeconomic groups. Approximately 50 million people in the United States are being treated for HTN. The prevalence of HTN is greater among blacks, in individuals who are overweight, and in people with a family history of HTN. HTN is one of the most significant morbidity and mortality risk factors associated with coronary heart disease, congestive heart failure, chronic renal failure, and stroke.

 ## PATHOPHYSIOLOGY
Essential Hypertension

Essential HTN occurs when there is an increased peripheral resistance caused by functional tightening and structural thickening of resistance vessels. Essential HTN occurs without evidence of other disease; it is a chronic elevation in BP to higher than 140/90 mm Hg, and the underlying cause is unknown. This type represents 90% to 95% of all cases being treated. This disease occurs in 15% of white adults and 30% of black adults in the United States.

Risk Factors

Age: risk progressively increases with age. Individuals older than 65 years of age are at significant risk.

Sex: men younger than 55 years are at greater risk than women of the same age. At 55 to 74 years of age, women are at a greater risk.

Family history: a family history of HTN or cardiovascular disease increases risk.

Other: cerebrovascular disease, diabetes mellitus, sedentary lifestyle, obesity, elevated serum lipid levels, high salt (sodium) intake, high caffeine intake, excessive consumption of alcohol, smoking, low socioeconomic status, and stress increase risks.

Secondary Hypertension

Secondary HTN develops secondary to a specific cause and occurs in 5% to 10% of individuals diagnosed with HTN. Kidney disease is the most common cause of secondary HTN (Table 15-4-1 provides a list of several causes).

Secondary HTN occurs before age 30 and after age 50. Renal artery stenosis and coarctation of the aorta are common in younger individuals. In older individuals, the sudden onset of secondary HTN is often associated with a renal artery atherosclerotic disease. Many of the conditions that cause secondary HTN can be corrected or alleviated by surgical or medical treatment.

Whether essential or secondary, HTN is subclassified by course progression as benign, malignant, or crisis.

Benign Hypertension

Benign HTN is a progressive mild, slow increase in BP over several years. The diastolic BP usually ranges between 90 and 120 mm Hg. Contrary to what the name implies, this type of HTN produces serious effects if untreated or undertreated. Endocrine disorders in essential or secondary HTN are more prevalent in individuals younger than age 45 and may be prolonged into the 50s. It occurs more often in men than in women. Vascular changes of the arteries are noted with accelerated arteriosclerosis and atheroma. The arterioles have hyaline thickening that causes open narrow lumina. Complications associ-

Table 15-4-1. Causes of Secondary Hypertension

Renal

Renal artery stenosis
Polycystic kidney
Acute glomerulonephritis
Renal failure
Renal vasculitis

Endocrine

Pheochromocytosis
Hyperaldosteronism
Cushing's syndrome
Hyperthyroidism
Hypothyroidism (myxedema)

Other

Estrogen use
Coarctation of the aorta
Preeclampsia/eclampsia

ated with benign HTN consist of hypertrophy of the left ventricles, heart failure, and cerebral hemorrhage (stroke) due to rupture of damaged arteries in 30% of cases. The kidney has varying degree of nephrosclerosis of less serious degree. The eyes have arterial narrowing and retinal exudate.

Malignant Hypertension

Malignant HTN is an accelerated form of HTN. Approximately 5% of hypertensive individuals have a rapid increase in BP, which, if untreated, results in death within 1 to 2 years. The clinical syndrome of malignant HTN includes severe HTN with a systolic BP of higher than 200 mm Hg or a diastolic BP of higher than 150 mm Hg. Vascular changes involve accelerated arteriosclerosis that causes intimal fibrous thickening, fibroid necrosis of the vessel wall, and thrombosis that affects the kidney and abdominal viscera. The main complications consist of renal failure, encephalopathy secondary to cerebral edema and hemorrhage, retinal hemorrhages, and exudates, with or without papilledema. The individual may have a history of a normotensive state or superimposed preexisting primary or secondary HTN.

Hypertensive Crises

A *hypertensive emergency* is an elevation of BP associated with target organ damage. BP should be controlled immediately (usually within 1 hour) to reduce the morbidity and mortality risks. Hypertensive crises are seen with the following conditions: encephalopathy, intracranial hemorrhage, left ventricular hypertrophy, aortic dissection, eclampsia or severe HTN associated with pregnancy, head trauma, extensive burns, unstable angina, and acute myocardial infarction. Treatment involves reducing the mean arterial pressure by no more than 25% to 30% within 2 hours. A diastolic BP of 100 to 110 mm Hg should be reached in 2 to 6 hours. From there, the BP should be lowered to normal levels over several days. A decline in BP that is too rapid may reduce blood flow and result in ischemia to vital organs such as the brain, heart, and kidneys. Individuals with hypertensive crises should be treated with appropriate intravenous antihypertensive therapy (i.e., nitroprusside, nitroglycerin, or labetalol) while the patient is in the intensive care unit. Frequent continuous monitoring of BP should be achieved with an intra-arterial line.

Hypertensive Urgency

Hypertensive urgency is an elevation of BP without evidence of target organ damage. BP should be brought under control within 24 hours. A decline in BP that is too rapid may lead to a greater degree of morbidity. The goal of therapy is to reduce the diastolic BP to 100 to 110 mm Hg during a 24-hour period. Treatment consists of the appropriate oral antihypertensive drug (i.e., clonidine, nifedipine, captopril, or labetalol) to achieve BP control.

Special Populations
Racial and Ethnic Population

The prevalence of HTN is greater in blacks and develops with more severe complications. Also, there is a higher mortality rate for stroke, heart disease, and HTN-related end-stage renal disease than in the general population. The higher incidence of complication may be contributed to inadequate treatment or to delayed treatment after BP has been elevated a long time and target organ damage is present. Blacks with higher cardiovascular risk factors and general response to reduced salt intake can benefit greatly from lifestyle modifications. American Indians have a prevalence of HTN that is the same as or higher than that of the general population. In Hispanics, BP is approximately the same as or lower than that of non-Hispanic whites, but there is a higher prevalence of obesity and type 2 diabetes mellitus. Asian Americans have a greater overall response to most antihypertensive drugs than whites.

Women

Oral contraceptives are one cause of secondary HTN in women. Women who take oral contraceptives have two to three times higher BP levels, especially if they are obese. Once the oral contraceptive is stopped, BP returns to normal in several months. Women who are 35 years of age or older and smoke cigarettes are at greater risk for HTN and are discouraged from taking oral contraceptives.

Pregnancy

Persistent high BP present before or at the twentieth week of gestation is considered to be chronic HTN (BP >140/90 mm Hg). The treatment goal is to minimize short-term risks of elevated BP to the mother while avoiding therapy that may cause harm to the fetus. Antihypertensive therapy drugs and diuretics taken before pregnancy are recommended for except angiotensin-converting enzyme inhibitors and angiotensin II receptor blockers. Methyldopa is recommended for women diagnosed with HTN during pregnancy. Beta-blockers with methyldopa use is safer in late stage of pregnancy. *Preeclampsia* is the development of HTN during pregnancy after the twentieth week of gestation and is accompanied by proteinuria (>300 mg/24 hr), edema, or both; coagulation abnormalities; renal and liver functions that may rapidly progress to eclampsia; and the convulsive phase. It may coincide as superimposed HTN (proteinuria after the 20th week of gestation) or preexisting chronic HTN.

Hormone Replacement Therapy

Research indicates that, in general, hormonal replacement therapy does not increase BP significantly in most women with or without HTN and has shown beneficial effects on overall cardiovascular risk factor profiles. However, a small percentage of women may have a rise in BP related to estrogen therapy, and it is advisable that all women on hormonal replacement therapy have their BP measured frequently after therapy has begun.

Older Individuals

Individuals age 60 or older commonly have primary HTN. They frequently develop isolated systolic HTN: systolic BP of 140 mm Hg or greater, and diastolic BP of 90 mm Hg or lower. Isolated systolic HTN reflects arteriosclerotic rigidity of large arteries. Some older individuals may have *pseudohypertension,* which is high-cuff BP measurements due to the inability of the cuff balloon to compress the calcified brachial artery. The Sixth Report of the Joint National Committee on Prevention, Detection, Evaluation and Treatment of High Blood Pressure (JNC VI) highly recommends that individuals who develop HTN after age 60 or are resistant to treatment be evaluated for identifiable causes of HTN, such as atherosclerosis renovascular HTN and primary aldosteronism. Lifestyle modification is recommended first, followed by pharmacologic therapy adjusted for the elderly at half the dosage used in younger individuals. In older persons with isolated HTN, diuretics such as hydrochlorothiazide are preferred.

 SIGNS AND SYMPTOMS

HTN is often asymptomatic and is called the *silent killer.* An elevation in BP is the most prominent and sometimes the only sign. The JNC provides a classification of BP for adults age 18 and older who are not taking antihypertensive drugs and not acutely ill. The classifications of BP is based on the average of two or more BP readings, obtained on two or more visits after an initial screening (Table 15-4-2).

When symptomatic, patients usually complain of occipital headaches frequent on awakening, dizziness, vertigo, visual problems, chest pain, dyspnea, claudication, malaise, sweating, and tremors.

Physical assessment may reveal the following:

Cardiac: point of maximal impulse may be laterally displacement; S3 and S4 sounds may be auscultated

Vascular: decreased peripheral pulses; bruits present at femoral, abdominal, or carotid vessels; peripheral edema

Neurologic: altered mental status, focal weakness and numbness, cranial nerve palsies (numbness at extremities, weakness at extremities, eyelid weakness, diplopia, decreased visual acuity)

Funduscopic: hypertensive retinopathy (arteriolar narrowing, focal arteriolar constriction, arteriovenous crossing changes, hemorrhage and exudate, disk edema)

Neck: carotid bruits, distended veins or enlarged thyroid gland thyroid bruits, thyroid nodules

Lungs: rales and evidence of bronchospasm

Table 15-4-2. Classification Schema of Blood Pressure

BLOOD PRESSURE CLASSIFICATION	DIASTOLIC (mm Hg)	SYSTOLIC (mm Hg)
Optimal (unusually low readings should be evaluated for clinical significance)	<80	<120
Normal	<85	<130
High-normal	85–89	130–139
Hypertension stage 1	90–99	140–159
Hypertension stage 2	100–109	160–179
Hypertension stage 3	110–119	180–209

If systolic and diastolic categories are different, the higher classification should be selected. For example, the patient with a blood pressure (BP) of 160/92 mm Hg should be classified as stage 2 hypertension, and the patient with a BP of 174/120 mm Hg should be classified as stage 3. Isolated systolic hypertension is defined as a systolic BP of >140 mm Hg with a diastolic BP of <90 mm Hg and appropriate staging. For example, a BP of 170/82 mm Hg is classified as stage 2 isolated systolic hypertension.

Adapted from *The sixth report of the joint national committee on prevention, detection, evaluation and treatment of high blood pressure.* (1997). Bethesda, MD: US Department of Health and Human Services, National Heart, Lung, and Blood Institute, National Institutes of Health, Publication No. 98-4080.

Abdomen: bruits, enlarged kidneys, masses, abnormal aortic pulsation
Secondary HTN: edema, truncal obesity, striae, hyperpigmentation, numbness at extremities, muscle weakness, foot ulcers, tachycardia

 DIAGNOSTIC CRITERIA

Blood Pressure

HTN is diagnosed when the systolic BP is higher than 140 mm Hg and the diastolic BP is higher 90 mm Hg (see Table 15-4-2) in the adult on at least three separate occasions, several weeks apart.

Routine Laboratory Tests

Routine laboratory tests are used to evaluate an individual's risk factors and the presence of target organ disease.
Renal studies: urinalysis, blood urea nitrogen, and creatinine values to determine renal involvement
Complete blood cell count: used to assess undiagnosed anemia, leukopenia, neutropenia, and polycythemia
Blood chemistry: potassium and sodium assessed for electrolyte imbalances; fasting glucose to identify the presence of diabetes mellitus
Serum lipid profile: fasting lipids, total cholesterol, high-density lipoprotein cholesterol, low-density cholesterol, and triglycerides used to assess for arthrogenetic risk factors

12-Lead Electrocardiography

The 12-lead electrocardiogram is used to determine whether the individual has myocardial ischemia, myocardial infarction, or hyperkalemia.

Optional Tests

Some optional tests are used to determine an individual's risk factor profile and comorbidities.
Limited echocardiography: to determine the presence of left ventricular hypertrophy
Renal testing: CT scan of adrenal glands; used to diagnose pheochromocytoma or adrenal tumors

 INTERVENTIONS

The major goal of the prevention and management of HTN is to reduce morbidity and mortality risks by the least intrusive method. The general approach of therapy is to reduce BP to less than 140/90 mm Hg. For essential HTN therapy, the main approach is to institute lifestyle modifications without or, if necessary, with antihypertensive drugs. The approach for secondary HTN is to identify and correct the underlying cause. The goal for both essential and secondary HTN is a normotensive state.

Clinical Evaluation

The evaluation of individuals with HTN encompasses three major objectives: (1) to identify known causes of high BP, (2) to assess the presence or absence of target organ disease or cardiovascular disease (see later), including the extent of disease and response to treatment, and (3) identify other cardiovascular risk factors or concomitant disorders that may define prognosis and guide treatment.

The medical history should include the following:

- Duration and levels of elevated BP history or symptoms of congestive heart disease, heart failure, cerebrovascular disease, PVD, renal disease, diabetes mellitus, dyslipidemia, other comorbid conditions, gout, or sexual dysfunction
- Family history of high BP, premature congestive heart disease, stroke, diabetes, dyslipidemia, or renal disease
- Symptoms suggesting causes of HTN
- History of recent change in weight, level of physical activity, and smoking or other tobacco use
- Dietary assessment—intake of sodium, alcohol, saturated fat, and caffeine
- History of prescribed and over-the-counter medications, herbal remedies, or illicit drugs that may raise or interfere with effective hypertensive drugs
- Results and adverse effects of previous antihypertensive therapy
- Psychosocial and environmental factors (e.g., family situation, employment status and working conditions, educational level) that may influence HTN control

Blood Pressure Assessment

Initial BP measurements on at least two subsequent visits after 5 minutes of rest and 30 minutes after smoking or ingestion of caffeine. Two or more BP measurements 2 minutes apart with the individual supine or seated and after standing for at least 2 minutes. Verification in the both arms (if values are different, the higher value should be used). Use appropriate BP cuff size (80% encircled around bare arm) and validated BP device. Obtain additional BP readings and take the average BP if the first two BP measurements differ by greater than 5 mm Hg.

Management by Risk for Cardiovascular Complications

Management for HTN should be individualized according to degree of BP elevation and stage, target organ disease, and clinical cardiovascular disease (Table 15-4-3).

Major risk factors: smoking, dyslipidemia, diabetes mellitus, age older than 60, men and postmenopausal women, men younger than 55 and women older than 65 with family history of cardiovascular disease

Target organ damage (TOD)/clinical cardiovascular disease (CCD): heart diseases, left ventricular hypertrophy, angina, or prior myocardial infarction; heart failure; stroke or transient ischemic attack; nephropathy; peripheral arterial disease; retinopathy

Once placed in the appropriate risk group for the appropriate BP stage, then specific treatment such as nonpharmacologic therapy (lifestyle modifications) and pharmacologic therapy (e.g., diuretics, angiotensin-converting enzyme inhibitors, beta-blockers) can be provided to achieve goal BP.

Goal BP consists of three categories:

- Risk group A (HTN with uncomplicated HTN): goal of less than 140/90 mm Hg

Table 15-4-3. Risk Stratification and Treatment

BLOOD PRESSURE STAGE (mm Hg)	RISK GROUP A (NO RISK FACTORS; NO TOD/CCD)	RISK GROUP B (AT LEAST 1 RISK FACTOR, NOT INCLUDING DIABETES; NO TOD/CCD)	RISK GROUP C (TOD/CCD AND/OR DIABETES, WITH OR WITHOUT OTHER RISK FACTORS)
High-normal (130–139/85–89)	Lifestyle modification	Lifestyle modification*	Drug therapy‡
Stage 1 (140–159/90–99)	Lifestyle modification (up to 12 months)	Lifestyle modification† (up to 6 months)	Drug therapy
Stages 2 and 3 (≥160/≥100)	Drug therapy	Drug therapy	Drug therapy

For example, a patient with diabetes and a blood pressure of 142/94 mm Hg plus left ventricular hypertrophy should be classified as having stage 1 hypertension with target organ disease (left ventricular hypertrophy) and with another major risk factor (diabetes). This patient would be categorized as stage 1, risk group C, and recommended for immediate initiating of pharmacologic treatment.

*Lifestyle modification should be adjunctive therapy for all patients recommended for pharmacologic therapy.

†For patients with multiple risk factors, clinicians should consider drugs as initial therapy plus lifestyle modifications.

‡For those with heart failure, renal insufficiency, or diabetes.

TOD/CCD, target organ disease/clinical cardiovascular disease.

Adapted from *The sixth report of the joint national committee on prevention, detection, evaluation and treatment of high blood pressure.* (1997). Bethesda, MD: US Department of Health and Human Services, National Heart, Lung, and Blood Institute, National Institutes of Health, Publication No. 98-4080.

- Risk group B (HTN with diabetes, renal failure, and heart failure): goal of less than 130/85 mm Hg
- Risk group C (HTN with renal failure with proteinuria greater than 1 g/24 hr): goal of less than 125/75 mm Hg

Nonpharmacologic Therapy

Nonpharmacologic therapy, such as lifestyle modifications, has been shown to be beneficial for the prevention and management of HTN. It has been shown to prevent or delay elevation of BP in individuals at risk or individuals who have high BP. Lifestyle modifications include the following:

Smoking Cessation. The patient should quit smoking to reduce cardiovascular risk.

Weight Reduction. Obesity increases BP. All individuals with HTN who are above desirable weight should be placed on a monitored weight reduction program, caloric restriction, and increased physical activity as part of their lifestyle modification.

Physical Activity. A physical exercise program is recommended to assist with weight loss and maintenance, improve functional health status, and reduce the risk of cardiovascular disease. BP can be reduced with moderate intense physical activity (40% to 60% of maximum oxygen consumption), such as 30 to 45 minutes of brisk walking at least three times a week.

Alcohol Consumption. Alcohol can elevate resistance to antihypertensive drugs and increase risk factors for high BP. The health care provider should obtain a detailed history of individuals who consume alcohol. To not raise BP, alcohol consumption should be limited to a maximum of 1 oz/day (equivalent to 2 oz of 100-proof whiskey, 8 oz of wine, or 24 oz of beer).

Dietary Intake. A reduction or restriction in salt may reduce the need for antihypertensive agents and reduce potassium loss if diuretics are administered. The maximum amount of sodium or sodium chloride should be 100 mmol/day (2.4 g of sodium or 6 g of sodium chloride). Potassium intake should be approximately 90 mmol/day. Dietary intake of calcium and magnesium is necessary for general health maintenance. Increased calcium has been shown to reduce BP in pregnant women. Reduced dietary fats and cholesterol intake should be maintained for general health status.

Included in the National Institutes of Health recommendations is the Dietary Approaches to Stop Hypertension (DASH) diet. The DASH diet is part of a clinical study funded by the National Heart, Lung, and Blood Institute. This is a combination diet that is rich in fruits, vegetables, and low-fat dairy foods and low in saturated and total fat. The DASH diet is based on the consumption of 2000 calories a day and has shown to lower BP.

Pharmacologic Therapy

Although lifestyle modifications are to begin for all patients, some may require pharmacologic therapy. Pharmacologic therapy is needed immediately for patients with stage 2 or 3 HTN. Pharmacologic therapy usually begins with low doses of diuretics or beta-blockers (see Chapter 12, Section 4 for the care and administration of the various antihypertensive medications).

BP should be monitored every 5 to 15 minutes or more frequently when intravenous antihypertensive medications are administered. For initial oral antihypertensive medications, evaluate BP every hour for 2 hours; frequency may decrease if the BP stabilizes. If BP remains elevated, continue to check 1 hour after every medication dose is administered.

Monitor mean arterial pressures. A pressure of more than 140 mm Hg may cause vascular alterations, resulting in sensory motor deficits. The goal is to achieve a mean arterial pressure of 70 to 110 mm Hg.

- Closely assess for hypotension.
- Assess for alterations in tissue perfusion.
- Assess neurologic status for focal deficits. These checks should be performed hourly during periods of crisis and initially after the initiation of drug therapy.
- Monitor the rate, rhythm, and character of peripheral and apical pulses to detect adverse effects on the myocardium and blood vessels.
- Assess renal status for evidence of decreasing renal perfusion. Intake and output should be closely monitored, as well as daily weight. Notify physician if urine output decreases to less than 0.5 mL/kg for 2 consecutive hours. Report weight gains of more than 1 kg (2.2 lb) in 24 hours. Also monitor serum blood urea nitrogen and creatinine levels (see Chapter 11, Section 5).

 COMMUNITY CARE

Clinical evaluation, medical history, and diagnosis are obtained as described earlier. Table 15-4-4 provides recommendation for follow-up based on initial BP measurements in accordance with the blood classification categories. All nonpharmacologic recommendations should be taught and reviewed.

Diet Therapy. Instruct the patient to read labels to identify hidden sources

Table 15-4-4. Follow-up Recommendations

INITIAL BLOOD PRESSURE		RECOMMENDED FOLLOW-UP
SYSTOLIC	DIASTOLIC	
<130	<85	Recheck in 2 years
130–139	85–89	Recommend lifestyle modifications and recheck in 1 year or less depending on evidence of cardiovascular risk and target organ damage
140–149	90–99	Recommend lifestyle modifications and confirm in 2 months or less
160–179	100–109	Clinically evaluate or refer to source of care within 1 month
≥180	≥110	Clinically evaluate or refer to source of care within 1 week

If systolic and diastolic categories are different, follow recommendations for the shorter time follow-up (e.g., 160/86 mm Hg indicates clinical evaluation or referral to a source of care within 1 month).

Adapted from *The sixth report of the joint national committee on prevention, detection, evaluation and treatment of high blood pressure.* (1997). Bethesda, MD: US Department of Health and Human Services, National Heart, Lung, and Blood Institute, National Institutes of Health, Publication No. 98-4080.

of additional sodium. Cholesterol and calorie sources should also be identified and reduced. The amount of meat on the plate should be no larger than the size of a deck of cards. Referral to a nutritionist may be necessary, especially to achieve weight reduction in overweight persons.

Physical Exercise. Identify exercise that fits the patient's lifestyle to ensure compliance. Walking, stretching while sitting, and water aerobics are some methods that may be helpful.

Medically supervised physical exercise programs (e.g., hospital-affiliated exercise programs) may be required for patients with heart disease.

Home Blood Pressure Monitoring. BP measurements should be obtained on a weekly basis at a regular time. Such measurements are helpful in monitoring true pressure changes, because they are obtained when the patient is more relaxed. Patients should report their readings on each visit to the health care provider. Review equipment and the correct use of the device.

Support. Patient and family members should be linked to the National Heart, Lung, and Blood Institute Information Center for current literature about the prevention of high BP and high blood cholesterol (800-575-WELL).

 PROGNOSIS

The prevention and treatment of HTN continue to represent a major health problem in the United States. HTN had declined from the 1970s to the 1990s with improved awareness, prevention, and treatment. During that time, the decline in HTN contributed to dramatic reductions in morbidity and mortality rates attributable to HTN. However, JNC VI noted that HTN awareness, treatment, and control rates have decreased since the JNC V report. Age-adjusted mortality rates for stroke and coronary heart disease that once were declining are now at a level plateau. Rates for end-stage renal disease and heart failure are rising.

 CLINICAL PEARLS

○ Obtain BP after a 5-minute rest with the appropriate size cuff and a calibrated or validated BP device.

- Set a clear goal of therapy based on the individual's risk. Control BP to below 140/90 mm Hg for those with uncomplicated HTN, 130/85 mm Hg for those with diabetes, and 125/75 mm Hg for those with renal insufficiency with proteinuria of greater than 1 g/24 hr.
- Educate individuals about HTN, and involve them in measurement and treatment.

NURSING PROBLEM/ DIAGNOSIS	NURSING INTERVENTIONS CLASSIFICATION (NIC)
Patient identification	Health screening
	Risk identification
Achievement of goal pressures	Self-modification assistance
	Cardiac precautions
	Teaching prescribed medication
	Exercise promotion
	Nutrition management
Prevention of target organ damage and cardiovascular disease/Effective therapeutic regimen management	Teaching disease process
	Smoking cessation assistance
	Self-responsibility facilitation
	Support system enhancement

Hypovolemic Shock

Section 5   Debra Pettack ■ Beverly George-Gay

 OVERVIEW

Hypovolemic shock occurs when there is insufficient circulating fluid volume in the vascular space to maintain adequate tissue perfusion. Intravascular volume depletion may be caused by internal or external blood loss or by fluid shifting out of the vascular space and into other fluid compartments (Table 15-5-1). Severity depends on the amount and rate at which the volume is lost, as well as on the patient's age and preexisting conditions.

 PATHOPHYSIOLOGY

The reduction in intravascular volume results in decreased venous return to the right side of the heart. Right and left ventricular filling pressures are reduced, decreasing stroke volume and cardiac output. As cardiac output diminishes, BP and tissues perfusion decrease. Consequently, oxygen and nutrients are poorly circulated at the tissue level, impairing cell function and leading to cell death.

Stages of Shock

1. **Initial stage:** Subtle changes may be occurring at the tissue level due to poor tissue perfusion. However, few clinical signs and symptoms are noted during this stage outside of a slight increase in heart rate.
2. **Compensatory stage:** This stage correlates with a total blood volume loss of 15% to 30%. The reduction in cardiac output that accompanies this stage initiates a set of compensatory responses.

▨ **Table 15-5-1.** Causes of Hypovolemic Shock

External Losses	
External hemorrhage (hemorrhagic shock)	Loss of whole blood due to trauma, surgical procedures, or coagulopathies. The most common cause of hypovolemic shock. Its severity may be classified according to the amount of blood lost.
Gastrointestinal losses	Gastrointestinal losses can occur from nasogastric suctioning, vomiting, diarrhea, ostomies, fistulas, or a reduction in oral intake (dehydration).
Renal losses	Excessive diuresis from diuretic administration, diabetes insipidus, Addison's disease, or osmotic diuresis from hyperglycemia.
Skin losses	These losses can occur from diaphoresis without adequate replacement, exudative lesions, or burn injuries.
Internal Losses	
Internal hemorrhage	This may occur in patients with hemothorax (as much as 3 L of blood can be sequestered in the pleural cavity), ruptured spleen or liver, fracture, and lacerations of great vessels.
Movement of intravascular fluid to interstitial space ("third spacing")	This is seen in patients with bacteremia, allergic reactions, thermal injuries, ascites, and generalized edema.

Neural Compensation. Baroreceptors and chemoreceptors on the carotid sinus and aortic arch detect the reduced cardiac output and send messages to the vasomotor center of the medulla, stimulating a sympathetic nervous system response. The sympathetic nervous system releases two catecholamines, epinephrine and norepinephrine, which increase heart rate and contractility; improve BP by causing arterial vasoconstriction and shunting blood from the kidneys, gastrointestinal tract, and skin to the heart and brain; augment venous return via venous vasoconstriction; and improve oxygenation by increasing respiratory rate and depth and relaxing bronchial smooth muscle.

Hormonal Compensation. Stimulation by the sympathetic nervous system in response to hypotension leads to the release of adrenocorticotropic hormone (ACTH), which causes glucocorticoids and mineralocorticoids to be produced. Glucocorticoids cause glycogen to be changed into glucose (glycogenolysis), thereby increasing blood glucose levels for energy. Mineralocorticoids increase intravascular volume by causing water to be reabsorbed in the renal tubules. The renin-angiotensin-aldosterone system is a part of hormonal compensation that is triggered by decreased renal blood flow. Renin is released from the juxtaglomerular apparatus in the kidneys in response to decreased renal perfusion. Renin reacts with angiotensin to produce angiotensin I, which forms angiotensin II as it circulates through the lungs. Angiotensin II is a potent vasoconstrictor that increases BP and improves venous return. Aldosterone and antidiuretic hormone are also released as a result of renin release. Both of these hormones cause the retention of sodium and water in an attempt to increase intravascular volume.

Chemical Compensation. Chemical compensation occurs as a result of the increased rate and depth of ventilation (hyperventilation) from sympathetic nervous system stimulation and leads to the development of a respiratory alkalosis. The loss of carbon dioxide due to hyperventilation causes vasoconstriction of cerebral blood vessels. This vasoconstriction coupled with already existing poor oxygenation leads to cerebral ischemia with resultant decreased level of consciousness, agitation, confusion, restlessness, or lethargy.

3. **Progressive stage:** This stage coincides with a 30% to 40% loss of volume as well as the loss of compensatory mechanisms and severe hypoperfusion ensues. Cells convert to anaerobic metabolism, and metabolic acidosis develops. In addition, capillary permeability increases as a result of histamine release, causing further deletion of intravascular volume. Blood thus becomes more viscous, and sludging occurs. Blood flow may be further impaired by alterations in coagulation. This phase is a vicious cycle that responds poorly to fluid replacement.

4. **Refractory (irreversible) stage:** During this stage, cell death is irreparable, and death is imminent. Severe acidosis and organ failure ensue as a result of inadequate tissue perfusion.

The American College of Surgeons Committee on Trauma has classified fluid and blood loss by volume that can be correlated to four stages:

Class I: blood loss of less than 750 mL or less than 15% of total blood volume

Class II: blood loss of 750 to 1500 mL or 15% to 30% of total blood volume

Class III: blood loss of 1500 to 2000 mL or 30% to 40% of total blood volume

Class IV: blood loss of more than 2000 mL or >40% of total blood volume

 ## SIGNS AND SYMPTOMS

Signs and symptoms vary according to the cause and stage of the shock (Table 15-5-2). Pulse, respiratory rate, and resting heart rate increase. Patients on beta-blockers are not able to mount a compensatory response and will not become tachycardic. Compensatory mechanisms prevent a significant drop in systolic BP until 30% of blood volume is lost, so hypotension is not an early sign of hypovolemia. Skin perfusion and urinary output decrease. Neck veins are nondistended. Eyeballs appear sunken. Dysrhythmias, mainly premature ventricular contractions, may be frequently noted, especially if there is underlying coronary artery disease.

Palpation of specific pulses can give an estimation of systolic BP. The presence of a palpable radial pulse indicates a systolic BP of at least 80 mm Hg; loss of a palpable radial pulse indicates the systolic BP has fallen below 80 mm Hg. A palpable femoral with the loss of the radial pulse indicates a systolic BP of approximately 70 mm Hg. A palpable carotid pulse with the loss of the radial and femoral pulse indicates a systolic BP of 60 mm Hg.

 ## DIAGNOSTIC CRITERIA

- A complete blood cell count identifies decreasing hemoglobin and hematocrit (see Chapter 11, Section 1). Hematocrit may increase falsely as the total volume of red blood cells appears to increase when plasma volume is lost, as seen in fluid shifting.
- Prothrombin and activated partial thromboplastin times should be monitored for prolongation, which may identify a coagulopathy.
- Arterial blood gas identifies decreased oxygen saturation and hypoxemia as perfusion to the tissues decreases.

Table 15-5-2. Signs and Symptoms Associated with Hypovolemic Shock

SIGNS AND SYMPTOMS	INITIAL STAGE	COMPENSATORY STAGE	PROGRESSIVE STAGE	REFRACTORY STAGE
Level of consciousness	Normal or slight restlessness	Restlessness, slight anxiety	Confusion, agitation	Unresponsive
Blood pressure	Normal, systolic blood pressure may be slightly elevated	Normal or systolic blood pressure may be slightly low, diastolic blood pressure slightly elevated	Decreased systolic and diastolic blood pressure	Severe hypotension
Heart rate	May be slightly increased (>100 beats/min)	Increased (>100 beats/min)	Increased (>120 beats/min)	Decreased
Respiratory rate	Normal rate, normal PaO_2	Increased rate (>20/min), decreased PaO_2, decreased $PaCO_2$	Increased and shallow, decreased PaO_2, decreased $PaCO_2$	Decreased and shallow
Skin	Normal, dry mucous membranes	Cool, clammy	Mottled	Cold pale, may be cyanotic
Peripheral pulses	Normal, capillary refill may be slightly delayed	Weak, thready Capillary refill >3 seconds	Weak, thready, and possibly absent	Weak, thready, and frequently absent
Urine output	Normal	Concentrated, <30 mL/hr	Scant (<20 mL/hr)	Scant to none
Pulse pressure	Normal (30–40 mm Hg)	Narrowed due to the rise in diastolic blood pressure	Narrowed	May be absent due to immeasurable lost diastolic blood pressure

- Serum electrolytes should be monitored. Depletions in potassium and sodium usually accompany gastrointestinal and renal fluid losses.
- Blood urea nitrogen and creatinine levels are altered. Blood urea nitrogen increases in response to less fluid and more solute in the blood in the case of plasma volume loss; creatinine is normal, so a ratio of blood urea nitrogen to creatinine will be more than 20 (see Chapter 11, Section 5). Creatinine will eventually raise as the kidneys become ischemic from decreased perfusion that occurs in the later stages.
- Imaging studies may be needed to assist in identifying the source of blood loss.
- Diagnostic peritoneal lavage may be performed in the unstable patient with possible abdominal injury to identify hemorrhage.

INTERVENTIONS

Management of hypovolemic shock includes locating and controlling the source of fluid loss and simultaneously restoring effective circulating volume. Management should be aimed at restoring and maintaining a systolic BP of 100 mm Hg or greater, hematocrit of 25% or greater, and a urine output of more than 50 mL/hr.

Oxygenation and Ventilation

Establishing and maintaining a patent airway with supplemental oxygen are of prime importance to increase oxygenation, thus combating tissue hypoxia and eventual cell death. Oral or nasopharyngeal airways and intubation and mechanical ventilation may be necessary. The goal should be to maintain a PaO_2 of more than 80 mm Hg. Monitor oxygen saturation and maintain an SaO_2 of more than 92%.

Blood Pressure Monitoring

BP monitoring by arterial line is preferred because vasoconstriction may alter auscultated cuff pressure sounds. Doppler devices are helpful. Mean arterial pressure should also be assessed; a pressure of 60 mm Hg or less indicates inadequate tissue perfusion and must be avoided.

Pulses

Carotid, radial, femoral, dorsalis pedis, and posterior tibial peripheral pulses should be assessed for rate, rhythm, quality, and character. Refer to signs and symptoms with correlation to BP.

Fluid Therapy and Volume Expansion

Fluid therapy is the mainstay of management for hypovolemic shock. Central venous access with a multilumen catheter is preferred for adequate volume replacement. If central access is not available, large-bore peripheral intravenous catheters of 16 or 18 gauge should be inserted. Smaller catheters may be needed if the patient is significantly vasoconstricted. Isotonic crystalloid therapy can be used initially, and blood and blood products are necessary for hemorrhage.

Crystalloids are readily available and inexpensive. However, they move freely from the intravascular space to the interstitial space. To maintain adequate intravascular volume, for every liter of blood loss, 3 L of crystalloid replacement is necessary. Lactated Ringer's solution and 0.9% normal saline are the crystalloid solutions of choice for hypovolemic shock. *Lactated Ringer's* solution is an isotonic solution that contains normal saline, potassium, calcium, and sodium lactate buffers (sodium lactate buffers are converted to bicarbonate in the liver), which help to maintain electrolyte balance and buffer acidosis. *Normal saline* (0.9%) also is isotonic but provides no electrolyte or bicarbonate protection. *Hypertonic saline* solutions such as 3%, 5%, or 7% saline exert a high osmotic pressure, causing extravascular fluid to be drawn into the intravascular space. Hypernatremia is a potential complication of this therapy. It is important to monitor closely for volume overload (pulmonary crackles, distended neck veins, and bounding pulses).

Colloids are solutions that contain large proteins or starches that increase intravascular osmotic pressure, thus keeping fluid in the intravascular space. Because colloids remain in the intravascular space longer than crystalloid, one third less volume of colloids is required. However, pulmonary edema and volume overload are potential complications. *Albumin* and *plasma protein fraction (Plasmanate)* are naturally occurring colloids but do not require type and cross-matching. These are preferred when volume loss is caused by loss of plasma rather than of blood, as in the case with burns or peritonitis. *Dextran* is a synthetic colloid that is used less frequently because it interferes with blood typing and clotting. Allergic reactions and renal damage are also associated with dextran. *Hetastarch,* which is also a synthetic colloid, carries the least risk for pulmonary edema. Clotting abnormalities may occur.

For **blood and blood product administration,** see Table 2-3-3.

Hypothermia should be avoided because it increases oxygen demand while decreasing oxygen binding capacity. It can contribute to the development of dysrhythmias and coagulopathies. Warm intravenous fluids with appropriate warmers before administration keep the patient appropriately covered.

Urine output should be closely monitored hourly with a urine meter. Urethral catheterization is contraindicated for patients with suspected urethral injury.

Pharmacologic Therapy

The primary treatment for hypovolemic shock is fluid therapy, but pharmacologic therapy may be needed, especially in the later stages.

Vasopressors such as epinephrine and norepinephrine cause vasoconstriction and increase venous return. These are used mainly with other types of shock (e.g., septic anaphylactic or neurogenic).

Dopamine may be administered at low dose (<5 μg/kg/min) to support renal blood flow. As renal blood flow is reduced owing to the shunting of blood to the vital organs, the risk of renal failure becomes high. Dopamine at low doses, often called "renal dose dopamine," may protect the kidneys from the complication of failure by dilating the renal arteries, thus enhancing flow. At 5 to 10 μg/kg/min, dopamine may be used to increase cardiac contractility, and at more than 10 μg/kg/min, dopamine can be used for vasoconstriction.

Sodium bicarbonate is used to treat severe acidosis with a pH less than 7.10. The pH should be monitored closely and therapy stopped once the pH reaches 7.25 to prevent rebound alkalosis.

Mechanical Therapy
Lower Extremity Elevation

Lower extremities should be elevated only slightly. Trendelenburg position should be avoided because it restricts diaphragmatic movement and may decrease BP even further by erroneously indicating to the baroreceptors that volume is available.

Pneumatic Antishock Garment/Military Antishock Trouser

The pneumatic antishock garment (PASG, or military antishock trousers [MAST]) is used in the treatment of hypovolemic shock associated with traumatic injury. It increases arterial pressure by compressing the vascular beds of the abdomen and lower extremities. It also acts as a tamponading device to stop bleeding and provides a splinting action for fractures. PASG use has diminished because it has not been shown to improve survival. Close cardiopulmonary, peripheral pulse, and device monitoring is essential to avoid complications.

 ## COMMUNITY CARE

Community care centers around initial assessment of the patient's airway, breathing, and circulation. Immobilization may be necessary if trauma is involved. Direct pressure can be applied to external sources of blood loss. Intravenous access and fluid resuscitation can be started with crystalloids for mild volume depletion. For severe volume depletion or if hemorrhagic shock is suspected, measures to transport the patient to the hospital should be taken.

 ## PROGNOSIS

The prognosis of hypovolemic shock depends on the stage of the shock state and the body's response to its compensatory mechanisms. It is usually good if identified in early stages. If compensatory mechanisms fail or treatment is not initiated, organ, tissue, and cellular ischemia ensues.

 ## CLINICAL PEARLS

○ A common error in the management of hypovolemic shock is failure to recognize it in its early stages, which are the signs of decreased peripheral perfusion.

○ Hypotension is *not* an early indication of shock; it is a late finding that occurs once compensatory mechanisms begin to fail.

○ Warm intravenous fluids whenever possible for use in fluid replacement.

○ If it is not possible to use type-specific blood, type O Rh-negative blood should be given to females of childbearing age. This will avoid sensitization and future complications with the Rh factor.

NURSING PROBLEM/ DIAGNOSIS	NURSING INTERVENTIONS CLASSIFICATION (NIC)
Diminished intravascular volume/Deficient fluid volume	Hypovolemic management Fluid resuscitation Shock management: volume
Ineffective tissue perfusion	Oxygen therapy Circulatory care Neurologic monitoring

Peripheral Vascular Disease

Section 6   Patricia Revolinski

 OVERVIEW

PVD is a progressive occlusive disease of the blood vessels outside of the heart. PVD includes blood vessel abnormalities that affect arteries, veins, or the lymph system, either singularly or in combination. It is usually a degenerative disorder, with more cases being identified as life expectancy increases. PVD manifests in a number of diseases (Table 15-6-1), which are discussed separately. However, the resultant sequela, ischemia, produces similar findings.

 PATHOPHYSIOLOGY

The function of the circulatory system is to transport nutrients, oxygen, electrolytes, and hormones to tissues, as well as to transport metabolic waste products away from tissues via the blood flow. Anything that impedes the transport of blood will result in damage to the tissue (ischemia) and diminished organ function and may progress to total loss of function.

Peripheral arterial disease is a chronic condition in which the lower extremities are deprived of nutrients due to arterial occlusion, either partial or total. It presents after the fifth decade of life and is prevalent in approximately 10% of persons older than age 70. Symptomatic disease is noted in approximately 1% to 2% of the adult population. A large number of patients with peripheral arterial disease also have carotid artery stenosis or coronary artery stenosis; some have both. The most significant risk factor is smoking; other factors include diabetes mellitus, HTN, and hyperlipidemia. The most common cause of impedance of blood flow in arteries is arteriosclerosis, and it most commonly manifests as atherosclerosis (see Chapter 14, Section 4).

Peripheral venous disease is the result of loss of patency of venous flow or incompetent valves. The most common manifestations of PVD in the venous system are DVT and varicose veins (see Chapter 15, Sections 3 and 9, respectively).

 SIGNS AND SYMPTOMS
Pain

This is the most frequent complaint and is more severe in arterial disease. The type and location of pain help to distinguish between arterial and venous

Table 15-6-1.   Peripheral Vascular Diseases

Arterial disease
   Atherosclerosis
   Thromboangiitis obliterans (Buerger's disease)
   Raynaud's syndrome
   Aneurysm
   Arteriovenous fistulas
   Arteritis
Venous disease
   Thrombophlebitis
   Venous stasis ulcers
   Varicose veins
   Pulmonary embolism

involvement. A sudden onset of severe pain is indicative of an acute arterial occlusion. The patient may report a sharp cramp-like pain, followed by weakness of the affected limb. The patient may report that he or she had to sit down, or fell down, as a result of the interruption of blood flow to the area.

Another type of pain characteristic of arterial involvement is *intermittent claudication,* which is pain that appears, usually in the calf, during exercise. The patient will report a cramping in the affected leg during some type of exercise and obtains relief only after resting the extremity. The pain is due to the muscle not receiving adequate oxygenation during the activity. Intermittent claudication is not a good index of the severity of the disease, because often the collateral circulation function to supply oxygen as long as it can and as such masks the disorder. The absence of intermittent claudication does not automatically rule out peripheral arterial disease. Patients may have limited walking as an accommodation to the disease, and as a result, they do not walk far enough to produce the ischemia.

Ischemic rest pain is another symptom that may indicate peripheral arterial disease. It usually occurs during sleep, affects the foot, and awakens the patient. It is a result of decreased perfusion to the tissues and is relieved only by the patient's movement of the extremity to increase perfusion.

Pain is rarely present in PVD of a venous origin, but if it is present, it is usually deep muscle pain. This pain is usually precipitated by standing for a long period and can be relieved by elevation of the affected limb. Homan's sign can be used to assess for DVT. The examiner extends the affected leg, places a hand on the knee, and places the other hand on the sole of the foot. The foot is then dorsiflexed. It the patient reports pain in the calf, this may indicate the presence of a DVT.

Edema

Edema is most frequently seen with venous involvement, although mild edema may accompany arterial disease. It is usually caused by venous stasis or orthostatic increases in hydrostatic changes resulting from prolonged sitting or standing. The edema associated with PVD in the venous system usually does not pit easily, and when the disease is chronic, the skin can become brawny and result in skin changes. These changes are due to the breakdown of extravasated red blood cells. This breakdown, along with increased interstitial fibrin, results in subcutaneous tissue inflammation and fibrosis. The lower legs and ankles are affected more often than the feet. Edema can also be present when there is lymph system involvement.

Skin Temperature

Cool skin may result from peripheral vasoconstriction in arterial occlusion due to diminished oxygen supply. Warmth over an area of the skin may reflect local inflammation, such as occurs in thrombophlebitis. In venous involvement, the skin is usually warm but may be cool to touch when edema is involved.

Skin Color

A bluish discoloration, or *cyanosis,* results from insufficient oxygenation. Rubor, a reddish-brown discoloration, is noted when the leg is in the dependent position, may be used to locate the damaged or dilated vessel in an arterial occlusion.

Skin Turgor

The skin may be dry and brittle if the decreased perfusion has been present for a long time. It may also have the appearance of being thin and shiny.

Skin Integrity

There may be ulcerations of the skin on the affected limb. An ischemic ulcer results from decrease in arterial perfusion. They manifest early with irregular edges and then progress until they form a crater-like appearance. They are very painful and deep. The base is usually black and may be gangrenous. This ulcer is usually found distal to the occlusion. Common sites include the tip of toes, toe webs, and heels.

Stasis ulcers, resulting from venous disruption, develop on the lower third of the leg, most often on the ankle—more specifically, the medial malleolus. They have a shallow, irregular shape with granulation tissue at the base. These are much less painful than arterial ulcers.

Nails and Hair

Nails may be brittle due to the lack of perfusion. This occurs after the condition has been present for a while. There may be loss of hair over the affected area.

Pulses

Pulses are rarely affected by venous disease, so it is usually a sign of arterial involvement if there is a change in the characteristic of the pulse. Pulses may be diminished, weak, or absent, depending on the degree of occlusion. The pulse is usually diminished distal to the occlusion. Pulses are graded on a scale of 0 to 4.

Muscles

The affected limb may be smaller owing to atrophy.

 # DIAGNOSTIC CRITERIA
Doppler Ultrasonography

Ultrasound waves are reflected back to the skin from vessels as a probe is passed over the skin. The patency of the vessel can be determined, and blood flow can be observed. It is used to determine whether there is an impedance in the movement of blood through the vessel.

Angiography

Contrast medium is injected into a blood vessel, allowing visualization of the circulatory system. The arteries are examined by arteriography, which involves injection of the medium into an artery. When a venogram is obtained, the contrast medium is injected into a large vein, usually an antecubital vein.

Digital Subtraction Angiography

This study allows direct arterial visualization without an arterial puncture. A peripheral vein is injected with contrast medium, and serial images are taken via a fluoroscope. A computer subtracts early images from later ones, removing all structures except the blood-filled arteries.

Magnetic Resonance Imaging

MRI is a minimally invasive technique that studies blood flow. The magnetic field aligns the charges on the blood components. As the components move along, they emit measurable radiofrequency signals. These signals are detected and recorded.

Segmental Plethysmography

This noninvasive test detects changes in blood flow through limbs by using BP cuffs and recording waveforms as the pressure is released. Alterations in waves gauge the severity of the disease.

Exercise Testing

Ischemia is measured by the exercise-induced claudication. True claudication is exhibited consistently by the same degree of exercise.

Ankle-Brachial Index

BP is measured at the ankle, using posterior tibial or dorsalis pedis pulse, and at the brachial artery. The ankle pressure value is then divided by the brachial artery pressure value. Resting pain will manifest with a value of less than 0.3; the normal value is more than 1.0. The ABI helps to determine the degree of ischemia.

 INTERVENTIONS

Assessment

1. Assess risk factors such as smoking, HTN, diabetes mellitus, hypercholesterolemia, hyperlipidemia, obesity, and family history.
2. Assess claudication using the pain scale of 0 to 10 to describe the severity, and administer analgesics as needed.
3. Palpate pulses to determine degree of arterial involvement.
4. Auscultate the aorta, iliac, and femoral arteries for bruits.
5. Inspect the extremities for size and symmetry, hair distribution, presence of edema, ulcerations, and skin color and temperature.
6. For to assess the upper extremities, the Allen test can be performed to measure patency of the palmar arch.

Lifestyle Changes

1. The patient should stop smoking.
2. If the patient is obese, he or she should lose weight.
3. Advise the patient to decrease saturated fat and cholesterol dietary intake.
4. Exercise that promotes emptying and filling of blood vessels, such as a walking program, should be increased.
5. Extremities must be kept warm to promote blood flow and hot water bottles and heating pads should not be used because they may cause burns. The decreased sensation in the affected limbs will increase the risk that a burn may occur. Checking the temperature of the water with a thermometer can reduce the risk of injury.
6. The patient should keep skin clean and dry and seek treatment for breaks in the skin or signs of ulcer formation.

Medical Management

1. BP is controlled to prevent further vascular damage. This is usually done through the use of thiazide diuretics.
2. Mild analgesics may be prescribed.
3. Pentoxifylline at 400 mg is taken orally three times daily to reduce claudication. It increases circulation and oxygen delivery by decreasing blood viscosity, increasing the flexibility of the erythrocytes, and preventing aggregation of red blood cells and platelets. It also has been shown to be effective in healing ulcerations.
4. Platelet inhibitors can decrease the complications of atherosclerosis.
5. Vasodilators, such as papaverine hydrochloride, can be used, although this is a controversial treatment that has not been proved to be useful.
6. Lipid-lowering agents, commonly referred to as statin drugs (lovastatin, pravastatin, simvastatin, atorvastatin), reduce serum cholesterol.
7. Thrombolytic agents, such as streptokinase, urokinase, and rtPA, reestablish blood flow after clot formation.
8. Anticoagulants, such as heparin and warfarin, prevent clot formation.
9. Medications should be administered to control diabetes.

Surgical Management

1. Bypass graft surgery restores blood flow via autologous vein or synthetic graft. This is usually reserved for patients with severe resting pain, persistent ulcerations, and gangrene.
2. Percutaneous transluminal balloon angioplasty compresses plaque in the arteries and increases blood flow in the presence of focal arterial obstruction.
3. Laser angioplasty allows obliteration of an occlusion using a fiberoptic catheter threaded to the site.
4. Endovascular stents can be implanted to stretch stenosed vessels and improve blood flow.
5. Rotating atherectomy disposes of plaque by pulverizing it with a rotating burr on the tip of a catheter. The particles are dispersed into the circulation.
6. Amputation of the affected limb is performed when other limb salvage methods have failed.

Nursing Management

1. Take a history and assess the risk factors, which include smoking, obesity, high-fat and -cholesterol diet, HTN, diabetes mellitus, positive family history, and sedentary lifestyle.
2. Assess pain characteristics to pinpoint the severity of the disease, including location, frequency, precipitating factors, and alleviating factors.
3. Inspect skin texture, interruptions in skin integrity, skin color, and nail bed changes.
4. Palpate pulses, and check skin temperature and degree of edema.
5. Measure capillary refill time.
6. Auscultate carotid, subclavian, and femoral arteries for bruits.
7. Monitor blood glucose values in diabetic patients and cholesterol levels in all patients.
8. Monitor clotting studies on patients receiving anticoagulant agents.
9. Encourage the patient to follow a smoking cessation program.

10. Encourage the patient to reduce weight by reducing the fat and choles-
    terol in his or her diet and to begin an exercise program of walking.
11. Encourage stress reduction techniques to reduce HTN.
12. Psychological support should be provided if needed to help the patient
    develop coping skills necessary to deal with a chronic illness.

 ## COMMUNITY CARE

Community care involves the prevention of the progression of disease and
includes smoking cessation, regular exercise, and the avoidance of prolonged
standing, with special attention to foot care and optimization of treatment of
comorbid conditions (e.g., diabetes mellitus, HTN, congestive heart failure, or
chronic obstructive pulmonary disease).

 ## PROGNOSIS

PVD is a chronic, irreversible process. Possible complications include pulmonary embolus, leg ulcers, and amputation. Approximately 10% of patients
require amputation within 5 years, with the incidence rising to 50% within the
diabetic population. Early detection and decreased risk factors may allow
patients to lead a more active life.

 ## CLINICAL PEARLS

○ Severe, sudden pain may be indicative of arterial occlusion and warrants
  immediate notification of a physician.
○ Avoid exposing the patient to extreme cold such as an ice pack, because it
  can result in peripheral vasoconstriction in an already compromised peripheral vascular system.
○ Avoid exposing the patient to warming blankets or hot soaks, because they
  can result in burns as the patient may have decreased sensation in the area.
○ Prevent the patient from sitting or standing for a prolonged time, because
  this can result in venous pooling.

NURSING PROBLEM/ DIAGNOSIS	NURSING INTERVENTIONS CLASSIFICATION (NIC)
Pain (peripheral ischemia)	Pain management
	Energy management
Ineffective tissue perfusion	Circulatory care
	Skin surveillance
	Self-modification assistance

Raynaud's Disease

Linda McCuiston

 ## OVERVIEW

Raynaud's disease is an intermittent, bilateral response of the fingers and
toes noted on the exposure to cold temperatures that leads to intense vasospasm

and vasoconstriction. Raynaud's phenomenon is a vasospastic, unilateral response of the fingers and toes that have vasospasm and vasoconstrictive characteristics similar to those of Raynaud's disease, with the cause being a secondary disease or disorder. Initially, Raynaud's disease usually involves all digits of the affected extremities bilaterally, whereas Raynaud's phenomenon usually involves a single digit and tends to be unilateral. The symptoms of Raynaud's disease are generally mild to moderate, whereas Raynaud's phenomenon produces moderate to severe symptoms. Raynaud's disease usually affects females who are between 16 and 35 years of age, whereas Raynaud's phenomenon usually occurs in either gender over 30 years of age. Raynaud's disease occurs in 70% to 80% of all cases of Raynaud disorders.

 PATHOPHYSIOLOGY

The cause of Raynaud's disease is idiopathic, but it is associated with exposure to cold temperatures or emotional stress. One theory portrays a defect in basal heat production that eventually decreases the ability of cutaneous vessels to dilate. However, Raynaud attacks are not confined to cold environments, because episodes may be precipitated by a breeze or on entering an air-conditioned area. In severe cases, classic Raynaud signs and symptoms may also occur at normal temperatures.

The following illustrates a similar theory regarding basal heat production. Raynaud's disease is more prevalent in females during their menstrual years owing to higher estrogen levels. Attacks are more likely when the core temperature is lowest during menstruation and postmenstrual periods. Likewise, attacks are less likely at the peak of ovulation, when core temperature is higher. Cutaneous blood flow is lower in females than in males, which may be due to differences in estrogen receptors on blood vessels, less muscle mass, or sympathetic tone.

Raynaud's phenomenon usually is due to a secondary disease or disorder and rarely is precipitated by emotional stress. Several diseases or disorders that are often associated with Raynaud's phenomenon include systemic sclerosis (scleroderma), rheumatoid arthritis, and systemic lupus erythematosus. Scleroderma is the most common connective tissue disease associated with Raynaud's phenomenon. Patients with an initial scleroderma diagnosis generally develop severe Raynaud's phenomenon in approximately 10 years, leading to digital infarcts or ischemic ulcers. This correlation may be due to damaged vascular endothelium and reduced blood flow, as well as to additional platelet activation. Raynaud's phenomenon has also been found frequently in patients with migraine headaches or variant angina.

In Raynaud's disease and Raynaud's phenomenon, the pathophysiology is the same. The small cutaneous arteries and arterioles of the fingers and toes are subjected to episodic vasoconstriction due to microvascular vasospasms. Typically, cold stimuli would produce only moderate vasoconstriction, but in Raynaud's disease, there is exaggerated vasoconstriction and vasospasm. On exposure to cold temperatures or stress, sympathetic stimulation causes increased release of norepinephrine, which in turn activates the alpha-2 adrenergic receptors in cutaneous arteries and veins, leading to vasospasms and vasoconstriction. Skin of the fingers, palms, knees, soles, and toes have a dense capillary bed and a liberal amount of arteriovenous shunts. It is believed that persons with Raynaud's disease may have an enhanced sensitivity, an excessive amount of alpha-2 adrenergic receptors, and an abnormally intense sympathetic vascular tone. On exposure to cold, the arteriovenous shunts close and cutaneous blood flow decreases. On rewarming, the shunts open and routine blood flow resumes.

First, the affected digits turn white at the tip extending to the palm due to vasospasm and resultant vasoconstriction. The pooling of deoxygenated blood during vasospasm and vasoconstriction causes the digits to turn blue, or cyanotic in appearance. Once the ischemia or vasospasm has stopped, reactive vasodilatation of skin vessels with resultant rapid resaturation of small amounts of blood occurs, and the skin becomes red or hyperemic. The vasospasm and resultant vasoconstriction episodes usually last several minutes but may continue for several hours. Perfusion of sufficient nutrition to the tissues throughout the capillary network usually remains adequate during an episode. This accounts for the lack of digital ulcers in Raynaud's phenomenon. However, patients with scleroderma and Raynaud's phenomenon may be unable to maintain nutrient perfusion during an attack, becoming prone to ulcerations and gangrene.

 ## SIGNS AND SYMPTOMS

The majority of patients experience only mild and infrequent vasospastic episodes with Raynaud's disease. During an episode, the fingers or toes become ischemic and blanched and turn white or pale, then blue or cyanotic, and then reddened or hyperemic. The red or rubor phase is considered to be extremely painful. The episodes of vasospasm are usually short in duration, lasting only a few minutes, or continuing for several hours in severe cases. The episodes tend to become more frequent and longer in duration.

The characteristics of Raynaud's disease include bilateral symmetry. Typically, the tip of the finger distal to the metacarpophalangeal joint is affected or the corresponding toes, or both. The fingers of the hand are usually affected rather than the thumb. In severe cases of Raynaud's phenomenon, the ears, nose, and tongue can be affected, whereas these areas would rarely be affected in Raynaud's disease.

Accompanying the color changes, other characteristics of Raynaud's include difficulty with fine motor movement and paresthesia, such as numbness, a sensation of coldness, stiffness, and throbbing. As with any ischemia, pain is a common characteristic of this vasospastic attack, particularly during the red phase and rewarming. If the attack is severe and lengthy, prolonged ischemia may lead to ulcers and gangrene of the digits.

 ## DIAGNOSTIC CRITERIA

History alone is considered adequate for diagnosis. The following depicts Raynaud's disease criteria:

- Exposure to cold temperatures or emotional stress produces the characteristic signs and symptoms.
- Involvement is bilateral and symmetric.
- Peripheral pulses are normal on palpation.

- Digital gangrene is absent or superficial.
- Signs and symptoms have been intermittently noted for 2 or more years without the identification of any other secondary condition, such as a connective tissue disorder.

 INTERVENTIONS

The goals of Raynaud's treatment are geared at symptomatic relief and the prevention of tissue damage. Usually, there is no prescribed treatment if the episodes are mild, because the symptoms are self-limiting. Avoidance of precipitating factors and reassurance are often sufficient. Attacks can be prevented by the use of heat preservation measures alone.

Conserve Heat

Patients should be taught to conserve heat by dressing warmly in layers and using thinsulate or lightweight warm clothing. In cold weather, affected patients should wear hats and mittens. Mittens are preferred over gloves, because the fingers are kept warmer by body heat. Reusable hand warmers and foot warmers are encouraged.

Medications

Usually, Raynaud's disease is not sufficiently detrimental for pharmacologic therapy to be necessary. Some patients with Raynaud's phenomenon may obtain relief of symptoms with low-dose nifedipine (Procardia). A few patients find that the adverse effects, such as fatigue, hypotension, reduced exercise tolerance, fluid retention, and heartburn, are more bothersome than the signs and symptoms of Raynaud's disease, thus after a prescribed trial, they elect to discontinue the medication. Calcium channel blockers, vascular smooth muscle relaxants, and vasodilators may be tried, but beta-blockers should be avoided, because they increase the severity of attacks.

Newer medications, such as iloprost (a prostacyclin analog), increase circulation and decrease pain. Other helpful medications may be cyclandelate (Cyclospasmol) and phenoxybenzamine (Dibenzyline). They are examples of vasodilators that can be used to prevent the characteristic vasoconstriction, vasospasm, and ischemia. Common side effects of vasodilators include headache, decreased BP, tachycardia, palpitations, dizziness (vertigo), fainting (syncope), drowsiness, weakness, and facial flushing.

Surgery

A sympathectomy surgical procedure may be necessary if signs and symptoms are severe. This involves cutting the sympathetic nerve fibers that cause vasoconstriction and may be helpful in the promotion of vasodilatation. By interrupting or dividing sympathetic nerves or their branches, vasodilatation is promoted, and the patient may have some improvement in status. Surgical sympathectomy should be avoided, if at all possible, because results are generally disappointing with only transient improvement.

Biofeedback

Biofeedback is a training technique that enables an individual to obtain an element of voluntary control over autonomic body functions. An electronic machine, which measures skin temperature, can "train" the patient to control this involuntary activity. Based on feedback or information received, a desired response of increasing skin temperature is learned when a specific thought or action produces the desired response. The patient is then weaned from the machine and can produce the desired response without the machine. Biofeedback can be used to increase skin temperature and help prevent vasospasm.

Guided Imagery

The use of guided imagery empowers patients to exert some control over their condition. Guided imagery is a technique that a patient can induce deliberately by recalling memories or visions of pleasant and desired "mental pictures." These visions may include a warm beach, beautiful mountains, or magnificent sunset. Images and thoughts are transmitted through the hypothalamus and limbic system in the brain via neurotransmitters. Neurotransmitters (norepinephrine and acetylcholine) affect peripheral and autonomic nervous systems to promote relaxation. Herbs and aromas, used in aromatherapy, can enhance the initial relaxation exercise. Patients can be taught to induce images independently to help reduce stress and prevent vasospasm.

Smoking Cessation

The nicotine in cigarettes stimulates the adrenal glands to produce epinephrine, which constricts blood vessels. Nicotine, tar, and carbon monoxide in cigarettes can irritate the endothelium of vessels, leading to vasospasm. The nurse should inform patients about the effects of smoking and that the cessation of or reduction in cigarette smoking leads to decreased vasoconstriction and improved circulation.

 COMMUNITY CARE

Assessment

1. Assess precipitating factors: age, sex, smoking, exposure to cold temperatures, and emotional stress.
2. Assess the patient for characteristics of Raynaud's: characteristic white, blue, and then red color pattern, as well as pain and paresthesia.
3. Assess involved area for differentiation between Raynaud's disease and phenomenon: unilateral or bilateral, and symmetry.
4. Assess for signs and symptoms of a secondary condition: stiffness and pain in joints on arising in the morning, thickening and atrophy of the skin, hypertrophy of the epidermis, and atrophic plaques with erythema.

Monitoring

1. Monitor the patient for needed instructions regarding episode management, such as rapid controlled rewarming. Rewarming may be accomplished by rapidly swinging the arms in a windmill motion, running warm water over hands, or blowing warm air from a hair dryer over the hands.
2. Monitor the patient who is on treatment with medications for side effects of postural hypotension, avoidance of alcohol, excessive exercise, and prolonged exposure to hot weather.

3. Monitor condition and treatment regimen if the patient has skin ulcerations for cleanliness, prescribed antimicrobial dressings, and required débridement or analgesics.
4. Monitor for severe complications, such as ulcerations and gangrene.

Prevention

1. Instruct the patient regarding the reduction of precipitating factors: smoking cessation, minimize exposure to cold temperatures, stress management, and relaxation techniques.
2. Instruct the patient regarding the avoidance of exposure to cold: provide adequate room temperature and blankets, warm layered clothing, hats and mittens, use of hand warmers and foot heaters, and use of insulated drinking glasses.
3. Instruct the patient regarding prescribed medication regimen.
4. Instruct the patient to avoid occupational trauma or occupations that involve the use of heavy vibrating tools, such as hand-held drills, grinders, polishers, riveters, pneumatic hammers, jackhammers, chain saws, and welding equipment. Caution patients, who are also subjected to repeated stress of the hands, regarding activities such as typing and playing the piano. In addition, caution patients who have excessive contact with cold temperatures, such as butchers or food preparers.
5. Instruct the patient to avoid medications or toxic substances that precipitate Raynaud's vasospastic episodes: over-the-counter cold medications (sympathomimetic agents), oral contraceptives, amphetamines, ergot, and cocaine.

PROGNOSIS

1. The prognosis for Raynaud's disease is varied.
2. Some patients gradually improve, some progressively deteriorate, and some remain the same.
3. Chronic recurrences of the disease may lead to atrophy of the surrounding skin and muscles in the affected area.
4. Ulceration and gangrene are rare.

CLINICAL PEARLS

○ Raynaud's disease occurs primarily in females (approximately 93%).
○ Rewarming the affected extremity may be done by rapidly swinging the arms in a windmill motion, running warm water over hands, or blowing warm air from a hair dryer over hands.
○ Biofeedback can be used to enable patients to control their skin temperature and prevent vasospasm.
○ The use of guided imagery empowers patients to exert some control over their condition. By using aromatherapy to initiate relaxation, the patient can deliberately induce desired "mental pictures" in guided imagery. Relaxation can produce relaxation and prevent vasospasm.
○ Quitting smoking has best outcome when multiple approaches are used at once.

NURSING PROBLEM/ DIAGNOSIS	NURSING INTERVENTIONS CLASSIFICATION (NIC)
Acute pain (vasospastic episodes) Ineffective tissue perfusion	Biofeedback Pain management Circulatory care Peripheral sensation management
Prevention of vasospastic episodes	Environmental management Skin surveillance Smoking cessation assistance

Thrombophlebitis

Section 8   Joanne M. Bullard

 OVERVIEW

Thrombophlebitis (also called *venous thrombosis*) is the most common venous disorder and may occur in either superficial or deep veins. It is an acute vascular condition in which the formation of a thrombus (*clot*) within a superficial or deep vein is associated with inflammation of the vessel wall. Superficial thrombophlebitis primarily occurs in the superficial veins of the upper extremities and the saphenous veins in the lower extremities, often occurring in varicose veins. In the lower extremities, the most common cause of superficial thrombophlebitis is related to varicose veins; in the upper extremities, the most common cause is related to intravenous therapy. Many factors are associated with an increased risk for the development of thrombophlebitis (Table 15-8-1). As many as 65% of all patients who receive intravenous therapy develop thrombophlebitis. The risk for serious complications of superficial thrombophlebitis is less than that of deep venous thrombophlebitis. *Phlebothrombosis* refers to the development of a thrombus without acute inflammation.

 PATHOPHYSIOLOGY

Virchow's triad, which consists of venous stasis, vascular endothelial injury, and hypercoagulability, is associated with thrombophlebitis. Venous stasis may occur in patients who are obese or have congestive heart failure. Venous stasis may also occur in patients who have been immobilized after surgical procedures, as a result of prolonged bed rest, or as a result of prolonged sitting, such as during travel. Vascular endothelial injury is caused by any trauma to the lining of the vein such as venipuncture, indwelling venous catheters, or the infusion of hypertonic or caustic solutions. Hypercoagulability may occur in patients with blood dyscrasias or malignant disease, on estrogen or steroid therapy, or who have systemic infections in which endotoxins are released. Hypercoagulability may also be caused by smoking.

Common sites of thrombus (clot) formation are the intima of the vein where trauma has occurred and in the valve cusp pockets where the blood flow is slowed and blood products accumulate. A thrombus is formed by a combina-

Table 15-8-1. Factors That Increase the Risk of Venous Thrombosis

Sugical procedures
    Orthopedic (especially knee and hip), thoracic, abdominal, genitourinary
Cancer
    Pancreas, lung, genitourinary tract, stomach, breast
Trauma
    Spinal cord injuries; fractures of the spine, pelvis, femur, tibia
Immobility (stasis)
    Congestive heart failure, acute myocardial infarction, stroke, bedrest
Pregnancy
    Particularly in the third trimester and the first month postpartum
Estrogen use
    Replacement or contraceptive
Hypercoagulable states
    Factor V Leiden; deficiencies of antithrombin III, protein C, or protein S; antiphospholipid
        syndrome; dysfibrinogenemia; myeloproliferative diseases; disseminated intravascular
        coagulation
Venulitis
    Thromboangiitis obliterans; Beçhet's disease; homocysteinuria
Other risk factors
    Intravenous therapy, varicose veins, prolonged sitting or standing, smoking

tion of aggregated platelets, red blood cells, and leukocytes enmeshed in fibrin. When the endothelial layer of the vein is injured or irritated, the normally smooth surface becomes roughened, providing a place for platelets to adhere. As platelets begin to adhere and aggregate, substances are released that stimulate the formation of fibrin. The fibrin surrounds the platelets, trapping blood cells and additional platelets and forming a thrombus that adheres to the vein wall. The thrombus may partially or completely occlude the lumen of the vein. Collateral circulation often compensates for this blockage when it occurs in superficial veins. A thrombus that partially occludes the vein may develop a segment, or "tail." The thrombus may dislodge or the tail may break off, causing an embolus. When a purulent infection develops within the lumen of a vein that is or had been cannulated, it is referred to as *suppurative thrombophlebitis*.

 SIGNS AND SYMPTOMS

Superficial Thrombophlebitis. Classic findings are localized pain, redness, edema, and warmth and tenderness over the affected vein. When palpated, the vein may be firm and cord-like. Linear, red streaks may also be present.

Suppurative Thrombophlebitis. Purulence may be at the intravenous cannula insertion site. Signs include redness, tenderness, and warmth, and symptoms are fever and leukocytosis. Often, no local signs are visible; a potential complication is septicemia.

 DIAGNOSTIC CRITERIA
Venography

- The venography (phlebography) is a procedure in which a radiopaque dye is injected into the vein and a series of radiographs (venograms) are taken.

Any obstruction to the flow of dye within the vein indicates the presence of a thrombus. A positive study confirms the diagnosis of thrombophlebitis.
- Rare complications of this test include cellulitis, thrombophlebitis, bacteremia, and embolism.
- A venography is contraindicated in patients who are allergic to iodine or have renal failure.

Duplex Ultrasonography
- Duplex ultrasonography is a noninvasive test that identifies any obstruction or reduced flow of blood to a specific area.
- Because ultrasonography is noninvasive, has no complications, and is sensitive and specific for the diagnosis of thrombophlebitis and DVT, it is usually the method of choice.

Plethysmography
- Plethysmography is a noninvasive test that provides a measurement of changes in the venous volume distal to the affected area indicating an occlusion.
- The sensitivity of this test, when used in obese persons, is greatly reduced.

^{125}I Fibrinogen Scan
- The ^{125}I fibrinogen scan is a radionuclear, noninvasive test that is used to identify thrombi in the veins of the extremities.
- It is useful in the study of established DVT and in the detection of early thrombi in persons who are at high risk for DVT.
- Disadvantages of this test are that: (1) DVT in the upper thigh cannot be detected because of normally occurring high quantities of fibrinogen in this area, (2) 24 hours must pass between the administration of the ^{125}I fibrinogen and the scan to test for increased uptake, and (3) the possibility of hepatitis transmission exists because the fibrinogen used for ^{125}I labeling comes from donated blood.
- False-positive results may occur if there is inflammation of the leg, such as superficial phlebitis or arthritis, because the fibrinogen also will go to areas of inflammation.

Blood Cultures
With superficial thrombophlebitis, blood cultures may be performed to rule out the presence of infection caused by *Staphylococcus* bacteria.

 INTERVENTIONS
Elevation
- Elevate the affected extremity above the level of the patient's right atrium to improve venous blood flow and to decrease venous pooling. Use of the knee gatch of the bed or placement of pillows under the knees may impede circulation and should not be done.
- If the patient is on bed rest, he or she should change position every 2 hours to reduce edema and to prevent skin breakdown.

Compression
- Apply warm, moist compresses to the affected area at least four times a day. Moist heat or use of an aqua-K pad will promote comfort by decreas-

ing venospasms and pain. Discontinue the compresses when the symptoms are relieved.

- Use antiembolic stockings (TED hose or compression stockings) as prescribed by physician. Each individual must be measured for the stockings to ensure a correct fit. Stockings may be removed for short periods (30 to 60 minutes) each day, usually during a bath.

Pharmacotherapy

- Nonsteroidal anti-inflammatory agents such as indomethacin (Naprosyn) may be administered to provide relief of symptoms. Concurrent use with warm, moist compresses is usually sufficient to provide relief from pain that accompanies superficial thrombophlebitis. Aspirin may be administered as an analgesic agent, also because of its antithrombotic properties, if the patient is not undergoing surgery or the aspirin will not cause clinical complications.
- Antibiotics are not usually used in the treatment of superficial thrombophlebitis unless there is an identified infection. In patients whose inflammatory response is a result of infection, antibiotic therapy for 7 to 10 days is usually sufficient. A longer course of therapy may be needed if there are complications.

Intravenous Line Maintenance in Hospital

- Monitor the intravenous catheter insertion site every 2 hours or more frequently during the infusion of intravenous fluids and medications.
- As recommended by the Centers for Disease Control and Prevention, change the peripheral intravenous catheter site every 48 to 72 hours and the intravenous tubing every no more frequently than every 72 hours unless the catheter is changed or clinically indicated.

 # COMMUNITY CARE

Assessment

1. Assess risk factors: intravenous catheters, intravenous therapy with caustic solutions such as chemotherapeutic agents or intravenous dye, varicose veins, direct trauma, smoking, and a recent history of travel in which the patient remained seated for a long time.
2. Assess for signs and symptoms of thrombophlebitis: warmth and redness; tenderness to touch over the affected vein; vein when palpated, firm and cord-like; red linear marks along the vein; edema.
3. Assess for any changes in tissue perfusion, peripheral pulses, capillary refill, skin integrity, and color; report any changes noted to the physician.

Monitoring

1. Assess for complications of superficial thrombophlebitis, such as infection, sepsis, and PE, which is rare with superficial thrombophlebitis.
2. Teach the patient to report any of the following: temperature of greater than 100.5°F (38°C), any shortness of breath, dyspnea, chest pain, or extreme anxiety.
3. As a result of the inflammatory process, the white blood cell count and the erythrocyte sedimentation rate may be elevated. The erythrocyte

sedimentation rate is elevated as a result of the inflammatory process because of a change in blood proteins that causes a clumping of red blood cells.

Prevention

1. Maintain strict aseptic techniques with intravenous therapy. Remove the catheter immediately if infiltration or contamination is suspected.
2. Explain to the patient the importance of keeping the affected extremity elevated at all times, of avoidance of sitting or standing in one position for long periods, and of avoidance of crossing the legs when sitting.
3. Discourage oral contraceptive use and smoking.

 PROGNOSIS

Superficial thrombophlebitis, with proper treatment, usually has no serious complications.

 CLINICAL PEARLS

o When starting an intravenous line, avoid veins that are susceptible to varicosities, thus decreasing the likelihood of phlebitis.
o Use an arm board to prevent the movement of intravenous cannula in veins in areas of joint flexion to prevent injury to the venous wall and the possibility of phlebitis.
o When a patient complains of a painful infusion, you may need to differentiate between early phlebitis and venospasm. Apply heat, and slow the rate of infusion. The heat dilates the vessel, increasing the blood flow and diluting the slowed intravenous solution, and the pain of the venospasm is relieved. If the pain is not relieved, consider early phlebitis and a change in the location of the intravenous site.

NURSING PROBLEM/ DIAGNOSIS	NURSING INTERVENTIONS CLASSIFICATION (NIC)
Ineffective tissue perfusion	Circulatory care Embolus precautions Skin surveillance Exercise promotion
Acute pain (inflammatory)	Heat/cold application Pain management

Varicose Veins

Section 9   Patricia Revolinski

 OVERVIEW

Varicose veins are veins that have become excessively tortuous and dilated. They can appear in any area affected by venous HTN but are most visible in the lower extremities. The affected veins are usually superficial. It is commonly considered to be a cosmetic disorder, but there can be some discomfort involved, as well as medical risks if deeper veins are affected. Estimates of incidence in the population have ranged from 2% to 15%, with most studies indicating a greater prevalence in women than in men. Varicosities are progressive, and the only real incidences of remission have been documented when the condition was aggravated by pregnancy, with some disappearance of dilatation after delivery.

In this section, the primary focus is on varicosities that affect the lower extremities.

PATHOPHYSIOLOGY

The function of a vein is to return blood to the heart from the capillary system. The venous system in the legs is composed of three components: deep veins, communicating veins, and superficial veins. Varicosities in the superficial veins are considered primary, whereas those in the deep or communicating veins are considered secondary. The *superficial veins* lie within the subcutaneous tissues, and the *deep veins* lie beneath the fascia and are surrounded by muscle. The *communicating veins* connect the superficial and deep veins and pierce the fascia to do so. The blood from the skin and subcutaneous tissues in the leg collects in the superficial veins and then is transported to the deep veins, via the communicating veins, for transport back to the heart. This is facilitated by the "calf pump," a mechanism by which the calf muscles contract with exercise, compressing the deep venous system and pumping the blood toward the heart. As the pressure rises in these veins, the valves in the communicating veins close. This prevents retrograde blood flow, as well as preventing the transmission of the pressure to the superficial system. In the deep veins, the pressure exerted by the fluid, known as *hydrostatic pressure,* can rise to 300 mm Hg, whereas in the superficial veins, it may rise to 150 mm Hg. When lying down, the pressure is as low as 15 mm Hg. As the patient stands, hydrostatic pressure is increased owing to the influences of gravity. The venous veins are capacitance vessels, which means that when the patient is relaxed, the veins are compressed. However, as the veins fill with blood, they become distended until they reach capacity. Once they are filled to capacity, any increase in volume will increase pressure.

Varicose veins can result from three pathophysiologic states: venous obstruction, venous valvular insufficiency, and calf muscle pump malfunction. *Venous obstruction* is most often a result of thrombophlebitis. When there is increased resistance to flow, the pressures will elevate and the valves will begin to malfunction. This may result in the increased volume and pressure being communicated to the superficial veins and result in varicose veins. Other sources of venous obstruction may be masses such as tumors, infection, or retroperitoneal fibrosis.

Valvular insufficiency may involve any or all of the venous systems in the leg. When the valves are incompetent, whether due to congenital or acquired causes, the result is high pressures being transmitted to the lower leg on standing. This pressure is not adequately relieved with exercise. Some manifestations of this abnormality include the absence of valves, which is rare; venous valve prolapse or floppy valves; dilation of valve rings affecting the function of the cusps; and incomplete closure of the cusps after prolonged dilation of the veins secondary to prolonged exposure to high venous pressures. Some causes of these prolonged elevations include arteriovenous fistulas, trauma, and DVT.

Finally, there can be failure of the *calf pump.* The muscles may not be strong enough to pump the blood out of the leg, such as occurs in the elderly, paraplegics, or traumatically injured or inactive, bedridden patients. Pathologic conditions that result in muscle fibrosis, such as muscular dystrophy and multiple sclerosis, may lead to failure of the calf pump. If the outflow is obstructed, there will be an increase in pressure, causing dilation of the veins. This is then transmitted to the communicating veins and on to the superficial veins and the surrounding tissue. *Venous stasis,* which is the cessation of the flow of the blood that results in prolonged contact of the blood with the vessel wall, can result in increased pressures or venous HTN in the legs. Varicose veins can result.

Typically, the affected veins are superficial leg veins and will appear as bluish, bulging, cordlike vessels just under the skin. It is not unusual for flooded capillaries, or *spider veins,* to surround the varicosity. This type of varicosity usually presents no medical risk, but the patient may seek treatment owing to some pain and disfiguring cosmetic effect. However, when the veins involved are part of the deep venous network of legs, the patient is at risk for blood clot formation. If this occurs in veins in the thighs or pelvis, the risk of PE, a life-threatening occurrence, is increased.

 ## SIGNS AND SYMPTOMS
Appearance

The only symptom of varicose veins may be simply the presence of dilated, bluish, ropelike veins. These most often occur in the saphenous system and manifest in the calves. Telangiectases may surround the affected vessel as well.

Pain

The patient may complain of dull leg aches and feelings of pressure, fatigue, and heaviness. This is caused by the increased blood volume in the affected veins. There may be a worsening of this pain before menstruation, related to increased circulating estrogen, which decreases venous tone. Nocturnal muscle cramps may occur as a result of venous stasis.

Edema

Leg edema is not a common problem with primary varicose veins and most often occurs with secondary varicose veins. Mild ankle edema may be present by the end of the day, due to the incompetence of the lower leg communicating veins. Post-thrombotic damage to deep veins can cause ankle and lower leg edema in patients who are less active.

Skin

Defective venous return from the lower limb, caused by varicose veins, can lead to venous ulcers, also known as *venous stasis ulcers.* These are usually present in secondary varicose veins. Itching may also be present over the affected vein.

 ## DIAGNOSTIC CRITERIA
Trendelenburg Test

Also known as the *retrograde filling test,* the Trendelenburg test is conducted to establish incompetent valve function and can be completed at the bedside.

A tourniquet is applied to the lower limb when the patient is lying down. After 1 minute, when the patient stands, if the veins below the tourniquet fill up, there is an incompetent pathway between the superficial and deep veins. The level of the compromised connection can be determined by repeating the test with the tourniquet at different levels. These tests are valuable in making management decisions in about 80% to 90% of patients with superficial varicose veins.

Venography

Venography is used to determine deep vein patency or adequacy. The patient has a tourniquet applied above the ankle and then reclines at a 45-degree angle while dye is injected into a vein. Then the leg is exercised by having the patient stand on the toes and down again several times. Radiographs are obtained while the leg is being exercised to determine the patency of the vein.

Doppler Ultrasonography

Ultrasound waves are reflected back to the skin from vessels. The patency of the vessel can be determined, and blood flow can be observed.

 INTERVENTIONS
Lifestyle Changes

1. Support stockings, compression bandages, or both are worn to promote drainage of veins and blood return to the heart.
2. Tight, restrictive clothing should be avoided, because it impedes venous drainage and increases hydrostatic pressure.
3. Obese patients are encouraged to reduce their weight.
4. Exercise is encouraged, especially walking at least three times per week.
5. Patients are advised to avoid prolonged standing to decrease venous pooling in the legs.

Surgical Management

Vein Ligation and Stripping. This procedure is used to remove a torturous vein that is causing discomfort or presents a higher risk for thrombophlebitis. It is the most common treatment of varicose veins. A distal incision, usually at the ankle, and a proximal incision, usually at the groin, are made in the affected leg. A wire is threaded through the lumen from distal to proximal site and then pulled back down distally, removing the vein with it. If there is excessive bleeding after a ligation procedure, apply direct pressure over the wound, elevate the leg, and notify the surgeon. Minimal bleeding can be controlled with elastic bandages.

Sclerotherapy. This is usually reserved for smaller varicosities or intradermal spider veins. Its use has been documented as far back as 1855, although there is some controversy regarding whether it is an effective treatment for varicosities. Various sclerosing agents are available, with hypertonic saline and sodium tetradecyl sulfate being two that are frequently used. The agent is injected directly into the vein, producing a sterile inflammation of the vein wall. It is believed that this results in occlusion of the lumen, causing the opposing surfaces to stick together. The vein then becomes a fibrosed cord and will become less prominent under the skin. This treatment was advocated to obliterate small varicose veins, telangiectases, and solitary varicose veins in the absence of main saphenous vein incompetence.

Follow-up Care

Both procedures are performed on an outpatient basis. Patients should wear compression stockings or dressing for the first 3 days after the procedure, and bathing is not recommended during this period. For vein ligation, have the patient keep the leg elevated for the first 24 hours while performing isometric leg exercises. Have the patient ambulate several minutes per hour after the first 24 hours, gradually increasing daily. Compression stockings should be worn for 8 to 12 weeks. For sclerotherapy, compression stockings should be worn during sleep for the next 2 weeks. Exercise should be avoided for the first 2 weeks after therapy; activities of daily living are permitted.

 COMMUNITY CARE

Assessment

1. Assess risk factors, including family history, obesity, and occupations that require prolonged periods of standing.
2. Inspect for dilated, ropelike veins and areas with spider veins.
3. Assess for interruptions in skin integrity that may be indicative of early venous ulcers.

Teaching

1. Teach the patient to report signs and symptoms of DVT, such as deep leg pain of sudden onset and leg warmth and swelling.
2. Have the patient avoid prolonged periods of standing.
3. Have the patient avoid sitting with legs crossed.
4. Support stockings must be applied and used appropriately.

Prevention

1. Encourage weight reduction where applicable.
2. Have the patient elevate the legs as much as possible throughout the day.
3. Have the patient begin a walking program.
4. Provide education about risk factors and their reduction.

 PROGNOSIS

Varicose veins are usually progressive in nature, and treatments are aimed at reducing the patient's anxiety over the disfiguring cosmetic effects of the veins and eliminating discomfort associated with them.

 CLINICAL PEARLS

○ Walking is thought to enhance the effect of sclerosing agents and is recommended 30 minutes after the procedure.
○ The patient should be cautioned that the sclerosed veins will look worse before they look better and can bruise 2 to 3 days after the procedure; this is normal.
○ The patient should be reminded to discontinue platelet-inhibiting drugs for 1 week before treatment.

○ When elastic wraps are used, the patient should be instructed to maintain a firm compression and to begin wrapping at the foot and end at the thigh.

NURSING PROBLEM/ DIAGNOSIS	NURSING INTERVENTIONS CLASSIFICATION (NIC)
Risk for ineffective tissue perfusion	Environmental management Embolus precautions Circulatory care
Acute pain (leg aches and cramps)	Environmental management: comfort Positioning
Postprocedural care	Bleeding precautions Teaching: prescribed activity/ exercise

Gastrointestinal—Lower

chapter **16**

Appendicitis

Section 1   Patricia B. Graham

OVERVIEW

Appendicitis is an acute inflammation of the *vermiform appendix,* the small finger-like pouch attached to the cecum of the colon. The appendix is about the thickness of a pencil, is from 2 to 6 inches long, and is usually located in the right iliac region, just below the ileocecal valve.

Appendicitis is the most common reason for abdominal surgery, and it occurs most frequently among individuals 30 years of age and younger. Males are affected more often than females, and teenagers are affected more often than adults. Diagnosis can be difficult, and in studies, patients undergoing emergency appendectomies were found to have a normal appendix 47% of the time. Diagnosis is even more difficult in women of childbearing age due to gynecologic disorders that mimic appendicitis.

Accurate diagnosis is important because if appendicitis is not diagnosed correctly, there is a risk of perforation. This is the probable reason for a high rate of unnecessary appendectomies. Physicians will choose to remove an appendix when symptoms are present rather than run the risk of a perforation.

PATHOPHYSIOLOGY

The appendix fills with food and empties into the cecum on a regular basis. Because it empties inefficiently and the lumen is small, it is prone to obstruction and vulnerable to infection. Inflammation occurs when the lumen is obstructed. Swelling occurs initially, and as the inflammatory process continues, it becomes hyperemic and covered with exudate. Without intervention, it may perforate. Although the cause of obstruction of the lumen remains controversial, obstruction from stool, neoplastic disease, adhesions, or foreign bodies are among the most accepted theories.

SIGNS AND SYMPTOMS

A classic series of events occurs in patients with appendicitis. Patients experience epigastric or central abdominal pain, followed by anorexia, nausea, and vomiting. The pain tends to move toward the right lower abdomen with rebound tenderness present. Abdominal tenderness on palpation is the most common, important, and reliable symptom. Tenderness is seen in the area of McBurney's point, which is located midway between the anterior iliac crest and the umbilicus in the right lower quadrant. Fever is next in the sequence (~100°F) and finally leukocytosis. A "shift to the left" in the leukocyte count (an increased number of immature white blood cells) is often seen, and a white blood cell count of higher than 20,000 may indicate perforation. Clinical signs that do not follow this sequence may be due to the anatomic variation of the location of the appendix.

In addition to leukocyte counts, C-reactive protein has been shown to be elevated in patients with acute appendicitis. In one study of 200 patients, an increase in leukocytes was an early marker of an inflamed appendix. C-reactive protein levels increased only after abscess formation or perforation.

 DIAGNOSTIC CRITERIA

A diagnosis of acute appendicitis is made on the basis of physical findings, leukocyte counts, C-reactive protein level, and appendiceal computed tomography (CT) scan. Appendiceal CT provides an accurate diagnosis in about 90% of cases.

 INTERVENTIONS

Because of the mortality rate associated with perforation, early diagnosis of appendicitis is imperative. The only therapy for appendicitis at the present time is surgical removal. After admission to the hospital, the patient is on nothing-by-mouth (NPO) restrictions in anticipation of surgery. An intravenous line may be started to replace fluids and electrolytes lost through vomiting. A nasogastric tube attached to suction may be inserted if vomiting remains a problem or if perforation is suspected. Patients should not receive laxatives or enemas because of the danger of perforation if appendicitis is present. If a firm diagnosis of appendicitis has been made, the physician may prescribe analgesics for pain. Because the sudden absence of pain may be an indication of perforation, analgesics may be withheld until surgery is performed. Antibiotics are initiated if perforation is suspected.

Appendiceal surgery may be divided into the following three types:

1. *Traditional open appendectomy:* the appendix is removed via a 3-inch incision in the lower right quadrant of the abdomen.
2. *Uncomplicated laparoscopic appendectomy:* several small incisions are made in the abdomen through which an endoscope is inserted. A cutting instrument is inserted through the endoscope, and the appendix is removed.
3. *Complicated appendectomy (in which perforation is present):* an open appendectomy is performed in which the incision may be much larger than 3 inches. Drains may be inserted and left in place for several days.

Postoperative care includes close monitoring of vital signs, observation for signs of infection and hemorrhage, management of postoperative nausea and vomiting or gastric suction, observation for the return of normal peristalsis, early ambulation, administration of antibiotics and analgesics, and regulation of intravenous fluids. Patients who undergo an uncomplicated laparoscopic appendectomy may be discharged on the day of surgery. Hospitalization length is about 3 days for a traditional uncomplicated appendectomy and about 7 days for a perforated appendix.

 COMMUNITY CARE

Community care for appendicitis is in large part education of the public about symptom recognition. Persons should be cautioned about the danger of using laxatives and enemas in the presence of abdominal pain or nausea and vomiting because of the danger of appendiceal perforation. Early discharge of patients who undergo a complicated appendectomy may require follow-up by a community-based nurse.

 PROGNOSIS

The prognosis for individuals undergoing an uncomplicated appendectomy is excellent, and they are usually able to resume normal activities very quickly. The prognosis is less favorable in cases of perforation. The rate of perforations remains at about 20% for all appendectomies performed. With proper treatment and follow-up, a patient with a perforated appendix can be expected to recover with no lasting effects, but recovery usually is longer than for an uncomplicated appendectomy. Mortality rates are 0.1% to 0.2% for nonperforated appendicitis and 3% to 5% for perforated appendicitis.

 CLINICAL PEARLS

○ Laxatives or enemas should not be used in the presence of abdominal pain or nausea and vomiting.
○ Appendiceal CT has about a 90% accuracy rate in the diagnosis of acute appendicitis.
○ Recovery time for a laparoscopic appendectomy is less than the time required for an open or a complicated appendectomy.
○ To properly assess rebound tenderness, depress the lower right abdominal quadrant. This elicits tenderness and muscle guarding. Keep the examining hand depressed, allowing the patient to get used to the pressure, and then suddenly release the pressure. This should cause a sudden increase in tenderness as voiced by the patient with an obvious grimace.

NURSING PROBLEM/ DIAGNOSIS	NURSING INTERVENTIONS CLASSIFICATION (NIC)
Presurgical pain/Acute pain Pain management Postsurgical management	Analgesic administration Postanalgesia care Infection prevention

Cirrhosis

Section 2   Veronica Njie

 OVERVIEW

Cirrhosis of the liver is the 10th leading cause of death in the United States. The death rate is 9.4 per 100,000 adults, which accounts for approximately 25,175 persons. Alcohol abuse is associated with 45% of the deaths. The liver is one of the most essential organs in the body. When it is diseased, multiple problems arise that, if not arrested, will result in death. In cirrhosis of the liver, the cells are scarred and damaged over a period of years, sometimes up to 30 years.

PATHOPHYSIOLOGY

In liver cirrhosis, the cells become grossly scarred (fibrosed). The number of functioning liver cells decreases progressively, and they are replaced with the scarred tissues. The change in scarred cells causes the structure to appear distorted. This abnormal structure of the liver causes an interruption of blood flow, leading to inability of the liver to perform its functions effectively and efficiently.

After the liver cells have progressed from normal to fibrotic, the condition becomes irreversible. Continuous assessment and monitoring are essential to identify complications early and to intervene promptly.

Regardless of the type of cirrhosis, the clinical course can be complicated with the following:

Portal Hypertension. This usually occurs as a result of interruption of the normal blood flow in the liver due to the scarred cells. This causes buildup of pressure within the portal circulatory system and backflow of venous blood to the gastrointestinal (GI), accessory, and other surrounding organs. This subsequently leads to esophageal, gastric, or rectal varices and splenomegaly. The esophageal varices are the most serious. The varices are due to congestion and increased pressure in the hepatic circulation causing enlargement and overdistention of the fragile blood vessels. This puts the individual at risk for rupture of the vessels and massive hemorrhage. The individual is also at risk for bleeding secondary to thrombocytopenia, which compounds the problem.

Ascites. This is caused by an accumulation of fluid in the abdomen. Low plasma protein levels combined with the sodium and water retention from excessive aldosterone make it worse.

Hepatic Encephalopathy. The liver is not able to convert ammonia into urea for excretion, which leads to accumulation of ammonia toxins in the blood. The ammonia crosses the blood-brain barrier and causes changes in level of consciousness, cognition, and motor function (see Table 16-2-1 for the changes and nursing assessment).

Spontaneous Bacterial Peritonitis. A bacterial infection that occurs in the abdomen due to the ascites. Usually there is no evidence of an actual infection, thus it is called "spontaneous."

Hepatorenal Syndrome. The cause of this syndrome is unknown. The normal function of the kidneys is affected, leading to manifestations of renal failure, such as oliguria or anuria, and elevated creatinine and potassium levels. In addition, the action of excessive aldosterone causes potassium retention.

Hepatocellular Cancer. Owing to the aberration of the liver cells, there is increased risk for the cells to become cancerous.

SIGNS AND SYMPTOMS

The liver has essential functions necessary to sustain life, including fat, protein, and carbohydrate metabolism; bile production and excretion; storage of vitamins and minerals; synthesis of clotting factors and coagulation regulation; and detoxification of drugs and substances. The manifestations seen in

Table 16-2-1. Assessment Findings in Hepatic Encephalopathy

CHANGES	NURSING ASSESSMENT
Level of consciousness	Drowsiness
	Stupor
	Coma
Cognition	Decrease in intellect
	Decrease in attention
	Change in behavior or personality
	Deterioration in decision-making ability
	Confusion
Motor function	Fatigue
	Lethargy
	Irritability
	Asterixis
	Abnormal positioning—decerebrate or decorticate posturing

This table provides changes in level of consciousness, cognition, and motor function and the concurrent assessment findings that may occur in individuals with hepatic encephalopathy if the process is not arrested.

liver cirrhosis are primarily a result of inability of the liver to perform these functions effectively and efficiently.

Altered Metabolism of Carbohydrate, Protein, and Fat. The liver is unable to perform glucogenesis, glycogenolysis, and glyconeogenesis for glucose metabolism; to synthesize amino acids and plasma proteins for protein metabolism; and to synthesize lipoproteins for fat metabolism. This results in GI symptoms. The increased pressure in the GI system also aggravates the symptoms.

Gastrointestinal Changes. These changes occur early and are usually common.

- Nausea and vomiting leading to weight loss
- Dyspepsia
- Change in bowel habits (diarrhea or constipation with melena)
- Abdominal pain (dull in the right upper quadrant/epigastric area)
- Enlarged spleen

Altered Synthesis of Clotting Factors and Blood Cells. Vitamin K is required to produce the clotting factors. Absorption of vitamin K, a fat-soluble vitamin, depends on fat absorption, which becomes compromised resulting in coagulation abnormalities. The enlarged spleen excessively sequesters and eliminates platelets, which results in bleeding tendencies. In cases in which cirrhosis is caused by alcohol abuse, the bone marrow becomes depressed resulting in decreased blood cell production. Together, thrombocytopenia, leukopenia, and anemia result.

Hematopoietic Changes

- Fatigue (due to anemia)
- Bleeding tendencies (e.g., easy bruising, bleeding gums)
- Risk for infection

Systemic Vascular Congestion. Pressure on gastrointestinal blood vessels from increased fluid accumulation and congestion within the liver causes backflow into the inferior vena cava, leading to elevated hydrostatic pressure and fluid retention.

- Portal hypertension
- Peripheral edema and ascites due to inability of the liver to synthesize albumin (compounded by excess aldosterone, leading to water and sodium retention)
- Varices: esophageal, gastric, and rectal (hemorrhoids)

Inability to Process Bilirubin. Bilirubin is a breakdown product of hemoglobin. It usually goes through the liver to be conjugated (direct bilirubin) and then is excreted in the duodenum as bile. This physiologic process results in normal dark brown stools. When the liver is diseased, bilirubin does not become conjugated. Instead, it remains in the bloodstream as unconjugated (indirect) bilirubin. The skin becomes jaundiced (yellowish). Excessive bilirubin excreted in the kidneys causes color changes in the urine. Bile salts are deposited under the skin, which causes pruritus.

- Jaundice
- Clay-colored stools
- Tea-colored urine
- Pruritus

Decreased Hormone Metabolism. The liver is unable to metabolize the hormones estrogen, testosterone, aldosterone, and antidiuretic hormone.

- Small dilated vessels (spider angiomas)
- Palmar erythema
- Menstrual irregularities
- Impotence
- Fluid and water retention

Inability to Detoxify Medications and Ammonia. The liver detoxifies ammonia and converts it to urea for excretion in the urine. In cirrhosis, the liver is unable to convert the ammonia to urea. The ammonia level rises in the bloodstream and crosses the blood-brain barrier, resulting in neurologic changes.

Neurologic Changes

- Agitation
- Behavioral changes
- Asterixis (uncontrollable flapping tremors of the arms and hands when the patient is asked to extend the upper extremities)
- Confusion
- Hepatic encephalopathy
- Coma

 DIAGNOSTIC CRITERIA

- **Complete blood cell count with differential:** decreased hemoglobin and hematocrit indicating anemia due to decreased nutritional intake or bleeding, thrombocytopenia secondary to decreased clotting factors, leukopenia due to depressed bone marrow
- **Electrolytes:** low sodium due to fluid excess, low potassium secondary to diuretics or poor nutritional intake
- **Coagulation studies:** prolonged bleeding time due to low protein and lack of vitamin K and the inability to synthesize clotting factors
- **Liver enzymes:** alanine aminotransferase (ALT), aspartate aminotransferase (AST), gamma-glutamyl-transferase (GGT), and alkaline phosphatase

elevated due to the release of enzymes as a result of damage to the liver tissues

- **Total, direct, and indirect bilirubin:** serum levels elevated in severe cirrhosis due to inability of the liver to process bile
- **Total protein and serum albumin:** low levels due to low nutritional intake and alteration in protein metabolism leading to ascites and peripheral edema
- **Ammonia:** elevated indicating seriousness of the individual's condition
- **Liver biopsy:** pathologic changes in liver cells; procedure confirms the diagnosis of cirrhosis; check coagulation studies before the procedure; vitamin K may be given before the procedure to decrease the potential for bleeding. After the liver biopsy, it is essential to
  1. Place the patient on the right side with a pillow under the costal margin for at least 6 to 8 hours to put pressure on the punctured site.
  2. Check the vital signs every 15 minutes for 1 hour, then every 30 minutes for 4 hours, and, if stable, every 4 hours for 24 hours.
  3. Assess for symptoms and signs of bleeding (low blood pressure, tachycardia, tenderness around biopsy site).
  4. Assess for pneumothorax (tachypnea, chest pain, shoulder pain, decreased breath sounds).
- **Esophagoscopy:** assess integrity of esophagus; will show if esophageal varices are present; best method to detect varices
- **Liver ultrasound:** evaluate the liver cells; any changes in the liver cells indicating cirrhosis will be visualized by this test

INTERVENTIONS
Conservative

The goal is to control manifestations and to provide comfort.
- The patient should rest to decrease metabolic demands.
- The patient should abstain from alcohol if indicated to reverse or prevent further damage.
- For nutrition, restrict sodium intake (<2 g/day); decrease fluid intake (1 L/day) or base on 24-hour intake and output; initially provide high-protein diet, as the individual's condition deteriorates as reflected in elevated ammonia level, restrict protein; provide high-calorie and low-fat diet; give adequate vitamins and minerals based on laboratory results; and provide total parenteral nutrition (TPN) if necessary.
- Monitor stools, emesis, and GI drainage for blood.
- Monitor vital signs to obtain baseline and then every 4 hours to monitor for signs of shock (restlessness, tachycardia, low blood pressure, tachypnea, decreased urine output, cold clammy skin).
- Record daily weights to monitor fluid overload, which is a gain of 2 lb or more per day ($\geq$1 L of fluid).
- Administer fluids or blood as ordered for replacement; albumin may also be given to maintain oncotic pressure and hence decrease edema and ascites.
- Provide gastric lavage with tap water or as ordered and monitor the effects.
- Assess for manifestations like asterixis indicating impending hepatic encephalopathy.

- Monitor laboratory values such as serum AST, ALT, GGT, and lactate dehydrogenase; direct and indirect bilirubin; and ammonia levels.

Pharmacologic

The goal in pharmacologic therapy is to prevent complications.

- **Antacids/H₂ antagonist:** to reduce gastric acidity
- **Diuretics:** to remove excess fluid and sodium and to resolve hypertension (e.g., furosemide [Lasix], spironolactone [Aldactone], which is the drug of choice because it is a potassium-sparing diuretic)
- **Vitamin K:** to assist in the synthesis of the clotting factors—thereby decreasing the risk of bleeding
- **Beta blockers:** to treat portal hypertension and to prevent esophageal bleeding
- **Lactulose and neomycin:** to eliminate ammonia through the stools and to reduce ammonia-producing bacteria, which subsequently minimizes the risk for hepatic encephalopathy
- **Sclerotherapy:** a sclerosing agent administered through an endoscope into the bleeding esophageal varices; causes thrombosis and eventually seals off the bleeding varices
- **Vasopressin:** can be administered intravenously or intra-arterially; produces vasoconstriction of the vessels of the varices; reduces portal pressure and stops the bleeding; should be used cautiously in patients with coronary artery disease
- **Balloon tamponade:** tube similar to the Sengstaken Blakemore tube inserted to apply pressure on the varices and thus arrest the bleeding

Surgical

The goal in surgical therapy is to correct complications or the causative problem depending on the type of cirrhosis.

- **Biliary:** to relieve obstruction
- **Paracentesis:** to remove excess fluid in the abdomen if conservative measures are unsuccessful or if ascites interferes with breathing
- **Vessel shunts:** shunts reduce variceal pressure by decreasing portal pressure and diverting the fluid to major blood vessels; examples include the Denver and portacaval and splenorenal shunts; splenorenal shunt the most widely used technique
- **Transplantation:** to replace diseased liver with a functioning viable liver

 COMMUNITY CARE

Assessment

- Assess for home care needs depending on the treatment interventions performed.
- Teach the patient and significant others about the importance of rest and skin care, diet regimen, signs and symptoms of complications, and drug treatment.
- Provide the patient with written instructions for all teaching provided.
- Advise the patient to not take any over-the-counter medications without the physician's consent.

Monitoring

- Follow-up with compliance with abstinence from alcohol.
- Monitor attendance at Alcoholics Anonymous meetings.
- Follow-up with laboratory results.

Prevention

- The patient should attend Alcoholics Anonymous to prevent relapse.
- The patient should avoid the risk of contracting hepatitis.
- The patient should avoid over-the-counter medications unless they are prescribed by a physician.

 PROGNOSIS

More than 50% of patients with cirrhosis without complications die within 5 years, and 70% to 95% die within 5 years after complications develop. The survival rate increases if the patient complies with treatment regimen and avoids hepatotoxic substances. Patients who receive a liver transplant for alcoholic cirrhosis have a 1-year survival rate of 85%, a 5-year rate of 70%, and a 10-year rate of 65%. Patients who receive a liver transplant secondary to bleeding varices have a 1-year survival rate of 79% and a 5-year rate of 71%.

 CLINICAL PEARLS

- The liver detoxifies most medications, including acetaminophen, hypnotics, sedatives, and barbiturates; therefore, extreme caution must be used if they have to be administered. Because the liver is not functioning effectively, the accumulation of these medications in the blood may lead to toxicity and death. Continuous (daily) monitoring of ammonia blood levels is essential so that lactulose dosage can be adjusted accordingly.
- Assess for occult or frank blood, which may indicate bleeding GI varices.
- Assess for asterixis early to determine baseline; then assess on every shift. The presence of asterixis indicates the seriousness of the condition and impending encephalopathy.
- There is a greater chance of reversing the damage if the individual stops drinking alcohol in the early stages of the disease.
- Closely monitor for bleeding after liver biopsy.
- Make sure that coagulation studies are normal before the liver biopsy. In most cases, the individual is administered vitamin K to prevent excessive bleeding during the procedure.

NURSING PROBLEM/ DIAGNOSIS	NURSING INTERVENTIONS CLASSIFICATION (NIC)
Imbalanced fluid volume	Fluid electrolyte management
	Hemodynamic regulation
Malnutrition	Nutrition management
Fatigue	Energy management
Risk of bleeding	Bleeding precautions

Food Poisoning

Section 3   Patricia B. Graham

 OVERVIEW

Approximately 76 million cases of foodborne diseases occur each year in the United States. According to the World Health Organization (WHO), illness from contaminated food is one of the most widespread health problems in the contemporary world. The problem is greatly under-reported because persons rarely seek medical help for GI illness. Foodborne disease is often mistakenly passed off as a virus or "stomach flu."

A large degree of foodborne illness is preventable through appropriate hand washing, food handling, refrigeration, and cooking.

 PATHOPHYSIOLOGY

There are five categories of foodborne illness agents.

1. **Bacteria** (responsible for two thirds of all outbreaks for foodborne illness in the United States)
2. **Viruses:** often found in untreated water, feces, or inadequately washed hands
3. **Parasites:** tapeworms, roundworms, and protozoa found in food and water
4. **Food toxins:** may be formed by microorganisms when food is stored at improper temperatures
5. **Unknown organisms:** classification for foodborne illness is used frequently because laboratory analysis was not conducted

 SIGNS AND SYMPTOMS

Signs and symptoms are often similar regardless of the organism, making the specific cause of foodborne illness difficult to identify. Some guidelines are given here.

Bacterial Organisms
Campylobacter

Onset: 1 to 7 days

Transmission: Campylobacter is the most frequently isolated pathogen mentioned on Foodnet sites (Foodborne Disease Active Surveillance Network), a component of the Centers for Disease Control and Prevention sites. This organism is the most commonly identified cause of diarrheal illness in the world. The bacteria live in the intestinal tract of healthy birds, and most raw poultry meat has *Campylobacter* on it.

Symptoms: nausea, abdominal cramps, diarrhea, fever

Associated foods: raw milk, undercooked poultry, raw poultry drippings, raw beef

Salmonella

Onset: 6 to 48 hours

Transmission: This bacterium is widespread in the intestines of birds, reptiles, and mammals. It can be spread to humans through a variety of foods of animal origin.

Symptoms: nausea, vomiting, diarrhea, abdominal cramps, fever, headache, chills

Associated foods: raw or undercooked meats, poultry, eggs, milk, dairy products, shrimp, salad dressing, cream-filled desserts, alfalfa sprouts

Escherichia coli *O157:H7*

Onset: 2 to 5 days

Transmission: E. coli O157:H7 lives in cattle and similar animals. It can produce a deadly toxin that causes illness and death. Illness follows the ingestion of food or water that has been contaminated with microscopic amounts of cow feces.

Symptoms: severe abdominal cramping, diarrhea (initially watery, then bloody), vomiting occasionally, low-grade to no fever

Associated foods: raw or undercooked ground beef, raw milk, some fresh produce, unpasteurized apple juice, alfalfa sprouts

Clostridium perfringens

Onset: 8 to 22 hours

Transmission: This organism grows where there is little or no oxygen. Foods in buffets, casseroles, and gravies are particularly susceptible and must be maintained above 140°F.

Symptoms: diarrhea, abdominal cramps, headache, chills

Associated foods: meat, poultry, stuffing, gravies, cooked foods held at inappropriate temperatures

Listeria

Onset: 2 days to 3 weeks

Transmission: contaminated cow's milk, cheese products; can grow slowly under refrigeration

Symptoms: fever, nausea, vomiting, diarrhea

Associated foods: soft cheese, deli meat, poultry, seafood, improperly refrigerated milk

Staphylococcus

Onset: 1 to 6 hours

Transmission: carried by humans in the nose and throat; produces a toxin that causes illness within a few hours

Symptoms: severe nausea, vomiting, diarrhea, abdominal cramps

Associated foods: custard, cream-filled baked goods, ham, tongue, cooked poultry, dressing, potato salad, cream sauces

Shigella

Onset: 12 to 50 hours

Transmission: infected person or food handler, contaminated foods, infected water

Symptoms: abdominal cramps; diarrhea with blood, mucus, or pus; fever; vomiting; chills

Associated foods: salads (tuna, chicken, potato, macaroni, shrimp), raw vegetables, untreated water

Clostridium botulinum

Onset: Can vary: 4 hours to 8 days

Transmission: underheated low-acid foods that are improperly processed or
  stored; botulism rare but very dangerous

Symptoms: nausea, vomiting, diarrhea, fatigue, headache, double vision,
  droopy eyelids, muscle paralysis, difficulty breathing; fatal in 3 days if
  not treated

Associated foods: low-acid foods improperly processed; often associated with
  home canning (green beans, etc.)

Viral Agents: Norwalk Virus

Onset: 24 to 48 hours

Transmission: untreated water, wells, recreational lakes, swimming pools,
  water on cruise ships, infected handlers

Symptoms: nausea, vomiting, diarrhea, abdominal pain, low-grade fever

Associated foods: water (see Transmission), shellfish, salad, raw or undercooked clams and oysters

Parasites

Parasites such as tapeworms and roundworms are present in food and water,
but they pose little threat in industrialized countries.

Food Toxins

Food toxins, one of which is *ciguatera,* are formed by microorganisms when
food is stored at improper temperatures. Ciguatera is a sporadic form of human
poisoning caused by the consumption of contaminated subtropical and tropical
marine finfish (e.g., barracuda, grouper, snapper, mackerel).

DIAGNOSTIC CRITERIA

Food poisoning or foodborne illness is diagnosed with specific laboratory
tests that identify the causative organism. For example, *Campylobacter, Salmonella,* and *E. coli* O157:H7 can be identified in stool cultures. Viruses are
more difficult because they are so small and difficult to culture. Because
persons with GI symptoms often do not report their illness, many cases of
foodborne illness go undiagnosed. The Centers for Disease Control and Prevention estimates that 38 cases of salmonellosis occur for every case that is
actually reported to health authorities.

Foodborne illness is often suspected when large numbers of persons develop
GI symptoms at the same time. The illness may then be traced to a common
food, and the diagnosis may be based on the symptoms experienced and the
time of onset of illness (see descriptions of organisms and symptoms later).

INTERVENTIONS

Many people self-treat the symptoms with antidiarrheal drugs, including
preparations such as bismuth subsalicylate (Pepto-Bismol). Care must be taken
in the administration of antidiarrheal drugs, because they may interfere with
elimination of the harmful agents from the body. Patients who become dehydrated through prolonged vomiting and diarrhea are at risk for electrolyte
imbalance and require intravenous fluid replacement until they are able to

retain fluids by mouth. If they can take fluids by mouth, preparations such as Pedialyte and Oralyte will help to replace the fluid and electrolyte losses. Gatorade does not replace the losses correctly in foodborne illness and should not be used. Antibiotics are not usually needed, and symptoms should disappear after 1 to 2 days. One instance in which antibiotics are useful is with traveler's diarrhea, which is frequently caused by invasive *E. coli, Shigella,* or *Campylobacter*; a combination of ciprofloxacin (Cipro) and loperamide (Imodium) has been shown to be effective with travelers. Persons with botulism will have to be treated with an antitoxin.

 COMMUNITY CARE

The major issue in community care for foodborne illness is prevention! Many communities recognize this and have programs in place in the schools and other facilities to educate the public about proper food handling. Regular inspections of restaurants and food-handling industries help to enforce the standards for keeping foods safe. Restaurant ratings are shared with the public, and individuals can choose not to eat at certain restaurants if their health practices are marginal. There are numerous Web sites that provide information about foodborne illness for consumers.

The International Food Information Council gives 12 food-handling tips to avoid foodborne illness:

1. Do not buy cans or jars with dents, cracks, or bulging lids.
2. Never eat raw meat, poultry, seafood, or eggs.
3. Cook raw meat, poultry, seafood, or eggs thoroughly to at least 165°F to kill any bacteria present.
4. Thoroughly reheat leftovers.
5. Promptly refrigerate cooked meat and poultry in small shallow containers. Remove stuffing from chicken and turkey and refrigerate separately.
6. Refrigerate perishable food immediately.
7. Store canned goods in a cool dry place and use within 1 year. Never store above the stove or in a damp area.
8. Do not thaw food on the counter at room temperature where bacteria can grow. Thaw in the refrigerator or microwave.
9. Keep work areas clean. Wash hands, utensils, and cutting boards in hot soapy water before preparing food and after handling raw meat or poultry.
10. Use a plastic or nonporous cutting board. Wash cutting boards in dishwasher or hot soapy water after use.
11. Keep pets away from food, cooking and eating surfaces, and equipment.
12. Do not take chances—if in doubt, throw it out!

 PROGNOSIS

The prognosis is good for most individual incidents of foodborne illness. The illness is often mild and will run its course within 1 or 2 days. For potentially severe illness such as botulism and infection with *E. coli* O157:H7, prompt diagnosis is necessary followed by immediate treatment, or death may occur.

On the larger scale, workers in any part of the food distribution chain need to become and remain diligent in the prevention of foodborne illness. In many instances, it is a matter of conscience: only the workers know whether they have washed their hands, but the results of not doing so can be devastating and can affect masses of individuals with a problem that is preventable.

 CLINICAL PEARLS

○ Foodborne illness is highly preventable through education and follow-through on the 12 food-handling tips.
○ Assess individuals who present with GI illness for foodborne illness and treat potentially dangerous forms.
○ Wash your hands!
○ When in doubt, throw it out!
○ Replace fluids lost through vomiting with electrolyte solutions (Pedialyte, not Gatorade)!

NURSING PROBLEM/ DIAGNOSIS	NURSING INTERVENTIONS CLASSIFICATION (NIC)
Deficient fluid volume	Diarrhea management
	Fluid/electrolyte management
Prevention	Surveillance
	Health education

Hepatitis

Section 4   Beverly George-Gay

 OVERVIEW

Hepatitis is inflammation of the liver. It can be caused by a number of factors, including drugs, chemicals, alcohol, and viral infections. *Toxic agent- and drug-induced hepatitis* is caused by the inhalation, ingestion, or parenteral administration of a number of pharmacologic and chemical agents that cause direct injury (hepatotoxic) to liver cells (Table 16-4-1). In *alcohol-induced hepatitis* (alcoholic hepatitis), alcohol causes the injury. It may occur concurrently with or as a precursor to cirrhosis (see Section 2). *Viral hepatitis*

Table 16-4-1. Hepatotoxic Agents

Erythromycin	Thiazide diuretics
Tetracycline	6-Mercaptopurine
Ketoconazole	Methotrexate
Zidovudine	Arsenic
Phenytoin	Carbon tetrachloride
Methyldopa	Chloroform
Propylthiouracil	Gold compounds
Halothane	Mercury
Isoniazide	Phosphorus
Sulfonamide	Anabolic steroids
Acetaminophen	

describes infections of the liver caused by viruses. Viral hepatitis can occur on an acute or, if lasting longer than 6 months, chronic basis. Six hepatitis viruses have been recognized: hepatitis A (HAV), B (HBV), C, (HCV) D (HDV), E (HEV), and G (HGV) virus. HAV and HEV are transmitted enterically. HBV, HCV, and HDV are transmitted parenterally. Acute viral hepatitis may also occur during the course of other viral infections, including human cytomegalovirus, Epstein-Barr virus, herpes simplex virus, yellow fever virus, coxsackievirus, and rubella.

Acute viral hepatitis is the most common cause of hepatitis. It affects young adults most commonly between the ages of 15 and 39 years. More than 90% of cases of acute viral hepatitis in the United States are caused by HAV, HBV, or HCV. Acute infection with HBV, HCV, and HDV can progress to chronic hepatitis. More than 5 million Americans have chronic hepatitis. It is the leading cause of chronic liver disease, liver cirrhosis, and liver cancer (Table 16-4-2 provides epidemiologic features).

 PATHOPHYSIOLOGY

After exposure to causative agents, there is widespread inflammation resulting in necrosis of hepatic cells. In viral hepatitis, the virus enters the host hepatocytes to replicate. A cell-mediated response results in hepatocyte lysis as host immune cells attack infected hepatocytes in attempts to eliminate the virus. Edema from the inflammatory process surrounding the bile canaliculi may obstruct bile flow, resulting in obstructive jaundice. Obstructive jaundice occurs when bile (with its conjugated bilirubin) accumulates in the liver and is forced into the bloodstream, resulting in hyperbilirubinemia. The increased plasma concentrations of bilirubin result in the discoloration of body tissues.

In mild cases of hepatitis, very little parenchymal damage occurs. Liver cells regenerate, and normal hepatic function returns in 2 to 5 months. Severe cases are associated with acute fulminant hepatitis. *Acute fulminant hepatitis* is a severe condition that occurs in a few patients with hepatitis. It is characterized by massive hepatic necrosis with the onset of coagulopathy or encephalopathy, or both, within 4 to 6 weeks of the onset of liver disease. It results in hepatocellular failure with a high mortality rate. *Chronic hepatitis* is characterized by persistent inflammation with abnormal liver functions for longer than 6 months. It can progress to liver cirrhosis.

Classifications of Viral Hepatitis

Hepatitis A. Formerly called *infectious hepatitis,* hepatitis A is caused by a small enterovirus containing RNA that enters the GI tract and replicates and then spreads to the liver, where it infects and multiplies in the hepatocytes. It has an incubation period of 15 to 45 days. The virus is excreted in the stool for 2 weeks before the onset of symptoms, so the patient is highly infectious at this time. Fulminant hepatitis occurs in 0.1% of cases, and there is no chronic form.

Hepatitis B. Formerly called *serum hepatitis,* hepatitis B is a more serious disease caused by a double-stranded DNA virus. The virus is transmitted to the liver parenterally, where it replicates in hepatocytes and sheds into the bloodstream. The blood becomes highly infectious. The incubation period ranges from 45 to 180 days. Fulminant hepatitis occurs in 1% of cases.

Table 16-4-2. Epidemiologic Virus Features

VIRUS	INCIDENCE	TRANSMISSION	RISK GROUPS	PCS
HAV	HAV accounts for 32% of reported cases of hepatitis in the United States. From 125,000 to 200,000 infections are reported annually, with 100 deaths per year due to fulminant hepatitis.	Fecal/oral, food/water	Household/sexual contacts of those infected, international travelers	No
HBV	Approximately 300,000 new cases are reported annually; of these, 90% will recover and clear the virus, and 10% will progress to a chronic state. About 1.25 million Americans have chronic HBV infection, with an estimated 4000 related deaths each year.	Blood, sexual, perinatal	Intravenous drug users, health care workers exposed to blood, sexually active heterosexuals and homosexual males, sexual/household contacts of those infected, hemodialysis patients	Yes
HCV	Annual new infections per year have declined from 242,000 during the 1980s to 36,000 by 1996 due to new therapies. An estimated 3.9 million Americans have been infected with HCV, of whom 2.7 million are chronically infected, resulting in about 8000 to 10,000 deaths per year.	Blood, sexual, perinatal	Intravenous drug users, health care workers exposed to blood, persons with multiple sex partners, sexual contacts of those infected, recipients of clotting factors before 1987 and transfusion before 1992, hemodialysis patients	Yes
HDV	The overall intravenous prevalence for HDV is low in the United States, largely restricted to intravenous drug users and those receiving clotting factors. A higher prevalence is noted in other countries: Italy, Eastern Europe, Colombia, Venezuela, Western Asia.	Blood, sexual	Same as for HBV	Yes
HEV	Virtually all cases of HEV infections in the United States have been reported among travelers returning from underdeveloped countries. Case-fatality rates are low except among pregnant women, in whom the rate may approach 20%.	Fecal-oral, fecally contaminated drinking water	International travelers	No
HGV	HGV is transmitted via blood transfusion and has been found to coexist with HCV. The prevalence is recognized as high worldwide, but it is associated with mild or no clinical illness.	Blood, other routes not well studied	Intravenous drug users, hemodialysis patients, transfusion recipients	No

HAV through HGV, hepatitis A through G virus, respectively; PCS, progression to chronic state.

Approximately 5% of patients fail to eliminate the virus completely and become persistently infected. Chronic infection may persist with minimal liver damage *(chronic persistent hepatitis)* or with aggressive parenchymal destruction *(chronic active hepatitis).* Persistent infection is associated with the development of hepatocellular carcinoma.

Hepatitis C. Formerly called *non-A non-B hepatitis,* hepatitis C is caused by an RNA virus that infects in a manner similar to HBV, but more than 85% of patients will develop chronic infection. Most HCV-infected persons are aged 30 to 49 years. Only 25% to 30% of HCV cases are symptomatic. Injected drug use accounts for 60% of HCV infections. The acute phase may be mild, so many individuals do not know that they are infected and serve as a source of transmission. Hepatitis C has an incubation period of 15 to 180 days. Forty percent of all cases of chronic liver disease are related to HCV. End-stage liver disease related to HCV is the most frequent indication for liver transplantation.

Hepatitis D. Called the *delta virus,* HDV is a defective RNA virus that requires the helper function of HBV to replicate. Therefore, it occurs only in patients infected with HBV. HDV infection can occur either as a coinfection with HBV or as a superinfection of persons with HBV infection. In persons with HBV/HDV coinfection, the risk of fulminant hepatitis increases. Of those with superinfection, 90% will develop chronic liver disease. Therefore, the addition of HDV increases the severity of liver disease in patients infected with HBV. The incubation period is approximately 21 to 140 days.

Hepatitis E. HEV is an enterically transmitted RNA virus with an incubation period of approximately 15 to 65 days. Infection is similar to HAV, with no chronic state. Infection is usually mild, resolving within a few weeks with no sequelae, except in pregnant women, in whom it can be fatal.

Hepatitis F. Viral particles found by an investigator in 1994 were presumed to cause hepatitis and were labeled "hepatitis F." These findings were never confirmed and may have been incidental. Therefore, hepatitis F is not confirmed, but its position in the nomenclature has been occupied.

Hepatitis G. Newly identified HGV is an RNA virus, classified as a flavivirus. The virus has been found to exist in blood and can be transmitted via transfusion. Infection is commonly subclinical, sometimes only identified by a transient increase in serum transaminases. Hepatitis G does not appear to cause chronic liver disease. The long-term disease significance has not been established.

 SIGNS AND SYMPTOMS

Most cases of hepatitis are asymptomatic. There is an incubation period for viral hepatitis that varies depending on the virus. Jaundice is the hallmark finding. Signs and symptoms when present can be classified into three phases. Peak infectivity occurs during the last few days of the incubation period and the beginning of acute symptoms.

Preicteric Phase. This phase precedes jaundice and may involve GI symptoms such as nausea, vomiting, diarrhea, and constipation. Upper respiratory symptoms may also be noted. Fatigue, malaise, anorexia, and low-grade fever are common. Food odors become offensive, and smokers often become repelled by the smell of smoke. Right upper quadrant pain and weight loss may be present.

Icteric Phase. This phase occurs with the appearance of jaundice. The GI symptoms frequently remain. Urine may be dark owing to the presence of bile, and pruritus may occur as a result of bile salts beneath the skin. The liver may become tender and enlarged (hepatomegaly). Splenomegaly may also occur.

Posticteric Phase. This recovery phase usually begins with the resolution of jaundice. Recovery of liver functions occurs within 2 to 4 months. It may take 2 to 6 months for diagnostic criteria to return to normal.

 DIAGNOSTIC CRITERIA

Viral hepatitis can be diagnosed by the presence of antigenic markers on the virus or on parts of the virus, from the antibodies (immunoglobulins [Igs]) that the body produces to combat the identified antigens (serologic markers), or both. A test that allows for the detection and quantification of viral concentrations by amplification was developed called the polymerase chain reaction (PCR) test. This test allows for the detection of the more recently identified hepatitis viruses.

Hepatitis A. Anti-HAV antibodies are diagnostic for hepatitis A. IgM class anti-HAV indicates recent or acute infection. However, risk for transmission during this time is low, because the virus is spread before the onset of symptoms. IgG class anti-HAV peaks during the recovery phase, provides long-term immunity, and indicates past exposure.

Hepatitis B. HBV has one surface antigen and two core antigens; the body produces antibodies against all three.

Hepatitis B Surface (Australian) Antigen. If present, hepatitis B surface (Australian) antigen (HBsAg) indicates the infectious state. The antibody to HBsAg, anti-HBs, indicates prior exposure and immunity.

Hepatitis B e-Antigen. Hepatitis B e-antigen (HBeAg), when present early, indicates a highly infectious state. Persistence indicates progression to chronic hepatitis. Anti-HBe, the antibody for HBeAg, indicates resolution of the acute illness.

Hepatitis B Core Antigen. Hepatitis B core antigen (HBcAg) is not useful as a serum marker because it is mainly found in liver cells. Anti-HBc, however, is the most sensitive indicator of hepatitis B. IgM class anti-HBc indicates recent infection, followed by IgG antibodies, which indicate chronic infection.

Hepatitis C. HCV can be detected with PCR testing. Anti-HCV antibodies can be detected, but the difference between acute and past infection cannot be distinguished.

Hepatitis D. Hepatitis delta antigen (HDAg) indicates acute infection. Anti-HDV IgM antibody indicates recent infection. IgG class indicates past infection.

Hepatitis E. HEV can be detected by PCR testing. Anti-HEV antibodies IgM class are diagnostic for acute or early HEV infection.

Hepatitis G. HGV can be detected by PCR testing.

Bilirubin. Levels are elevated during the preicteric period. Urine bilinogen levels may also be elevated. Total serum bilirubin is divided into two forms: *direct (conjugated) bilirubin,* which is primarily excreted through the GI tract, and *indirect (unconjugated) bilirubin,* which circulates freely primarily in the bloodstream. Increased amounts of conjugated bilirubin enter the bloodstream as a result of obstructive jaundice. Unconjugated bilirubin rises due to hemoglobin breakdown during hemolytic conditions. Urinary output of urobilinogen (an end product formed by the action of bacteria on conjugated bilirubin) is increased. Bile appears in urine when serum bilirubin levels reach higher than 2 mg/dL, increasing urine bilirubin levels (normal: direct bilirubin, 0 to 0.3 mg/dL; indirect bilirubin, 0.1 to 1.0 mg/dL; urobilinogen, 0.1 to 1.1 U/dL or 0.5 to 4.0 mg/24-hr specimen; urine bilirubin <0.02 or negative).

Serum Transaminases (or Liver Enzymes or Aminotransferases). These are indicators of liver cell inflammation and necrosis and are highly elevated in viral hepatitis. They usually rise before the onset of jaundice. AST and ALT are the most specific enzymes (normal: AST, 8 to 20 U/L; ALT, 4 to 46 U/L).

Prothrombin Time and Activated Partial Thromboplastin Time. These may be prolonged owing to liver cell damage, because the liver is responsible for synthesizing clotting factors (see Chapter 12, Section 2).

Complete Blood Cell Count. A leukocytosis and monocytosis may occur with an increase in large atypical lymphocytes.

Viral Load Testing. Measures the serum viral particle concentration. Used to decide on and monitor the response to pharmacologic therapy for viral hepatitis.

INTERVENTIONS
Supportive Care

Interventions for drug-, toxic agent–, or alcohol-induced hepatitis involve removal of the causative factors with supportive care. For acute viral hepatitis, the goals are to reduce symptoms with the return of normal liver functions and to prevent transmission. Patients who are hospitalized have severe disease or fulminant hepatic failure.

Rest. Rest allows the liver to regenerate, prevents undue fatigue, and decreases metabolic demand. Bed rest with light ambulation may be needed. Institute measures to prevent complications of prolonged bed rest (see Table 21-2-1 and Chapter 15, Section 3). If the fatigue level increases, assess for progression of liver dysfunction or inadequate caloric intake.

Fluid Maintenance. Encourage intake of 3000 mL/24 hr if not contraindicated. Monitor for signs of dehydration (increased thirst, orthostatic hypotension). Intravenous fluids may be needed in severe cases of vomiting. Fluids also decrease dermatologic side effects. Electrolytes should be monitored and replaced as needed.

Bleeding Precautions. Monitor for decreases in hemoglobin and hematocrit, which may indicate bleeding. Monitor urine and feces for occult blood. Monitor prothrombin time and activated partial thromboplastin time for prolongation. Teach the patient to use soft-bristle toothbrushes and electric razors. Report prolonged bleeding, bluish-purple discolorations, and nose bleeds.

Nutrition. A high-carbohydrate, low-fat diet is usually recommended. The carbohydrates provide calories for the much-needed energy and prevent further weight loss. Fat intake should be low because bile may not be available to digest it. Protein intake should be high to assist in healing but may be restricted during symptomatic phases because the ability of the liver to metabolize protein byproducts is impaired. Vitamin supplements are usually recommended. Vitamin K may be required if prothrombin time and activated partial thromboplastin time are prolonged.

Pruritus Management. Avoid the use of soaps and alkaline products. Oil-based lotions (Alpha-Keri) are soothing. Antihistamines are helpful but must be used with caution at low doses because they are cleared by the liver. Keep nails short and smooth. If the patient is confused or obtunded, soft mittens may have to be applied to prevent scratching. Teach the patient to avoid hot baths and tight-fitting clothing.

Pharmacologic Therapy

Antiemetics. These agents are useful in patients with nausea and promote food intake. Be alert to drugs that may be toxic or have prolonged actions when liver functions are impaired, such as prochlorperazine (Compazine). Monitor the environment for odors that are offensive to the patient.

Antiviral Therapy. This is useful for chronic forms of viral hepatitis. It requires considerable commitment by both the patient and health care provider. Interferon alfa is an injectable antiviral agent that has been mildly successful in the treatment of chronic hepatitis B and C. It is used in combination with ribavirin (an oral antiviral agent) with better results. Combination therapy is now preferred to monotherapy. Absolute contraindications to interferon alfa alone or in combination with ribavirin include pregnancy, psychosis/suicidal ideation, myocardial infarction/cardiac dysrhythmias, and renal insufficiency (creatinine clearance <50 mL/min). Monitor complete blood cell count closely throughout therapy because interferon alfa has a depressive effect on the bone marrow. Irritability, weight loss, thinning hair, and diarrhea may also occur, but these are reversible with cessation of therapy. Combination therapy may result in anorexia and nausea and vomiting. Antiviral therapy is considered successful with normalization of ALT levels and loss of virus detection by PCR testing.

Surgical Management

Liver transplantation has been a successful treatment for chronic active hepatitis and for fulminant hepatic failure for several years. As with any transplant, it requires the availability of the cadaveric organ and life-long immunosuppression. Living-donor liver transplantation is a more recent option for adults with fulminant hepatitis; a right liver lobe is transplanted. This procedure is riskier for the donor, but results have been positive.

 COMMUNITY CARE

Most cases of hepatitis are self-limiting and are managed in the community. Patients should be taught to monitor for signs of worsening disease in the case of a relapse or for fulminant disease; signs include altered mental status, fluid retention, ascites, bleeding, and hypoglycemia. Close follow-up should be maintained for at least 1 year past the acute phase to monitor liver function tests and serologic markers, to assess disease progression to the chronic state, and to prevent complications.

Bleeding precautions, nutritional therapy, and pruritus management should be taught and reinforced as described earlier. Over-the-counter medications must be avoided (Table 16-4-1), especially acetaminophen. Alcohol should be avoided during and up to 6 months after acute hepatitis. Referral to drug and alcohol treatment programs is needed for patients with these problems.

Prevention of Transmission

- Teach and reinforce proper hand-washing techniques.
- Do not share personal items such as toothbrushes, razors, and linen.
- Sex should be avoided or condoms should be used diligently until test results are negative.

Pharmacologic Prophylaxis

Hepatitis A vaccine is recommended for travelers to underdeveloped countries and places where sanitation is unsatisfactory and for household contacts of acute cases. Immune globulin is used for short-term protection after exposure.

Hepatitis B vaccine protects 90% to 95% of healthy people from contracting hepatitis B. The Centers for Disease Control and Prevention recommends universal vaccination for all infants. Health care workers and sexual partners of chronic carriers should also be vaccinated.

 PROGNOSIS

The prognosis for patients with hepatitis is generally good, with an overall mortality rate of approximately 1%. Most patients recover completely within 3 months. Fulminant hepatitis occurs in a few patients with a mortality rate of 25% to 90%.

Chronic liver disease is the 10th leading cause of death in the United States among adults. It accounts for 1% (~25,000) of all deaths annually. Chronic hepatitis accounts for more than 40% of chronic liver diseases (see Table 16-4-1 for additional information on prognosis).

 CLINICAL PEARLS

- Tattoo application does not appear to be a risk factor for chronic viral hepatitis.
- Signs of fulminant hepatitis include altered mental status, fluid retention, ascites, bleeding, and hypoglycemia.
- Acute infection with HBV, HCV, and HDV can progress to chronic hepatitis.
- Combination therapy with interferon alfa and ribavirin is preferred to monotherapy for the treatment of chronic viral hepatitis.
- Therapy with interferon alfa can produce bone marrow depression, so complete blood cell count should be monitored throughout therapy.
- Be alert for medications that provide comfort measures because they may have toxic or prolonged actions in a patient with an impaired liver.

NURSING PROBLEM/ DIAGNOSIS	NURSING INTERVENTIONS CLASSIFICATION (NIC)
Fatigue	Energy management
Anorexia	Nutrition management
	Fluid/electrolyte management
Transmission prevention	Health education
	Health screening
	Sexual counseling

Inflammatory Bowel Disease

Section 5   Diane Anthony Manghram ▪ Beverly George-Gay

 OVERVIEW

Crohn's disease (CD) and ulcerative colitis (UC) are both inflammatory bowel diseases (IBDs) that result from a complex multifactorial interplay among immune, genetic, and environmental factors. Similarities between the two involve chronic recurrent episodes of acute inflammation characterized by diarrhea, fecal urgency, and weight loss, with periods of remission.

The causes for IBD (both CD and UC) are unknown. Theories of causation include the following:

- *Environmental agents:* more common in industrial countries; smoke and dietary substances may play a role
- *Infectious agents:* mucosal changes similar to infectious diarrhea, but no pathogen has been found
- *Genetic factors:* a familial tendency and a high concordance in twins
- *Immunologic factors:* may involve self-antibodies and other factors, because other immune-related disorders are usually present

Risk factors for IBD consist of family history of the disease. It is prevalent in twins and those of Jewish descent and among white populations. It is more common in industrial countries. The relative risk is higher in smokers. The prevalence is equal in men and women. The age of onset for CD is usually 10 to 30 years, and for UC it is 10 to 40 years, but it can occur at any age for both.

The prevalence of CD is estimated at 20 to 40:100,000 population, with an increase that may be related to more accurate reporting. UC affects approximately 70 to 150:100,000 population in the United States.

 PATHOPHYSIOLOGY

CD is a slowly progressive disabling inflammatory disorder that affects the GI tract. Inflammation affects some segments, leaving other segments healthy and creating "skip" lesions on the intestinal wall. This discontinuous pattern distinguishes CD from UC. Most lesions are deep with cobblestone projections of inflamed tissue. Healing lesions result in fibrous scarred tissue, which may cause obstruction. Lesions penetrate the entire depth of the intestinal wall, often producing fistulas. Fistula formations may occur between loops of intestines or extend into the anal and perianal areas (bladder, rectum, or vagina). Inflammation and intestinal wall changes and fistula formation result in malabsorption, which produces symptoms that range from mild to severe depending on the areas affected.

Lesions can occur anywhere in the GI tract, but they usually localize to certain regions. Disease of the terminal ileum is most common (40% of patients), colonic disease affects 30% of all patients, small bowel disease affects 30% of patients, and upper GI disease (stomach, esophagus, and duodenum) affects only 5% of patients.

UC is a chronic inflammatory disorder that affects the mucosal and submucosal layers of the walls of the colon and rectum. The site of involvement usually begins in the rectum and extends continuously throughout the extent of the colon, sometimes involving the terminal ileum. The affected mucosa becomes hyperemic and edematous with a dark red, velvety appearance and the development of abscesses. Ulcers develop in the submucosal layers due to small erosions from ruptured abscesses and tissue necrosis of the mucosa. The intestinal lumen narrows owing to edema and thickening of the muscularis mucosa. Mucosal destruction produces diarrhea with varying amounts of blood and purulent mucus. Loss of mucosal surface area prevents water reabsorption, resulting in large amounts of watery diarrhea.

Complications

Complications for both CD and UC include toxic megacolon, perforation, and cancer. In *toxic megacolon,* inflammation extends into the muscularis, inhibiting the ability of the colon to contract. This causes significant colonic distention and may result in perforation. Toxic megacolon is often seen in UC patients and rarely seen in CD patients. *Perforation* is a common complication of both diseases. In CD, perforations result from lesions that penetrate all layers of the bowel wall, creating fistula tracts into the peritoneum. Perforations in UC are usually due to toxic megacolon. In either case, perforation results in peritonitis (see Chapter 16, Section 9), which can be life threatening. Patients who have UC for longer than 10 years have an increased incidence of *colon cancer.* The incidence decreases for patients with CD, but it remains higher than that of the general population.

 ## SIGNS AND SYMPTOMS

Patients with IBD have a clinical course of periods of remissions and exacerbations. Findings will vary depending on the region involved. Some patients have mild symptoms and no physical findings, whereas others have severe symptoms. Nonbloody diarrhea is the most common symptom of CD, accompanied by weight loss and abdominal pain. Anemia with resultant complaints of fatigue and fever are common. As the disease progresses, anorexia, malnutrition, fever, and more systemic manifestations occur.

The cardinal symptom of UC is bloody diarrhea. Symptoms depend on disease severity.

Approximately 60% of individuals with UC have mild UC. Diarrhea consists of semiformed stools that contain a small amount of blood. Remissions may last for weeks to months; no other systemic manifestations may occur. In moderate UC, bloody diarrhea occurs four or five times a day, with abdominal cramp, fatigue, anorexia, weight loss, and intermittent fever. The abdominal cramps may awaken individuals at night and are relieved by defecation. Severe UC has an acute onset and rapid course and affects 15% of individuals with UC. Diarrhea is a major symptom that is usually profuse and bloody, occurring anywhere from 10 to 20 times per day. Dehydration and weight loss usually occur due to fluid loss, bleeding, and inflammation. Various complications, such as obstruction caused by edema, strictures, and fibrosis, are commonly associated with this form. Perforation may occur but is rare in UC.

Extraintestinal and systemic symptoms of IBD commonly involve every system in the body and are seen more commonly in CD than in UC. Systemic complications result from malabsorption of needed vitamins and minerals and include arthritis, iritis, skin lesions, liver disease, and renal stones. Nutritional deficiencies occur, such as weight loss, iron deficiency anemia, folate deficiency, hypokalemia, hypoalbuminemia, dehydration, osteomalacia, and deficiency in vitamins B, C, and D. These are more common in CD.

Peripheral arthritis, or arthralgia, is a common symptom that occurs in 4% to 23% of patients with IBD. It affects the joints of the upper and lower extremities (e.g., hips, ankles, wrist, and elbows). Liver findings, such as cholelithiasis, fatty liver, cirrhosis, and cholangitis, are seen in 4% to 5% of patients. Kidney stones and urethral obstruction occur in approximately 4% to 23% of patients. Aphthous ulcerations are small ulcers located in the mouth that commonly appear during severe attacks of the IBD as well with nutritional deficiencies associated with underlying bowel disease.

Ocular system involvement occurs in approximately 4% to 10% of patients as uveitis (inflammation of the middle layer of the eye wall) or episcleritis (inflammation of the outer coating of the eye). Both problems may cause sensitivity to light, blurred vision, pain, and redness of the eye. Other ocular problems include corneal ulcerations and retinopathy. Keratopathy (a corneal abnormality with white deposits at the edge of the cornea) is seen in CD, without pain or visual loss and requiring no treatment, and dry eyes may occur, possibly due to vitamin A deficiency.

Two classic cutaneous manifestations are erythema nodosum and pyoderma gangrenosum. *Erythema nodosum* manifests as reddened areas without breakdown located on the front of the legs below the knees or on the arms. This occur in 1% to 10% of patients with CD and 1% to 5% of patients with UC. *Pyoderma gangrenosum* is an ulcerative skin lesion that occurs on the legs and is associated with early IBD. Approximately 5% of patients with UC and 1% of patients with CD develop this problem.

DIAGNOSTIC CRITERIA

Blood Tests

- **Complete blood count:** to identify anemia, leukocytosis, and thrombocytosis for both diseases
- **Electrolyte studies:** may identify imbalances as well as renal alterations; hypokalemia due to losses by diarrhea is common; hypoalbuminemia may also be noted due to protein malabsorption
- **Erythrocyte sedimentation rates**: elevated; measures the presence of active inflammation or infection; used to monitor response to therapy
- **Liver function tests:** abnormal findings may be suggestive of pericholangitis
- **Nutritional status**: nutrition laboratory test results (albumin, prealbumin, transferrin) are low
- **Stool examination**: occult (hidden) blood often present in CD and frequently present in UC; frank blood frequently in UC; stools for parasites, *Clostridium difficile* toxin, ova, and parasites examined to rule out bacterial causes of colitis
- **Sigmoidoscopy**: flexible sigmoidoscope used to view the rectum and sigmoid colon; useful for initial diagnosis and obtaining biopsy sample; avoid cathartics and enemas in patients with UC before tests as these will exacerbate the condition
- **Colonoscopy:** to diagnose and determine the extent of colonic disease; necessary to obtain biopsy samples, which differentiate CD from UC

through histologic examination; also screens for colon cancer in patients with long-term colonic CD; contraindicated during acute flare-ups or in CD when there are known fistulas or deep ulcerations present, as hemorrhage or perforation may result

- **Barium enema**: to identify intestinal wall irregularities, which assists in diagnosis; less sensitive in mild disease states; double-barrel technique is more sensitive and has become the standard for evaluating patients with colitis; in acutely ill patients with severe colitis, the cleansing enemas that normally precede this procedure can cause toxic megacolon and should be avoided
- **Upper GI and small bowel series**: to diagnose upper GI CD, stricture, fistulas, loss of smooth mucosa, prominent undermined ulcers, skip lesion areas, and narrowed lumen; performed in patients with suspected UC to exclude the diagnosis of CD
- **Upper GI endoscopy (gastroscopy):** for diagnosis and biopsy of suspected upper GI CD
- **CT with oral contrast medium:** to define abdominal mass and abscess; to identify abdominal fistulas or any suspected complications
- **Abdominal radiographs:** to define colonic distention in acute severe disease; also used when barium enema and colonoscopy are contraindicated

INTERVENTIONS

The goals of treatment for IBD are the induction and maintenance of remission, prevention of disease complications, and optimization of surgical outcomes.

Blood, Fluid, and Electrolyte Management

Fluid and electrolyte losses from diarrhea or fistula drainage are corrected by intravenous replacement. In severe cases of colitis, the patient is placed on NPO status because even clear liquids can stimulate colonic activity. Intake, output, and daily weight measures are obtained to closely assess fluid gains and losses. Closely monitor for hypotension. Electrolyte levels should be monitored daily. Assess for signs of alterations, especially hypokalemia. Replace electrolytes as prescribed (see Chapter 11, Section 3). Monitor for rectal bleeding, and assess hemoglobin and hematocrit for decreases. Monitor stools for gross and occult blood. Replace blood and blood products as prescribed (see Chapter 2, Section 3).

Pharmacologic Therapy

Pharmacologic therapy reduces inflammation, treats infection, and aims to alleviate symptoms. Classes of medications used to perform these functions include aminosalicylates, glucocorticoids, immunosuppressants, and antibiotics. Antidiarrheal agents may be used with caution. Therapy with more than one of these agents is required.

Aminosalicylates are drugs derived from salicylic acid. They are used in the acute treatment of IBD and to maintain remission of symptoms in mild to moderate UC and in CD after acute symptoms have been managed.

Sulfasalazine (Azulfidine): gradually increase dosage to minimize adverse effects. Common adverse reactions are nausea, vomiting, diarrhea, abdominal pain, serum sickness, and drug fever.

Mesalamine (Asacol, Pentasa, Rowasa): used in the acute treatment of active small bowel CD and for maintenance therapy in both CD and UC. Available in rectal suppository and rectal enema suspension. Adverse reactions to mesalamine oral preparation include diarrhea, dizziness, nausea, rhinitis, abdominal pain, abdominal cramps, unusual tiredness, weakness, and vomiting. Adverse reactions to mesalamine rectal preparation include headache, dizziness, fatigue, malaise, abdominal pain, cramps, diarrhea, nausea, pancreatitis, itching, rash, urticaria, hair loss, wheezing, and fever.

Olsalazine (Dipentum): indicated for pancolitis and maintenance of remission in patients intolerant of sulfasalazine. Adverse reactions include diarrhea, abdominal pain, abdominal cramps, nausea, headache, skin rash, erythema nodosum, second-degree heart block, and dyspepsia.

Glucocorticoids relieve symptoms of IBD through their anti-inflammatory actions on the GI mucosa and are used for the induction of remission but not for maintenance.

Prednisone (Aristocort, Deltasone, liquid prednisone): indicated as a primary treatment for acute exacerbations of moderate to severe disease. Taper prednisone dose over a 2-month period once remission is achieved. Adverse reactions are dose and drug dependent; insomnia, hypertension, edema, GI irritation, hyperglycemia and carbohydrate intolerance, pancreatitis, hirsutism, and acute adrenal insufficiency may occur with increased stress. Sudden withdrawal may be fatal. Do not give steroids to patients with septic complications, abscess, or fistulas.

Immunosuppressants are used to induce and maintain remission of IBD.

Infliximab (Remicade): a new chimeric IgG_{1K} monoclonal antibody indicated for moderate to severe IBD to reduce the signs and symptoms in individuals who have an inadequate response to conventional therapy. Also used for the treatment of individuals with fistulizing CD for reduction in the number of draining enterocutaneous fistulas. Adverse reactions include hypertension, hypotension, tachycardia, involuntary muscle contractions, paresthesia, vertigo, acne alopecia, eczema, fungal dermatitis, constipation,, dyspepsia, flatulence, intestinal obstruction, arthralgia, arthritis, myalgia, dyspnea, peripheral edema, malaise, diarrhea, and urinary tract infections.

Azathioprine (Imuran): used in the treatment of UC and CD for individuals dependent on corticosteroids, for fistulous disease, and for the maintenance of remission. Approximately 3% of individuals incur an adverse reaction, usually a few weeks after starting the drug. Common signs and symptoms are pyrexia, nausea, emesis, diarrhea, hypotension, oliguria, tachycardia, maculopapular rash, urticaria, vasculitis, erythema multiforme, and erythema nodosum. These reactions may be caused by release of cytokines induced by azathioprine. Symptoms clear within 24 hours of discontinuation of the drug.

6-Mercaptopurine (6-MP, Purinethol): primarily indicated for fistulous disease. Drug onset of action takes 2 to 6 months.

Methotrexate (Folex, Rheumatrex): can promote short-term remission in patients with CD, thus reducing the need for glucocorticoids. Common adverse reactions include severe leukopenia, ulcerative stomatitis, nausea, abdominal distress, malaise, undue fatigue, chills and fever, dizziness, and decreased resistance to infection. Give folic acid supplementation (folic acid 1 to 2 mg/day) to decrease stomatitis and GI side effects.

Cyclosporine: for severe IBD unresponsive to glucocorticoids. Also used as short-term adjunctive therapy during the delayed onset of action of other immunosuppressants. Adverse reactions include leukopenia, thrombocytopenia, tremor, gum hyperplasia, nausea, vomiting, diarrhea, nephrotoxicity, hirsutism, elevated cholesterol levels, and infections.

Antibiotics may be used to limit secondary infections and excessive bowel flora and to control suppurative complications.

Metronidazole (Flagyl): for colonic, fistulous disease. Adverse effects include nausea, headache, anorexia, vomiting, diarrhea, epigastric distress, abdominal cramping, and constipation. *Ciprofloxacin* (Cipro) may be an alternative.

Antidiarrheal agents are used as supportive therapy to reduce fluid loss and cramping.

Diphenoxylate-atropine (Lomotil): useful in individuals with nontoxic diarrhea. Caution should be used with antidiarrheal agents in those with severe colonic disease to decrease the risk of toxic megacolon.

Loperamide (Imodium, Imodium A-D): antimotility agents may also be used. This agent may precipitate toxic megacolon.

Other Pharmacologic Agents

Vitamin B_{12} injection (anacobin, betalin, cyanocobalamin): indicated for extensive ileal disease or prior ileal resection.

Cholestyramine: bile acid–binding resin to treat bile salt–induced diarrhea.

Surgical Therapy

Surgery is reserved for major complications of CD such as obstruction, pyogenic abscess, fistula unresponsive to medical therapy, perforation, toxic megacolon, cancer, refractory disease, and severe hemorrhage. Surgery may consist of partial bowel resection; however, in CD there is a recurrence rate of 50% to 70% over a 5-year period. With total colectomy and ileostomy, the recurrence rate is slightly lower.

In UC, surgery is indicated for colon perforation, toxic megacolon, or severe disease unresponsive to intensive inpatient medical therapy. Surgical treatment is usually curative for patients with UC, but it leaves the patient with some form of ileostomy.

Surgical Procedures

Segmental Colectomy. The affected segment of the colon is removed, and the remaining portions are anastomosed.

Total Proctocolectomy with Permanent Ileostomy. The colon, rectum, and anus are removed. The terminal end of the ileum is brought out through the lower right quadrant of the abdomen, forming a stoma. This requires an ostomy collection device (see Chapter 3, Section 3).

Total Proctocolectomy with Continent Ileostomy. An internal pouch, called a "Kock pouch," is constructed from approximately 30 cm of distal ileum. A nipple valve outlet is created and is brought through to the abdominal wall lying flush with the skin. No ostomy bag device is required. A small dressing or adhesive strip is used to cover the stoma. A catheter is inserted into the nipple valve approximately four times a day for emptying. Nipple valve failure occurs in up to 40% of patients. This is contraindicated in CD patients owing to the potential disease recurrence.

Total Colectomy and Ileoanal Reservoir. The colon and rectal mucosa are removed, a temporary loop ileostomy is created, and an ileal reservoir or pouch is constructed and is anastomosed to the anal canal. Two to 3 months later, the loop ileostomy is rejoined, restoring fecal continuity. The pouch acts to accommodate and store fecal contents. It takes 3 to 6 months for adaptation, which may result in a decrease in the number of stools from 17 to 20 to 4 to 8 per day. This is contraindicated in patients with CD.

Postoperative Management

Nasogastric suction is maintained until bowel sounds resume, at which time the diet may be advanced from clear liquid. Monitor the incision site for infection and provide aseptic care. Monitor stools for color and consistency. Bloody stools may be a sign of anastomosis rupture. Monitor fluid and electrolytes closely, because significant amounts of fluid can be lost from the ileostomy. Intravenous fluids and electrolyte replacement will be needed. Fecal drainage should thicken slightly as diet progresses.

Nutritional Therapy

Proper nutritional support is an important aspect of care for individuals with IBD. Most individuals with moderate to severe disease are malnourished. Malnourishment is a result of decreased nutrient intake associated with the inflammatory process and with significant malabsorption, maldigestion, or catabolic effects of the disease process. Diet modification may be indicated in moderate illness to decrease diarrhea and abdominal cramps.

Ingestion of adequate amounts of proteins and calories is necessary to counterbalance catabolic influences of active inflammation and steroid therapy. Nutritional supplements (oral) are indicated for malnutrition. Enteral nutrition or TPN is indicated for nutrition during severe unresponsive disease. TPN may be required for bowel rest during severe attacks.

Low-residue (low-fiber) foods are used to decrease bowel frequency, because they reduce the amount of fecal material in the lower intestinal tract. Some low-residue foods are non–whole grain breads and cereals, nonfried smoked or pickled meats, and strained fruits and vegetables. Teach the patient to avoid nondigestible carbohydrates such as foods containing sorbitol. Avoid foods that cause diarrhea during an acute attack, such as raw fruits, raw vegetables, caffeine, and spicy foods. Avoid medications containing sorbitol. Consult a nutritionist for dietary advice.

COMMUNITY CARE

Community care for IBD involves the evaluation and definition of disease extent and the adjustment of therapy made with assessment and physical examination.

- Regular assessment of symptoms (e.g., weight, pain, diarrhea, hemoglobin, and erythrocyte sedimentation rates) every 3 to 6 months for individuals with stable disease
- Endoscopy and further images for sign and symptom changes
- Annual liver function test for individuals with CD
- Vitamin B-12 level checked in individuals with ileal disease or ileal resection

- Folate level should be checked in individuals taking 5-amino salicylate; give such patients folic acid supplementation
- Endoscopy (for UC and CD) or barium enemas (for UC) if major complications are suspected or if there is lack of expected response to therapy and changes in signs and symptoms
- Medication adjustment (e.g, tapering and discontinuation of steroids)
- Evaluation and management of extraintestinal health problems related to UC by health care specialists (e.g., ophthalmologist, gastroenterologist, physical therapist)
- Annual surveillance for colon cancer beginning 12 to 15 years after the onset of left-sided disease and at the first 8 years after onset of pancolitis
- Emotional support is recommended; approximately 90% of patients diagnosed with chronic illness will have a period of depression in the course of their illness

 PROGNOSIS

CD responds well to therapy, but most patients will require surgery at some point during the course of the disease. Surgery is not curative because the disease commonly recurs. Mortality rates increase with the duration of disease, probably ranging from 5% to 10%. Most deaths are caused by peritonitis or sepsis.

Mortality rates for an acute attack of severe UC are less than 5%. Mortality rates increase when the entire colon is involved, the age of onset is greater than 60, and toxic megacolon develops. For chronic UC, relapse occurs in 75% to 85% of individuals after treatment. Colectomy is required in an average of 20% of individuals, but colectomy is usually curative treatment. Colon cancer risk is the most important risk factor affecting long-term prognosis. Left-sided colitis and ulcerative proctitis have a favorable prognosis with a probably normal life span with therapy.

 CLINICAL PEARLS

○ The patient and health care providers should work closely together to develop the patient's plan of care. The majority of patients with IBD are well educated because of the nature of the disease and the many attempts made to find the special combination of drugs to achieve remission.
○ Scales of Disease Activity Indices (e.g., Crohn's Disease Activity Index) are helpful tools to measure disease severity and quality of life for those who have chronic IBD.
○ Annual cancer surveillance (e.g., colonoscopy with biopsies for dysplasia) is recommended for individuals with chronic IBD at risk for cancer 8 years after the onset of pancolitis or 12 to 15 years after the onset of left-sided colitis.
○ Adjustment of therapy may be imperative and is often made by assessment and physical examination after the initial evaluation and definition of the extent of the disease.
○ There is no universal prescription for CD treatment; it is tailored to the location and extent of the disease.

○ The extent of the disease does not reflect the severity of the symptoms. Severe symptoms may involve only a segment of the colon, whereas pancolitis may have mild symptoms.

○ Colostomy may be indicated as corrective surgery for UC.

○ Many patients with chronic disorders experience emotional imbalance and require emotional supportive care.

NURSING PROBLEM/ DIAGNOSIS	NURSING INTERVENTIONS CLASSIFICATION (NIC)
Diarrhea	Diarrhea management Fluid/electrolyte management Medication management
Acute pain	Pain management Environmental management: comfort
Malnutrition/Imbalanced nutrition: less than body requirements	Nutrition consultation Teaching: diet therapy Total parenteral nutrition administration

Hernias

Section 6   Patricia B. Graham

 ## OVERVIEW

A hernia is a weakness in the abdominal muscle through which a segment of bowel or other abdominal structure protrudes. The weakness can be congenital or acquired or can result from a postoperative defect in the muscle wall of the abdomen. Ninety percent of all hernias are located in the inguinal region. Hernias are usually asymptomatic, although they can strangulate. Patients usually present with the simple complaint of a bump or a lump on the abdomen.

 ## PATHOPHYSIOLOGY

Hernias result from a defect in the integrity of the muscle wall and increased abdominal pressure. Defects in the muscle wall are a result of weakened collagen or widened spaces at the inguinal ligament. The muscle weakness may be inherited or a result of the aging process. Increases in abdominal pressure as a result of pregnancy, obesity, distention, ascites or coughing, straining, or heavy lifting can be contributing factors.

Inguinal Hernia. The inguinal hernia is the most common type of hernia and occurs three times more frequently in men than in women. Inguinal hernias can be classified as indirect inguinal hernia, in which the hernia is caused by a weakness in the abdominal wall opening through which the spermatic cord emerges in men and the round ligament emerges in women. The hernial sac, which contains intestine or omentum, will extend down through the inguinal canal and onto the scrotum or labia. Inguinal hernias can also be classified as direct inguinal hernia, in which the hernial sac protrudes through a weak point in the abdominal wall. This type of hernia is more common in the elderly.

Femoral Hernia. Femoral hernias occur when the intestines descend through the femoral ring. This occurs more frequently in women and can easily result in strangulation.

Umbilical Hernia. The umbilical hernia occurs due to a weak rectus muscle or failure of the umbilical opening to close at birth.

Ventral (Incisional) Hernia. Ventral hernias occur as the result of a weak abdominal incision. Pressure from the abdomen on the incision wall causes protrusion of part of the gut. This is most commonly seen in obese patients, those with multiple surgical incisions in the same area, or those with poor wound healing.

All hernias can be further classified as:

Reducible Hernia. A reducible hernia can be returned to the abdominal cavity with gentle pressure when the patient is in a supine position.

Irreducible (Incarcerated) Hernia. The hernial sac is larger than the opening through which it protrudes and cannot be reduced or placed back in the abdominal cavity.

Strangulated Hernia. Blood supply to the herniated area is cut off and necrosis of the bowel can result. This is a medical emergency and requires immediate surgical intervention.

 SIGNS AND SYMPTOMS

Patients with hernias are usually asymptomatic unless the hernia becomes incarcerated or strangulated. However, hernia repairs are often made to avoid the possibility of strangulation. In addition to the inability to reduce the hernia, a patient with a strangulated hernia usually experiences abdominal pain, nausea and vomiting, distention, fever, and tachycardia. Elderly patients may have a strangulated hernia without pain but often have nausea, vomiting, and sometimes mental confusion. Emergency surgery is the treatment for strangulation because of the danger of bowel obstruction and necrosis.

 DIAGNOSTIC CRITERIA

Hernias are directly observed or may be palpated. In the male patient, an inguinal hernia may be palpated by having the examiner place his or her finger in the scrotum above the testes and invaginate the scrotal skin. The examiner's finger should follow the spermatic cord. With the finger in the inguinal canal or against the external inguinal ring, the patient is instructed to cough or strain. If a hernia is present, a sudden bulging against the finger will be felt by the examiner. The examination should be performed on both the left and right side. If the hernia is not reducible and the patient is experiencing abdominal pain, nausea, and vomiting, emergency surgery should be performed as soon as possible.

 INTERVENTIONS

Nonsurgical management of inguinal hernias is possible as long as the hernia is not incarcerated. After the hernia is reduced, the patient may wear a *truss,* which is a firm pad held in place with a belt. The truss holds the abdominal contents in place and prevents the hernia from protruding. The truss must be properly fitted, and the patient must be instructed to not use the truss or attempt to reduce a hernia when it has become incarcerated.

A reducible hernia requires no intervention, but the patient must be taught to notify the physician if there is a change in his or her condition. If it becomes impossible to reduce the hernia or the patient experiences abdominal pain, nausea, or vomiting, the physician should be notified. If the patient is to use a truss, he or she should be shown how to use it. Proper fitting is necessary and should be done by a qualified person. The truss should not be used if the hernia becomes irreducible.

Surgical repair is the treatment of choice for hernias, although there is considerable discussion in the literature regarding the best surgical approach. Methods include the laparoscopic approach, the Shouldice (open) method, and the Lichtenstein (open) method. Laparoscopic repair is considered favorable by British surgeons when performed by experienced laparoscopists on healthy patients. They note that visceral or vascular injury is a serious concern when laparoscopic repair is the method of choice. In a study of 121 patients who had an open repair, followed by a recurrence or the development of a new hernia, 97% of the patients reported that the laparoscopic procedure was associated with significantly less pain.

Nursing interventions for patients undergoing surgical repair depend on the type of anesthetic agent used and the type of procedure performed. Either local or general anesthesia may be used in any of the procedures.

Laparoscopic surgery is usually performed on an outpatient basis. The patient must be instructed to take nothing by mouth for 8 hours before the surgery and to arrange to have a support person to escort him or her home and to assist at home after surgery. Depending on the surgeon's preference, the patient may be instructed to administer an enema the night before or the morning of surgery. The surgical procedure may be done under local or general anesthesia. After surgery, the patient will remain in the outpatient area until recovered from the anesthesia.

Postanesthesia care involves close observation, monitoring of vital signs, administration of analgesic agents, and management of postoperative nausea and vomiting, if present. Because most laparoscopic patients will be discharged on the day of surgery, the nurse must be sure the patient is sufficiently recovered from the effects of anesthesia and that teaching regarding home care is complete.

Patients should be instructed to decrease activities for 5 to 6 days, to avoid heavy lifting, and to avoid straining at bowel movements. Scrotal swelling may occur after surgery and can be very painful. Elevation of the scrotum on a rolled towel and application of an ice pack may be helpful. Urinary retention may also be a problem. Fluids should be encouraged and the patient instructed to watch for bladder distention. Wound infection is rare, but the wound should be inspected for redness, tenderness, or discharge. Teach the patient to report these symptoms immediately.

Open surgical repair requires 1 to 3 days of hospitalization. Ambulation should begin on the day of surgery, and the patient should be encouraged to move about throughout the postoperative period. Analgesics may be given every 3 to 4 hours. Patients who undergo a hernia repair should not cough, so lung expansion is promoted through frequent position change, deep breathing, and early ambulation. After surgery, the patient should not strain at defecation, so stool softeners or mild laxatives may be prescribed. Some patients experience difficulty in voiding. Male patients should be assisted to stand to void, and a high fluid intake should be encouraged. Regular activities may be resumed within about 1 week with avoidance of straining or lifting for about 2 weeks.

If incarceration or strangulation has occurred, the hospitalization period is expected to be longer. If bowel obstruction or necrosis has occurred, more extensive surgery may be required; this can include a bowel resection or temporary colostomy. In such cases, the patient is expected to require nasogastric suction, intravenous therapy, and antibiotics in addition to the postoperative care described earlier. Information on postoperative care for bowel resection and colostomy care is given in Chapter 3, Section 3.

 COMMUNITY CARE
Prevention

Although hernias result from a defect in the muscle wall, they can sometimes be prevented by avoiding situations that require heavy lifting or straining. If there are family tendencies toward the development of hernias, these individuals should be particularly careful. Once a hernia has been discovered, individuals can be taught to care for it to avoid strangulation. Lifting and straining should be avoided, and if a truss is to be used, the patient should be taught appropriate use. Patients must be informed about the signs and symptoms of incarceration and advised to seek medical assistance quickly if these signs appear.

Community Follow-up

Because patients undergoing hernia repair are discharged soon after surgery, they may need some follow-up care by the home health nurse (see Nursing Interventions).

 PROGNOSIS

The prognosis is good for persons undergoing herniorrhaphy. Postoperative infections are rare, and persons usually return to full activity within days. The possibility for recurrence exists both at the same site or at new sites.

 CLINICAL PEARLS

○ A reducible hernia requires no intervention.
○ Patients with existing hernias should be taught to avoid lifting and straining to avoid the possibility of strangulation.
○ Laparoscopic hernia repair is the method of choice in the United States.
○ Postoperative hernia repair patients should avoid lifting or straining for about 2 weeks.

NURSING PROBLEM/ DIAGNOSIS	NURSING INTERVENTIONS CLASSIFICATION (NIC)
Strangulation prevention/Risk for ineffective tissue perfusion Postsurgical management	Environmental management Teaching: disease process Positioning Fluid management Wound care

Intestinal Obstructions

Section 7　　　　　　　　　　　　　　　　　　　　　　　　　Bridget Odom

 OVERVIEW

The bowel plays a major role in the absorption of GI secretions and electrolytes that pass through the intestinal lumen. Intestinal obstruction creates a block to the forward passage of the bowel contents. Causes of intestinal obstruction range from inflammatory conditions to malignant lesions. The obstruction may occur at any point along the course of the small or large intestine. Regardless of the cause or the location of the obstruction, the pathophysiologic process is essentially the same. Diagnosis is based on the characteristics of the symptoms, physical examination, and laboratory and imaging findings. Management strategies include surgical, medical, and nursing interventions with the common goal of relieving the obstruction, minimizing complications, and improving the outcome of the patient.

 PATHOPHYSIOLOGY

When an intestinal obstruction is present, GI secretions and gas accumulate, increasing intraluminal pressure and abdominal distention. As the pressure increases, circulation and viability of the bowel wall are affected, leading to ischemia and necrosis. Stasis of intestinal contents encourages bacterial overgrowth that may translocate to the lymph nodes and systemic organs, resulting in septicemia. If bacteria gains access to the peritoneal cavity, this may lead to a fatal peritonitis.

Intestinal obstructions are classified as either mechanical or functional disorders. The majority of obstructions are *mechanical,* due to blockage of the intestinal lumen by a lesion. The lesion may be intrinsic (located within the lumen) or extrinsic (external to the lumen, but pressing on the lumen wall). Obstructions are further classified as simple (i.e., interference with passage of intestinal contents only), closed loop (i.e., a section of bowel is looped over itself), or strangulated (i.e., circulation to the bowel wall is occluded leading to ischemia). Two examples of conditions that carry a high risk of strangulation are *volvulus* and *intussusception.*

A *functional* obstruction is a failure of motility, in the absence of an obstructing lesion. The lumen remains patent, but peristalsis is inhibited. The impaired intestinal motility is thought to be related to increased sympathetic activity in the GI tract. A common example of a functional obstruction is the

Table 16-7-1. Causes of Intestinal Obstruction

MECHANICAL	FUNCTIONAL
Adhesions	Paralytic ileus
Hernias	Intestinal spasms
Extraintestinal masses (e.g., pregnancy, tumors)	Electrolyte imbalances
Volvulus	Spinal cord injury
Intussusception	Toxic megacolon
Diverticular disease	Drugs (e.g., anticholinergics, opiates,
Colorectal cancer	chemotherapeutic agents)
Gallstones	Low flow syndromes
Bezoars	Sepsis
Fecal impaction	Idiopathic

ileus that occurs as part of the normal postoperative process. Table 16-7-1 summarizes other causes of mechanical and functional bowel obstruction.

Intestinal obstructions may be partial or complete. When the bowel is partially obstructed, movement of intestinal activity is slowed or compromised. Total occlusion of the bowel lumen and obstipation occur with a complete obstruction.

Small Bowel Obstruction

Postoperative adhesions account for 50% to 70% of small bowel obstructions. Hernias are the second leading cause, accounting for 25% of cases; up to one third of hernias contain strangulated bowel. When the obstruction is located high in the small bowel, the predominant problem is loss of GI contents, due to vomiting and extravasation of intestinal fluid into the peritoneal cavity. In a low small bowel obstruction, accumulation of intestinal contents results in significant abdominal distention. In 24 hours, up to 8 L of GI secretions can accumulate. Although the small intestines can distend to significant proportions, the increasing intraluminal pressure will eventually affect bowel wall viability.

Large Bowel Obstruction

Malignant lesions account for more than 50% of large bowel or colon obstructions. The majority of these neoplasms are adenocarcinomas. The most common site of obstruction is the sigmoid colon. If the ileocecal valve is competent, the cecum cannot decompress the fluid and gas into the small bowel. The increasing distention of the cecum has the potential for perforation if measures are not taken to relieve the pressure. If the ileocecal valve is incompetent, the intestinal contents will decompress into the small intestines.

 SIGNS AND SYMPTOMS
History
Assess for the following:
- Previous abdominal surgeries
- Changes in weight and bowel habits
- Blood in stool
- History of IBD
- Use of drugs that affect the GI tract

Physical Findings

Abdominal distention occurs as the intestinal fluid, gas, and swallowed air accumulate proximal to the obstruction. Obstructions high in the small bowel may result in little or no distention. Marked distention is seen with distal small bowel or large bowel obstructions

Abnormal bowel sounds are heard on auscultation. Hyperactive bowel sounds, or borborygmi, heard proximal to the obstruction are a result of increased waves of peristalsis during early obstruction. Hypoactive bowel sounds may be heard distal to the obstruction due to diminished intestinal contents. Bowel sounds are absent over the obstruction site.

Abdominal pain is attributed to the pressure of peristalsis as the bowel tries to push its contents past the obstruction. The pain is usually described as episodic, colicky, or crampy. The pain may subside as intestinal motility decreases. Small bowel obstruction pain tends to be located in the epigastric or umbilical regions. Pain associated with colon obstruction is noted in the lower abdomen. Pain that is constant and localized may indicate strangulation or peritonitis. Pain that occurs after eating may indicate a partial obstruction.

Rebound tenderness may indicate peritoneal irritability when accompanied by muscle guarding and rigidity. This may occur with perforation or necrotic bowel.

Vomiting occurs as the sequestering of fluid increases above the point of obstruction. Gastric outlet obstructions result in early vomiting of clear gastric contents or undigested food. Obstructions located high in the small bowel produce bilious emesis. Obstructions distal in the small bowel may have a feculent smell, due to the proliferation of bacteria in the stagnant intestinal contents. True fecal vomiting is rare and occurs when the ileocecal valve is incompetent.

Fluid and electrolyte disturbances occur due to fluid accumulation, vomiting, and third space losses. If the obstruction is high in the small intestine, metabolic alkalosis may develop with loss of hydrogen ions. When the obstruction is lower in the intestine or prolonged, metabolic acidosis may occur with loss of bicarbonate ions. Signs of dehydration are evident, including decreased urine output, orthostatic hypotension, tachycardia, tachypnea, poor skin turgor, and dry mucous membranes. Hypovolemic shock becomes an inevitable consequence.

Constipation may be the only sign of a large bowel obstruction during the early stages. Keep in mind that patients with complete bowel obstruction may still have bowel movements during early obstruction, as they evacuate contents of the bowel distal to the obstruction. Partial obstruction may permit the continued passage of small amounts of stool, frequently manifested as diarrhea.

 DIAGNOSTIC CRITERIA

Laboratory studies, imaging techniques, and other pertinent procedures may assist in confirming the diagnosis of intestinal obstruction.

Laboratory Values

Laboratory data will not identify a specific diagnosis but will assist in identifying causative factors and associated complications.

- Electrolytes: hyponatremia and decreased chloride ion (Cl^-) levels may indicate dehydration. Hyponatremia is seen with vomiting and nasogastric suctioning. Reduced magnesium ions (Mg^{2+}) occur with diarrhea; elevated Mg^{2+} may occur with dehydration. Hypokalemia may result with any loss of GI secretions. A rapid decline in electrolyte values may be seen with fluid resuscitation, due to the dilutional effect.

- **Complete blood cell count and differential:** used to detect anemia and signs of infection. A significant increase in the band neutrophils, or a left shift, is an indicator of significant infection, inflammation, or tissue necrosis. Elevated hemoglobin and hematocrit may indicate hemoconcentration or loss of plasma volume.
- **Blood urea nitrogen:** elevation may indicate dehydration, renal dysfunction, or blood in the GI tract.
- **Osmolality:** serum levels are elevated with dehydration and decreased with overhydration.
- **Serum amylase, alkaline phosphatase, creatine kinase, or lactate dehydrogenase:** elevation may indicate intestinal obstruction or ischemia.
- **Arterial blood gas:** evaluate for presence of metabolic acidosis or alkalosis.

Imaging

- **Abdominal films** (upright, supine, and lateral decubitus): will provide information related to the presence, level, and cause of obstruction, confirming the diagnosis.
- **CT scan or contrast studies:** may identify obstructive lesions such as diverticulitis or volvulus. These studies may be indicated if the plain abdominal film is nondiagnostic or the patient presents with atypical symptoms. Barium studies are avoided in patients with suspected colon obstruction, due to potential impaction. Barium studies can be performed in patients with small bowel obstructions.
- **Doppler ultrasound:** may be performed to assess for absence of intestinal vascular blood supply, an indicator of strangulation.

INTERVENTIONS

Fluid management is initiated with aggressive fluid and electrolyte resuscitation. The type and amount depends on the level of obstruction and the duration. Fluid restoration is initially accomplished with normal saline in patients with no electrolyte abnormality. Normal saline is the fluid of choice for the treatment of metabolic alkalosis. Lactated Ringer's is not indicated because the lactate is converted to bicarbonate, potentially worsening the alkalosis. Treatment for metabolic acidosis may include sodium bicarbonate. Third space fluid must be treated as fluid loss to the body because it is no longer available in the intravascular space. Alternate fluid choices (i.e., colloids or hypotonic saline) may be indicated in specific situations.

TPN may be indicated for patients who are NPO for prolonged periods.

Intestinal decompression with nasogastric or long nasointestinal tubes is initiated early. Nasointestinal tubes may be used with obstructions due to CD or partial bowel obstructions and as a temporary measure with small bowel obstructions before surgery. Their purpose is to decrease the distention; they do not treat the obstruction. Because nasointestinal tubes decompress only the small intestines, a nasogastric tube may still be required for stomach decompression. Repeat abdominal films are ordered to monitor the progress of treatment. Once the patient is pain free, the tube may be clamped, while monitoring for signs of recurrent obstruction.

Nasointestinal tubes have no real place in the management of large bowel obstruction other than preoperative decompression of the proximal distended bowel. Data suggest no advantage of nasointestinal tubes over nasogastric tubes for the resolution of small bowel obstruction.

Enteral stenting is a relatively new technique used for temporary or long-term decompression. This procedure may be indicated for patients who are poor surgical candidates or have nonoperable malignant obstructions or as a temporary measure before surgical correction. Stent placement is accomplished with fluoroscopy, endoscopy, or a CT-guided procedure. Perforation, migration, and restenosis are rare, but major, complications. Minor complications include abdominal pain and transient rectal bleeding.

Large bowel decompression for obstructions may be accomplished with enemas or rectal tubes or by removing the fecal impaction. Sigmoidoscopy or colonoscopy may be therapeutic in decompressing a sigmoid or cecal volvulus.

Pharmacologic management of bowel obstruction depends on the cause and other contributing factors. Systemic broad-spectrum antibiotic therapy provides coverage for both aerobic and anaerobic organisms commonly found in the GI tract. Antibiotics may be instilled directly into the peritoneal cavity. Other medications used in the management of bowel obstruction are listed in Table 16-7-2.

Nursing Interventions

The following interventions summarize the routine nursing care of the patient:

- Assess frequently for signs of worsening obstruction (disappearance of bowel sounds, fever, hypotension, and signs of sepsis, peritonitis, and strangulation).

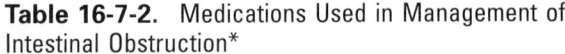

Table 16-7-2. Medications Used in Management of Intestinal Obstruction*

CATEGORY	AGENT	ACTION
Motility enhancers	Metoclopramide Erythromycin	Stimulate motility
Antiemetics	Hydroxyzine Promethazine Prochlorperazine Ondansetron Haloperidol	Relieve symptoms of nausea and vomiting; some agents may provide analgesic effect
Antisecretories	Octreotide Scopolamine	Reduce gastrointestinal secretions, decreasing abdominal distention
Anti-inflammatories	Dexamethasone Methylprednisolone	Decrease edema, improving intestinal transit
Antispasmodics	Scopolamine Loperamide	

*Pharmaceutical reference should be consulted for dose and route of administration and for additional indications and contraindications.

- Measure abdominal girth at its largest circumference.
- Record accurate intake and output, including all fluid gains and losses.
- Monitor vital signs closely, including central venous and pulmonary artery pressures, when applicable.
- Check for signs of dehydration, including decreased skin turgor, dry mucous membranes, tachycardia, and decreasing urine output.
- Note color, consistency, and frequency of bowel movements.
- Monitor daily weights.
- Provide DVT prophylaxis, including the use of sequential compression devices, antithrombotic hose, and early ambulation.
- Assess for fecal impaction, and administer gentle enemas as prescribed.
- Provide wound and stoma care.
- Provide tube and drain care.
- Provide pulmonary toilet treatment.
- Elevate the head of the bed to improve ventilation and to minimize the risk of aspiration.
- Abdominal distention may elevate the diaphragm, impairing ventilation.
- Provide judicious pain management, while avoiding masking the signs and symptoms of strangulation.
- Patient and family education should be provided.
- Psychosocial support may be necessary.

Surgical Interventions

The majority of patients presenting with complete obstruction require surgical intervention. Surgical options include laparatomy, lysis of adhesions, detorsion, reduction of hernias, resection of gangrenous bowel, and bypass of the obstruction. Right and transverse carcinomas are treated with resection and a primary anastomosis. Operations for lesions on the left side of the colon include colon resection with primary anastomosis or a staged procedure; this typically involves performing a colostomy to relieve the distention and to provide a temporary fecal outlet. A segment of the bowel is resected with an anastomosis. Once the anastomosis is healed, the colostomy is closed.

The abdominal incision may be left open due to the massively distended bowel or when spillage of intestinal contents has occurred, to avoid wound infection. Some patients may undergo a "second look" exploratory laparotomy a few days after the initial procedure to assess bowel viability.

Surgery is usually not an option for patients with functional bowel obstructions. Patients with end-stage carcinomas may not be suitable candidates for surgery.

Partial bowel obstructions are treated medically initially but may require surgical intervention if they become complete or no improvement is seen with medical management.

 COMMUNITY CARE

The goal of community care is to assist the patient and the family in the transition from care provided by the health care professional in the hospital setting to care in the home environment. This is accomplished through the following:

- Discharge planning geared to meet the individual needs of the patient
- Patient and family education

- Case manager or home health nurse referral as indicated
- Assessment of need for hospice or respite care referrals
- Ostomy association and cancer support groups

 PROGNOSIS

Patients with simple obstructions have morbidity and mortality rates similar to those of other patients undergoing uncomplicated abdominal surgeries. Nearly half of all deaths from small bowel obstruction occur in patients with strangulation. There are reports of high rates of recurrence of small bowel obstructions due to adhesions.

Patients with large bowel obstructions are likely to have a higher mortality rate due to the fact that the obstructions are often the result of carcinoma. There is a poor prognosis for patients with advanced age, multiple sites of obstruction, and a history of radiation or chemotherapy treatment.

 CLINICAL PEARLS

- The elderly may be unable to mount a significant fever or leukocytosis.
- Ask the patient if his or her abdomen is distended; he or she may be the best judge of an increasing abdominal girth.
- Always auscultate the abdomen before percussion and palpation, to avoid altering bowel sounds.
- Emesis can occur without nausea.
- The venous carbon dioxide level can be substituted for bicarbonate to evaluate for the presence of metabolic acidosis or alkalosis.
- Doubling the serum sodium value provides a quick assessment of osmolarity.
- Opioid analgesics may be avoided due to their constipating effect.
- Use a spray bottle filled with cold water as an oral mister (ice chips contribute to electrolyte washout and lemon glycerin swabs dry the mucosa).

NURSING PROBLEM/ DIAGNOSIS	NURSING INTERVENTIONS CLASSIFICATION (NIC)
Acute pain (abdominal)	Pain management Analgesic management
Fluid deficit/Deficient fluid volume	Fluid/electrolyte management
Imbalanced nutrition	Nutrition therapy

Obesity

Section 8   Patricia B. Graham

 OVERVIEW

Obesity is defined as body weight 15% to 20% or more above ideal weight for height, gender, and age. Others define it as a body mass index (BMI) above 27 (see Chapter 9, Section 1 for calculation of BMI). *Morbid obesity* is defined as being more than 100 lb above ideal body weight or having a BMI above 40. *Obesity* and *overweight* are terms that are often used interchangeably, but they refer to different conditions. *Overweight* is an increase in body weight for height compared with a reference standard. Well-developed athletes may appear overweight due to their increased muscle mass. In contrast, *obesity* refers to an excess amount of body fat. The normal amount of body fat for men is 15% to 20% of body weight, and for women, it is 18% to 32%. Obese young men have body fat of greater than 22%; obese young women have body fat of greater than 25%.

The distribution of body fat is also an issue when considering the relationship of obesity to health risks. A waist-to-hip measurement ratio of 0.95 in men and 0.80 in women with excess fat concentrated at the waist and abdomen carries a higher health risk than when fat is more evenly distributed. Studies have shown that increased abdominal fat is related to stroke, insulin resistance, hyperinsulinemia, and diabetes mellitus.

The relationship between weight and death is U shaped, with higher levels at the low end (<19) as well as at the high end (>25). Researchers caution against interpreting this finding to mean that lean weight is harmful because of other confounding factors. Individuals with prolonged illness may have experienced massive weight loss, and smokers may be lean but have higher risks for cardiovascular disease and death.

Cultural differences are reflected in the prevalence of obesity. Obesity is substantially higher among African Americans, Hispanic Americans, Asian Americans, Pacific Islanders, Native Americans, Native Hawaiians, and Native Alaskans than in whites.

 PATHOPHYSIOLOGY

Maintenance of weight indicates a balance between energy intake (food and drink) and energy expenditure (exercise and activity). In both children and adults, excess energy intake leads to increases in both lean body mass and adipose tissue. Studies have identified leptin as a key factor in weight regulation in mice, but its applicability to human obesity is still under study. Leptin appears to send a message to the brain signaling that the body has stored sufficient fat and should stop eating. In obese individuals, it is suggested that the body does not receive the signal to stop eating. Evidence suggests that energy balance and body weight are regulated not only by the hormonal action of leptin but also by the interaction of leptin and insulin with the hypothalamus.

 SIGNS AND SYMPTOMS

The signs of obesity include an excess of body weight for height and the presence of fatty tissue. In adults, with the exception of those involved in muscle building, substantial gains in weight are in large part fat. Some practitioners define obesity as having a BMI over 27; others view it as beginning at 25 with some increasing health risks seen at values of 22 and 23. A large or increasing abdominal circumference is usually caused by excess fat, once ascites and tumors have been ruled out.

 DIAGNOSTIC CRITERIA

Most clinicians consider a BMI above 25 as overweight, a BMI above 30 as obese, and a BMI above 40 as morbidly obese. Individuals who are 100 lb above their ideal weight may be candidates for surgical intervention if they have not responded to other weight loss programs.

 INTERVENTIONS

Weight loss through dietary control is the safest means of eliminating obesity. However, if the individual is to be successful, he or she must have the motivation to maintain a restricted but balanced diet over a lengthy period of time. Weight loss is achieved by establishing a balance between energy intake and energy expenditure. Nutritionally balanced diets provide about 1200 calories a day. Eliminating 1000 calories per day will result in a weight loss of approximately 2 lb/wk. Unbalanced diets that eliminate or restrict a major nutrient such as carbohydrate have not been shown to increase weight loss beyond the caloric restriction imposed.

Drugs that suppress the appetite have been used with some success but should be used in conjunction with a comprehensive weight reduction program. Certain weight reduction drugs have come under heavy criticism, and some have been removed from the market because of dangerous side effects. In addition, when the drugs were discontinued, patients quickly returned to their starting weight.

Surgical treatment of obesity is considered for individuals who are more than 100 lb above their ideal body weight and who have been unsuccessful with traditional weight loss programs. Gastric bypass (stomach stapling) and vertical banded gastroplasty are the procedures of choice. In *gastric bypass surgery,* the proximal section of the stomach is transected to form a small pouch with a small gastroenterostomy stoma. In *vertical banded gastroplasty,* a double row of staples is applied along the lesser curvature of the stomach (Fig. 16-8-1). A small stoma is created at the end of the staples by adding a circle of staples or a band of polypropylene mesh. Weight loss after these procedures maximizes in 18 to 24 months.

A nasogastric tube is placed and maintained in the immediate postoperative period and is removed once bowel sounds return. Clear liquids can then be started and advanced slowly as tolerated by the patient. In the early postoperative period, the obese patient should be ambulated to reduce the risk of atelectasis, pneumonia, and deep venous thrombosis (DVT).

 COMMUNITY CARE
Prevention

Teaching about the importance of diet and exercise should begin in early childhood. Children will learn to like healthful snacks if they are encouraged and provided. Healthful dietary patterns at home will help to lay the foundation for eating patterns in later life. Parents should stress regular meals at a regular time of day at the same place. Meals should be eaten sitting down, at the table, and not in front of the television or while doing other things. Older children involved in multiple activities should learn to pick and choose wisely, particularly on days when they are relying on fast food. Food should not be used as a reward, or one food group, such as dessert, valued above another.

Exercise should be encouraged both during and after school. If school physical education programs are reduced in a cost-cutting measure, children

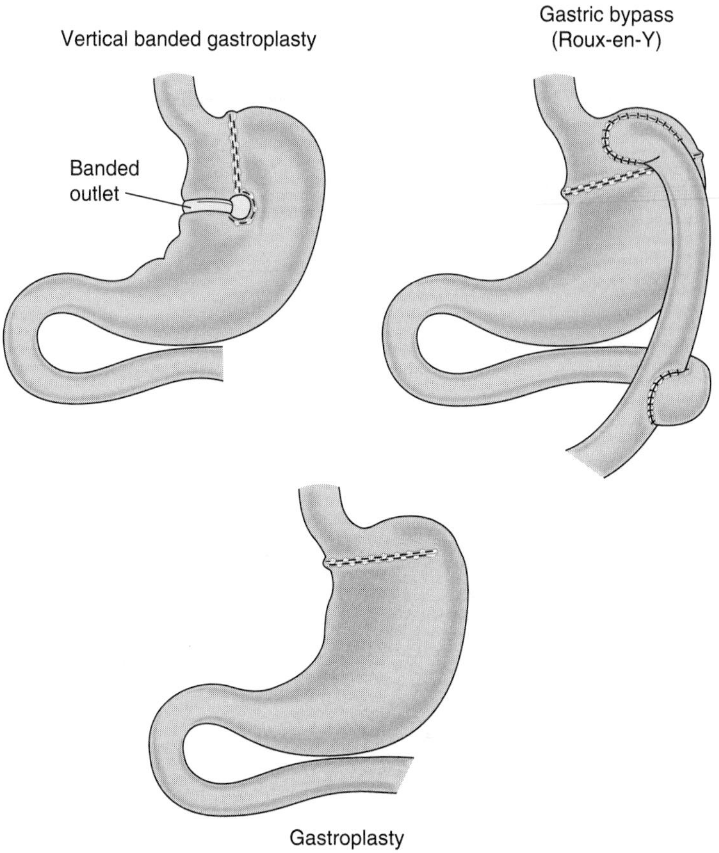

Vertical banded gastroplasty

Gastric bypass
(Roux-en-Y)

Banded
outlet

Gastroplasty

Figure 16-8-1. Surgical procedures for obesity.

should be encouraged to find other means of exercise, such as walking to school, walking at lunch time, or playing ball after school. Time in front of the television and on the Internet should be carefully monitored by parents and balanced with physical activity.

Weight Loss Programs

Weight loss programs abound in most communities and are usually available for both adults and adolescents. Care should be taken to select a program that provides a healthful balance of regular foods and does not focus on fads or the elimination of entire food groups.

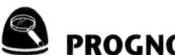 PROGNOSIS

Despite ongoing research into the causes and treatment of obesity, achieving a balance between food intake and energy expenditure remains the mainstay of the treatment of obesity. Medications that have been approved for weight loss do not work for all individuals and on average induce only a modest weight loss. Most overweight individuals can successfully lose weight, but the majority regain that weight within 5 years. Surgical treatment, appropriate only for the severely obese, can have substantial procedure-related morbidity rates.

As research continues, it is hoped that more effective treatments for obesity will be found. The best hope for resistance to weight gain and achievement and maintenance of weight loss is increased physical activity in conjunction with a healthy diet.

 ## CLINICAL PEARLS

o Obesity can usually be avoided by finding the right balance between energy intake and energy output.
o Mortality rates increase significantly with a BMI of 25 or above.
o Weight loss programs should be designed around balanced meals with good nutritional value.
o Persons taking drugs to lose weight will usually regain the weight when the drug is stopped.

NURSING PROBLEM/ DIAGNOSIS	NURSING INTERVENTIONS CLASSIFICATION (NIC)
Obesity/Imbalanced nutrition: more than body requirements	Weight reduction assistance Weight management

Peritonitis

Section 9   Timothy Wren ▪ Kathleen Wren

 ## OVERVIEW

Peritonitis is an inflammation of the peritoneum. This inflammation can be acute or chronic. Acute causes of peritonitis include inflammation arising from: (1) abdominal organ infection, such as pancreatitis or salpingitis (inflammation of the fallopian tubes); (2) intraperitoneal blood due to internal bleeding (ruptured ectopic pregnancy, aneurysmal leak); or (3) irritating substances released from ruptured or penetrated organs (bile leakage from liver trauma or digestive juice leakage due to ulcer rupture). Acute infection may also arise from the contamination of peritoneal dialysis fluids and supplies or bacterial invasion of ascites fluid during chronic liver failure. Chronic peritonitis is rarer, and causes are often related to tuberculosis or a longstanding irritation in the abdominal cavity (retained foreign body).

 ## PATHOPHYSIOLOGY

Peritonitis results when the peritoneal membranes become inflamed. Peritoneal membrane inflammation causes fluid to leak from the abdominal organs into the abdominal cavity. Bacterial contamination can occur directly through leakage of intestinal contents and its normal flora. It can also result from disruption of intestinal wall integrity, leading to leakage of normally present bacteria (normal flora) from the intestinal lumen into the abdominal cavity. As a result of trauma, bacteria and organisms normally present on the skin can enter the abdomen directly with the puncturing object. Last, infection can spread from an originating source such as the fallopian tubes. As bacteria or infecting organisms multiply in the abdominal cavity, organ tissues become more inflamed and edematous. Exudate and abscess formation results from the cytotoxic products of organism activity as well as the cellular byproducts of bacterial, fungal, and white blood cell death. Thus, the peritoneal fluid becomes filled with cellular debris, white blood cells, protein, and blood. The inflammatory process results in pain, tenderness, and decreased motility of the intestinal tract, although increased motility resulting in diarrhea may occur during the initial stages.

SIGNS AND SYMPTOMS

Peritonitis is caused by many conditions and may arise from many different areas of the abdomen. Thus, presenting signs and symptoms are related to the pathophysiologic process responsible for the inflammation and the organs involved.

Causes

Common causes of peritonitis follow.

Trauma

- Penetrated bowel
- Ruptured spleen
- Fractured kidney
- Lacerated liver

Perforation

- Ruptured appendix
- Ruptured diverticulum
- Eroding tumor masses
- Ruptured duodenal ulcer
- Ruptured ectopic pregnancy

Internal Bleeding

- Leaking or ruptured aneurysm
- Bleeding ulcer
- Ruptured ectopic pregnancy

Organ Infection

- Salpingitis
- Pelvic inflammatory disease
- Pancreatitis
- Ascites fluid infection
- Contamination of peritoneal dialysis solution or catheter access device

Organ Infarction

- Strangulated hernia
- Small bowel obstruction
- Mesenteric artery embolus

Common Signs and Symptoms

Nausea and Vomiting

This is a frequent sign and symptom, despite specific causative factor, and most likely due to the bowel becoming inflamed and decreased peristalsis.

Fever

Centrally mediated effect of the body meant to destroy invading bacteria. Temperature increase is aimed at denaturization of bacterial proteins, leading to cell death.

Pain

As the structures in the abdomen become inflamed, they also become swollen and distended, often causing pain. The pain may start as localized and mild, but it quickly becomes severe. The abdomen becomes very rigid and guarded, resulting in the characteristic "board-like" abdomen. These are the classic symptoms of peritoneal irritation. Often, the patient will assume the fetal position and refuse any attempts at movement. Inflammation and the resultant pain process may be diminished or absent in patients with nerve disorders, those taking anti-inflammatory medications (steroids) or narcotics, and those with immune compromise.

Dehydration

Inflammation and decreased peristalsis result in third space losses into the intestinal tract and into the abdominal cavity as well. Nausea limits oral intake. Vomiting results in direct fluid loss.

 DIAGNOSTIC CRITERIA

Diagnosis usually consists of three parts: physical examination, blood tests, and radiography. More extensive procedures, such as ultrasonography or perito-neal lavage, may assist in the diagnosis and treatment of more difficult cases.

On *physical examination,* the abdomen is rigid and firm to the touch. Rebound tenderness may be present. The patient may have a fever, be con-fused, and have signs of hypovolemic shock, such as low blood pressure, increased pulse rate, and tachypnea.

Radiographic examination may reveal the presence of free air in the abdo-men, indicative of intestinal rupture. The presence of tumors or foreign bodies may indicate possible sources of irritation, infection, or inflammation.

Complete blood cell counts may help in the estimation of blood or fluid loss. An elevated white blood cell count with a leftward shift reflects infection. Cultures of the peritoneal fluid sample determine the presence of bacteria and direct antibiotic therapy. A white blood cell count above 200/mm^3 in peritoneal fluid is indicative of infection.

Ultrasonography, a noninvasive alternative to exploratory surgery, assists in pinpointing the cause of peritonitis when patient history and physical examina-tion may be inconclusive. Peritoneal lavage also may be used to detect bacteria, blood, white cells, bile, and vegetable fibers in peritoneal fluid. The presence of white blood cells and vegetable fibers is indicative of inflammation. Free blood and bile in peritoneal fluid are irritating and may help pinpoint the cause of peritonitis. Culture and sensitivity of the contaminating organism are useful in antibiotic coverage.

 INTERVENTIONS

Peritonitis treatment commonly involves a combination of surgery and antibiotics. Surgery is often required to remove toxic matter (bacteria, abscesses, blood, stool), isolate the source of the problem, and repair a compromised viscus, if needed. Antibiotic therapy to combat the bacterial invasion can then be prescribed based on culture results obtained during surgery. The patient may require intravenous fluid resuscitation, stomach and bowel decompression via a nasogastric tube, and pain medication. The patient should also be placed on NPO restrictions with strict intake and output recordings. Prolonged NPO restrictions may necessitate the institution of TPN therapy.

Patients receiving peritoneal dialysis frequently encounter problems with peritonitis. It is estimated that peritoneal dialysis patients experience an episode of peritonitis every 12 to 18 months. For peritonitis related to peritoneal dialysis, replacing the access device and giving antibiotics both systemically and directly into the intraperitoneal cavity constitute the usual intervention.

Last, it is not uncommon for patients with severe liver disease to develop peritonitis due to bacterial contamination of the ascites fluid. Many of these patients will present with only mild abdominal pain and a change in mental status. Early treatment of peritonitis in liver failure patients is essential, because mortality rates are extremely high if diagnosis and treatment are delayed. Paracentesis and antibiotic therapy provided in response to the culture and sensitivity are the mainstays of treatment. Prophylactic antibiotics are administered to susceptible liver patients, such as those undergoing invasive procedures and hospitalization. Long-term survival is poor in liver patients who develop peritonitis due to the underlying disease state.

Nursing Care

Initial nursing assessment should include review of the patient's medical history and progression of the problem. The patient's hydration status may be evaluated by skin turgor, urine output, amount and frequency of emesis, vital signs, and reports of fluid intake. Urine color can provide clues to fluid status. Dark yellow to brown urine is indicative of dehydration.

In addition, the presence of fever and its characteristics (constancy, cycles, sweats, chills) should be evaluated. Pain assessment using a visual analog method ("Rate your pain on a scale of 1 to 10") will help guide analgesic therapy. Instructions on abdominal splinting should be provided.

Only after information gathering and other assessments are complete is a careful, gentle physical examination of the abdomen performed. The nurse should anticipate a rigid abdomen. Very gentle pressure is adequate for the detection of rebound and direct tenderness. Often, assessment of bowel sounds (with the stethoscope) and abdominal palpation can be completed simultaneously.

Again, assessment of mental status throughout the nursing assessment is important, because a change in mental status may be the only indication of peritonitis in patients with preexisting or coexisting liver failure.

Many patients with peritonitis require surgical intervention to correct the underlying cause. Postoperative recovery may be prolonged as the patient recovers from infection. Normalization of the temperature and heart rate along with decreasing abdominal pain suggests resolution. Ambulation and a slow institution of oral intake (diet) will assist in returning normal bowel function.

 COMMUNITY CARE

As patients are discharged home, nurses must reinforce the importance of completing oral antibiotic therapy. Postoperative instructions should include avoidance of lifting objects in excess of 10 lb. Patients should also understand the signs and symptoms of infection, such as fever, chills, pain, increased heart rate, and increased body temperature. Peritoneal dialysis patients should understand and be able to demonstrate the application of aseptic principles as they perform their dialysis procedures. Patients with underlying liver failure disease should be instructed in the use of prophylactic antibiotic coverage during invasive procedures and hospitalizations. They should also be cautioned to seek early treatment for local infections.

 PROGNOSIS

Peritonitis is a serious condition that requires prompt, emergency intervention. Successful recovery is dependent on correction of the underlying cause, responsiveness to antibiotic therapy, immune system functioning, age, and underlying patient health status. The elderly and those with compromised wound healing and immune system functioning and end-stage renal or hepatic disease experience higher mortality rates. The development of sepsis is ominous.

 CLINICAL PEARLS

○ Signs and symptoms of peritonitis may be blunted in patients receiving narcotic, anti-inflammatory, immunosuppressive, and chemotherapeutic agents.
○ Signs and symptoms of peritonitis may also be blunted in patients with immune compromise, such as patients with acquired immunodeficiency syndrome or cancer.
○ In liver failure patients, sometimes the only indication of peritonitis is a change in mental status.

NURSING PROBLEM/ DIAGNOSIS	NURSING INTERVENTIONS CLASSIFICATION (NIC)
Acute pain (abdominal)	Analgesic administration
	Pain management
Dehydration/Deficient fluid volume	Fluid/electrolyte management
	Nutrition therapy
Risk for sepsis/Risk for infection	Infection protection
	Medication administration
	Surveillance
	Wound care

chapter 17

Gastrointestinal—Upper

Cholelithiasis and Cholecystitis

Section 1   Ethlyn Gibson

OVERVIEW

The two most common diseases of the biliary tree are *cholelithiasis* (stone formation in the gall bladder) and *cholecystitis* (inflammation of the gallbladder). These conditions may occur alone but usually occur simultaneously. Gallstones are becoming more common in the United States, affecting an estimated 20 million adults. Approximately 500,000 cholecystectomies are performed annually. Gallstones are usually found in individuals older than age 20, with a high incidence in Pima and Chippewa people, white women, and African Americans.

Clinical conditions that may predispose to gallstones include diabetes, obesity, cirrhosis, ileal disease or resection, cancer of the gallbladder, and pancreatitis. Cholecystitis usually results from obstruction of the cystic duct from gallstones (acute calculous cholecystitis); however, in a few patients, it results from stasis, bacteria, or sepsis (acute acalculous cholecystitis).

PATHOPHYSIOLOGY

The pathophysiology of gallstones depends largely on the following factors: the type of stone, the stone's location within the ductal system, and whether the occurrence is acute or chronic. Gallstones are classified as: (1) cholesterol stones, (2) pigment stones, and (3) mixed stones. Cholesterol stones are the most common type and occur most often in women. Pigment stones are present in approximately 30% of those presenting with gallbladder disorders. They consist primarily of calcium bilirubinate. Mixed stones are a combination of pigment and cholesterol stones.

The exact cause of gallstone formation is unclear. Contributing factors may include:

- *Supersaturation* of bile with cholesterol. Bile is composed mainly of water, with other components including cholesterol bile salts and pigments. Cholesterol alone is insoluble in water; it must be combined with other components (e.g., bile salts) to remain in solution. When bile salts are insufficient to maintain cholesterol in solution, cholesterol crystals form.
- *Bile stasis.* This occurs when gallbladders have not contracted normally in response to a meal and the bile sits and they become thick and concentrated. This occurs in patients on prolonged total parenteral nutrition (TPN). Approximately 50% of these patients develop "sludge" (a mucus gel composed of calcium bilirubinate and cholesterol crystals) in the gallbladder by week 6 of TPN therapy. Gallstones frequently occur during periods of fasting or dieting, during which there is a lack of stimulus for the gallbladder to contract.

595

- *Nucleation.* A nucleus (nidus) is formed of agents such as bacteria, bile, pigments, cellular debris, and calcium salts. Additional substances aggregate around this nucleus, forming a stone.
- *Genetics* may be a factor, as evidenced by increased prevalence in Pimas and Chippewas.

Some stones may form and pass through the ducts without causing clinical manifestations (asymptomatic cholelithiasis). Symptomatic cholelithiasis occurs when stones intermittently become lodged in the cystic duct, causing biliary colic (episodic pain in the right upper quadrant or epigastric area). The pain usually occurs after meals, especially high-fat meals, as a result of increased intraluminal pressure when the gallbladder attempts to contract to release bile (a normal response to food entering the duodenum) against the obstructing stone.

Cholecystitis develops as stones become impacted within the cystic duct, causing unyielding obstruction, edema, distention, and inflammation of the gallbladder. In chronic cholecystitis, gallstones remain, causing recurrent obstructions and producing changes in the gallbladder wall from recurrent edema and inflammation. The muscular coat becomes fibrous, and the gallbladder functions less effectively.

Complications

Edema and distention of the gallbladder walls decrease blood supply, resulting in patchy areas of necrosis and gangrene. Perforation of these areas can then occur. Bile leakage through these perforations into the peritoneum results in peritonitis. Abscess formation may also occur if secretions from the ruptured gallbladder are confined by omentum or other adjacent organs (e.g., colon, stomach, duodenum, pancreas).

Stone migration from the gallbladder to the common bile duct (CBD) may cause *cholangitis* (acute CBD inflammation). The presence of gallstones in the CBD is called *choledocolithiasis.* CBD stones are a major source of morbidity in patients with symptomatic gallstone disease. Stone migration to the ampulla of Vater can cause pancreatitis.

 SIGNS AND SYMPTOMS

Most patients with *cholelithiasis* are asymptomatic. The patients who are symptomatic experience biliary colic. Biliary colic begins abruptly and can last from minutes to 4 hours. The pain usually starts after a meal but can start several hours after a meal as well as at night. The pain may subside abruptly or gradually as the stone is passed or returns to the gallbladder.

Cholecystitis may cause the patient to present with tenderness in the right upper quadrant, epigastrium, or both. The biliary pain differs from that of cholelithiasis, because it is caused by inflammation and can last for several days. The patient also reports nausea and vomiting, intolerance of fatty foods, flatulence, bloating, and other upper abdominal sensations. *Jaundice,* caused by blocked bile flow into the duodenum, is seen in 20% of patients. Bile accumulates in the liver, from where it can be forced into the bloodstream, resulting in hyperbilirubinemia. Steatorrhea (fatty stools) results from a lack of bile in the duodenum, which prevents fat breakdown. Stools may be clay-colored, because of a lack of bile in the duodenum.

Physical assessment may reveal a positive Murphy sign. To elicit this sign, the examiner palpates the right subcostal area while having the patient take a deep breath. A positive Murphy sign occurs if the patient complains of extreme tenderness and stops breathing on inspiration. Rebound tenderness and guarding may be signs of peritoneal involvement.

DIAGNOSTIC CRITERIA

Diagnosis of biliary disease may be made from clinical manifestations (i.e., location of pain, nausea, vomiting, and abdominal guarding) along with the following tests.

- *Ultrasound* of the gallbladder and biliary tree is diagnostic for stones in the gallbladder. The sonogram shows: (1) cholelithiasis, (2) focal tenderness over the gallbladder (sonographic Murphy's sign), (3) thickening of the gallbladder wall by more than 3 mm, and (4) distention of the gallbladder lumen by more than 5 cm. Ultrasound is relatively insensitive for detecting stones in the CBD.
- *Serum amylase and lipase* are evaluated to determine the presence of pancreatitis.
- *White blood cell (WBC) count* is elevated in 85% of patients.
- *Serum bilirubin and alkaline phosphatase* levels may be elevated in biliary disease.
- *Flat-plate radiograph* of the abdomen can reveal an enlarged gallbladder; gallstones may contain enough calcium to be visible on film.
- *Oral cholecystogram.* Oral contrast allows for imaging of the gallbladder through the accumulation of dye in the bile. This is done to assess the gallbladder's ability to fill and excrete bile, as well as to identify stones.
- *Hepato-iminodiacetic acid (HIDA) scans.* Injected radioisotopes travel through the liver and biliary system. With normal bile circulation, the gallbladder is seen within 30 minutes. If the cystic duct is obstructed, the gallbladder cannot be visualized. This test is 98% sensitive for acute cholecystitis.
- *Endoscopic retrograde cholangiography* (ERC). The CBD is endoscopically examined for stones. A new procedure that is a modification of endoscopic retrograde cholangiopancreatography (ERCP). A small flexible fiberoptic endoscope is passed through the mouth and advanced into the duodenum. From here, a cannula is inserted through the sphincter of Oddi and the ampulla of Vater and into the CBD, and contrast material is injected and x-rays are obtained. ERC also enables removal of visualized stones at this time. ERC carries a 3% to 10% risk of pancreatitis.
- *Endoscopic ultrasound* is useful for detecting CBD stones without the risk of pancreatitis, but does not allow for stone removal. It may be performed before laparoscopic cholecystectomy to rule out CBD stones in suspected cases.
- *ERCP.* This test evaluates the CBD and pancreatic duct when associated pancreatic disease is suspected. It is similar to ERC except that the cannula enters only the ampulla of Vater. ERCP carries a risk of pancreatitis.
- *Percutaneous transhepatic cholangiography* (PTC). If ERC cannot be performed, PTC may be done. In this test, a very thin needle is passed through the abdomen into the bile ducts, dye is injected, and radiographs are taken. This test is associated with significant morbidity.

- *Magnetic resonance cholangiography* (MRC). This noninvasive test is extremely sensitive for detecting CBD stones. It may be used to rule out or locate CBD stones in suspected cases before gallbladder removal by laparoscopy.
- *Computed tomography (CT) scan.* Advanced techniques in CT scanning may identify the location and type of stone.
- *Isolation of microorganisms* in bile obtained during an endoscopic procedure. *Escherichia coli*, *Streptococcus*, and *Salmonella* are often isolated.

INTERVENTIONS

Prophylactic cholecystectomy for asymptomatic gallstones may be recommended in high-risk populations, including American Indians, morbidly obese persons, and persons with diabetes mellitus. Cholecystectomy is the standard recommendation for all patients with symptomatic gallbladder disease (including cholecystitis) for the relief of biliary pain and prevention of major complications.

Nonsurgical management may be obtained for those who cannot tolerate surgery, but is usually associated with stone recurrence. Nonsurgical management involves radiologic extraction, dissolution therapy, laser therapy, and extracorporeal shock wave lithotripsy.

Symptomatic Management

Opioid analgesics or nonsteroidal anti-inflammatory drugs (NSAIDs) may be used depending on the severity of the pain (see Chapter 12, Section 1). Anticholinergics or antispasmodics may also be used to decrease ductal tone and spasm. Antiemetics may provide relief of nausea and vomiting. If pruritus occurs from jaundice, cholestyramine (a bile salt-binding agent) may be prescribed. Calamine- or antihistamine-containing lotions and Alpha-Keri baths may be soothing.

A low-fat diet is recommended to reduce gallbladder stimulation. Foods to avoid include whole milk, butter, ice cream, fried foods, gravies, nuts, and pastries. A reduced-calorie diet may also be recommended for an obese patient.

Food and fluids may be withheld with placement of a nasogastric tube for decompression in patients with severe nausea and vomiting. Fluid and electrolytes must be closely monitored and replaced as needed. Gastric acid suppression therapy helps to prevent stress ulcers.

Nonsurgical Management
Endoscopic Retrograde Cholangiography

ERC allows for stone extraction from the CBD through the endoscope (see Diagnostic Criteria). In endoscopic sphincterotomy, the endoscope is placed in the same manner as for ERC. But the cannula apparatus allows for an incision into the sphincter of Oddi by electrocautery, allowing stones to pass freely into the duodenum, relieving obstruction.

Oral Solubilizing Agents

Ursodeoxycholic acid (UDCA) (ursodiol [Actigall]) and chenodiol are agents that contain a natural bile acid that slowly dissolves small uncalcified (radiolucent) gallstones over a period of 1 to 2 years. These agents are well tolerated, but mild transient diarrhea may occur in some patients. They require a functioning gallbladder, and are typically effective in 50% of patients.

Chemical Solvent Dissolution

This outpatient procedure uses monoctanoin, a cholesterol stone-dissolving solution (solvent). Patients must have symptomatic gallstones that are mostly cholesterol by composition as determined by specialized CT scan. The solvent is administered into the gallbladder via a catheter. The solvent is removed, but the catheter may be kept in place for a few days for later removal. While at home, the patient keeps the catheter taped to the skin; the catheter does not normally affect the patient's daily activities or work. Complete dissolution occurs in approximately one third of those treated.

Percutaneous Endoscopic Laser Lithotripsy

This procedure is effective for all types of stones. A laser probe inserted via a gallbladder catheter is used to apply short bursts of laser energy to fracture the stones into small pieces, which are then passed out of the gallbladder. This procedure is usually reserved for high-risk patients with noncholesterol stones.

Extracorporeal Shock Wave Lithotripsy

In extracorporeal shock wave lithotripsy (ESWL), shock waves generated outside the body are focused on the gallstones to fracture them into smaller fragments and "sand," which can then be dissolved more efficiently by oral agents. ESWL is useful for cholesterol stones. It is not effective for more than three stones or for large stones. A functioning gallbladder is required. ESWL necessitates sedation and may require analgesia for postprocedure tenderness. Biliary colic can occur as fragments pass through the bile duct into the intestine.

Antibiotics

Broad-spectrum antibiotic coverage may be required for the treatment of enteric organisms.

Surgical Management

Laparoscopic Cholecystectomy

This remains the treatment of choice for symptomatic gallstones. Hospital stays are typically less than 24 hours, pain level is minimal, and postoperative convalescent period is short. First, 4 to 5 L of carbon dioxide (CO_2) gas is injected into the abdomen to create a pneumoperitoneum. This separates the abdominal wall from the organs so that the gallbladder can be visualized. With the patient under general anesthesia, a video telescope and instruments are introduced into the abdomen through four or five small incisions and used to visualize, decompress, and remove the gallbladder. The patient is typically hospitalized for 1 to 2 days and requires a recovery time of 1 to 2 weeks. Possible contraindications to this procedure include cirrhosis, coagulopathy, pancreatitis, morbid obesity, and severe cardiorespiratory insufficiency. Conversion to an open procedure may be necessary because of multiple adhesions or an inability to visualize the bile ducts secondary to inflammation and edema.

Postoperative care involves monitoring for Kehr's sign (i.e., radiation of pain to the right shoulder), which can occur from diaphragmatic irritation from retained CO_2 gas. It is relieved by placing the patient in Sims' (side-lying) position. Pain is usually minimal because no muscles are cut and is relieved with oral analgesia. Incisional drainage should be scant, and bowel sounds should be present.

Open Cholecystectomy

In this procedure, the gallbladder is removed through an open incision and the cystic duct and its vessels are ligated. This procedure usually requires 3 to 5 days of hospitalization and 4 to 5 weeks of recuperation. A modification of this procedure is an open minimally invasive cholecystectomy, which involves 1 to 3 days of hospitalization and allows return to full activities in 2 weeks.

If CBD stones were identified radiographically, then exploration of the CBD with stone extraction is performed. CBD exploration usually leaves the frail duct edematous, necessitating T-tube placement to prevent obstruction of flow as bile continues to be produced.

A *T-tube* is a drain with the crossed part of the "T" placed in the CBD and the long end brought through a stab wound in the skin and connected to a drainage bag. Bile flows into the drainage bag, allowing the CBD to heal. T-tubes also facilitate the removal of residual stones and allow access for radiologic examination. T-tube drainage decreases as swelling subsides, allowing bile to drain unobstructed into the duodenum. (See Chapter 3, Section 4 for information on T-tube management.)

Postoperative care may involve nasogastric tube management and IV fluid administration until bowel sounds return. Bowel sounds should return in 24 to 72 hours. Teach the patient to avoid lifting anything weighing more than 10 lb, which puts a strain on the incision, for the first 4 postoperative weeks.

Common complications of cholecystectomy, both open and laparoscopic, include bile duct obstruction from stone retention, disruption of the ducts, and pancreatitis (see Chapter 17, Section 3). Symptoms of obstruction from retained stones include jaundice, dark yellow-brown urine, and clay-colored stools. Retained stones may be relieved by ERC with sphincterotomy or open exploration. Ductal disruption allows bile leakage; it requires surgical repair and T-tube placement. Bile leakage or other complications should be suspected in any patient who does not progress satisfactorily. The patient should be taught to look for and report local signs of infection (i.e., redness, swelling, drainage from incision sites) and signs and symptoms of peritonitis (i.e., fever, severe abdominal pain, and chills).

Cholecystostomy

In cholecystostomy, a catheter is placed into the gallbladder to enable drainage of pus and stones. This may be done if gallbladder removal is too dangerous because of severe infection and inflammation.

Choledochostomy

This procedure involves opening the CBD for stone removal and placing a T-tube in the CBD.

The gallbladder is not essential for life. Thus its removal may have little or no effect on digestion. Bile continues to be produced by the liver and is stored in the CBD, which enlarges to accommodate this function. Some patients may experience loose stools, gas, and bloating, but most require no dietary restrictions after gallbladder removal.

 COMMUNITY CARE

Community care involves ongoing teaching that targets various treatment options. The community team comprises the patient, physician, dietician, and community health nurse. A cooperative extension agent as well as a consultant from a state-funded nutrition program, can also be a valuable asset to the team, to assist in nutrition and meal planning for the patient and family.

Patients choosing nonsurgical interventions need teaching on the following subjects:

- Dietary considerations: Baseline nutritional assessment; low-fat diet for first few days after an acute episode
- Medications: Analgesics, antibiotics, oral bile acids; dicyclomine HCl (Bentyl) or nitroglycerin to decrease spasms and relax smooth muscles, thus decreasing abdominal pain
- Vital sign monitoring: Temperature elevation, which may indicate inflammation and/or infection

Those choosing surgical treatment need the following teaching:

- Dietary considerations: Advance to clear liquids, then to a full, soft diet; note tolerance before discharge to home
- Preoperative teaching: Surgical procedure, pulmonary toileting, diet
- Postoperative teaching: Pain control, analgesics, antibiotics, prevention of infection, resuming diet

Dietary consultation is ongoing and is valuable in decreasing the recurrence of acute cholelithiasis. The dietician or cooperative extension agent can help the patient and family recognize the benefits of a low-fat diet for all. The patient will also need teaching about reading food labels to help maintain a low-fat diet.

Typical high-fat foods to avoid should be reviewed with the patient and family. These foods may include:

- Gravies with fat and cream
- Whole-milk products
- Sausage, bacon, hot dogs
- Fried foods (e.g., hamburgers, French fries)
- Butter, cooking oils

The physician or another health care provider may review weight-reduction strategies with the patient as needed.

 PROGNOSIS

The prognosis for patients with cholelithiasis and cholecystitis is favorable, given the various surgical and nonsurgical treatments. Patients should be encouraged to monitor dietary fat intake, not only to help decrease the incidence of gall bladder disease, but also to help stem the growing epidemic of diabetes. Gallbladder disease affects the same ethnic minority groups as diabetes, and the major culprit in both is the excessive fat content of the typical American diet. Gall bladder disease provides health care practitioners with an opportunity to promote health interventions early, to decrease the need for the 500,000 cholecystectomies performed annually in this country.

 CLINICAL PEARLS

○ Address any patient anxiety related to changes in nutritional status.
○ Identify lifestyle, cultural, and psychosocial factors that affect the patient's dietary choices.
○ Encourage the patient to set realistic goals for dietary changes and/or weight loss.
○ Assess the patient's level of pain (acute of chronic) and encourage the patient to use various methods for pain relief.
○ Teach the patient to avoid a high-fat diet to decrease pain.
○ Encourage the patient to take pain medication during a pain crisis.
○ Encourage the patient to monitor temperature when pain occurs; this may indicate infection/inflammation.

NURSING PROBLEM/ DIAGNOSIS	NURSING INTERVENTIONS CLASSIFICATION (NIC)
Biliary pain	Pain Management
	Nutritional Counseling
	Teaching: Prescribed Medication
	Surveillance
Post-surgical management	Fluid and Electrolyte Management
	Tube Care: Gastrointestinal
	Incision Site Care
	Infection Protection

Hiatal Hernia

Section 2   Colette L. McKinney

 OVERVIEW

Although the exact prevalence of hiatal hernia is unknown, it is the most common abnormality of the gastrointestinal (GI) tract in Western countries. Hiatal hernia tends to be more common in women, but incidence in both sexes increases with advancing age. Approximately half of the U.S. population older than 50 years of age has some evidence of hiatal hernia.

 PATHOPHYSIOLOGY

Hiatal hernias are classified into four types on the basis of clinical presentation and management.

Sliding (Type I) Hernia

A sliding hiatal hernia is characterized by the extension of the distal esophagus and gastroesophageal (GE) junction into the thoracic cavity through the hiatus (Fig. 17-2-1). This upward movement occurs because of a lax phrenoesophageal ligament. A congenital short esophagus, weakening of the diaphragmatic muscles at the GE junction, or trauma can contribute to the development of sliding hernias.

GER and esophagitis are also associated with this type of hernia. This is because the hernia lowers the resting pressure of the lower esophageal sphincter (LES), allowing backward flow of gastric contents into the esophagus.

Paraesophageal (Type II) Hernia

A paraesophageal hiatal hernia is a true herniation of the stomach fundus into a mediastinal hernia sac while the GE junction remains anchored in its normal position below the diaphragm (see Fig. 17-2-1). Reflux is uncommon, because the GE junction is not disturbed; however, a portion of the stomach above the diaphragm causes congestion of blood flow and can lead to gastritis and ulcer formation. A large hernia may press on the mediastinum, producing angina-like pain or dyspnea. The hernia sac and gastric mobility can lead to

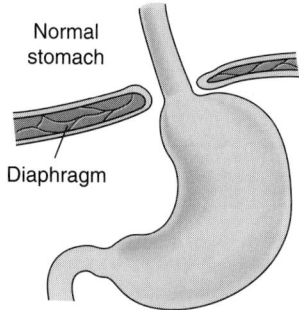

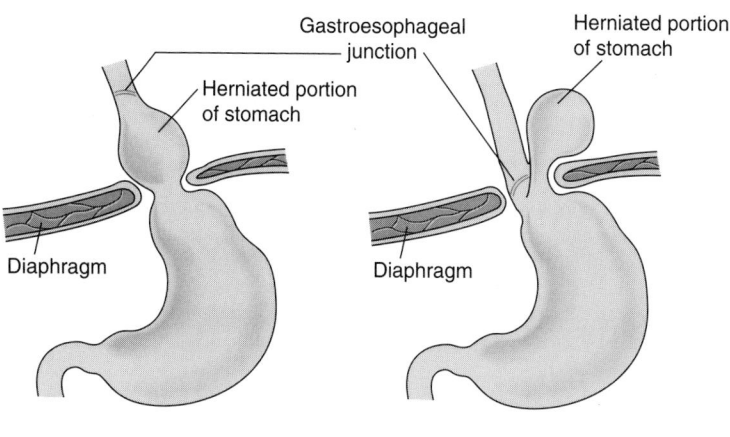

Figure 17-2-1. Sliding and rolling hiatal hernias.

obstruction, gastric volvulus, or strangulation, resulting in life-threatening conditions. Infarction of the hernia sac and perforation can cause massive bleeding.

Mixed (Type III) and Type IV Hernias

A mixed hernia develops when a paraesophageal hernia enlarges and the GE junction is pulled above the diaphragm. Because both the stomach and the GE junction are in the chest, reflux may be present, as may other symptoms and complications of paraesophageal hernia (e.g., obstruction). A type IV hernia develops with a large paraesophageal hernia when other viscera (e.g., colon, small intestine, spleen, pancreas) enter the hernia sac.

 ## SIGNS AND SYMPTOMS

Sliding (Type I) Hernia

Inappropriate relaxation of the LES causing GER is the most common clinical manifestation of a sliding hernia, although the patient may be asymptomatic. LES pressure can be influenced by dietary factors (e.g., caffeine), increased abdominal pressure (in, e.g., obesity and pregnancy) or pharmacologic agents (e.g., diazepam). Reflux symptoms in sliding hiatal hernia can appear as heartburn or substernal or epigastric pain (angina characteristics).

Although GER is a common treatable cause of chest pain, a cardiac or pulmonary cause should be excluded first. Thus, extensive and costly workups may be unavoidable. Excessive coughing, ascites, tight clothing, bending, or improper posture accentuates the discomfort. Increased intra-abdominal pressure caused by recumbent positions accentuates discomfort and also increases the risk of nocturnal aspiration and resultant bronchitis or pneumonitis.

Complications

If reflux is allowed to continue, the protective mucosal barrier of the esophagus starts to break down, triggering an inflammatory response. Esophageal shortening, bleeding, and stricture formation are associated with chronic inflammation. The most worrisome complication of inadequately treated GER is Barrett's esophagus (replacement of the normal lining of the esophagus with columnar epithelium), which increases the risk of cancer.

Other complications include iron deficiency anemia and nocturnal aspiration, leading to bronchitis or pneumonitis.

Paraesophageal (Type II) Hernia

Signs and symptoms of paraesophageal hernias result from an anatomic defect rather than physiologic changes. Reflux usually is not associated with paraesophageal hernias, because the LES remains below the diaphragm. Often these patients are asymptomatic, which allows the hernia to enlarge undetected. Large hernias can cause palpitations, dyspnea, and epigastric or substernal pain, caused by pressure exerted on the mediastinum.

Complications

Development of ulcers in the supradiaphragmatic stomach (Cameron's ulcers), along with vascular engorgement secondary to venous occlusion, can lead to bleeding, melena, and various degrees of iron deficiency anemia. Because the bleeding is slow and insidious, the patient may not be aware of the anemia until symptoms cause him or her to seek medical attention. Other complications associated with paraesophageal hernias include obstruction, perforation, intrathoracic stomach, and gastric volvulus resulting from lack of gastric mobility and laxity of the ligaments.

Gastric volvulus is an acquired rotation of the stomach of 180 degrees or more, resulting in a closed-loop obstruction. It most often occurs as a complication of a paraesophageal hernia and is life-threatening because of possible incarceration, necrosis, and hemorrhage of strangulated blood vessels in the GI tract. Respiratory compromise, caused by a significant mediastinal shift of abdominal organs (particularly the stomach), is most common in infants and the elderly, who already have limited pulmonary reserve. Chronic gastric volvulus develops slowly over time and may be asymptomatic. Gastric volvulus should be suspected in patients with dysphagia or abrupt onset of abdominal pain, nausea, or vomiting.

Mixed (Type III) and Type IV Hernias

Mixed (type III) and type IV hernias are a combination of sliding and enlarged paraesophageal hernias; therefore, signs, symptoms, and complications are also a combination of those of sliding and paraesophageal hernias. Signs and symptoms include reflux (regurgitation), heartburn, substernal or epigastric pain, dyspnea, palpitations, melena, low LES pressure, and prolonged pH monitoring score above 20 (see Diagnostic Testing). Complications include esophageal shortening, bleeding, iron deficiency anemia, strangulation, perforation, incarceration, necrosis, obstruction, gastric volvulus, Barrett's esophagus, herniation of abdominal organs (in type IV hernia), nocturnal aspiration, ulceration, strictures, and mediastinal pressure.

 DIAGNOSTIC CRITERIA

An ordinary upright *chest radiograph* confirms the diagnosis of a paraesophageal hiatal hernia by revealing a retrocardiac air fluid level. An *upper GI study* with barium swallow confirms the diagnosis and identifies the type of hernia by determining the location of the GE junction and abdominal organs and by detecting reflux, if present. The absence of contrast in the thorax does not rule out the diagnosis of paraesophageal hernia, however. A tight orifice may prevent the contrast medium from filling the herniated portion of the stomach.

Upper GI endoscopy enables identification and location of the GE junction and evaluation of acquired short esophagus and mucosal changes that suggest reflux. This enables both visualization and biopsy for histologic assessment, which cannot be done in a barium swallow.

A CT scan is usually not necessary for a diagnosis but can help distinguish a hernia from an abdominal mass. Other procedures that are not used routinely include esophageal manometry and prolonged pH monitoring.

Esophageal manometry measures LES pressure and is used to evaluate patients with suspected reflux. This test is not performed for a true paraesophageal hernia; in this case, results would be normal, because the GE junction remains anchored in its normal position.

Prolonged pH monitoring evaluates the frequency and duration of reflux over a 12- to 24-hour period. Based on the percentage of time that the pH is below 5, the number of GER episodes, the duration of the longest episode, and the number of episodes lasting longer then 5 minutes yields a computerized score. A score above 20 is abnormal and indicative of GER.

 INTERVENTIONS

Diet and Lifestyle Changes

Diet and lifestyle changes are usually the bases of managing hiatal hernia. Avoidance of smoking and alcohol are remediable lifestyle issues that should be addressed. Smoking, alcoholic beverages, and caffeine decrease LES pressure, allowing for reflux. Sleeping with the head of the bed elevated, correcting posture, avoiding tight-fitting clothes, and eating small frequent meals may help to relieve some symptoms.

Because obesity increases intraabdominal pressure and severity of symptoms, diet modification should focus on weight reduction, as needed. Other diet and lifestyle modifications include those recommendations for gastroesophageal reflux disease (GERD) (Table 17-2-1).

Although these recommendations reduce symptoms, they may not necessarily correct the problem. Medical management is likely needed.

Pharmacotherapy

Medical treatment is an integral part of reflux management. Symptoms of reflux are managed effectively in 90% of patients when pharmacotherapy is added to conventional behavior modifications.

 Table 17-2-1. Diet, Lifestyle, and Pharmacologic Recommendations for Treating Gastroesophageal Reflux Disease

Diet	Avoid caffeine (e.g., chocolate, coffee, tea, cola).
	Avoid medications containing caffeine (e.g., Vivarin, Excedrin).
	Eat four to six small meals daily.
	Avoid lying down 2 to 3 hours after eating.
	Avoid snacking 2 to 3 hours before bedtime.
	Eat a high-protein, low-fat diet (stimulates gastrin release).
Lifestyle	Avoid constrictive clothing or belts, heavy lifting, and working in a slouched or bent position.
	Eliminate or reduce nicotine-containing products (e.g., smoking, smokeless tobacco).
	Reduce body weight if obese.
Pharmacologic	Avoid drugs that decrease lower esophageal sphincter pressure:
	• Calcium channel blockers
	• Alpha-adrenergic antagonists
	• Progesterone
	• Diazepam
	• Tricyclic antidepressnts
	• Beta-adrenergic agonists
	• Anticholinergics
	• Theophylline
	Avoid drugs that cause direct esophageal mucosal injury:
	• Alendronate
	• Nonsteroidal anti-inflammatory drugs
	• Potassium chloride tablets
	• Aspirin
	• Quinidine
	• Tetracycline
	• Iron salts

Although antacids play a part in the initial therapy, histamine-receptor antagonists (e.g., ranitidine, cimetidine, famotidine, nizatidine) and proton pump inhibitors (e.g., omeprazole, lansoprazole) have become the mainstays of medical therapy. Histamine-receptor antagonists and proton pump inhibitors are both antisecretory agents that reversibly inhibit acid secretion and elevate serum gastrin levels. They are effective in both gastric and duodenal ulcers. Patients with mild-to-moderate reflux are usually treated with histamine-receptor antagonists. Those with more severe symptoms are given proton pump inhibitors, which have a longer duration of action than histamine-receptor antagonists. If these two agents fail to provide adequate relief, a prokinetic oral agent (e.g., cisapride) may be added.

A health history must include identification of any drug that affects LES pressure or promotes gastric ulceration. Table 17-2-1 lists agents that decrease LES pressure and that cause direct esophageal mucosal injury. These agents must be avoided or used judiciously.

Surgical Management

Although surgical correction of a sliding hernia is not mandatory treatment, failure of conservative methods and medical therapy should warrant consideration of surgery to prevent associated complications. Asymptomatic patients with paraesophageal hernias who are good surgical candidates are generally advised to have surgery. Because the risk of surgical complications increases with age and with other preexisting health problems, good clinical judgment is essential. Life-threatening complications of paraesophageal hernias (e.g., gastric volvulus) provide a rationale for surgical intervention, regardless of the severity of symptoms.

Failure to relieve symptoms of reflux led to the development of an antireflux procedure. The three most frequent antireflux repairs performed are Nissen fundoplication, Hill gastroplexy, and Belsey Mark IV fundoplication; in these procedures, the common goal is to recreate a competent antireflux barrier. The transabdominal approach is preferred because it is more protective of the abdominal organs. However, the transthoracic approach may be required in certain cases (e.g., extreme obesity).

Nissen fundoplication (in which the stomach fundus is wrapped around the lower esophagus at the GE junction) is the most commonly used procedure for repairing sliding hernias because of its effectiveness in relieving the symptoms of GER. Laparoscopic fundoplication has become a suitable alternative to an open procedure in selected cases. In terms of recovery and perioperative morbidity, the laparoscopic approach is favored and further fuels the enthusiasm for early surgical intervention. Dysphagia can develop if the wrap is too tight; bloating can result if the wrap is too long. An esophageal surgeon with experience in laparoscopic techniques can safely and successfully perform the procedure, thereby decreasing complications and hospital stay.

 COMMUNITY CARE

Although hiatal hernia is a common abnormality, determining its incidence is difficult, because many persons are asymptomatic and hernias are often incidental findings. The availability of effective over-the-counter medications (e.g., Pepcid AC, Zantac) may affect a person's decision to seek medical advice. A person may not be aware that a hernia is the cause of his or her heartburn and thus may not explore options for surgical management. Delaying medical advice could lead to possible complications or life-threatening conditions such as anemia or perforation. On the other hand, over-the-counter medications may be appropriate for selected patients who can be managed adequately with them. However, it is essential that persons be aware that medical advice should be sought if symptoms of reflux are not relieved or if they find themselves taking more and more of the same medication for relief.

Avoiding the use of agents that decrease LES pressure may not always be the best decision. For example, although diazepam lowers LES pressure, for some patients a good night's sleep may be far more important than any potential problems associated with decreased LES pressure.

 ## PROGNOSIS

There is general agreement that paraesophageal hernias should be repaired selectively, especially in good surgical candidates, to avoid serious complications such as gastric volvulus and the high mortality rate associated with incarceration. Complications of esophagitis in sliding hernias are expected in 33% of all symptomatic patients. Although the risk of developing Barrett's esophagus is only 7% to 10%, this premalignant condition increases the risk of adenocarcinoma 30- to 40-fold above that in the general population. Cameron's ulcers develop in approximately 7% of paraesophageal hernias; bleeding and anemia stemming from ulceration occur in 20% of cases. Complications associated with hiatal hernias can be virtually eliminated with appropriate recognition, diagnosis, and management.

 ## CLINICAL PEARLS

○ Surgical repair is appropriate for selected patients.
○ Surgical repair of a sliding hiatal hernia should be considered for patients with related problems, those at risk for developing complications, and those for whom medical therapy has failed.
○ Surgical repair should also be considered for patients who cannot afford or do not wish to take lifelong medication, and for those who are noncompliant.
○ A true paraesophageal hernia must be distinguished from a mixed hernia, especially when surgery is being considered.
○ All patients who present with noncardiac chest pain should be followed up with either endoscopy or barium swallow to rule out the presence of a hiatal hernia so that appropriate therapy may be initiated.
○ Patient complaints of choking, coughing, or wheezing during the night are often misdiagnosed as asthma.
○ Nocturnal aspiration should be considered in patients with recurrent episodes of asthma, bronchitis, or pneumonitis, because patients will not necessarily complain of reflux if they are asymptomatic.
○ In patients presenting with acute onset of abdominal pain, nausea, or vomiting, gastric volvulus should be considered.
○ Patients with acute volvulus may present with a history of inability to swallow food and high gastric obstruction.

NURSING PROBLEM/ DIAGNOSIS	NURSING INTERVENTIONS CLASSIFICATION (NIC)
Risk for complications	Nutritional Counseling Smoking Cessation Assistance Self-modification Assistance

Pancreatitis

Section 3   Nancy Stark

OVERVIEW

The pancreas is responsible for the production and secretion of enzymes and hormones that promote the digestion of fats, proteins, and carbohydrates in the metabolism of sugars. Inflammation of the pancreas, or pancreatitis, has acute and chronic forms. Pancreatitis occurs in response to various precipitating factors. Whatever the precipitating factor, an abnormal premature activation of the pancreatic enzymes initiates the process of organ autodigestion.

PATHOPHYSIOLOGY

The pancreas is an accessory organ of the GI system that has exocrine and endocrine functions. The acini cells of the exocrine pancreas produce the enzymes amylase, lipase, proelastase, trypsinogen, chymotrypsinogen, and phospholipase. The enzymes are secreted in an inactive form by the pancreas into the duodenum, where they mix with intestinal contents and become activated. In the intestine, the activated enzymes digest protein, fats, and carbohydrates.

The alpha, beta, and delta cells of the endocrine pancreas produce insulin, glucagon, and somatostatin, respectively. These hormones are then secreted into the blood supply and influence the metabolism of the body's sugars.

Multiple factors can contribute to the development of pancreatitis. The most common precipitating factors (accounting for 80% of cases) are biliary tract disease (e.g., gallstones) and alcoholism. Other precipitating factors include infections, trauma, stomach or biliary tract surgery, prescription drugs (e.g., NSAIDs, estrogens, sulfonamides, thiazide diuretics), hyperlipidemia, and heredity. In some cases, no precipitating factors are identified. Alcoholism is the most common cause of chronic pancreatitis.

Several theories are proposed to explain the preactivation of pancreatic enzymes. One theory suggests that causative agents initiate toxins that alter the normal pancreatic metabolic and secretory processes. A second theory suggests that reflux of duodenal contents containing activated digestive enzymes into the pancreas occurs. A third theory proposes that a gallstone obstructs the ampulla of Vater and allows for bile reflux back into the pancreas, resulting in enzyme activation within the pancreas. Yet another theory promotes pancreatic ductal hypertension resulting in outflow obstruction as a possible cause.

Common to all of these theories is the fact that the organ's digestive enzymes are prematurely activated within the pancreas and the process of autodigestion is initiated. Autodigestion causes inflammation that results in edema, hemorrhage, and necrosis of the pancreatic duct and its surrounding tissues.

Acute pancreatitis may be clinically classified as mild or severe. In mild acute pancreatitis, there is minimal interstitial edema with no organ system failure. The pancreas usually remains normal before and after the attack. Patients usually improve in 48 to 72 hours with supportive care. Severe acute pancreatitis is accompanied by necrosis, organ failure, and increased mortality. It is characterized by rupture of the pancreatic ducts and spillage of pancreatic enzymes into the peritoneum, resulting in a chemical peritonitis and systemic inflammation.

Chronic pancreatitis is an ongoing inflammatory disorder characterized by varying degrees of irreversible damage and ultimately loss of function. Fat digestion is affected most severely.

 SIGNS AND SYMPTOMS

The most common complaint of patients with acute or chronic pancreatitis is *abdominal pain*. In acute pancreatitis, the pain is severe and isolated in the epigastric region and may radiate to the back. The abdominal pain is generally constant and does not fluctuate in intensity or subside for any periods. The pain may worsen with the ingestion of food or alcohol. Nausea and vomiting are other common findings. Additional findings may include anorexia, dehydration, jaundice, low-grade fever, and weakness.

The patient with chronic pancreatitis may present with dull epigastric pain and weight loss in the presence of normal eating habits and appetite. Symptoms of diabetes (e.g., increased thirst, hunger, and urination) are associated with chronic pancreatitis. Steatorrhea, resulting from inadequate digestion of fats, may also be present.

The inflammation of severe acute pancreatitis may progress to multiple organs. Patients may experience pleural effusion, abdominal rigidity, and ascites. Oliguria, tachycardia, and hypotension may be signs that a shock state is developing. Inflammation, renal failure, adult respiratory distress syndrome, and myocardial depression can occur. Pancreatic hemorrhage, a rare finding, manifests as *Cullen's sign* (bluish discoloration of the periumbilical region) or *Grey-Turner's sign* (bluish discoloration of the flanks).

Abdominal inspection may reveal distention. There are decreased or absent bowel sounds on auscultation. The area over the pancreas is dull to percussion. Guarding, rebound tenderness, and mass may be detected by palpation. Rebound tenderness is associated with a more advanced stage of pancreatitis and indicates inflammation from spillage of enzymes into the peritoneal cavity.

Patient history usually reveals one of the following risk factors, which should be investigated:

- Previous gallstones or biliary disease
- Alcohol ingestion, including amount, frequency, and duration
- Previous episodes of pancreatitis or abdominal pain
- Current prescription drug regimen
- Recent blunt or penetrating trauma

- Recent gastric or biliary surgery
- Recent GI tests (e.g., ERCP or endoscopy)
- Recent infections

 DIAGNOSTIC CRITERIA

The diagnosis of pancreatitis is based on patient history, clinical findings, laboratory studies, and radiographic and imaging findings.

Laboratory Values

The following tests are used in the diagnosis of pancreatitis.

Serum Amylase. Normal amylase level is 60 to 180 Somogyi units/dL. Amylase is a commonly used indicator in the diagnosis of pancreatitis. Serum amylase levels are elevated to 3 to 5 times normal within 6 to 8 hours after the onset of symptoms. The level remains elevated for 24 to 72 hours.

Serum Lipase. Normal serum lipase level is 13 to 141 Somogyi units/L. Lipase is a more specific indicator of pancreatitis. Lipase levels elevate within the first 24 to 48 hours after symptom onset. Levels remain elevated for 5 to 7 days.

Urine Amylase. Normal urine amylase level is 35 to 260 Somogyi units/hr or 260 to 950 Somogyi units/24 hr. The urine amylase level rises within 6 to 8 hours of symptom onset and remains elevated for 7 to 10 days.

Additional Laboratory Values

The following tests are not specific to the diagnosis of pancreatitis but can be useful tools in assessing causative factors for the disease and associated complications.

Serum Glucose. Transient mild elevations of serum glucose may be seen early in acute pancreatitis. Persistent hyperglycemia may be indicative of pancreatic necrosis in more advanced acute pancreatitis. In chronic pancreatitis, hyperglycemia could indicate the onset of diabetes mellitus.

White Blood Cell (WBC) Count. WBCs may be moderately elevated in association with an infectious process in pancreatitis.

Serum Potassium. Nausea and vomiting are symptoms of pancreatitis. In a patient who has experienced vomiting, serum potassium level may be low. A patient whose disease has progressed to a necrotizing state may have elevated levels.

Serum Calcium. Low calcium levels may be seen 2 to 3 days after disease onset. As serum albumin (see Chapter 9, Section 1) levels decrease, reductions in serum calcium will occur, because 50% of calcium (see Chapter 11, Section 3) is bound to albumin. Hypoalbuminemia is usually related to poor digestion of nutrients.

Hematocrit. Hematocrit may be low because of the hemoconcentration related to fluid sequestration.

Liver Enzymes. Levels of liver enzymes may be elevated from biliary tract disease or from alcohol ingestion.

Radiologic Procedures

Abdominal Films. Abdominal x-rays are used to identify accumulations of gas, ileus, ascites, or dilatation of the small intestine in proximity to the pancreas.

Abdominal Ultrasound. Ultrasound can define fluid, tumor, masses, stones, fistulas, pseudocysts, abscess, and organ enlargement. Ultrasound is used to rule out the blockage of pancreatic secretions by gallstones, to determine the size of the CBD and its contents, and to detect and localize fluid collection.

Computed Tomography Scan. CT scans are used to visualize the pancreas and surrounding structures and define tumors, abscesses, and space-occupying lesions. The most common CT finding in pancreatitis is pancreatic enlargement. The second most common finding is phlegmon (a solid mass of inflamed pancreas with patchy areas of necrosis).

Magnetic Resonance Imaging. Magnetic resonance imaging (MRI) can visualize the pancreas and surrounding structures.

Endoscopic Retrograde Cholangiopancreatography. ERCP is used when direct visualization of the pancreatic ductal system is necessary. The test can reveal strictures, obstruction, intraductal stones, and ductal dilatation.

 INTERVENTIONS

Management of the patient with pancreatitis focuses on relief of symptoms, supportive care, rest of the pancreas, and complication management. This section discusses treatment goals for acute and chronic pancreatitis and for an acute exacerbation of chronic pancreatitis.

Elimination of Oral Intake

Nasogastric suction is used for patients with consistent vomiting, gastric distention, or ileus. It is also used to reduce contents entering the small intestine, which reduces the stimulation of pancreatic secretions. Oral intake should be stopped and not resumed until symptoms abate. Nutritional support must continue with the initiation of intravenous (IV) fluid therapy. TPN may be necessary for patients who develop a complicated course and do not recover quickly.

Fluid and Electrolyte Replacement

Assessment for clinical signs of dehydration coupled with accurate intake and output measurement is needed. IV fluids or colloids are administered to restore intravascular volume. Electrolyte replacement is often needed. Calcium, potassium, and magnesium levels should be monitored, with supplemental replacements provided as needed. Glucose should also be monitored, with sliding-scale insulin coverage used for hyperglycemia.

Pain Management

Abdominal pain is the most common symptom of pancreatitis, and pain control is a crucial aspect of management. A standard pain intensity scale should be used to ensure consistent assessment and evaluation. Analgesics (e.g., Demerol) are administered for pain control via a patient-controlled analgesia (PCA) pump. Alternative pain control measures (e.g., imagery, relaxation, massage) may also be used. Morphine is usually avoided, because it is believed to cause spasm of the sphincter of Oddi. Like all mu-agonist opioids, meperidine affects the sphincter of Oddi. All opioids, including meperidine, can increase smooth muscle tone in the biliary tract, causing constriction, decreased biliary flow, and increased bile duct pressure and resulting in biliary and pancreatic duct spasm.

Some believe that because pancreatic pain is often resistant to opioid therapy, morphine may be a better choice because it has no toxic ceiling or metabolites, as meperidine does. Meperidine is still most commonly recommended for the relief of abdominal pain associated with pancreatitis.

Treatment of the Causative Agent

Identifying and modifying the causative agent can help prevent further attacks. Patients who use alcohol chronically or excessively should stop drinking and be referred for counseling and treatment. If gallstones or CBD disease is the causative factor, then cholecystectomy (see Section 1) should be performed.

Prevention of, Monitoring for, and Treatment of Complications

Assess vital signs, perform a physical examination, evaluate laboratory test values, and monitor intake and output. Patients with acute pancreatitis who develop pseudocyst, abscess, or hemorrhagic complications may require surgical intervention, including lavage, drainage, and débridement.

Other Interventions

Pancreatic extracts (pancreatin, pancrelipase) may be administered orally to prevent malabsorption in a patient with chronic pancreatitis.

Surgical treatment in chronic pancreatitis may be performed to relieve intractable pain, facilitate pancreatic drainage, or resect diseased portions of the organ.

Prophylactic antibiotic use is necessary in severe acute pancreatitis to reduce the risk of septic complications and improve the likelihood of survival. Broad-spectrum antibiotics may be used to treat infection or abscess.

Endocrine function may be affected, most commonly in chronic pancreatitis, necessitating insulin replacement therapy and blood glucose monitoring.

 COMMUNITY CARE

The goals of community care are to:
- Help the patient achieve and maintain a healthy lifestyle.
- Encourage compliance with the treatment plan.

The following are suggestions to facilitate achievement of the recommended goals:

- Causative factors precipitating the disease should be determined and the patient and family educated about the factors.
- If excessive alcohol use was a causative factor, the patient should be referred for counseling and treatment by substance abuse experts.
- Annual health screenings and evaluations should be encouraged. An exercise regimen and stress management techniques should be developed and implemented.
- Nutrition and diet management counseling should be offered. High-protein, high-carbohydrate, low-fat diets are encouraged.
- Patient and family education regarding the signs and symptoms of pancreatitis should be reinforced and reporting of any signs or symptoms encouraged. Teaching about known complications (e.g., diabetes) should be provided.

• The need for home health support and referral to community agencies is assessed.

 PROGNOSIS

In 85% to 90% of patients with acute pancreatitis, the disease is self-limiting and subsides within 3 to 7 days after the initiation of treatment. Complications that can cause morbidity and mortality include renal failure, infection, abscess, fistula or pseudocyst formation, adult respiratory distress syndrome, and shock. The overall mortality rate for acute pancreatitis is 10%. Patients who develop hemorrhagic pancreatitis have a mortality rate of 50%.

A tool used to predict the severity and outcome in acute pancreatitis is Ranson's prognostic signs (Table 17-3-1).

 CLINICAL PEARLS

○ There is no gold standard or single diagnostic laboratory indicator for pancreatitis. The most common laboratory tests used in the diagnosis of pancreatitis are serum amylase and lipase levels.

○ The pain associated with pancreatitis is often described as radiating to the back. The pancreas is a retroperitoneal organ.

○ Abdominal pain associated with pancreatitis is generally not relieved by vomiting.

○ One supportive measure to relieve abdominal pain associated with pancreatitis is to have the patient sit up and lean slightly forward. Lying down flat can often aggravate the pain.

○ In patients with acute pancreatitis, auscultate the left lower lobes of the lungs, because a left-sided pleural effusion is a possible complication of pancreatitis.

○ Noting the time from onset of symptoms is important. A patient who did not present for treatment until several days after the onset of symptoms could have a normal serum amylase level. An elevated serum amylase level

Table 17-3-1. Ranson's Prognostic Signs for Predicting Severity in Patients with Acute Pancreatitis

At admission or diagnosis
• Age over 55 years
• White blood cell count over 16,000/mm^3
• Blood glucose over 200 mg/dL
• Serum lactate dehydrogenase over 350 U/L
• Serum aspartate transaminase over 250 sigma-frankel units %

During the initial 48 hours
• Hermatocrit falls more than 10%
• Blood urea nitrogen rises to greater than 5 mg/dL
• Serum calcium level is below 8 mg/dL
• Arterial oxygen (Pao$_2$) is below 60 mm Hg
• Base deficit is greater than 4 mEq/L
• Estimated fluid sequestration is more than 6000 mL

Mortality predications associated with Ranson's prognostic signs
• Three to five signs: 10%–20% mortality
• More than six signs: 50% or greater mortality

is not necessarily indicative of pancreatic disease. Serum amylase can be elevated in a number of disease states, including salivary gland dysfunction, tumors of the ovary and lung, intestinal obstruction, and biliary tract disease.

NURSING PROBLEM/ DIAGNOSIS	NURSING INTERVENTIONS CLASSIFICATION (NIC)
Acute pain	Analgesic Administration
	Pain Management
Fluid and electrolyte replacement/Deficient fluid volume	Fluid/Electrolyte Management
	Intravenous Therapy
	Vital Sign Monitoring
Elimination of oral intake	Gastrointestinal Intubation
	Nutrition Management
	Total Parenteral Nutrition (TPN) Administration

Peptic Ulcer

Section 4   Maryjo Gerlach

 ## OVERVIEW

Approximately 25 million persons in the United States suffer from peptic ulcer disease (PUD), and every year there are approximately 500,000 new cases. PUD is now attributed to three major causes: NSAIDs, hypersecretory states (e.g., Zollinger-Ellison syndrome), and chronic *Helicobacter pylori* infection.

The rate of PUD has declined since 1982, as practitioners have become more knowledgeable about the correlations between PUD and *H. pylori* infection, and with the advent of multidrug (anti-infective agents, antisecretory agents, and antacids) treatment protocols. Approximately two thirds of the world's population is infected with the *H. pylori* bacterium. In the United States, the organism is most prevalent in older adults, African Americans, Hispanics, and persons of lower socioeconomic status.

 ## PATHOPHYSIOLOGY

PUD involves disorders of the upper GI tract caused by the corrosive actions of acid and pepsin on the GI mucosa. These disorders can range from slight mucosal injury to severe ulceration and can occur in the esophagus, stomach, or duodenum. The duodenum is the most common location, followed by the stomach.

Peptic ulcers form when corrosive gastric juices penetrate the gastric mucosal barrier or spill into the proximal duodenum. Once the mucosal barrier is penetrated, these agents cause destruction of the unprotected epithelial cell membrane and eventual erosion of the epithelial wall.

The cause of *ulcerogenesis,* or ulcer development, is multifactorial. A balance exists between factors that naturally protect the gastric mucosa (defensive factors) and those that contribute to mucosal injury (aggressive factors).

There are four defensive factors that prevent ulceration. First, a layer of mucus is produced by cells of the GI mucosa that coats and protects the gastric epithelium. Second, the secretion of bicarbonate by the epithelial cells maintains a slightly alkaline mucosal environment. Third, blood flow to the GI epithelium assists in the renewal of epithelial cells as they rapidly regenerate. Finally, prostaglandins contribute to increased blood flow by causing vasodilatation. Adequate submucosal blood flow is essential to maintain epithelial and mucosal cells. Ischemia leads to cell injury and loss of defense mechanisms.

Factors that make the mucosa more susceptible to the injurious actions of acid and pepsin include *H. pylori* infection, aspirin and NSAID use, smoking, and alcohol.

H. pylori **Infection.** *H. pylori* is a gram-negative bacillus that resides in the submucosal space. Reports suggest that up to 90% of persons with duodenal ulcers and 70% of persons with gastric ulcers have *H. pylori* infection. Research is ongoing to determine the actual mechanisms through which *H. pylori* promotes or activates ulcer formation. Its presence allows acid and pepsin to penetrate the epithelial cells. In addition, the organism itself produces urease, an enzyme that converts gastric urea to carbon dioxide and ammonia, both of which are irritating to the gastric mucosa.

Humans are believed to be the primary reservoir for the *H. pylori* organism. Once a person is infected, possibly in early childhood, the organism may live for years without causing any symptoms of clinical illness. *H. pylori* is most likely spread person to person, through fecal-oral and/or oral-oral routes. Research continues to identify transmission routes and to determine why some persons develop PUD and others remain disease-free.

Aspirin and NSAIDs. These drugs strip away the surface mucus, allowing acid and pepsin to penetrate into the epithelial layers.

Smoking. PUD develops twice as often in smokers than in nonsmokers. Smoking is also related to poor ulcer healing and increased rates of recurrence.

Alcohol. Alcohol is a potent stimulator of acid secretions.

Zollinger-Ellison Syndrome. Zollinger-Ellison syndrome is a condition caused by the development of gastrin secreting tumors of the pancreas. Gastrin is a hormone that causes the release of hydrochloric acid and pepsin. In this syndrome excessive amounts are released leading to peptic ulceration.

Gastric ulcers and duodenal ulcers are distinct entities that share the common elements of decreased mucosal defenses or increased gastric acid secretion. *Gastric ulcers* are less common than duodenal ulcers and occur more often in persons over age 65, especially in women. Persons with gastric ulcers are at increased risk for gastric carcinoma.

Duodenal ulcer formation is associated with hypersecretion of acid. Increased acid production may result from increased stimulation of the vagus nerve due to physiologic or psychological stress, hyperplasia of the gastric parietal cells, or possibly from genetic influences. This can overwhelm the gastric defense mechanisms. The two groups at greatest risk are children and persons in the fifth decade of life.

Complications of PUD include hemorrhage, obstruction, and perforation. Hemorrhage occurs in approximately 20% of patients with duodenal ulcers. Perforation affects 2% to 3% of patients with duodenal ulcers, penetrating into the peritoneal cavity most commonly and into the liver, colon, and biliary tract less commonly.

 SIGNS AND SYMPTOMS

Epigastric pain, including nocturnal episodes, is frequently described as gnawing or burning and is present in 80% to 90% percent of patients. Pain itself is not a specific enough symptom to provide a definitive diagnostic criterion, however. The pain is frequently relieved by ingesting food or antacid (especially when associated with duodenal ulcer) but may recur when the stomach empties 2 to 4 hours later. In patients with gastric ulcers, food intake may intensify pain because of the local irritation to the gastric mucosa. Other, less common symptoms may include nausea, vomiting, belching, bloating, and anorexia.

For some persons, especially chronic NSAID users, painless bleeding may be the first signs of an ulcer. If bleeding is extensive, hematemesis (vomiting of bright red blood), hematochezia (stools containing bright red blood), or melena (stools containing dark blood) may be present.

 DIAGNOSTIC CRITERIA

Upper Endoscopy

This is the procedure of choice for inspecting the mucosal surfaces of the esophagus, stomach, and duodenum to detect possible irritation, inflammation, erythema, pallor, or atrophy. An endoscope is placed through the esophagus to visualize any pathology in the upper GI tract. Endoscopy also enables biopsy to detect *H. pylori* or malignancy.

Upper Gastrointestinal Series

An upper gastrointestinal (UGI) series with barium contrast medium allows for x-ray visualization of possible pathology and may be definitive for persons with uncomplicated dyspepsia (heartburn). Direct endoscopic visualization of any existing pathology is preferred. It is impossible to differentiate benign ulcers from malignant ulcers through imaging.

Testing for H. pylori Infection

H. pylori may be diagnosed by serological tests, a breath test, or with biopsy. *Serology* is an inexpensive test that is useful in measuring *H. pylori*-specific IgG antibodies to detect infection. The test is simple and can be performed in an office or clinic setting. Serology tests are useful when a biopsy for the rapid urease test is not possible.

The *breath test* detects active infection by measuring the amount of labeled carbon in exhaled air following ingestion of either ^{13}C (nonradioactive) or ^{14}C (radioactive) urea. In the presence of *H. pylori*, urea is hydrolyzed to the labeled bicarbonate and ultimately to labeled carbon dioxide (CO_2). The labeled CO_2 is then measured in the expired air. Preferred follow-up is no sooner than 4 weeks after antibiotic therapy.

The rapid urease test (*Campylobacter*-like organism test, CLO test) involves obtaining a biopsy of gastric tissue by endoscopy. The tissue sample is placed in an agar gel, containing gastric urea. If present, the *H. pylori* organism produces urease as gastric urea is metabolized. A distinctive color change occurs within several hours or after up to 24 hours, depending on the concentration of the bacterium in the tissue sample. False-negative results can occur if the concentration of the bacterium in the particular tissue sample is absent or low. The test itself is inexpensive; however, the tissue samples must be obtained through endoscopy.

Mucosal biopsy is essential for histologic examination. Samples are obtained at the same time that the rapid urease test samples are collected. If result of the rapid urease test is negative, the pathologist can examine the tissue samples for the presence of *H. pylori* and also visually inspect the status of mucosal tissue. Tissues may be cultured; however, this is a complex procedure, and results may take a long time to determine.

Routine Laboratory Studies

Complete blood count (CBC) and hematocrit are most valuable in determining possible complications associated with PUD, such as anemia related to acute or chronic blood loss from a bleeding ulcer. Elevated WBC count may be indicative of ulcer perforation from an inflammatory response. Expect an elevated serum amylase level if the ulcer has penetrated the pancreas. Cultures are time-consuming and expensive and are useful only if bacterial sensitivity is required before treatment.

INTERVENTIONS

Drug Therapy

The purpose of drug therapy in treating PUD is to reduce symptoms by neutralizing or suppressing acid secretion, to enhance healing, and to prevent ulcer recurrence (Table 17-4-1). Acid suppression is achieved by H_2 blockers or proton pump inhibitors. Other drugs provide a milieu that supports healing of the ulcer.

Antibacterial agents are the only definitive treatment to eradicate *H. pylori*. Therapy regimens for *H. pylori* infection consist of 10 to 14 days of antibiotics plus a proton pump inhibitor or Bismuth. Bismuth, normally listed as an antidiarrheal, actually acts topically on bacteria, disrupting the cell wall and leading to bacterial cell lysis and death. Multiple antibiotics are necessary to reduce resistance. Cost, compliance, side effects, and drug interactions affect the choice of regimen used.

Triple therapy in 14-day courses has the best eradication rate (up to 94%) of all regimens. Proton pump inhibitor (PPI)-based triple therapy includes:
- Omeprazole or lansoprazole
- Clarithromycin
- Metronidazole or amoxicillin
  Bismuth subsalicylate–based triple therapy includes:
- Bismuth
- Metronidazole
- Tetracycline

Nutritional Support

There is no specific ulcer diet. Individualizing the diet to the patient's needs is paramount. Experimentation with a variety of foods is essential to determine foods that cause indigestion, pain, or other GI symptoms.

Food acts as a buffer. Research has determined there is little difference in the pattern of gastric acid secretion whether the person eats three meals or eats smaller, more frequent meals. Milk, coffee (caffeinated and decaffeinated), and alcohol can significantly increase gastric acid levels. Byproducts of protein digestion as well as calcium stimulate the release of gastrin and hence the amount of gastric acid secretion. Alcohol can damage the gastric mucosa.

Milk-alkali syndrome is a metabolic alkalosis that occurs with the simultaneous use of antacids and milk. This may cause a rebound increase in gastric acid secretion. An additional problem of hypercalcemia occurs with the use of calcium-based antacids (calcium carbonate; e.g., Tums). Hypercalcemia can predispose to the formation of kidney stones, especially in elderly persons.

Surgical Interventions

Surgery may be indicated for complicated ulcer disease, although the need has declined significantly with the development of curative drug therapy for *H. pylori*. The following procedures are commonly performed.

Vagotomy and Antrectomy. The trunks of the vagus nerve are transected, inhibiting gastric acid secretion. The antrum (distal portion) of the stomach is then removed. GI motility is reestablished by suturing the remaining stomach to the proximal duodenum (Billroth I anastomosis), or to a loop of the jejunum (Billroth II anastomosis). These procedures carry a very low recurrence rate but higher mortality and morbidity rates than in other procedures. For gastric ulcers not located in the pyloric region, only antrectomy is necessary.

Vagotomy and Pyloroplasty. Proximal gastric vagotomy carries the lowest risk for complications, but the highest ulcer recurrence rate ($\sim 10\%$). This partial vagotomy procedure denervates only the acid-secreting portion of the stomach, sparing the vagus nerve branches that innervate the antrum. Thus, pyloroplasty (remodeling of the pylorus) is not necessary.

See Chapter 9, Section 3, for information on postoperative dietary management.

COMMUNITY CARE

Assessment

- Obtain a history and assess for risk factors, including long-term NSAID ingestion for treatment of arthritis.
- Assess for signs and symptoms of PUD: epigastric pain, nausea, and vomiting. Note the role of food and/or antacids in relief pattern.
- Assess for signs of painless bleeding in chronic NSAID users.
- Assess for signs and symptoms of advanced PUD: hematemesis, hematochezia, or melena.
- Follow-up endoscopy is needed to document the healing of gastric ulcers and to rule out gastric cancer.
- Assess compliance with drug therapy, as indicated by absence of symptoms.
- Assess for side effects of medication therapy (see Table 17-4-1).

Monitoring

Assess for complications of PUD:

- Bleeding: "Coffee ground" emesis, hematemesis, hematochezia, and/or melena

Table 17-4-1. Drug Therapy for Peptic Ulcer Disease

DRUG, CLASSIFICATION, ACTION	NURSING IMPLICATIONS
Antibiotics (eradicate *H. pylori* infection) Bismuth (Pepto-Bismol) Metronidazole (Flagyl) Tetracycline (Achromycin V) Amoxicillin (Amoxil) Clarithromycin (Biaxin)	• Used in combination to prevent resistance (may be given in combination with omeprazole). • Take as prescribed for full course of therapy (14 days). • Bismuth causes harmless black coloration of the tongue and stool (may cause difficulty in detecting melena); it increases the risk of salicylate toxicity (do not take with other salicylates such as aspirin). Bismuth is also available in combination with ranitidine (ranitidine bismuth citrate) under the brand name Tritec. Tritec is used in several of the treatment regimens for *H. pylori*. • Antibiotic resistance and patient noncompliance are the major reasons for treatment failure.
Histamine 2 (H₂)-receptor antagonists (decrease HCl production by blocking histamine receptors on parietal cells) Cimetidine (Tagamet) Famotidine (Pepcid) Nizatidine (Axid) Ranitidine (Zantac)	• Take as prescribed. Dosing may be qid, bid, or once daily at bedtime. Bedtime doses are advised, because acid secretion peaks between 10 PM and 2 AM. • Cimetidine and ranitidine to a lesser degree inhibit hepatic drug metabolism and can increase levels of other drugs (e.g., warfarin, phenytoin, theophylline, and lidocaine). • Note central nervous system effects: confusion, hallucinations, and lethargy, especially in the elderly. • Do not administer concurrently with antacids, to ensure proper absorption (can give 1 hour before or 2 hours after antacids). • Be aware that these products are available over-the-counter (OTC); dosage is 1/2 the strength of prescribed dosages.

Proton pump inhibitors (suppress HCl secretion from parietal cells)

Omeprazole (Prilosec)
Lansoprazole (Prevacid)

- Used in conjunction with antibiotics for *H. pylori* eradication.
- May inhibit hepatic drug metabolism; monitor serum drug levels of warfarin, phenytoin, and diazepam.
- Preparations are enteric-coated; do not give with milk or milk products.

Mucosal protectant (coats surface of ulcer crater, protects against HCl and pepsin)

Sucralfate (Carafate)

- Give 30 minutes to 1 hour before meals and 1 hour before antacids.
- The drug is activated to form ulcer protectant in the presence of acid. Sucralfate forms a complex with pepsin (proteolytic enzyme), rendering it inactive. Constipation is a common side effect.

Antisecretory agent (prostaglandin analog, stimulates secretion of mucus and bicarbonate, maintains mucosal blood flow, suppresses gastric secretion)

Misoprostol (Cytotec)

- Beneficial in preventing nonsteroidal anti-inflammatory drug–induced ulceration.
- Contraindicated during pregnancy; can cause birth defects.
- Diarrhea is a common dose-related side effect.

Antacids (neutralize gastric acid, provide pain relief)

Aluminum hydroxide
Magnesium hydroxide
Calcium carbonate

- Use with caution in patients with hypertension or heart failure.
- Use magnesium-based antacids with caution in patients with renal insufficiency.
- Aluminum antacids can cause constipation.
- Magnesium antacids may cause diarrhea.
- Calcium antacids given concurrently with milk or milk products may lead to milk-alkali syndrome.
- To ensure proper drug absorption, do not administer other medications within 1 hour of any antacid.
- Since H₂ receptor antagonists have been available, antacid therapy is considered outmoded.

- Pain: Sudden, severe, generalized abdominal pain (may signal perforation)
- Peritonitis: Rigid, quiet abdomen with rebound tenderness, leukocytosis, slightly elevated serum amylase level (less than twice normal), hypotension (later, following peritonitis)

Assess for signs of gastric outlet obstruction (edema or narrowing of the pyloric area): abdominal fullness after meals, vomiting 1 to several hours after meals, and vomitus containing partially digested food. Teach the patient to report any of following: acute epigastric/abdominal pain, hematemesis, hematochezia, and melena.

A follow-up breath test should follow drug therapy to document *H. pylori* eradication.

Prevention

- Reinforce teaching about understanding PUD process, drug regimen, and complications associated with noncompliance.
- Teach the importance of handwashing to prevent the spread of *H. pylori* as well as the importance of eating food that is thoroughly cooked and drinking water from only clean, safe sources.
- Teach the importance of follow-up visits to the health care provider after eradication of *H. pylori* to rule out gastric cancer and gastric lymphoma.
- Teach the importance of curtailing the use of nicotine, alcohol, and caffeine-containing foods and beverages.
- Teach the patient to eat three meals a day and to avoid eating foods that increase GI symptoms.
- Teach the patient to avoid the use of NSAIDs and aspirin.
- Teach the patient to avoid stress and to use coping mechanisms that have been effective in the past.

 PROGNOSIS

Because 90% of ulcers are now known to be caused by *H. pylori* infection, the infection may be eradicated with combination drug therapy. With proper treatment, 80% of patients do not experience ulcer recurrence.

 CLINICAL PEARLS

○ PUD caused by *H. pylori* is a curable infection. Eradication of PUD is possible with a 14-day course of combination therapy with anti-infective agents and an antisecretory agent (e.g., omeprazole).
○ Noninvasive diagnostic tests (e.g., the ^{13}C and ^{14}C breath tests) are 94% to 98% sensitive and specific for *H. pylori*.
○ Administration of NSAIDs for more than 7 days may increase the risk of GI bleeding.
○ Relief of pain and eradication of PUD can be a powerful stimulus to encourage the patient to comply with drug therapy for *H. pylori* infection, despite whatever transient drug side effects may occur during the 14 days of treatment.
○ In the treatment of *H. pylori* infection, bismuth (Pepto-Bismol) is used for its topical bacteriocidal and antidiarrheal properties.
○ Antacids are outdated in the current treatment of PUD.

NURSING PROBLEM/ DIAGNOSIS	NURSING INTERVENTIONS CLASSIFICATION (NIC)
Acute pain	Medication Management
	Teaching: Prescribed Medication
Prevention	Teaching: Disease Process
	Vital Sign Monitoring
	Smoking Cessation Assistance

Endocrine

Diabetes Mellitus

Section 1   Ethlyn Gibson

OVERVIEW

Diabetes mellitus (DM) is the fourth leading cause of death in the United States. Sixteen million Americans have DM, and approximately half are undiagnosed because the disease may be asymptomatic until complications develop. DM is the leading cause of end-stage renal disease, blindness, non-traumatic amputations, and impotence. Patients with DM are two to four times more likely to develop a heart attack or stroke than those without DM.

DM is a chronic metabolic disease in which there is an absolute deficiency of insulin or resistance to its metabolic actions. This lack of insulin causes the body to be unable to process food into energy. When this occurs, the glucose in food remains in the blood, causing hyperglycemia to develop.

DM is classified as type 1, type 2, gestational, and other conditions associated with DM, including endocrinopathies related to hyperglycemia, drug- or chemical-induced hyperglycemia, and infection-associated and genetic syndromes accompanied by an increased incidence of DM. These classifications are different disease entities but share the symptoms and complications of hyperglycemia (high blood glucose).

Impaired glucose tolerance, formerly known as "borderline diabetes," is a degree of hyperglycemia that may precede DM.

PATHOPHYSIOLOGY

Type 1 DM, present in 10% of patients, is caused by pancreatic beta cell destruction and results in absolute insulin deficiency. The rate of beta cell destruction varies but is usually rapid in infants and children and slow in adults. Onset may occur at any age but most commonly occurs before age 30. Weight loss, polyuria, and polydipsia may develop rapidly at onset. Insulin therapy is essential for survival.

Type 2 DM, accounting for 90% of persons with DM, is caused by a combination of insulin resistance and relative insulin deficiency. It usually occurs in patients older than 30 years of age but is becoming more prevalent in adolescents because of the increased incidence of obesity in this population. Approximately 75% of persons diagnosed with type 2 DM are classified as obese. Insulin may be required to help control glucose elevations but is not necessary for survival.

Both type 1 and type 2 DM are associated with metabolic, vascular, and neuropathic complications. These complications result from underlying defects in the body's handling of carbohydrates.

The **metabolic syndrome** includes delays in glucose-induced insulin secretion, impaired insulin-mediated glucose uptake, and ineffective intracellular glucose transport.

Diabetic ketoacidosis (DKA) is one of the more acute and serious metabolic disturbances occurring in DM. Incidence is highest in adolescents with type 1 DM and older adults with type 2 DM. The hallmark signs of DKA are dehydration, metabolic acidosis (low serum bicarbonate), ketosis, and ketonuria. Patients with DKA usually present with hyperglycemia (plasma glucose above 250 mg/dL) but may present with normoglycemia. Goals of treatment include: (1) correcting metabolic acidosis, (2) correcting fluid and electrolyte imbalance, (3) providing adequate insulin to lower plasma glucose and prevent ketosis, and (4) preventing further complications of treatment.

Hyperosmolar nonketotic coma syndrome (HNKC) is another serious metabolic complication commonly seen in older adults with type 2 DM. These patients present with severe dehydration and elevated blood glucose level, but minimal ketosis and acidosis. Plasma glucose level typically exceeds 600 mg/dL with marked hyperosmolality (serum osmolality above 340 mOsm/L of water) and blood urea nitrogen (BUN) above 60. General treatment principles are the same as for DKA.

The **vascular syndrome** includes an accelerated arteriosclerosis affecting large blood vessels, which can result in heart attack, stroke, and peripheral vascular disease, and affecting small vessels, which can result in retinopathy and nephropathy.

The **neuropathic syndromes** are believed to develop secondary to the thickening of the walls of the endoneural arterioles that supply the nerve, resulting in neural ischemia and a segmental demyelination process. Diabetic neuropathies affect both the peripheral and autonomic nervous systems.

SIGNS AND SYMPTOMS

The following signs and symptoms are usually, but not always, present with hyperglycemia:

- Increased urination (polyuria): Sugar pulls water from the cells of the body. More water is filtered through the kidneys and more urine is made in an attempt to rid the body of excess sugar. The person may become dehydrated from this process. Electrolytes are lost to this osmotic diuresis and dehydration.
- Increased thirst (polydipsia): Because the sugar is pulling water from the body the person experiences increased thirst.
- Increased hunger (polyphagia): Because the cells are unaware the sugar is on the "other side of the door," they feel starved for food. They send a message to the person to eat, and constant hunger may develop.
- Weight loss: Since the body is unable to store or use sugar for energy, weight loss may occur. The body also begins to break down fat and muscle stores as it continues to lose sugar through urine.
- Weakness and fatigue: These symptoms are caused by the lack of available energy. Just as a car that runs out of gas is unable to function, the body is unable to perform even the simplest task without sugar for energy.
- Blurred vision: Elevated sugar levels cause sugar to collect and cause swelling in the lens of the eye, resulting in visual changes. These are reversible with control of the glucose levels. It is important to wait 6 to 8 weeks after the blood sugar has normalized before having an eye exam for glasses.

- Other problems: Numbness and tingling around the mouth, tongue, fingers and distal extremities due to hyperglycemia. Increased infections, including yeast and wounds that are slow healing, also due to elevated serum blood glucose.

Table 18-1-1 compares common versus panic signs and their immediate interventions for hypoglycemia and hyperglycemia.

 DIAGNOSTIC CRITERIA

Because early diagnosis and treatment of DM may decrease morbidity and mortality, screening should be used in asymptomatic, high-risk individuals (Table 18-1-2). Criteria for the diagnosis of DM include:

- Symptoms of DM plus a casual plasma glucose concentration greater than or equal to 200 mg/dL (11.1 mmol/L). Casual refers to any time of the day, unrelated to meals.
- Fasting plasma glucose greater than or equal to 126 mg/dL (7.0 mmol/L). Fasting is defined as 8 hours or more without caloric intake.
- Two-hour plasma glucose greater than or equal to 200 mg/dL (11.1 mmol/L) during performance of an oral glucose tolerance test (OGTT). The OGTT should be performed following World Health Organization (WHO) criteria, which specify a glucose load containing the equivalent of 75 g of anhydrous glucose dissolved in water.

 INTERVENTIONS

Studies have shown that the most effective way to manage DM is from a team approach. The team includes the patient, physician, nurse educator, dietician, and others as needed to include ophthalmologists, podiatrists and mental health professionals, and family members. The overall goal is for treatment to achieve blood glucose levels as low as possible without increasing risk for hypoglycemia.

The American Diabetes Association's current recommendations are targeted at achieving a fasting plasma glucose level below 130 mg/dL (7.2 mmol/L) and glycosylated hemoglobin (HgA_{1c}) below 7%. Important factors to consider when developing a treatment plan include the patient's age, life expectancy, other health problems, home and family situations, educational background, intelligence, and motivation.

The most important element of the treatment plan is teaching the patient self-management skills including:

- Pathophysiology: An understanding of the primary type of DM.
- Meal planning: Basic nutrition guidelines and limitations on sugar intake (see Chapter 9, Section 3).
- Self-monitoring blood glucose (SMBG) with record keeping: Frequency of testing and interpretation of results (see Chapter 4, Section 4).
- Type 1 and 2: Insulin use with adjustment and supplementation guidelines
- Type 2: Review of the prescribed medication regimen, which may include oral agents, an oral agent/insulin combination, or bedtime insulin
- Sick day and DKA management (in type 1 DM) and hyperglycemic hyperosmolar nonketotic coma (HHNK)
- Hypoglycemia prevention and treatment: An understanding that a blood

glucose value below 60 mg/dL requires immediate administration of non-diet soda, orange juice, or glucose tablets

- Exercise precautions: The need to test blood glucose before exercise and an understanding of how exercise may lower insulin or medication requirements
- Chronic complications, with screening guidelines to detect early disease (e.g., annual eye, feet, and dental examinations)
- Ongoing monitoring, with glycosylated hemoglobin twice per year
- Foot care: An understanding of the need for daily care to decrease the risk of injury, early detection of problems, and early treatment of problems (e.g., routine care: inspection, washing, application of lotion, care of nails, corns and/or calluses); properly fitted socks and shoes; the importance of never going barefoot.

Treatment for patients with type 1 and type 2 DM needs to target the primary processes that contribute to the pathogenesis of the disease: insulin deficiency and insulin resistance. Treatment for type 1 DM targets the total or near-total deficiency in endogenous insulin secretion. The goal of therapy for type 1 DM is precise replacement of insulin secretion. Treatment for type 2 DM targets insulin resistance and deficient insulin secretion. Treatment recommendations for type 2 DM begin with lifestyle changes (diet and exercise) and includes oral agent monotherapy, then multidrug therapy if monotherapy fails, and often inclusion of insulin.

Oral agents that target insulin secretion include:
- Sulfonylureas (glyburide, glimepiride)
- Short-acting insulin tropic agents (meglitinides)

Oral agents that target insulin resistance include:
- Biguanides (metformin)
- Thiazolidinediones (pioglitazone, rosiglitazone)
- Alpha-glucosidase inhibitors (e.g., acarbose, miglitol)

Insulin therapy for type 1 and type 2 combination includes:
- Rapid-acting insulin analogues (e.g., Lispro)
- Long-acting insulin analogues (e.g., NPH, Lente)
- Premixed insulin formulations

See Chapter 12, Section 9 for details on these agents.

 COMMUNITY CARE

Social factors and family functioning play important roles in facilitating the patient's response to self-care management. Families and communities can help foster independence and self-reliance through active support. Studies have found that in a person with DM, the perception of supportive behavior is predictive of compliance with the self-care regimen. Social and community support have been found to have a positive effect on outcomes in self-care management.

 PROGNOSIS

The prognosis for persons with DM is bright. Care must involve the comprehensive team approach that incorporates all members of the team to reduce mortality, morbidity, and associated health care costs. The team should

Table 18-1-1. Common and Panic Signs of Hypoglycemia and Hyperglycemia

TYPE	SIGNS OF HYPOGLYCEMIA	INTERVENTIONS FOR HYPOGLYCEMIA
Common	Sweatiness Shakiness Irritability Cold, clammy skin Nervousness Weakness Tachycardia Nausea Blurred vision	If patient is awake and alert: • Administer an oral form of a rapidly absorbed carbohydrate (CHO): 4 oz. fruit juice (e.g., orange, grape, apple), 3 graham crackers, 8 oz milk, 5–7 Lifesaver candies, 2–3 small pieces of candy, or 1–2 teaspoons of honey, sugar. • Retest blood glucose level and repeat oral intake of CHO until glucose level $\geq$ 110 mg/dL is obtained. • The patient should have a snack or meal within 30 minutes. If acarbose (Precose) or miglitol (Glyset) was taken with sulfonylurea, the glucagon or glucose (oral or IV) must be given, because these drugs prevent the digestion and absorption of oral carbohydrates in the gastrointestinal tract.
Panic	Loss of consciousness Seizures Confusion, disorientation	If the patient cannot swallow or is unconscious, glucagon or parenteral glucose must be given immediately. At home: • Glucagon is given intramuscularly or subcutaneously (the usual dose is 0.5–1 mg). • If glucagon is unavailable, 15–20 g of glucose gel may be inserted into the buccal cavity. • Once consciousness is regained, provide oral intake of CHO. In the hospital: • Administer 20–50 g of 50% glucose IV push as bolus. • Depending on the cause, the patient may need IV fluid hydration and/or inotrophic drugs to maintain circulation.

628

TYPE	SIGNS OF HYPERGLYCEMIA	INTERVENTIONS FOR HYPERGLYCEMIA

Common	Increased appetite (polyphagia)
	Increased thirst (polydipsia)
	Frequent urination (polyuria)
	Fatigue
	Headaches
	Blurred vision
	Dry, itchy skin
	Poor wound healing
	Flu-like achiness
		If blood glucose level is > 200 mg/dL
		• Assess fluid balance:
		  if fluid volume deficit: first correct with IV of 0.9% normal saline as ordered by physician to prevent hypovolemic shock, then treat hyperglycemia as ordered.
		  if fluid volume adequate: a short-acting insulin is prescribed by a *sliding scale* one-time dose.
		For HHNK or DKA
		• Fluid replacement: 0.9% or 0.45% normal saline at a rate of 1–2 L/hr for first 2–4 hr, then as ordered by physician.
		• After blood glucose reaches 250–300 mg/dL, saline IV fluids are changed to 5% dextrose. Regular insulin may be given by IV bolus or continuous infusion doses determined by glucose levels until glycemic control is attained. Blood glucose and potassium levels should be checked every hour during insulin infusion.

Panic	Blood glucose level >240 mg/dL Nausea Weakness Vomiting Hypotension Fruity or alcohol breath smell Ketones in urine Decreased level of consciousness Coma	

Courtesy of Joanne Bullard.

Table 18-1-2. Screening Criteria for Asymptomatic, Undiagnosed Individuals

1. Test starting at age 45; repeat at 3 year intervals if results are normal.
2. Test at a younger age or repeat the test more frequently if the patient has one or more of the following risk factors:
   - Obesity (≥120% of desirable body weight or body mass index ≥27 kg/m²)
   - A first-degree relative with diabetes
   - Member of high-risk ethnic population (e.g., African American, Asian, Hispanic, or Native American)
   - History of gestational diabetes or delivery of an infant weighing >9 lb
   - Hypertension (≥140/90 mm Hg)
   - High-density lipoprotein (HDL) cholesterol level ≤35 mg/dL and/or triglyceride level ≥250 mg/dL
   - A history of impaired glucose tolerance or impaired fasting glucose (fasting plasma glucose ≥110 mg/dL but ≤126 mg/dL on previous tests)

Adapted from Report of the Expert Committee on the Diagnosis and Classification of Diabetes Mellitus. *Diabetes Care* 20:1183–1197. Copyright 1997 by American Diabetes Association.

collaborate with the patient and develop a plan of care tailored for the patient's individual needs and lifestyle. Optimal glycemic control and achievement of near euglycemia should be the goals of treatment.

Long-term results of the Diabetes Control and Complications Trial (DCCT) on type 1 DM, as well as the United Kingdom Prospective Diabetes Study (UKPDS) and the Japanese Kumamoto Study, reflect that intensive therapy aimed at tight glycemic control does help reduce long-term complications in persons with DM. The goals should include screening in high-risk groups, individualizing multiple-agent regimens in persons with type 2 DM, and promoting SMBG for ongoing evaluation. Health care costs for DM will continue to rise if these are not the goals of treatment. Early detection is still the cornerstone of optimum treatment and reduction of devastating long-term complications that drain the health care system and decrease the productivity of the American workforce.

 CLINICAL PEARLS

○ Communicate with other members of the comprehensive team, who can provide valuable information for planning care.
○ Identify early lifestyle, cultural, and psychosocial factors that may impede optimal care.
○ Encourage the patient to set initial treatment goals for better compliance and motivation.
○ Involve family members in the patient's plan of care.
○ Inspect the patient's feet and footwear. Show the patient how to check his or her feet using a mirror for inspection and to put the hands inside shoes to check for problems.
○ Instruct the patient to wash the hands under warm water before performing finger sticks for SMBG, to help improve circulation and increase blood flow, and to stick fingers on the side to obtain a better drop of blood.
○ Remember that the patient is not the problem; DM is the disease that requires effective treatment and management.

NURSING PROBLEM/ DIAGNOSIS	NURSING INTERVENTIONS CLASSIFICATION (NIC)
Hyperglycemia Risk for complications	Hyperglycemia Management Hypoglycemia Management Environmental Management Peripheral Sensation Management Surveillance
Patient teaching/Deficient knowledge	Medication Management Nutritional Counseling Teaching: Disease Process Health System Guidance

Hyperparathyroidism

Section 2   Suzanne Marnocha

OVERVIEW

Hyperparathyroidism is extremely rare; one estimate of incidence is 0.1% of the population. Hyperactivity of the parathyroid gland leads to abnormal accumulation of calcium, resulting in dysfunction in most body systems. Quality of life and activities of daily living (ADL) are affected as calcium accumulates in the kidneys and impairs renal function. Osteoporosis develops in the long bones, causing pain and leading to fractures. Gastrointestinal (GI) problems develop and lead to chronic epigastric pain. Central nervous system (CNS) changes occur leading to changes in personality, confusion, and even coma. If left untreated, hypercalcemia can become fatal, usually from cardiac dysrhythmias.

PATHOPHYSIOLOGY

Hyperparathyroidism is an abnormal endocrine condition characterized by hyperactivity of any of the four parathyroid glands with excessive secretion of parathyroid hormone (PTH), increased reabsorption of calcium from the skeletal system, and increased absorption of calcium from the kidneys and GI system. This condition is classified as primary, originating in one or more of the parathyroid glands, or secondary, resulting from an abnormal hypocalcemia-producing condition in another part of the body that causes compensatory hyperactivity of the parathyroid glands.

The most common causes of primary hyperparathyroidism are single adenomas (85%), hyperplasia of multiple glands (12% to 22%), and carcinoma of the parathyroid gland (3%). Primary hyperparathyroidism may also occur in a familial pattern from an autosomal dominant trait in 10% to 15% of all cases.

In hyperparathyroidism, PTH levels are elevated, and excessive bone reabsorption and renal reabsorption of calcium produce hypercalcemia. Most affected persons do not require emergency treatment for their hypercalcemia but rather need some form of treatment to prevent accelerated bone loss.

Hypercalcemia is also associated with the abnormal increase in PTH after a successful renal transplantation. As the new kidney starts to work, the parathyroid glands become hyperplasic and produce excessive amounts of PTH from 6 to 24 months.

 ## SIGNS AND SYMPTOMS

The signs and symptoms associated with hyperparathyroidism vary and, as stated earlier, may be absent. Manifestations reflect abnormalities in calcium levels. As many as 75% of patients with hyperparathyroidism are asymptomatic, and hypercalcemia is noted only when serum calcium is measured for other reasons. Hypercalcemia in primary hyperparathyroidism produces dysfunction in most body systems. In the kidneys, tissues calcify and calculi form. Initially, polyuria is seen; if left untreated, renal failure eventually occurs. Osteoporosis develops from bone demineralization, causing increased susceptibility to fracture and pain. Synovitis and pseudogout (chondrocalcinosis) often occur.

CNS effects may include abnormal behavior, confusion, psychosis and even coma. GI effects may include chronic, penetrating abdominal pain associated with pancreatitis or ulcer formation. Patients with severe hypercalcemia are predisposed to pancreatitis, probably related to the deposition of calcium in the pancreatic ducts. Hypercalcemia may also lead to duodenal ulcer disease from increased gastric acid secretion, promoted by calcium's effect on the parietal cells of the stomach. Decreased gastric emptying leads to anorexia and nausea. Constipation may result from calcium's effect on smooth muscle and nerve conduction, as well as from dehydration.

Cardiovascular manifestations may include hypertension from increased cardiac inotropy and increasing systemic vascular resistance. Other cardiovascular changes include syncope from bradycardia and varying degrees of heart block. The appearance of such dysrhythmias is directly related to the serum calcium level. As the calcium level rises, the heart rate drops, and heart blocks develop.

Renal calculi are particularly troublesome. The combination of three variables—hypercalciuria, alkaline urine, and hyperphosphatemia—predisposes to the formation of calcium stones, particularly in the renal pelvis or renal collecting ducts. Calcium stones are associated with infection and resultant impaired renal function. Alopecia is an unpleasant side effect.

 ## DIAGNOSTIC CRITERIA

The diagnosis of primary hyperparathyroidism is made by elevated serum levels of PTH, calcium, chloride, and alkaline phosphatase with abnormally low levels of magnesium and phosphorus. Radiographs of the long bones reveal changes characteristic of osteoporosis.

 ## INTERVENTIONS

Reduction of Serum Calcium Level

General interventions are directed toward reducing serum calcium levels. This may be achieved by increasing excretion of calcium in the urine, inhibiting bone resorption of calcium, reducing the intake of nutritional calcium, blocking intestinal calcium absorption, or enhancing formation of calcium complexes. More severe forms of hypercalcemia cause dehydration associated with abdominal cramping and diarrhea. The patient requires IV rehydration with an isotonic solution such as 0.9% sodium chloride (NaCl) at 200 mL/ hour until the intravascular volume is replaced. The volume expansion with isotonic saline dilutes the plasma calcium, increases the glomerular filtration rate, and increases renal calcium excretion. The patient requires close monitoring during this period to detect fluid volume excess. Serum calcium level can be expected to decrease by 2 to 3 mEq/L over 8 to 24 hours. Simultaneous use of furosemide and NaCl increases excretion of calcium and fluid.

If this is not acceptable, or if furosemide is ineffective, then a different regimen may be tried. Possibilities include biphosphonates, mithramycin, calcitonin, glucocorticoids, and phosphate salts. The biphosphonates (e.g., etidronate [Didronel], pamidronate [Aredia]) are relatively new compounds that work by inhibiting the activity and number of osteoclasts. This inhibits bone reabsorption, which decreases serum calcium level. These drugs are useful when a bone-absorbing disease, such as breast cancer, causes the hypercalcemia. Plicamycin (Mithracin) is an antineoplastic agent that works by limiting the bone reabsorption seen in malignancies; however, this drug has toxic side effects to both the liver and kidneys. In more severe cases of hypercalcemia, peritoneal or hemodialysis may be needed.

Surgical Management for Symptomatic Hyperparathyroidism

When the underlying cause is primary hyperparathyroidism, partial or complete parathyroidectomy is the treatment of choice. Single or multiple adenomas are surgically excised. Surgical removal of the affected gland or glands is considered curative. If all four glands are affected, three are removed and portions of the fourth gland are implanted in the forearm. If other pathology is causing the hyperparathyroidism, up to one half of the tissue might need to be excised. Complications of surgery include hypocalcemia (see Chapter 11, Section 3), vocal cord paralysis and hematoma formation.

Conservative Management for Asymptomatic Patients

When the hypercalcemia is non–life-threatening (for the asymptomatic patient), conservative measures may be used. Ensure an adequate fluid intake (2.5 to 3 L/day) to avoid volume depletion, and eliminate any drugs that may contribute to hypercalcemia (e.g., thiazide diuretics, vitamin D preparations, and calcium-containing antacids). Instruct patients to avoid calcium-rich foods, including dairy products and dark-green, leafy vegetables.

 COMMUNITY CARE

Asymptomatic patients require careful monitoring of clinical symptoms and serum calcium levels. Patients should be seen twice a year for the evaluation of blood pressure, serum calcium level and bone mass. Serum calcium levels should not exceed 11.5 mg/dL. These patients must avoid dehydration, immobilization, excessive dietary intake of calcium and vitamin D, and the use of loop or thiazide diuretics. Patient teaching includes information about avoiding calcium-rich foods and increasing fluid (see Interventions).

Postsurgical patients should be monitored for hypocalcemia and tetany. Some patients may require calcium and vitamin D supplementation.

For patients with the familial form of hyperparathyroidism, genetic screening is available for their family members.

 PROGNOSIS

The prognosis for hyperparathyroidism is good with early detection and treatment of the underlying cause. The surgical success rate is about 90% for the initial procedure. The condition can be life-threatening if serum calcium levels are extremely high (above 13.5 mg/dL) because of cardiac dysrhythmias.

 CLINICAL PEARLS

○ A serum calcium level above 13.5 mg/dL can produce life-threatening cardiac dysrhythmias.
○ Calcium-rich foods include dairy products and dark-green, leafy vegetables.
○ Isotonic saline solution at 200 mL/hour should cause serum calcium to decrease by 2 to 3 mEq/L over 8 to 24 hours.
○ Mobilization and full activity can promote hypocalcemia.
○ Inactivity can foster hypercalcemia.

NURSING PROBLEM/ DIAGNOSIS	NURSING INTERVENTIONS CLASSIFICATION (NIC)
Hypercalcemia	Electrolyte Management: Hypercalcemia
Deficient knowledge	Teaching: Disease Process

Hyperthyroidism

Section 3   Suzanne Marnocha

 OVERVIEW

Hyperthyroidism has many causes and is characterized by hyperactivity of the thyroid gland. The gland is usually enlarged and secretes excessive amounts of thyroid hormones. This causes acceleration of the body's metabolic processes.

 PATHOPHYSIOLOGY

Elevation of the thyroid hormone T_3 results in a hypermetabolic state with increased oxygen consumption by all body tissues. Thyroid hormones in excess act as pseudo-catecholamines, inducing a sympathetic nervous system–like response. Negative feedback induced by elevated thyroid hormones may result in deficiencies of other hypothalamic and pituitary hormones.

Graves' disease, the most common form of hyperthyroidism, is characterized by a goiter and exophthalmos. Graves' disease is seven to nine times more common in women than men. The cause is unknown but is thought to be related to an autoimmune disorder. Clinical presentation usually follows infection, physical stress, or an emotional crisis.

Thyroid storm is a rare but dangerous worsening of the thyrotoxic state. In this complication, also known as acute hyperthyroidism or acute thyrotoxicosis, a generalized extreme hypermetabolic state occurs in response to excessive levels of circulating thyroid hormone. The condition may develop spontaneously but more often occurs in individuals who have undiagnosed or undertreated Graves' disease. This is most common when there is associated stress, including surgeries or infections. The synergistic effect of catecholamines predominates, and the hypermetabolic state accelerates.

Another form of hyperthyroidism, known as *apathetic hyperthyroidism*, is more insidious. This is most often identified in older patients who demonstrate a single symptom. Rather than presenting with a generalized hypermetabolic state in which temperature, heart rate, and neurologic functions are accelerated, the patient with apathetic hyperthyroidism may only demonstrate tachycardia at rest, or weight loss, or muscle fatigue, or depression. The cardiac signs are the most life-threatening, and the patient may present with congestive heart failure. It is quite common for patients to develop uncontrolled atrial fibrillation, as demonstrated by an irregular rhythm greater than 100 beats/minute. This profile is especially dangerous in the elderly patient and requires aggressive, yet careful treatment.

 SIGNS AND SYMPTOMS

The manifestations of hyperthyroidism can be discussed by body system. Cardiovascular findings include palpitations, increased cardiac output, tachycardia, hypertension, dysrhythmias (atrial fibrillation), and angina. Pulmonary problems are manifested by dyspnea and crackles, especially if congestive heart failure develops. CNS signs and symptoms include tremors, insomnia, mood swings, diaphoresis, heat intolerance, restlessness/irritability, weakness and fatigue, personality changes and hyperkinesias. GI symptoms include weight loss, hyperactive bowel sounds, and diarrhea. The basal metabolic temperature may be elevated.

The most common manifestation of hyperthyroidism is goiter. A goiter is generalized hyperplasic enlargement of the thyroid gland and appears as a bulge in the front of the neck. It may be nodular, cystic, or fibrous on palpation, and a bruit may be auscultated.

The patient may also exhibit exophthalmos with eyelid retraction. Characterized by abnormal protrusion of the eyeballs, exophthalmos is associated with Graves' disease as well as other conditions causing the contents of the eye sockets to bulge (e.g., tumor, intraocular hemorrhage, trauma to the intraocular muscles).

 DIAGNOSTIC CRITERIA

Significantly suppressed TSH levels are the best indicator of primary hyperthyroidism (Table 18-3-1). A radioactive iodine uptake (RAIU) study is required for all patients in a thyrotoxic state. Diffuse uptake can confirm the diagnosis. Free T_4 (unbound to thyroid-binding proteins) levels are usually increased.

 INTERVENTIONS

The initial treatment of hyperthyroidism is determined by the degree of metabolic hyperactivity that the patient is experiencing. If the diagnosis is

▌ **Table 18-3-1.** Tests of Thyroid Function

TESTS OF THYROID FUNCTION	NORMAL VALUES	HYPOTHYROIDISM	HYPERTHYROIDISM
Thyroid-stimulating hormone	0.5–5.0 µU/mL	Elevated or decreased	Elevated or decreased
T_4 (L-thyroxine)	4.5–10.9 µg/dL	Decreased	Elevated
T_3 (tri-iodothyronine)	60–181 ng/dL	Not usually performed	Elevated
Calcitonin	Male 3–26 ng/L Female 2–17 ng/L	Not usually performed	Not usually performed

based on mild symptoms and positive blood tests, then treatment involves antithyroid drugs (e.g., propylthiouracil, methimazole, carbimazole). This medical management is followed by the surgical removal of the thyroid tissue or radioactive iodine therapy (Table 18-3-2).

Surgical Management

Near-total thyroidectomy removes up to 90% of the thyroid. A small amount of tissue is left to allow for adequate regeneration. Complications include recurrent laryngeal nerve damage, hypocalcemia, bleeding, and infection. The patient then becomes hypothyroid and needs life-long thyroid hormone replacement (see Section 5).

Radioactive Iodine Therapy

This is the therapy of choice for Graves' disease. It is performed on an outpatient basis with low-dose radioactivity, and no radiation safety precautions

▌ **Table 18-3-2.** Therapies in Hyperthyroidism

TREATMENT	MECHANISM OF ACTION	COMMENTS
Antithyroid drugs	Inhibits thyroid peroxidase	Relieves symptoms within a few days, with remission within 6 months to 2 years.
Methimazole (Tapazole)	Inhibits peripheral conversion of thyroxine (T_4)	
Propylthiouracil		
Radiation	Ablation therapy	Leaves the patient permanently hypothyroid within 3–6 months, requiring lifelong thyroid replacement.
Radioactive iodine (RAIU or ^{131}I)	Taken up by the thyroid and used in hormone synthesis; radioactivity (beta emission) destroys follicles over time	Common therapy in the U.S.
Beta-blockers (e.g., propranolol)	Symptomatic improvement until the patient is euthyroid	Contraindicated for patients with hyperactive airway disease or low cardiac output.
Calcium channel blockers (e.g., diltiazem)		
Thyroidectomy (total or subtotal)	Surgical removal of thyroid tissue	Common; expect in patients with large goiters.

are needed. One treatment is effective in 75% of cases. Radioactive iodine is contraindicated during pregnancy.

Treatment for Thyroid Storm

Treatment for a patient experiencing thyroid storm involves sustaining the primary body functions of airway, breathing, and circulation. Supplemental oxygen is delivered to meet the increased metabolic demands. Excessive circulating thyroid hormone augments the beta-receptors that are sensitive to catecholamines, thus enhancing myocardial excitability. Beta-blocking drugs are useful in controlling dysrhythmias and tachycardia. The drug of choice is propranolol; however, if the patient has hyperactive airway disease or congestive heart failure, propranolol many worsen the condition.

In addition to the emergency measures, the patient needs to be started on an antithyroid drug (e.g., propylthiouracil, methimazole, or carbimazole), because maximum drug effect is not reached for 7 to 14 days.

The patient is hyperthermic and needs a nonaspirin antipyretic and frequently, a cooling blanket. (Aspirin is contraindicated, because it increases circulating T_4 levels, potentiating the storm.) If beta-blocker therapy fails, the next class of drugs to try is calcium channel blockers (e.g., verapamil), to control the tachydysrhythmias.

Once the crisis has passed, definitive therapy (e.g., surgical removal of the thyroid gland or radioactive iodine therapy) is required.

 COMMUNITY CARE

The critical factor to be aware of is that this disease is more common in women. Any signs and symptoms merit a high index of suspicion for thyroid storm. The patient must be followed closely within the health care system to avoid potential crisis.

Thyroid hormone levels should be monitored until stabilized. For a patient receiving hormone replacement therapy, thyroid hormone levels are monitored biannually or annually.

 PROGNOSIS

Hyperthyroidism is treated effectively with medications and surgical removal of the thyroid gland. Untreated hyperthyroidism will likely progress to thyroid storm. Thyroid storm is considered a medical emergency. This condition affects virtually every system in the body and so mandates admission to a critical care unit for close monitoring and intervention. If the condition is left untreated, death can occur within 2 hours.

 CLINICAL PEARLS

○ Graves' disease is a common form of hyperthyroidism and is more common in women. In many cases, clinical signs and symptoms are been misinterpreted as "nervousness," and the patient goes untreated.

○ When treating a patient in thyroid storm, remember the ABCs. Provide supplemental oxygen, auscultate for crackles, obtain IV access, and administer a beta-blocking agent to slow the heart rate and interfere with catecholamine conversion. Monitor and treat hyperthermia with non–aspirin-containing drugs.

NURSING PROBLEM/ DIAGNOSIS	NURSING INTERVENTIONS CLASSIFICATION (NIC)
Metabolic hyperactivity	Energy Management Teaching Prescribed Medication Nutrition Therapy
Perioperative management (thyroidectomy) Deficient knowledge	Incision Site Care Airway Management Teaching: Disease Process

Hypoparathyroidism

Section 4   Suzanne Marnocha

 OVERVIEW

Primary hypoparathyroidism is extremely rare and usually the result of an autoimmune disorder. Secondary hypoparathyroidism occurs most commonly as a result of surgical removal of the parathyroid gland or its irradiation. Both result in absent or decreased PTH secretion.

PTH normally acts to raise serum calcium levels by increasing the absorption of calcium from the bone and GI tract, increasing the activation of vitamin D, and increasing the reabsorption of calcium in the kidneys. Without PTH, hypocalcemia ensues.

 PATHOPHYSIOLOGY

PTH deficiency is most commonly associated with surgical removal of the parathyroid glands for adenoma resection. Hypocalcemia usually results when surgery involves the total removal of glandular tissue, radical neck dissection for laryngeal cancer, or a near-total thyroidectomy. Temporary hypocalcemia may be seen from 1 to 5 days after surgery if less permanent damage has occurred. This transient hypocalcemia may also result from a reduction in blood supply during surgery, gland suppression after removal of an adenoma, or intraoperative release of calcitonin.

Hypoparathyroidism may also result from hypomagnesemia. Once serum magnesium levels return to normal, PTH secretion does as well. Hypomagnesemia is related to chronic alcoholism with malnutrition.

Some researchers have found that there is a deficiency of PTH in patients with acute pancreatitis. When acute pancreatitis develops, the fatty acids combine with calcium ions to form soaps. This causes a decrease in serum calcium concentrations. Between 40% and 75% of patients with acute pancreatitis develop hypocalcemia. Other causes of hypocalcemia include magnesium abnormalities, alkalosis, inadequate vitamin D, malabsorption syndromes, infusion of citrated blood, certain drugs, alcoholism, and sepsis.

 SIGNS AND SYMPTOMS

The signs and symptoms associated with hypoparathyroidism are related to hypocalcemia and the associated neuromuscular irritability. Neuromuscular

effects include laryngeal spasm, tremor, hyperreflexia, paresthesias, and tetany. *Tetany,* a hallmark finding, is characterized by cramps, convulsions, and seizures. During physical examination, tetany may be demonstrated by *Chvostek's sign* (ipsilateral contraction of the facial muscles elicited by tapping the facial nerve anterior to the ear) or *Trousseau's sign* (carpal spasm produced by pressure ischemia of the nerves in the upper arm during inflation of a blood pressure cuff above the systolic blood pressure for 3 to 5 minutes).

Cardiovascular findings include hypotension, bradycardia, congestive heart failure, and prolonged Q-T interval. These effects result from impaired contractility, vasodilation, and conduction abnormalities associated with hypocalcemia. The CNS may also be affected, resulting in lethargy, depression, psychosis, hyperirritability, and seizures. Head hair loss may also occur.

 ## DIAGNOSTIC CRITERIA

Total serum calcium level is low (5 to 7 mg/dL). Ionized (i.e., free, unbound to protein) calcium level is also low (see Chapter 11, Section 3). Ionized calcium truly determines the amount of available calcium and is preferred to serum calcium. Serum phosphorus level is elevated (7 to 12 mg/dL). Serum albumin and serum magnesium levels, as well as parathyroid function, should be evaluated.

 ## INTERVENTIONS

Serum calcium levels must be checked every 8 to 12 hours after neck surgery—more frequently if symptoms of paresthesias, tetany, or laryngeal spasm are present. In patients with symptomatic hypocalcemia, treatment with IV calcium salts (e.g., calcium gluconate, calcium chloride) is imperative. Whenever possible, calcium should be administered through a central line, because it is extremely irritating to veins and can also cause tissue sloughing. Calcium must be given cautiously to patients undergoing digitalis therapy, because it potentiates the effect of digitalis and may precipitate dysrhythmias. During parenteral calcium therapy, electrocardiogram (ECG) monitoring is instituted and the serum calcium level is monitored every 4 to 6 hours.

Patients with chronic hypocalcemia may be treated with oral forms of calcium. Calcium carbonate is the least expensive and most widely used form. Calcium replacements must be used cautiously in patients with severe hyperphosphatemia, because the calcium and phosphate may precipitate in the soft tissues. To prevent this, patients should be given phosphate-binding medications such as aluminum hydroxide. Vitamin D, in the form of calcitriol (the agent of choice) or ergocalciferol is also required in hypoparathyroid disorders.

 ## COMMUNITY CARE

Patients must be followed closely during the postsurgical period, with periodic serum ionized calcium blood samples and clinical examinations for evidence of hypocalcemia, including neuromuscular irritability associated with tetany. Patients should be taught to recognize the signs of hypercalcemia and hypocalcemia, especially while calcium and vitamin D dosages are being adjusted. Serum and urine calcium levels should be monitored every 3 months.

PROGNOSIS

The prognosis for hypoparathyroidism is good if severe hypocalcemia is prevented. However, in a patient with unrecognized hypocalcemia, the condition can progress. Tetany can lead to laryngeal spasms and death.

CLINICAL PEARLS

○ Serum calcium is bound to albumin. Low serum albumin level may lead to hypocalcemia. In turn, severe malnutrition may lead to hypocalcemia and should be investigated. Severe alcoholics often fall into this category and have an accompanying hypomagnesemia. Severe hypomagnesemia alone (<1 mg/dL) inhibits PTH secretion.

○ Rapid infusions of blood products may result in hypocalcemia. All packed red blood cells (PRBCs) are preserved with citrate. Calcium binds with citrate and may result in hypocalcemia, especially when the PRBCs are infused rapidly. Ionized calcium levels must be monitored.

○ Early signs of tetany may be present on examination. Watch for unusual flapping of the wrist when measuring blood pressure. This may be Trousseau's sign, which occurs when the arm is slightly ischemic in the presence of hypocalcemia. (This may not occur until the blood pressure cuff has been inflated for several minutes.) Watch for other evidence of muscle twitching (e.g., unusual nose twitching) that may have been overlooked.

○ When a patient is in an acidotic state, the total serum calcium level may be low but the patient may be asymptomatic, because more calcium is in the ionized state. When the pH returns to normal (7.35 to 7.45), signs and symptoms of hypocalcemia may become apparent.

○ Treatment for tetany varies depending on the cause. It may include the administration of vitamin D, calcium, or PTH. In a patient who has sustained parathyroid gland damage, lifelong PTH replacement may be needed.

NURSING PROBLEM/ DIAGNOSIS	NURSING INTERVENTIONS CLASSIFICATION (NIC)
Hypocalcemia	Electrolyte Management: Hypocalcemia
Deficient knowledge	Teaching: Disease Process

Hypothyroidism

Section 5   Suzanne Marnocha

OVERVIEW

Hypothyroidism is characterized by decreased activity of the thyroid gland. It may be caused by surgical removal of all or part of the gland, overdose with antithyroid medication, decreased effects of thyroid-releasing hormone (TRH) secreted by the hypothalamus, decreased secretion of thyroid-stimulating hormone (TSH) by the pituitary gland, or atrophy of the thyroid gland itself.

Effects of hypothyroidism include weight gain, mental and physical lethargy, skin dryness, constipation, arthritis, bradycardia, hypotension, depressed muscular activity, goiter, and overall slowing of the body's metabolic processes. Left untreated, hypothyroidism leads to myxedema and death.

 ## PATHOPHYSIOLOGY

Deficient production of thyroid hormones T_3 and T_4 by the thyroid gland results in the clinical state called hypothyroidism. Hypothyroidism can be primary, a consequence of thyroid gland failure, or secondary, a result of hypothalamic-pituitary gland failure. The most common cause of primary hypothyroidism is Hashimoto's thyroiditis, which is believed to be an autoimmune condition that produces antibodies that target thyroid tissue. Two other common causes of primary hypothyroidism are ablative therapy in the treatment of hyperthyroidism and endemic iodine deficiency. The latter is not a major concern in North America because of the institution of iodized salt.

Secondary hypothyroidism results from the pituitary's failure to synthesize adequate amounts of TSH. Postpartum pituitary necrosis and pituitary tumor are the most common causes of secondary hypothyroidism.

Hypothyroidism develops insidiously and often goes unrecognized. A stressor usually causes a life-threatening exacerbation of the disease. Stressors may include infection, drug toxicity, digitalis, sedatives, hypovolemia or hypervolemia, surgery, emotional or physical stress, autoimmune disease, or long-term illness. These stressors inhibit thyroid hormone production or function and ultimately disturb metabolic balance. Individuals develop a hypometabolic state with a resulting decrease in metabolic rate. The decrease in thyroid hormone can lead to excessive TSH production and goiter.

 ## SIGNS AND SYMPTOMS

Hypothyroidism generally affects all body systems and occurs insidiously over months or years. The decrease in thyroid hormone reduces energy and heat production by lowering metabolic rate. This is why patients present with many vague signs and complaints. Unfortunately, hypothyroidism is often mistaken for other problems. Many patients with hypothyroidism complain of forgetfulness and even changes in personality; in elderly persons, these findings may be mistakenly attributed to dementia or depression.

Common findings may be discussed by body system. Cardiovascular findings include bradycardia, hypotension, edema, and congestive heart failure. Neurologic findings may include personality changes, fatigue, lethargy, confusion, somnolence, and coma. GI effects include constipation, anorexia, and weight gain. Musculoskeletal alterations include weakness and joint pain. Loss of libido and impotence are reproductive findings. Integumentary changes include alopecia, loss of the outer third of the eyelid, and dry, coarse skin. Ophthalmic concerns include exophthalmos, periorbital edema, and drooping eyelids. Other changes include deepening of the voice, cold intolerance, goiter, and enlargement of the tongue.

Severe, long-standing hypothyroidism is termed *myxedema*. This condition is characterized by alterations in connective fibers and tissues that produce nonpitting, boggy edema of the hands, feet, and face. The tongue becomes thickened, with resultant slurred speech and hoarseness.

Severe forms of this condition may lead to *myxedema coma*, a medical emergency. The patient suffers pronounced hypothermia without a normal shivering response, along with hypoventilation, hypotension, hypoglycemia, and lactic acidosis.

 DIAGNOSTIC CRITERIA

The diagnosis of hypothyroidism is confirmed by evaluation of thyroid hormone levels (see Table 18-3-1). Two of the hormones produced by the thyroid gland are forms of thyroxin. Triiodothyronine (T_3) contains three iodine atoms in a molecule; L-thyroxin (T_4), four iodine atoms. Adequate iodine intake is necessary for the continuing formation of T_3 and T_4. Adult reference values are 75 to 195 ng/dL for T_3 and 4 to 12 μg/dL for total T_4. The third thyroid hormone is calcitonin. It lowers the plasma calcium level by inhibiting mobilization of calcium from the bone. Calcitonin levels are usually measured only for known or suspected cases of medullary carcinoma of the thyroid.

TSH is secreted by the anterior lobe of the pituitary gland to control the release of thyroid hormone. This substance is necessary for the growth and function of the thyroid gland. Also referred to as thyrotropin, TSH has a diurnal variation, with the lowest levels found at 10 AM and the highest levels found between 10 PM and 11 PM. Acutely ill patients may have different patterns. Adult reference values for TSH are 0.5 to 5.0 μU/mL).

In addition to the alterations in TSH, T_3, and T_4, other laboratory anomalies in hypothyroidism may include hyponatremia and hypoglycemia.

 INTERVENTIONS

Immediate treatment is required for the patient with myxedema coma, a manifestation of severe, untreated hypothyroidism. Care is directed toward supporting the airway and supplying adequate oxygen. Intubation and ventilatory support may be required to correct hypoventilation and hypercarbia. The concurrent hypovolemia necessitates careful volume expansion while monitoring all cardiovascular parameters, to avoid contributing to the dilutional hyponatremia that can accompany myxedema coma. Hypothermia usually is treated by slowly rewarming the patient with blankets. Rapid rewarming will trigger vasodilation and further hypovolemia.

For simple primary hypothyroidism, the patient is given levothyroxine (Synthroid), a synthetic preparation of T_4, to replace the deficient hormone. The synthetic hormone acts exactly as natural T_4; the goal is to normalize TSH level, not suppress it. Because hypothyroidism is a chronic health problem, levothyroxine must be taken for life. If the hormone is stopped, the patient's quality of life will be greatly affected. The usual dosage varies for each patient and is adjusted according to blood levels of TSH.

 COMMUNITY CARE

The most important issue to be aware of is how common hypothyroidism is and how it is often confused with other medical and psychological problems.

The nurse in the community should have a high index of suspicion for hypothyroidism in any patient who exhibits the characteristic signs and symptoms. The overall prevalence of hypothyroidism is about 1% in females and somewhat lower in males; incidence is much higher in elderly persons. In the elderly, many of the symptoms may be absent, and thus there must be increased reliance on thyroid function tests.

Once therapeutic levels of hormone replacement therapy have been met, TSH levels should then be monitored biannually or annually.

 PROGNOSIS

The prognosis for uncomplicated hypothyroidism is very good. Once hypothyroidism is detected, treatment should begin immediately with daily oral synthetic supplementation. If undetected and untreated, hypothyroidism can lead to myxedema coma with severe compromise of basic life functions.

 CLINICAL PEARLS

○ Have a high index of suspicion for hypothyroidism when assessing older adults with any of the characteristic signs and symptoms of the disorder.

○ A patient should not change brands of thyroid supplement without first checking with the physician. There is great variability in dosages among "natural" or desiccated forms of oral thyroid supplements.

○ Although myxedema coma and thyroid storm are opposing diagnoses of thyroid dysfunction, they share three common clinical findings: altered mental status, altered thermoregulation, and a precipitating event or illness.

○ A patient with preexisting evidence of coronary artery disease should be monitored closely during adjustment of oral thyroid supplement dosage. This medication can lead to a marked increased in cardiac output, with a resulting increase in myocardial oxygen demand. This could lead to angina in a vulnerable patient.

NURSING PROBLEM/ DIAGNOSIS	NURSING INTERVENTIONS CLASSIFICATION (NIC)
Metabolic hypoactivity	Teaching: Prescribed Medication Environmental Management: Comfort Nutrition Management
Deficient knowledge	Teaching: Disease Process

chapter 19

Neurologic

Alzheimer's Disease

Section 1   Ann Kolanowski

OVERVIEW

Alzheimer's disease (AD) is a progressive, degenerative brain disorder of insidious onset. The disease proceeds in stages during which the individual exhibits a loss of intellectual and cognitive abilities and behavioral changes that severely impair social and occupational functioning. Approximately 4 million Americans have AD and more than 70% of these individuals live at home. Currently, there is no cure for AD.

PATHOPHYSIOLOGY

AD is characterized by the presence of: (1) neuritic plaques, dense beta-amyloid protein deposits outside and around nerve cells in the brain, and (2) neurofibrillary tangles, twisted strands of tau proteins inside brain cells. Beta-amyloid is toxic to neurons, causing inflammation, the release of free radicals, and increased transport of choline across nerve cell membranes. The latter mechanism depletes intracellular stores of choline.

Tau proteins help to bind and stabilize microtubules, the cell's internal support structure. In AD, the microtubules collapse, resulting in twisted strands of fiber, leading to malfunctioning communication between cells.

The disease process begins in the entorhinal cortex, which is part of the hippocampus, a structure important in memory formation located on the inner surface of the temporal lobe (Fig. 19-1-1). From here, the disease progresses to the cerebral cortex, where it affects the temporal and parietal lobes. These areas of the brain are involved in language, reasoning, and way-finding.

In regions affected by AD, neurons degenerate or die and lose their connections (synapses) with other neurons. The disease process causes cerebral atrophy, widened sulci, lateral ventricular enlargement, and narrowed convolutions.

AD has no known cause, although there is evidence of a link between the disease and defective genes on four chromosomes: 1, 14, 19, and 21. The apo E4 gene on chromosome 19 has been linked to an increased risk of late-onset AD, the most common form of the disease. Other research has demonstrated a link between AD and low levels of acetylcholine (ACh), a neurotransmitter critical in memory formation. The risk of AD rises exponentially with age, doubling for each decade after age 65.

SIGNS AND SYMPTOMS

AD is a variable disease with symptoms progressing at different rates in different individuals. Several scales can be used to measure the progression of

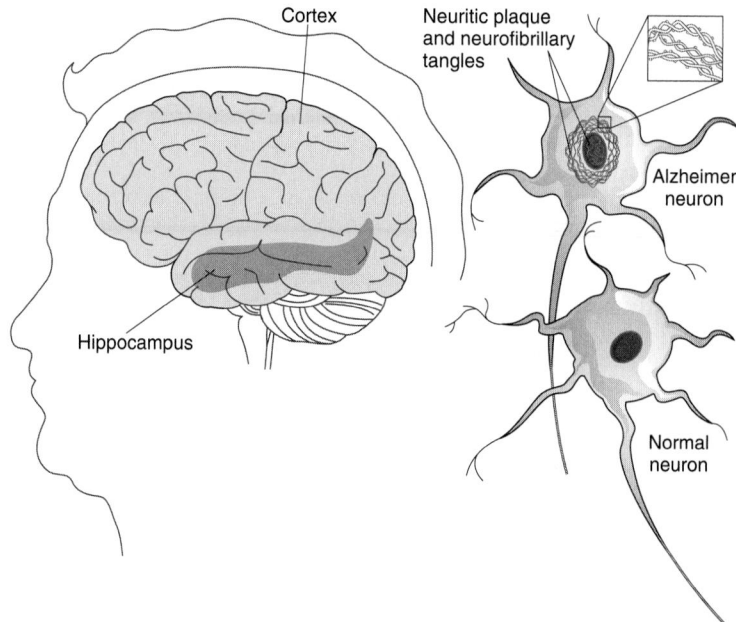

Figure 19-1-1. Neuron changes in Alzheimer's disease.

symptoms. Most sources divide the disease into three stages: mild, moderate, and severe.

Mild Symptoms
- Short-term memory loss
- Disorientation
- Difficulty with word-finding
- Loss of interest, passivity
- Difficulty with problem solving

Moderate Symptoms
- Agitation, anxiety
- Wandering
- Difficulty with activities of daily living (ADL)
- Sleep disturbances
- Personality changes

Severe Symptoms
- Loss of speech (aphasia)
- Incontinence
- Total dependence in ADL

 DIAGNOSTIC CRITERIA

There is no specific test for AD; it can be diagnosed only on postmortem examination. "Possible" AD and "probable" AD can be diagnosed with

85% to 90% accuracy using criteria established by the National Institute of Neurological and Communicative Disorders and Stroke and the Alzheimer's Disease and Related Diseases Association.

Recommended criteria for establishing a diagnosis include the following:

- Patient history: Past and present patient/family medical history; onset of symptoms and rate of progression; medications; psychological and functional problems
- Diagnostic tests: Complete blood count (CBC), glucose, blood urea nitrogen (BUN), electrolytes, liver function, thyroid profile, vitamin B_{12}, and folate
- Radiologic studies: Chest radiograph, computed tomography (CT) scan, magnetic resonance imaging (MRI), and positron emission tomography (PET) scan
- Neuropsychological tests: Mental status examination, Hachinski ischemic rating scale, functional assessment, and other neuropsychological test batteries that include measures of memory, language, praxis, and general cognitive functions

It is important to establish a diagnosis early, because 20% of persons who present with symptoms have treatable disease that mimics dementia. These potentially reversible conditions include depression, drug reactions, metabolic deficiencies, head injury, and cerebrovascular accident.

INTERVENTIONS

Interventions for patients with AD are adapted according to the stage of disease and individual needs. Several broad goals guide care.

Obtain an Adequate Assessment

The patient's preserved functional and cognitive strengths and weaknesses are carefully assessed. The nurse needs this information so that interventions can support deficits and build on remaining strengths. Helpful tools include mental status examinations and functional assessments (i.e., ADL).

Promote Quality of Life

The cognitively impaired patient's dignity and independence must be maintained and excessive disabilities prevented. The nurse should encourage the patient and family to continue hobbies and other activities that they find pleasurable. Activities should be kept simple and routine. The patient's ability to engage in potentially dangerous activities (e.g., driving, cooking) should be assessed frequently, with care taken to restrict these activities only when necessary.

Facilitate Daily Activities

Ample, appropriate sensory stimulation should be provided. Some suggestions include listening to music, tending to plants or pets, and engaging in physical activity. The use of large clocks, calendars, and signs for bathrooms and other areas help maintain orientation. Instructions for bathing or dressing should be given one step at a time. Clothes should be laid out in the order in which they are to be put on. Velcro fasteners instead of buttons and laces may be helpful. A smock or apron may be appropriate for a messy eater. Milk should be avoided for a patient who drools or has breathing problems. Snacks may be made available for a patient who likes to nibble.

Promote Safety

As the disease progresses, it becomes necessary to "safety proof" the environment to prevent accidents. Door alarms alert caregivers to possible elopement. The local police department should be given a description of a high-risk eloper. An article of the patient's unwashed clothing should be kept available to aid canine tracking. Stove knobs may need to be removed or car keys hidden to prevent injury. Fall prevention is important for a high-risk individual, especially one taking psychotropic drugs. Throw rugs should be eliminated, and lighting should be adjusted in areas of heavy traffic.

Physical restraints should be avoided, because they erode the patient's remaining capabilities and can be a cause of serious injury, including death by strangulation. Psychotropic drugs should be given at the smallest doses possible, and their use should be monitored to prevent adverse effects, such as tardive dyskinesia.

Facilitate Communication

The nurse should face the patient when speaking and use short, simple sentences. If the patient's language skills are deficient, gestures can be used to communicate. The nurse should avoid challenging or disagreeing with a distraught patient. The use of touch can be comforting. "Either/or" choices should be provided when appropriate. Verbal prompts when asking the patient to do something may be helpful.

Prevent or Treat Incontinence

The patient should be toileted every 2 hours. Adequate fluid intake should be maintained, taking into consideration cardiac or renal problems that may coexist with AD. Indwelling (Foley) urinary catheters should be avoided. Visual aids may help the patient find the bathroom. Clothing with elastic waistbands or Velcro fasteners and plastic covers for furniture may also be helpful.

Respond to Behavioral Problems (Agitation, Aggression, Wandering)

A log can be maintained to help identify the patient's behavioral triggers (i.e., who, what, when, where, why). These triggers should be removed whenever possible. The nurse should maintain a calm, reassuring approach and avoid arguing with the patient. Desirable behavior should be reinforced. The patient exhibiting a dementia behavior can be distracted and the behavior replaced with a more desirable one.

Provide Respite Care

In AD, the family caregiver is the "second patient." It is important to provide support and respite to prevent caregiver health problems. The Alzheimer's Association is an excellent resource, as are other community agencies (see Community Care).

Coordinate Hospice Care

AD is a terminal illness, and caregivers go through a series of losses as the disease progresses. It is important for the nurse to be sensitive to the grief response that caregivers experience and to mobilize the necessary end-of-life care and support.

Monitor Medical Interventions

Drug interventions fall into two broad categories: biomedical treatments and symptom management. Biomedical treatments are aimed at replacing ACh and counteracting the effects of beta-amyloid. Drugs such as donepezil (Aricept) and tacrine act by inhibiting acetylcholinesterase, an enzyme that breaks down ACh. Estrogen prevents the formation of beta-amyloid and acts like an antioxidant. Vitamin E is also an antioxidant and helps remove free radicals released in the presence of beta-amyloid. Nonsteroidal anti-inflammatory drugs (e.g., ibuprofen) are thought to counter the inflammatory process caused by beta-amyloid. The use of many of these drugs in treating AD is in experimental stages, and results vary.

Antipsychotic and antidepressant agents are often prescribed for behavioral symptoms such as agitation and depression. These drugs should be initiated only after other nonpharmacologic interventions have proved ineffective, and their effects must be closely monitored.

 COMMUNITY CARE

Because more than 70% of all persons with AD reside in the community and are cared for by family members, supporting these informal caregivers is of paramount importance. Local chapters of the Alzheimer's Association offer support groups for caregivers and may provide day or respite care for the afflicted. Other services that reduce caregiver burden and support quality of life include Meals on Wheels, senior transport services from the local area Agency on Aging, and homemaker services.

The patient's family may need the help of a social worker when making arrangements for nursing home placement. Many nursing homes have designated units for patients with dementia. These units are designed for the special needs of this population and have staff trained to respond to problems that arise during the course of the disease.

 PROGNOSIS

AD has no cure. The average length of survival from diagnosis is 4 to 8 years, but some individuals live as long as 20 years with the disease. Death usually results from pneumonia. Despite these statistics, quality of life can be improved with proper nursing care and medical attention.

 CLINICAL PEARLS

○ Caregivers need to be flexible and adjust expectations to fit the patient.
○ Respite care should be arranged to help the patient's family deal with the burden of AD.
○ Caregivers promote patient dignity by presenting options whenever possible.
○ The family is a valuable source of information on the patient's past preferences and behavior.

NURSING PROBLEM/ DIAGNOSIS	NURSING INTERVENTIONS CLASSIFICATION (NIC)
Communication difficulties	Dementia management
Self-care deficit	Self-care assistance
Risk for injury, wandering (safety)	Dementia management, environmental management, surveillance
Caregiver role strain	Caregiver support, health system guidance

Cerebrovascular Accident

Section 2   Lori Schumacher

 ## OVERVIEW

Cerebrovascular accident (CVA), also known as stroke, is a focal neurologic dysfunction caused by decreased blood flow to a vascular territory in the brain. The term "brain attack" is used to promote urgency in seeking care, as associated with "heart attack." CVA is the third leading cause of death and the leading cause of disability in the United States. Each year, approximately 700,000 new strokes occur, with an estimated cost of more than 40 billion dollars.

CVA is classified as ischemic or hemorrhagic. *Ischemic* strokes account for 80% to 85% of all strokes; the remaining 15% to 20% of strokes are *hemorrhagic*. CVA may also be classified by the manner by which it develops. *Progressive stroke* (or *stroke-in-evolution*) develops over a period of 1 to 3 days, during which time symptoms worsen until the maximum deficit is reached. *Completed stroke* occurs when the maximum deficit is identified at the time of symptom onset.

Risk factors for CVA have been identified as modifiable, nonmodifiable, and other factors (Table 19-2-1).

 ## PATHOPHYSIOLOGY
Ischemic Stroke

Ischemic stroke results from complete or partial occlusion of one or more cerebral blood vessels secondary to thrombus formation or embolization. Thus ischemic strokes can be subclassified as thrombotic or embolic. When blood flow is impeded, ischemia occurs. Left untreated, the ischemia leads to infarction and necrosis of nerve cells, producing neurologic deficits. Cerebral edema develops within minutes of the insult to the neuronal cells, peaks within 2 to 4 days, and contributes to neurologic deficits. Ischemia may possibly be reversed with pharmacologic agents.

The occlusion seen in *thrombotic strokes* usually results from the narrowing of the lumen of the vessel, as seen in atherosclerosis. Significant atherosclerotic plaques in the carotid arteries can be assessed as carotid bruits. *Embolic strokes* result from occlusion by an embolus that commonly originates in the heart because of atrial fibrillation.

If the obstruction is lysed by the normal fibrinolytic mechanisms before

Table 19-2-1. Risk Factor for Stroke

NONMODIFIABLE	MODIFIABLE	OTHER FACTORS
Age	Hypertension	Obesity
Gender	Diabetes mellitus	Migraines
Race	Cardiac disease	Oral contraceptive use
Earlier stroke or transient ischemic attack	Abnormal serum lipid levels	Hypercoagulability states
Asymptomatic carotid artery stenosis	Cigarette smoking	
Heredity	Excessive alcohol intake	
	Drug abuse	

Adapted from Hock, N.H. (1999). Brain attack: The stroke continuum. *Nursing Clinics of North America*, 34(3), 691.

permanent damage occurs, the associated neurologic deficit will resolve completely. This type of episode is called a *transient ischemic attack* (TIA). Focal neurologic symptoms associated with TIAs last an average of 2 to 15 minutes but no longer than 24 hours. TIAs serve as warning signs of thromboembolic disease and carry a significant risk for subsequent stroke. They are most commonly associated with thrombotic strokes. A focal deficit that lasts more than 24 hours but resolves in days to weeks is considered a *reversible ischemic neurologic deficit.*

Hemorrhagic Stroke

Hemorrhagic stroke may result from a ruptured aneurysm, subarachnoid hemorrhage, vascular malformation, intracerebral hemorrhage, or traumatic brain injury. The most common cause of intracranial hemorrhage is chronic hypertension. Once hemorrhage has occurred, there is an immediate increase in intracranial pressure (ICP) owing to the accumulating blood. The increased ICP causes an ischemic cellular response that produces cerebral edema and compromises cerebral perfusion pressure. If untreated, possible herniation of brain tissue and death may occur.

 SIGNS AND SYMPTOMS

The signs and symptoms of stroke depend on the location of the cerebral vessel involved and severity of the insult (Table 19-2-2). Signs and symptoms vary according to the cerebral hemisphere affected:
- Left-sided stroke: Right-sided hemiplegia, expressive and receptive aphasia, intellectual impairment, and defects in the right visual fields
- Right-sided stroke: Left-sided hemiplegia, spatial-perceptual deficits, denial, impulsive behavior, poor judgment, and defects in left visual fields

Focal neurologic deficits persist for more than 24 hours. Nonfocal symptoms (e.g., headache, vomiting, altered level of consciousness [LOC], cranial nerve palsies) suggest increased ICP.

 DIAGNOSTIC CRITERIA

The first step in diagnosing stroke is *determining the time of symptom onset*, especially if the patient has had an ischemic stroke and is a candidate for thrombolytic therapy. A complete patient history is obtained, and physical and neurologic examinations are performed. The *neurologic examination* should use the National Institutes of Health Stroke Scale (NIHSS) to assess for impairment and stroke severity. The NIHSS scores LOC, gaze, visual disturbances, facial palsy, motor function, and sensory and language dysfunction. It is a predictor for discharge disposition. Neurovascular examination should focus on orthostatic blood pressure measurements, cardiac auscultation, and possibly 12-lead electrocardiography (ECG), carotid auscultation for bruits, palpation of neck and facial pulses, and fundoscopic examination. A *CT scan* without contrast can determine whether brain pathology such as a tumor or hemorrhage is present. *Laboratory studies* for hematology, chemistry, and coagulation are analyzed to detect bleeding disorders or other conditions that mimic stroke.

After the initial diagnosis has been made, other diagnostic studies that may be done include a brain MRI, magnetic resonance angiography (MRA), carotid duplex, cerebral angiography, echocardiography, and transcranial Doppler. MRA, carotid duplex, and transcranial Doppler permit noninvasive evaluation of the intracranial vasculature. Cerebral angiography is an invasive and reliable method of assessing the cerebral vasculature. Finally, a complete cardiology workup may be performed because of the possibility of cardiogenic emboli.

 ## INTERVENTIONS

Ischemic and hemorrhagic stroke have the potential to affect multiple body systems. Interventions related to specific clinical problems are listed in Table 19-2-3.

Transient Ischemic Attacks and Ischemic Stroke

Education stresses prevention and includes risk factor identification, lifestyle modifications, adherence to treatment plans, identification of early signs and symptoms, and actions to take if symptoms occur.

Pharmacologic therapy includes antiplatelet, anticoagulant, antithrombolytic, and neuroprotective agents:

- For TIAs or minor ischemic stroke: Aspirin (ASA), or clopidogrel (Plavix) if the patient is hypersensitive to ASA, to prevent recurrence
- For progressing ischemic stroke: Heparin IV, then warfarin
- For complete embolic stroke: Heparin IV, then warfarin (to prevent cardiogenic emboli in chronic atrial fibrillation)
- For completed thrombotic stroke: ASA or ticlopidine (Ticlid)

Surgical interventions may include *carotid endarterectomy,* a procedure that may be performed with the goal of preventing TIA and stroke. Carotid endarterectomy involves an incision into the carotid artery and the removal of plaque. *Carotid bypass surgery* involves placing a graft to bypass the occluded carotid artery using a saphenous vein or synthetic graft, to restore circulation on a patient with a narrowed extracranial artery.

Early emphasis on *rehabilitation* must begin as soon as possible to assist the patient in making an optimal recovery.

Thrombolytic Therapy

The goal of management for any stroke patient is to maximize neurologic function. The advent of thrombolytic therapy has made it possible to dissolve the occlusion and reestablish blood flow to an ischemic brain before infarction

Text continued on page 655

Table 19-2-2. Signs and Symptoms of Cerebrovascular Accident according to the Vessel and Vascular Region Affected

VASCULAR REGION	AREAS AFFECTED	SIGNS AND SYMPTOMS
Carotid Region		
Internal carotid artery syndrome	Provides blood supply to the forebrain	Paralysis of the contralateral face, arm, and leg
		Sensory deficits
		Aphasia
		Apraxia, agnosia, and unilateral neglect
		Homonymous, hemianopsia
Middle cerebral artery syndrome	Frontal lobe	Hemiplegia
	Parietal lobe	Sensory impairment
	Temporal lobe	Aphasia
	Corpus striatum	Homonymous hemianopsia
	Internal capsule	
	Thalamus	
Anterior cerebral artery syndrome	Internal capsule	Contralateral foot and leg paralysis
	Medial and lateral surfaces of the hemisphere	Sensory deficits of the toes, foot, and leg
		Impaired gait
		Flat affect
		Cognitive impairment
		Urinary incontinence
Vertebrobasilar Region		
Vertebral artery syndrome	Brain stem	Dizziness
	Cerebellum	Nystagmus
		Dysphagia and dysarthria
		Pain
		Ipsilateral numbness and weakness
		Staggering gait and ataxia
		Clumsiness
Basilar artery syndrome	Medial temporal lobe	Quadriplegia
	Occipital lobe	"Locked-in" syndrome (complete paralysis with intact cortical function)
	Corpus callosum	Weakness

Syndrome	Location	Signs/Symptoms
Anterior inferior cerebellar artery syndrome	Pons Cerebellum Inner ear	**Ipsilateral side** Paresis of lateral conjugate gaze Horner's syndrome Cerebellar signs **Contralateral side** Impaired pain sensation Impaired temperature sensation
Posterior inferior cerebellar artery syndrome	Lateral portion of the medulla	Nausea and vomiting Dysphagia and dysarthria Horizontal nystagmus Cerebellar signs Loss of pain and temperature sensation
Posterior cerebral artery syndrome	Cerebral peduncle Thalamus Upper brain stem	**Peripheral area** Homonymous hemianopsia Memory deficits Preseveration Severe visual deficits **Central area** Thalamus involvement Cerebral peduncle involvement Brain stem involvement
Deep Cortical Syndrome **Putamenal hemorrhage**	Internal capsule	Contralateral hemiplegia Contralateral hemisensory deficits Hemianopsia Slurred speech
Thalamic hemorrhage	Thalamus	Contralateral hemiplegia Contralateral hemisensory deficits Deficits of vertical and lateral gaze
Pontine hemorrhage	Pontine	"Locked-in" syndrome Deficits in lateral eye movement
Cerebellar hemorrhage	Cerebellum	Occipital headache Dizziness Ataxia Vertigo

Table 19-2-3. Common Problems and Interventions in Stroke Patients

PROBLEM	INTERVENTION
Increased intracranial pressure Sensorimotor disability/immobility	(See Chapter 7, Section 2) • Provide range-of-motion exercises. • Ensure correct positioning of the flaccid extremity. • Use support hose and sequential inflation devices. • Assess for deep vein thrombosis and signs and symptoms of pulmonary embolus. • Administer low-dose heparin (See Chapter 12, Section 2). • Assess skin integrity. • Provide a specialty bed if needed. • Refer to physical therapy/occupational therapy. • Involve the family in care. • Ensure adequate nutrition and hydration.
Dysphagia	• Assess swallowing ability and the presence of a gag reflex. • Implement aspiration precautions. • Maintain a patent airway. • Assess respiratory status and signs and symptoms of aspiration pneumonia. • Consult a speech therapist and dietitian. • Ensure adequate nutrition, and possibly provide a feeding tube. • Monitor intake and output. • Educate the patient and/or family.
Incontinence	• Assess for appropriateness of urinary catheter (use only if necessary). • Implement a bladder/bowel training program. • Assess for urinary tract infection, a drug- or diet-related problem (e.g., diarrhea), or fecal impaction.
Unilateral neglect	• Provide a safe environment. • Implement falls protocol. • Refer for occupational therapy. • Promote the patient's involvement in care. • Provide patient/family education.
Communication deficit	• Assess for aphasia and/or dysarthria. • Consult a speech therapist. • Utilize alternative communication methods. • Utilize prescribed exercises. • Provide patient/family education.
Poststroke depression	• Assess for signs and symptoms of depression. • Administer an antidepressant as ordered. • Provide patient/family education.
Cognitive dysfunction	• Assess for short- and long-term memory loss, altered insight, judgment, and reasoning skills. • Arrange for a speech therapist evaluation. • Arrange for a neuropsychologist evaluation.

Adapted from Wojner, A.W. (1998). Neurovascular disease. In M.R. Kinney, S.B. Dunbar, J. Brooks-Brunn, N. Molter, & J.M. Vitello-Cicciu (Eds.), *AACN clinical reference for critical care nursing* (4th ed.). Philadelphia: CV Mosby.

Hickey, J. (1997). Stroke and other cerebrovascular diseases. In *The clinical practice of neurological and neurosugical nursing* (4th ed.). Philadelphia: JB Lippincott.

occurs, provided that the patient meets the established criteria. *Inclusion criteria* include:

- Symptom onset of less than 3 hours
- Clinical diagnosis of ischemic stroke with measurable deficit on NIH stroke scale
- Older than age 18
- No evidence of cerebral hemorrhage on a CT scan
  Exclusion criteria include:
- Stroke or serious head trauma within the past 3 months
- Systolic blood pressure above 185 mm Hg, diastolic blood pressure above 110 mm Hg (values that require aggressive treatment)
- Conditions that could suggest or precipitate parenchymal bleeding (e.g., seizures, major surgery within the past 14 days, gastrointestinal or urinary tract hemorrhage, lumbar puncture within the past 7 days)
- Serum glucose level below 50 mg/dL or above 400 mg/dL; international normalized ratio (INR) of 1.7; platelet count below 100,000/mm^3.
- Rapidly changing neurologic signs or minor symptoms
- Recent myocardial infarction
- Treatment with heparin (IV or SC) within the past 48 hours and an elevated prothrombin time (PTT)
- A woman of childbearing age with a positive pregnancy test.

Recombinant tissue plasminogen activator (rt-PA) is a thrombolytic drug approved for treatment of acute ischemic stroke. The dosage of rt-PA is dependent on patient's weight and is calculated as follows: patient's weight in kg $\times$ 0.9 mg = dose of rt-PA to be given (not to exceed 90 mg).

Of the total rt-PA dose, 10% is given as an IV bolus over 1 to 2 minutes and the rest is infused over 1 hour. After administration, the patient is monitored in an intensive care unit for 24 hours. If the patient is outside the timeframe for receiving rt-PA or does not meet the criteria for rt-PA administration, then management will involve the interventions discussed earlier.

Hemorrhagic Stroke

The acute management of a patient who has sustained a hemorrhagic stroke focuses on managing ICP. Depending on the severity and location of the hemorrhage, discharge planning and early focus rehabilitation should begin as soon as the patient is hemodynamically and neurologically stabilized. To protect the brain from delayed cerebral arterial spasm after subarachnoid hemorrhage or ruptured aneurysm, neuroprotective agents (e.g., calcium antagonists [e.g., nimodipine], *N*-methyl-D-asparate [NMDA] antagonists, and free-radical scavengers are used.

Clinical problems and interventions related to hemorrhagic stroke are outlined in Table 19-2-4.

 ## COMMUNITY CARE

Community education should focus on the fact that stroke is an emergency and that "time is brain." Good teaching reinforces risk factors and lifestyle modifications. It covers the importance of follow-up visits to a health care provider to assess for and treat hypertension and diabetes mellitus; the need to monitor cholesterol levels; the details of pharmacologic therapy; and how to recognize early signs and symptoms of stroke.

Table 19-2-4. Hemorrhagic Stroke: Common Problems and Interventions

PROBLEM	INTERVENTION
Hydrocephalus	• Assess for signs and symptoms of increased intracranial pressure (ICP). • Monitor ICP readings and CPP. • Manage ventriculostomy if present. • Provide patient/family education.
Fluid and electrolyte imbalance	• Monitor intake and output. • Monitor laboratory results. • Administer fluids and medications as prescribed and indicated. • Provide patient/family education.
Cardiac dysfunction	• Monitor cardiac rhythm. • Assess and monitor hemodynamic readings. • Administer medications to ensure optimal perfusion.
Seizures	• Implement seizure precautions. • If seizure occurs, assess the type and duration. • Administer anticonvulsant medication as ordered. • Monitor serum drug levels. • Provide patient/family education.
Vasospasm	• Administer nimodipine as ordered. • Administer "triple H" therapy: hypertension, hypervolemia, and hemodilution. • Use transcranial Doppler ultrasonography to measure cerebral blood flow. • Monitor hematocrit levels and administer fluids and albumin as ordered.

Adapted from Wojner, A.W. (1998). Neurovascular disease. In M.R. Kinney, S.B. Dunbar, J. Brooks-Brunn, N. Molter, & J.M. Vitello-Cicciu (Eds.), *AACN clinical reference for critical care nursing* (4th ed.). Philadelphia: CV Mosby.

Hickey, J. (1997). Stroke and other cerebrovascular diseases. In *The clinical practice of neurological and neurosugical nursing* (4th ed.). Philadelphia: JB Lippincott.

 PROGNOSIS

Stroke is the third-leading cause of death in the United States. It affects more than 700,000 people every year and is the major cause of serious disability in adults. Most recovery occurs within the first few weeks after the stroke. Death usually occurs from respiratory compromise (aspiration pneumonia) and brainstem compromise (increased ICP, herniation, or brainstem hemorrhage).

 CLINICAL PEARLS

○ Intracerebral hemorrhage is more common in the elderly; subarachnoid hemorrhage is more common in the young.
○ The brain is vulnerable to ischemic injury. It is only 2% of the total body's mass but depends on a continuous supply of oxygen and glucose to function and receives 20% of the cardiac output to meet these demands.

- A carotid stroke usually presents with weakness in the arm rather than the leg.
- Weakness in the arm and leg suggests a capsular or brainstem stroke.
- A patient's lack of awareness of a stroke usually indicates that the stroke occurred in the nondominant hemisphere.
- Headache is unusual with ischemic stroke. Sudden, severe headache usually suggests a subarachnoid hemorrhage. Headache preceding the stroke by weeks or more suggests a brain tumor.
- The risk of stroke doubles with high hemoglobin levels.
- Hypoglycemia and hyperglycemia may manifest focal neurologic signs that mimic stroke.

NURSING PROBLEM/ DIAGNOSIS	NURSING INTERVENTIONS CLASSIFICATION (NIC)
Prevention: community awareness of early intervention and reduction of risk factors	Environmental Management: Community Risk Identification Health Education Health Screening
Acute care	Cerebral Perfusion Promotion Circulatory Care Neurologic Monitoring Nutrition Therapy
Impaired cognitive function	Activity Therapy Communication Enhancement Environmental Management
Impaired physical function	Self-Care Assistance Exercise Therapy: Ambulation Environmental Management: Safety

Guillain-Barré Syndrome

Section 3   Lori Schumacher

OVERVIEW

Guillain-Barré syndrome (GBS) is an acute neurologic disorder that affects the sensory, motor, and autonomic nervous systems. The incidence of GBS is 1 to 2 cases per 100,000. GBS occurs worldwide during all seasons and affects all age groups equally. It has an unknown etiology and is characterized by rapidly progressing weakness and paresthesias in ascending order.

PATHOPHYSIOLOGY

The etiology of GBS is unknown, but it is thought to be triggered by a viral infection occurring in the previous 1 to 4 weeks. The most common acute infections identified with GBS include:

- Viral pneumonia
- Upper respiratory infection
- Gastrointestinal infections

- Cytomegalovirus
- Epstein-Barr virus (mononucleosis)
- Recent flu vaccine/viral immunization

The viral infection probably initiates an autoimmune attack against the myelin sheaths of both cranial and spinal nerves. Lymphocytes, macrophages, and immune complexes infiltrate the myelin specifically between the nodes of Ranvier, causing edema and eventual demyelination. When the myelin sheath is destroyed, the underlying axon is exposed and can be permanently damaged or detached from the cell body. Demyelination causes loss of nerve impulse conduction, which results in paralysis. If the protective Schwann cells surrounding the axons remain intact, then myelin can be regenerated. The process of remyelination and regeneration occurs gradually; maximum improvement with or without permanent deficits may take up to 2 years. Usually, GBS is a self-limiting disease that subsides in reverse order.

 SIGNS AND SYMPTOMS

The onset of GBS is usually heralded by paresthesias in the distal extremities. A few days later, ascending weakness begins in the lower extremities. The weakness progresses symmetrically up to the trunk and arms. The progression of weakness may take hours to days.

GBS progression has three phases. The acute onset phase begins with first definitive symptom (i.e., paresthesias or weakness) and ends when no new symptom or deterioration occurs. It lasts for 1 to 3 weeks. During the plateau period, there is no further progression of neurologic symptoms. This period lasts from several days to 2 weeks. During the recovery phase, remyelination and axonal regeneration occur, and strength returns in a descending pattern. This takes up to 2 years.

Motor, sensory, and autonomic deficits as GBS progresses vary in severity. Common manifestations are as follows. *Motor (extremities) dysfunction* includes progressive ascending weakness beginning in the legs and moving to the trunk, arms, neck, and face, along with diminished or absent deep tendon reflexes. *Motor (respiratory) dysfunction* includes respiratory failure from fatigue and weakness of the intercostal muscles and diaphragm, decreased cough effort, decreased oxygen saturation, respiratory acidosis, and decreased forced vital capacity (<10 to 15 mL/kg).

Sensory dysfunction includes tingling or numbness in the legs and arms; heightened sensitivity to touch; and back, flank, and thigh pain with muscle tenderness.

Autonomic dysfunction includes cardiac dysrhythmias, orthostatic and paroxysmal hypertension, sweating dysfunction, paralytic ileus, urinary retention, and syndrome of inappropriate antidiuretic hormone secretion (SIADH).

Cranial nerve dysfunction mainly affects two nerves:

- CN VII (facial): Inability to smile, frown, whistle or suck through a straw
- CN IX (glossopharyngeal): Dysphagia

GBS does not affect level of consciousness or cognition. The patient is aware of everything happening to him or her.

 DIAGNOSTIC CRITERIA

The diagnosis of GBS is made from history, clinical observation, and diagnostic studies. A history of a recent viral infection and course of the

Table 19-3-1. Interventions for Autonomic Dysfunctions

AUTONOMIC DYSFUNCTION	INTERVENTION
Cardiac dysrhythmias	Institute cardiac monitoring.
	For severe bradycardia, administer atropine as prescribed, consider a pacemaker.
	For tachycardia administer beta-blockers or alpha-adrenergic blockers.
Hypotension	If the patient is orthostatic, do not leave him or her sitting; requires gradual elevation of the head.
	Administer fluid boluses and vasopressors as prescribed.
Hypertension	Administer an antihypertensive medication, e.g., nitroprusside (Nipride) or phentolamine (Regitine).
Paralytic ileus	Insert a nasogastric tube.
	Monitor for abdominal distention.
	Monitor bowel sounds.
Urinary retention	Insert an indwelling Foley-catheter.
Dysphagia	Provide nutritional support via enteral feedings.
	Evaluate swallowing ability to prevent aspiration.
Syndrome of inappropriate antidiuretic hormone (SIADH)	Monitor fluid balance.
	Monitor electrolyte values, especially sodium.

illness will be revealed. Clinical observation includes the findings listed in Table 19-3-1. Neurologic examination reveals the characteristic motor, sensory, and autonomic deficits. The two diagnostic studies performed to aid diagnosis of GBS are cerebrospinal fluid (CSF) analysis and electromyography (EMG).

CSF analysis reveals elevated protein level without elevated white blood cell (WBC) count. This occurs several days after the onset of symptoms and peaks between 4 and 6 weeks later.

In EMG, a concentric needle electrode is inserted into a muscle to record the electrical activity of the muscle as it contracts and rests. In GBS, EMG reveals slowed or blocked nerve conduction velocities.

 INTERVENTIONS

Plasmapheresis

Plasmapheresis is generally used for patients with severe GBS with respiratory muscle involvement. For maximum effectiveness, it is initiated within 7 to 14 days after the onset of GBS. Plasmapheresis is done in an effort to remove the antibodies responsible for GBS. It is usually performed every 1 to 2 days for a total of three to four treatments.

Plasmapheresis has proven effective in reducing mechanical ventilation and hospitalization time. Disadvantages of plasmapheresis include high cost and the risk of intravascular line sepsis.

Respiratory Support

Respiratory failure is common in GBS because of the progressive muscular weakness. Therefore, careful monitoring of respiratory status is essential. Between 20% and 30% of patients will need intubation and mechanical ventilation to maintain adequate oxygenation. Usually, respiratory failure is anticipated; therefore, the patient is monitored closely. When forced vital capacity falls below a predetermined level (15 mL/kg), the patient is electively intubated. Ventilatory support is provided until respiratory function improves to the point at which the patient can be weaned from the ventilator. Sometimes this may take time, in which case a tracheostomy is done to facilitate the weaning process and decrease the risk of pneumonia.

The last important aspect of respiratory support is prevention and monitoring for the development of pneumonia, which is a common complication of GBS. Interventions include frequent suctioning, turning, repositioning, and chest physiotherapy.

Autonomic Dysfunction

Because autonomic symptoms (e.g., cardiac dysrhythmias, blood pressure variations) are common in GBS, the patient must be monitored continuously to detect problems (e.g., heart block, hypotension, hypertension) early and initiate treatment promptly. Common interventions are outlined in Table 19-3-1.

Intravenous Immunoglobulin

Intravenous immunoglobulin (IVIg) has proved as effective a therapy as plasmapheresis. IVIg therapy is administered daily for 2 weeks. Advantages of IVIg are that it is simpler to deliver and less expensive than plasmapheresis. One disadvantage of IVIg therapy is the possible transmission of viral infection (e.g., human immunodeficiency virus [HIV]).

General Nursing Management

Because of the long duration of GBS, the patient needs astute nursing assessment and supportive care throughout the course of the illness, as well as care aimed at preventing complications that arise from immobility and altered nutritional status. Common problems and interventions associated with immobility and nutrition are listed in Table 19-3-2.

 COMMUNITY CARE

Assessment

Obtain a history of recent viral infections and vaccinations. Determine any pattern of symptom onset. Establish a baseline of neurologic symptoms; assess for weakness and monitor for progression.

Monitoring

Monitor the progression of weakness. Assess for respiratory compromise and the development of pneumonia. Monitor for increasing muscle strength in reverse order from the progression of weakness.

Prevention

Prevent complications of immobility: skin breakdown, musculoskeletal problems (e.g., contractures, muscle wasting), and respiratory problems (e.g., pneumonia).

 PROGNOSIS

An estimated 80% to 90% of patients with GBS make a full recovery or a recovery with some residual disabilities. Death occurs in approximately 5% of cases, primarily from impaired respiratory function.

Table 19-3-2. Common Problems and Interventions for Patients with Guillain-Barré Syndrome

PROBLEM	INTERVENTIONS
Respiratory • Ineffective breathing pattern • Ineffective airway clearance	• Assess respiratory status. • Monitor for respiratory difficulties. • Administer oxygen, if ordered. • Monitor arterial blood gas values and pulse oximetry readings. • Be prepared for possible intubation.
Nutrition: Less than Body Requirements • Decreased weight and muscle mass • Weakness and fatigue • Inability to wean from the ventilator	• Initiate feedings early; consult with a speech therapist. • Consult a dietician. • Provide adequate nutrition based on the patient's specific requirements. • Weigh the patient daily.
Immobility • Deep vein thrombosis; pulmonary emboli • Alteration in skin integrity • Impaired functional abilities	• Administer low-dose heparin or low molecular weight heparin to prevent deep vein thrombosis and pulmonary emboli. • Apply a pneumatic compression device to the lower extremities. • Ensure frequent turning and repositioning. • Provide skin care. • Perform range-of-motion exercises. • Progress activity gradually. • Arrange for physical therapy and occupational therapy consults. • Consider a specialized bed or mattress to prevent skin breakdown.

 CLINICAL PEARLS

○ Paresthesia is usually the initial symptom and occurs a few days before the onset of weakness, and is the most common presenting symptom.

○ Corticosteroids have proved to be ineffective in treating GBS.

○ In addition to respiratory impairment, there are two life-threatening complications of GBS: pain and psychological trauma.

NURSING PROBLEM/ DIAGNOSIS	NURSING INTERVENTIONS CLASSIFICATION (NIC)
Risk for respiratory failure Risk for ineffective breathing pattern Risk for progression of deficits	Respiratory Monitoring Airway Management Oxygen Therapy Neurologic Monitoring Activity Therapy Circulatory Care Nutrition Therapy
Autonomic complications	Vital Sign Monitoring Hemodynamic Regulation Fluid Management

Meningitis

Section 4   Lori Schumacher

OVERVIEW

Meningitis is defined as the inflammation and infection of the subarachnoid space and the meninges. It usually involves adjacent brain tissue, spinal cord, and CSF. Meningitis is predominately bacterial in origin; the annual incidence of bacterial meningitis is 2.5 to 3.5 cases per 100,000 population. Meningitis may also be of viral, fungal, or parasitic origin. Seasonal outbreaks of meningitis occur, with increased incidence in the spring, fall, and winter and a decline in the summer.

PATHOPHYSIOLOGY

The pathophysiology of meningitis varies slightly depending on the origin. *Bacterial meningitis* is caused by bacteria entering the subarachnoid space from an adjacent structure such as the sinuses or bloodstream. Common organisms associated with bacterial meningitis include:

- Streptococcus pneumoniae
- Neisseria meningitidis (meningococcal)
- *Haemophilus influenzae*

Initially, the bacteria invade the subarachnoid space, which is very vascular, inciting the migration of massive numbers of neutrophils. The neutrophils engulf and destroy the bacteria, producing inflammatory exudate within the subarachnoid space. The exudate causes congestion in the brain, particularly of the ventricles, which leads to edema, possible hydrocephalus, increased ICP, and advancement to brain tissue ischemia.

Viral meningitis is caused by invasion of the central nervous system (CNS) by a virus from a generalized viral infection through the respiratory tract, gastrointestinal tract, or genitourinary tract or through skin inoculation. Common viruses associated with viral meningitis include:

- Enteroviruses (coxsackievirus, echovirus)
- Mumps virus
- Adenoviruses
- Herpes simplex virus types 1 and 2
- Epstein-Barr virus
- HIV
- Arboviruses
- Influenza virus types A and B

The course of viral meningitis depends on the specific causative virus. Some viruses remain dormant in the nervous system for years before producing symptoms, whereas others cause a chronic, progressive infection.

Fungal meningitis most often affects patients who are immunocompromised. *Candida albicans* is the most common causative pathogen.

SIGNS AND SYMPTOMS

Regardless of the cause, meningitis has three classic signs and symptoms: fever, headache, and neck stiffness. The headache is of sudden onset and involves the frontal or occipital areas. Fever is usually above 104°F (40°C) in bacterial meningitis and below 104°F (40°C) in viral or fungal meningitis.

Bacterial and viral meningitis have three phases of clinical manifestations: prodromal, meningitic, and recovery. Signs and symptoms of each phase, as well as complications, are outlined in Table 19-4-1. The time frame for each phase varies depending on the cause.

 DIAGNOSTIC CRITERIA

The diagnosis of meningitis is made from history, clinical observations, and diagnostic studies. Gathering a history of recent infections is important, especially those involving the respiratory tract, ears, and sinuses. Clinical observations include a complete physical and neurologic examination, which will reveal the symptomatology of meningitis.

The primary study performed to diagnose meningitis is *CSF analysis*, with the sample obtained through lumbar puncture. CSF analysis accurately determines whether the meningitis is bacterial or viral in origin (Table 19-4-2). *WBC count* reveals leukocytosis with a predominance of neutrophils and bands in bacterial meningitis. Other studies that may aid with diagnosis include blood

 Table 19-4-1. Clinical Manifestations of Bacterial and Viral Meningitis

BACTERIAL	VIRAL
PRODROMAL	
• Muscle pain, backache	• Fever
• Lethargy	• Malaise
• Respiratory infection, pneumonia	• Sore throat
• Otitis media	
MENINGITIC	
• Severe frontal/occipital headache	• Headache
• Neck stiffness (nuchal rigidity)	• Photophobia
• Photophobia	• Drowsiness
• Purpuric or petechial skin rash	• Neck stiffness
• Positive Kernig's and Brudzinski's signs	• Kernig's sign
• Impaired level of consciousness	• Skin rash
• Focal or generalized seizures	• Parotitis
• Cranial nerve dysfunction	• Diarrhea
• Increased intracranial pressure	• Myalgia
	• Fever <40°C
RECOVERY	
• Depends on the infectious agent and treatment	• 7–14 days
COMPLICATIONS	
• Shock	• Febrile seizures
• Thrombocytopenia	• Syndrome of inappropriate antidiuretic hormone (SIADH)
• Disseminated intravascular coagulation	
• Syndrome of inappropriate antidiuretic hormone (SIADH)	
• Acute bacterial endocarditis	

Table 19-4-2. Cerebrospinal Fluid Analysis for Bacterial and Viral Meningitis

CEREBROSPINAL FLUID CHARACTERISTICS	BACTERIAL MENINGITIS	VIRAL (ASEPTIC) MENINGITIS
Appearance	• Turbid • Cloudy	• Clear • Sometimes turbid
Cells	• Increased white blood cells (>1000 mm³) • Mainly polymorphonuclear neutrophils	• Increased white blood cells (300 mm³) • Mostly mononuclear
Protein level	• 100–500 mg/dL	• Normal or slightly increased
Glucose level	• <40 mg/dL	• Normal
Smear and culture	• Bacteria present	• No bacteria present • Virus may be detected by special technique
Pressure on lumbar puncture	• Elevated (>180 mm of water pressure)	• Variable

culture (positive in 50% of cases), nose and throat cultures, chest radiograph, and skull and sinus x-rays.

 INTERVENTIONS

Intravenous antibiotic therapy is initiated immediately for bacterial meningitis. Treatment consists of a 10- to 14-day course of drugs that cross the blood-brain barrier. Ampicillin plus ceftazidime or ceftriaxone (third-generation cephalosporins) are recommended. Vancomycin is added if a penicillin-resistant strain of *S. pneumoniae* is the known or suspected causative organism. Penicillin G is recommended for meningococcal meningitis; ceftazidime and ceftriaxone are alternatives for patients who are allergic to penicillin. For uncomplicated viral meningitis, interventions include supportive care with fluids, rest, and pain relief. Nursing management for patients with meningitis is outlined in Table 19-4-3.

 COMMUNITY CARE

Certain types of meningitis (e.g., *Neisseria* meningitis) must be reported to the Public Health Department, and anyone in contact with this person needs prophylactic treatment. Teach the importance of completing the prescribed medication regimen. The need for long-term management is rare, because when treated promptly, meningitis has no permanent neurologic sequelae.

 PROGNOSIS

Prognosis depends on several factors. Early identification of the causative organism and prompt initiation of treatment is imperative. The patient's age is also important. Usually, neonates and elderly patients have a very poor prognosis. Finally, the presence of underlying diseases also can complicate patient

Table 19-4-3. Nursing Management of the Patient with Meningitis

KEY POINTS	RESPONSIBILITIES
Maintain airway, ventilation, oxygenation	Maintain a patent airway: • Position to promote drainage of secretions • Suction • Aspiration precautions Maintain adequate oxygenation and ventilation: • Administer oxygen as ordered • Assess respiratory status • Assess for signs and symptoms of dyspnea and cyanosis
Neurologic status	• Assess neurologic status for changes. • Assess for signs of meningeal irritation (e.g., stiff neck, Kernig's sign, Brudzinski's sign). • Provide a quiet, darkened environment and maintain the patient on bedrest. • Institute seizure precautions. • Monitor for signs of increased intracranial pressure (e.g., widening pulse pressure, bradycardia, respiratory variations).
Vital signs	• Assess frequently. • If the patient is febrile, administer antipyretics, give tepid baths, use a cooling blanket, remove excess clothing, and maintain a cool room temperature. • Observe for signs of adrenal insufficiency (meningococcal meningitis): hypotension, respiratory collapse, petechial rash.
Pain	• Elevate the head of the bed 30 degrees. • Maintain a quiet, darkened environment. • Administer analgesics (e.g., acetaminophen, codeine).
Nutrition	• Provide adequate nutrition. • Monitor intake and output.
Treat infection	• Administer antibiotics. • Administer antivirals.
Prevent transmission of disease	• Maintain good handwashing technique. • Maintain respiratory isolation/airborne precautions for meningococcal meningitis (see hospital infection control guidelines).
Skin care	• Provide good skin care; give special attention to bony prominences. • Reposition every 2 hours. • Maintain good body alignment.

management and affect the prognosis. The overall mortality rate for meningitis is approximately 25%.

 CLINICAL PEARLS

○ Signs of meningeal inflammation may or may not be present in elderly persons. Instead, confusion and obtundation may be the presenting signs.

○ Meningococcal meningitis often produces a diffuse rash that becomes petechial or purpuric before the meningitis is suspected or diagnosed.

○ The classic, acute presentation of meningeal symptoms may not be evident in persons who are immunosuppressed or taking antibiotics.

NURSING PROBLEM/ DIAGNOSIS	NURSING INTERVENTIONS CLASSIFICATION (NIC)
Actual infection	Medication Administration: Parenteral Infection control
Neurologic deterioration	Neurologic monitoring
Headache, neck discomfort	Analgesic Administration Environmental Management: Comfort

Multiple Sclerosis

Section 5   Lori Schumacher

 OVERVIEW

Multiple sclerosis (MS) is a chronic progressive disease of the CNS. It affects approximately 350,000 persons annually, occurs during the most productive years of life, and is more common in women. The disease course of MS is unpredictable, and chronic system problems accumulate, making the prognosis uncertain for each individual.

 PATHOPHYSIOLOGY

MS occurs in a genetically susceptible person as the result of an abnormal autoimmune response. Stimulation of the immune system by an infection or environmental event (e.g., stress) causes immune cell activation, resulting in inflammation. The inflammation produces lesions or scarring of the myelin sheaths. Mild inflammation allows for regeneration of the sheaths. Severe inflammation ultimately causes separation or permanent destruction of the sheaths, leaving sclerotic plaques. These plaques occur on the optic nerves and the white matter structures of the nervous system: brainstem, cerebrum, cerebellum, and spinal cord. Scarring of the myelin sheath slows or blocks conduction of the nerve impulses, producing the neurologic symptoms associated with MS.

 SIGNS AND SYMPTOMS

The signs and symptoms of MS vary depending on the areas of the brain and spinal cord affected and on where the patient is on the continuum of this progressive disease. Most commonly reported signs and symptoms of MS include extremity muscle weakness (primarily in the lower extremities and may be greater on one side), fatigue, paresthesias in one or more extremities, decreased sensory sensation in one or more extremities, tremors, coordination and balance difficulties, cognitive changes, visual changes or loss of vision, paralysis, spasticity, neuralgic pain, bladder and bowel dysfunction, and sexual dysfunction. Other problems may result or evolve from these symptoms; these commonly include reduced ability to perform activities of daily living (ADL), problems associated with immobility (e.g., falls, skin breakdown, contractures), and psychosocial concerns (e.g., depression, social isolation, loss of independence, role changes).

 DIAGNOSTIC CRITERIA

The diagnosis of MS is made primarily from clinical observation, patient history, and a complete neurologic examination. Currently, there is no specific radiographic or laboratory test used to diagnose MS. Radiographic and laboratory tests are used to confirm the clinical impression of MS. Neurologic examination findings that aid in the diagnosis of MS include:

- Spasticity and/or hyperreflexia
- Babinski's sign
- Dysmetria or tremor
- Nystagmus
- Diplopia
- Impaired position sense
- Lhermitte's sign
- Facial weakness
- Impaired touch or temperature sensation
- Decline in intellectual and cognitive function

Procedures

MRI of the brain or spinal cord is the most sensitive radiographic study for detecting the characteristic lesions of MS and ruling out other diseases that imitate MS. MRI is positive in 90% of persons with MS. Three lesion characteristics support the diagnosis of MS:

- The lesions border the lateral ventricles.
- The lesions are greater than 0.6 cm in diameter.
- The lesions tend to be found in the posterior fossa.

Evoked potential studies also aid the diagnosis of MS. These studies show delayed neuronal impulses in the CNS, reflecting the plaques throughout the nervous system.

CSF analysis may also be useful in diagnosing MS. The finding of two or more oligoclonal bands suggests MS. CSF analysis also may show slightly elevated protein levels and immunoglobulin G (IgG), as well as kappa light chains.

 INTERVENTIONS

Management of MS involves symptomatic treatment, acute relapse treatment, and treatment to reduce relapse frequency. Symptomatic treatment is described in Table 19-5-1.

Acute relapse of MS is determined by the presence of disabling symptoms with neurologic impairment. Currently, this is managed with high-dose intravenous corticosteroid therapy, usually methylprednisolone 0.5 to 1 g/day for 3 to 7 days. The patient is then placed on an oral prednisone taper, with the length of the course determined by the physician based on the severity of the relapse.

Treatment to reduce the frequency of relapse includes the use of one of three approved immunomodulating drugs: interferon beta-1b (Betaseron), interferon beta-1a (Avonex), or glatiramer acetate (Copaxone). These medications are thought to alter the immune system and control the immunologic

Table 19-5-1. Symptomatic Treatment

SYMPTOM	TREATMENT/INTERVENTION
Fatigue	• Energy conservation: frequent rest periods, moderate exercise, use of assistive devices (scooters) • Cooling techniques (air-conditioning) • Occupational therapy • Amantadine (Symmetrel) • Pemoline (Cylert), methylphenidate (Ritalin) • Antidepressants
Spasticity	• Physical therapy • Oral medications: baclofen, tizanidine, dantrolene sodium, diazepam, clonazepine • Surgically implanted intrathecal baclofen pump • Nerve blocks • Surgery to cut tendons or block nerves
Bladder dysfunction	**Urinary tract infection** • Antibiotic therapy • Adequate fluid intake **Failure to store** • Anticholinergic agents (oxybutynin, hyoscyamine sulfate, and propantheline bromide) • Avoid diuretics, caffeine, aspartame, and alcohol • Timed/scheduled voiding **Failure to empty** • Intermittent catheterization • Indwelling catheter **Combined dysfunction** • Intermittent self-catheterization • Anticholinergic medication • Indwelling catheter
Bowel dysfunction	**Constipation** • Adequate fluids • Bulk-forming agents • Stool softeners • Oral stimulants • Mild laxatives • Suppositories/enemas **Diarrhea** • Medications to decrease gastrointestinal motility • Bulk-forming supplements • Monitoring electrolytes • Monitoring weight • Appropriate skin care **Involuntary bowel** • Bowel training • Anticholinergics • Suppositories
Pain	**Primary pain** • Tranquilizers • Antidepressants **Secondary pain** • Pinpointing the cause of pain • Application of moist, moderate heat • Massage • Physical therapy • Analgesics • Nonsteroidal anti-inflammatory drugs • Cyclobenzaprine for back spasms

cascade that normally causes demyelination in MS. All three of these medications are given by self-injection subcutaneously or intramuscularly (Table 19-5-2).

 ## COMMUNITY CARE

Assess for signs of infection from corticosteroid use, and report any such signs to the physician. Assess for signs and symptoms of depression and anxiety, which are common in patients with MS. Report these, especially any suicidal ideations. Watch for other complications from corticosteroid use: severe mood changes, epigastric distress, change in stool color or blood in stool, mental status changes, and decreased or blurred vision.

Reinforce that flu-like symptoms are common when receiving beta-interferon injections, especially during the first months of treatment.

Teach the importance of avoiding factors known to exacerbate MS:

- Excessive exertion or fatigue
- Infections
- Hot baths
- Overheating
- Exposure to cold or excessive chilling
- Fever
- Emotional stress
- Pregnancy

Preventing or Reducing Complications

MS is a chronic disease, and it is important that the patient and family be actively involved in its management. Encouraging the patient to take an active role in self-monitoring and a positive attitude will help to promote a sense of wellness and appreciation for life.

Patient and family teaching should focus on understanding the disease process, the prescribed medication regimen, side effects of medications, and potential complications of MS. Teach the importance of follow-up visits to health care providers for continued evaluation of the disease process and treatment regimen. Also teach prophylactic measures to prevent urinary tract infections: hippuric acid, vitamin C, and dietary modifications (e.g., cranberry juice).

 ## PROGNOSIS

MS is a disease with no known cure. The prognosis depends on the course that the disease takes. Exacerbating and remitting MS usually has a mild course and manageable symptoms, but chronic and progressive MS is associated with a steady decline, complications, and debilitations that ultimately lead to death.

 ## CLINICAL PEARLS

- MS is based on clinical diagnosis and cannot be diagnosed based on a single episode of neurologic dysfunction.
- MRI scans can be normal in a patient with MS, and other conditions can exhibit white matter abnormalities similar to those in MS.
- MS patients may have normal neurologic examination findings while in remission.

Table 19-5-2. Immunomodulation Drugs: Frequency and Route

DRUG	TYPE OF MULTIPLE SCLEROSIS	FREQUENCY	ROUTE	SIDE EFFECTS
Interferon beta-1b (Betaseron)	Relapsing remitting	Every other day	Subcutaneous	• Fever • Fatigue • Flu-like symptoms • Depression • Injection site reactions
Interferon beta-1a (Avonex)	Relapsing forms	Every week	Intramuscular	• Fever • Fatigue • Flu-like symptoms
Glatiramer acetate (Copaxone)	Relapsing remitting	Every day	Subcutaneous	• Facial flushing • Chest tightness (Both lasting less than 15 minutes, with no electrocardiogram changes)

∘ In the early phases of MS, symptoms may be attributed to a psychological problem, thus delaying diagnosis.

NURSING PROBLEM/ DIAGNOSIS	NURSING INTERVENTIONS CLASSIFICATION (NIC)
Prevention/Reduction of complications/Effective therapeutic regimen management	Teaching: Disease Process Environmental Management Health System Guidance
Acute exacerbation	Medication Administration Neurologic Monitoring Exercise Therapy: Muscle Control
Progressive deterioration	Energy Management Activity Therapy Medication Management Self-Care Assistance

Myasthenia Gravis

Section 6   Lori Schumacher

 OVERVIEW

Myasthenia gravis (MG) is a chronic autoimmune disease that is characterized by fatigue and muscle weakness. MG affects 5 in 100,000 population (or about 25,000 people) in the United States and typically occurs during the most productive years of life. The disorder is most common in women age 20 to 40; men tend to develop MG in their 50s.

 PATHOPHYSIOLOGY

MG is a chronic autoimmune disease that affects the neuromuscular junction (NMJ). In MG, an autoimmune process causes antibodies to attack ACh receptor sites on the endplates of muscles in the NMJ. ACh is a neurotransmitter that transmits impulses from the nerve to the skeletal muscle. Without the receptor site, ACh has nowhere to attach; thus the impulse never reaches the skeletal muscle, and muscle contraction does not occur. Factors that trigger the autoimmune response are unknown; however, almost all patients with MG have thymus gland abnormalities that sensitize T cells. This triggers continual stimulation of B cells to produce anti-ACh antibodies.

Normally, ACh is degraded in the NMJ as part of the termination phase of synaptic transmission. MG is treated with drugs that prevent the degradation of ACh at the NMJ, in an attempt to allow ACh to be available for use by the few remaining receptor sites. These drugs are called cholinesterase inhibitors, or anticholinesterase agents.

Myasthenic crisis is a complication that requires emergent respiratory support and intensive care monitoring. Myasthenic crisis develops suddenly from a precipitating event, such as an infection, certain medications (Table 19-6-1),

Table 19-6-1. Common Medications That May Exacerbate Myasthenia Gravis or Cause Crisis

Cardiac drugs	Verapamil, beta-blockers
Antibiotics	Aminoglycosides, polymyxins, tetracyclines
Other	Phenytoin, chlorpromazine

or failure to follow the prescribed drug regimen. In myasthenic crisis, rapidly developing extreme muscle weakness results in swallowing difficulties and respiratory fatigue with potential failure. A common monitoring parameter for this complication is vital capacity; when vital capacity falls below a predetermined value (e.g., 1000), elective intubation is usually performed.

 SIGNS AND SYMPTOMS

Most often, the patient complains of fatigue and muscle weakness that improve with rest. The severity of weakness and the muscles involved vary and fluctuate among patients. Weakness of the eye muscles occurs in 90% of patients and is usually the first sign of MG. Signs and symptoms of ocular weakness include ptosis and diplopia. The presentation of generalized weakness varies and may include any or all of the following:

- Arm weakness; difficulty holding the arms above the head
- Difficulty holding the head up
- Leg weakness after walking or climbing stairs
- Absent reflexes
- Sensory abnormalities
- Coordination abnormalities
- Jaw weakness with chewing
- Dysarthria, slurred or garbled speech
- Dysphagia
- Expressionless face
- Rapid, shallow breathing

MG is sometimes classified as ocular or generalized. MG can be exacerbated by factors such as emotional stress, physical stress, concurrent illness, infection, surgery, thyroid disturbance, menstrual cycle, pregnancy, alcohol, and medications such as polymyxin antibiotics, tetracyclines, aminoglycosides, narcotics, sedatives, phenothiazines, barbiturates, tranquilizers, and antiarrhythmic agents.

 DIAGNOSTIC CRITERIA

The diagnosis of MG is made primarily from clinical observations, patient history, and a complete neurologic examination. The most common and conclusive diagnostic laboratory test is the *edrophonium chloride test* (also known as the *Tensilon test*). The Tensilon test involves administering IV edrophonium, a short-acting anticholinesterase agent. This usually produces a significant, temporary improvement in strength in patients with MG. Other diagnostic tests for MG include an EMG, CT, or MRI scan of the chest, and ACh receptor antibody serum levels. In EMG, repetitive muscle stimulation produces reduced muscle potential amplitude and delayed neuromuscular transmission in patients with MG. A CT or MRI scan of the chest reveals abnormalities of the thymus gland. ACh receptor antibody serum level is elevated in 80% to 90% of patients with MG.

 INTERVENTIONS

MG is treated with medications, plasmapheresis, immunoglobulin therapy, or surgery. The main therapeutic goals are to control symptoms and optimize function. Usually, alleviation of all symptoms is not possible, but some patients do enjoy periods of complete or partial remission.

Pharmacotherapy

Medications used in MG symptom and disease management include immunosuppressants and cholinesterase inhibitors (anticholinesterase agents) (Table 19-6-2). Commonly used *immunosuppressants* include prednisone, azathioprine (Imuran), and cyclophosphamide (Cytoxan). Immunosuppressants alter antibody production and suppress the autoimmune process.

Anticholinesterase agents, including neostigmine, pyridostigmine (Mestinon), and ambenonium, manage symptoms of MG by inhibiting the destruction of ACh, thus enhancing transmission of an impulse at the neuromuscular junction. ACh is the neurotransmitter not only for skeletal muscle, but also for muscarinic receptors on various organs of the parasympathetic nervous system and the sweat glands.

Overdose or toxic levels of anticholinesterase agents can produce a life-threatening complication known as *cholinergic crisis*. Similar to myasthenic

 Table 19-6-2. Common Medications Used in Myasthenia Gravis Symptoms and Disease Management

MEDICATION	USES	COMMON SIDE EFFECTS
Anticholinesterases Neostigmine Pyridostigmine (Mestinon) Ambenonium	• Control symptoms • Optimize function	**Muscarinic** • Abdominal cramping • Diarrhea • Increased peristalsis • Increased salivation • Increased perspiration • Blurred vision • Bradycardia **Nicotinic** • Muscle twitching • Weakness • Fatigue
Immunosuppressants Prednisone Azathioprine (Imuran) Cyclophosphamide (Cytoxan)	• Control symptoms • Improve symptoms • Produce remission	• Fluid retention • Hyperglycemia • Nausea • Vomiting • Gastric ulcers • Bone marrow suppression • Osteoporosis • Hepatotoxicity

crisis, cholinergic crisis is characterized by extreme respiratory muscle weakness or paralysis. This occurs from excessive amounts of ACh in the NMJ, which keeps the motor end plates in a constant state of depolarization, effectively causing depolarizing neuromuscular blockade. High doses also produce CNS depression with resulting respiratory depression. Other symptoms of cholinergic crisis caused by excessive muscarinic stimulation include bradycardia, hypotension, increased salivation, sweating, and severe weakness. Cholinergic crisis may develop slowly or rapidly. Treatment includes IV atropine to relieve muscarinic side effects, monitoring for respiratory difficulties, supporting ventilation (with mechanical ventilation as needed), and withholding anticholinesterase medications until the crisis is resolved.

Plasmapheresis

The goal of plasmapheresis in treating patients with MG is to produce short-term immunomodulation. In plasmapheresis, plasma is removed from the serum, the pathogenic antibodies are filtered out, and albumin or fresh frozen plasma is returned to the patient. After plasmapheresis, many patients experience decreased symptoms. Plasmapheresis is usually performed three to four times over 8 to 10 days to remove a majority of antibodies. Plasmapheresis is done to stabilize patients in crisis or those not responding adequately to medication.

Immunoglobulin Therapy

Intravenous immunoglobulin (IVIg) is used as a short-term therapy. IVIg has naturally occurring antibodies that react specifically to the antigens that cause MG. IVIg has been shown to improve symptoms within 4 to 5 days in 70% of patients with MG.

Surgery

Thymectomy may be performed in patients with hyperplasia of the thymus gland. Thymectomy has been shown to produce an 85% remission rate in patients who do not have thymus tumors. Some patients experience complete remission of symptoms, whereas others have partial remission, allowing for reduced medication use.

 COMMUNITY CARE

Long-term care involves monitoring for the progression of weakness and for long-term side effects of immunosuppressant therapy (e.g., fluid retention, hyperglycemia, gastric ulcers, osteoporosis).

Except during myasthenic crises, patients with MG live in the community. Patient teaching includes the following points:

- Set priorities, plan ahead, and pace oneself to avoid undue fatigue.
- Provide for adequate rest periods throughout the day.
- Provide frequent eye care to prevent corneal abrasions.
- Wear a Medic-Alert bracelet.
- Take medications with a cracker to decrease incidence of nausea or gastric irritation.
- Take medications on time to optimize their effectiveness. Take cholinesterase inhibitors 30 to 45 minutes before eating to ensure sufficient strength to chew and swallow food.

- Do not take any over-the-counter medications without the physician's permission.
- Eat slowly and follow a soft diet if difficulty swallowing occurs.
- Understand the actions, dosages, and possible side effects of all prescribed medications.

 PROGNOSIS

MG has no known cure. The prognosis can range from good (in mild forms of MG) to poor (in severe forms of MG), with death occurring from respiratory muscle weakness and general debilitation.

 CLINICAL PEARLS

○ Some 80% of patients with MG have an abnormality of the thymus gland, either hyperplasia or tumor.
○ About 89% of patients with MG have antibodies against ACh receptors.
○ Patients usually present with complaints of specific muscle weakness, not generalized fatigue.

NURSING PROBLEM/ DIAGNOSIS	NURSING INTERVENTIONS CLASSIFICATION (NIC)
Risk for ineffective breathing pattern	Respiratory Monitoring Airway Management Oxygen Therapy Mechanical Ventilation
Prevention/Reduction of exacerbation/Effective therapeutic regimen management	Environmental Management: Community Teaching: Disease Process Teaching: Prescribed Medication
Progressive weakness	Neurologic Monitoring Activity Therapy Circulatory Care Self-Care Assistance Health System Guidance

Parkinsonism

Section 7   Lori Schumacher

 OVERVIEW

Parkinson's disease (PD) is a chronic, degenerative movement disorder that affects the basal ganglia, which is responsible for muscle tone and voluntary movement. PD is the most common movement disorder seen in clinical practice; incidence is 20 per 100,000 population. The onset usually occurs in adults between age 40 and 70, peaking in the mid-50s. PD can be idiopathic (i.e., with no demonstrable cause identified), referred to as primary, or acquired (caused by conditions such as infection, intoxication, and even head trauma, as in the case of Muhammad Ali), called secondary PD. PD caused by infection is rare. PD caused by intoxication with chemicals (e.g., carbon monoxide) or by drugs (e.g., chlorpromazine, prochlorperazine, thioridazine, haloperidol, methyldopa) resolves rapidly once the chemical is removed or the drug is stopped.

PATHOPHYSIOLOGY

The substantia nigra is one of a group of structures that make up the basal ganglia, which normally produces and stores dopamine. Dopamine is an inhibitory neurotransmitter that supports impulse transmission throughout the structures of the basal ganglia. With the help of dopamine and other neurotransmitters (e.g., ACh), the basal ganglia controls balance and coordination, regulates muscle tone, and fine-tunes voluntary movement. In PD, the dopamine-producing cells of the substantia nigra degenerate; as a result, significantly decreased levels of dopamine are available for the basal ganglia. On autopsy, dopamine levels in the brains of patients with PD are less than 10% of the levels found in the normal brain. PD upsets the normal balance between inhibitory (dopamine) and excitatory (ACh) neurotransmitters. The dopamine deficit reduces inhibitory effects on movement in the basal ganglia, allowing for a relative abundance of ACh and producing increased excitatory effects. The overexcitement of the basal ganglia produces a dysfunction of the extrapyramidal (pathways between the cortex, basal ganglia, and cerebellum) motor system, resulting in tremor, rigidity, and unstable movements. The amount of cell loss in the substantia nigra directly correlates with the severity of the signs and symptoms.

SIGNS AND SYMPTOMS

Cardinal signs include gradual slowing of voluntary movements (bradykinesia), increased muscle tone (rigidity), unstable gait, and resting tremor. The initial symptoms of PD are often vague and attributed to the aging process. Eventually the symptoms interfere with the person's ability to perform normal independent functions. The signs and symptoms of PD can be divided into major and secondary manifestations (Table 19-7-1).

DIAGNOSTIC CRITERIA

The diagnosis of PD is a clinical one, made from history and observation with the presence of two or more cardinal signs. There are no definitive laboratory tests. If PD is suspected, the patient may be given antiparkinsonian medication and monitored for a response; a decrease in symptoms verifies the diagnosis.

INTERVENTIONS

Treatment goals for PD include reducing or alleviating symptoms, optimizing the quality of life, and preventing complications. These goals are accomplished by assessment and monitoring for neurologic deterioration, pharmacologic therapy, home health services, dietary modifications, patient and family education, and referrals to physical, speech, and occupational therapists.

Table 19-7-1. Manifestations of Parkinson's Disease

CLINICAL MANIFESTATION

Major manifestation	• Coarse tremor of the hands that is present at rest, improves with movement, and is absent during sleep • Pill rolling (thumb moves rhythmically back and forth on the palm) • Muscle rigidity or stiffness • Akinesia/bradykinesia (difficulty initiating movement and then moves very slowly) • Stooped gait, with small, shuffling steps that accelerate almost to a trot • May fall forward (propulsion) or backward (retropulsion)
Secondary manifestation	• Fine motor difficulty, e.g., progressively smaller handwriting, difficulty dressing and buttoning clothing, clumsiness • Monotonic, soft, whisper-like voice that becomes more muffled • Expressionless face • Staring with decreased blinking • Fatigue during activity • Cognitive decline: memory deficits, unable to make a decision, depression • Dysphagia, drooling • Excessive perspiration • Constipation • Orthostatic hypotension • Urinary hesitation and frequency

Pharmacologic Therapy

Pharmacologic therapy for PD (Table 19-7-2) may take days to weeks to become therapeutic. *Anticholinergic agents* are useful in early disease and very useful in patients with tremor. They have no effect on hypokinesia. They may be used in combination therapy with dopaminergic agents in later stages of the disease. Anticholinergics may cause confusion in older patients and should be avoided. Common side effects include dry mouth, constipation, and blurred vision. Urinary retention may occur in men. Monitor for signs of closed-angle glaucoma (see Chapter 24, Section 3).

Dopaminergic agents are used as monotherapy in early disease and mid-course therapy. Combination therapy should be initiated before increasing dosages. These agents can cause significant side effects, including anorexia, vomiting, dizziness, and orthostatic hypotension. Dyskinesia may occur with high doses or with prolonged therapy. Prolonged therapy may produce psychological side effects, such as visual hallucinations, vivid nightmares, and paranoid delusions. These symptoms usually improve with dosage reduction. Cardiac dysrhythmias may occur. Efficacy of therapy may be enhanced by taking the medication before meals or by reducing dietary protein intake, especially at breakfast and lunch. (Amino acids compete with levodopa for transport into the brain.) Dosing after meals will also help to minimize nausea and vomiting.

Amantadine, used alone or in combination with an anticholinergic agent, may improve mild symptoms with little side effects. Its effectiveness may be only transient, however.

Table 19-7-2. Pharmacologic Treatment in Parkinson's Disease

MEDICATION	PURPOSE	ACTION
Anticholinergic agents Trihexyphenidyl (Artane) Benztropine (Cogentin)	At the onset of functional impairment, used for the relief of tremors in early disease.	Assists in normalizing the imbalance of cholinergic/ dopaminergic neurotransmission by blocking access of acetylcholine in the basal ganglia.
Dopaminergic agents Levodopa	Treats rigidity and bradykinesia	Natural precursor of dopamine
Dopamine agonists Bromocriptine (Parlodel) Pergolide	Provide benefit and assist with decreased fluctuation of motor response to L-dopa	Directly stimulates dopamine receptors
Other: Monoamine oxidase B (MAO) inhibitor Selegiline (Eldepryl)	Slows Parkinson's disease; increases response to L-dopa	Slows the underlying disease process by blocking the catabolism of central dopamine
Amantadine (Symmetrel) Can be classified as an antiparkinsonian agent (originally classified as an antiviral agent)	Sometimes helpful for mild parkinsonism, in early disease.	Promotes the synthesis and release of dopamine from the remaining dopamine terminals.

Diet

Dietary considerations include increased fluid and fiber to reduce constipation caused by pharmacologic therapy. Increased calcium intake can help maintain existing bone structure. Reduced protein intake is recommended.

Surgery

Surgical interventions used to reduce or alleviate PD symptoms include thalamectomy, pallidotomy, deep brain stimulation, and fetal nigra transplantation. *Thalamectomy* is a stereotactic procedure that localizes a group of cells within the thalamus and destroys them by freezing, radiation, electrical coagulation, or ultrasonography. A thalamectomy is performed to help reduce or alleviate rigidity and intractable tremor of PD.

Pallidus pallidotomy is a stereotactic procedure that localizes and places a lesion on the globus pallidus of the basal ganglia. This procedure is done to reduce or alleviate tremor and improve motor function.

Deep brain stimulation is a stereotactic procedure in which an electrode is implanted into the brain and connected to a pacemaker. Electrical impulses provide depolarization blockade to the overactive globus pallidus, thus reducing or relieving severe tremors.

Fetal nigra transplantation is investigative therapy involving implanting embryonic dopaminergic neurons into the striatum of the patient with PD. This procedure aims to improve motor symptoms without dyskinesias.

COMMUNITY CARE

Assess for signs and symptoms of further neurologic deterioration. These include problems with mobility from tremors and rigidity (putting the patient at high risk for injury), confusion, visual hallucinations, paranoia, dementia, and sleep disturbances.

Because PD is a chronic disease that is most frequently managed in the home, it is important that the patient and family be actively involved in management. Reinforce patient teaching, including:

- Understanding the disease process
- The prescribed medication regimen
- Side effects of medications
- Potential complications of PD
- The possible need for small feedings of soft, ground food if dysphagia occurs
- The need to participate in an exercise program
- Available community resources
- The importance of follow-up visits to the health care provider for continued evaluation of the disease process and treatment regimen
- The patient's home environment needs to be evaluated for potential safety dangers, such as throw rugs, poor lighting, and assistive devices (handrails in bathroom).

 PROGNOSIS

The prognosis for PD has improved with advances in treatment. With proper treatment, a person with PD has the potential to live a normal lifespan. The clinical course of PD varies but decline usually happens over several years.

 CLINICAL PEARLS

- MRI and CT scans are usually normal in patients with PD.
- Symptoms of PD are not evident until 80% of the dopamine-producing cells become damaged.
- Depression is common in patients with PD (affecting more than 50%) and sometimes occurs before PD is diagnosed.

NURSING PROBLEM/ DIAGNOSIS	NURSING INTERVENTIONS CLASSIFICATION (NIC)
Impaired physical mobility	Activity Therapy Fall Prevention Medication Administration Surveillance: Safety
Deficient knowledge of disease process	Teaching: Disease Process Family Involvement Teaching Prescribed Medication Nutrition Management
Community referral	Health System Guidance

Seizures

Section 8   Lori Schumacher

 OVERVIEW

Seizures are sudden, rapid, and repeated depolarizations or uncontrolled electrical discharges of the neurons in the cerebral cortex that interfere with normal function. These alterations may involve sensory, motor, autonomic, or psychic manifestations with a change in the level of arousal, all of which are usually temporary.

Seizures are the second most common neurologic disturbance. Nonrecurring seizures are not in themselves a specific disease entity. Rather, they are symptoms of disease that can result from an acute neurologic illness or a neurologic procedure. These seizures do not recur once the illness is treated. When seizures are recurrent, epilepsy is diagnosed.

Epilepsy is a common neurologic condition affecting approximately 1% of the U.S. population, or more than 2 million people. Each year, approximately 120 of 100,000 people seek medical attention for a newly recognized seizure, and 50 of 100,000 people are diagnosed with epilepsy.

The etiology of epilepsy is unknown in 70% to 75% of cases, called *idiopathic* (or *primary*) epilepsy. The remaining cases, known as *symptomatic (or secondary)* epilepsy, result from biochemical or pathologic causes or from posttraumatic cerebral irritation. Common predisposing factors include the following:

Biochemical
- Fluid and electrolyte disturbances
- Hypoxia
- Acidosis
- Toxin and chemical exposure (heavy metals)
- Drug overdose and withdrawal (cocaine, alcohol)

Pathologic
- CNS infections: meningitis, encephalitis, brain abscess, opportunistic infections from acquired immunodeficiency syndrome
- Brain tumors
- Genetic trait
- Fever
- Cerebrovascular disorders: stroke, hemorrhage, aneurysms, arteriovenous malformations

Post-Traumatic Head Trauma
Trauma and substance abuse are the most common diagnoses accompanying secondary epilepsy in young adults. New-onset secondary epilepsy in older adults is often related to neoplasm, stroke or trauma. Idiopathic epilepsy usually appears during childhood, adolescence, and young adulthood.

In the past, difficulty in understanding seizures existed because of imprecise definitions of terms. Today, an international classification system for both seizures and epilepsy aids understanding, diagnosing, and treating the disorders and improving outcomes for seizure patients.

 PATHOPHYSIOLOGY

A seizure occurs from an irritable neuron in the cerebral cortex that rapidly depolarizes and discharges. Adjacent neurons are recruited, and these also

begin to depolarize and discharge. Clinical symptoms of a seizure are not always evident but become so when a sufficient number of neurons discharge abnormally. Rapid depolarization and discharge of the neurons places metabolic demands on cells, leading to depletion of oxygen and glucose stores. Decreased oxygen and glucose in the brain leads to increased cerebral blood flow in an attempt to meet the brain's increased metabolic demands.

When the glucose and oxygen levels are depleted, neurons turn to anaerobic metabolism, which produces cellular lactic acid. Increased lactate levels produce a further energy debt, which may progress to cellular exhaustion and destruction. Seizure activity can increase oxygen demand by about 60%, with an approximate 250% increase in cerebral blood flow. Hypoxemia or hypoglycemia resulting from the increased metabolic rate may trigger respiratory or cardiac arrest.

Status epilepticus is a life-threatening condition defined as continuous seizure activity lasting for more than 30 minutes. If the seizure(s) are uncontrolled, secondary brain injury can occur.

 SIGNS AND SYMPTOMS

Seizures can be classified as partial, generalized, or status epilepticus. Each of these three categories can be further delineated according to the clinical presentation (Table 19-8-1). A seizure has three phases. When a patient is experiencing a seizure, it is important that the nurse be able to identify the phase so that appropriate interventions may be performed.

Preictal Phase

The *preictal phase* occurs before actual seizure activity. In this phase, the patient may experience an *aura* before the onset of a seizure. An aura may be a visual, auditory, gustatory, or visceral experience (e.g., metallic taste in the mouth, the sensation of seeing flashing lights). A patient's auras are usually the same each time and predictable. Other clinical manifestations of the preictal phase may include confusion, nausea, headache, and feelings of depression.

Ictal Phase

The *ictal phase* is the actual seizure. During this phase, it is important for the nurse to assess which type of seizure the patient is experiencing (see Table 19-8-1). The autonomic nervous system is stimulated during the seizure, producing tachycardia, increased blood pressure, diaphoresis, salivation, and incontinence. Another important aspect of this phase is altered level of consciousness.

Postictal Phase

The *postictal* phase immediately follows a seizure. During this phase, the patient may experience lethargy, muscle soreness, headache, aphasia, or Todd's paralysis. Todd's paralysis, which may occur after a partial or generalized seizure, is a temporary focal weakness or paralysis that may last up to 48 hours. During this phase, the patient should be assessed for possible injuries to the head, tongue, or extremities that may have occurred during the seizure.

 DIAGNOSTIC CRITERIA

The cause of a seizure needs to be determined if possible. A precise patient history should be obtained that includes clinical presentation of the seizure,

Table 19-8-1. Classification of Seizures

CLASSIFICATION		CLINICAL MANIFESTATION
Partial (arises from a localized/focal area in the brain)	**Simple partial** (also known as jacksonian seizures) Originate in the motor cortex of the frontal lobe	• No loss of consciousness • Focal twitching of arm or leg and spreads • Difficulty speaking • Visual, auditory, or olfactory hallucinations • Feeling or a sense of doom
	Complex partial Originate in the temporal lobe and involves the limbic system	• Consciousness is impaired • May begin as a simple partial seizure and progress • No memory of any behavior • Lip smacking • Chewing • Picking at clothes • Lasts a few seconds to a few minutes • Patient may have brief confusion after seizure
Generalized (involves both hemispheres at onset)	**Partial** **Absence** (also known as petit mal)	• May progress to generalized seizure • Sudden onset and termination • Brief loss of consciousness (3–30 seconds) • Eyes: stare or roll upward • Eyelids twitch • No postictal state • May be viewed as inattention • Unable to talk • Motor movement stops during seizure • Most common in children
	Myoclonic	Brief, rapid jerking of one or more muscle groups Lasts 1–2 seconds Common around time of awakening Consciousness is usually preserved

Atonic	Loss of muscle tone
	Drop attack; person suddenly drops to the floor
	Consciousness is usually preserved
Clonic	Rhythmic jerking of muscle groups
Tonic	Stiffening of muscle groups
Tonic-clonic	Onset is bilateral
Tonic—first phase	Entire seizure lasts less than 2 minutes
Clonic—second phase	Consciousness is impaired
	Postictal lasts minutes to hours, initially in a deep sleep, followed by a period of lethargy and confusion
	Tonic
	All muscles become rigid
	Extension of extremities and arching of the back
	Shrill cry (from tightening of thoracic muscles)
	Cessation of breathing momentarily
	Jaw snaps shut (tongue may be bitten)
	Urinary and/or fecal incontinence may occur
	Last 10–30 seconds
	Clonic
	Violent muscular jerking
	Hyperventilation
	Frothing of the mouth
	Diaphoresis
	Rolling of the eyes
	Facial grimaces
	Lasts 30–60 seconds
Status epilepticus	Continuous or recurring seizures without recovery
	More than 30 minutes in duration

surrounding events, and medical history. Careful physical examination, neurologic examination, and diagnostic testing are needed. Blood work may be obtained to evaluate for electrolyte abnormalities (e.g., decreased serum sodium), toxicology screen (e.g., cocaine, alcohol), and anticonvulsant drug levels (to assess therapeutic level). A CT scan or MRI may be performed to identify any structural abnormality (e.g., tumor, intracranial hemorrhage) that may have caused the seizure. Electroencephalography (EEG) identifies patterns of abnormal electrical activity in the brain and may help identify the particular type of seizure or epilepsy so it can be treated appropriately. Finally, a lumbar puncture, if not contraindicated, can be done to collect CSF for analysis for CNS infection.

INTERVENTIONS

The underlying condition, if identified, should be treated. For instance, if an electrolyte abnormality exists or if anticonvulsant medication levels are subtherapeutic, then corrections must be made. Protecting the patient from injury and observing for complications are the primary goals for intervening during a seizure. Establish the time, note the duration, and describe the movement and activity of the seizure. Assess neurologic status throughout. Usually, seizure precautions are initiated for a patient with a history of seizures.

Seizure Precautions

Seizure precautions are safety measures implemented to help protect the patient from injury during a seizure. These measures consist of padding the side rails of the bed, ensuring that the side rails of the bed are up, the bed is kept in the lowest position, suction equipment is at the bedside, an airway and oxygen are available at the bedside, and the call light is within reach.

During a seizure, the following measures should be followed:
- If the patient is out of bed, lower him or her to the floor.
- Remove glasses, if present.
- Loosen any constrictive clothing.
- Do not force anything into the patient's mouth.
- Do not restrain the patient's movements; just guide him or her to prevent injuries, particularly of the head.
- Stay with patient during seizure and monitor duration and manifestations exhibited

During the postictal phase, the following measures should be observed:
- Position the patient on the side to facilitate draining of secretions.
- Maintain a patent airway; suctioning to prevent aspiration or oxygen may be needed.
- Allow the patient to sleep.
- Monitor vital signs.
- Orient the patient on awakening.

Pharmacotherapy

Short- or long-term pharmacotherapy may be needed to control or manage seizures. Short-term medications are used to control or stop seizures. Usually, a short-acting sedative, such as lorazepam (Ativan) or diazepam (Valium), is administered. Seizure control is generally accomplished with a longer-acting medication, such as phenytoin (Dilantin) or phenobarbital. Certain medications, used alone or in combination with other anticonvulsant medications, may be needed for specific types of seizures. Pharmacotherapy is individualized for each patient (Table 19-8-2). Thus, patient education is essential to ensure understanding of the medication, dosage schedule, and possible side effects to improve patient compliance and outcomes. (Chapter 12, Section 6 provides more information on anticonvulsant medications.) Teach the importance of taking medication on a schedule. Noncompliance with anticonvulsant medications leads to subtherapeutic levels, which can precipitate a seizure.

Surgery

Patients with epilepsy that cannot be managed or controlled with medication and those with refractory epilepsy are candidates for epilepsy surgery. The most common type of epilepsy surgery is a temporal lobectomy, removal of the temporal lobe from which the seizures are originating. The benefits of temporal lobectomy can be dramatic; up to 90% of patients experience significant improvement in seizure control, with 68% becoming seizure free and 24% experiencing improved seizure control.

Vagal Nerve Stimulation

Vagal nerve stimulation (VNS) is used in patients with refractory epilepsy in whom surgery is not feasible or has not been effective. VNS involves surgically implanting a generator with an electrode attached to the vagus nerve. The generator is then individually programmed to deliver bursts of electrical stimulation to the vagus nerve. The generator may also be triggered on demand using a magnet when the person has a warning of an oncoming seizure or the seizure is witnessed. The most common side effects of VNS are hoarseness and cough, both of which tend to decrease over time.

 COMMUNITY CARE

Reinforce teaching of seizure precautions and prescribed medications. Assess compliance with and side effects of anticonvulsant therapy. Once the

Table 19-8-2. Seizure Medications

SEIZURE TYPE	FIRST-LINE MEDICATION	ADJUNCTIVE AGENTS
Tonic-clonic	Phenytoin Carbamazepine Valproic acid	Phenobarbital Primidone Lamotrigine
Absence	Ethosuximide Valproic acid	Benzodiazepines Lamotrigine Acetazolamide
Myoclonic	Valproic acid Benzodiazepines	Lamotrigine
Tonic/atonic	Valproic acid Benzodiazepines	Lamotrigine
Focal (partial)	Carbamazepine Phenytoin Valproic acid	Gabapentin Lamotrigine Phenobarbital/primidone

From Fovary, N, & Wyllie, E. (1999). Epilepsy. In *Textbook of clinical neurology*, (p. 1081). CG Goetz and EJ Papper (Eds.). Philadelphia: WB Saunders.

patient is seizure free for at least 2 years with normal EEG findings, a medication taper may be attempted.

Lifestyle changes must include proper rest, a well-balanced diet, and stress management. Teach the importance of follow-up visits to health care provider to monitor, treat, and evaluate the seizure disorder.

 PROGNOSIS

Because of epilepsy-related accidents, people with epilepsy have a higher death rate than the population at large. Sudden death occurs most frequently in patients age 20 to 40 with history of seizures.

 CLINICAL PEARLS

○ Tongue blades are no longer used during the ictal phase of a seizure, because the tongue cannot be swallowed during a seizure, and attempting to insert a tongue blade can cause broken teeth and injury to the lips and tongue.
○ Decreased sodium levels are a common cause of seizures.
○ Sometimes an EEG may be normal with simple partial seizures.
○ Oral contraceptives usually do not exacerbate seizures.

NURSING PROBLEM/ DIAGNOSIS	NURSING INTERVENTIONS CLASSIFICATION (NIC)
Prevention/Effective therapeutic regimen management	Seizure Precautions Teaching: Disease Process Teaching: Prescribed Medication Health System Guidance
Acute seizure activity	Seizure Management Fall Prevention Medication Administration: Parenteral

Spinal Cord Injury

Section 9   Lori Schumacher ■ Beverly George-Gay

 OVERVIEW

Spinal cord injury (SCI) is a physically and emotionally devastating problem. The estimated annual number of persons with SCI in the United States is approximately 30 to 40 per million per year (with 10,000 new cases each year). SCI primarily affects males age 16 to 30. Most cases result from motor vehicle accidents, and more than 50% of SCIs involve the cervical spine. The costs of caring for persons with SCIs vary according to the severity of injury. Many advances have been made in the realms of emergency management, pharmacology, acute care, and rehabilitation.

SCI is classified by the American Spinal Injury Association (ASIA) as tetraplegia or paraplegia. *Tetraplegia* is impairment or loss of sensory or motor function to the cervical cord segment, resulting in impaired function of the arms, legs, trunk, and pelvic organs. The level of injury is above cervical spine level 6 (C-6).

Paraplegia is impairment or loss of sensory and/or motor function to the thoracic, lumbar, or sacral cord segments, resulting in impaired function of the legs, trunk, or pelvic organs depending on the level of the injury. The arms are spared.

 PATHOPHYSIOLOGY

The pathophysiologic changes occurring in SCI can be classified as primary and secondary injuries. Primary injury occurs at the time of mechanical insult and shortly thereafter. Secondary injury occurs hours after the insult, allowing for a window of time during which treatment can be initiated to halt further damage and decrease the extent of disability. Transection caused by either primary or secondary injury can be complete or incomplete (Table 19-9-1) and results in permanent damage.

Primary Injury

The primary injury produces small perivascular hemorrhages, particularly in the gray matter of the cord, causing ischemia and infarction. Frank tissue damage results in permanent loss of function. Edema may produce transient loss of function that is restored once the edema is resolved or may produce secondary injuries. Vertebral injuries provide the mechanism for the actual physical damage. Mechanisms of vertebral injury include hyperextension, hyperflexion, vertical compression (shattering), and rotational forces. These mechanisms cause injury to the cord by *compression,* which can result in ischemia to the area being compressed. Compression can be the result of a contusion, laceration, or an actual tear in neural tissue from penetration by an object (e.g., a bone fragment), usually resulting in permanent damage.

Hemorrhage into the neural tissues usually does not cause permanent damage. However, the area from which the blood supply has been lost does suffer ischemia and necrosis.

Secondary Injury

Secondary injury occurs minutes to hours after the primary injury. White matter edema develops, impairing microcirculation of the cord and causing

 Table 19-9-1. Complete versus Incomplete Spinal Cord Injury

INJURY	DESCRIPTION
Incomplete	Sensory and motor function is partially preserved below the level of injury.
	• These injuries manifest in a variety of patterns according to the predominant area of the cord involved.
	• Evidence of voluntary motor function or sensation below the level of injury qualifies as an incomplete SCI.
	• Voluntary contraction of the anal sphincter on a digital examination confirms this injury.
Complete	Sensory and motor function is lost below the level of injury because of complete disruption of neural tissue.

further ischemia. Global infarction develops 8 hours after injury from the release of various immune mediators, vasoactive substances, and cellular enzymes. It is at this point that necrosis and paralysis become irreversible. The hemorrhages from the initial insult enlarge to occupy one or two levels above and below the point of impact.

SIGNS AND SYMPTOMS

A clinical manifestation occurring in both complete and incomplete injuries is *spinal shock*. This is the temporary but complete loss of motor, sensory reflex, and autonomic function below the level of the injury. It results from the loss of input from higher cerebral centers to the spinal cord. Symptoms include loss of pain and temperature sensation and proprioception, flaccid paralysis, impaired thermoregulation, and paralytic ileus. Spinal shock usually occurs at the time of injury but may take up to 1 week to develop. It typically lasts for 7 to 20 days. Resolution is identified by the return of reflexes; flaccidity is replaced by spasticity.

Neurogenic shock, a form of distributive shock, occurs with cervical or upper thoracic SCI from loss of sympathetic nervous system control, allowing the parasympathetic system to act unopposed. Symptoms are related to the overriding parasympathetic influence. Hypotension results from global vasodilation due to loss of vasoconstrictor tone. Bradycardia (heart rate below 60 beats/min) results from inhibition of baroreceptor response. Loss of thermoregulation occurs from the loss of vasomotor tone in cutaneous blood vessels. Neurogenic shock may develop 60 minutes after injury and can persist for up to several weeks. It is managed in the intensive care unit.

Motor and sensory impairment in *complete SCI* depend on the level and mechanism of injury. Symptoms also vary as edema increases or resolves. Table 19-9-2 lists symptoms according to the level of the SCI.

Incomplete injuries follow certain patterns manifested more commonly in the following syndromes.

Central Cord Syndrome. Motor and sensory loss is more pronounced in the upper extremities than in the lower ones. This syndrome most commonly affects the central portion of the cervical cord.

Anterior Cord Syndrome. This is the most common syndrome causing loss of motor function and loss of temperature and pain sensation below the level of injury. Proprioception (position) and motion sense, touch, and vibration remain intact.

Brown-Séquard Syndrome. This results from the hemisection of the cord. It causes ipsilateral (on the same side as the injury) loss of voluntary motor function, sense of touch, vibration, and proprioception. Pain and temperature sensations are lost contralaterally (on the opposite side of the injury).

Conus Medullaris Syndrome. This syndrome produces flaccid bowel and bladder, and sexual dysfunction. Impaired motor function in the lower extremities can occur.

Complications

Autonomic dysreflexia (or hyperreflexia) is a potentially life-threatening complication that can occur in tetraplegics most often after spinal shock and neurogenic shock have resolved. It can affect any patient with an injury at T-

Table 19-9-2. Signs and Symptoms Associated with Level of Spinal Cord Injury

LEVEL OF SPINAL CORD INJURY	MOTOR FUNCTION	SENSORY FUNCTION	RESPIRATORY FUNCTION	BOWEL AND BLADDER FUNCTION
C 1–4	Motor function lost from neck down	Loss of sensory function from the neck down	Loss of involuntary and voluntary respiratory function	No bowel or bladder control
C 5	Loss of motor function below the upper shoulders; able to control head	Loss of sensation below the clavicle; head, shoulders, part of forearms and lateral aspects of the arms may have sensation	Involuntary respiratory function intact (diaphragm), but loss of voluntary respiratory function	No bowel or bladder control
C 6	Loss of all function below the shoulders; able to extend wrists	Loss of sensation below the clavicle but increased arm and thumb sensation	Involuntary respiratory function intact, but loss of voluntary respiratory function	No bowel or bladder control
C 7	Loss of motor control to portions of arms and hands; able to extend at the elbow	Loss of sensation below the clavicle but middle finger sensation	Involuntary respiratory function intact, but loss of voluntary respiratory function	No bowel or bladder control
C 8	Loss of motor control to portions of arms and hands; able to squeeze hands and extend fingers	Loss of sensation below the chest and portions of hands (with little finger sensation)	Involuntary respiratory function intact, but loss of voluntary respiratory function	No bowel or bladder control
T 1–6	Loss of motor control from the mid-chest down	Loss of sensation below the mid-chest area	Involuntary respiratory function intact; possibly some loss of voluntary respiratory function	No bowel or bladder control
T 6–12	Loss of motor control below the waist	Loss of sensation below the waist	No impairment of respiratory function	No bowel or bladder control
L 1–3	Loss of most motor control of legs and pelvis	Loss of sensation of lower abdomen and legs	No impairment of respiratory function	No bowel or bladder control
L 3–4	Loss of motor control of portions of the lower legs	Loss of sensation of portions of the lower legs	No impairment of respiratory function	No bowel or bladder control
L 4–S 5	Variable loss of motor function	Variable loss of sensation	No impairment of respiratory function	Possibly impaired bowel or bladder control

689

8 or above. Manifestations include a sudden episode of hypertension (up to 300 mm Hg systolic), headache, bradycardia (heart rate of 30 to 40 beats/minute), sweating with flushing above the level of injury, and piloerection (goose bumps). It is caused by noxious stimuli from below the level of injury to the spinal cord to which the sympathetic nervous system responds inappropriately. A distended bladder or rectum is the most common precipitating stimulus. Treatment focuses on removing the stimulus and managing blood pressure. Untreated hypertension may cause seizures and cerebral or retinal hemorrhages.

Pressure ulcers, deep vein thrombosis, urinary tract disorders, and increased susceptibility to respiratory diseases are also common in these patients.

 DIAGNOSTIC CRITERIA

A spinal radiograph is obtained early to establish the level and extent of injury. A CT scan provides better detail of the soft tissue injury. MRI is done if the patient has an incomplete injury or neurologic deficit with evidence of fracture identified by x-ray or CT scan.

Somatosensory evoked potential (SEP) testing is used to determine the extent of injury and to establish a prognosis. In SEP, a peripheral nerve is stimulated from the arm or leg below the level of injury. The message is traced along a neural pathway to centers in the brain. The message is absent in the patient with complete injury, as information is unable to pass the area of injury, and altered in the patient with incomplete injury.

 INTERVENTIONS

The care of the patient with SCI is divided into phases: accident scene, emergency department, acute care, and rehabilitation. At the scene of the accident, the top priorities are assessing the airway, breathing, and circulation and immobilizing the neck to prevent any further movement of the spine until the patient can be medically evaluated in the emergency department.

In the emergency department, a detailed history is obtained and a complete neurologic and physical examination is done. The patient is kept immobilized and assessed for life-threatening problems such as hypotension, bradycardia, and hypovolemia that may result from spinal shock. High-dose IV methylprednisolone is given to prevent or reduce secondary injury. It should be initiated within 3 hours of injury for best results but can be initiated up to 8 hours after injury. The methylprednisolone dosage is a 30 mg/kg IV bolus followed by a continuous infusion of 5.4 mg/kg for 23 hours.

Depending on the mechanism of injury to the spinal cord, immobilization may be surgical (e.g., spinal fusion, rod placement) or nonsurgical (e.g., halo vest, brace, traction). Decompression may be necessary to relieve compression or remove bone fragments. Typical problems that occur during the acute care phase are outlined in Table 19-9-3. Once the patient is physiologically stabilized, then the focus becomes a multidisciplinary team approach to ready the patient for rehabilitation.

 COMMUNITY CARE

Specialized SCI rehabilitation centers are available for patients following the acute phase. These centers focus on the retraining of physiologic processes,

Table 19-9-3. Acute Care Problems and SCI

PROBLEM (ACTUAL OR POTENTIAL)	INTERVENTIONS
Respiratory • Depends on level of injury • Hypoxia • Aspiration • Atelectasis • Pneumonia	• Provide intubation and ventilation (if long-term, possibly tracheostomy). • Institute pulse oximetry. • Provide chest physiotherapy. • Provide suctioning. • Teach "quad" coughing technique. • Provide incentive spirometry, if applicable.
Cardiovascular • Spinal shock • Deep venous thrombosis • Autonomic dysreflexia	• Assess for signs of hypotension and bradycardia. • Assess calves for deep vein thrombosis. • Use antiembolism stockings and compression devices. • Administer subcutaneous heparin. • Assess for hypertension, bradycardia, pounding headache, flushed face and neck, and cold lower extremities. • Remove noxious stimuli.
Gastrointestinal • Decreased peristalsis • Abdominal distention • Alteration in nutritional intake • Altered bowel function	• Insert a nasogastric tube. • Meet caloric needs; depending on the level of injury, may need enteral or parenteral nutrition. • Institute a bowel training/management program.
Genitourinary • Altered urinary elimination • Urinary tract infections • Sexual dysfunction	• Monitor intake and output. • Provide intermittent catheterization. • Institute a bladder training/management program. • Provide information about sexual function.
Skin • Alteration in skin integrity	• Reposition every 1 to 2 hours. • Assess for skin breakdown.
Activity • Immobility • Orthostatic hypotension • Spasticity	• Advance activity as tolerated. • Use an abdominal binder; wrap the lower extremities. • Provide range-of-motion exercises. • Assess for and remove noxious stimuli. • Administer antispasmodic agents.

with emphasis on occupational and physical therapy. Mechanical devices such as electronic wheelchairs and portable ventilators are available and funded by the state and federal government.

Dysreflexia cards should be carried at all times. These simply explain the syndrome for the lay public, and give simple instructions on management should an episode occur. Many homes and businesses are handicap accessible or are being converted to comply with the Americans with Disabilities Act. Many associations are available as resources.

 PROGNOSIS

The mortality rate for acute SCI has dropped from about 80% in the 1940s to about 6% today. The average lifespan is 30 to 40 years after SCI. The major cause of death in patients with SCI is pneumonia.

 CLINICAL PEARLS

○ "Tetraplegia" is the contemporary term for "quadriplegia" used more often in the clinical setting.

○ If signs of autonomic dysreflexia are noted, assess for bladder distention and check the urine drainage device for obstruction. Then check the bowel for stool or impaction.

○ During the patient's coughing and deep-breathing exercises, assist by performing the "quad assisted-cough" technique. Have the patient take two deep breaths. On the third breath, during inspiration, place the heel of your hand between the patient's umbilicus and diaphragm. Then have the patient cough while you push down and up.

○ Global infarction occurs 8 hours after injury, thus high-dose methylprednisolone must be administered before this occurs.

NURSING PROBLEM/ DIAGNOSIS	NURSING INTERVENTIONS CLASSIFICATION (NIC)
Risk for autonomic dysreflexia	Dysreflexia Management Cerebral Perfusion Promotion Urinary Elimination Management Bowel Management
Impaired physical mobility	Positioning: Neurologic Positioning Pressure Management Circulatory Care Environmental Management: Safety
Deficient knowledge about disability and resources	Anxiety Reduction Health System Guidance Support Group Teaching: Individual

Psychosocial Health

chapter 20

Alcohol Withdrawal Syndrome

Section 1   Lori Schumacher

 OVERVIEW

Chronic consumption of alcohol may lead to the development of alcohol withdrawal syndrome (AWS) in a hospitalized patient. An estimated 10 to 20 million Americans display alcohol dependence, which contributes to many alcohol-related illnesses and deaths each year. If hospitalized, these patients have the potential to experience symptoms of AWS, resulting in complicated hospitalization, increased length of stay, and increased use of health care services.

 PATHOPHYSIOLOGY

When alcohol is consumed, it is rapidly absorbed from the gastrointestinal tract, circulated throughout the body, and metabolized by the liver. Alcohol causes central nervous system depression, liver disorders (cirrhosis), nutritional disorders, and gastrointestinal disorders (pancreatitis). Alcohol tolerance develops because of the central nervous system's adaptive mechanisms. AWS occurs when there is a sudden withdrawal from a prolonged intake of alcohol. Usually, symptoms of AWS begin within 8 hours to several days of the last drink. Within 48 hours, symptoms usually either subside or progress. Delirium tremens (DTs) usually occurs within 4 days of the onset of AWS.

 SIGNS AND SYMPTOMS

Signs and symptoms correlating with blood alcohol concentration are listed in Table 20-1-1. Intoxication occurs when the blood alcohol level exceeds 150 mg/dL. The initial signs and symptoms of AWS include:

- Tremor
- Craving for alcohol
- Insomnia
- Vivid dreams
- Anxiety
- Irritability
- Headache
- Restlessness
- Tachycardia
- Sweating
- Nausea and vomiting

DTs may occur as AWS progresses; signs and symptoms include:

- Clouding of sensorium

693

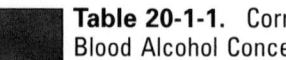 **Table 20-1-1.** Correlation of Signs and Symptoms with Blood Alcohol Concentrations

BLOOD ALCOHOL CONCENTRATION (mg/dL)	SIGNS AND SYMPTOMS
50–150	• Euphoria or dysphoria • Shy or brazen • Friendly or disagreeable • Impaired concentration • Impaired judgment • Sexual inhibitions
150–250	• Slurred speech • Ataxic gait • Blurred vision, diplopia • Nausea • Drowsiness • Tachycardia • Mood swings
300	• Stupor, may be combative at times • Incoherent speech • Vomiting • Heavy breathing
400	• Coma
500	• Respiratory cessation • Death

Adapted from Burst, J. M. (1993). Alcoholism. In Carlson & Geheb (Eds.), *Principles and practice of medical intensive care*. Philadelphia: WB Saunders.

- Hallucinations (auditory, visual, tactile, or any combination)
- Seizures
- Autonomic hyperactivity (e.g., tachycardia, hypertension, increased temperature)

DIAGNOSTIC CRITERIA

The diagnosis of AWS or identification of the potential for AWS is based on history, clinical observation, and laboratory studies. A history of alcohol consumption is obtained, and a screening questionnaire may be administered to assess the patient's risk for AWS. The CAGE screening questionnaire inquires about potential problems of high alcohol intake and diagnosis of problem drinking through four questions:

1. Have you felt you should *c*ut down on your alcohol consumption?
2. Have people *a*nnoyed you by criticizing your drinking?
3. Have you felt *g*uilty about your drinking?
4. Have you ever had a drink first thing in the morning to steady your nerves or get rid of a hangover (an *e*ye opener)?

A positive alcohol consumption history and one or more affirmative CAGE responses suggest that the patient is at risk for AWS.

Clinical observation includes assessing and monitoring for signs and symptoms of AWS. A urine or serum toxicology specimen may be collected on admission, especially if the patient was involved in an accident or other trauma. A positive ethanol toxicology result also suggests that the patient is at risk for AWS.

 INTERVENTIONS

Clinical assessment and monitoring is the primary intervention for patients considered to be at risk for AWS. Of the various assessment scales available for monitoring these patients, the Clinical Institute Withdrawal Assessment for Alcohol (CIWA-A) scale is the most commonly used. The CIWA-A scale rates the severity of symptoms associated with AWS, including tremor, tachycardia, hypertension, diaphoresis, nausea/vomiting, fever, agitation, confusion, sleeplessness, hallucinations, and seizures. A patient's CIWA-A score guides monitoring and aids early identification of more severe symptoms that may indicate the need for prophylactic medications, such as lorazepam.

Despite preventive efforts, however, a patient with AWS may develop DTs. If this occurs, treatment focuses on treating the symptoms and preventing complications. Symptoms are treated with benzodiazepines, sedatives, anticonvulsants, beta-adrenergic blockers, and antipsychotics. Supportive care for AWS may include administering thiamine, folate, calcium, magnesium, and phosphates and ensuring adequate fluid intake to help maintain normal cell function.

 COMMUNITY CARE

Assessment
- Obtain an alcohol consumption history and note the date and time of the patient's last drink.
- Assess for signs and symptoms of AWS.

Monitoring
- Monitor for signs and symptoms of AWS (may use the CIWA-A scale).
- Assess the patient's response to medications administered and interventions performed.

Prevention
- Provide community education about the effects of alcohol abuse and the development of AWS.
- Screen, identify, and counsel patients with alcohol-related problems.

 PROGNOSIS

In the United States, alcohol is involved in 10% of all deaths. The mortality rate is 50% higher in persons who consume six or more drinks per day. Mortality for DTs is estimated at 5% to 15%.

 CLINICAL PEARLS

- Alcohol accounts for approximately 65% of cases of acute and chronic pancreatitis.
- Various medical and mental health complications may coexist with AWS.
- Alcoholism is a disease that can be fatal if left untreated.
- Not all patients with AWS exhibit the same symptoms.

○ Regular alcohol consumption gradually builds tolerance, with increasing amounts of alcohol needed to get the initial euphoric effect.

NURSING PROBLEM/ DIAGNOSIS	NURSING INTERVENTIONS CLASSIFICATION (NIC)
Alcohol withdrawal	Substance use treatment: alcohol withdrawal
Risk for delirium tremens	Delirium management
Deficient knowledge about alcoholism and resources	Anxiety reduction
	Health system guidance
	Support group
	Teaching: individual

Depression

Section 2   Susan Rick

 ## OVERVIEW

Depression has been called the number one mental health problem in the United States. This common disorder has a lifetime prevalence of about 15%, perhaps as high as 25% in women. Profound feelings of sadness, hopelessness, and helplessness not only have negative effects on the individual and his or her family but also cause significant economic losses because of increased morbidity, mortality, and treatment costs.

Although depression may occur at any age, it often begins in youth or middle age, when a person is at his or her productive peak. The clinical consequences are varied and often critical. Depression is the most common contributing factor to suicide, with rates as high as 20% to 30%. The risk of suicide is especially high for persons with a history of suicide attempts, psychotic features, or concurrent substance abuse. Premature death from general medical conditions has also been linked to depression.

 ## PATHOPHYSIOLOGY

Several factors have been proposed to explain the development of a major depressive episode. Neurotransmitters, particularly norepinephrine and serotonin, have been implicated. It is thought that depression may result from poor regulation of these transmitters rather than from simply a decrease in their amounts. Other neurotransmitters thought to play a role in depression include acetylcholine, dopamine, and gamma-aminobutyric acid.

Laboratory findings are not specific for diagnosing a major depressive episode. However, sleep electroencephalogram (EEG) abnormalities are evident in as many as 90% of the patients diagnosed with depression. Another test that has demonstrated abnormalities is the dexamethasone suppression test. A plasma cortisol level above 5 mg/dL is considered positive for depression; however, false-positive results are not uncommon. Functional and structural brain imaging tests, evoked potential studies, and waking EEGs have also demonstrated some abnormalities in patients with depression.

Studies have shown evidence of genetic transmission of depression. First-degree relatives of persons with major depression have about twice the risk of developing this disorder as does the rest of the population.

Depressive episodes occur approximately twice as often in women as in men. The symptoms appear to worsen several days before the onset of menses. Childbirth may also precipitate a major depressive episode, as may other psychosocial stressors, such as death and divorce.

Various psychological theories offer possible insight into the development of a major depressive episode. Cognitive theorists, such as Aaron Beck, suggest that stressful events activate negative cognitions, which result in information-processing errors. These errors may become habitual, and the resulting pattern of negative, affective, and behavioral responses may lead to depression.

Behavioral theorists assume that depression is a learned response, related to inadequate social skills and resulting in negative social interactions. This promotes low self-esteem, and depression becomes a conditioned response.

Interpersonal theory suggests that real or perceived losses may lead to a depression. This is true, particularly in persons with dependency needs, who have additional interpersonal and environmental stressors.

Psychoanalytic theories have also been postulated to explain the development of depression. Three areas are noted to be of particular importance. Anger turned inward against oneself, the experience of a major loss, and the continued presence of internal conflicts are offered as explanations of the development of this mood disorder.

 ## SIGNS AND SYMPTOMS

Individuals with major depressive episodes experience a profound sense of sadness, hopelessness, and loss of pleasure. They also experience at least four additional symptoms. These may include:

- Changes in weight
- Alterations in sleep and psychomotor activity
- Decreased energy
- Feelings of worthlessness or guilt
- Difficulty thinking
- Difficulty concentrating or making decisions
- Recurrent thoughts of death or suicide

In some individuals, the depression may be exhibited in a more somatic way. Complaints of body aches and pains replace direct discussion of sad or hopeless feelings. When children or adolescents are depressed, they may be seen as irritable rather than sad.

Thought patterns of depressed individuals are often impaired. Inability to concentrate and make decisions and altered ability to remember names and events are not uncommon. Feelings of hopelessness and guilt may evolve to thoughts of suicide.

Sleep pattern disturbances are also common, and psychomotor changes may be present. For example, the person may pace in an agitated fashion or may demonstrate a slowing of activity (psychomotor retardation). Decreases in general energy level and sexual interest are often associated with depression. Even the smallest tasks of daily living may become burdensome.

According to the DSM IV criteria, signs and symptoms of a major depressive episode are similar, if not identical, to those associated with specific medical conditions, such as hypothyroidism. These signs and symptoms should be applied to the identification of a major depressive episode, except when they are clearly representative of a general medical condition.

 DIAGNOSTIC CRITERIA

According to the DSM IV, criteria for a major depressive episode include five (or more) of the following symptoms present during the same 2-week period and representing a change from previous functioning; at least one of the symptoms is either depressed mood or a loss of interest or pleasure:

- Depressed mood most of the day, nearly every day, as indicated by either subjective report (e.g., feels sad or empty) or observation made by others (e.g., appears tearful)
- Diminished interest or pleasure in all, or almost all, activities most of the day, almost every day (as indicated by either subjective account or observation by others)
- Significant weight loss when not dieting or weight gain (e.g., a change of more than 5% of body weight in a month), or decrease or increase in appetite almost every day
- Insomnia or hypersomnia almost every day
- Psychomotor agitation or retardation almost daily (observable by others, not merely subjective feelings of restlessness or being slowed down)
- Fatigue or loss of energy almost daily
- Feelings of worthlessness or excessive or inappropriate guilt (which may be delusional) almost every day (not merely self-reproach or guilt about being sick)
- Diminished ability to think or concentrate, or indecisiveness, almost daily (either by subjective account or as observed by others)
- Recurrent thoughts of death (not just fear of dying), recurrent suicidal ideation without a specific plan, or a suicide attempt or a specific plan for committing suicide.

The signs and symptoms cause clinically significant distress or impairment in social, occupational, or other important areas of functioning. They are not caused by the direct physiologic effects of substance abuse, a general medical condition (e.g. hypothyroidism), or mood-incongruent delusions or hallucinations. They cause significant impairment of functioning and are not better accounted for by bereavement with symptoms persisting longer than 2 months.

 INTERVENTIONS

Once a patient is diagnosed with a major depressive episode, health and safety needs must be clearly identified and monitored.

Screening

To optimize safety and allow for a complete assessment, a depressed patient may be treated on an inpatient basis. This is particularly important if the patient poses a danger to himself or herself or to others. Diagnostic tests may rule out any underlying organic cause. Information from both the patient and those close to him or her may be used to complete an accurate health history and psychological profile. The nurse should note any self-care deficits that may be present. The patient's plan of care needs to address issues related to safety, exercise, nutritional requirements, sleep pattern disturbances, hygiene, and spiritual and psychosocial needs. Interventions should be specifically designed not only to ensure safety, but also to promote self-esteem and social interaction. During all interactions with the patient, the nurse must remain hopeful, while avoiding excessive cheerfulness.

Safety

Safety is a primary concern. Untreated persons with a depressive disorder are at a 25% to 30% risk of suicide. In a direct and caring manner, the nurse must ask and determine whether or not the patient is having thoughts of suicide. If the patient indicates that suicide is an option, whether or not he or she has developed an actual plan, this must be considered a serious threat to safety that merits hospitalization.

Self-destructive behavior is an ongoing concern in the hospitalized depressed patient. The patient must be physically searched for weapons and harmful materials and carefully monitored to prevent any form of self-injurious behavior. Even if the patient's threat of suicide is seen as a manipulative gesture, it must be treated seriously, as suicide is sometimes the result.

Pharmacotherapy

Pharmacotherapy for the treatment of major depression has been available for more than 4 decades and has provided significant relief for many individuals. Effects usually become evident after 2 to 6 weeks of therapy, as therapeutic levels are achieved. More recently introduced agents, including bupropion (Wellbutrin) and the selective serotonin reuptake inhibitors (SSRIs), such as paroxetine (Paxil) and sertraline (Zoloft), are better tolerated and as effective as the earlier tricyclic antidepressant (TCA) drugs, which are now considered second-line agents.

Most clinicians choose SSRIs as the first-line treatment for major depression. These drugs act specifically on the neurotransmitter serotonin, preventing its reuptake. Fluoxetine (Prozac), the first available SSRI, is still considered by many to be the most effective. Fluoxetine may cause transient agitation and anorexia but is less likely to cause sedation. Other popular SSRIs include sertraline (Zoloft), which is most associated with gastric distress, and paroxetine (Paxil), which is more likely to cause sedation. Unfortunately, SSRIs are associated with anorgasmia and other sexual dysfunction.

For individuals who fail multiple medication trials, two older classes of medications may be used: TCAs and monoamine oxidase inhibitors (MAOIs). Nortriptyline (Aventyl, Pamelor) and desipramine (Norpramin) have become the most popular TCA agents. TCAs block reuptake of neurotransmitters, primarily serotonin and norepinephrine, at the presynaptic neurons. Their side effect profile, however, includes sedation, dry mouth, blurred vision, weight gain, and possible cardiovascular effects (e.g., dysrhythmias). Thus, a baseline electrocardiogram is often recommended. When discontinuing TCA therapy, the dosage must be tapered to minimize withdrawal symptoms (e.g., nausea, vomiting, sweating, and headache).

MAOIs, such as phenelzine (Nardil) and tranylcypromine (Parnate), are less frequently chosen, because they pose a risk of hypertensive crisis if the patient ingests items with a high tyramine content, such as bananas, aged cheese, vermouth, chianti, pickled and smoked meats, soy sauce, tap beer, brewer's yeast tablets, and sauerkraut. Thus, adherence to a dietary guideline is necessary to ensure safety during MAOI therapy.

Atypical antidepressants, including bupropion, nefazodone (Serzone), and venlafaxine (Effexor), are newer antidepressants that act similarly to SSRIs but have no adverse effects on sexual function. Of concern, however, are increased seizure risk with bupropion, hypotensive effects with nefazodone, and dose-related hypertension with venlafaxine.

Natural products and herbal remedies have gained some recognition in the treatment of depression. These products need not be approved by the U.S. Food and Drug Administration, and their claims of effectiveness are not necessarily drawn from scientific study. For example, St. John's wort has become popular in the treatment of depression, but conflicting evidence exists to substantiate claims of its effectiveness.

Patients on antidepressants should be monitored closely for adverse reactions. Patients must be educated about the specific dosing schedule and warned that these drugs can be lethal when taken in overdose or in combination with alcohol or other medications.

Hypotension is a serious adverse effect of many antidepressant agents. This is of particular concern for elderly patients. Another common adverse effect of many antidepressants is decreased libido or erectile dysfunction. This occurs in up to 33% of patients taking SSRIs.

Selection of a specific antidepressant agent may be influenced by a history of positive response and consideration of possible side effects. Combined drug therapy may be used to treat some depressive episodes, particularly those that are associated with psychosis or are resistant to other treatments.

Antidepressant treatment should be maintained for at least 6 months or longer, depending on the severity of symptoms. Several studies indicate that maintenance antidepressant medication appears to be safe and effective for chronic depression. When antidepressant therapy is discontinued, the dosage should be tapered over 1 or 2 weeks.

Psychotherapy

Psychotherapy may be used in combination with pharmacotherapy to effect a more positive outcome. Some evidence supports that combined psychotherapy plus pharmacotherapy is superior to either of these treatments alone. Psychotherapy may be interpersonal, behavioral, brief psychodynamic, or family-oriented in approach. The length of psychotherapy is influenced by the severity of the depression and the specific therapeutic approach. Psychoanalytic-oriented therapy may be open-ended and long term, continuing for several years. Cognitive therapy and behavior therapies focus on developing adaptive and positive actions and are of a brief and fixed duration, making them more cost-effective. Interpersonal therapy usually consists of 12 to 16 weekly sessions, during which the patient and therapist examine interpersonal problems thought to be perpetuating the depressive symptoms.

Alternatives to Drug Treatment

Electroconvulsant therapy (ECT) may be used in some cases where pharmacotherapy has proved ineffective or not tolerated by the patient. It is often used for patients with a psychotic disorder and when symptoms demand rapid treatment. This relatively safe procedure involves low-energy electrical stimulation of the brain to induce a seizure lasting approximately 1 minute. During the procedure, the patient is anesthetized with a short-acting general agent, such as sodium thiopental. The patient is given a neuromuscular blockade with succinylcholine, administered 100% oxygen, and monitored continuously until spontaneous breathing returns.

It is thought that the ECT-induced seizure causes neurobiologic changes. The effects are not fully understood, but brain chemistry is altered in some manner, providing relief from depressive symptoms. Treatments may be given two to three times a week; six to ten procedures are generally considered necessary. These may be given on either an inpatient or an outpatient basis.

The patient must sign a consent for ECT and should be educated as to the course of treatment, as well as possible adverse effects. Family members need to know that the patient will seem sedated after the treatment. The patient should be given nothing by mouth for 8 hours before the procedure. Atropine may be administered to reduce secretions.

The patient is monitored carefully during and after the ECT procedure to ensure that vital signs remain stable. Adverse reactions may include disorientation, headache, muscle pain, and possible cardiac dysrhythmias. The risks of anesthesia (e.g., central nervous system depression and aspiration) are also of concern. The most notable adverse effect is memory loss. This is usually transient and resolves within a few days.

The patient is monitored closely. If ECT is given on an outpatient basis, once vital signs are stable, the patient can be transported home. The patient should not be allowed to drive, however.

 COMMUNITY CARE

Assessment

- Assess risk factors, both psychological (e.g., recent loss or trauma) and possible genetic or physical predisposition to a major depressive episode.
- Assess for the psychological symptoms that would be associated with depression, for example, feelings of sadness, hopelessness, worthlessness, loss of pleasure and ability to concentrate, and thoughts of self-injurious behavior, suicide, or death. (Safety is of primary importance.)
- Assess for physiologic signs and symptoms of depression, such as weight loss or gain, psychomotor retardation, agitation, insomnia or hypersomnia, and loss of energy.
- Assess the patient's compliance with prescribed pharmacologic therapy. Question the patient regarding the administration of medication. Make sure that the patient understands that it may take several weeks before the actual positive effects of the medication are noted.
- Assess the patient's support system and knowledge of the depressive disorder and its significant symptoms and treatments.

Monitor

- Monitor the patient's depressive symptomatology and response to treatment. Monitor the patient's compliance with treatment.
- Assess for side effects of pharmacologic therapy.

- Carefully monitor for evidence of self-injury. If this is present, hospitalization may be necessary to ensure the patient's safety.

Prevention
- Identify people with an increased risk for depression, that is, those with a genetic predisposition or history of mood disorders.
- Offer people at risk for depression support and education about the disease. Encourage them to seek appropriate treatment.

 PROGNOSIS

Recurrence of major depressive episodes is common. Approximately 50% to 60% of persons with a single episode of major depressive disorder can expect to have a second episode. After discharge from the hospital, 25% of patients experience a recurrence within the first 6 months, 30% to 50% within the first 2 years, and 50% to 75% within 5 years.

Ongoing pharmacologic treatment reduces relapse rates. In one 3-year follow-up study, the mean time to relapse was 45 weeks without antidepressant drug therapy, compared with 124 weeks with antidepressant therapy.

Mild episodes, the absence of psychotic symptoms, a short hospital stay, and presence of family and social support are good prognostic indicators.

 CLINICAL PEARLS

○ Depressive episodes may occur in major depressive disorders and bipolar 1 disorder. Clinically, these disorders are distinguished by the patient's history and course of the disease.

○ Some groups are at increased risk for depression. For example, African Americans are less likely than Hispanics or whites to suffer from major depression.

○ About two thirds of all depressed persons consider suicide, but only 10% to 15% may actually commit the act. Ensuring the safety of people experiencing depression must be of primary importance.

○ Adequate patient education on the use of antidepressant medication is critical to successful treatment. It must be stressed that addiction to these medications does not occur and that several weeks of therapy may be needed before symptoms improve.

NURSING PROBLEM/ DIAGNOSIS	NURSING INTERVENTIONS CLASSIFICATION (NIC)
Depression/Hopelessness	Support system enhancement Mood management Self-esteem enhancement
Risk for suicide	Suicide prevention Surveillance: safety
Deficient knowledge of resources	Health system guidance

Drug Overdose and Poisoning

Section 3   Diana Davis Rovira

 OVERVIEW

Drug overdose can result from a variety of both legal and illegal substances. Substances considered legal include alcohol, household products, pesticides, aspirin, acetaminophen, prescription medications, nonsteroidal anti-inflammatory drugs, and cough and cold medications. Illegal substances include cocaine, heroin, amphetamines, phenmetrazine, and prescription medications prescribed for another individual.

Each year, between 1.5 and 2 million exposures to potential poisons are reported to poison control centers throughout the world. Approximately 700 people die of poisoning each year, as reported to poison control centers. Approximately 5000 people die each year of suicide poisoning from solids, liquids, gases, or vapors. Another 1500 people die each year of poisoning of undetermined cause; whether these are intentional or unintentional is unknown.

Cleaning products are the most common substances involved in accidental human exposure. Analgesics cause the greatest number of deaths from poisoning. The toxic ingestion of illicit substances (most commonly, cocaine, heroin, and inhalants) is also common.

 PATHOPHYSIOLOGY

If the concentration of a chemical in the tissues does not exceed a critical level, then the effects of the toxic ingestion are usually reversible. *Local toxicity* is an effect occurring at the site of first contact between a biologic system and a toxicant; an example is a chemical burn. *Systemic toxicity* is the effect occurring after the absorption and distribution of a toxicant. Most toxins affect one or two organs. It is important to know that a target organ for toxicity is not always where the substance accumulates. Major organ systems affected, listed in order of frequency, are the central nervous system, cardiovascular system, blood and hematopoietic organs, visceral organs (e.g., liver, kidneys, lungs), and the skin. Bone and muscles are least affected. The physiologic effects of an overdose depend on the substance involved.

 SIGNS AND SYMPTOMS

Signs and symptoms of illicit drug use depend on the substance ingested and can range from euphoria and analgesia to central nervous system depression. Signs of overdose of hallucinogens, sedatives, and opiates may include disorientation, decreased respirations, bradycardia, hypotension, and coma. Overdose of stimulants may produce hyperactivity, dilated pupils, tremor, tachycardia, hypertension, seizures, and paranoia.

Clinical manifestations of poisoning depend on the substance ingested. Common effects include dehydration, hypotension, hyperpyrexia, mental status changes, tachycardia or bradycardia, pulmonary edema, and acute tubular necrosis. Signs of poisoning include nausea and vomiting, diarrhea, constipation, anorexia, stomatitis, metallic taste, skin rash, hair loss, diaphoresis, wheezing, peripheral neuropathy, tremors, paralysis, and headache. These also depend on the substance ingested.

 DIAGNOSTIC CRITERIA

Urine and blood studies (and rarely gastric contents for toxic screen) for acetaminophen, aspirin, and alcohol level are indicated specifically in all patients who have taken an intentional overdose.

A complete blood count should be obtained to assess for anemia or signs of infection. Serum electrolyte levels should be assessed for abnormalities, which may be correctable with intravenous (IV) fluids or supplements and glucose for hypoglycemia or hyperglycemia.

Prothrombin and partial thromboplastin times may be evaluated to assess for bleeding abnormality. Liver function tests may be done to assess liver damage and to obtain baseline values on admission. Blood urea nitrogen and creatinine levels help evaluate renal perfusion and function. Arterial blood gas evaluation detects acidosis or hypoxemia.

A chest radiograph is important as a baseline study in patients with evidence of aspiration. A baseline electrocardiogram is important in patients who have taken an overdose of tricyclic antidepressant agents. A pregnancy test should be performed on all women of childbearing age.

Tests for levels of specific substances (e.g., iron, mercury, digitalis, theophylline, lead, arsenic) should also be obtained depending on the situation.

 INTERVENTIONS
Assessment
History

Be sure to note the source of information about the patient's substance ingestion: the patient, a family member, a friend, emergency medical personnel, or a bystander. A description of the event includes the location and time, the substance(s) involved, the type of container that the substance was in, the amount ingested, and signs and symptoms exhibited. If the patient had been detained by law enforcement for substance use, suspect body packing or body stuffing in an attempt to get rid of evidence. Ascertain whether there is a regular pattern of alcohol and substance use. In substance users and abusers, suspect polydrug abuse, which is far more common than single drug or alcohol use alone. Attempt to obtain collateral reports of substance use patterns from significant others.

Obtain a past health history. Use the mnemonic AMPLE: *a*llergies, *m*edications (including prescription and over-the-counter; also ask about tetanus immunization), *p*ast illnesses (medical and surgical), *l*ast meal eaten (time, quantity, type), and *e*vents preceding ingestion.

Obtain a social history from the patient's partner, spouse, housemates, roommates, significant others, or contact person. Inquire about occupation, education, and whether or not there are dependents or children. Find out about religious preference; sometimes a minister or hospital chaplain can be helpful in these situations. Investigate financial considerations; for example, does the patient have the ability to maintain income and insurance coverage? If so, was this a precipitating factor in the overdose?

Other important information to note in the history are the patient's height and weight and, in women of childbearing age, date of last menstrual period to determine the potential for pregnancy.

Examination

Primary Survey. This is a rapid assessment (30 seconds to 2 minutes) that simultaneously identifies and manages life-threatening alterations. It focuses on assessing the ABCs: airway, breathing, circulation (see Chapter 1, Section 4). Early consultation with a poison control center is essential after the ABCs are established.

Secondary Survey. A complete physical examination is begun as soon as the primary survey and emergency life-saving interventions are completed. A patient suspected of body stuffing or body packing needs to be monitored for cardiovascular compromise in intensive care. Take a nonjudgmental and honest approach when assessing symptoms, and determine the precise amount of drug ingested. Vital signs are widely variable, depending on the compound.

Inspection. Inspect all areas of the skin and mucous membranes for needle marks (especially between toes) or abscesses.

Monitoring

Monitor core temperature and manage hypothermia and hyperthermia. *Monitor cardiac rhythm* and manage dysrhythmias and hypovolemia with IV crystalloids, as needed. Pressor agents such as dopamine will not work in a hypovolemic patient.

Monitor respiratory status using pulse oximetry. If respirations are deemed not adequate, hyperventilate with a bag-valve-mask and 100% oxygen followed by intubation. One-hundred percent oxygen may be considered an antidote for carbon monoxide poisoning. *Do not* rely on partial pressure of oxygen or oxygen saturation values to detect carbon monoxide poisoning.

Monitor the environment for items that could be used for self-inflicted injury. Implement suicide precautions if appropriate.

Pharmacotherapy

To rule out hyperglycemia as a cause of coma, 50% dextrose may be administered IV. Thiamine, 100 mg IV, may be ordered to prevent precipitation of Wernicke-Korsakoff syndrome.

Naloxone 2 mg may be given IV, intramuscularly, or endotracheally to antagonize narcotics. Smaller doses (0.1 or 0.2 mg) are given to opioid-dependent patients who are not apneic, to avoid withdrawal. Naloxone is used routinely in patients with central nervous system or respiratory depression (with respiratory rates below 12 breaths/min) and who have a low likelihood of opioid addiction or polydrug addiction. The drug's half-life is 30 minutes; symptoms may recur after that period, indicating the need for a continuous infusion. See Chapter 12, Section 1 for more information on naloxone.

Do not administer physostigmine (Antilirium), analeptics (e.g., amphetamines, caffeine), or flumazenil routinely until the toxic agent is identified and the use of these drugs is warranted.

Provide a known antidote, if any. If no antidote is available, maintain vital functions, remove the toxic substance, and limit the absorption of any remaining substance.

Strategies for Toxin Removal
Orogastric Lavage

This procedure is done to eliminate unabsorbed toxins. It is usually performed in the emergency department rather than the intensive care unit.

Indications. Orogastric lavage is generally accepted instead of emesis in comatose patients, except in cases of caustic ingestion where a chemical injury has occurred. Common substances that cause caustic injury include acetic acid (found in permanent wave solutions), ammonia (found in common household cleaning products), phosphorus (used in matches and fireworks), benzalkonium chloride (used in detergents), oxalic acid (found in disinfectants and bleach), formaldehyde, iodine (found in antiseptics), and sulfuric acid (found in batteries and drain cleaners).

Management of Caustics. Intubate the patient if necessary. Examine the patient for splash injuries to the skin and eyes. If there are no signs of visceral perforation and the patient can swallow, dilute the toxicant with cool milk or tap water; do not administer an emetic or perform gastric lavage.

Procedure for Gastric Lavage. If the patient is unable to protect the airway, intubate and inflate the cuff. Use a 36- to 40-French tube, which is large enough to remove particulate matter. Pass the tube orally to prevent epistaxis and trauma to the nasal mucosa. To keep the patient from biting the tube, an oral airway may be placed. After verifying tube placement in the stomach, place the patient in the left lateral decubitus position with the head lower than the feet, attach the lavage funnel to the end of the orogastric tube, and administer 150 to 200 mL (in adults) of tap water or normal saline solution. In some protocols, a catheter-tipped syringe is used to irrigate and withdraw the fluid until it is clear. Allow the tube to drain by gravity. Monitor for complications of aspiration, esophageal or gastric perforation, and laryngospasm.

Contraindications for Lavage. Lavage is contraindicated in hemorrhagic diathesis, nontoxic ingestion, and ingestion of sharp materials and drug packets.

Emetics

Ipecac syrup is the emetic of choice for home first aid; it is rarely recommended for emergency department use. This induces vomiting through local activation of peripheral sensory receptors in the gastrointestinal tract and stimulation of the chemoreceptor trigger in the central vomiting center of the brain. Vomiting usually begins in 20 minutes, occurs at least three times, and lasts about 30 to 60 minutes.

Implications. Do not give ipecac with milk, which may slow action. Ipecac may be inactivated by activated charcoal. In the emergency department, gastric lavage is preferable if gastric emptying is required.

Signs of Toxicity. Toxicity may be indicated by protracted vomiting, diarrhea, seizures, cardiac toxicity, and neuromuscular weakness.

Activated Charcoal

Activated charcoal absorbs drugs and other chemicals through ionic binding and molecular forces. Absorption begins within 1 minute after administration. It should be administered after several liters of gastric lavage produce a clear effluent. Activated charcoal is mixed with water or a cathartic (e.g., magnesium citrate, magnesium sulfate, sorbitol) to form a slurry and is administered orally or through a nasogastric tube. Contraindications to cathartics include paralytic ileus, diarrhea, abdominal trauma, intestinal obstruction, and renal failure.

Whole-Bowel Irrigation

Whole-bowel irrigation is done with polyethylene glycol and electrolytes for oral solution, given orally or by nasogastric tube for 4 to 6 hours until the effluent is clear. This works by clearing the entire gastrointestinal tract without inducing emesis or causing a fluid and electrolyte disturbance.

Indications. Whole-bowel irrigation is indicated to remove sustained-release drugs, slow-dissolving substances (e.g., iron tablets, paint chips), and "crack" vials and drug (e.g., cocaine, heroin) packets ingested for smuggling purposes. It is not used to remove rapidly absorbed drugs, liquids, parenterally administered drugs, or caustics.

Complications. Possible complications of whole-bowel irrigation include rectal itching and vomiting.

Contraindications. Whole-bowel irrigation is contraindicated in patients with ileus, bowel obstruction, bowel perforation, or gastrointestinal bleeding.

Hemodialysis, Hemoperfusion, and Hemofiltration

Three other methods may be used to clear toxic substances from the blood. *Hemodialysis* involves the dialysis of soluble substances and water from the blood by diffusion through a semipermeable membrane. Hemodialysis also corrects for metabolic acid-base disturbances, hyperkalemia, and fluid overload.

Hemoperfusion involves passing blood through columns of absorptive material, such as activated charcoal, to remove toxic substances from the blood. This procedure is better than hemodialysis for clearing blood of substances that bind to plasma proteins.

Hemofiltration is a process similar to hemodialysis in which blood is dialyzed using ultrafiltration and simultaneous reinfusion of physiologic saline solution. Hemofiltration is mostly experimental; however, it can be used to remove larger molecules, such as aminoglycoside antibiotics. Hemofiltration can be used after the other two techniques are performed to prevent a rebound of toxic levels. However, dialysis is most commonly done. Hypotension makes all three techniques difficult to use.

Referrals

Make appropriate referrals for detoxification management. Refer the patient to self-help groups as applicable.

 COMMUNITY CARE

Assessment

About 90% of poison exposures occur in the home; about 3%, in the workplace. Table 20-3-1 lists the 10 most common substances. Almost 70% of poison exposures are classified as *general* (undefined). The remaining 30% can be classified as follows:

- Environmental (2.5% of total), including any passive nonoccupational exposure resulting from contamination of air, water, or soil

Table 20-3-1. The 10 Most Common Substances in Human Poison Exposure

RANK	SUBSTANCE
1	Cleaning substances
2	Analgesics
3	Cosmetics
4	Plants
5	Cough and cold drugs
6	Animal bites
7	Pesticides
8	Topical preparations
9	Foreign bodies
10	Food poisoning

From Litovitz, T. L., Felberg, L., Soloway, R. A., et al. (1995). 1994 annual report of the American Association of Poison Control Centers Toxic Exposure Surveillance System. *American Journal of Emergency Medicine 13*, 551–597.

- Occupational (2.2%), occurring as a direct result of being in the workplace or on the job
- Therapeutic error (4.6%), an unintentional deviation from a proper therapeutic regimen that results in the wrong dose, incorrect route, or wrong substance
- Unintentional misuse (3.6%), the unintentional use of a nonpharmaceutical substance, such as a household cleaning product or yard/lawn product
- Food poisoning (2.2%), suspected or confirmed ingestion of contaminated food
- Suspected suicide (7.7%), exposure to a toxic substance resulting from inappropriate use for reasons that are suspected to be self-destructive
- Bite or sting (3.6%), including jellyfish stings
- Intentional misuse (1.4%), the improper use of a substance for reasons other than pursuit of a psychotropic effect

Identification of Poison Control Centers. In the United States there is no single national number that an individual can call for information on poisoning. According to the American Association of Poison Control Centers (AAPCC), each state has its own poison control center(s). The AAPCC web page (http://www.aapcc.org/) provides links to locate the nearest poison control center but does not provide information on what to do in a poisoning emergency. The web page states specifically to call 911 if a victim has collapsed and is not breathing.

 PROGNOSIS

With early identification and management, poisonings are generally well managed. For substance abuse, recovery is a long-term process with many relapses.

 CLINICAL PEARLS

○ If the patient becomes symptomatic while in police custody, suspect body stuffing with cocaine unless proved otherwise.

○ Partial pressure of oxygen and oxygen saturation levels are not reliable in carbon monoxide poisoning.
○ Obtain appropriate blood samples before starting IV fluids.
○ Do not delay treatment while awaiting laboratory results.

NURSING PROBLEM/ DIAGNOSIS	NURSING INTERVENTIONS CLASSIFICATION (NIC)
Hypoventilation due to central nervous system depression/ Ineffective breathing pattern	Airway management Substance use treatment: overdose
Cardiovascular instability	Fluid management Dysrhythmia management
Detoxification	Substance use treatment: drug withdrawal Substance use prevention Substance use treatment

Mental/Emotional Abuse

Section 4   Patricia Rickli

 OVERVIEW

Emotional abuse is only one form of domestic/family violence. The terms "abuse," "maltreatment of others," and "domestic violence" are often used interchangeably in discussions of destructive behavior that takes place within relationships. In addition to emotional abuse, other major categories of abuse include physical violence, sexual violence, neglect, and economic maltreatment. Emotional abuse can occur alone or with physical and sexual abuse.

Violence is a significant public health problem in the United States and was addressed as a specific area of concern in the *National Objectives of the Year 2000*. Violence occurs across all age groups, socioeconomic levels, educational levels, professions, ethnic backgrounds, and religions. Domestic violence is often not reported by the victim because of fear and embarrassment. Emotional abuse is present in each episode of physical and sexual abuse. In addition, emotional abuse may occur as the only type of abuse.

Abuse may be found in opposite-sex or same-sex relationships. Abuse may also be inflicted by a teenager on parents, especially by a son on a single-parent mother. In 90% of cases, a man is the perpetrator/abuser and a woman is the victim; however, in some cases, a woman is the perpetrator/abuser and a man is the victim. Because most victims of abuse are female, in this section a female victim is discussed.

In the United States, a woman is battered every 15 seconds. An estimated 35% of women seen in emergency departments are victims of abuse, yet only 5% to 10% of those seen are identified as victims. In 1990, it was estimated that there were 4 million incidents of abuse of women treated at a cost of approximately $50 million.

The occurrence of physical abuse can be described using the framework of the "cycle of violence." This cycle has three phases: tension building, acute battering, and loving. During the tension-building phase, the abuser exhibits behaviors of power and control of the victim. The behaviors include anger, frequent arguments, criticizing the victim, and blaming the victim for anything that goes wrong. The victim tends to believe the negative, critical, and blaming comments made by the abuser. The victim believes that if she changes her behavior, she can decrease the abuser's anger and prevent the abuse. The stress and tension escalate, culminating in acute battering. The battering incident is followed by the third phase, which is characterized by kind and loving actions by the abuser toward the victim or by the absence of anger and tension. The abuser may promise that such abuse will never happen again. The victim wants to believe these promises and may feel safe. Unfortunately, the professional literature reflects that abuse tends to become more frequent and intense over time.

While physical abuse is an episodic event, emotional abuse is a constant style used by the perpetrator/abuser in relating to the victim. Emotional abuse destroys the victim's self-esteem and impairs her ability to act independently, to feel deeply, and to forge emotional bonds with others. Self-esteem is defined as how a person views her personal worth and her level of regard for herself. Self-esteem is influenced by the actions of others toward oneself, and also by genetic and environmental factors. Conditions that promote positive self-esteem include feeling loved and respected, having control over one's life and ability to influence others, feelings of security, and the ability to achieve expectations.

Characteristics of abusers and characteristics of victims have been identified. Characteristics of men who are abusers include feelings of inferiority, insecurity, and powerlessness. To deal with these feelings of low self-esteem, they may use violence to feel that they are powerful and in control. The best predictors of a man's becoming an abuser are a history of violence and a personality that includes the need to control others, extreme jealousy, and possessiveness. The abuser may be well respected in the community and appear self-confident but feel inferior in his role as a husband.

Characteristics of female victims include holding a traditional view of the "woman's role," a passive attitude, approval-seeking from men, and low self-esteem. The women believe that they deserve to be abused and that the abuse is their fault. They experience feelings of guilt, fear, hopelessness, and depression. Such feelings result in an inability to identify options and to perform problem solving. They are often isolated from family and lack social support. They may live with the threats of the abuser that he will harm them and the children if they try to leave the relationship.

 PATHOPHYSIOLOGY

A clear biologic model for the cause of violence has not been identified. The development of aggression and violence is best understood by considering biologic, psychosocial, and environmental influences.

Biologic factors have been studied in the area of neurophysiologic disorders and biochemical factors. Research has linked violent behavior to temporal lobe epilepsy, tumors in the area of limbic system and temporal lobe, trauma to the brain, encephalitis, and damage to the amygdaloidal nucleus. Biochemical factors that have been implicated in violent behavior include hormonal dysfunctions found in hyperthyroidism and Cushing's disease. The neurotransmitters epinephrine, norepinephrine, dopamine, acetylcholine, and serotonin have been studied for a possible role in inhibiting or contributing to violent behavior.

Psychosocial factors include learning and socioeconomic factors. Learning influences the expression of aggressive behavior and violence. Role modeling and operant conditioning are two types of learning that relate to violence. Research into socioeconomic influences on violence has found that the incidence of violence is higher in poverty areas. It is thought that conditions associated with poverty (e.g., disruption of families, unemployment, and deprivation) are factors contributing to increased incidence of violence.

Environmental factors that have been studied in relationship to aggression include crowding, heat, presence of alcohol and drugs, and availability of firearms. Crowding has been implicated in increasing violence. Moderately uncomfortable temperature has been found to increase violence, whereas extremely hot temperatures are associated with decreased violence.

Specific factors can be identified in abuse-prone families. Upbringing and increased stress are considered important factors in the development of abusive patterns in families. The factor of upbringing includes being exposed to physical punishment and seeing violent conduct in the home. The violent parent is the role model, and the child may make a connection between love and violence. Emotional abuse from a parent may involve setting unrealistic goals and then criticizing and berating the child when the child does not reach these goals. The child grows up feeling worthless and may attempt to deal with feelings of inferiority and the need to protect himself by being hostile to and distrustful of others. He views people who are the objects of his abuse as "out to get me." The factor of increased stress becomes important when a person who feels inferior is faced with a crisis. The crisis increases the feelings of inferiority and low self-esteem, which may lead to an abusive incident.

 ## SIGNS AND SYMPTOMS

Signs of physical abuse include bruises, scars, cuts, facial injuries, and sprains. Look for signs of old injuries, because the victim may be seeking care for a problem not related to violent abuse. The abuser may not allow the victim to seek treatment after an episode of abuse. Symptoms commonly associated with physical and emotional abuse include headache, fatigue, back pain, gastrointestinal upset, anxiety, and insomnia. The signs and symptoms of emotional abuse may be subtle. The victim may act in a passive way, make only limited eye contact with the health care professional, and be reluctant to answer questions.

Low self-esteem is a characteristic found in both the abuser and the victim. It is useful to consider the defining characteristics of three North American Nursing Diagnosis Association (NANDA) nursing diagnoses related to self-esteem: self-esteem disturbance, chronic low self-esteem, and situational low self-esteem. The defining characteristics of these diagnoses can be viewed as signs and symptoms; they include self-negating verbalization, expressions of shame/guilt, evaluation of oneself as unable to deal with events, rejection of positive feedback and exaggeration of negative feedback about oneself, hesitancy to try new things, frequent lack of success in work or other life events, and nonassertive/passive behavior.

Keep in mind that a person who has experienced chronic abuse and severe trauma may repress his or her feelings and thus not show the behavioral manifestations associated with low self-esteem.

 DIAGNOSTIC CRITERIA

The Abuse Assessment Screen, developed by the Nursing Research Consortium on Violence and Abuse, is a very useful tool for identifying domestic violence. The screening tool comprises five main questions:

1. Have you ever been emotionally or physically abused by your partner?
2. Within the past year, have you been hit, slapped, kicked, or otherwise physically hurt by someone?
3. Since you have been pregnant, have you been hit, slapped, kicked, or otherwise physically hurt by someone?
4. Within the past year, has anyone forced you to have sexual activities?
5. Are you afraid of your partner or anyone in questions 1 through 4?

 INTERVENTIONS

It is important that the nurse be aware of the risk factors associated with abuse so that early identification can be made. These risk factors include presence of psychiatric illness, substance abuse, grief after death of a loved one, isolation, lack of support system, homelessness, previous violent behavior, chronic unemployment, weapons, history of runaways, single car accidents, and psychosomatic complaints.

It is also important that the nurse be aware of her or his own beliefs regarding domestic violence. These beliefs may interfere with the ability to recognize signs and symptoms. For example, a nurse may ignore the signs of domestic violence in a patient who is the wife of a prominent man in the community because he or she may think that domestic violence occurs only in families of low socioeconomic classes. Another belief that can block communication and interfere with intervention is the idea that abuse is the victim's fault. The nurse's reactions toward patients who present with signs of abuse may include anger toward the abuser, feeling helpless to improve the situation for the victim, fear that the abuser will be violent in the health care agency, and discomfort because the nurse may also be a victim of domestic violence.

The most important intervention is to ensure the victim's safety. Observe both verbal and nonverbal communication. If the abuser is present, find a way to spend time alone with the victim. Do not place the victim in jeopardy by asking her questions or giving her information on shelters in the presence of the abuser. Try to think of an "errand" or a task you can ask the abuser to perform so that you can get the victim alone.

When you are alone with the victim, use the assessment scale described earlier. Write the phone number of a shelter or crisis hotline where the abuser is not likely to notice the information, such as on the back of a wallet photo that the woman has in her purse. Give information on the cycle of violence, emphasizing that the episodes usually increase in intensity and frequency over time. Help the victim learn how to recognize signs of escalating stress in the abuser and to formulate an exit plan. You may also want to consult with or refer the victim to a mental health professional.

 COMMUNITY CARE

Several factors in the community influence violence. The attitude that "events in the family are private" serves to perpetuate family violence. Neighbors can become aware of actions of other families. The community needs to be aware of early indicators of possible domestic violence. Community resources for education and support of high-risk families are essential to prevent domestic violence. Community health nurses and school nurses can play a major role in the success of prevention programs.

Prevention occurs on three levels: primary, secondary, and tertiary. Primary prevention involves activities aimed at preventing domestic violence. Examples of primary prevention activities include developing a neighborhood watch program, teaching people how to improve personal safety, and teaching about such topics as parenting and coping with stress.

Secondary prevention activities are aimed at minimizing the effects of domestic violence through early intervention. Teaching families more effective communication patterns, effective parenting techniques, and coping strategies to deal with stress may help decrease episodes of violence. The nurse can work with community agencies to help establish screening programs to identify families in which domestic violence occurs. Support groups and psychotherapy groups can be established in outpatient settings. Self-help groups such as Alcoholics Anonymous, Alanon, Alateen, and Adult Children of Alcoholics may be helpful for families struggling with alcohol abuse.

Tertiary prevention involves interventions when there is an established pattern of abuse. The priority is the safety of each family member. The nurse can refer family members to appropriate individual, group, or family therapy.

Safe homes and shelters can be found in most major cities. The shelters provide physical safety as well as emotional support, legal assistance, employment counseling, and assistance in locating child care services and housing. Professional staff and volunteers work together to provide the needed services.

 PROGNOSIS

Without intervention, abuse almost never diminishes and almost always escalates. Each episode further erodes the self-esteem of the victim. With treatment, abusers can change their behavior. Victims of abuse can also learn new behaviors and successfully leave the abusive relationship. For changes to occur, the abuser must recognize that he can choose to respond with violence or choose to learn acceptable responses to his stress. Also, the victim must recognize that she does not deserve abuse and that the abuse is not her fault.

If treatment is not effective, the frequency and intensity of abuse may increase over time to a point where it results in serious injury to or death of the victim. Thus, it is essential that violence or the risk for violence be recognized early.

 CLINICAL PEARLS

○ A victim of abuse is at the greatest risk for injury when leaving the relationship.

- One out of ten abused women attempts suicide.
- A victim may leave many times before leaving for the final time.
- Battering usually increases during pregnancy.
- Pregnant teenagers have a higher incidence of abuse than pregnant adults.
- The most important intervention is to address issues related to safety.
- Encourage the victim to establish an exit plan.
- Three key risk factors for predicting violence are past history of violence, diagnosis, and current behaviors.
- Suspect that violence accompanies emotional abuse if the explanation does not match the injury seen.
- Internet resources include http://www.domestic-violence.org/ and www.ndvh.org/.

NURSING PROBLEM/ DIAGNOSIS	NURSING INTERVENTIONS CLASSIFICATION (NIC)
Acute management of the abused	Abuse protection Crisis intervention Emergency care Self-esteem enhancement
Management of undesirable behaviors	Counseling Anger control assistance Environmental management: violence protection Support group

Suicidal Ideation

Section 5   Patricia Rickli

 OVERVIEW

Approximately 30,000 people in the United States commit suicide each year. During any given 1-hour period, approximately 100 people in the United States attempt suicide. According to statistics from 1996, suicide is the ninth leading cause of death in the United States. Suicidal behaviors occur in all ages, socioeconomic classes, ethnic groups, and in both genders. Suicide has been identified as a significant public health problem by the World Health Organization and the U.S. Surgeon General.

Any nurse, regardless of specialty, may come in contact with a person experiencing suicidal ideation. Depression may accompany chronic physical illness, chronic pain, insomnia, and loss of function or role resulting from changing health status. Patients are often admitted to the general medical-surgical areas with physical problems that are secondary to alcohol abuse; these patients, along with those who have a secondary diagnosis of alcoholism, account for about 50% of successful suicides. Another group of patients at high risk is battered women.

All nurses must be able to recognize risk factors and clues that may indicate that a patient has a high potential for suicidal behavior. It is believed that loss of life can be prevented through education that focuses on suicide awareness, recognition of risk factors and warning signs, and early intervention.

PATHOPHYSIOLOGY

Suicide is not a diagnostic category but is rather a behavior that can be seen in a variety of diagnoses. Predisposing factors to suicidal behaviors include internalized anger; feelings of hopelessness, desperation, guilt, shame, and humiliation; a history of aggressive and violent behavior; developmental stressors; sociologic influences; genetic factors; and neurochemical factors. An estimated 30% to 70% of completed suicides are related to depression. Suicide is the leading cause of premature death in persons with schizophrenia. Because depression and schizophrenia greatly increase the risk of suicide, this section focuses on the psychobiology associated with those two diagnoses.

During the 1990s, deemed the "Decade of the Brain" by the 101st U.S. Congress, the biologic basis of behavior and mental illness became a research priority. Traditionally, the etiology of behavioral disturbances has focused on either the nature (biologic) or nurture (psychodynamic) view. Such an approach has made only limited contributions to the understanding of human behavior and mental illness. The biologic and psychodynamic bases of behavior need to be studied in concert instead of taking an either/or approach.

Neuroimaging has advanced our understanding of the function and the anatomy of the brain. Computed tomography (CT) scanning and magnetic resonance imaging (MRI) are used to study anatomic structures. The CT scan provides a three-dimensional view. CT scans of persons with schizophrenia and mood disorders (depression and bipolar) reveal nonspecific abnormalities. MRI studies done on persons with schizophrenia reveal such abnormalities as larger ventricles, cortical atrophy, and smaller temporal lobe and hippocampus. Positron-emission tomography (PET) and single photon emission computed tomography (SPECT) allow the noninvasive study of brain function and metabolic activity. Consistent finding in persons with schizophrenia include enlarged lateral ventricles and decreased cerebral blood flow and glucose utilization in the prefrontal cortex.

Neurotransmitters play a key role in the hypothesis of a biologic basis of specific psychiatric conditions. Mechanisms include decreased levels of norepinephrine, dopamine, and serotonin in depressive disorders; dopamine hyperactivity in schizophrenia; and increased levels of norepinephrine and decreased gamma-aminobutyric acid (GABA) in panic disorder. One theory links decreased serotonin level with suicidal behavior. Another theory related to suicidal behavior is that suicide-prone patients have increased numbers of serotonin-2 receptors in the brain and platelets.

The advances in neuroscience provide evidence that mental illness does have a biologic basis. Such findings help to decrease the stigma associated with psychiatric illness and improve treatment modalities.

No laboratory tests are definitive in establishing the diagnosis of depression and schizophrenia. In schizophrenia, abnormal laboratory findings may be related to side effects of prescribed medications, such as decreased granulocytes, or may be related to behaviors of the illness (e.g., drinking excessive amounts of water, which results in electrolyte imbalance). The dexamethasone suppression test (DST) is used by some clinicians as a screening tool for depression. The test has 90% specificity and 45% sensitivity. DST results have been found to be inconsistent and seem to be affected by age and gender. Excessive cortisol levels following the DST are also found in persons with anorexia nervosa and alcoholism.

About 50% of patients with moderate to severe depression exhibit hyperactivity of the hypothalamic-pituitary-adrenal (HPA) axis. The patient is given a dose of dexamethasone at night, and the cortisol level is measured in the morning. If the morning cortisol level is not excessive, then HPA axis function is considered normal.

SIGNS AND SYMPTOMS

Approximately 80% of persons completing suicide have given warnings and clues (overt or covert; verbal or nonverbal) that they were planning to commit suicide. Unfortunately, family and other associates often ignore the warnings or just do not believe that the person is serious.

A person may give away prized possessions, make sure that financial affairs are in order, and make comments along the line of "I won't be here when you get back." Clues also include decreased contact with family and friends. The person may also drop out of usual activities. The person may experience the loss of the ability to experience pleasure in activities that were once enjoyable. Listen for clues that indicate that the person views the situation as unbearable or hopeless.

DIAGNOSTIC CRITERIA

Depression has been identified as a factor in as many as 70% of completed suicides. Depression also is related to suicide attempts. It is estimated that about 10% of people seeking medical care also have coexisting depression. The depression is often not observed and thus is not treated. Untreated depression may have serious implications in terms of increased chronic illness and in incidence of suicide.

One tool for evaluating suicidal patients is called the SAD PERSONS scale. This scale lists 10 major risk factors for suicide. The patient receives one point for each factor present. The total number of points is associated with general guidelines for intervention. The 10 risk factors are as follows:

Sex. Males are at higher risk than females.

Age. Persons younger than 19 years of age and 65 years of age and older are at greatest risk.

Depression. Symptoms of depression are present in 35% to 80% of suicides.

Previous attempt. Previous attempts were made by 65% to 70% of those who complete suicides.

ETOH (alcohol). Other drugs are also used heavily; 65% of suicides involve alcohol.

Rational thinking loss. People with psychosis are at higher risk than the general population.

Social support lacking. A lack of relationships and connections with organizations increases the risk.

Organized plan. A specific plan that includes date, method, and the means is an obvious risk factor.

No spouse. Single, widowed, or divorced persons are at greater risk than the married population.

Sickness. Persons with chronic, debilitating illness are at greater risk.

Additional risk factors include being unemployed and having financial problems.

INTERVENTIONS

Caring for a person who is experiencing suicidal ideation or has made a suicidal attempt presents a great challenge for the nurse. Patients with suicidal behaviors are encountered not only by psychiatric nurses in mental health treatment settings, but also by nurses in various other settings, including intensive care units, emergency departments, general medical-surgical units, gynecologic and obstetric services, primary care clinics, pediatric and adolescent services, geriatric services, women's shelters, homeless shelters, and occupational/industrial settings.

Common emotional responses of the nurse when caring for a person with suicidal ideation or attempts include anxiety, irritation, avoidance, and denial. A nurse working with a suicidal patient may realize that she or he also has thoughts of suicide at times. Such a realization may make the nurse feel anxious and vulnerable. The nurse's response to a patient who has made numerous suicide attempts may be irritation. This may be a product of the nurse not understanding that the patient feels desperate and hopeless and lacks the coping skills and level of self-esteem necessary to deal with the situation. The nurse's irritation may be expressed directly through negative comments (e.g., "Quit wasting my time when I have patients who want to live to take care of") or sarcasm, or indirectly by avoiding the patient because the nurse does not know what to say. Denial may be in response to the nurse's inability to believe that a person would actually commit suicide. This denial can keep the nurse from identifying clues to suicidal risk.

The critical factor is to not miss the clues that may indicate risk of self-injury or suicide. The nurse who picks up clues that are of concern should discuss them with the primary care provider and a mental health professional who can further assess the patient's risk. A formal referral to a mental health professional may be needed. Whereas every nurse specialist is not equipped to do a complete assessment of suicide risk, every nurse does have the skills and the responsibility to identify clues of danger.

The ability to establish a professional relationship, to use active listening, and to communicate effectively is fundamental to the process of nursing. The quality of the database developed when taking a patient history and performing a nursing assessment depends on the patient's trust in the nurse. Active listening that focuses on both verbal and nonverbal components of the communication helps the nurse understand the patient's message and not just the words. Listen for statements and be aware of body language that may indicate hopelessness and the inability to cope with the present situation any longer. Hopelessness and poor self-esteem increase the risk of suicidal behavior. The information that the patient shares is related to his or her feeling that the nurse is interested and shows empathy. Be careful to not give a response that can make the person feel even more hopeless. Avoid such social phrases as "Things will get better"; "Cheer up—things can't be that bad"; or "Don't be talking about ending your life; you have so much to live for." Often such comments increase the patient's feelings of hopelessness, because he or she feels unable to communicate the depth of his or her despair.

Again, be aware of your own feelings in response to a patient who has engaged in suicidal ideation or attempts. The nurse's negative attitude toward a patient who has engaged in self-injury will adversely affect the care given. A critical, judgmental attitude by the nurse may serve to further decrease the patient's self-esteem and increase the risk of suicide.

A patient's direct or indirect comments about death should be investigated. The patient will most likely perceive the nurse's questions as an indication that the nurse is trying to understand the patient's desperation to obtain relief from an unbearable situation. For example, for a patient who recently lost his wife and has stated that he just cannot imagine life without her, an appropriate question would be "Have you thought about joining her?" If the patient's response hints that suicidal ideation is present, the nurse needs to directly ask the question, "Are you thinking about harming yourself?"

The nurse should strive to identify the message that the patient is sending, not just the actual words. For example, if the person says, "I don't think things will ever get any better," an appropriate response by the nurse would be "Are you saying you are in a hopeless situation? Are there any options that you can identify to help in this situation?" The nurse will use the knowledge of risk factors to identify areas to explore. Risk factors include marital status (single persons are twice as likely as married persons), gender (more women than men attempt suicide, but more men than women succeed), age (adolescents and people older than 65 years of age are at highest risk), presence of psychiatric illness, history of previous attempts, and family history of suicide. If a patient indicates that he or she is thinking of suicide, the nurse must refer that patient to a mental health professional for an in-depth assessment of suicide risk.

 ## COMMUNITY CARE

The evolution of treatment services for crisis intervention and mental illness has involved self-help/advocacy groups, identification of community needs, and legislation at the national level. The National Alliance for the Mentally Ill (NAMI) is a very active advocate group for family members of persons with mental illness. NAMI provides services to patients and families, supports research related to cause and treatment, and works to decrease the stigma associated with mental health issues. NAMI also works with suicide prevention and provides support for survivors of suicide.

Suicide, like mental illness, carries a stigma. For community-based programs of suicide prevention to be effective, the misinformation regarding suicide needs to be corrected. Accurate information will help decrease the stigma associated with suicide and increase the involvement of the community in programs. Attitudes that interfere with suicide prevention include the erroneous belief that nothing can be done, the belief that suicide is a crime that merits a punitive approach, and the belief that serious depression is a character defect rather than a disease with biologic factors. Common myths regarding suicide that need to be corrected include the following:

- A person who talks about suicide will not commit suicide.
- A person thinking seriously about suicide does not give clues.

- Only people with depression kill themselves.
- Asking a person if he or she is suicidal will put the idea in his or her head.
- A person who has made a serious suicide attempt will not try again.
- A person attempting suicide is completely intent on dying.

The nurse, as a member of the community, can help the community identify attitudes that are obstacles to suicide prevention, be aware of the resources, and request that public officials support programs that focus on mental health.

 PROGNOSIS

Suicidal behavior can be prevented and treated. The prognosis is related to the effectiveness of treatment for the coexisting condition such as depression, alcohol/substance use disorders, schizophrenia, chronic pain, and feelings associated with significant losses.

 CLINICAL PEARLS

○ Suicide is a behavior that can be prevented.
○ Know the risk factors associated with suicidal behavior—depression, previous attempt, use of alcohol or other drugs, and chronic debilitating disease with pain.
○ Some 80% of completed suicides have given verbal and nonverbal clues.
○ Always share your concerns of suicidal risk with team members.
○ View any attempt as a cry for help, and approach the patient with empathy rather than sarcasm or hostility.

NURSING PROBLEM/ DIAGNOSIS	NURSING INTERVENTIONS CLASSIFICATION (NIC)
Risk for suicide	Suicide prevention Behavior management: self-harm Anger control Support group
Depression (see Section 2)	

chapter 21

Musculoskeletal

Arthritis and Joint Replacement

Section 1 Selma Brophy ■ Beverly George-Gay

 OVERVIEW

Arthritis means "inflammation of the joints." It is usually accompanied by pain and often changes in structure. Arthritis may have an autoimmune component as well. This section deals primarily with rheumatoid arthritis (RA) and osteoarthritis (OA), the two major forms of arthritis in adults.

OA is extremely prevalent, affecting about 20 million Americans. It is estimated that one third of all adults have radiographic evidence of OA in the weight-bearing joints. Although OA can be found in any age group, the incidence increases with age, and men are affected more than women.

RA affects approximately 6 million Americans (1% to 2% of the population), 75% of whom are women. It can be found in any age group but is most commonly seen in women of childbearing age (Fig. 21-1-1).

 PATHOPHYSIOLOGY
Osteoarthritis

OA, also called *degenerative joint disease*, is a degenerative disease characterized by the progressive loss of articular cartilage in mobile joints, most commonly weight-bearing joints. Degeneration of the articular cartilage results in wear on the bone and irritation of bone against bone due to lack of cartilage buffering. OA is primarily noninflammatory and may be classified as idiopathic (primary) or secondary. Secondary OA is due to trauma, overuse, infection, or congenital joint abnormality.

Rheumatoid Arthritis

RA is a chronic systemic inflammatory disorder affecting the joints and most commonly results in nonsuppurative synovitis, which often progresses to degeneration of the articular cartilage and immobility of the joint. Other tissues and organs affected by RA include the skin, the blood vessels, the heart, the lungs, and the muscles. In RA, inflammation is the primary process, and degeneration is secondary. The exact cause of RA remains unknown; however, current research suggests an immune mechanism that is determined genetically. An antibody (rheumatoid factor [RF]) against self has been found in 80% of all patients and is believed to trigger the inflammatory response in genetically susceptible persons.

 SIGNS AND SYMPTOMS

Arthritis may have a variety of signs and symptoms, which may include fatigue, pain (chronic or acute), decreased mobility, decreased function of affected joints, weakness, anorexia, fever, redness, and swelling.

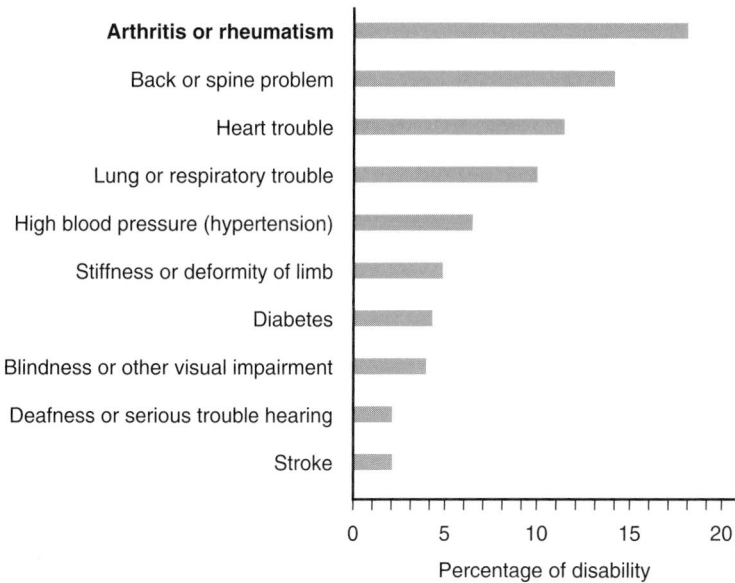

Figure 21-1-1. Leading causes of disability among persons aged 15 years and older in the United States (1991–1992).

Osteoarthritis

The onset of OA is insidious, with joint stiffness (usually in the neck or the back) progressing to joint pain (affecting the knees and the hips). Physical examination may reveal a knobby appearance of the digits. Heberden's nodes are an enlargement of the distal interphalangeal joint, and Bouchard's nodes are an enlargement of the proximal interphalangeal joint. Thumb bases may be tender and squared off. Small effusions, tenderness, and crepitus may be noticed at the knees. Range of motion may be limited significantly at the hip. The feet may reveal enlarged bunion joints. There are usually no systemic findings.

Rheumatoid Arthritis

The course of RA most often begins insidiously but may begin abruptly. It is usually progressive with exacerbations and remissions. Musculoskeletal symptoms include joint tenderness, swelling, and pain, usually symmetrical. Joint stiffness occurs on arising in the morning (lasting more than 1 hour) and following periods of inactivity, but it improves with activity. Joints commonly affected include the proximal interphalangeal joints, the metacarpophalangeal joints, the metatarsophalangeal joints, the wrists, the ankles, and the knees. Disease progression may lead to joint deformity and disability. Muscle atrophy and tendon destruction around the affected joints may cause one articular surface to slip or sublux past the other. Ulnar deviation is a characteristic deformity in which the fingers are flexed and turned toward the ulna. Swan-neck and boutonnière deformities of the fingers may also develop.

Nonspecific symptoms include malaise, fatigue, weight loss, anorexia, muscle weakness, and low-grade fever.

Extra-articular symptoms may also be noted, most commonly rheumatoid nodules. These are firm, nontender subcutaneous masses found over extensor surfaces or articular regions. They occur in up to 50% of patients. Other extra-articular symptoms include pleural effusion, pericarditis, vasculitis, compression neuropathies, Sjögren's syndrome (dry eyes and dry mouth due to decreased lacrimal and salivary gland secretions), episcleritis, and scleritis.

DIAGNOSTIC CRITERIA
Osteoarthritis

No specific tests or markers are available for OA. Radiography may reveal narrowing of the joint space, spur formation, sclerosis, and cystic erosions. Radiographic findings are present in 85% of patients older than 65 years of age. Synovial fluid, when aspirated, is noninflammatory.

Rheumatoid Arthritis

RA can be diagnosed from the presence of four or more of the following criteria, as classified by the American Rheumatism Association (the first four criteria must be present for at least 6 weeks):

1. Morning stiffness in and around joints lasting more than 1 hour before maximum improvement.
2. Soft tissue swelling of three or more joint areas (including right and left proximal interphalangeal, metacarpophalangeal, wrist, elbow, knee, ankle, and metatarsophalangeal joints).
3. Swelling of at least one wrist, metacarpophalangeal, or proximal interphalangeal joint.
4. Simultaneous symmetrical swelling in joints listed in criterion 2.
5. Subcutaneous rheumatoid nodules.
6. Presence of RF.
7. Radiologic erosions or periarticular osteopenia, or both, in hand or wrist joints.

Laboratory Tests

Rheumatoid Factor. RF is an immunoglobulin that appears in serum and synovial fluid several months after the onset of clinical disease. False-positive results can occur in the presence of other systemic diseases, however, and the test for RF is negative in up to 20% of cases. The normal value is less than 30 IU/mL.

Erythrocyte Sedimentation Rate. The erythrocyte sedimentation rate will be increased because it is an indicator of inflammation. It is also useful for monitoring the severity of disease. The normal value in an adult female is 20 to 30 mm/hr; in an adult male, the normal value is 15 to 20 mm/hr.

Synovial Fluid. Synovial fluid may be cloudy, milky, or dark yellow and may contain inflammatory cells.

Antinuclear Antibody. Antinuclear antibodies are antibodies produced by the body against its own DNA. A positive test response characterizes autoimmune disease.

Complete Blood Count. The complete blood count may reveal anemia due to chronic inflammation. The white blood cell count may or may not be increased.

Immunoglobulins. Hypergammaglobulinemia will be present, strongly suggesting an autoimmune process.

Radiography. Joint films will reveal soft tissue swelling and articular osteoporosis early in the disease process. Later, juxta-articular erosions and joint space narrowing will be noted.

 INTERVENTIONS

Interventions are based on the development of a suitable therapeutic regimen that promotes self-management. *Patient education that is understandable and culturally acceptable* is essential to success.

Pain and Symptom Management

Pain is frequently the presenting problem prompting an individual to seek treatment. Pain control and management are key to the implementation of other goals. Owing to the usual chronic nature of the pain and the probability of pain with movement, pain assessment is the first step in management.

Pain assessment includes evaluation of the following: (1) onset and duration of the pain, (2) characteristics of the pain, (3) movements and activities that increase pain, (4) methods used to control pain at home, (5) alternative or complementary therapies used, (6) effectiveness of pain management techniques, (7) activities or functions that are compromised because of pain, (8) the relationship of pain to the current problem (i.e., swollen joint), and (9) cultural beliefs regarding chronic disease pain. Patients with arthritis may at some point try alternative or complementary therapies or practices. Some of these practices may enhance standard treatment, whereas others may be of little or no value. A careful, nonjudgmental, sensitive health history including use of alternative therapies is essential to planning nursing interventions.

Pain management techniques include medication, application of heat or cold, massage, positioning, relaxation techniques, and reduction of fatigue.

Medications

Various medications are used for RA. More aggressive combination therapy is advocated over the use of single drug therapy, which was common in the past. The most common categories are nonsteroidal anti-inflammatory drugs (NSAIDs) and disease-modifying antirheumatic drugs.

Nonsteroidal Anti-inflammatory Drugs. NSAIDs are used for pain relief and have the added benefit of decreasing inflammation. These drugs have no effect on the underlying disease. Examples include ibuprofen, naproxen, ketoprofen, and diflunisal.

Disease-modifying Antirheumatic Drugs. Disease-modifying antirheumatic drugs alter the progression of RA. Because they can be toxic, frequent laboratory and physical evaluations of the skin and of liver, renal, bone marrow, and gastrointestinal function are required. They can be subclassified into two groups: slow-acting antirheumatic drugs and immunosuppressants.

Slow-acting Antirheumatic Drugs. Slow-acting antirheumatic drugs are used to alter the disease course and may arrest the progression of joint degeneration. They take weeks to months to show benefit, however. This delayed action must be explained to the patient to ensure continued compliance. Side effects include intense rashes with pruritus, stomatitis, nausea and vomiting, diarrhea, renal toxicity, and decreased blood counts. These drugs are often discontinued because of toxicity. Examples include gold compounds, antimalarial agents (e.g., hydroxychloroquine), penicillamine, and sulfasalazine.

Immunosuppressants. Immunosuppressants are used to restrain the autoimmune process. Side effects include bone marrow suppression, gastrointestinal ulceration, hepatic fibrosis, and pneumonitis. *Methotrexate is considered the first-choice drug for active RA* and results in rapid improvement. Other drugs in this group include azathioprine and cyclophosphamide.

Other Drugs. *Cyclooxygenase-2* (COX-2) inhibitors (celecoxib and rofecoxib) are also used. Cyclooxygenase is an enzyme required for the synthesis of mediators of the inflammatory response. COX-2 inhibitors are effective for the management of OA and have fewer side effects than NSAIDs.

Salicylates (aspirin, choline magnesium trisalicylate, salsalate) can be used for pain relief.

Corticosteroids (prednisone) are used for their anti-inflammatory and immunosuppressive effects, which can be topical, oral, or injected into the joints.

Antibiotics are used for patients with arthritis associated with infection, such as Lyme disease.

Application of Heat or Cold

Application of heat may be useful in reducing pain, stiffness, and muscle spasm. Heat can be applied in the form of baths, showers, or moist compresses, especially for larger joints. Paraffin dips are sometimes used for finger and wrist involvement. Applications of paraffin for 20 minutes are most beneficial.

During phases of the acute inflammatory process, application of cold may be tried. The use of heat or cold *must* be evaluated on an individual basis. Patient teaching must include information about the safe use of heat or cold, especially if there is any potential for impaired sensation.

Massage

Gentle massage may prove helpful for some individuals. Massage should not be strenuous, nor should it be painful. Massage should be performed over muscles, *not* joints.

Positioning

Positioning to maintain maximum mobility is very important. Many people who have arthritis are reluctant to move if it hurts; however, nonmovement can result in further loss of function and mobility.

Relaxation Techniques

Various relaxation techniques can be used, such as muscle relaxation, guided imagery, self-hypnosis, and distraction. It is important to evaluate the capability and the willingness of the individual to use these techniques before considering them.

Reduction of Fatigue

Reduction of fatigue is another major component of nursing intervention. Fatigue reduction involves planning activities to avoid strain (e.g., rearranging usual routines to accommodate periods when the patient has less pain or is less tired). Another fatigue-reducing technique is energy conservation (e.g., pacing activities, delegating activities that are too difficult, and prioritizing activities, or deciding which are most important to accomplish). The patient needs to take a very active role in planning for these techniques to be successful.

Maintenance of Functioning, Joint Mobility, and Functional Status

Maintenance of functional status is one of the most important goals of therapy. The focus is on what the patient is able to do. When necessary, assistive devices (e.g., canes, walkers, splints, braces, reaching devices, or chair lifts) are provided to extend function. Assistive devices in conjunction with medical therapy can improve functional status and help the patient to maintain a measure of independence.

One area that is frequently overlooked is sexual function. For patients who are sexually active, a sensitive exploration of how to maintain healthy sexual expression can be most important. A discussion of planning for sexual expression may include information about pain control, the time of day when function is optimal, the use of warm baths or showers to decrease stiffness, and the use of alternative positions.

Exercise and Physical Therapy

Exercise is one of the keys to maintaining mobility and function. The goal of exercise is to maintain or increase flexibility, muscle tone, circulation, and function. It may be necessary to consult with a physical therapist to plan a workable exercise program. Most individuals find it helpful to take a pain control medication 30 minutes before exercising. Patients with arthritis may require either group or individual support to continue exercise programs. Regular physical activity is recommended to maintain normal muscle strength, joint structure, and joint function in arthritis, especially in OA.

Prevention of Complications

Positioning and exercise are critical to maintaining function. Regular supervision is necessary to monitor or treat any other concomitant problems that may exacerbate the rheumatic symptoms. Injuries, infections, and other medical problems should be treated promptly. Arthritis increases the risk of development of osteoporosis, especially in women. Calcium, vitamin D, and hormone replacement therapy may be necessary (see Chapter 21, Section 4).

Another component in the prevention of complications is awareness of the possibility of depression (see Chapter 20, Section 2). Depression can accompany any chronic disease state and can compromise even the most excellent therapeutic regimen.

Appropriate Nutritional Practices

One of the problems commonly associated with arthritis is obesity. Obesity can place additional stress on affected joints and can impair mobility. It is a complex problem requiring both education and long-term support to manage additional lifestyle changes. Other nutritional problems can lead to decreased energy. There is no specific diet for arthritis, but overall nutrition should be maintained.

Surgical Intervention

Synovectomy. Synovectomy (removal of the synovial membrane) may be used as a prophylactic measure in RA to alleviate pain. It does not restore function.

Tenosynovectomy. Tenosynovectomy (surgical reconstruction of an inflamed tendon sheath) is used most frequently on hands to restore function.

Osteotomy. Osteotomy involves cutting the bone and redirecting the lines of force and weight bearing. This is used as an alternative to joint replacement (see later) for individuals who are 50 years of age or younger.

Arthrodesis. Arthrodesis involves the fusing or the joining together of bone to provide joint stability, relieve pain, and increase function. It is most useful on the wrists.

Joint Replacement. Joint replacement (arthroplasty) is the reconstruction of a joint or the replacement of a joint with an endoprosthesis. It is an elective procedure indicated for joint pain that has failed to respond to medication or that is increasing, for inability to perform activities of daily living, and for severely destroyed joint surfaces. Joint replacement can be performed on elbows, knees, shoulders, phalangeal finger joints, hips, ankles, and feet. It offers the patient with various forms of arthritis a significant decrease in pain with an increase in mobility. Patient understanding and compliance are crucial to an effective outcome, because physical therapy, exercises, and weight control maintenance are responsibilities that fall on the patient. Teaching begins in the preoperative period.

Total Hip Replacement and Total Hip Arthroplasty. In addition to the treatment of patients with RA and OA, total hip replacement may be used for fractures of the hip. Once the prosthesis has been placed, a drain is inserted. Management issues involve neurovascular assessment, pain, and blood loss. Prevention of prosthesis dislocation, infection, and deep vein thrombosis (DVT) is a primary nursing intervention. Care should also involve the prevention of the complications of immobility.

Neurovascular Assessment. Peripheral neurovascular injury can occur not only from the surgical procedure but also from immobilization devices. A neurovascular assessment (see Chapter 21, Section 2) of the affected hip should be obtained preoperatively and should be compared with the postoperative assessment. The affected hip should also be compared with the unaffected hip.

Blood Loss. Because blood loss during the procedure may be significant, autologous blood is collected weeks before the procedure (which is elective) and is used to replace blood lost during surgery. Blood and fluid accumulation in the wound may provide a site for infection. The drain put in during the procedure avoids this complication. Drainage amounts to 200 to 500 mL in the first 24 hours postoperatively and decreases to 30 mL or less on the second postoperative day, at which time drains are removed. Greater volumes must be reported. The nurse should assess how bloody the drainage is and the amount of drainage on the dressing. Autologous blood may be collected through the drainage tube through a filter into an autotransfusion container (see Chapter 2, Section 3). Use of an anticoagulant is required. Collection time is limited to 6 hours.

Pain. Pain is often managed with patient-controlled analgesia, epidural narcotics, or ketorolac (Toradol) during the first 24 to 48 hours, after which oral analgesics may be used. Increased pain should be reported. Pain management is imperative for appropriate rest and compliance (see Chapter 12, Section 1).

Dislocation. Signs of dislocation include shortening of the leg; increased pain and swelling at the surgical site, resulting in immobilization; and a reported "popping" feeling in the hip. If dislocation occurs, a second operation (revision arthroplasty) will be required. Internal rotation of the leg, adduction of the leg, and greater than 90 degrees of flexion (hyperflexion) of the hip will cause dislocation and must be avoided for 4 to 6 weeks postoperatively. An abduction pillow (or two or three pillows between the legs) may be used to keep the leg abducted, especially while sleeping and turning. Adduction is also avoided by teaching the patient never to cross the legs, to avoid bending forward to retrieve something from the floor, and to use assistive devices (long-handled reachers) for dressing and picking things up. The use of raised toilet seats, high-back chairs, and recliners helps prevent hip hyperflexion.

Muscle-strengthening physical therapy is employed to allow return to normal function and activities and to prevent dislocation. Physical therapy is started on the first postoperative day with ambulation and weight bearing for those with cemented prostheses. Weight bearing may be restricted for those with cementless prostheses for several days. Therapy continues throughout the recovery period, which may last 3 to 6 months.

Infection. Indications of wound infection include restricted hip motion, sensations of hip pressure, fever, pain, swelling, local warmth, and discharge. Because infection may result in removal of the prosthesis, prophylactic antibiotic therapy is initiated preoperatively and is continued for 3 to 5 days.

Deep Vein Thrombosis. Patients undergoing lower extremity arthroplastic procedures are in the highest-risk category for developing DVT. Without prophylaxis, the incidence of DVT after total hip arthroplasty is 40% to 50% (see Chapter 15, Section 3). A significant number of these patients will develop pulmonary emboli. DVT prophylaxis (see Chapter 15, Section 3) may involve anticoagulation with standard heparin, low-molecular-weight heparin (enoxaparin), or warfarin (see Chapter 12, Section 2). Low-dose heparin and aspirin have not been found to be efficacious and are not used in this patient population. Anticoagulation may continue for up to 6 weeks after joint replacement, depending on the patient. Pneumatic devices, antiembolic stockings, hourly ankle circle exercises, foot pumping (while awake), and ambulation are all required to reduce the risk of DVT (see Chapter 15, Section 3). Other exercises demonstrated by physical therapists to improve circulation and muscle tone should be continued at home.

Total Knee Replacement/Total Knee Arthroplasty. Total knee replacement is the replacement of arthritic or diseased femoral condyles, tibial plateau, and possibly patella with prosthetic components. Total knee replacement may be done bilaterally. Wound drains are usually placed, and a pressure dressing is applied. Neurovascular assessment of the affected leg, pain, and blood loss is similar to that for total hip replacement. Prevention of prosthesis loosening is a primary intervention. Interventions for the prevention of infection and DVT are similar to those for total hip replacement.

Blood Loss. Postoperative drainage ranges from 200 to 400 mL in the first 24 hours and decreases to less than 25 mL by 48 hours.

Dislocation. If the knee is dislocated, abduction is not necessary. The knee is immobilized with a commercially prepared immobilizer or a posterior splint after surgery, which keeps the knee extended. The device is worn at all times except during flexion exercises; it is especially important during ambulation. A continuous passive motion device is usually started on the first postoperative day, depending on the amount of drainage. The device accelerates healing by keeping the prosthetic knee in motion to prevent scar tissue formation, by increasing the range of motion, and by maintaining muscle strength. Continuous passive motion machines can be used 4 to 20 hours per day, depending on the needs of the patient. The device is preset to flex and extend the knee joint at certain degrees (20 to 30 degrees of flexion and 10 degrees of extension initially) and at a certain number of cycles per minute. The goal is to increase range of motion progressively to reach flexion of 90 degrees and total extension. Proper padding and positioning should be ensured.

Pain. Pain is managed with patient-controlled analgesia, intramuscular medications, or oral therapy.

Infection. Prophylactic antibiotic therapy is initiated preoperatively and is continued for 1 to 2 days.

Deep Vein Thrombosis. Without prophylaxis, the incidence of DVT after TKA is up to 70% (see Chapter 15, Section 3).

 ## COMMUNITY CARE

Arthritis is usually a chronic disease that requires management by the patient in the community. The nurse must teach self-management of all interventions discussed previously. Care of the patient should be reviewed, and he or she should be monitored for complications.

Patients receiving medications must be frequently re-evaluated for drug toxicity. They must avoid any over-the-counter drugs that have not been cleared by the health care professional.

Many alternative therapies are available. Research studies either have not been done or have shown no benefit for many of these therapies. These alternative options should be reviewed with the health care provider before use.

The Arthritis Foundation (www.arthritis.org) is a very useful resource for these patients.

 ## PROGNOSIS

Arthritis is a chronic condition that has no cure. Untreated, the various arthritic conditions can lead to decreased mobility, quality of life, and functional status. The major goals of treatment are to maintain or improve joint mobility and function, manage or control pain, and improve quality of life.

 ## CLINICAL PEARLS

○ A careful, sensitive, unrushed assessment is crucial to providing quality care.
○ Socioeconomic and cultural factors *must* be considered in planning adherence to treatment regimens.
○ Patient education is a necessity!
○ It is extremely important to discuss the need to maintain medication regimens. Prematurely discontinuing medications can lead to complications.
○ Quality care depends on *collaboration* and *cooperation* with the individual who has a chronic condition.

○ Spiritual resources are important.
○ A sexual history should be obtained when function and mobility are impaired.

NURSING PROBLEM/ DIAGNOSIS	NURSING INTERVENTIONS CLASSIFICATION (NIC)
Chronic pain	Pain management
	Analgesic administration
	Heat/cold application
Impaired physical mobility	Exercise therapy: joint mobility
	Teaching: prescribed activity, exercise
Postsurgical management	Circulatory precautions
	Peripheral sensation management
	Positioning
	Infection protection
	Exercise therapy

Fractures

Section 2   Linda McCuistion

 OVERVIEW

Fractures occur in all age groups, with the highest incidence in males 15 to 24 years of age and in elderly persons, especially females older than 65 years of age. Adequate bone healing is affected by the patient's age and general condition, fracture location and reduction, circulation, immobilization, and remobilization.

 PATHOPHYSIOLOGY

The causes of fractures include direct or indirect force, torsion, muscle spasms, and bone disease.

A *closed* (or *simple*) fracture is a bone fracture in which the skin remains intact without external injury. In an *open* (or *compound*) fracture, a fractured bone penetrates the skin but may or may not protrude through it. When the skin is broken, soft tissue injury and blood loss usually occur from the sharp, jagged bone edges.

Several types of fractures are characterized by their fracture line, including complete and incomplete fractures. Examples of complete fractures are the following: *oblique*, a diagonal break across the bone axis or at a 45-degree angle; *transverse*, a break directly across the axis of the bone; *spiral*, a complete break that partially encircles the bone; and *comminuted*, a break splintered into multiple fragments, usually as a result of crush injuries.

Examples of incomplete fractures are a skull fracture and a *greenstick* fracture, which is more common in children than adults owing to their bone composition. In the greenstick fracture, the more flexible bone shaft is bent and cracked but is not completely broken.

Bone Healing

The process of bone healing involves five stages (Fig. 21-2-1). The first stage, which begins immediately after injury and lasts approximately 1 day, is called the *hematoma formation* stage. Immediately after a fracture, bleeding usually occurs from ruptured vessels in the bone, the torn periosteum, and the surrounding soft tissue. The immediate bleeding coagulates to form a hematoma or a clot around the injured site. This mesh of fibrin safeguards the damaged bone and acts as a scaffold for the ingrowth of capillary buds and fibroblasts.

The second stage of bone healing, called *cellular proliferation*, lasts 2 to 6 days. The fibroblasts from the periosteum and the nearby connective tissue enter the injured site and change into fibrous connective tissue or granulation tissue. White blood cells migrate into the injured area to contain the inflammation by phagocytosing the red blood cells and tissue debris.

The third stage of bone healing is called *callus formation* and lasts approximately from days 6 to 10. Osteoblasts invade the clot and the granulation tissue to form a soft tissue or provisional callus around the injured site. The granulation tissue changes into callus, which is composed of newly formed cartilage and bone matrix. This newly formed callus is strong enough to hold bones together but is not strong enough to bear weight.

Next is the *callus ossification* stage, lasting 2 to 10 weeks. New rigid bone and cartilage are dispersed into the soft tissue callus, and calcium salts are deposited into it. This causes rigid calcification forming a permanent callus.

The last stage, *consolidation with remodeling*, may last 2 months to 1 year. Bone tissue overgrowth and excess calcium are remolded to normal bone contour by osteoclastic activity.

 SIGNS AND SYMPTOMS

The major symptom of a fracture is pain, which is usually immediate. Fracture pain is generally continuous and very severe on movement. The

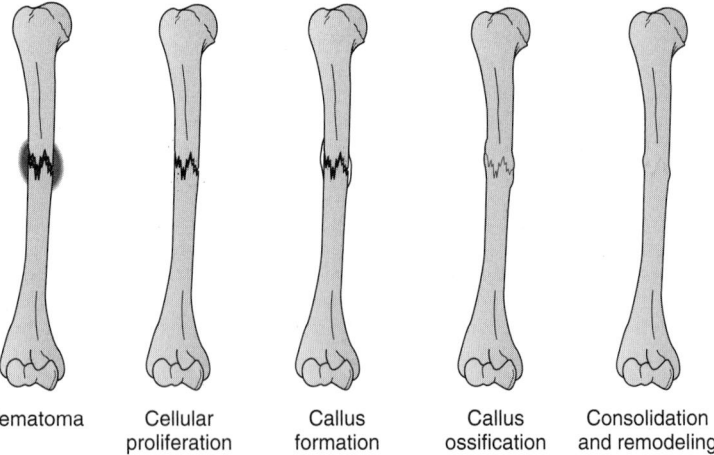

| Hematoma | Cellular proliferation | Callus formation | Callus ossification | Consolidation and remodeling |

Figure 21-2-1. Stages of bone healing.

severity usually increases until the fracture site is splinted and protected. An injured patient with a fracture may also experience tenderness on palpation. Bone pain is usually due to stretching, swelling, and rubbing of the periosteum.

A change in bone alignment resulting in a deformity may be a sign of bone fracture. If the break involves an arm or a leg, the extremity may have internal or external rotation, angulation, or displacement, or the affected limb may be shorter than the matching extremity owing to overlapping or telescoping of bone fragments. Abnormal movement may be present as a result of instability of the broken bone.

Other symptoms of a fracture include paresthesia or abnormal sensations owing to nerve injury from a pinched or severed nerve. Crepitus, which may be noted on movement, is a grating sound or sensation caused by jagged bone ends rubbing together. The patient with a fracture usually experiences muscle spasms resulting from sudden involuntary muscle contractions, which are stimulated by nerve irritation. Edema may also be present after a fracture and is caused by the extravasation of blood into tissues, resulting in accumulation of serous fluid at the injury site and contributing to a discolored appearance.

 ## DIAGNOSTIC CRITERIA

When the nurse obtains the trauma history, the patient usually describes hearing or feeling the bone break. Physical examination may reveal edema, deformity, crepitus, moveable bone fragments, muscle spasms, or ecchymosis. The most common diagnostic aid in determining the location of a fracture and the extent of trauma is radiography. A complete set of x-ray films is needed to evaluate the fracture site adequately.

Computed tomography, bone scanning, and magnetic resonance imaging are also used to visualize fractures and soft tissue damage. A computed tomographic scan detects fractures of complex structures (e.g., hip, pelvis) and compression fractures of the spine. A gallium bone scan is helpful in detecting small bone fractures, delayed or nonhealing fractures, infection, or avascular necrosis. Magnetic resonance imaging detects vertebral and skull fractures as well as soft tissue damage. If a stress fracture is suspected but is not seen on the radiograph, a bone scan or magnetic resonance imaging may be used to diagnose the fracture. If nearby soft tissue trauma is present, arteriography may be necessary to determine associated vascular damage. If a large amount of blood has been lost, hemoglobin and hematocrit values can be obtained to determine the amount of blood loss.

 ## INTERVENTIONS

The immediate goal of fracture intervention is to regain alignment, which is achieved by means of fracture reduction. Further goals are to retain alignment to allow for the healing process, to restore function, and to prevent further tissue injury and complications. Alignment is maintained by immobilization of the reduced fracture site, which is accomplished by means of traction or casting. Function is restored by the use of rehabilitative exercises.

At the trauma or accident site, the patient with a suspected fracture should be assessed for deformity, shortening of the extremity, limited or abnormal movement, pain, swelling, diminished neurovascular status, discoloration, soft tissue damage, or crepitus. To ensure a complete neurovascular assessment, follow the "7 P's" (see Nursing Management). When a fracture is suspected, the site should be splinted immediately to provide immobilization and to prevent movement of the injured part before the victim is moved. One should never try to elicit crepitus by moving an injured body part because it may cause further damage. Elevation decreases swelling, and applications of cold decrease bleeding and pain. See Chapter 1, Section 4 for first aid care.

If medical equipment is available at the injury scene, oxygen may be administered to ensure adequate tissue oxygenation. Also, attainment of venous access for the provision of fluid replacement needs immediate attention.

Medical Management

Fracture Reduction

Fracture reduction is the replacement of fractured bones into their normal anatomic position. Realignment of fractured bone fragments is achieved by means of either open or closed reduction or traction. A fracture should be reduced as soon as possible because swelling tends to increase for 6 to 12 hours after an injury. The localized soft tissue swelling at the fracture site may become inelastic, making reduction more difficult.

Open Reduction. Open reduction is indicated when closed reduction cannot be accomplished or has failed. It may also be preferred because it allows early use of a joint or an extremity. Open reduction involves surgery with direct visualization of the injury. Open reduction with internal fixation to stabilize the fracture and promote bone healing should be performed within 24 to 48 hours in medically stable patients. Unstable patients require stabilization before surgery for safety reasons. Contraindications to open reduction include excessively weakened bones, in which fixation devices cannot be secured; severely damaged surrounding soft tissue, such as in burns; medical conditions that preclude anesthesia; active infection; or osteomyelitis.

Prophylactic antibiotics should be administered within 2 hours of a fracture and should be continued for at least 24 hours. Heparin may be administered for DVT prophylaxis. Additionally, deep breathing, turning if allowed, adequate fluids, and compression stockings are used for the prevention of thromboembolism.

Closed Reduction. Closed reduction is indicated for patients who are unable to tolerate open reduction. This method involves realignment of the broken bones without direct visualization. Closed reduction may be accomplished by means of manual manipulation or reduction traction. Immobilization of the broken fragments must be performed to retain alignment and allow for proper healing. Inadequate immobilization can lead to a shifting of the realigned bones with resultant delayed or abnormal union. Bearing weight on the injured extremity too soon may disrupt the bone healing stages and cause new bleeding. Additionally, bearing weight too soon in the provisional soft callus stage may cause malformation and deformity.

Reduction Traction. Reduction traction may also be performed to reduce a fracture by applying a pulling force, which realigns broken bone. This is used for patients (e.g., the elderly) who are unable to undergo open reduction because of the dangers associated with surgical anesthesia. In some cases, closed reduction may cause additional fractures in fragile bones, requiring an alternative method of reduction.

Fracture Immobilization

Casting. After a fracture occurs, a cast splint is applied initially. A cast splint is a half cast, made up of solid casting material usually placed on the underside of the injured extremity, with an elastic bandage encircling the protected area and securing the half cast in place. While immobilizing the affected area, the cast splint allows the injured soft tissue to swell and expand.

After the danger period for swelling (usually 12 to 24 hours) has passed, a rigid cast that completely encircles the injured part is usually applied more securely to support and immobilize the fracture site. Casting material may be plaster of Paris or fiberglass. A plaster cast takes approximately 10 minutes to set or take shape and dries slowly over 1 to 3 days. Care of the plaster cast involves keeping it dry. If a plaster cast becomes wet, strength and integrity are lost. The plaster cast is very heavy and may cause equilibrium problems in a frail patient.

Special handling of a plaster cast is necessary. The initial cast is described as "green" and has not yet thoroughly dried. If the cast is handled improperly with the fingertips, indentations may be pressed into the cast and may cause areas of pressure under it. Therefore, a wet cast should be handled with the palms of the hands. Another possible cause of pressure areas is placement of a green cast on a hard surface. Care should be taken to place a newly applied cast on a pillow or a soft surface.

The fiberglass cast dries quickly, usually in less than 20 minutes when aided by ultraviolet light, and is very lightweight. This newer, more expensive cast may be immersed in water and will not lose its shape. After being immersed, however, the fiberglass cast must be dried thoroughly or skin maceration may occur underneath it. Use of a blow dryer on a cool setting is usually sufficient to dry the fiberglass cast thoroughly.

Windowing or bivalving of a cast is done when visualization of an injured site is required or on cast removal. If an infection is suspected, direct access to the injured site via a cast window is necessary for visualization and treatment. In bivalving, a cut is made along the lateral portions of the cast, and the top half is removed, allowing more extensive visualization of an affected extremity. When the cast cutter is being used, the patient will feel vibration and pressure, but the oscillating motion of the tool is designed to avoid cutting the patient's skin. The padding under the cast may then be cut with scissors and removed.

Traction. Traction employs a system of weights and pulleys attached to the patient's body. It may be used to reduce a fracture, to maintain alignment of bone fragments during healing, to decrease muscle spasms, and to prevent or correct deformities. Either skin or skeletal application methods can be used.

Skin Traction. Skin traction is the application of a traction apparatus to skin or soft tissue. This treatment is usually employed for less than 3 to 4 weeks. In skin traction, the pull of weight is exerted directly on the skin. Therefore, skin conditions, such as a rash, dermatitis, lacerations, an open wound, or allergy to the adhesive, would be contraindications to skin traction. Additional contraindications include poor circulation (e.g., peripheral vascular disease) or diabetes mellitus. Because the pull of the weight applied to skin or soft tissue may result in damage, the maximum weight for skin traction is less than 5 to 8 pounds.

Skeletal Traction. Skeletal traction is a pull exerted directly on the skeleton.

It not only exerts a longitudinal pull but also controls rotation. Usually, a pin is inserted perpendicular to the long axis of the bone, and weights are attached to produce the required pull. Because bone is stronger than soft tissue, up to 20 to 30 pounds of weight may be used for skeletal traction for as long as 3 or 4 months. This treatment is achieved via insertion of a Steinmann pin or a Kirschner wire, which is connected to a holder or a bow and then to the ropes and a free-hanging pulley system. Both the Steinmann pin and the Kirschner wire are round stainless steel rods. Although the Kirschner wire is a thin wire of 0.7 to 1.6 mm, the Steinmann pin has a larger diameter, 2 to 4.8 mm.

Pin Tract Infection

Pin care is an important nursing intervention for a patient in skeletal traction. Monitor the pin site for infection every 8 hours, noting purulent drainage, warmth, pain, and fever. Pin care should be done as often as prescribed or at least once a shift. The pin sites should be assessed for irritation, redness, swelling, tenderness, and drainage. After gloving, the nurse should cleanse the site beginning from the insertion site outward in a circular motion using sterile cotton-tipped applicators and the cleansing solution of hydrogen peroxide, alcohol, or povidone-iodine (Betadine), as prescribed by the physician or hospital policy. Separate applicators should be used for each pin site to prevent cross-contamination. Betadine or antibiotic ointment is applied only if ordered. Some ointments react with certain metals of the traction pins and may also increase bacterial growth by providing a moist environment. If any drainage is noted, the physician should be notified, who may order a culture to detect infection. Because patients have a tendency to touch their injured site, the nurse should instruct them to avoid touching the pin sites to prevent infection.

Types of Traction

Buck's traction is the most common type of skin traction applied to the affected lower extremity to relieve muscle spasms or to immobilize or reduce a fracture. Buck's traction may be applied by placing commercial skin traction strips on both sides of the lower leg (laterally and medially). Next, an elastic wrap, such as an Ace bandage, is applied to ensure that the strips remain in place. A newer form of Buck's traction apparatus is a foam boot, which is secured around an injured leg with Velcro straps. A footplate is attached to the traction apparatus and to weights at the foot of the bed via a rope-and-pulley system. Buck's traction is generally used when traction is needed for less than 72 hours.

Russell's traction may be either a skin or a skeletal application to the affected lower extremity. It is especially useful in reducing an intertrochanteric fracture of the femur. Russell skin traction is applied with a Buck's apparatus plus a knee sling, which suspends the knee in midair. Russell skeletal traction usually uses a Steinmann pin through the proximal tibia with a knee suspension and double-pulley system. The double-pulley system exerts a pull equal to double the weight used. For example, if the weight of a double-pulley system is 10 pounds, the pull exerted is 20 pounds.

Straight skeletal traction or running traction is applied with a Kirschner wire or a Steinmann pin inserted through the bone distal to the fracture and perpendicular to the long bone axis. The pulley apparatus is attached to the pin on each side of the bone, and a pull is exerted on the skeleton by the weight. This results in a pull on the fractured extremity to regain alignment of and treat joint contractures.

Balanced suspension traction uses a Thomas splint with a Pearson attachment. With this traction variation, the patient is able to move more freely in bed while the affected extremity is supported. Suspension allows the patient's fractured part to "float" over the bed, which facilitates bedpan use and bed linen changes with minimal disturbance of the fracture.

Side-arm traction can be used for immobilization of fractures or dislocations of the upper arm and the shoulder. The shoulder is abducted 90 degrees from the body and is externally rotated. The elbow is flexed 90 degrees and is held perpendicular. In side-arm traction, the involved pressure sites are the scapula, the axilla, and the elbow.

Overhead or 90–90 traction may be used for immobilization of either an arm or a leg fracture or dislocation. The proximal injured extremity is placed perpendicular to the body. Joints of the extremity are flexed 90 degrees. The distal injured extremity is parallel to the body and rests in a supporting sling. The hand or the foot must be kept fully supported by the sling or the footplate. If either the hand or the foot is allowed to droop, circulatory impairment or contractures may develop. Pressure sites include the scapula and the coccyx.

An *external fixation device* is commonly used to stabilize the reduction of a comminuted fracture. Several pins are inserted into the fractured bone as a scaffold to hold bone fragments together securely. The main complication of an external fixation device is infection secondary to the multiple entrance sites into the body.

Manual traction is a temporary method of traction applied with the hands. It may be used during cast application, traction apparatus adjustment, or weight removal.

Traction must be continuous, unless the physician specifies otherwise. Any disruption of traction, especially skeletal traction, may further damage the fracture site. *Countertraction* must be sufficient for the traction to be effective. The patient's body weight and the bed position often supply the required countertraction to any type of traction; however, additional countertraction is sometimes needed to keep the patient from sliding to the foot of the bed. In Russell's traction, the added countertraction is achieved by elevating the foot of the bed on 6-inch blocks or by placing the bed in Trendelenburg's position. Good body alignment must be maintained for the patient in traction to maintain the appropriate line of pull. *Ropes and weights must be free of friction.* Ropes must be kept in the center of the pulley. Weights should hang freely and should not rest on a chair, the bed, or the floor. The knots used in the traction system must not be caught in the pulley system or entangled in the bed linen.

Nursing Management

Nursing management of a fracture involves the prevention of complications and the restoration of independent function. The keys to preventing complications are close monitoring and preservation of neurovascular status.

Neurovascular Compromise

Excess pressure from bandages, traction devices, casts, or dressings can lead to swelling, which can cause neurovascular impairment and irreparable soft tissue damage. Nerve impairment alone is usually due to compression and excess pressure on peripheral nerves. The nerve most commonly injured by traction is the peroneal nerve. The peroneal nerve is located nearest the surface just below the lateral head of the fibula. With damage of the peroneal nerve, the patient may develop footdrop.

Application of cold and elevation of a fractured extremity above heart level reduce swelling and may prevent further complications. Inclusion of the "7 P's" ensures a thorough neurovascular assessment.

1. Pain—the main symptom of circulatory impairment
2. Pallor—sometimes cyanosis
3. Paralysis—the patient's inability to move extremities
4. Paresthesia—abnormal sensations in the affected extremity, such as tingling, numbness, prickling, or increased sensitivity
5. Pulselessness—pulse quality and rate
6. Puffiness—swelling at the affected site
7. Poikilothermia—cool skin temperature

Compare the injured part with the opposite extremity whenever possible to assess skin color, movement, pulse quality, puffiness, and skin temperature. Also, evaluate capillary refill by performing the blanching test.

Nerve Assessment

Because nerve impairment is very serious, the function of pertinent nerves should be assessed frequently. The peroneal nerve should be evaluated for any type of lower extremity traction. To assess sensation, the nurse should stroke the web space between the great and second toes of the affected extremity. To determine peroneal nerve function on movement, the nurse should instruct the patient to dorsiflex the affected foot. To evaluate tibial nerve function on movement, the nurse should instruct the patient to plantar flex the affected foot. Additionally, by noting the sensation on the ulnar side of the little finger, the ulnar nerve may be assessed. The ability to abduct the little finger is evidence that the ulnar nerve movement function is intact. If sensation or function is decreased or absent, the nurse should notify the physician immediately.

Vascular Assessment

Because many fracture complications are related to impaired circulation, the nurse should assess the patient's circulation frequently. Initially, circulatory status should be evaluated every 15 minutes, progressing to every 4 hours. Proximal and distal pulses need to be monitored. Color and temperature of the skin and capillary refill need to be assessed. The injured part should be evaluated for edema, pain, paresthesia, and mobility. The patient should be taught to report promptly any changes in paresthesia, such as numbness or tingling. Homans' sign and calf tenderness are indications of DVT. If Homans' sign is positive, one should NOT repeat it, because a blood clot might be dislodged. Although Homans' sign is not definitive, it does provide valuable data.

Progression of Activity

Immobilization holds the bone in place, promotes healing, relieves pain, prevents rotation and shearing, and maintains reduction. The fracture needs to be immobilized, however, not the patient. When moving or turning the patient in bed, the nurse should provide support of the joint above and below the fracture site; muscle spasms may be caused by grasping the belly of a muscle, such as the calf. The patient progresses to ambulation as quickly as possible to avoid complications of immobility. See Table 21-2-1 for the complications

Table 21-2-1. Complications of Immobility

COMPLICATION	CAUSE	PREVENTION
Thrombus formation	Prolonged bed rest leads to decreased circulation and allows clot formation; slings or other types of traction apparatus may damage the vessel intima and also promote clot formation	Range of motion or isometric exercises, antiembolism hose, and pneumatic compression devices to stimulate circulation Avoid smoking and caffeine to prevent vasoconstriction Promote adequate hydration Prophylactic anticoagulation may be needed
Pulmonary embolus	Same as for thrombus formation	Same as for thrombus formation
Orthostatic hypotension	Vascular muscle weakness from prolonged bed rest	Range of motion or isometric exercises as often as possible
Atelectasis	Inadequate ventilation due to decreased chest expansion from bed rest	Deep breathe, cough, and use incentive spirometer at least every 2 hours
Hypostatic pneumonia	Inadequate ventilation due to decreased chest expansion; creates pulmonary environment for bacterial growth	Deep breathe, cough, and use incentive spirometer at least every 2 hours
Urinary tract infection	Prolonged bed rest in recumbent position and gravity allow urine buildup in kidney pelvis; also, dehydration may contribute	Instruct client to drink at least 8 glasses of water per day
Constipation	Prolonged bed rest leads to decreased peristalsis; also analgesics and other medication decrease peristalsis	Instruct client to drink at least 8 glasses of water per day Increase fiber in diet Use stool softeners or laxatives as needed
Muscle atrophy	Disuse of muscles	Range of motion or isometric exercises
Joint contractures	Disuse of joints leads to shortening of tendons and ligaments	Range of motion exercises as often as treatment will allow
Osteoporosis	Without the stress of weight bearing on bone periosteum, bone resorption occurs at a greater rate and calcium is lost, which results in weaker bones	Range of motion or isometric exercises Tensing or tightening of muscles in the thigh and buttocks helps maintain muscle function and strength, which are important in ambulation
Emotional depression	Forced inactivity and uncertainty of prognosis lead to emotional depression	Explain procedures to client; encourage questions and verbalization of feelings Promote independence Facilitate communication between other pertinent health team members (e.g., clergy, counselor)
Renal calculi	Calcium is resorbed from bones owing to lack of movement resulting in increased level outside the bone which contributes to calcium crystal formation in the urine	Instruct client to drink at least 8 glasses of water per day

of immobility and prevention methods. Mobilization of the patient by means of an adequate exercise regimen increases circulation, promotes healing, and assists in restoring function. Usually, physical therapy is necessary to remobilize the fractured area properly.

Pain Management

Pain management is a major part of the nursing care of patients with fractures. When pain is controlled, the patient can exercise with greater ease (see Chapter 12, Section 1).

Analgesics. The patient may require narcotic analgesics initially. Later, NSAIDs become very useful and are effective with 6- to 8-hour dosing.

Complications of Fractures

Compartment Syndrome. Compartment syndrome, also known as *Volkmann's contracture*, is considered a medical emergency because neuromuscular damage may be irreversible within 6 hours of compression. Compartment syndrome is due to excessive pressure from tight bandages, bleeding into tissue, or trauma due to injury or surgery. Excess pressure impairs circulation, which leads to ischemia and muscle infarction. Ischemic muscle tissue releases histamine, which increases capillary permeability and allows plasma proteins to leak into the interstitial fluid space. Continued leaking leads to further edema.

Compartment syndrome usually develops within 2 hours to 6 days of excessive compression, with the initial sign being diminished pulse. As the swelling continues to affect the neurovascular status, pain, paresthesia, pallor, cool skin, and loss of function develop. Decompressive fasciotomy may be needed to relieve the excessive pressure caused by soft tissue swelling. Compartment syndrome usually occurs in the hand, and, if uncorrected, fibrous scar tissue replaces muscle, tendons, and nerves, resulting in the typical claw hand deformity. When compartment syndrome is suspected, a continuous monitoring system may be needed to measure invasively the compartment pressure readings and to detect the syndrome at an early stage.

Fat Embolus. A fat embolus is a potentially fatal complication and most often occurs after a fracture of the pelvis or the long bones. This complication usually occurs 1 to 3 days after an injury or surgery. Mechanical and biochemical theories explain its cause. In the mechanical theory, manipulation of bone fragments allows a release of fat from the yellow bone marrow, which floats in the circulation as an embolus. The biochemical theory is concerned with the alteration of lipid metabolism owing to trauma, resulting in the formation of fat globules that float in the blood vessels.

Signs and symptoms of this complication reflect a triad of central nervous system (CNS), pulmonary, and skin involvement. The CNS signs and symptoms include confusion, tachycardia, tachypnea, fever, lethargy, and an altered mental status. Lung involvement leads to dyspnea, restlessness, wheezes, and rales. The patient usually states that he or she cannot breathe or is smothering. Skin involvement includes the classic symptom of petechiae, usually present on the face, the neck, the axilla, the conjunctiva, and the soft palate.

A fat embolus may be prevented by moving high-risk patients only minimally. Important nursing interventions include identifying high-risk patients and monitoring them for early signs and symptoms of fat emboli. Thorough assessment of respiratory status, lung auscultation, and monitoring of arterial blood gases and vital signs may help detect this complication as soon as possible. Once detected, fat embolus may be treated with corticosteroids and adequate hydration treated with albumin, a volume expander.

Gas Gangrene. Gas gangrene and tetanus are complications that usually occur with open contaminated wounds. *Clostridium perfringens, Clostridium novyi*, and *Clostridium septicum* are the responsible organisms in gas gangrene, which is a severe infection of the skeletal muscle. Signs include local edema, severe pain, crepitus of soft tissue from vesicles filled with a watery fluid and gas, tachycardia, fever, and a coppery skin color. Treatment involves surgical débridement, antibiotics, and hyperbaric oxygen; amputation may be necessary.

Skin Breakdown. Skin breakdown is usually caused by irritation caused by a traction device or by a reaction to tape or foam. Also, if there is not enough countertraction, the patient is pulled to the end of the bed by the weights, exerting a shearing force on the skin. Shearing forces could cause damage to the skin over bony prominences.

Skin Assessment. It is imperative to maintain intact skin and to prevent unnecessary problems for the patient in traction. By using adequate countertraction, the nurse should keep the patient from sliding to the foot of the bed via a shearing force. To limit any excess jostling and movement of the patient, bed linen should be changed beginning with the unaffected side. By changing bed linen on the affected side of the bed last, the clean linen may be pulled through with minimal patient movement. If the patient is able, he or she should be encouraged to assist in this process by pulling up on the overhead trapeze, allowing easy removal of linen. The patient should be encouraged to eat and drink meals high in protein and vitamin C to promote healing and to maintain nutrition of healthy skin. Back care should be given every 2 hours. Special mattresses (air-filled or high-density foam of 4-inch minimal thickness) may be used to prevent pressure ulcers.

Tetanus. Tetanus, caused by *Clostridium tetani*, is a neurologic condition with an onset of 3 to 14 days after exposure, usually at the time of injury. Tetanus may be localized if only the nerves supplying affected muscles are affected. When toxins enter the lymphatics and the bloodstream, the condition becomes generalized. Tetanus is characterized by increased muscle tone and spasms. Laryngospasm, dysphagia, twitching, irritability, restlessness, stiffness, muscle rigidity (lockjaw or opisthotonos), weakness, paralysis, diaphoresis, and ileus are common. Treatment includes antibiotics, an antitoxin, physical therapy to prevent contractures, fluids, and nutrition therapy. Muscle relaxants (e.g., diazepam, benzodiazepine, lorazepam, and midazolam) are used to control muscle spasms. Ventilatory support may be required for laryngospasms.

This condition lasts 4 to 6 weeks, with increased tone and spasms lasting for months. Recovery from tetanus is usually complete without residual sequelae, but the condition is entirely preventable with immunization.

Avascular Necrosis. In avascular necrosis, the bone loses its blood supply and becomes necrotic. Avascular necrosis is associated with femoral intracapsular fractures, which disrupt the blood supply to the femoral head. When the blood supply to the femoral head is impaired and the anterior and posterior retinacular arteries are severed, it is difficult to supply the femoral head with the required nutrition. The femoral head then becomes ischemic and necrotic. The devitalized bone may collapse and be reabsorbed.

Signs and symptoms of avascular necrosis include pain and limited movement. On diagnostic radiography, calcium loss and structural collapse may be noted. To treat avascular necrosis, the bone must be revitalized with bone grafts or surgical procedures, including prosthetic bone replacement or arthrodesis.

Delayed Union. Delayed union denotes healing that is slow. It may be due to inadequate immobilization, infection, poor circulation, or poor nutrition. Electrical stimulation and bone grafts have proven to be effective in the promotion of bone healing. Another method is osteoinduction, which involves substances such as platelet-derived growth factor or peptide-signaling molecules.

Nonunion. Nonunion indicates the absence of firm union of bone fragments. This may be due to a gap between bone fragments caused by excess traction or soft tissue caught between the fragments. Malunion indicates that the bone fragments have healed in an abnormal alignment.

Hemorrhage. Hemorrhage may also be a complication of fractures. Hemorrhage can result from excessive bleeding at the site of injury, damage to internal organs or tissue, or surgical repair. Signs and symptoms include excessive bright red drainage, which indicates active external bleeding. Indications of bleeding (external or internal) include changes in heart rate, blood pressure, and respiration. Generally, the heart rate and respirations are increased and the blood pressure is decreased.

Management of the patient with hemorrhage includes direct pressure if active bleeding is visible. Frequent monitoring of vital signs after trauma or surgery until they are stabilized within normal limits is necessary. This aids in the detection of internal bleeding. Hemoglobin and hematocrit values need to be monitored and, when abnormal, reported to the physician.

 COMMUNITY CARE

The patient should be monitored for signs and symptoms of neurovascular impairment: pain, pallor or cyanosis, diminished or absent pulse, edema, coolness of skin, paresthesia (e.g., numbness, tingling), capillary refill time of greater than 3 seconds, and inability to move. The effectiveness of analgesia should be assessed. Asepsis should be used in caring for patients with open wounds to prevent infection.

The patient should be instructed regarding how to prevent fractures (e.g., use of sturdy nonslippery shoes). He or she should also be informed about important signs and symptoms to report, such as infection (e.g., fever, redness, and warmth at the site), unusual pain, or a cast that feels too tight.

The psychological impact of immobility on the patient in traction should be assessed. When a patient is confined to a limited space for an extended period of time, he or she should be observed for confusion, disorientation, anger, and hostility.

Prolonged or excessive pressure on the elbows, the scapula, the coccyx, the Achilles tendon, and the medial and lateral aspects of the knee and the ankle should be monitored. The nurse should also look for complications of immobility, such as pressure ulcers, muscle atrophy, contractures, constipation, pneumonia, atelectasis, thromboembolus, DVT, anorexia, urinary calculi, and depression. Circulatory impairment should be prevented by encouraging the patient to perform hourly active exercises with moveable joints and isometric exercises for injured areas that cannot be moved. Deformity should be prevented by maintaining proper positioning of the affected extremity and the traction device.

The nurse should provide information regarding the specific fracture site, the expected healing time, and the degree of immobility. The patient needs to be instructed about the treatment regimen, potential complications, crutch walking, and symptoms to report to the physician. If a cast is required, the patient should be taught about the exothermic sensation felt on application, the daily cast care, and the peculiar sensations felt on removal of the cast. It is also important to inform the patient about the stages of bone healing and the importance of non–weight bearing during the early stages.

 PROGNOSIS

The prognosis is usually good for patients with fractures. Factors affecting healing include accurate fracture reduction, proper immobilization, adequate circulation, and early remobilization. If any of these factors is absent, the prognosis may be worse. Also, the patient's age, the fracture location, and the patient's general condition affect the healing process. The elderly may heal more slowly. A fracture in a weight-bearing extremity may take longer to heal. Healthy patients with adequate nutritional status heal more quickly than malnourished, emaciated patients.

 CLINICAL PEARLS

○ In the emergency management of a fractured bone, the nurse should move the suspected fracture site as little as possible and should use a padded splint that is longer than the fractured bone.

○ Immediately after an injury, the patient should not be allowed to move or "test" the injured part. This will help avoid eliciting crepitus, which could lead to soft tissue damage.

○ Elevation (above the level of the heart) and applications of cold to the injured body part are important nursing interventions to reduce swelling.

○ The "7 P's" (pain, pallor, paralysis, paresthesia, pulselessness, puffiness, and poikilothermia) should be used in checking neurovascular status to prevent complications and irreparable soft tissue damage.

○ The joint should be supported above and below the fractured site when moving or turning the patient to promote stability and to avoid muscle spasms and disruption of the healing process.

○ Cast splints are used initially after a fracture to allow for expansion from expected swelling (6 to 12 hours after trauma) and to prevent neurovascular impairment.

○ A green cast should be handled with the palms of the hands, not the fingertips, to prevent pressure areas under the cast.

○ Plaster casts need to be kept dry to maintain their integrity and support. A plaster cast may be covered with plastic wrap to maintain dryness when bathing or using a bedpan.

○ The patient should be instructed not to scratch or place any objects under the cast, because this may cause a break in the skin with a resultant skin ulcer. Cool air from a hair dryer may relieve itching.

○ Fiberglass casts may be immersed in water but must be dried thoroughly to prevent skin maceration.
○ Rest is the best treatment for a hairline stress fracture.

NURSING PROBLEM/ DIAGNOSIS	NURSING INTERVENTIONS CLASSIFICATION (NIC)
Acute pain	Analgesic administration
	Pain management
	Heat/cold application
Impaired physical mobility	Traction/immobilization care
	Exercise therapy: ambulation; joint mobility
Prevention of complications	Surveillance
	Vital sign monitoring
	Circulation precautions
	Cast care: maintenance

Gout

Section 3   Linda McCuistion

 OVERVIEW

Gout is a metabolic disorder caused by supersaturation of serum uric acid, which may later form crystals that are deposited in joints and surrounding tissue. The first metatarsophalangeal joint is affected in 75% of cases. Other frequently affected areas are wrists, fingers, ears, elbows, knees, and Achilles tendon. Gout is found in all countries and ethnic groups, with approximately 2 million Americans being affected. The first gout attack usually occurs between 40 and 60 years of age. There seems to be a genetic basis, because 85% of cases occur in families with a known tendency toward this disorder. Furthermore, gout occurs in males 95% of the time.

 PATHOPHYSIOLOGY

Gout is a metabolic disorder due to hyperuricemia, an excessive amount of serum uric acid. This can result from either overproduction or underexcretion of uric acid. Uric acid is an end product of purine metabolism. Ineffective purine metabolism may also explain excess uric acid levels. The normal amount of uric acid excretion in urine is 250 to 750 mg/day.

Underexcretion is the cause of gout in 90% of cases. "Underexcreters" usually excrete less than 200 mg/day of uric acid, and "overproducers" usually produce much more than 800 mg/day. When uric acid levels rise above 7 mg/dL, the uric acid forms monosodium urate monohydrate crystals. These needle- or rod-shaped crystals are deposited in the tissues surrounding the joints, such as synovial fluid or articular cartilage. The deposits of urate crystals irritate joint linings and lead to inflammation. Formed deposits, called *tophi*, are usually located in peripheral joints.

Gout has four stages. The first stage is known as *asymptomatic hyperuricemia*. In this stage, uric acid levels are greater than 7 to 10 mg/dL, without other significant signs and symptoms. Because uric acid levels normally increase after puberty for males, asymptomatic hyperuricemia usually begins in this gender during adolescence. In females, this phenomenon is delayed until after menopause, because estrogens tend to increase renal excretion of uric acid. Because uric acid levels normally increase after menopause, postmenopausal females have an increased risk of developing gout, especially if they are also taking thiazide diuretics. This stage can last for decades, with only 20% to 25% of patients progressing to the second stage.

The second stage is called *acute gouty arthritis*. In this stage, hyperuricemia is greater than 10 mg/dL, and albuminuria is greater than 100 mg/day. This supersaturation of uric acid in plasma and body fluids leads to urate crystal deposits in joints and surrounding tissue. The urate crystals tend to form in cooler parts of the body, such as fingers, toes, or feet. Usually, the metatarsophalangeal joint or the great toe is involved. Often, the first attack is monarticular. As the attacks begin to occur more frequently, they become polyarticular and last longer. The body's immune system attacks the crystals and treats them as foreign substances. Polymorphonuclear leukocytes (PMLs) permeate the joint and phagocytize the urate crystals. Phagocytosis by PMLs results in the death of PMLs and release of lysosomal enzymes, as well as other inflammatory mediators, into surrounding tissues. This inflammatory response makes the affected joint extremely painful, red, hot, and swollen. Limited motion is also present. Accompanying symptoms are fever, increased erythrocyte sedimentation rate, and increased number of white blood cells. (Leukocyte count is usually greater than 11,000/mm.) The second gouty attack usually occurs at least 1 year after the first. Recurrent attacks increase in frequency over a period of years.

The third stage is called the *intercritical* stage. Throughout this stage, patients are without symptoms. The time period for this stage may be months to up to 10 years with appropriate treatment. If the patient is not treated, however, the interval between attacks is usually less than 1 year.

Chronic gout or chronic tophaceous gout is the fourth stage, which may develop 10 years or more after the first attack. In this stage, chronic inflammation from urate crystals leads to persistent pain or an aching stiffness, as well as joint swelling and tophi. Tophi are monosodium urate crystals that develop because of the insolubility of urates. Tophi are commonly deposited in synovial membranes, cartilage, soft tissues, tendons, and other tissues surrounding joints. Chronic gout attacks tend to have a rapid onset and may develop over a few hours. Without effective pharmacologic treatment, acute attacks may occur every few weeks.

Factors contributing to a gouty attack include a diet high in purines, poor eating habits, dehydration, trauma, emotional stress, alcohol intake, and certain medications. Foods with high purine content include sardines, herring, liver, goose, venison, mussels, kidney, meat soups, and sweetbreads. A diet high in purines can lead to a gout attack if inborn faulty metabolism is present; otherwise, there is not necessarily a direct relationship. Poor eating habits may precipitate a gout attack, because plasma uric acid levels are increased during starvation. Therefore, meals should be eaten at regular intervals. Dehydration triggers an acute gouty attack as well as kidney stones owing to the increased concentration of serum uric acid. Both trauma and emotional stress stimulate the body's stress response and lead to fluid retention outside the vascular system, mimicking dehydration. Alcohol has a direct relationship, because it causes both overproduction and underexcretion of uric acid. A patient prone to gout should especially avoid beer, because it has high guanosine content, which catabolizes beer into uric acid. Any form of alcoholic beverage increases the uric acid level by accelerating the breakdown of intracellular adenosine triphosphate. Hyperuricemia is a common side effect of cyclosporine (Neoral); therefore, patients who have undergone organ transplants and are taking cyclosporine should be carefully monitored. Patients with obesity, renal disease, hypertension, or hyperlipidemia have a greater tendency to develop gout. If gout is untreated, tophi accumulate and may cause irreversible joint damage.

 ## SIGNS AND SYMPTOMS

The local inflammatory characteristics of gout initiate excruciating pain, joint edema, warmth, redness, extreme sensitivity, and limited joint movement. Fatigue, chills, fever (38°C to 39.5°C [100°F to 103°F]), and an increased white blood cell count also accompany gout. An acute attack often occurs at night and awakens the patient because of excruciating pain. Gout pain is often too intolerable to endure even the weight of bed linen.

In later stages, tophi are present. Common sites for tophi include the helix of the ear, the hands and the feet, the olecranon bursa, the extensor surface of the forearm, the infrapatellar bursa, and the Achilles tendon, and they may even be found in the aorta or the heart valves. Patients with tophi tend to have gouty attacks with more frequency and severity. Tophi are not painful but may restrict joint movement and cause deformities. On examination, tophi are cream-colored or reddened nodules that are firm and moveable.

 ## DIAGNOSTIC CRITERIA

Generally, a history and a physical examination provide enough data for the diagnosis of gout. The finding of an elevated serum uric acid level of greater than 7.5 mg/dL may contribute to the diagnosis but is not definitive, because the level may be normal at the time of an attack. The normal uric acid level is 2.4 to 6 mg/dL in females and 3.4 to 7 mg/dL in males. A definitive diagnostic parameter is the discovery of urate crystals in the synovial fluid of an affected joint. Most rheumatology specialists recommend arthrocentesis or aspiration of affected joints; however, many primary care physicians believe that this approach is neither necessary nor practical. Siegel, Alloway, and Harris write that it is important to make an accurate definitive diagnosis of gout via aspiration of synovial fluid to confirm the presence of monosodium urate crystals in a joint. This test will accurately differentiate gout from coincidental hyperuricemia, OA, RA, calcium pyrophosphate dihydrate deposition (pseudogout), and spondyloarthropathies, which may mimic gout. Differential diagnosis would prevent patients from receiving gout medication unnecessarily. A radiograph may show urate deposits in the joints or the tophi, but only in later stages.

INTERVENTIONS

Three management goals for acute painful gouty attacks are to reduce uric acid production, increase renal excretion of uric acid, and prevent recurrent attacks. NSAIDs, antimitotics, corticosteroids, and analgesics provide drug therapy for acute gout. Usually, no treatment is indicated in the asymptomatic hyperuricemic stage because crystals are unformed and the patient is without symptoms.

Nonsteroidal Anti-inflammatory Drugs

In the second stage of acute gouty arthritis, NSAIDs are administered to decrease inflammation in and surrounding the joints. Indomethacin (Indocin) is particularly successful in the treatment of acute gout and is a first-line drug because it produces fewer adverse effects than other NSAIDs. Indomethacin was the first NSAID to be used for gout, but others are also effective, including ibuprofen (Motrin), naproxen (Naprosyn), sulindac (Clinoril), piroxicam (Feldene), ketoprofen (Orudis), and tolmetin sodium (Tolectin). NSAIDs relieve inflammation quickly if taken soon after the onset of symptoms. Initially, a loading dose of 150 to 300 mg three times daily is given for 5 to 7 days; the dose is lowered as pain decreases. Treatment continues until pain has subsided for 48 hours, then drug administration is tapered off quickly over 2 to 3 days. Adverse effects associated with NSAIDs include gastrointestinal distress (nausea, vomiting, diarrhea, anorexia), headache, vertigo, syncope, fatigue, insomnia, drowsiness, psychic disturbances (hallucinations, depression, depersonalization), gastrointestinal ulceration, hemorrhage, perforation, aplastic anemia, agranulocytosis, inhibited platelet aggregation, hypersensitivity, toxic hepatitis, hypertension, and renal function impairment. Adverse effects of NSAIDs are more pronounced in the elderly. Contraindications to NSAIDs are peptic ulcer disease, renal or liver dysfunction, anticoagulation therapy, and poorly compensated congestive heart failure.

Xanthine Oxidase Inhibitors

In the chronic stage of gout, treatment is directed at the reduction of serum uric acid levels. Allopurinol (Zyloprim) is currently the only available inhibitor of uric acid synthesis given in gout management. This drug inhibits the enzyme xanthine oxidase, thereby blocking the production of uric acid. Xanthine oxidase converts hypoxanthine to xanthine and xanthine to uric acid. The dose of allopurinol is 300 mg/day. Adverse effects of allopurinol include rash, nausea, vomiting, diarrhea, abdominal discomfort, drowsiness, headache, vertigo, bone marrow depression, and hepatotoxicity. Xanthine oxidase inhibitors should be used cautiously in patients with hepatic or renal impairment, in patients with a history of peptic ulcer, and in those with bone marrow depression.

Uricosuric Agents

Uricosuric agents, such as probenecid (Benemid) and sulfinpyrazone (Anturane), are administered in hyperuricemic cases of chronic gout, which are due to underexcretion of uric acid. Uricosuric agents promote excretion of uric acid by blocking renal tubular reabsorption. The dose of probenecid is 500 to

1000 mg two times a day, whereas the dose of sulfinpyrazone is 50 to 400 mg two times a day. With uricosuria, the patient's fluid intake needs to be increased to at least 3000 mL/day to promote uric acid excretion and to prevent kidney stones. Uric acid levels should be less than 5 mg/dL. By reducing the uric acid level to less than this amount, body storage of urate is depleted; therefore, formation of tophi and renal damage are prevented. Adverse effects of uricosuric agents include flushing, rash, headache, dizziness, nausea, vomiting, anorexia, aggravation of peptic ulcer, urinary frequency, renal calculi, and blood dyscrasias. Patients should be instructed to avoid alcohol when taking uricosuric agents. Also, taking uricosuric agents in divided doses along with food prevents gastrointestinal upset. Contraindications to uricosuric therapy include blood dyscrasias and low-dose salicylate therapy. Low-dose salicylates inhibit the action of uricosuric agents and account for a significant number of treatment failures. Uricosuric agents should be used cautiously in patients with a history of peptic ulcer and renal impairment.

Antimitotic Agents

Colchicine is the oldest treatment for gout. Colchicine decreases the inflammatory response by inhibiting a phagocytic response to urate crystals. It causes neutrophils to block the release of chemotactic factor, reduces mobility and adhesion of PMLs, and inhibits production of leukotriene. By inhibiting the inflammatory response, colchicine generally eliminates pain in 48 hours in an acute attack. Colchicine decreases gouty signs and symptoms dramatically and rapidly. The usual loading dose is 1 mg, followed by 1 tablet of 0.6 mg every 1 to 2 hours until diarrhea, nausea, or vomiting develops. A maximum dose of 8 mg is allowed. The most common adverse effects are nausea, vomiting, abdominal cramping, and diarrhea. Intravenous administration should be used cautiously because it may lead to tissue necrosis from intravenous line infiltration, bone marrow suppression, renal failure, disseminated intravascular coagulation, and death. Cimetidine and erythromycin potentiate the effects of colchicine and make it more toxic. Ineffective once an attack has been present for several days, colchicine should be taken at first warning of an acute attack. Patients should drink at least 2 L of fluid daily to prevent urinary stone formation. Antimitotic agents should be used with caution when the patient also has renal, hepatic, or cardiac disease.

Corticosteroids

Corticosteroids are used for gout only when other medications are ineffective or contraindicated; however, they are very potent and suppress the inflammatory response. If needed, prednisone (Deltasone), 20 to 50 mg/day, is given for 3 to 5 days, then tapered over 1 to 2 weeks. Intra-articular injections of methylprednisolone (Solu-Medrol) are useful if there is polyarticular involvement or if the patient is not able to take oral medication. The intra-articular dose is individualized to the involved joint. A toe joint may require only 5 to 20 mg, whereas a knee would require 20 to 60 mg. Adverse effects of corticosteroids include nausea, vomiting, headache, euphoria, psychosis, sodium and water retention, and peptic ulcer. Corticosteroids should be administered with caution in patients with renal impairment or peptic ulcers.

Opioid Analgesics

The analgesics used in gout are codeine and meperidine (Demerol). These analgesics bind with the same receptors as endogenous opioid peptides to produce relief of pain. The oral dose of codeine is usually 30 to 60 mg, and the dose of Demerol is 50 to 100 mg every 4 hours as needed for pain. Adverse effects include rash, nausea, vomiting, constipation, sedation, euphoria, disorientation, dizziness, hypotension, paradoxical CNS stimulation, and respiratory depression. These analgesics are contraindicated in patients with severe renal and liver impairment.

Surgery

Surgery may have to be performed for very large tophi deposits that interfere with daily functioning or joint movement. Except for the occasional removal of tophi, surgery for gout is unnecessary.

Nursing Management

The primary focus of nursing management is pain relief and mobility. These interventions include rest, joint immobilization, and local application of cold to reduce pain in an acute attack. Joint rest should be maintained until at least 24 hours after resolution of an acute gouty attack to prevent urate mobilization and joint inflammation. If the joint is acutely inflamed (e.g., red and hot), application of heat should be avoided, because this would increase the inflammatory process. If a patient is overweight, weight reduction is desirable, because blood uric acid levels are higher in overweight people. The nurse should teach the patient and significant others about the disease process, its signs and symptoms, and the treatment regimen.

COMMUNITY CARE

Assessment

- Assess the history and precipitating factors: gender, age, trauma, previous gouty attack, dietary history (e.g., high-purine diet, poor diet and eating habits, dehydration, alcohol use), emotional stress, obesity, and medication history (e.g., low-dose salicylates).
- Assess the patient for presenting signs and symptoms of gout: excruciating pain (assess the extent of pain by having the patient rate the pain on a scale of 0 to 10); a red, hot, swollen joint with stiffness, limited motion, and nodules; and systemic characteristics, such as fever and increased erythrocyte sedimentation rate and white blood cell count.
- Assess the patient for possible contraindications to medication: blood dyscrasias (detected via complete blood count), renal impairment (detected via blood urea nitrogen and creatinine levels), hepatic impairment (detected via liver function tests), cardiac disease, bleeding ulcers, or hypersensitivity.

Monitoring

- Monitor patient compliance with the treatment regimen: hydrating with at least 3000 mL of fluids per day, taking medication at the prescribed dose and frequency, checking uric acid levels, and observing the frequency of gouty attacks.

- Monitor the patient for common potential adverse effects of drug therapy: rash, dizziness, headache, intolerable gastrointestinal distress (e.g., nausea, diarrhea), renal dysfunction (detected from increased creatinine and blood urea nitrogen levels and from dilute or frothy urine), bone marrow suppression (detected from the complete blood count), bleeding ulcers (e.g., bruising; detected from the prothrombin time), or hypersensitivity (e.g., rash). Hypersensitivity occurs more frequently in patients taking ampicillin, amoxicillin, or thiazide diuretics.
- Monitor the patient for the possible complications of gout, which include kidney stones (detected from blood in the urine and painful urination).

Prevention

- Instruct the patient regarding the management of an acute gouty attack: Maintain bedrest for at least 24 hours after resolution of the attack; protect the inflamed joint by using a bed cradle; attain a position of comfort by elevating the affected extremity on a pillow.
- Instruct the patient to avoid purine foods: organ meats (e.g., liver, kidneys, sweetbreads), luncheon meats, herring, sardines, anchovies, bouillon, broth, gravies, nuts, yeast, peas, oatmeal, spinach, asparagus, cauliflower, and mushrooms.
- Instruct the patient regarding safety: Take medications with meals to avoid gastrointestinal distress, and use caution when driving or performing activities that require alertness.
- Instruct the patient to avoid medications that elevate uric acid levels by blocking renal excretion of uric acid: salicylates (aspirin) in low doses, most thiazide diuretics, diazoxide (Hyperstat), acetazolamide (Diamox), levodopa (Larodopa), nicotinic acid, cyclosporine, and ethambutol (Myambutol).

 PROGNOSIS

The prognosis is good for patients with gout when it is successfully managed by means of avoidance of precipitating factors and drug therapy. Early diagnosis and pharmacologic treatment can prevent tophi.

 CLINICAL PEARLS

- Acute gout attacks may be prevented by adhering to the medication regimen, avoiding medications that promote uric acid imbalance (e.g., salicylates, thiazide diuretics, diazoxide, acetazolamide, levodopa, cyclosporine, ethambutol, and loop diuretics), hydrating adequately (with at least eight glasses of water per day), avoiding excessive dietary purines and all alcohol, eating at regular intervals, and avoiding starvation and crash dieting.
- The most common medications for acute gout attacks are NSAIDs, especially indomethacin (Indocin), and colchicine to reduce the inflammatory response.
- The most common medications for chronic gout attacks are allopurinol (Zyloprim), a xanthine oxidase inhibitor that inhibits uric acid production, and probenecid (Benemid), a uricosuric, which increases uric acid excretion.
- Nonpharmacologic measures include the use of a bed cradle to protect joints from the weight of the bed linens, elevation of joints, and application of cold to decrease inflammation and pain.

NURSING PROBLEM/ DIAGNOSIS	NURSING INTERVENTIONS CLASSIFICATION (NIC)
Gouty pain	Analgesic administration
	Pain management
	Heat/cold application
Impaired physical mobility	Environmental management
Hyperuricemia	Teaching: prescribed diet
	Teaching: prescribed medication
	Fluid management

Osteoporosis

Section 4   Cecilia Tiller

 OVERVIEW

Osteoporosis causes the skeleton to weaken and the bones to break under the slightest strain or during routine activity. Normally, skeletal mass is constantly undergoing a process called *remodeling*. During this process, osteoclasts remove or resorb old bone tissue, and osteoblasts replace bone tissue or form new tissue. During youth, bones grow in both length and density. During the adolescent years, maximum height is reached, and bones continue to grow more dense. Between the ages of 20 and 40 years, bone reaches its maximum density. After that, an imbalance in the normal cycle of bone resorption and formation occurs; bone loss becomes greater than bone formation.

After bone mass peaks, usually by the age of 40, age-associated losses occur at a rate of about 1% each year. Women may experience a 3% to 5% loss during the 5 years after menopause. Lifetime losses may reach 30% to 40% of peak bone mass in women and 20% to 30% in men. One in two women and one in eight men are at risk of a fracture owing to osteoporosis.

 PATHOPHYSIOLOGY

Skeletal mass is usually maximal by the age of 35 and begins to decline in women after the age of 40 and in men after the age of 50, when the rate of new bone formation does not equal the rate of bone resorption. In the normal remodeling process, osteoclasts in the bone marrow migrate outward to digest the bone surface and thus form an erosion cavity. Osteoblasts and other mononuclear cells enter the cavities and over the next 3 to 4 months rebuild the bone.

In osteoporosis, the osteoclasts continue their normal process of erosion; however, the osteoblasts do not act normally and do not fill the cavities. After menopause, the bone turnover rate increases. The osteoclasts make deeper erosion cavities, and the osteoblasts cannot rebuild the bone. Thus, the bones become porous, lose mass and strength, and become very fragile and easy to break.

 SIGNS AND SYMPTOMS

Osteoporosis is known as the silent disease because the condition is seldom detected until a wrist, hip, or vertebral fracture occurs. Clinical signs such as

Table 21-4-1. Risk Factors for Osteoporosis

Female gender	Diet low in calcium
Thin and/or small frame	Use of corticosteroids, anticonvulsants, thyroid medications
Age >40 years	
Postmenopausal status (natural or surgical)	Low testosterone levels in men
Family history of osteoporosis	Inactive lifestyle
Abnormal absence of menstrual periods	Cigarette smoking
Anorexia or bulimia	Excessive use of alcohol
Oral contraceptive use for more than 5 years (unconfirmed)	White or Asian race, although African Americans and Hispanic Americans are at risk as well
Medical diseases: endocrine diseases and neoplasms	Participation in highly competitive athletics

height loss, kyphosis, and minimal traumatic fractures suggest that the disease is present. Early diagnosis and detection of low bone mass density (BMD) in those at risk of osteoporosis are important. Risk factors that predispose to osteoporosis are presented in Table 21-4-1. A diminished quality of life can result from these fractures or from recurring fractures. Therefore, prevention is vital.

DIAGNOSTIC CRITERIA

Diagnosis of osteoporosis is made from a review of the risk factors and measurements of BMD. A thorough history and physical examination followed by diagnostic evaluation are necessary. Because osteoporosis can begin before menopause, women should be screened at the age of 40. The American College of Obstetricians and Gynecologists and the American College of Physicians recommend that menopausal women at risk of osteoporosis undergo BMD measurement before beginning any treatment. BMD should also be calculated in premenopausal women who report significant risk factors.

Bone Mass Density

Several noninvasive tests can be used to determine BMD, such as nuclear scanning and radiographic techniques. Scintigraphy, a form of nuclear scanning, is an important imaging technique that is sensitive in the detection of stress fractures and bone metastases. It can also assess suspected injury that is difficult to see on plain films. This technique can determine the age of fractures to help identify osteoporosis and to uncover other causes of pain. The dual-energy x-ray absorptiometry (Dexa) scan is probably the most reliable; however, all techniques are accurate in detecting low BMD.

Biochemical Markers

Biochemical markers may also be assessed to help identify osteoporosis and to rule out other diseases. Biochemical markers of bone remodeling can track both formation and resorption and are a less expensive means of measuring BMD. Markers that indicate bone resorption include urine tests (for calcium, hydroxyproline, hydroxylysine, pyridinoline, deoxypyridinoline, and N-telopeptide of cross-linked type I collagen) and serum tests (for plasma tartrate-resistant acid phosphatase). Markers that indicate bone formation include serum alkaline phosphatase, serum bone-specific alkaline phosphatase, procollagen 1 extension peptides, and osteocalcin.

 INTERVENTIONS

The main objectives of osteoporosis treatment are to increase bone mineral density and to decrease the risk of fractures. Interventions are most effective when started in the asymptomatic period, which requires early identification of those at risk.

Estrogen

Estrogen is the principal treatment for all perimenopausal women. Estrogen reduces osteoclast activity, which decreases bone loss and thereby reduces fractures and prevents loss of height. Estrogen treatment, also known as hormone replacement therapy—although still controversial—has been found to have other benefits. It helps reduce the risk of myocardial infarction, improves vasomotor symptoms, and helps maintain moist membranes.

Many women cannot tolerate the side effects of estrogen (e.g., uterine bleeding, breast swelling and tenderness, and weight gain) and discontinue therapy. The ideal minimum dose for prevention and reduction of bone loss is unknown. Studies indicate that lower doses of estrogen therapy are better than no estrogen therapy in the prevention of bone loss. Women who decline hormone replacement therapy should be encouraged to make lifestyle changes to counteract their risk factors.

Dietary Supplementation

Adequate calcium and vitamin D are needed for healthy bone maintenance. Patients should be encouraged to supplement their diets with calcium and vitamin D. All postmenopausal women and men older than 65 years of age should take 1000 to 1500 mg/day of calcium and 400 to 800 IU/day of vitamin D, regardless of other prescribed medications that they may be taking.

Exercise

Weight-bearing and routine exercise (e.g., walking) promotes higher levels of BMD. A walk for 20 to 30 minutes every day or for 1 hour three times a week is recommended.

Programs that persuade women to adopt long-term changes in behavior can be very beneficial in preventing osteoporosis.

Pharmacologic Therapy

Several drugs have been approved for prevention of osteoporosis. These pharmacologic agents, coupled with prevention education, provide a variety of options. Raloxifene (Evista) is thought to rebuild bone; however, it needs further study. Bone changes occur slowly, so that BMD measurements every 12 to 18 months are adequate to evaluate the effects of pharmacologic treatment.

Alternative Therapies

Herbal medications, meditation, and acupuncture are gaining attention and are becoming widely used by the general public. Lay publications advertise the benefits of alternative therapies; however, their efficacy has not been well studied. Alternative therapies may be harmful or even fatal. Nevertheless, many women would rather take herbal preparations than estrogen. Some of the most common herbal therapies used by women are the following:

- Black cohosh (*Cimicifuga racemosa*), also called black snakeroot, rattleweed, rattleroot, or squawroot
- Chaste tree berry (*Vitex agnus-castus*), also called Monk's pepper
- Evening primrose (*Oenothera biennis*), also called fever plant, field primrose, night's willow herb, or king's cure.

 COMMUNITY CARE

Assessment

- Take a history and assess for risk factors.
- Assess the place of residence for risks of falling (throw rugs, cluttered walkways, poor lighting, stairs).
- Assess dietary practices; especially look for calcium intake.

Monitoring

- Assist the woman in accepting and coping with menopause and the physical changes that occur with age.
- Use anticipatory guidance, counseling, and referral as necessary, depending on the woman's response to menopause and aging.
- To improve bone structure, encourage dietary and exercise habits that enhance health and slow the aging process.

Prevention

- Begin diet and exercise programs for the prevention of osteoporosis in adolescence.
- Provide information to women about estrogen replacement therapy and alternatives to allow for informed decision-making.
- Promote good health habits, exercise, and avoidance of alcohol and tobacco in adolescents to prevent problems in later years.

 PROGNOSIS

Osteoporosis is not curable; however, steps can be taken to prevent bone loss. Both women and men can make lifestyle changes to reduce their risk factors for osteoporosis. Early detection of the potential for osteoporosis is a major step in preventing the life-threatening fractures that could occur. Individuals at risk can minimize the health consequences of osteoporosis by changing their diet, exercise, and medication practices. Those who suffer fractures may find their lives greatly altered and may experience suffering and pain.

 CLINICAL PEARLS

- All postmenopausal women should take 1000 to 1500 mg/day of calcium and 400 to 800 IU/day of vitamin D.
- Walking for 20 to 30 minutes every day or for 1 hour three times a week reduces the risk of bone loss.
- Taking calcitonin in the evening may minimize the flushed feeling that may occur.

○ Alendronate (Fosamax) should be taken with a full glass (6 to 8 ounces) of water at least 30 minutes before or after other food or drink and preferably within 2 hours of dairy products, antacids, or mineral supplements.

○ After Fosamax has been taken, the patient should be encouraged to remain in an upright position for at least 30 minutes and until after eating.

NURSING PROBLEM/ DIAGNOSIS	NURSING INTERVENTIONS CLASSIFICATION (NIC)
Risk of fracture/Injury	Environmental management: safety
	Surveillance
	Exercise promotion
	Nutrition management
Prevention of bone loss/Effective therapeutic regimen management	Risk identification
	Teaching: disease process
	Teaching: prescribed diet
	Activity therapy

Systemic Lupus Erythematosus

Section 5   Pamela Cook

 OVERVIEW

Systemic lupus erythematosus (SLE) is a chronic inflammatory autoimmune disease of vascular and connective tissue that may involve any system or organ. The etiology is unknown. It causes the body to attack its own tissues, resulting in localized or generalized inflammation, permanent cellular damage, and death. Research has verified genetic, immunologic, hormonal, and environmental factors that induce or perpetuate the disease. The incidence is 1 in 2100, with a female predominance approaching 90%. The disease is more common and more severe in African Americans, Afro-Caribbeans, Asians, Native Americans, Hispanics, and Puerto Ricans (a 14:1 ratio). The peak incidence in women is in the 20-to-39 age group, with a median age of 37 to 50. SLE develops later in men, with a median age of 50 to 59. The clinical signs and symptoms vary in severity and depend on the organ systems involved (Table 21-5-1). The objective of treatment is to decrease inflammation, thus slowing tissue damage and disease progression.

The survival of patients with SLE has improved remarkably; in the 1990s, there was a 90% 10-year survival rate, with 20-year rates approaching 70%. The most common causes of death are active disease, infections, glomerulonephritis, vascular events, and CNS dysfunction. SLE is not infectious or contagious, nor is it a type of cancer or malignancy or related to acquired immunodeficiency syndrome. SLE can be mild with few symptoms or very severe with extreme symptoms and periods of exacerbations and remission, depending on the systems affected. Mild cases can become more serious if left untreated.

 PATHOPHYSIOLOGY

This disease appears in two forms: discoid (cutaneous) lupus erythematosus and SLE. Discoid lupus is a chronic skin condition characterized by a raised,

Table 21-5-1. Clinical Manifestations of Systemic Lupus Erythematosus

SYSTEM/ ORGAN	CLINICAL SIGNS AND SYMPTOMS	PREVALENCE
Hematologic	Anemia, leukopenia, thrombocytopenia	100
Musculoskeletal	Joint pain, swelling, fibrosis	90
Skin	Vasculitis, rash, raised areas, scaling	85
Renal	Proteinuria, glomerulonephritis	50
Central nervous	Seizures, depression	50
Pulmonary	Pleural effusion, pneumonia	46
Cardiovascular	Percarditis, myocarditis, arrhythmias	25
Gastrointestinal	Nausea, dyspepsia, diarrhea, ulcers	21

Adapted from Cotran, R., Kumar, V., & Collins, T. (1999). *Pathologic basis of disease.* Philadelphia: WB Saunders.

red, scaly rash, most commonly seen on the face, with a characteristic red butterfly distribution over the cheeks and the bridge of the nose. Lesions may be single or multiple, are generally asymmetrical, and may persist for months. Patients with this type of lupus usually have normal internal organs. SLE is an internal form of the disease characterized by inflammation of varying forms and intensity of the internal organs, such as the kidneys, the heart, the lungs, and the joints. Clinical manifestations depend on the organs involved.

A genetic predisposition to the disease is evidenced by its clustering in families, especially among identical twins, and in certain ethnic groups. Defects in the regulation of the immune response system leading to the development of antibodies against one's own tissues have been linked to the major histocompatibility complex genes and the human leukocyte antigen complex.

An imbalance in sex hormone levels has been suggested to play a role in the development of the disease. Androgen hormones appear to protect against SLE, and estrogen hormones seem to favor its development. The imbalance in the two hormones may lead to an increase in the number of helper T cells and a decrease in the number of suppressor T cells, leading to the development of autoantibodies.

Environmental factors, such as exposure to radiation or to certain chemicals, have been linked to the development of lupus or to exacerbation of the disease. Certain drugs, as outlined in Table 21-5-2, may induce antinuclear antibodies at a much higher frequency, causing a lupus-like syndrome.

Recent studies have determined that SLE is primarily T cell dependent because it begins with the failure of helper T cells to moderate the immune reaction. This failure allows autoantibodies to react with the DNA of the antigen and to form multiple DNA immune complexes in the serum, which are deposited in the basement membranes of capillaries, particularly those of the kidneys, heart, skin, brain, and joints.

SIGNS AND SYMPTOMS

The clinical signs and symptoms vary in type and intensity (see Table 21-5-1). Common universal symptoms are malaise, fatigue, weight loss, and a low-grade fever (99.5°F to 100.5°F), usually in the late afternoon. Symptoms are associated with the organ system involved.

Table 21-5-2. Drug-Induced Lupus Erythematosus

KNOWN TO IMPOSE RISK	CLASSIFICATION
Procainamide (Pronestyl)	Antiarrhythmic
Quinidine (Quinaglute)	Antiarrhythmic
Hydralazine (Apresoline)	Antihypertensive
Chlorpromazine (Thorazine)	Antipsychotic
Carbamazepine (Tegretol)	Anticonvulsant
Isoniazid (INH)	Antibiotic
Penicillamine (Cuprimine)	Anti-inflammatory
Sulfasalazine (Azulfidine)	Anti-infective

Adapted from Lahita R.G., Pisetsky D.S., & Wallace D.J. (1998). Lupus: high stakes diagnosis, broad treatment options. *Patient care 32*(4): 101–123.

Hematologic

Hematologic disorders may manifest as anemia (<13 g/100 mL for males, <11 g/100 mL for females), leukopenia (<4000/mL on two or more occasions), or thrombocytopenia (<100,000/mm). The disorders are secondary to the reaction of autoimmune antibodies to red blood cell antigens, or they may be caused by other reasons (e.g., blood loss, renal insufficiency, and side effects of medications).

Musculoskeletal

Arthralgia and arthritis are common manifestations of SLE. Approximately 90% of all persons with SLE complain of joint pain, swelling, tenderness, and stiffness on movement.

Skin

A wide range of skin lesions occurs in patients with SLE, which can be acute or chronic, simple or complex. The most familiar manifestation is a red rash or flush across the bridge of nose and on the cheeks, giving the appearance of a butterfly pattern (commonly triggered by sunlight). An erythematous rash accompanied by raised areas, hives, and scaling may occur over the neck, the chest, and the upper and lower extremities. Mucus membrane involvement may result in ulcers in the mouth, the nose, and the vagina, but these are usually painless.

Renal

Forty to fifty percent of patients with SLE develop deposits of anti-DNA autoantibodies in the kidneys. The deposits cause poor excretion of waste products such as nitrogen, which accumulates and produces untoward symptoms of decreased motor ability and confusion. Mesangial lupus glomerulonephritis, the mildest form of nephritis, occurs when deposits form in the intercapillary mesangial matrix. A focal lesion occurring in the glomeruli is known as focal proliferative glomerulonephritis. Diffuse proliferative glomerulonephritis is the most serious complication, leading to pulmonary hypertension and renal insufficiency. Proteinuria (>35 g/24 hr urine) increases incrementally with nephritis and reflects the extent of involvement of the peripheral glomerular capillary loops. Other symptoms are gross hematuria, oliguria, and edema.

Neurologic

Nervous system dysfunction is present in 40% to 50% of patients with SLE. The symptoms are related to acute vasculitis caused by the fibrinoid deposits in the vessel walls, which thicken the lumen and impede blood flow, leading to strokes, hemorrhage, or blood clots in the brain. Temporary seizures, depression, unusual worry, headache, excitability, nervousness, transient paralysis, stroke, and other forms of cognitive impairment are common.

Pulmonary

Pulmonary involvement in SLE occurs in 20% to 40% of patients. Pleuritis or pleural effusion is most common. Less common are pneumonitis, pulmonary hypertension, and pulmonary embolism.

Cardiovascular

Pericarditis is the most common cardiac manifestation, occurring in up to 30% of patients with SLE. Symptoms include chest pain, fever, dry cough, dyspnea, peripheral edema, and possible friction rub. Myocarditis, endocarditis, resting tachycardia, valvular abnormalities, and symptoms similar to pericarditis are other manifestations. Alteration of collagen and subendothelial thickening of small vessels may obstruct the flow of blood in the extremities, leading to infection and possibly gangrene. Hypertension may occur secondary to lupus nephritis.

Gastrointestinal

Feelings of nausea, dyspepsia, diarrhea, constipation, vomiting, and abdominal pain are sometimes associated with SLE. These symptoms can also be related to the medications prescribed for treatment, such as antimalarial drugs, NSAIDs, corticosteroids, and immunosuppressives. The symptoms may be so severe that they may imitate acute appendicitis or kidney stones.

DIAGNOSTIC CRITERIA

Diagnosis is based on a comprehensive subjective and objective assessment and on analysis of laboratory studies, because no single test can diagnose lupus in everyone. Assessment includes obtaining information about past history, family medical history, exposure to chemicals, occupation, past and current medications, use of tanning beds, exposure to unshielded fluorescent lights, and psychosocial issues. Because recent studies have found that the leaking of silicone into the breast tissue can lead to SLE, questions pertaining to breast implants should be explored.

To assist practitioners in diagnosing SLE, the American College of Rheumatology devised a set of criteria including 11 clinical findings (Table 21-5-3). To be considered as having SLE, the patient must demonstrate the serial or simultaneous presence of at least 4 of the 11 findings. In addition to the history and the examination, various serologic tests are used in diagnosis.

Fluorescent Antinuclear Antibody Test

The fluorescent antinuclear antibody (FANA) test has positive results in more than 95% of patients with SLE because the antinuclear antibodies found in the cells of patients with various connective tissue diseases are larger and

Table 21-5-3. American College of Rheumatology Diagnostic Criteria

CRITERION	DEFINITION
1. Facial rash on the cheeks	1. Erythematous, flat, raised, "butterfly pattern"
2. Discoid rash	2. Raised patches, scaling, scarring
3. Sensitivity	3. Rash develops after exposure
4. Mouth or nose lesions	4. Usually painless
5. Arthritis	5. Swelling or inflammation of several joints
6. Renal disorders	6. Persistent proteinuria >0.5 g/dL Presence of cellular casts and RBCs in urine
7. Neurologic disorders	7. Seizures, psychosis
8. Pleuritis or pericarditis	8. Pleuritic pain or rub
9. Hematologic disorders	9. Hemolytic anemia, thrombocytopenia, leukopenia
10. Immunologic disorders	10. Positive anti-DNA and anti-Sm antigen test results, false-positive for syphilis
11. Presence of antinuclear antibody	11. Abnormal titer, >1:80

From Lahita, R.G. (1999). *Systemic lupus erythematosus* (3rd ed.). San Diego: Academic Press.

offer a more discrete (shaggy, speckled, homogeneous) fluorescence display. Certain medications such as hydralazine (Apresoline), procainamide (Pronestyl), and corticosteroids may create a positive FANA result.

Antinuclear Antibody Panel

When FANA results are positive in a patient with clinical findings of SLE, an antinuclear antibody panel should be obtained to determine the type of antinuclear antibody circulating in the blood. The panel includes anti-DNA, anti-Sm, anti-U1RNP, anti-Ro/SSA, and anti-La/SSB. The presence of anti-DNA and anti-Sm antibodies provides strong evidence for the diagnosis of SLE and against the diagnosis of drug-induced SLE. The higher the titer (>1:10), the greater the degree of inflammation. Although the anti-DNA antibody test is highly specific for SLE, a positive test occurs in only 40% to 50% of people with SLE. The anti-DNA level increases with nephritis; therefore, anti-DNA status is helpful in monitoring progression of the disease.

The anti-Sm test is slightly less useful because 60% of patients with SLE will have negative tests. It can be helpful in diagnosis because it is specific for the disease and is rarely positive in other rheumatic conditions or connective tissue diseases. The anti-Ro/SSA should be tested in pregnant women because its presence indicates a risk of neonatal lupus. Sometimes an enzyme-linked immunosorbent assay will be ordered instead of an FANA panel because it is easy to perform, readily measured, and less labor intensive.

Complement Level

Complement is a term used to describe 20 specific serum globulin proteins, identified by letters and numbers, that are activated in the inflammatory response. C3 and C4 are two of the nine major complement proteins that bind with antigen-antibody complexes for the purpose of lysis. When the number of complexes increases, more complement is used for lysis, depleting the amount available in the blood. Therefore, C3, C4, and CH50 complement levels will be decreased in a patient with SLE or an altered hemolytic system. The C3 value will be less than 55 mg/dL, the C4 value will be less than 11 mg/dL, and the CH50 value will be less than 40 mg/dL.

Coombs' Test

The direct antiglobulin test (direct Coombs') is used to detect abnormal coating of red cells with antibody globulin (IgG). The IgG antibody is one of five classes of immunoglobulins produced by the B cells to neutralize an antigen and to precipitate lysis. In patients with SLE, there is increased activation of B cells, which secrete an increased number of Ig-secreting cells into the peripheral blood. It is never normal for circulating red blood cells to be coated with antibody, so a negative finding would be to discover no antigen-antibody reaction. Some drugs such as methyldopa (Aldomet), phenytoin (Dilantin), and penicillin may cause positive results, as will some illnesses such as pneumonia, leukemia, and hemolytic anemia.

INTERVENTIONS

The goal is to control the disease by preventing active inflammation, relieving the symptoms during an acute phase, and forcing the disease into remission. Potential nursing diagnoses include: (1) deficient knowledge related to the disease process, treatment regimen, medications, and health promotion, and (2) risk for infection related to a compromised immune system. Nursing interventions include encouraging patients to do the following.

Nutrition

- Follow a well-balanced diet of carbohydrates, protein, fats, and calories that is low in sodium intake, especially for patients with hypertension and nephritis.
- Consume a low-fat, low-lipid diet to prevent exacerbation of the disease.
- Avoid consumption of alfalfa sprouts and saturated fats, because these can induce lupus and may exacerbate the disease process.
- Read nutrition labels.

Exercise/Rest

- Develop regular sleeping habits, ideally 8 to 10 hours of sleep a night.
- Prioritize and space activities of daily living to conserve energy and prevent fatigue.
- Participate in regular periods of exercise balanced by rest periods. Strengthening and toning will keep the joints in working order and will increase muscle strength and endurance.
- Promote exercise without placing excessive strain on the joints and the muscles by following an aquatic exercise program.
- Call to determine the availability of local aquatic programs, which the Arthritis Foundation has developed at YMCAs.

Sun/Ultraviolet Light

- Avoid the sun during peak hours of 10 AM to 3 PM because it has an impact on the epidermal DNA, promoting an inflammatory response and exacerbation of current skin problems.

- Use sunscreens with a protection factor (SPF) of at least 25 on a year-round basis.
- Tint the windows in the car, and avoid sun lamps, tanning booths, and unshielded fluorescent lights.
- Wear protective clothing such as a wide-brimmed hat, white and light-weight fabrics, long sleeves, pants, and protective sunglasses specifically coated to block ultraviolet rays.
- Avoid snow and water skiing because the sun is reflected from water and snow.
- Avoid discotheques, color television sets, halogen lamps, and photocopier machines.
- Avoid certain medications that may cause a photoallergic or a phototoxic reaction (e.g., tetracyclines, phenytoin, sulfa-containing agents).

Skin

- Inspect the skin daily for open areas, rashes, or other signs of infection.
- Cleanse with a mild soap, use mild shampoos, dry by patting versus rubbing, and take cool baths to decrease discomfort and scaling of the skin.
- Avoid powder, irritating perfumes, and other drying agents.
- Use hypoallergenic cosmetics that contain moisturizers.
- Avoid harsh household chemicals and cleansers.

Immunizations

- Immunizations with weakened live (attenuated) organisms (e.g., polio, measles, mumps, rubella) produce a very mild case of the disease to stimulate production of antibodies to protect against the disease. They have not been established as being safe in patients who are taking high doses of steroids or cytotoxic therapy because they can exacerbate the disease and the vaccine may be ineffective.
- Immunizations with killed vaccines (e.g., pneumococcus, influenza, tetanus) are generally regarded as safe but may be ineffective for those taking immunosuppressive agents.
- Avoid immunizations during immunosuppressive therapy and at least 3 months after therapy has been discontinued.

Contraception

- Discuss pregnancy with the practitioner before becoming pregnant; women with SLE have a 60% risk of experiencing a lupus flare-up during pregnancy.
- Successful pregnancies with good outcomes can occur, provided that there is minimal organ involvement (especially renal, CNS, and cardiopulmonary systems).
- Female or pregnant patients with active SLE and renal disease or who take more than 20 mg/day of prednisone have an increased risk of a preterm birth.
- Review contraception options: a diaphragm or a sponge with contraceptive jelly or foam, a progestational agent, or a contraceptive device used by the partner is recommended.
- Use a low dose of an oral estrogen-containing contraceptive in mild lupus, unless there is marked lipidemia, hypertension, or a history of thrombotic events.
- Visit the gynecologist twice as often.

Stress

- Determine life stressors, coping strategies, and additional strategies to eliminate or cope with stressors.
- Join the Lupus Foundation of America or the Arthritis Foundation.
- Realize that during an acute phase, you may be homebound (weak and fatigued); use the telephone and the Internet as support networks.
- Ask for help when needed; make sure that family members have realistic expectations of the disease.

Flare-ups

- Review the signs and symptoms that may suggest an acute flare-up or an increase in severity of the disease.
- Discuss potential triggering factors and the relationship between these and flare-ups, and call the practitioner immediately when symptoms occur.

Lifestyle Change

- Abstain from smoking and avoid second-hand smoke. Smoking impairs oxygenation, raises blood pressure, and can exacerbate the disease.
- Avoid alcohol because of kidney involvement and medication effects.

Osteoporosis

- Undergo a bone density test to determine the degree of osteoporosis. The patient with SLE has additional risks secondary to high-dose glucocorticoid therapy and physical inactivity. Promote exercise to prevent further bone loss.
- Take a minimum of 1000 mg/day of calcium. Calcium is poorly absorbed while on glucocorticoid therapy.
- If postmenopausal, take a low dose of estrogen to prevent the development of osteoporosis.

Pharmacologic Modalities

NSAIDs such as indomethacin (Indocin), naproxen (Naprosyn), or ibuprofen (Motrin) are used to control mild inflammation (arthritis, myalgia, arthralgia) and fever. They should be taken with food. Side effects include gastrointestinal distress, anemia, thrombocytopenia, headache, and abdominal pain. These drugs should be used with caution in patients with stomach ulcers and should be avoided in those with lupus nephritis because they can cause impairment of renal function. Because NSAIDs can interact with diuretics, beta-blockers such as propranolol, cardiac glycosides such as digitoxin, and antidepressants such as lithium, all medications must be reviewed before these agents are recommended. The nurse should closely supervise any patient on warfarin (Coumadin) for bleeding and should ensure that the patient understands the need to avoid aspirin when taking NSAIDs.

Corticosteroids

Prednisone (Deltasone) and fludrocortisone (Florinef) are used to suppress inflammation and to treat internal changes caused by lupus.

Topical. Fluorinated forms, such as betamethasone dipropionate 0.05% (Diprolene) and clobetasol propionate 0.05% (Temovate), are stronger than non-fluorinated forms (hydrocortisone). The fluorinated form should not be used on the face for more than 2 weeks at a time because cutaneous side effects may occur. Ointments should be used for dry skin and creams for oily. The ointment form is most effective, and fluorocarbon-propelled sprays are least effective. Side effects are bruising, striae, and acne. The cream form should be used sparingly because systemic absorption may occur.

Oral. Prednisone (Deltasone) is commonly used because it does not require hepatic metabolism. Side effects are changes in physical appearance, acne, easy bruising, moon facies, hypertension, gastrointestinal bleeding, and diabetes. Diabetic patients need to assess their blood sugar more often, and patients with hypertension must assess their blood pressure frequently and restrict their sodium intake. Oral prednisone should be taken at mealtime or with a snack to prevent gastric irritation. The medication should be protected from light. The drug should be tapered rather than discontinued abruptly, because this may cause an adrenal gland crisis. Alcoholic beverages should be avoided because they increase stomach irritation. The patient should wear a medical alert bracelet or carry identification tags when receiving long-term steroid therapy.

Antimalarial Drugs

Hydroxychloroquine (Plaquenil) and chloroquine (Aralen) reduce exacerbations and decrease inflammation by increasing the pH of cells, making them more basic versus acidic and turning off the antigen process. These drugs are useful in managing skin, joint, and muscle symptoms; fever; and fatigue. They should not be used in those with organ involvement (e.g., heart, lungs, or kidneys) because clearance from the body increases the risk of side effects and causes the skin to yellow. Retinal toxicity can occur, so a baseline ophthalmologic examination should be performed. These drugs should be avoided in patients with preexisting ophthalmic conditions. Side effects are bloating, diarrhea, and nausea.

Immunosuppressive Drugs

Azathioprine (Imuran) and cyclophosphamide (Cytoxan) are effective in lupus nephritis and severe SLE. It takes 3 months for the full effect to occur. The side effects are gastrointestinal distress, bone marrow depression, nausea, cramps, weight loss, alopecia, and amenorrhea. These drugs are contraindicated in patients with hepatic impairment. A complete blood count and liver function tests should be obtained before starting these agents. Immunosuppressive drugs suppress positive reactions to tuberculin skin tests, *Candida*, and mumps. Female patients are advised not to become pregnant for up to 4 months after the medication is discontinued because of the drug's mutagenic potential.

 COMMUNITY CARE

Assessment

- Obtain biographical data (e.g., gender, age, race, culture, occupation).
- Determine the reason for seeking care (i.e., chief complaint, location and characteristics of symptoms, severity, precipitating events, and aggravating and alleviating factors, including home remedies, herbal preparations, and over-the-counter and prescription medications).

- Note the present health status (i.e., perceived level of health, current medications, health promotion activities, dietary patterns, weight gain or loss, fatigue, and energy level).
- Elicit the past health history (childhood illnesses, chronic illnesses, previous surgeries, and obstetric history).
- Inquire about the family history. Trace back two generations to determine if there were any autoimmune disorders, kidney diseases, or neurologic or musculoskeletal disorders.
- Review the systems (general, dermatologic, otolaryngologic, mammary, cardiovascular, neurologic, respiratory, gastrointestinal, urinary, reproductive, and musculoskeletal).
- Determine what environmental factors are present (occupation, hazards in place of employment or home, recent or past travel outside the country, use of tanning beds, home location, and chemical exposure).
- Note the patient's psychosocial status (significant relationships, hobbies, demands, recent changes or stressors, coping strategies, and habits).

Monitoring

- Order laboratory and diagnostic studies (liver function tests, complete blood count, renal studies, chest radiography, bone density testing).
- Observe for any skin ulcerations.
- Ensure compliance with the treatment regimen.
- Determine if there are any side effects of the medication.

Prevention

The patient should do the following:

- Manage stress.
- Avoid fad diets; maintain a well-balanced diet.
- Find a support group to assist in living and coping with the disease.
- Strive for regular exercise and adequate rest.
- Follow the prescribed regimen for control of hypertension, diabetes, and cardiovascular diseases.
- Avoid and prevent pregnancy until disease activity has subsided.
- Stop smoking, and maintain body weight of less than 120% of ideal weight.

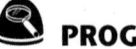 **PROGNOSIS**

Today, the 10-year survival rate for patients with lupus is approximately 90%, and the 20-year survival rate is 70%. The major causes of morbidity and mortality are glomerulonephritis (in 60% to 76%), nervous system dysfunction (in 50%), and infections due to *Staphylococcus*, *Escherichia coli*, and fungal organisms (in 19% to 50%). The presence of renal disease at the onset, measured by means of serum creatinine or urine protein excretion, is by far the most important predictor of poor outcome. Patients with systolic blood pressure consistently greater than 145 mm Hg in combination with a serum blood urea nitrogen level of greater than 40 mg/dL have the poorest prognosis.

During the next decade, the goal is disease remission and even to find a cure. Currently, experimental medications, antileprosy agents (dapsone and thalidomide), antiviral agents (interferon), and vasodilators (prostaglandin E_1) have been found to produce improvement in disease activity. Other treatments in the experimental phase are anti–T cell antibody injections, plasmapheresis followed by intravenous cyclophosphamide, and transplantation of bone marrow stem cells.

 CLINICAL PEARLS

○ Sunlight may trigger the appearance of the red rash or flush across the bridge of the nose and on the cheeks (called the butterfly rash).
○ Alfalfa sprouts and diets high in saturated fats may exacerbate the disease process. A low-fat diet is preferred.
○ Sunscreens with an SPF of at least 25 should be worn year-round.
○ Topical corticosteroids come in ointment and cream forms. Use ointments for dry skin and creams for oily skin.

NURSING PROBLEM/ DIAGNOSIS	NURSING INTERVENTIONS CLASSIFICATION (NIC)
Risk for infection	Infection protection Infection control Surveillance Teaching: prescribed medication
Arthralgia (joint pain)	Pain management Exercise therapy: joint mobility
Fatigue Risk for flare-ups/Effective therapeutic regimen management	Energy management Exercise promotion Nutrition management Immunization/vaccination administration Teaching: disease process

chapter 22

Immunologic

Human Immunodeficiency Virus

Section 1

Debora Burkett Nutt

 OVERVIEW

Human immunodeficiency virus (HIV) is a retrovirus that attacks the body's immune system. HIV is characterized by a long interval between initial infection and the onset of serious symptoms leading to acquired immunodeficiency syndrome (AIDS). This latency period can last 10 to 15 years. Over time, HIV destroys the helper T cells (CD4 cells) that help fight infection. Persons who have AIDS usually develop opportunistic infections. They die of these infections because the immune system is unable to fight the microbes, viruses, or bacteria that cause these illnesses.

At the end of 2000, 36.1 million people worldwide were living with HIV/AIDS. Of these, 34.7 million were adults and 1.4 million were children younger than 15 years of age. In the United States, the Centers for Disease Control and Prevention (CDC) estimates that 800,000 to 900,000 people are living with HIV infection, one third of whom do not know that they have the infection. About 40,000 new HIV infections occur annually in the United States—70% in men and 30% in women.

 PATHOPHYSIOLOGY

The HIV virus is spread in several ways. The most common route is through sexual contact with an infected partner. The virus enters the body through the vagina, vulva, penis, rectum, or mouth during sexual contact. HIV is often spread among intravenous (IV) drug abusers through the sharing of needles or syringes that are contaminated with tiny quantities of blood.

Before 1985, HIV could be spread through blood transfusions or blood components. Since then, all blood and blood products are routinely screened for HIV, and new heat-treating techniques for blood have significantly reduced the risk of acquiring HIV from blood products.

A woman can transmit the HIV virus to her fetus during pregnancy and to her infant during birth and breast-feeding. The incidence of such transmission can be reduced to 1% with zidovudine (AZT) therapy during pregnancy, labor, and delivery. The preferred method of delivery is caesarean section, and the infant is treated with AZT during the first 6 weeks of life.

The HIV virus uses reverse transcriptase to alter the normal flow of genetic material. After the virus enters the body, it invades cells with the CD4 antigen. Once the virus is inside the cell, it sheds the protein coat and uses reverse transcriptase to convert viral RNA to viral DNA. The new viral DNA mixes with the host cell DNA and is duplicated during the normal process of cell division. Within the cell, the virus can be latent, can infect daughter cells during host replication, or can replicate and cause lysis of the host cell as the virus seeks to invade other cells.

The primary cells affected by the HIV are the CD4 cells. HIV also infects macrophages and certain cells of the central nervous system. The CD4 cells are important in normal immune system function. They recognize foreign antigens and infected cells and activate antibody-producing B cells. They also activate the phagocytic activity of monocytes and macrophages. The loss of CD4 cells leads to the immunodeficiency characteristic of HIV and AIDS.

The clinical course of HIV infection is divided into seven stages:

1. Viral transmission
2. Primary HIV infection (acute retroviral syndrome)
3. Seroconversion
4. Asymptomatic chronic infection with or without persistent generalized lymphadenopathy (PGL)
5. Symptomatic HIV infection (previously known as "AIDS-related complex" [ARC] and more recently referred to as "stage B" according to the 1993 CDC classification)
6. AIDS (AIDS indicator conditions according to the 1993 CDC criteria or a CD4 cell count below 200/mm^3)
7. Advanced HIV infection, characterized by a CD4 cell count below 50/mm^3.

 SIGNS AND SYMPTOMS

Many people do not develop symptoms of HIV infection. Some exhibit flu-like signs and symptoms within 1 to 2 weeks after exposure. These early signs and symptoms include fever, headache, malaise, and enlarged lymph nodes (easily felt in the neck or groin). Often these are overlooked as possible signs and symptoms of HIV and instead are attributed to flu or viral illness. Although the person is asymptomatic, the virus is still replicating and deteriorating the CD4 cells.

As the immune system weakens and deteriorates, late signs and symptoms develop. These may include large swollen lymph nodes, lack of energy, weight loss, frequent fever and night sweats, persistent or frequent yeast infections (oral or vaginal), persistent skin rashes or flaky skin, pelvic inflammatory disease, and short-term memory loss.

The CDC has established a classification system based on the clinical conditions associated with HIV infection and AIDS. In category A, patients have primary HIV infection with no or only minor signs and symptoms of mild viral disease. This category includes asymptomatic HIV infection, persistent generalized lymphadenopathy, and acute HIV infection with accompanying illness or history of acute HIV infection. In category B, patients have an increased incidence of infectious and malignant complications that are attributed to HIV infection and a dysfunctional immune system. This category includes bacterial infections (e.g., endocarditis, meningitis, pneumonia, sepsis), fungal infections (including vaginal or oropharyngeal candidiasis that is recurrent and unresponsive to therapy), fever or diarrhea (lasting longer than 1 month), cervical dysplasia/carcinoma, hairy leukopenia of the oral mucosa, herpes zoster involving two episodes or more than one dermatome, pelvic inflammatory disease, peripheral neuropathy, listeriosis, and tuberculosis. In category C, patients experience serious, life-threatening complications related to the severe immunodeficiency. The following conditions are indicators of AIDS: systemic fungal and protozoal infections, including candidiasis (of the bronchi, trachea, esophagus, or lungs), coccidioidomycosis, cryptococcosis, histoplasmosis, cryptosporidiosis, toxoplasmosis, and *Pneumocystis carinii* pneumonia (PCP); viral infections (e.g., herpes and cytomegalovirus); malignancies (e.g., Kaposi's sarcoma and lymphoma); bacterial infections (e.g., *Mycobacterium avium* complex or *Mycobacterium* tuberculosis); HIV encephalopathy; and wasting syndrome.

 ## DIAGNOSTIC CRITERIA

The diagnosis of HIV is made by detecting HIV antibodies in the blood. It may take 6 to 12 weeks for the body to develop antibodies to HIV.

Enzyme-linked immunosorbent assay (ELISA) is the initial screening test for HIV in adults, adolescents, and children older than 18 months. The ELISA can produce false-negative results if done before 12 weeks after exposure to HIV, before seroconversion has taken place. The ELISA is 99% accurate for patients in whom exposure to HIV occurred more than 12 weeks earlier. If results are positive, the test should be repeated. After a second positive ELISA, a Western blot test should be done.

The Western blot test reveals the reactivity of antibodies with HIV-specific proteins that have been separated by electrophoresis. This test is expensive and is used to confirm a positive ELISA or verify a suspected false-negative ELISA.

The diagnosis of HIV can also be based on a positive result of a detectable quantity of any of the following virologic (nonantibody) tests: HIV nucleic acid (DNA or RNA) detection (DNA polymerase chain reaction [PCR] or plasma HIV-1 RNA); HIV p24 antigen test, and HIV isolation (viral culture). Serum p24 antigen can be detected after infection but before antibodies to HIV develop and also later when the patient becomes ill. This test is used to measure viral replication.

 ## INTERVENTIONS
Pharmacologic Management

Pharmacologic management of the HIV-infected patient has two primary goals. The first goal is to suppress the infection, decrease symptoms, and prolong the patient's life. The second goal is to treat opportunistic infections and malignancies.

Table 22-1-1 lists the mechanisms of action and nursing implications for drugs commonly used to treat HIV infection. The antiretroviral agents known as *nucleoside reverse transcriptase inhibitors (NRTIs)* act by interrupting the early stage of the virus making copies of itself. A subclass of drugs in this category, nucleoside analogs, works by inhibiting HIV reverse transcriptase, the enzyme responsible for viral replication by competitive inhibition and termination of DNA elongation. In essence, they slow the spread of HIV in the body and delay the onset of opportunistic infections. Specific nucleoside analogs include zidovudine (AZT, Retrovir), didanosine (ddI, Videx), zalcitabine (ddC, Hivid), stavudine (d4T, Zerit), lamivudine (3TC, Epivir), and aba-

Table 22-1-1. Medication Therapy for Human Immunodeficiency Virus

DRUG CATEGORY	DRUG ACTIONS	NURSING IMPLICATIONS
Nucleoside reverse transcriptase inhibitors (NRTIs) or nucleoside analogs Zidovudine (Retrovir, AZT) Didanosine (Videx) Zalcitabine (Hivid) Stavudine (d4T, Zerit) Lamivudine (3TC, Epivir) Ziagen (Abacavir, 1592U89) Adefavir dipivoxil (Preveon) Lamivudine/zidovudine Retrovir/epivir (Combivir)	Inhibits HIV reverse transcriptase by competing for binding with the natural enzymes; inhibits HIV DNA synthesis	• These drugs can cause bone marrow suppression, requiring therapy breaks or administration of bone marrow growth factors. • Monitor complete blood count. • Instruct the patient to take the medication on an empty stomach. • Monitor for signs and symptoms of superinfections (e.g., furry tongue, mouth lesions, vaginal or rectal itching, thrush).
Protease inhibitors Saquinavir (SQV, Invirase, Fortovase) Ritonavir (Norvir) Indinavir (Crixivan) Nelfinavir (Viracept) Amprenavir (Agenerase) Lopinavir/Ritonavir	Inhibits the activity of HIV protease, preventing cleavage and maturation of the HIV polypeptides	• These drugs can cause gastric intolerance such as cholecystatic disease or pancreatitis and diarrhea.
Nonnucleoside reverse transcriptase inhibitors (NNRTIs) Nevirapine (Viramune) Delavirdine (Rescriptor) Efavirenz (Sustiva, DMP-266)	Binds directly with HIV reverse transcriptase to inhibit HIV replication	• These drugs can produce multiple drug interactions. • Keep the drug refrigerated at all times. • Instruct the patient to take the drug on an empty stomach. • Rashes are very common. • Transient neurologic adverse effects, such as dizziness and headache, may occur.

cavir (Ziagen). These drugs can have serious side effects. They can cause depletion of red and white blood cells, leading to anemia with increased risk of infection, inflammation of the pancreas, painful nerve damage, lactic acidosis, and severe hepatomegaly (enlarged liver) with steatosis (fatty liver).

A second class of drugs approved for treating HIV infection is the *protease inhibitors.* These drugs interrupt virus replication at a later step in the viral life cycle. They inhibit the activity of HIV proteases and prevent the cleavage of viral polyproteins into functional proteins in HIV-infected cells. Drugs in this class include saquinavir (SQV, Invirase), ritonavir (Norvir), indinavir (Crixivan), amprenavir (Agenerase), and nelfinavir (Viracept). Common side effects associated with protease inhibitors include nausea, diarrhea, gastrointestinal symptoms, and drug interactions.

A third class of drugs known as *nonnucleoside reverse transcriptase inhibitors (NNRTIs)* acts by binding to the actual reverse transcriptase, inhibiting HIV replication. The major drugs in this class are delavirdine (Rescriptor), nevirapine (Viramune), and efavirenz (Sustiva, DMP-266). The primary side effect is rash. Transient neurologic effects, such as dizziness and headache, may also occur. These drugs can be taken in combination with nucleoside analogs and protease inhibitors.

Because the HIV virus can become resistant to single therapy regimens, combination therapy is necessary to effectively suppress the virus. This usually involves a combination of three drugs. Research has proved that the highly active antiretroviral therapy (HAART) protocol is a major factor in reducing the number of deaths from AIDS. HAART is a combination of triple drug therapy that includes drugs from two or all three classes. This combination therapy can be given to newly diagnosed HIV patients, as well as patients with AIDS.

Prophylaxis: It is recommended that all HIV-infected patients receive pneumococcal influenza, hepatitis B, and Hemophilus influenza B vaccines. A patient with a positive PPD is started on isoniazid (INH). When a patient's CD4 cell count falls below 200/mm^3, then prophylactic treatment for PCP is started with trimethoprim-sulfamethoxazole (TMP-SMX). A patient with a CD4 cell count below 50/mm^3 is started on prophylactic treatment for *Mycobacterium avium* complex with clarithromycin or azithromycin. Table 22-1-2 provides more information on treating opportunistic infections.

Nursing Care

Nursing care for HIV-infected patients varies depending on the stage of the disease. In the early stages, it is important to provide patient teaching about prevention, health maintenance, knowledge of drug side effects, symptoms of potential complications and psychosocial support. During the later stages, care focuses on treating symptoms along with providing ongoing psychosocial support and physical care.

Prevention includes encouraging the patient to discuss the diagnosis with his or her sexual partner(s). This may be difficult because of feelings of guilt or anger related to the diagnosis. The major preventive measure during sexual contact is the use of latex condoms. Limiting concurrent sexual partners is also recommended. A patient who uses IV drugs should be encouraged to discuss the diagnosis with his or her drug partners and to always use a clean needle. It is recommended that all pregnant women be tested for HIV, so that an infected mother and fetus can be identified and treated during pregnancy. The patient should be taught to notify all health care providers of his or her HIV status.

Patients are taught about routine immunizations aimed at preventing other disease complications. Routine follow-up for physical examination and laboratory testing are important to monitor disease progression. Laboratory tests at this time include measurement of viral load as well as CD4 cell counts. An expert panel from the International AIDS Society-USA has issued the following guidelines for testing:

- Take two different viral load measurements 2 to 3 weeks apart to determine a baseline measurement.
- Repeat this every 3 to 6 months along with CD4 counts to monitor the viral load and CD4 count.
- Repeat the test 4 to 6 weeks after starting or changing antiretroviral therapy to determine the effect on viral load.

maintenance strategies emphasize physical exercise, diet, stress management, and knowledge of side effects of drug therapy as well as future potential complications. Physical exercise is important to overall physical and mental health. It improves health by increasing lung capacity, energy, and circulation and improving sleep, appetite, and bowel activity. Nutrition is important in maintaining the immune system. The patient needs to maintain an adequate weight by eating a high-calorie, high-protein diet. Ways to do this include using food supplements and eating between meals. Stress-reduction activities include adequate sleep and rest and regular exercise. Other possible stress-reduction strategies include meditation, visualization, and biofeedback. Another important factor in reducing stress is through social interactions with friends and family, as well as spiritual and religious activities.

In-hospital nursing care focuses on progression of HIV. The nurse should assess for the following potential problems that are related to disease advancement.

Mental Status Changes. Loss of short-term memory, altered behavior and mood patterns, disorientation, and impaired judgment and decision-making ability may occur. These effects are related to central nervous system infections and intracranial lesions. The nurse should reorient the patient and assist with appropriate decision-making functions while reducing any sensory stimulation. A safe environment must be ensured, because the patient may be at risk for falls.

Infection. Signs of infection include elevated temperature and abnormally high or low white blood cell count. Infection results from altered immune response. It should correlate inversely with CD4 cell count. The nurse monitors the patient's temperature and laboratory values for abnormal changes.

Skin Integrity. Skin problems (e.g., pigmentation changes, turgor, irritation, blisters, and rash) are associated with poor nutritional status and other complications, such as herpes or Kaposi's sarcoma. Skin care is aimed at keeping skin clean and dry. Rashes are treated with topical creams as needed.

Activity Intolerance. Fatigue, dyspnea with activity, and weakness with activity commonly occur. The nurse should monitor functional status and promote daily activity with planned rest periods to help the patient maintain strength. This is a sign of overall health.

Nutritional Status. Problems may include difficulty swallowing, loss of appetite, and poor intake compared to output. This can result from oral candidiasis and other complications. The nurse monitors the patient's weight and laboratory values to evaluate nutritional status. In concert with the dietician, the nurse then recommends a proper diet and meal supplements for the patient. The patient needs a diet with high-protein and high-calorie foods.

Bowel Activity. Diarrhea commonly occurs from medications or gastrointestinal infection. The patient should avoid caffeine, which stimulates peristalsis. Send stool specimens to the laboratory for culture and identification of *Clostridium difficile* and ova and parasites. Diarrhea is treated with loperamide (Imodium) or diphenoxylate (Lomotil) as long as there is no blood in the stool and no source identified from laboratory tests, and if the patient is afebrile. Fluid and electrolytes are monitored and replacement provided as needed (see Chapter 11, Section 3).

Psychosocial Isolation. To combat feelings of depression, withdrawal, and apathy, the nurse should provide a supportive, comforting environment.

Table 22-1-2. Pharmacologic Management of AIDS Complications

COMPLICATION	PROPHYLAXIS	PREFERRED TREATMENT
Pneumocystis carinii pneumonia (acute inflammation of the lungs characterized by nonproductive cough and dyspnea)	Trimethoprim/sulfamethoxazole PO (1 double-strength tab/day, or 1 double-strength tab, 3 times a week)	Trimethoprim 15 mg/kg/day plus sulfamethoxazole 75 mg/kg/day Po or IV for 21 days (Typical oral dose of TMP-SMX is 2 double-strength tabs, tid.)
Aspergillosis (an acute invasive pulmonary infection)		Amphotericin B 1.0–1.5 mg/kg/day
Oropharyngeal candida (thrush) (white creamy plaques on the inflamed base of the palate, buccal mucosa, or tongue)	Maintenance: Nystatin 500,000 U gargled 5 times a day; clotrimazole oral troches 10 mg 5 times a day; Fluconazole 100 mg/day PO or 200 mg 3 times a week.	Fluconazole 100 mg/day PO; clotrimazole oral troches 10 mg 5 times a day; nystatin 500,000 U gargled 5 times a day
Vaginitis (characterized by itching, redness, and white discharge)	May require continuous treatment	Intravaginal miconazole suppository 200 mg for 3 days or cream (2%) for 7 days; clotrimazole cream (1%) for 7–14 days or tablets, 100 mg/day for 7 days, 100 mg/day for 2 or 3 days, or 500 mg single dose; fluconazole 150 mg single dose PO
Cryptococcal meningitis (marked by fever, headache, nausea and vomiting, visual changes, stiff neck, cranial nerve deficits, and seizures)	Maintenance: Fluconazole 200 mg/day PO	Amphotericin B 0.7 mg/kg/day IV for 10–14 days, plus/minus flucytocine 100 mg/kg/day PO, then fluconazole 400 mg/day for 8–10 weeks
Cryptococcosis without meningitis (pulmonary, disseminated, or antigenemia)	Maintenance: Fluconazole 200 mg/day	Itraconazole 200 mg PO bid or 100 mg oral suspension/day for 6–10 weeks
Histoplasmosis (a type of fungal infection caused by *H. capsulatum* with symptoms of fever, weight loss, SOB, and dyspnea)	Maintenance: Itraconazole 200 mg PO bid	Amphotericin B 0.5–1.0 mg/kg/day IV for 7–14 days; itraconazole 300 mg PO bid for 3 days, then 200 mg PO bid of 100 mg oral suspension bid
Coccidioidomycosis (a systemic fungal infection marked by fever, dyspnea, nonproductive cough, and chest films with diffuse nodular infiltrates)	Maintenance: Fluconazole 400 mg/day	Amphotericin B 0.5 mg/kg/day IV for 8 weeks, total dose 2–2.5 g

770

Condition	Treatment	Treatment
Mycobacterium tuberculosis	Maintenance: 1. INH/RIF daily or 2–3 times a week for 18 weeks 2. INH/RIF 2–3 times a week for 18 weeks 3. INH/RIF/PZA/EMB (or SM) 3 times a week for 4 months	Induction: 1. INH/RIF/PXA/EMB (or SM) daily for 2 months 2. INH/RIF/PZA/EMB (or SM) daily for 2 weeks, then 2–3 times a week for 6 weeks. 3. INH/RIF/PZA/EMB (or SM) 3 times a week for 8 weeks
Mycobacterium avium complex (MAC) bacteremia (most common systemic bacterial infection in AIDS producing fever, night sweats, weight loss, and diarrhea)	Clarithromycin 500 mg PO bid, or azithromycin 1200 mg q week	Clarithromycin 500 mg PO bid plus ethambutol 15 mg/kg/day PO plus/minus rifabutin 300 mg/day PO
Herpes simplex (viral infection that should be considered with any chronic nonhealing ulcer with symptoms of orolabial, genital, or rectal infection)	Acyclovir 400 mg PO bid or famciclovir 125–250 mg PO bid or valacyclovir 500 mg PO bid or 1 g day Recurrent: Acyclovir 400 mg PO tid or 800 mg PO bid or famciclovir 125 mg PO bid or valacyclovir 500 mg PO bid, all given for 5 days	Initial (mild): Acyclovir 400 mg PO tid or famciclovir 250 mg PO tid or valacyclovir 1 g PO bid, all given for 7–10 days Refractory (severe): Acyclovir 15 mg/kg/day IV for at least 7 days
Herpes zoster (a common pathogen that causes shingles, disseminated skin involvement, postinfectious vasculitis, or visceral disease)	Varicella zoster immune globulin (ZVIG) 5 vials (6.25 mL) within 96 hours of exposure Maintenance: Acyclovir, famciclovir, valacyclovir PO in doses in next column	Dermatomal: Acyclovir 800 mg PO 5 times a day for at least 7 days (until lesions crust) or famciclovir 500 mg PO tid or valacyclovir 1 g PO tid Ophthalmic nerve: Acyclovir 30–36 mg/kg/day IV for at least 7 days Acyclovir-resistant strains: Foscarnet 40 mg/kg IV q 8 h or 60 mg/kg q 12 h
Cytomegalovirus retinitis (viral infection affecting the eyes with symptoms of decreased visual acuity, presence of floaters or visual field cuts)	Prophylaxis: Generally not recommended Maintenance: Foscarnet 90–120 mg/kg/day IV, ganciclovir 5–6 mg/kg day IV for 5–7 days or 1000 mg PO tid, cidofovir 5 mg/kg IV every other week; intraocular ganciclovir release device every 6 months plus oral ganciclovir 1 g PO tid	Foscarnet 60 mg/kg IV q 8 hr or 90 mg/kg IV q 12 h for 14–21 days; ganciclovir 5 mg/kg IV bid for 14–21 days; intraocular ganciclovir release device (Vitrasert) every 6 months plus/minus oral ganciclovir 1 g PO with meals tid; cidofovir 5 mg/kg IV each week for 2 weeks, then 5 mg/kg IV for 2 weeks plus probenecid, 2 g PO 3 hr before each dose, 1 g PO at 2 hr and 8 hr postdose

COMMUNITY CARE

The diagnosis of HIV can be devastating. Eventually, the patient becomes unable to work, which leads to problems with health care coverage. The U.S. health care system is focused on acute care, with minimal emphasis on long-term care for terminal illness. Only limited state and federal funds are available to assist with the care of terminal illness in the varying phases of symptom control. Once a patient reaches the endpoint of the disease, family and friends sometimes are not available for support. There comes a time when the patient becomes unable to care for himself or herself. Options for long-term care include residential care, home care services, and hospice. Health care professionals involved with case management can improve these services if they are knowledgeable about the different service providers.

 PROGNOSIS

AIDS is a chronic, progressive, and terminal illness caused by HIV. During 2000, AIDS caused an estimated 3 million deaths, including 1.3 million women and 500,000 children younger than 15 years of age. As of June 1999, 438,795 deaths from AIDS had been reported to the CDC. AIDS is now the fifth leading cause of death in the United States for people who are 25 to 44 years of age.

 CLINICAL PEARLS

○ A diagnosis of HIV does not mean that the person has AIDS.
○ AIDS is the end-stage of HIV infection, characterized by CD4 count below 200/mm^3 and the presence of opportunistic infections.
○ With new combinations of antiretroviral therapy, HIV can remain in the latent stage for 10 to 20 years.

NURSING PROBLEM/ DIAGNOSIS	NURSING INTERVENTIONS CLASSIFICATION (NIC)
Prevention	Health education
	Health screening
	Teaching: safe sex
	Environmental management: community
	Behavior management: sexual
	Sexual counseling
Risk for opportunistic infection/ Risk for infection	Infection protection
	Respiratory monitoring
	Surveillance
	Immunization/vaccination administration
	Oral health maintenance
	Exercise promotion
Poor nutrition/Imbalanced nutrition less than body requirements	Nutrition therapy
	Nutrition monitoring
	Nutrition counseling

Allergies

Section 2   Patricia S. Preston

 OVERVIEW

More than 20% of the American population has some form of allergic disease. Two factors contribute to the development of allergy: genetic predisposition and environmental exposure.

The direct cost of care for allergic disorders is more than 18 billion dollars annually. Besides the direct and indirect cost to the nation, allergies can negatively affect an individual's quality of life. Even the most benign form of allergy, allergic rhinitis, has been shown to correlate with poorer scores on tests designed to measure quality of life. On the other end of the spectrum, two forms of allergic disease, asthma and anaphylaxis, can be life-threatening.

 PATHOPHYSIOLOGY

Allergy results from an exaggerated or inappropriate response of the immune system to antigens that do not present a threat to the body. There are four types of allergic reactions:

- Type I: immediate type (IgE and mast cell mediated)
- Type II: non-IgE antibody mediated
- Type III: immune complex mediated
- Type IV: Delayed type (cell mediated)

Type I Reactions

Type I, or immediate, hypersensitivity reactions usually occur within 30 minutes of exposure to an allergen. Allergic rhinitis and asthma are examples of type I allergic reactions. The most dramatic and dangerous type I reaction is anaphylaxis, which usually occurs within minutes of exposure. Anaphylactoid reactions are also in this category, but they differ from anaphylaxis in that they are less severe, more easily reversed with antihistamines, and are not IgE mediated.

Late-phase reactions complicate the picture. These reactions can occur 4 to 6 hours after an immediate hypersensitivity response. Unlike in immediate allergic reactions, histamine is not responsible for the symptoms in late-phase responses. Therefore, antihistamines cannot prevent or alleviate a late-phase response.

Pathophysiology of Type I Reactions

Antigen, IgE, and mast cells are the main components of a type 1 allergic reaction. Exposure to an antigen leads to the formation of IgE antibodies specific to that antigen. These IgE antibodies attach themselves to receptors located on the walls of mast cells. This attachment sensitizes the mast cells to the particular antigen, which is now referred to as an allergen.

On subsequent exposures, the allergen binds to IgE attached to mast cell walls. This initiates an antigen–antibody reaction. In this reaction, the wall of the mast cell disintegrates and releases its contents—histamine, chemotactic factors, interleukin, and arachidonic acid—into the circulation. These products of mast cell degeneration are directly and indirectly responsible for creating the complex of symptoms seen in allergic disorders.

Histamine. Histamine increases vascular permeability, stimulates vasodilation, and contributes to smooth muscle contraction. Histamine's effect on the vasculature leads to edema of the mucous membranes and skin, as well as increased mucus secretion (causing nasal congestion and drainage), hives, and bronchoconstriction.

Chemotactic Factors. Chemotactic factors attract leukocytes, which further enhance the inflammatory response. Once the effect of histamine wears off, the leukocytes attracted by the chemotactic factors cause further inflammation.

Arachidonic Acid Derivatives. Leukotrienes and prostaglandins derive from the breakdown of arachidonic acid. Leukotrienes cause bronchoconstriction, increased vascular permeability, and vasoconstriction. Prostaglandins inhibit platelet aggregation and cause vasodilation.

Interleukins. Interleukins are cytokines. Cytokines are responsible for regulating the growth, development, and activation of the immune response. For example, interleukin-3 (IL-3) and interleukin-4 (IL-4) regulate IgE secretion.

Types II, III, and IV Reactions

The complement system is another important mediator in allergic reactions, and it plays a major role in type II and type III reactions. Once activated, complements bind to mast cells, attract neutrophils and phagocytes, and lyse cell membranes. Type II and type III reactions result from antibody–antigen reactions, but these reactions do not involve IgE. The clinical manifestations of a type II reaction can be similar to those of a type I reaction, such as in a transfusion reaction, or different, as in autoimmune disorders, in which the antibodies target the host protein.

In type III reactions, the complement cascade is initiated by the creation of immune complexes formed from the binding of circulating antigens and antibodies. Because the formation of immune complexes is a common and beneficial event in many disease processes, other host and antigenic factors contribute to a type III reaction. These reactions result in problems such as nephritis, iritis, and synovitis.

In type IV (delayed) reactions, manifestations of the allergy occur days after exposure. This is the only type of hypersensitivity that results primarily from cell-mediated (specifically T cell) immunity. Skin testing for tuberculosis exposure, for example, uses a type IV reaction. The body has difficulty eliminating mycobacterium, and thus attempts to "wall it off." When an immunocompetent person is exposed to tuberculosis, antibodies to the mycobacterium are formed. Therefore, when the mycobacterium is introduced intradermally (e.g., as in the Mantoux test), a reaction occurs at the injection site within 48 to 72 hours. Contact dermatitis (e.g., from poison ivy) is another example of this type of reaction.

 SIGNS AND SYMPTOMS
Type I Reactions
Allergic Rhinitis

Allergic rhinitis is the term describing the constellation of upper respiratory symptoms that result from allergen exposure. Allergens commonly implicated in allergic rhinitis include grass, weed and tree pollen, dust mites, molds, and dander from household pets and cockroaches.

Signs and symptoms of allergic rhinitis include watery, itchy eyes; thin, clear to yellow nasal discharge; sneezing; itching of the soft palate and nose; allergic shiners; nasal crease; pale, boggy nasal turbinates; cobblestoning of the posterior pharynx; and dry, hacking cough, usually a side effect of postnasal drainage.

Anaphylaxis

Anaphylaxis is a life-threatening, multiorgan manifestation of allergy resulting from a massive release of mediators from mast cells and basophils that cause widespread vasodilation and other manifestations. These reactions most often follow injection or, less often, ingestion of the allergen. Certain foods (e.g., legumes and shellfish), insect bites and stings, and medications (particularly antibiotics) are the most common causes of anaphylaxis. Penicillin is the most common cause of fatal anaphylaxis in the United States.

Anaphylactic reactions can begin with seemingly benign symptoms, such as flushing, warmth, tingling of the extremities, a lump in the throat, and a feeling of impending doom. When the major organs are affected, the following symptoms and signs may be seen:

- Skin: pruritus, urticaria, angioedema
- Cardiovascular: palpitations, hypotension, tachycardia, syncope, vascular collapse, and shock
- Respiratory: congestion, dyspnea, wheezing, stridor, asphyxiation
- Gastrointestinal: abdominal bloating, diarrhea, vomiting

Urticaria (Hives)

Urticaria is an allergic reaction involving the superficial portion of the dermis. Symptoms include pruritus and rash. The pruritus can be intense. Urticaria lasting 6 weeks or less is considered acute and occurs more commonly in children and young adults. Signs include a rash characterized by well-circumscribed wheals with raised borders and light centers, along with localized, nonpitting edema. These lesions can occur anywhere on the body but are most commonly seen on the extremities, face, and external genitalia.

Angioedema

Angioedema is similar to urticaria but involves the deeper layer of the dermis. The edema extends beyond circumscribed lesions, commonly affecting areas of loose connective tissue such as the lips, face, eyelids, mucous membranes, and tongue, although it can occur anywhere. Swelling in the upper airway, such as in the larynx, may compromise airflow and lead to respiratory distress and arrest.

Atopic Dermatitis

Another cutaneous manifestation of allergy is atopic dermatitis, also referred to as eczema. Atopic dermatitis may not appear until hours or days after exposure to an allergen, but it is considered a type I reaction because it results from IgE binding and mast cell degeneration. It is an inflammatory skin disorder in which edema occurs between keratinocytes and the epidermis, thus giving the skin a spongy appearance.

The main symptom of atopic dermatitis is pruritus. Signs include dry, scaly patches that are commonly found on the flexor surfaces of the extremities but can be located anywhere on the body. Intense scratching of these areas can cause them to take on a thickened, leathery appearance (lichenification). Secondary bacterial infections, usually caused by *Staphylococcus*, are common.

Asthma

Asthma results from hyperresponsiveness of the bronchi. This increased responsiveness causes narrowing and obstruction of the airways in response to various stimuli. Reversal of the airway obstruction is achieved either through medical intervention or spontaneously.

Signs and symptoms include shortness of breath, coughing, wheezing, and possibly respiratory distress. Lung function tests reveal decreased forced expiratory volume in 1 second (FEV_1) and forced vital capacity.

Other

Ingestion of certain foods or medications (see Anaphylaxis) can lead to allergic reactions. These are usually manifested in the gastrointestinal tract by nausea, vomiting, abdominal pain, and diarrhea. Contact with certain substances (e.g., latex or poison ivy) can cause allergic dermatitis. Contact dermatitis is a type IV allergic reaction.

DIAGNOSTIC CRITERIA

Various tests can help establish a diagnosis of allergy. An increase in total IgE level and eosinophilia are often present in allergic disease, but their absence does not necessarily rule out allergy. Skin tests and the radioallergosorbent (RAST) test are used to identify the specific allergens that invoke the allergic reaction in the patient.

Skin Testing

Skin testing is considered the gold standard for diagnosing allergies. The skin-prick test involves introducing an antigen directly into the epidermis by pricking the skin with an instrument impregnated with the antigen. Because mast cells are abundant in the dermis, the epidermal introduction of an antigen produces a localized skin reaction in persons sensitized to it.

No reaction should occur in response to the diluent, but the histamine, because of its intrinsic inflammatory capabilities, should cause a reaction even in nonallergic individuals. The positive control is placed to ensure that the patient's immune system is adequate. Many factors can lead to a lack of response to the positive control; the most common is recent antihistamine use. The patient should be advised to discontinue short-acting antihistamines for 2 to 3 days before the test. A patient taking a long-acting antihistamine must discontinue use up to 1 to 2 weeks earlier.

Blood Testing

The RAST test is a blood test used to identify allergies. This test measures levels of allergen-specific IgE in the blood. RAST testing is significantly more expensive than skin testing and thus is reserved for special cases, such as for a person with such extensive eczema so as to make skin testing impossible.

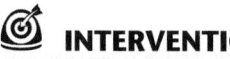 INTERVENTIONS
Anaphylaxis

Many patients believe that if they took a medication in the past without any adverse effects, they will never experience any adverse reactions to that medication. This is not the case, however. As discussed earlier, previous exposure not only provides no guarantee against anaphylaxis but is also necessary, because sensitization to an antigen must be established before a hypersensitivity response can occur.

Remembering three basic concepts can decrease the incidence of anaphylactic shock and help minimize its adverse outcomes: prevention, awareness, and preparation.

Prevention

Injection is the route most commonly linked to anaphylaxis, and antibiotics (particularly penicillin and beta-lactam inhibitors) are the most common triggers. Before any intramuscular (IM) or IV medication is given, all known drug allergies must be verified with the patient.

The patient should be told what medication he or she is being given immediately before administration. This may prompt the patient to recall a previous adverse reaction to that medication.

A patient who has experienced an anaphylactic or other significant allergic reaction should be encouraged to remove all remaining triggers from the home and taught how to use an Epi-pen, a device for home use that delivers a subcutaneous (SC) dose of epinephrine in an emergency situation.

Awareness

The early warning signs of anaphylaxis vary. Some people get a "funny feeling," whereas others may have little warning before shock develops. Complaints of itching, shortness of breath, dizziness, nausea, and diaphoresis should raise the possibility of ensuing anaphylaxis. The patient should report any of these symptoms immediately.

If a patient starts to experience any of the early warning signs of anaphylaxis, all medications should be stopped. The patient's condition should be closely monitored, but treatment should be initiated before the condition becomes critical. In the absence of an immediate adverse reaction, the patient should still be monitored for up to 30 minutes after an injection, to guard against the possibility of a delayed anaphylaxis.

Stridor, acute respiratory distress, wheezing, hypotension, cardiac arrhythmias, shock, seizures, and loss of consciousness are signs of a life-threatening reaction that requires immediate treatment.

Almost 20% of persons who have an anaphylactic event experience a recurrence of symptoms up to 8 hours after the initial event. This late-phase response may be prevented by administering corticosteroids. Unlike antihistamines, which inhibit the immune response by blocking the action of the mediators, corticosteroids indiscriminately suppress the immune response. This is important, considering that histamine does not play a role in late-phase reactions. Even with the administration of corticosteroids, observation of at-risk patients is recommended for 6 to 8 hours after the anaphylactic episode.

Preparation

When an anaphylactic reaction occurs, early recognition and rapid response are essential. The treatment goal is to maintain cardiac and respiratory function. Epinephrine in an aqueous solution of 1:1000 (1 mg/mL) administered IV, IM, or SC, is the most effective treatment. The recommended adult dosage is 0.2 to 0.5 mL IM or SC. This can be repeated every 10 to 15 minutes, up to a total of 1 mg.

Epinephrine should be given at the first sign of an anaphylactic reaction. Having epinephrine that is not outdated and syringes for both SC and IM injection in an easily accessible location decreases response time and increases the chance of the patient's survival.

Other medications are commonly used to supplement the treatment of anaphylaxis. For example, an IM antihistamine, usually diphenhydramine 1 to 2 mg/kg, is routinely given to block the continued release of histamine.

If there is any evidence of respiratory involvement, especially if respiratory distress is evident, oxygen should be administered through a nasal cannula.

IV access should be established to allow for the administration of medication and fluids, if necessary. Resuscitation equipment should be readily available.

Asthma (See Chapter 13, Section 1)
Allergy Immunotherapy

In cases where allergen avoidance and medication do not provide adequate control of symptoms, or after an episode of anaphylaxis from an insect bite or sting, allergy immunotherapy (AI) is indicated. AI is accomplished by administering frequent injections of the allergen in very low doses. Initially, the patient receives two to three low-dose injections per week. Slowly, the dosage of the allergen is increased until a maintenance dose is reached. From that point, the patient receives maximum levels of the allergen at 2-week intervals over a period of years.

Because of the risks inherent in injecting an allergic person with the offending allergen, accurate preparation and administration of the injection is essential. As with any injection, the risk of adverse reactions and anaphylaxis not only exist, but also may be magnified with AI. Many people underestimate the risks of allergy injections. This poor understanding may come in part from the fact that for years, patients were allowed to administer their own allergy injections at home. This policy has long been rescinded, and the current standard of practice is that no one should receive an allergy injection without resuscitation equipment and trained medical personnel readily available.

 COMMUNITY CARE

Although it remains unclear whether allergen avoidance can prevent allergic disease, avoidance remains a cornerstone of allergy treatment. Obviously, certain allergens (e.g., pollen) cannot be avoided, but for other allergic conditions, such as food or drug allergies, avoiding the trigger is the only way to avoid the reaction. Prevention of anaphylaxis also relies on allergen avoidance.

Recently, many products aimed at allergy-proofing the home have been developed. Mattress and pillow covers and special carpet cleaners can diminish exposure to dust mites. Dehumidifiers and high-efficiency particulate air filtration systems decrease mold spore production and dust mite populations.

Sometimes lifestyle changes are sufficient. Putting indoor pets outside and keeping them there can greatly improve the quality of life for a person allergic to dog or cat dander. It may be inconvenient for a family to put their pets outside, but this simple intervention can significantly enhance the health of a family member with animal allergies. Modifying the home environment in these ways can have a positive effect on patients with allergic disorders.

PROGNOSIS

Untreated, persons with asthma experience a dramatic and steady decline in FEV_1 compared to persons without asthma. The mortality rate of asthma is 0.1% annually but rises to 3.3% in patients who experience episodes of status asthmaticus.

Up to 50% of children with asthma are no longer symptomatic when they reach adulthood. The absence of allergic rhinitis and early development of asthma are good prognostic indicators. Severe asthmatic disease in childhood increases the likelihood of persistent disease.

Approximately 20% of children with allergic rhinitis are asymptomatic as adults.

CLINICAL PEARLS

- Allergic disorders are prevalent. These disorders have a significant impact on health care expenditures, lost time at work and school, and quality of life (and can even be fatal).
- The allergic response involves an allergen binding with IgE that has attached itself to a mast cell. This causes the mast cell to degranulate and spill into circulation the substances responsible for the symptoms of allergy.
- The most common trigger for an anaphylactic reaction is medication injection. Before giving any injection, always check with the patients about their allergies and have epinephrine readily available. After giving an injection, monitor the patient for 20 to 30 minutes afterwards for any untoward reactions.
- Anaphylaxis should be treated initially with 1:1000 epinephrine 0.2 to 0.5 mL, administered IV, SC, or IM. IM injections of antihistamines can also help reverse the process. Supplemental oxygen and IV fluids may also be necessary.

NURSING PROBLEM/ DIAGNOSIS	NURSING INTERVENTIONS CLASSIFICATION (NIC)
Acute respiratory distress/ Ineffective breathing pattern	Airway management Ventilation assistance
Anaphylaxis	Shock management
Prevention of allergic responses/ Effective therapeutic management	Allergy management Shock prevention

Cancer and Solid Tumors

Section 3   Phyllis G. Peterson

 OVERVIEW

Cancer is the second leading cause of death in the United States, behind cardiovascular disease. Cancer may be seen in any age group, but tends to occur most often in the elderly and is comparatively rare in children and young adults. The main cause of cancer death for both sexes in the United States is lung cancer. The second most common diagnosed malignancy is cancer of the breast in women and prostate cancer in men.

The incidence and mortality associated with cancer varies widely depending on the type of cancer, age of the individual, presence of immunosuppression, and stage of the disease at the time of diagnosis. Other factors influencing survival rate include socioeconomic status and access to health care. Cancer incidence appears to be increasing, possibly because of improved methods of detection and diagnosis. It is encouraging to note that survival rates are also increasing, probably because of diagnosis at earlier stages, when the cancer is more amenable to treatment and improved methods of therapy.

 PATHOPHYSIOLOGY

Cancer is a malignant disease resulting from a sequence of cellular genetic aberrations that lead to abnormal cell proliferation, unchecked growth, and invasion of healthy surrounding tissue. Cancer cells also possess the unique ability to spread to other areas of the body.

Cancer is classified according to the organ system in which it begins, although it is actually a disease that starts on a cellular level (Table 22-3-1). Cancers arise in the body as a result of abnormal activity of cell genes that are responsible for the regulation and control of cell growth and reproduction. The malignant process begins in cells that were originally normal but were altered by oncogene activity.

Growth patterns and behaviors of cancer cells are very different from normal cells. Normal cells have a distinct shape, nucleus, and recognizable

---

Table 22-3-1. Tumor Nomenclature

Carcinomas that arise in epithelial tissues may include the following terms:
- Adeno: cancers arising from glandular epithelium
- Organ of origin is also included
- Squamous: cancers arising from squamous epithelium

Sarcomas originating in connective tissue
- Osteo: arising from bone
- Chondro: arising from cartilage
- Lipo: arising from fat
- Rhabdo: arising from skeletal muscle
- Leiomyo: arising from smooth muscle

Hematologic malignancies arise from hematopoietic stem cells and are classified according to:
- Cell type
- Cell maturity

characteristics; in contrast cancer cells tend to have an increased number of mitotic figures (indicative of increased cell division), an irregular cell shape, and loss of normal function and properties commonly seen in the tissue of origin.

Cancer cells have the ability to invade and destroy normal tissue, and may secrete hormone-like substances that lead to metabolic and electrolyte disturbances. These cells may spread to distant sites in the body via the lymphatics or the blood stream. In addition, some tumors secrete angiogenesis factors that cause the host to grow new blood vessels to feed the tumor cells, permitting growth of the mass and increasing the risk of metastatic disease.

Although the precise cause of cancer is unknown, many different factors are thought to contribute to the malignant evolution of what was originally a normal cell line. Hereditary and genetic tendencies may have a significant influence on the development of cancer, as in familial adenomatous polyposis (FAP). Individuals with FAP develop many polyps in the colon at an early age and eventually develop colon cancer. Thus, in these individuals, prophylactic colectomy is often recommended before age 30. Other disorders that carry a high risk for cancer include retinoblastoma, neurofibromatosis, and Fanconi's anemia.

Certain forms of cancer, including some types of breast cancer, appear to have familial patterns of occurrence. This may be linked to common genes, environmental factors, or both. Familial cancer seems to be associated with the absence of groups of genes that prevent cancer.

Viruses play a role in the development of cancer. Individuals with HIV infection have a significantly increased risk of unusual forms of cancer that are not typically seen in the general population. Positive correlations have also been seen between the human papilloma virus and cervical cancer, and Epstein-Barr virus and Burkett's lymphoma.

It is likely that cancer development is also related to cell mutations that occur as a result of exposure to biological, chemical, and environmental factors. These factors include ionizing radiation, industrial exposure to chemicals and heavy metals, exposure to unbound asbestos, a compromised immune system, and exposure to plant and microbial agents, such as cytotoxic chemotherapy. Cigarette smoking is a causative factor in 30% of all cancer deaths.

SIGNS AND SYMPTOMS

Cancer is usually asymptomatic in the early stages. As the disease progresses, it may cause a variety of symptoms, depending on the nature and location of the tumor. Pain is one of the most common symptoms associated with cancer. With advancing disease, the tumor mass may interfere with the function of vital organs or obstruct or infiltrate sensitive structures such as nerves and visceral organs. Tumor infiltration may also cause painful inflammatory processes and indirectly result in infection, which then further escalates the pain cycle.

Particularly with hematopoietic malignancies, such as leukemia and lymphoma, tumor infiltration of the bone marrow may result in varying degrees of bone marrow failure. Leukopenia may then cause decreased resistance to infection. Thrombocytopenia may cause serious bleeding episodes. Anemia is a common finding associated with malignant disease. In addition to marrow infiltration, causes of anemia include chronic blood loss, malnutrition, and defective iron utilization. Thrombocytopenia and leukopenia are significant sources of mortality and morbidity in cancer patients. Anemia has an adverse impact on quality of life and may also result in other complications, such as congestive heart failure in the compromised patient.

Fatigue is one of the most common symptoms associated with malignant disease. The underlying cause of fatigue is poorly understood.

The syndrome of cachexia is one of the most distressing problems faced by patients with cancer. Cachexia is a severe form of malnutrition characterized by anorexia, severe weight loss, emaciation, and overall poor quality of life.

 DIAGNOSTIC CRITERIA

Because almost any tissue in the body may undergo a malignant transformation, many different methods can be used to establish a diagnosis of cancer. Ultimately, to establish an accurate diagnosis, a piece of the suspect tissue must be surgically excised and microscopically examined. In the case of palpable masses or skin lesions, this is readily accomplished by a biopsy or minor surgical procedure. For certain tumors, surgery may also be helpful in establishing the stage of the disease.

Confirming the diagnosis of cancer is more problematic in the absence of an external lesion or palpable mass. When patients present with abnormal physical findings suggestive of cancer (e.g., unusual fatigue, unexplained weight loss, and night sweats), the diagnosis of cancer may need to be ruled out. Diagnostic tests depend on the patient's signs and symptoms. A complete blood cell count with differential may be drawn to evaluate hematopoietic function. Radiologic examinations, such as computed tomography scans, magnetic resonance imaging, and ultrasonography may be used to detect space-occupying lesions and changes in bony architecture. Even after radiologic examination has established the presence of a questionable lesion, a specimen of that tissue must still be examined microscopically to confirm the diagnosis of cancer.

 INTERVENTIONS

Because cancer is often a lethal disease, interventions must include the elimination of modifiable risk factors known to contribute to carcinogenesis, as well as aggressive screening and early detection of the disease. In most cases, therapy is more successful for early-stage malignant disease.

Cancer treatment is directed toward cure, control, or palliation. The major treatment modalities for cancer are surgery, radiation, and cytotoxic chemotherapy. Depending on the patient's physical status and tumor type, a combination of these modalities may be used, particularly if there is hope of achieving a cure or prolonged survival. Because cancer therapy has many side effects and toxicities, patients require extensive education, monitoring, and follow-up care to decrease the risk of complications.

Primary Prevention and Early Detection

Cancer is thought to be preventable, at least in part. Research indicates that if all measures known to be effective in cancer prevention were implemented, then cancer incidence would decrease by two thirds. Health promotion measures directed toward cancer prevention must be made available to the general public. Nurses have a responsibility to help individuals eliminate modifiable risk factors, such as tobacco and exposure to environmental agents that promote carcinogenesis. Other risk factors known to promote the development of certain cancers include multiple sexual partners (particularly at an early age) and obesity.

Mortality and morbidity associated with cancer may be significantly reduced with early detection of the disease. Effective screening and self-examination play a vital role in the early detection and treatment of cancers of the skin, breast, cervix, mouth, prostate, and testes.

Surgery

Surgery plays a vital part in the diagnosis, staging, and treatment of malignant disease. It is the treatment of choice for localized disease and may be curative if the disease is in an early stage. In some situations, surgery also may be used to prevent the development of cancer in high-risk individuals. Examples of this approach include prophylactic mastectomy in women with a strong family history of breast cancer and the removal of colon polyps to prevent the development of neoplasms.

Other roles of surgery include cytoreduction for large, bulky tumors, salvage therapy for progressive disease, and palliation of distressing symptoms in advanced disease. Surgery is also useful in combination with other therapies, including chemotherapy and radiation.

Drug Therapy

Chemotherapy is the preferred treatment for many different types of malignancies. It is the primary treatment modality for hematolymphatic diseases, such as lymphoma and leukemia. It is also indicated for the treatment of solid tumors with metastatic disease and malignancies located in certain areas of the body, such as the central nervous system, that may not be treatable by other therapies.

As with other modalities, the goal of chemotherapy is to achieve a cure. When cure is no longer realistic, chemotherapy may also be used to control disease and to palliate distressing symptoms. Most chemotherapeutic agents are cytotoxic and act to either kill tumor cells or interfere with their ability to replicate and create more malignant cells.

Chemotherapeutic agents are classified according to their chemical structure and their activity within the cell cycle (Table 22-3-2).

To increase the possibility of cure, most chemotherapeutic agents are given as combination therapy involving two or more drugs. In combination therapy, agents with different mechanisms of action and cellular toxicities are chosen to increase the tumor cell kill and decrease toxic and adverse reactions. Chemotherapeutic agents may be given by various routes: oral, IV, arterial, intrathecal, intracavitary, intravesicular, intraperitoneal, and topical. Because these drugs are considered hazardous substances, special care must be taken when handling them as well as excreta from patients undergoing treatment. In addition, special precautions must be taken when discarding chemotherapy waste products such as bags, tubing, and syringes.

The duration of chemotherapy is highly variable and is a function of the stage and type of malignant disease being treated, as well as the patient's

Table 22-3-2. Cancer Chemotherapy Classifications

CLASSIFICATION	MECHANISM OF ACTION	COMMON SIDE EFFECTS
Antimetabolites	Active in S phase; interferes with DNA synthesis	Myelosuppression; nausea, vomiting, diarrhea, and mucositis
Vinca alkaloids	Active in late G_2 phase; also in M phase. Prevent cell division and replication	Myelosuppression, nausea, neurotoxicity, paralytic ileus
Epidophyllotoxins	Arrest cells in premitotic phases of the cell cycle; interfere with cellular metabolism	Myelosuppression, nausea, vomiting, anorexia, orthostatic hypotension
Taxanes	Inhibit cell division; active in G_2 and S phases	Myelosuppression, alopecia, peripheral neuropathy, hypersensitivity reactions
Camptothecins	Active in S phase; damage DNA	Myelosuppression, diarrhea, alopecia
Alkylating agents	Damage DNA strands, interfere with DNA replication	Myelosuppression; hyperuricemia
Antitumor antibiotics	Inhibit DNA and RNA synthesis	Myelosuppression, nausea, vomiting, diarrhea, alopecia, mucositis
Hormonal agents	Interfere with hormone receptors in all phases of the cell cycle	Fluid retention, electrolyte imbalances; hyperglycemia, changes in secondary sexual characteristics

From Oncology Nursing Society (1999). *Cancer Chemotherapy Guidelines* (2nd ed.). Pittsburgh, PA: Author.

overall health status. Poor performance status, debilitation, or compromised function of the heart, lungs, kidneys, or liver may necessitate a decrease in dosage or may rule out chemotherapy as a treatment option.

Radiation Therapy

Radiation therapy uses ionizing radiation to kill malignant cells. Not all tumors are sensitive to radiation. A radiation-sensitive tumor is one that can be killed by a dose of radiation that can be safely tolerated by surrounding healthy tissue. To decrease the toxic effects associated with radiation, the prescribed dose is usually given in divided, or fractionated, doses over a period of several days.

Radiation therapy has many different uses in cancer treatment. In some cases, radiation therapy may be curative, particularly in early-stage disease. Other indications include:

- Combination therapy in conjunction with surgery or radiation
- Alternate treatment for patients who are unable to undergo surgery
- Treatment of sanctuary sites within the body that are at high risk for metastatic disease
- Treatment of oncologic emergencies, such as increased intracranial pressure
- Palliation of distressing symptoms

Radiation therapy may be delivered either internally or externally. Teletherapy is the delivery of radiation from a source outside the body. Brachytherapy is the delivery of radiation from a source placed inside a body cavity. Because patients receiving brachytherapy are radioactive, nurses and other health care providers who come in direct contact with these patients must take care to limit their exposure.

Toxicity associated with radiation therapy is a function of the dose delivered and the area of the body radiated. This toxicity may be short-term or long-term in nature. For example, because a significant amount of hematopoiesis in adults occurs in the sternum, ribs, and pelvis, radiation to these areas may result in myelosuppression. Depending on the level of myelosuppression, treatment may be delayed to allow for bone marrow recovery. In some cases, damage to vital organs by radiation may be permanent. Late or delayed effects of radiation therapy may be seen in almost every body system, including the nerves and bones (Table 22-3-3).

Patients receiving radiation therapy must be taught self-care measures to deal with its side effects. Skin affected by radiation therapy must be cleansed with a gentle soap and patted dry. Lotions and emollients used on the area must be approved by the radiation therapist, because some agents may affect how the radiation is delivered to and absorbed by the targeted area. A patient who has received radiation to the oral cavity requires specialized dental care, particularly if the salivary glands have been adversely affected. To decrease the incidence of radiation-induced dental caries, the patient should be taught to perform daily fluoride treatments.

Radiation-induced enteritis should be treated with supportive measures, including a bland diet low in roughage and fiber. Severe cases may require bowel rest and support with hyperalimentation. Radiation-induced myelosup-

Table 22-3-3. Acute and Late Effects of Radiation Therapy

SITE OF EXPOSURE	ACUTE RESPONSE	LATE RESPONSE[a]
Skin	Loss of epidermal layer; redness, swelling, itching and weeping	Fibrosis, atrophy, a permanently "tanned" appearance
Gastrointestinal tract	*Mouth:* dryness, ulceration, pain, changes in taste perception, loss of appetite	Permanent destruction of salivary glands, radiation induced dental caries, osteonecrosis of the jaw, fibrosis; permanent taste alterations
	Stomach: sloughing of epithelial layer, nausea, vomiting	Ulceration, necrosis, obstruction
	Intestines: sloughing of intestinal villi, malabsorption of nutrients, diarrhea	Ulceration, necrosis, obstruction
Genitourinary tract	*Kidneys*	Radiation nephritis, renal failure
	Bladder: urinary urgency, cystitis, ulceration	Fibrotic, contracted bladder
Bone marrow	Pancytopenia: complete recovery usually occurs within 2–6 weeks	Anemia
Lungs	Pneumonitis: may be fatal if 75% or more of lungs is involved	Fibrosis; restrictive lung disease
Gonads	Temporary sterility or possible mutations in low doses	Permanent sterility in both sexes from high-dose of radiation therapy
Eyes	Lens opacity	Cataracts

[a]Severity of the late response is a function of the dose of radiation received.

pression may also require supportive measures, such as protective isolation, transfusion therapy with red blood cells and platelets, and careful monitoring for evidence of side effects and complications.

Assessment

Before the start of therapy, all patients require a comprehensive physical assessment. Special care must be taken to verify normal organ function and rule out the possibility of coexisting disease or infection, which may compromise a patient's ability to safely withstand the rigors of treatment. Depending on the treatment regimen used, organ-specific toxicities, including cardiomyopathy, pulmonary fibrosis, and renal and hepatic damage, may occur.

During treatment, careful evaluation and monitoring are mandatory to detect toxic and adverse effects. A complete blood count with differential is one of the most readily obtained and most effective measures of immune status. Cancer therapy may lead to a decline in neutrophils, the specialized white blood cells that are the body's first line of defense against infection. Depending on the severity of neutropenia, protective measures may be required to decrease the risk of possibly lethal infections. (See Chapter 10, Section 3 for information on protective isolation.) Other laboratory tests that should be monitored include blood chemistry panel, serum albumin level, and liver function tests. Before discharge, the patient must be taught how to decrease the risk of contracting infections from the home environment, as well as how to monitor for evidence of infection (Table 22-3-4).

Other toxicities commonly associated with chemotherapy (e.g., nausea, vomiting, anorexia, stomatitis) may have a significant impact on nutritional status and fluid and electrolyte balance. Before discharge, the patient should be taught measures to manage nausea and anorexia at home. A patient who is unable to maintain adequate fluid intake may require IV hydration and correction of electrolyte imbalances. Dehydration and uncorrected electrolyte imbalances may lead to renal insufficiency and permanent renal damage.

Uncontrolled nausea and vomiting persisting more than 24 hours in an adult require immediate medical intervention. Most patients respond favorably to rehydration and aggressive therapy with IV antiemetics. A dietary consult may be helpful in some situations, depending on the severity of the problem. All patients should have their weight monitored at least twice a week. Intake and output measurements may be indicated to validate adequate fluid intake and hydration. In severe cases, therapy may need to be interrupted, or the patient may need supportive care with IV hyperalimentation.

 COMMUNITY CARE

Assessment

Initial evaluation of all patients, regardless of their medical history, should include possible risk factors for malignancy. Modifiable risk factors include a history of tobacco use, excessive alcohol use, sun exposure at an early age, multiple sexual partners at an early age, and obesity. Nonmodifiable risk factors include a positive family history of cancer, age, race, and gender. Occupational exposure may also be a risk factor for cancer. High-risk occupations include those that entail exposure to petrochemical compounds, heavy metals, and unbound asbestos. Patients who fall into a high-risk category

Table 22-3-4. Patient Education for Management of Chemotherapy Side Effects

INSTRUCTION	RATIONALE
For Infection Prevention	
Take your temperature orally at least once a day, preferably in the evening. Immediately report temperature of 100.4 °F or higher to the physician.	Small temperature elevations with no other symptom may be the only indication of early infection in the immunocompromised individual.
Avoid cuts and potential sources of injury. Wear protective gloves when in a risky situation, such as doing dishes by hand. Use a soft toothbrush when cleaning teeth. Protect the lower extremities from injury; wear shoes and protective clothing when appropriate. Treat all cuts and abrasions immediately with a disinfectant and antibiotic ointment, unless instructed otherwise by your physician.	Maintaining the integrity of the skin and mucous membranes helps protect the body from numerous pathogens in the environment. Patients with immunocompromise require prompt, vigorous treatment when exposed to potential sources of infection.
Avoid direct contact with pets and animals. Under no circumstances have direct contact with animal excreta, such as litter boxes and bird cages.	Organisms found in and on animals may be pathogenic to the immunocompromised individual. Animal bites and scratches may be a significant hazard and pose a high risk of serious complications.
Avoid uncooked/raw food or food that has been kept warm for long periods.	These items are likely to be heavily contaminated with bacteria that may be hazardous for the immunocompromised individual.
Avoid crowds and direct contact with people with contagious illnesses such as colds and flu. Avoid contact with children who have recently been exposed to childhood diseases or have recently received a childhood immunization.	Viruses may cause significant morbidity in immunocompromised individuals.
For Nausea and Vomiting	
Eat frequent small bland meals served at room temperature.	Bland foods are less likely to cause nausea. Cool or room-temperature foods are less aromatic and thus less likely to cause nausea. Smaller, more frequent portions will help overcome problems associated with early satiety due to chemotherapy.
If nausea is a problem, take an antiemetic ½ hour before scheduled mealtimes.	Improves comfort and ability to tolerate meals. Judicious use of antiemetics will help decrease the risk of developing a conditioned aversion to food.
If antiemetic is unsuccessful in controlling nausea, consult the health care provider for alternate choices.	Other antiemetics may offer better control of nausea.
If possible, have someone else cook and serve food.	Decreases exposure to cooking odors which may contribute to nausea.
If not medically contraindicated, gentle exercise may decrease nausea and improve appetite.	This provides an improved sense of well-being, personal control over circumstances.
If adequate intake is a problem, select foods and snacks that are high in protein and calories.	Protein-rich foods aid tissue repair. Calories provide energy.

should be counseled to modify their risk factors as much as possible and to engage in thorough screening practices. Patients with a previous history of cancer should be regularly assessed for evidence of recurrence, so that appropriate treatment measures may be initiated as soon as possible.

All patients should be assessed for evidence of cancer. Constitutional symptoms (e.g., unexplained weight loss, fever, bleeding episodes, night sweats) may be indicative of an occult malignancy. The American Cancer Society has also identified seven warning signs for cancer:

- Change in bowel or bladder habits
- A sore that does not heal
- Unusual bleeding or discharge
- Thickening or lump in breast or elsewhere
- Indigestion or difficulty swallowing
- Obvious change in a wart or mole
- Nagging cough or hoarseness

Monitoring

A patient undergoing active treatment for cancer requires close medical and nursing follow-up and evaluation. Carefully evaluate the patient's understanding of self-care measures and compliance with treatment regimens, particularly if care is being provided in the outpatient setting. Some patients may require periodic reviews of self-care measures, including activity restrictions, and signs and symptoms indicating the need for medical intervention. Assess for treatment-associated complications, including infection, bleeding, nausea, vomiting, and electrolyte imbalances.

Assess for evidence of progressive disease:

- *Neurologic and central nervous system.* Changes in neurologic status may be indicative of metastatic disease. Decreased level of consciousness, abnormal cranial nerve function, and paralysis may indicate the growth of a space-occupying lesion within the central nervous system.
- *Respiratory.* Respiratory symptoms, including respiratory failure, generally indicate invasion of the lungs by metastatic disease.
- *Hematologic.* Anemia, leukocytosis, leukocytopenia, and thrombocytopenia may indicate that the bone marrow is infiltrated with tumor cells.
- *Obstruction.* Blockage of an organ or hollow organ may indicate tumor growth.

Prevention

Promote primary prevention of cancer in all populations. Teach and promote the elimination of high-risk behaviors and avoidance of contributing factors (e.g., sun exposure). Provide teaching on healthy habits (e.g., a low-fat diet, regular exercise) that may decrease the risk of malignancy.

Secondary prevention involves careful screening for cancer while it is still in early (and more likely curable) stages. Special attention should be paid to high-risk populations. Examples of screening measures include Pap tests for women age 18 and older, flexible sigmoidoscopy for men and women age 50 and older, and breast self-examination.

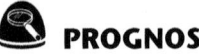 **PROGNOSIS**

Without treatment, cancer is almost uniformly fatal. With treatment, survival rates vary depending on the tumor type, stage, grade, and characteristics of the host. Survival rates also vary in different populations, which may be reflective of genetic differences as well as access to health care. Overall survival rates for cancer have improved significantly since the turn of the century. With the possible exception of breast cancer, a malignancy is considered to be cured if there is no clinical evidence of disease 5 years after completion of treatment.

 CLINICAL PEARLS

○ Certain forms of cancer may have familial patterns of occurrence. Individuals at risk for these forms should undergo regular screening for cancer.
○ Elimination of common risk factors, such as tobacco use and unprotected sun exposure, could significantly decrease the incidence of cancer.
○ Cancer is most treatable and curable while in the early stages. Effective screening and secondary prevention measures can decrease the mortality and morbidity associated with cancer.
○ Initial decisions on the treatment modality for cancer can decrease or eliminate other treatment options later in the course of the disease. The initial treatment should be chosen carefully, weighing all relevant factors.
○ Persons with impaired immune system function should be aware of the risk of infection from devices such as hearing aids, from venipuncture or venous access, and from exposure to persons with colds or flu.
○ Patients undergoing active treatment for cancer require careful evaluation, monitoring, and follow-up before, during, and after treatment to decrease the incidence and severity of treatment-related complications.

NURSING PROBLEM/ DIAGNOSIS	NURSING INTERVENTIONS CLASSIFICATION (NIC)
Acute/chronic pain	Pain management
	Analgesic administration
Infection/Risk for infection	Infection protection
Fatigue	Energy management
	Bleeding precautions
	Nutrition therapy

chapter 23

Hematologic

Anemia

Section 1   Judy Kaye ■ Mia Smitt

 OVERVIEW

Anemia is a disorder of the erythrocytes, or red blood cells (RBCs), characterized by inadequate oxygen-carrying capacity of the blood. It involves a decrease in the total number of circulating RBCs or a decrease in the quality or quantity of hemoglobin (Hgb), which carries oxygen. A low reticulocyte count indicates a state of decreased RBC production, whereas a high reticulocyte count indicates a state of increased RBC destruction. Anemia is present in adults when the hematocrit is below 41% in males and 37% in females. Anemia may be classified according to RBC size (mean corpuscular volume [MVC]) and color.

 PATHOPHYSIOLOGY

Anemia results from a reduction in the total number of circulating RBCs or a decrease in the quality or quantity of Hgb. Anemia usually results from: (1) decreased RBC production due to nutritional deficiencies (e.g., iron, vitamin B$_{12}$, folic acid) or bone marrow abnormalities, (2) blood loss, (3) impaired RBC maturation, or (4) RBC destruction (i.e., hemolysis). The different types of anemia have specific different causes. Table 23-1-1 lists types, pathophysiologic mechanisms, and causes of anemia.

 SIGNS AND SYMPTOMS

Signs and symptoms can vary with the severity of the anemia and comorbid conditions (e.g., heart disease, chronic obstructive pulmonary disease). Signs and symptoms can include any of the following: dizziness, headache, irritability, difficulty concentrating or sleeping, cold intolerance, syncope or vertigo, fatigue, pallor, anorexia, indigestion, and nausea. Women may have amenorrhea, and men may experience impotence or decreased libido. When Hgb falls below 7.5 g/dL, resting cardiac output rises with increased heart rate and stroke volume. The patient may complain of chest pain with chronic conditions and shortness of breath. A patient with vitamin B$_{12}$ deficiency anemia may exhibit neurologic changes.

 DIAGNOSTIC CRITERIA

Table 23-1-1 presents information on diagnosing anemia.

 INTERVENTIONS

Because the patient with anemia is easily *fatigued,* the patient needs to conserve energy by adjusting activities to provide periods of rest and adequate

Table 23-1-1. Anemia Classifications, Pathophysiology, and Diagnosis

TYPE	PATHOPHYSIOLOGY	CAUSE	SPECIFIC DIAGNOSIS
Macrocytic normochromic anemia (large, abnormally shaped RBCs but normal color)	*Pernicious anemia:* Lack of B_{12} (cobalamin) and abnormal DNA and RNA synthesis results in cell death.	Deficiency of intrinsic factor; hereditary autoimmune disorder	Low serum B_{12} Schilling test indicating poor B_{12} absorption
	Folate deficiency anemia: Lack of folate results in premature cell death.	Dietary folate deficiency: alcoholism, anorexia, inadequate fresh fruit and vegetable intake	Low folate level
Microcytic hypochromic anemia (small abnormal RBCs with pale color)	*Iron-deficiency anemia:* Lack of iron for hemoglobin production	Chronic blood loss; dietary iron deficiency; dysfunction in iron metabolism; chronic hemoglobinuria	Low plasma iron; high TIBC; low ferritin; low transferrin; high free erythrocyte protoporphyrin
	Sideroblastic anemia: Heme is not incorporated into protoporphyrin to synthesize hemoglobin.	Congenital or acquired dysfunction of iron metabolism in RBCs. Acquired dysfunction can result from drugs or toxins.	High bilirubin; increased or normal free erythrocyte protoporphyrin; high plasma iron ferritin and transferrin; excessive sideroblasts on bone marrow biopsy
	Thalassemia: Synthesis of globin chains (alpha or beta) is impaired.	Genetic defect of globin synthesis	Hemoglobin electrophoresis demonstrates the characteristic trait
Normocytic normochromic anemia (normal RBC size and color; destruction or depletion of normal RBCs)	*Posthemorrhagic anemia:* Blood is lost.	Acute or chronic hemorrhage; reticulocytes are not seen.	Normal or low hemoglobin and hematocrit but elevated reticulocyte count
	Hemolytic anemia: Mature RBCs are lysed.	Any condition that increases the fragility of erythrocytes	Low Hbg and Hct low with elevated reticulocyte count
	Sickle cell anemia: An abnormal cell shape results from abnormal hemoglobin synthesis, which leads to chronic hemolytic anemia.	Congenital autosomal recessive disorder	Hemoglobin electrophoresis; microscopic sickled RBCs
	Anemia resulting from chronic diseases: RBC survival is reduced and the bone marrow fails to compensate.	Chronic infection or inflammation, cancer, and liver disease; anemia of chronic renal failure is more severe.	Low hemoglobin and hematocrit; low iron; low TIBC; slightly high bilirubin; reticulocytes initially increased, then decreased
Aplastic anemia	*Pancytopenia:* Production of all blood cells has stopped.	Intrinsic stem cell defect, growth factor defect, and immune suppression of marrow; drug toxicity	Pancytopenia; neutrophils $<500/\mu L$; platelets $<200,000/\mu L$; reticulocyte count $<1\%$; marked hypocellular bone marrow $<20\%$

RBC, red blood cell; TIBC, total iron-binding capacity.

sleep. Shortness of breath and tachycardia may indicate decreased cardiac output; the patient may need supplemental oxygen. Transfusions also may be necessary.

If the patient is *anorexic,* eating frequent small meals may be helpful. Foods rich in iron, protein, and minerals can help elevate Hgb in anemia related to *nutritional deficiencies,* especially iron deficiency anemia. Iron-rich foods include liver, meat, eggs, whole grains, legumes, enriched bread and cereals, and dark-green vegetables. Folic acid is available in liver, leafy green vegetables, and legumes and should be emphasized in dietary teaching for a patient with folate deficiency. Daily vitamin and iron supplements are usually indicated. The patient should be informed of the possible side effects of iron therapy, including constipation, gastric distress, and dark, tarry stools. Adequate hydration, increased intake of fruits and vegetables, and use of stool softeners or laxatives may help alleviate constipation.

Folic acid and vitamin B_{12} replacement may be indicated to treat anemias involving these deficiencies. Cyanocobalamin (vitamin B_{12}) is initially given intramuscularly until the Hgb value returns to normal, and is then given intranasally. The patient needs to understand that B_{12} replacement is a lifelong therapy. Neurologic changes resulting from B_{12} deficiency (e.g., tingling or paresthesias in the hands and feet, gait disturbances from a loss of position sense, irritability, bladder and bowel dysfunction, delirium) may be reversed if they have existed for less than 6 months.

In *thalassemia,* iron absorption is greatly increased and accumulates resulting in iron overload. Regular consumption of tea may decrease intestinal iron absorption. However, iron chelation therapy is usually necessary for these patients.

Anemia resulting from uremia in chronic renal failure may be treated with erythropoietin, available as epoetin alfa and administered by subcutaneous injection. This therapy is very expensive, however.

Because anemia causes *cold intolerance,* the patient may need adjustment of environmental temperature, warm clothing, and extra blankets at night. The patient should be cautioned to avoid electric blankets, heating pads, and extremely hot baths, to prevent skin damage resulting from increased sensitivity to heat. Extra attention should be given to protecting the skin, which is prone to damage because of decreased oxygen supply related to low Hgb. *Nails* may become brittle and in iron deficiency may become spoon shaped from impaired epithelial growth. Referral to a podiatrist may be indicated.

Assessment for *acute or chronic bleeding* is important. Stools, urine, and gastrointestinal drainage or emesis are tested for microscopic blood. Blood transfusions may be necessary. Blood component infusion must be done slowly and monitored carefully to prevent congestive heart failure. A patient with hemolytic anemia is at increased risk for transfusion reaction.

Splenectomy is the treatment of choice in *hereditary spherocytosis* and may be helpful in thalassemia. Referral for genetic counseling may be appropriate for a patient with a genetically linked type of anemia.

 # COMMUNITY CARE

Untreated anemia may be fatal; therefore, patient and family education on the disease process, treatment, and when to call the health care professional is mandatory. Anemia also tends to be a chronic or recurrent condition that necessitates lifestyle changes, including dietary modifications and replacement therapies. The patient needs specific teaching regarding nutrition, food lists, meal plans, and supplemental medications.

Identification of any contributing socioeconomic factors (e.g., limited education or financial resources) should prompt referrals to home health agencies, public health departments, or other social and community agencies. If alcoholism is the cause of the anemia, the patient should be referred to a behavioral counselor and Alcoholics Anonymous.

A patient with neurologic deficits resulting from vitamin B_{12} deficiency may require assistance and attention to safety. Referrals to occupational and physical therapy may be indicated. Follow-up laboratory tests and examinations are necessary. The patient's work and home environments should be assessed for possible exposure to toxins or drugs known to impair RBC production or shorten RBC lifespan.

 ## PROGNOSIS

Prognosis depends on the type and cause of anemia. Untreated anemia may be fatal, but this is rare. Most patients, even those with chronic or genetically related anemia, live a long, normal life with corrective therapy. Bone marrow transplant may cure aplastic anemia.

 ## CLINICAL PEARLS

- Iron deficiency anemia is the most common cause of anemia worldwide. Incidence is highest in young children, women of childbearing age, and elderly persons.
- Thalassemia-alpha is the most common cause of microcytic anemia and is most common in people of African or Asian ancestry. The beta form is the most common type of thalassemia in persons of Mediterranean descent (i.e., Italians, Greeks, Arabs, and Jews).
- Iron metabolism is balanced between absorption and a loss of 1 mg/day. Pregnancy upsets the iron balance, because requirements increase to 2 to 5 mg/day during pregnancy and lactation. Normal dietary iron intake cannot meet this additional need, and iron supplements are required during pregnancy and lactation.
- Chronic aspirin use can cause occult blood loss and iron deficiency anemia without a structural lesion or gastrointestinal bleeding. Although gastrointestinal bleeding is the most common cause of iron deficiency anemia, other possible causes include menorrhagia, other uterine bleeding, and repeated blood donations.
- Meticulous skin, nail, and mouth care are necessary because of reduced oxygen delivery to the skin and nails and the predisposition to stomatitis.
- Treatment with folate alone may mask vitamin B_{12} deficiency anemia without treating the neurologic deficits that result from myelin degeneration in the dorsal and lateral columns of the spinal cord and cerebral cortex.
- Coexisting deficiencies of other vitamins and iron-containing enzymes can produce complications. Therefore, the patient should be evaluated for vitamin deficiencies and given a multivitamin supplement as indicated.

NURSING PROBLEM/ DIAGNOSIS	NURSING INTERVENTIONS CLASSIFICATION (NIC)
Fatigue Nutrient deficiency Diminished oxygen-carrying capacity/ineffective tissue perfusion	Energy management Nutrition management Blood product administration Oxygen therapy

Leukemia

Section 2　　　　　　　　　　　　　　　　　　　　　　　　　Judy Kaye

 OVERVIEW

Leukemia is a malignancy of the blood-forming organs and blood that causes an uncontrollable proliferation of leukocytes, or white blood cells (WBCs)—mainly granulocytes, lymphocytes, and monocytes. Virchow termed this WBC disorder "leukemia" to describe the reversal of the usual ratio of RBCs to WBCs. The leukemic cell is not able to mature, fight infection, and respond to normal regulatory mechanisms. The bone marrow becomes overcrowded with immature, undifferentiated "blast" cells, resulting in decreased production and impaired function of normal blood cells.

Leukemia affects males more often than females; annual incidence is 13.2 per 100,000 in males and 7.7 per 100,000 in females. Some 70% of leukemias affect adults, most commonly chronic lymphocytic leukemia (CLL) and acute myelocytic leukemia (AML). More than half of all leukemias occur in people over age 60.

Although 60% to 80% of adults with AML will achieve remission, long-term survival is in the 20% to 40% range. For all types of acute leukemia, the mortality rate in the U.S. is approximately 7 per 100,000. African Americans have a lower mortality rate than whites.

 PATHOPHYSIOLOGY

Leukemia is classified according to the type of immature blast cell present and according to the course of the disease. There are four broad classifications:

- Acute lymphocytic (lymphoblastic or lymphogenous) leukemia (ALL)
- CLL (chronic lymphocytic)
- AML (myeloblastic or myelogenous)
- Chronic myelocytic (myelogenous) leukemia (CML)

The myelocytic leukemias are also termed granulocytic; for example, chronic granulocytic leukemia (CGL) and acute granulocytic leukemia (AGL).

Acute leukemias are characterized by impaired WBC differentiation, resulting in a massive accumulation of immature blast cells. Because ALL and AML involve the earlier stages of hematopoiesis (cell proliferation, maturation, and regulation) that result in a more acute disease, WBCs are poorly differentiated. Approximately 80% of cases of ALL arise from the B cell line, with the ALL antigen CD-10 present. T cell lineage accounts for 15% to 20% of cases of ALL, with the antigens CD-5, CD-7, or CD-10 present. A few (<5%) lack either B or T cell origin and are called null cell ALL. ALL is uncommon in adults.

AML is the most common acute leukemia in adults. Although the etiology is unknown, AML is most strongly associated with toxins, congenital disorders (e.g., Down's syndrome), hematologic disorders, and other types of cancer. AML is classified into seven subsets, based on the line of differentiation and maturity of the cells. AML is primarily an adult disease with a median age of 50 years. Coagulation disorders are common, and a positive disseminated intravascular coagulation (DIC) profile may be present.

CLL and CML have a more insidious onset than the acute leukemias and are often discovered during a routine examination. More than 90% of people with CML have the Philadelphia chromosome, a clonal maturation involving a transposition of chromosome 9 and the short arm of chromosome 22 that may appear up to 6 years before elevated WBC count is detected. CML has three progressive stages: (1) stable (3 to 4 years), (2) accelerated (6 to 24 months), and (3) acute or blast crisis (8 to 16 weeks). CML is predominantly a disorder of adults, but can also affect children. CLL mainly affects older adults.

CLL is the most common form of adult leukemia, with 95% of cases occurring in persons over age 50. It is twice as common in males as in females. CLL is classified as stage 0 to IV based on physical findings and laboratory findings. Prognosis is determined by the clinical stage, but people may live 20 to 30 years with early-stage disease. Adults can live for decades with monitoring and supportive care.

SIGNS AND SYMPTOMS

Fatigue, malaise, bleeding, bruising, anemia, infection, and bone pain are common signs and symptoms in most leukemias. The different types may have different initial presentations. Patients with AML usually present with fatigue and weakness secondary to anemia and weight loss due to cachexia. Hematuria, melena, epistaxis, petechiae, and ecchymoses are manifestations of the abnormal bleeding. Fever and infections result from neutropenia and increased numbers of immature WBCs. Night sweats occur in 50% of these patients because of an increase in tumor necrosis factor and interleukin-1 stimulation. Dental problems may arise from gingival swelling and mucocutaneous ulcers. Bone and joint pain may arise from the overpacked marrow; this is more common in children. DIC may occur, particularly in AML. Leukemic infiltrates can be seen in the optic fundus.

CML may be asymptomatic in the chronic phase, which generally lasts from 2 months to 5 years. WBC count is usually above 10,000/mm^3 but below 50,000/mm^3. Weight loss, decreased exercise tolerance, night sweats, early satiety, and left upper abdominal quadrant fullness or pain from splenomegaly or sternal tenderness also occur. The initial presentation during the early stages can vary; fatigue, night sweats, and low-grade fever are common. Other signs and symptoms include complaints of abdominal fullness and an elevated WBC count discovered incidentally. The accelerated phase, lasting from 6 to 24 months, is associated with fever in the absence of infection, bone pain, and splenomegaly. The blast crisis phase lasts for 8 to 16 months, during which the patient may experience bleeding and infection related to bone marrow failure.

The signs and symptoms of ALL are usually of abrupt onset. As in AML, these may include malaise, fatigue, bone and joint pain, bleeding, and easy bruising. Headache is a common complaint. Patients usually present with pallor, petechiae, ecchymoses, and lymphadenopathy. Splenomegaly and hepatomegaly may be mild or severe. A mediastinal mass (usually with sternal tenderness) typifies a T cell subtype, whereas bulky abdominal nodes are usually indicative of a B cell subtype. In 10% of patients, headache and cranial nerve palsies indicate central nervous system infiltration. Some 50% of patients have meningeal leukemia.

 DIAGNOSTIC CRITERIA

Complete blood count with differential reveals decreased hemoglobin, RBC count, and hematocrit. Total WBC count is usually elevated but may vary from low to high (see Chapter 11, Section 2). Platelet count is usually below 100,000/mm³ and may be below 25,000/mm³ in some cases. The presence of blasts in a peripheral smear is a finding indicative of leukemia. (Normally, few to no immature cells are found in peripheral or circulating blood; immature cells are found in the blood marrow.) A peripheral smear may also help classify the type of leukemia:

- ALL: Significant presence of immature lymphocytes (lymphoblasts)
- AML: Presence of immature myelocytes (myeloblasts)
- CLL: Lymphocyte count above 5000/mm³, accounting for 75% of the total WBC count
- CML: Presence of myeloblasts

Bone marrow aspiration reveals increased numbers of lymphoblasts or myeloblasts.

 INTERVENTIONS

A patient with leukemia has overwhelming physical and psychological needs. He or she is at great risk of death from either bleeding or infection and requires precautions to prevent injury and exposure to microorganisms. Adequate nutrition is a challenge because of anorexia, stomatitis, and gastrointestinal disorders exacerbated by chemotherapy and radiation therapy.

Pain may be significant and cause physical as well as psychological distress. Pain-relief medications and complementary and alternative therapies (e.g., music therapy, relaxation techniques, massage) have proved effective. Cachexia and alopecia from chemotherapy can threaten the patient's self-image. Wearing a scarf or wig may help boost the self-image of a patient with alopecia.

The fear of impending death may cause distress, necessitating psychological as well as spiritual support. Psychosocial and family support, as well as spiritual care, are important aspects of care that facilitate coping.

Radiation therapy and chemotherapy vary somewhat according to the phase and type of leukemia. Table 23-2-1 provides an overview of common therapies for the four major types of leukemia.

Corticosteroids may be used to control leukocytosis and cytopenia mediated by the immune response. Side effects of chemotherapy are treated with agents to minimize gastric upset, stomatitis, diarrhea, and constipation as needed. Blood transfusions may be indicated.

Table 23-2-1. Leukemia Therapies

AML (treatment duration usually 6 months)	• *Induction chemotherapy:* cytosine arabinoside (Ara C) for 7 days and an anthracycline such as daunorubicin, doxirubicin, or mitoxantrone for 3 days Bone marrow biopsy and aspirate on the 14th day; repeat induction treatment if residual leukemic cells
	• *Postremission therapy:*
	    Consolidation: very high doses of same drugs for induction
	    Intensification: different drugs than for induction
	• *Allogenic bone marrow transplant* in first remission (60% survival long-term)
	• *Autologus stem cell transplant*

ALL (2-year treatment duration with 18 months of maintenance therapy)	• *Induction therapy:* vincristine, prednisone, and L-asparaginase plus an anthracycline (daunorubicin, doxorubicin, or mitoxantrone) Complete remission occurs in 70%–75% of cases. • *CNS prophylactic/prevention of meningeal leukemia:* cranial radiation and intrathecal methotrexate • *Postremission therapy:* same drugs as induction with or without the addition of methotrexate plus 6-mercaptopurine
CML	• *Chronic and accelerated phase:* palliative with oral agents, such as hydroxyurea, busulfan, and interferon-alpha • *Blast crisis:* treated like AML • *Allogeneic bone marrow transplant:* potential cure in the chronic phase.
CLL	• *Early stage:* observation for lymphocytosis • *Symptomatic patients:* oral alkylating agents (chlorambucil or cyclophosphamide) or fludarabine or cladribine • *Radiation* to bulky painful sites • *Splenectomy* if severe pain and thrombocytopenia occur • Gamma globulin to decrease the number of infections

ALL, acute lymphocytic leukemia; AML, acute myelogenous leukemia; CLL, chronic myelogenous leukemia.

 COMMUNITY CARE

The patient needs to be taught about the nature of the disease, the prescribed treatment regimen, and side effects of therapies. Some chemotherapy and radiation therapy is conducted on an outpatient basis. Thus, the patient may be at home when side effects occur. The patient needs to be taught signs and symptoms of infection and bleeding and instructed on when to contact the health care provider. The patient and family should be helped to identify successful coping strategies used in the past and also members of their social support network. The effectiveness of their social support network should be assessed and members from the patient's faith community involved to facilitate coping. Expressions of spirituality have been shown to have a direct inverse relationship to depression in people dealing with the stress of illness and should be encouraged when possible.

 PROGNOSIS

Acute Myelogenous Leukemia (AML)

Incidence increases with age. It will be fatal in months if untreated. Remission is 70 to 80% with aggressive therapy. Long-term survival is 25 to 30%.

Acute Lymphocytic Leukemia (ALL)

This is uncommon in adults. ALL accounts for 80% of childhood leukemias. Remission rate is 60 to 80% with aggressive therapy. Long-term survival is 40%.

Chronic Myelogenous Leukemia (CML)

Higher incidence is seen with males and increased age. Stable phase is 3 to 4 years, the accelerated phase is 6 to 24 months, and blast crisis lasts 8 to 16 weeks.

Chronic Lymphocytic Leukemia (CLL)

Most common in older adults. CLL has a slow chronic course. In 90% of cases, the person is over age 50 years. CLL is twice as common in males. Prognosis varies according to clinical stage, but many patients live normal lives for over 10 years. Some have lived 30 years.

 CLINICAL PEARLS

○ In acute leukemia, the WBCs are primarily immature cells, whereas in chronic leukemia, the WBCs are more mature or differentiated cells.

○ The effectiveness of pain relief medications can be maximized by using alternative and complementary therapies, such as massage therapy, music therapy, and pet therapy.

○ A patient's personal spirituality enhances feelings of control, purpose and meaning, and power. Spiritual activities should be encouraged to facilitate coping and decrease depression. Social support from the patient's faith community should be maximized.

○ The potential for infection is a major issue for patients with leukemia. The WBC count often is very low, predisposing the patient to opportunistic infections that the immune system cannot combat effectively. The patient must be instructed to immediately report fever. Vomiting, diarrhea, malaise, and fatigue may be symptoms of therapies or of infection and need to be evaluated.

○ Adequate nutrition is a problem for many patients with leukemia. Anorexia, nausea, and fatigue impact appetite and decrease the intake of foods and fluids. Chemotherapeutic agents can alter taste and affect the gastric mucosa. Small, frequent meals and the addition or deletion of favorite seasonings may enhance the palatability of foods. Meticulous oral care and the prompt treatment of stomatitis will help ensure adequate nutrition and hydration.

○ Bleeding can be a life-threatening complication of leukemia and its treatment. Activities such as contact sports should be avoided to reduce the risk of injury. Epistaxis usually can be controlled by applying firm pressure to both nostrils with the patient in an upright position. Avoid rectal temperatures and medications. Avoid injections when platelet count is low. Platelet transfusions may be ordered.

○ Some patients undergo splenectomy to reduce the burden on abdominal and respiratory organs. The spleen tends to become enlarged from the storage of leukemic and normal cells. Appropriate patient teaching should always be provided before hospital discharge and during follow-up appointments.

○ Family teaching and support are critical components of care. The nurse is often the best resource for information and support.
○ Fatigue is a major problem in leukemia. Activities must be spaced throughout the day, with frequent rest periods to help the patient conserve energy.

NURSING PROBLEM/ DIAGNOSIS	NURSING INTERVENTIONS CLASSIFICATION (NIC)
Diminished oxygen-carrying capacity	See Section 1
Risk for infection	Infection protection Immunization/vaccination administration
Risk for injury	Surveillance: safety
Fatigue	See Section 1

Sickle Cell Disease

Section 3   Judy Kaye

 OVERVIEW

Sickle cell disease is a genetically linked (autosomal recessive) anemia caused by a structural variation within the hemoglobin characterized by sickle-shaped RBCs. There are four major sickling disorders, each of which has a specific inheritance pattern:

• Sickle cell disease (also called sickle cell anemia)
• Sickle cell trait
• Sickle cell-hemoglobin disease
• Sickle cell beta-thalassemia disease

Sickle cell disease is the most common genetic disorder in the United States. It affects about 50,000 African Americans. The incidence is 1 in 400 births of African American children; approximately 8% of the African Americans carry the sickle cell gene. The disease also affects other populations, including those from Asia Minor, India Minor, Central Africa, and countries adjacent to the Mediterranean and Caribbean Seas.

Over time, this chronic hemolytic anemia affects most organs. The anemia causes jaundice, pigment gallstones, splenomegaly, and poor-healing ulcers in the lower extremities. The accelerated hemolysis increases marrow space in developing bones, leading to the classic enlargement of the frontal portion of the skull.

The chronic anemia may become life threatening when severe anemia is caused by hemolytic or aplastic crisis. These recurrent disabling painful attacks, known as *sickle cell crises*, occur throughout the person's life.

The most dreaded, recurrent, and common sickle cell crisis is the *infarctive* crisis. It is often accompanied by excruciating pain and fever. Infarction may occur in the bones, muscles, lungs, spleen, intestines, and brain. Young children may sustain cerebral infarction with permanent neurologic deficits. By adulthood, repeated episodes may produce abnormal development of bones and

Table 23-3-1. Inheritance and Hemoglobin Distribution

GENOTYPE	DIAGNOSIS AND TYPE OF HEMOGLOBIN	PARENTAL PATTERN
AA	Normal—HbA	Neither parent has HbS.
AS	Sickle trait—HbAS	One parent has HbS.
SS	Sickle cell disease (anemia)—HbSS	Both parents have HbAS and carry the sickle trait.

damage to the heart, kidneys, liver, spleen, lungs, or eyes. The person is predisposed to infections because of dysfunctional spleen, leukocytes, and macrophages. In addition, vascular occlusion may result in prolonged, painful priapism in males.

 PATHOPHYSIOLOGY

Sickle cell anemia is marked by a defect in the B chain of the Hgb molecule, with an abnormal substitution of a single amino acid. A recessive gene (Table 23-3-1) transmits sickle hemoglobin (HbS). In sickle cell disease, sickling occurs in the homozygote when Hgb is deoxygenated. One HbS molecule interacts with another, causing a curved deformity in cell shape that resembles a sickle. In sickle cell trait, in which less HbS is present, in the heterozygote there is little tendency for the cells to sickle except in the presence of significant hypoxia.

Once the sickled cells are formed, they obstruct flood flow in the microcirculation, producing localized tissue hypoxia and infarctions. The Hgb of the sickled cell has less affinity for oxygen and thus releases oxygen molecules more readily than does normal Hgb, compounding the problem. A painful sudden crisis results from vessel occlusion and can affect almost any part of the body.

There are four types of crisis:
- Infarctive, caused by vascular occlusion
- Hemolytic, associated with increased destruction of the defective erythrocytes
- Sequestration, caused by massive pooling of blood in the spleen or liver
- Aplastic, associated with infection or folic acid deficiency

Sickle cell anemia eventually affects most body organs and tissues, with common sites being the abdomen, chest, and joints. Chronic damage to liver, spleen, heart, and kidneys as well as other organs results from sluggish blood flow, especially in the renal medulla in the hypertonic environment. Chronic hyperbilirubinemia resulting from the breakdown of Hgb often leads to pigment stones in the gallbladder. Cerebral infarctions and retinal detachment can also occur suddenly. There is no known cure for the disease.

 SIGNS AND SYMPTOMS

Pale skin and mucous membranes, associated with low Hgb and moderately severe normocytic normochromic anemia, are present. A classic finding is enlargement of the frontal portion of the skull, resulting from marrow space increases in developing bones. The hand-foot syndrome is generally the earliest manifestation of the disease, caused by damage to rapidly growing small bones and feet by microinfarctions at age 3 to 20 months. This syndrome is characterized by low-grade fever, pain, and swelling of the hands and feet.

Scleral icterus due to excessive bilirubin and "corkscrew" retinal conjunctival vessels related to congestion by sickled cells are seen on ophthalmic examination. The urine may appear dark brown to orange, and cholecystitis may result from pigmented gallstones developing from increased bile pigment. Cardiac murmurs associated with cardiomegaly may be auscultated. The liver may be easily palpated with hepatomegaly. Splenomegaly generally develops early in life, during which time the spleen is the major site of hemolysis. In later life, however, the spleen is usually nonpalpable, because it is eventually destroyed by repeated infarcts. Fulminating sepsis may develop because of functional asplenia and is a leading cause of death. Scarring or ulcers may be seen on the lower extremities, especially around the ankles.

Sickle cell crisis is marked by severe pain and fever and loss of function in the area of infarction. The pain is throbbing and of sudden onset. The crisis typically lasts between 1 and 10 days. Physical assessment reveals tenderness and swelling over the sites of infarction. Osteomyelitis should be considered when the patient complains of bone and joint pain. Aseptic necrosis of the femoral head is common. The frequency of sickle cell crisis varies from every few weeks to every few years.

DIAGNOSTIC CRITERIA

Initial examination should include complete blood count, reticulocyte count, and Hgb electrophoresis. Diagnostic studies reveal anemia with a fluctuating Hgb level of 5.5 to 9.5 g/dL. However, Hgb electrophoresis is necessary to confirm diagnosis. Reticulocytes, leukocytes, and platelet counts may be elevated. Increased indirect bilirubin and urine urobilinogen levels occur from chronically increased hemolysis. Serum bilirubin level can climb to dangerously high levels (>340 μmol/L or >20 mg/dL).

Abnormal liver function tests may indicate hepatic infarction, transfusion-related hepatitis, or biliary disease. Increased serum creatinine, proteinuria, hematuria, and fixed specific gravity of 1.010 indicate that renal damage has occurred.

Radiographic bone films may reveal abnormal bone formation with increased marrow space. Aseptic necrosis of the femoral head commonly occurs by young adulthood and is the major cause of crippling in adult patients. Salmonella osteomyelitis should always be differentiated when the patient complains of joint and bone pain.

INTERVENTIONS

Treatment is supportive, because there is no cure. Oxygen should be administered to reduce sickling and to improve oxygen delivery to ischemic tissues. Intravenous fluids for hydration, analgesics for pain, antibiotics for infection, and correction of acidosis are necessary.

The frequency of painful episodes is one criterion for determining disease severity. Codeine preparations are given for mild to moderate pain, but hydromorphone, morphine, or oxycodone is needed to manage more severe pain.

Morphine is the drug of choice for acute painful episodes that last more that 24 hours. Fentanyl and other anesthetics are a last resort.

Oral folic acid is given to prevent folate depletion, and erythropoietin may be given to stimulate RBC production. Many patients tolerate a Hgb level below 7 g/dL. However, if the patient becomes symptomatic, blood transfusion may be necessary. Heptavax vaccine may be given as early as age 6 months if frequent transfusions are planned.

IV hypotonic solutions are administered to enlarge the RBCs in an attempt to minimize sickling. IV hydration is important; the goal is to reduce the abnormal HbS level to below 1.0% and to mobilize sickled cells before complete infarction occurs. Hydroxyurea, commonly used to treat polycythemia vera, has also been used with some success both alone and in combination with erythropoietin. Hydroxyurea increases the level of fetal hemoglobin (HbF), which has a sparing effect on sickled RBCs and may decrease episodes of painful crises and reduce the need for blood transfusions. Experimental treatments include bone marrow transplant and gene therapy.

Osteomyelitis is treated with antibiotics. Leg ulcers are managed by elevating the leg and applying compresses with cleaning oxidants. Débridement, topical antibiotics, absorbents, porous dressings, and collagen matrix wrappings with skin grafting may be necessary. Bed rest is mandatory to promote healing.

Patient education and genetic counseling are imperative. The patient is taught to avoid situations that precipitate crises, such as infections, cold exposure, severe physical exertion, and dehydration.

Priapism occurs in approximately 40% of men and should be managed initially with sedation, analgesia, local cooling, walking, transfusion, and hydration. If these measures are not effective, spinal anesthesia and needle aspiration of blood from the corpora cavernosa may be attempted. Counseling and psychological support are needed to allay fears, embarrassment, and concerns about future sexual function.

Retinopathy can eventually lead to blindness; regular ocular examinations should be conducted. Glaucoma is often triggered by trauma.

 COMMUNITY CARE

Teaching the patient self-care measures for home and work is central to the management of this chronic disease. The importance of adequate nutrition must be emphasized, with special attention given to folic acid, iron, protein, vitamins, and minerals. The patient should be instructed to avoid exposure to cold, strenuous exercise, exertion at high altitudes, and scuba diving. Avoiding smoking and exposure to smoke is vital to maintaining good oxygenation. Arrange for home oxygenation equipment if needed and teach the patient and family about its use.

Teach the patient to inspect the feet and legs regularly and to avoid wearing knee-high hose or anything with restrictive bands. Careful trimming of the toenails, frequent application of gentle lotion, and elevation of the legs several times a day are important preventive measures. Instruct the patient to report signs of skin breakdown to the health care provider.

Facilitate referrals to support groups and for genetic counseling. Help the patient and family identify successful coping strategies used in the past and evaluate their quality of life. Assess their satisfaction with social support and involve members from the patient's faith community to support spirituality and reduce stress.

 PROGNOSIS

Sickle cell disease evolves into a chronic multisystem disease that begins as early as 4 to 6 months of age. Multiple organs are affected throughout the life span. The leading cause of death is bacterial infection. Myocardial infarction, chronic lung disease, chronic renal failure, and stroke are also common. Some patients may live full lives, reaching age 60 to 70; for other patients, however, the disease results in death between age 20 and 40. This emphasizes the importance of regular evaluation and careful monitoring.

 CLINICAL PEARLS

○ Important interventions center on oxygenation, fluid administration, and pain management.
○ Education about the disease process, signs and symptoms, and triggers for sickle cell crisis is mandatory.
○ Genetic counseling and information on disease transmission should be provided.
○ Support groups, community agencies, and spiritual support are important resources.

NURSING PROBLEM/ DIAGNOSIS	NURSING INTERVENTIONS CLASSIFICATION (NIC)
Fatigue	See Section 1
Diminished oxygen-carrying capacity/Ineffective tissue perfusion	See Section 1 Fluid administration
Risk for injury	Surveillance: safety

chapter 24

Sensory

Cataracts

Section 1   Karen Harris

 OVERVIEW

A cataract is opacity or clouding of the eye's lens that can lead to reduced or lost vision. Cataracts may develop slowly over years or may progress rapidly depending on the type and etiology. Cataract is the third-leading (after arthritis and heart disease) cause of disability in older adults and the most common cause of age-related visual loss. Approximately 50% percent of individuals between age 65 and 74 and 70% of those age 75 and older develop cataracts. Statistics show that cataract is the most common cause of visual impairment as well as the third most common cause of preventable blindness in the United States.

The cause of most cataracts is unknown; they are probably the result of the aging process and present as a gradual visual impairment. However, a cataract may be caused or accelerated by an eye injury, eye inflammation, certain disorders, or as a side effect of certain medications.

 PATHOPHYSIOLOGY

Cataracts present as several different types and can result from various causes, including certain illnesses (e.g., diabetes mellitus, uveitis, ocular trauma), long-term use of certain drugs (e.g., glucocorticoids), prolonged sun exposure, and radiation therapy.

The most common type of cataract is related to aging and is referred to as *senile cataracts.* These cataracts usually develop bilaterally, with each eye progressing independently. One eye is commonly more compromised. Visual impairment may or may not progress at the same rate in both eyes. This can happen over many years or in some cases within a matter of months. The three common types of senile cataracts are classified by their location within the lens.

The *nuclear cataract* (also known as immature cataract) is associated with myopia. The nucleus of the lens is opaque whereas the cortical areas remain clear. As the cataract progresses over time, the patient develops increasing nearsightedness.

The *cortical cataract* (known also as mature cataract) is distinguished by opacification of the entire lens. Research indicates that individuals with excessive sun exposure are more likely to develop cortical cataracts than are those with limited sun exposure.

The *posterior subcapsular cataract* occurs in front of the posterior capsule. It generally develops in younger individuals and is associated with prolonged corticosteroid use, inflammation, or trauma. Near vision is usually affected, and the patient may complain of sensitivity to glare from strong sunlight or headlights from oncoming vehicles.

Other factors, including genetics, can affect a person's risk of developing cataracts.

 SIGNS AND SYMPTOMS

In the early stages, a cataract may not cause a problem. The cloudiness may affect only a small part of the lens. However, over time, the cataract has the potential to grow and cloud more of the lens. Although many people develop cataracts bilaterally, cataracts do not spread from one eye to another. The most common symptoms include:

- Painless cloudy or blurred vision
- Problems with light, with patient complaints of dim surroundings, increased sensitivity to light (e.g., headlights at night seem too bright), and light scattering
- Faded colors and color shifting (as the aging lens becomes more absorbent at the darker end of the spectrum)
- Poor night vision
- Decrease in visual acuity
- Double or multiple vision (which may resolve as the cataract grows)
- Frequent changes in eyeglasses or contact lenses
- Myopic shift and astigmatism

These signs and symptoms may also indicate other eye problems. A patient exhibiting any of these should be assessed by an eye care professional.

 DIAGNOSTIC CRITERIA

The Snellen visual acuity test measures how well an individual can see at various distances. A decrease in visual acuity is directly proportional to the density of a cataract.

Slit-lamp examination (using a special microscope) provides magnification and establishes the degree of cataract formation. However, the degree of lens opacity does not always correlate with the patient's functional status.

Tonometry is a standard test that measures intraocular pressure (IOP; fluid pressure inside the eye). Increased pressure may also be a sign of glaucoma.

Direct or indirect ophthalmoscopy and ocular examination allow the examiner to visualize and determine the presence of cataracts. *Perimetry* examination evaluates the scope or extent of the peripheral visual fields.

Pupil dilatation uses eyedrops to widen the pupil. This allows the examiner to see more of the lens and retina and look for other eye problems.

 INTERVENTIONS
Surgery

In the early stages of a cataract, vision may improve by using different eyeglasses, magnifying lenses, or stronger lighting. If these measures do not help, then surgery is the only effective treatment. The cloudy lens is removed and may or may not be replaced with a substitute lens. The current trend is to perform the surgery as a same-day procedure. Surgical procedures include the following.

Extracapsular Cataract Extraction

In this procedure, the anterior lens capsule and cortex are incised and removed, leaving the posterior capsule intact. A posterior chamber intraocular lens (IOL) is generally implanted in place of the patient's own lens. If an IOL is not implanted at the time of surgery, the patient may be fitted later for prescriptive glasses or contact lenses. This procedure is appropriate for patients of all ages and is the most common cataract-correction surgery in the United States.

Intracapsular Cataract Extraction

This procedure involves removal of the entire lens and the intact capsule. This is done by cryoextraction, in which the moist lens sticks to an extremely cold metal device for easy and safe removal with low traction. This procedure is rarely performed today; it has been replaced by extracapsular cataract extraction and phacoemulsification.

Phacoemulsification

This procedure involves mechanically breaking up (emulsifying) the lens by a hollow needle that vibrates at ultrasonic speed. This is combined with aspiration and irrigation of the emulsified pieces from the anterior chamber of the eye.

Intraocular Lens Implantation

IOL implantation serves as an alternative to vision correction. A synthetic lens is implanted to accommodate distance vision. Calculations are predetermined for the actual prescription of the lens before implantation. Many types of lenses are available; these should be discussed by the patient and ophthalmologist. Intraocular implantation may be an attractive alternative for individuals who cannot wear cataract glasses or contact lenses. Also, unlike glasses or lenses, the implanted lens cannot be lost or damaged. This procedure does carry the risk of complications, however, including pain and inflammation of some eye structures.

Preparation for Surgery

The nurse orients the patient and explains the planned procedure to help decrease anxiety. The patient should be instructed not to touch or rub the eyes, to decrease contamination and reduce the risk of injury. Conjunctival cultures should be obtained as requested, using aseptic technique.

Postoperative Care

After recovering from anesthesia, the patient should receive verbal and written instructions on how to protect the operative eye. Medications should be given to promote comfort. The nurse assesses for nausea and vomiting, sudden onset of restlessness, and increased pulse rate. The patient is cautioned against excessive coughing or sneezing, rapid movement, and bending to prevent increased IOP. The patient is encouraged to ambulate and resume activities of daily living as soon as possible. The patient is also urged to wear sunglasses while outside and patches at night to protect the operated eye from injury. Any eye or brow pain should be reported, because this may indicate a serious complication that requires immediate attention.

Administration of Eye Medication

The patient is taught how to self-administer eye medications as directed. The patient is instructed to bring all eye medications to the follow-up appointment with the ophthalmologist to allow adjustment of dosages or changes in the medication regimen. What will not be used can then be discarded by the health care professional so as to prevent confusion for the patient.

COMMUNITY CARE

Promotion of Home Care/Education

Once at home, the patient should be forewarned to continue to wear a protective eye patch for the next 24 to 48 hours after surgery. This helps to prevent accidental rubbing or poking. This first patch is usually removed at the first follow-up visit.

Eyeglasses should be worn during the day, followed by an eye patch at night for the next 4 to 6 weeks. Sunglasses should be worn while the person is outdoors during the day to protect the sensitive eye from direct sunlight.

The patient should gradually increase normal activities in the first few days after surgery. Any restrictions should have been specified before discharge from the hospital. The patient should continue to avoid activities that cause straining (e.g., defecation) or heavy lifting.

Minimal morning discharge, redness, and an itchy sensation are expected for a few days after surgery. A clean wet cloth may be used to blot the eye discharge. Pain is not normal and should be reported promptly.

Health Maintenance and Illness Prevention

With continuous improvement in cataract surgical procedures, the goal is to transition the patient from a clouded or opaque lens to excellent unaided distance vision. The patient should be advised that cataract surgical procedures increase the likelihood of retinal detachment and instructed to contact the surgeon if dots or floaters appear in the visual field.

The patient should know that there is usually a 6- to 12-week period after surgery in which the eyes adjust to visual changes. Temporary corrective lenses are usually worn for the first 6 weeks after surgery, and a prescription for permanent lenses is determined about 6 to 12 weeks after surgery.

Family and friends should offer encouragement during this period. The adjustment period can be very frustrating. The patient should be told that individuals with IOL implants experience more rapid visual improvement than those waiting for glasses or contact lenses. However, some patients who undergo extracapsular extraction can develop a secondary membrane in the posterior lens capsule, causing decreased visual acuity.

The patient should be informed that with permanent glasses, the perceived image is about one-third larger than that seen before the formation of cataracts. The patient is taught to look through the center of the corrective glasses and to turn the head as necessary to look to the side, because peripheral vision is significantly distorted. With contact lenses, magnification is increased by only 5% to 10%, but peripheral vision is not affected.

Some patients are not considered good candidates for contact lenses. For example, a patient with tremor in the hands may have difficulty applying lenses, and a patient who cannot maintain good general hygiene may be prone to irritation or infection.

The patient should know that with the implantation of IOLs, eyeglasses may not be required for distance vision but probably will be needed for reading and writing. The patient should be informed that it might be necessary to relearn space dimensions, especially while walking and using stairs. Daily activities, such as reaching for items on a table and pouring liquids, require adjustment.

 PROGNOSIS

There is no nonsurgical treatment to cure cataracts. The prognosis is generally good. Surgery improves vision in 95% of affected individuals. Ongoing studies are investigating ways to stop progression of cataracts, such as the use of vitamin C and other antioxidants.

 CLINICAL PEARLS

○ Cataracts may result from injuries to the eye, exposure to excessive heat and sun, or inherited factors.
○ Most cataract cases are senile cataracts, which result from the normal aging process.
○ Blurred vision and dimmed vision are usually the first symptoms of cataract. The patient may notice that he or she needs brighter light for reading.
○ Continued clouding of the lens may cause double vision.
○ The only known effective treatment for cataract is surgical removal of the lens. The procedure of choice is extracapsular lens extraction.
○ After cataract extraction, the loss of the natural lens is compensated for by either intraocular implantation of a permanent artificial lens (either during cataract surgery or later), special eyeglasses, or removable contact lenses.
○ Cataract surgery is usually done on an outpatient basis under general anesthesia.
○ Preoperative and postoperative nursing care is minimal. The greatest challenge is the patient's adjustment to visual changes, eyeglasses, or contact lenses, and the ability to maintain independence.
○ When caring for a patient with impaired vision, always identify yourself clearly when approaching the patient and strive to minimize distractions.

NURSING PROBLEM/ DIAGNOSIS	NURSING INTERVENTIONS CLASSIFICATION (NIC)
Decreased visual perception	Environmental management Surveillance: safety
Risk for postoperative eye injury	Eye care Contact lens care

Conjunctivitis

Section 2 Gigi Robison

 OVERVIEW

Conjunctivitis, also called "red eye" or "pink eye," is the most common eye infection in the United States. The conjunctiva is continually exposed to many microorganisms and environmental agents that can cause eye infections. Conjunctivitis may occur secondary to systemic disease or other ocular disorders.

 PATHOPHYSIOLOGY

Conjunctivitis is an inflammation or redness of the conjunctiva characterized by vascular dilation and exudate formation. It can be caused by infection, allergic reaction, or physical agents, or can be secondary to systemic or ocular diseases.

Conjunctivitis can affect one eye or both eyes. It is often spread by direct contact with the ocular discharge and can be easily transmitted to others during close physical contact.

Infectious Etiologies

Acute Bacterial Conjunctivitis. It is highly contagious and uncommon in adults. The most common causative organisms are *Staphylococcus aureus, Hemophilus influenzae,* and *Streptococcus pneumoniae.*

Chronic Bacterial Conjunctivitis. *Staphylococcus aureus* is the most common causative organism identified, because of its ability to colonize the eyelids.

Hyperacute Bacterial Conjunctivitis. The causative organism in this entity is commonly *Neisseria gonorrhoeae.* This is also the causative organism of gonorrhea, a sexually transmitted infection of the genitals and urinary tract. The gonococcal organism may occasionally affect the eye, causing blindness if not treated.

Chlamydial Keratoconjunctivitis. Two types of conjunctivitis are caused by the *Chlamydia trachomatis* organism: trachoma and adult inclusion conjunctivitis. This organism is a modified gram-negative bacterium that is an obligate intracellular parasite. It is transmitted by sexual contact and can infect the genital tract, the respiratory tract, and the eye.

Trachoma. *Chlamydia trachomatis* (serotypes A to C) is the causative agent in trachoma, which is a major cause of blindness worldwide. Trachoma begins with the sudden onset of inflammation of the conjunctiva. Next, follicles form under the conjunctiva, the eyelids become scarred, and granulations form on the inner surface on the eyelids. Then corneal vascularization (pannus) and infiltration of the cornea can occur. The entire cornea may eventually become involved, with eventual loss of vision. Trachoma can result in conjunctival scarring, keratitis, and blindness.

Adult Inclusion Conjunctivitis. The causative organism, *Chlamydia trachomatis* (serotypes D to K), is also responsible for genital tract disease in adults. The eye is usually involved from accidental contact with genital secretions. Therefore, this disease occurs most frequently in sexually active young adults.

Viral Conjunctivitis. Viral infections that can affect the eye include colds, acute respiratory infections, and viral diseases such as measles, herpes simplex, and herpes zoster. Many cases of conjunctivitis are caused by adenovirus type 3. One common form of conjunctivitis, epidemic keratoconjunctivitis, occurs in adults, is very contagious, and is caused by adenovirus types 8 and 19. Visual loss is more likely to be a complication with this type of conjunctivitis because of corneal subepithelial infiltrates. The disease usually lasts for 1 to 2 weeks.

Noninfectious Etiologies

Allergic Conjunctivitis. This is triggered by airborne allergens, such as pollen, grass, air pollutants, smoke, occupational irritants, dust, dander, mold, and topical medications (including eye solutions for persons who wear contact lenses). It is an acute process that is IgE mediated and results in the degranulation of conjunctival mast cells and the release of allergic mediators, such as histamines.

Three other forms of conjunctivitis include irritative conjunctivitis, conjunctivitis due to systemic disease, and conjunctivitis due to ocular disease.

 SIGNS AND SYMPTOMS

Two prominent features of conjunctivitis are hyperuremia (redness) of the conjunctiva and exudate (discharge) formation. Persons with acute conjunctivitis do not experience any visual impairment (e.g., blurring) and exhibit normal pupil size, pupillary reaction to light, and IOP. Other signs and symptoms of each type of conjunctivitis are outlined below. Although conjunctivitis usually begins in one eye, it can quickly spread to the other eye by contamination of the person's hands or of personal items, such as washcloths, towels, or handkerchiefs.

Acute/Chronic Bacterial Conjunctivitis. This type is marked by acute onset with diffuse conjunctival redness, modest mucopurulent discharge deposited on the lashes and corners of the eyes, with lids sealed shut in the morning, and with swelling, mild pain/discomfort, burning, itching, a sensation of a foreign body in the eye, tearing, and photophobia. A slightly enlarged preauricular node may be present.

Hyperacute Bacterial Conjunctivitis (*Neisseria gonorrhoeae*). This type presents with copious purulent discharge associated with marked lid swelling, beefy red appearance, and conjunctival edema. The globe may be extremely tender, and a preauricular node is usually present. This is considered an ophthalmologic emergency, because corneal involvement may rapidly lead to perforation.

Chlamydial Keratoconjunctivitis

Adult Inclusion Conjunctivitis. Signs and symptoms include acute redness, chronic unilateral or bilateral mucopurulent discharge, irritation, photophobia (sensitivity to light), and follicular conjunctivitis with mild keratitis. A nontender preauricular node may be present.

Trachoma. Trachoma presents with the sudden onset of conjunctivitis, and can result in conjunctival scarring, corneal vascularization (pannus), keratitis, and blindness. If the cornea is involved, photophobia may develop.

Viral Conjunctivitis. Symptoms vary from mild to severe and may include redness, copious watery discharge and scanty exudates, sticky eyelids in the morning, mild itching, and photophobia. Preauricular nodes are present in most cases, and a scratchy foreign body sensation in the eye may be reported. Epidemic keratoconjunctivitis is marked by unilateral conjunctival redness, pain, tearing, and an enlarged preauricular lymph node. This syndrome runs a 1- to 2-week course and is often accompanied by subepithelial corneal infiltrates.

Allergic Conjunctivitis. Signs and symptoms include conjunctival edema, redness, bilateral itching, tearing, photophobia, burning, a feeling of grit in the eye, and manifestations of associated systemic allergy. Mucous discharge may occur in severe cases.

Irritative Conjunctivitis. Unilateral or bilateral irritation is seen.

 DIAGNOSTIC CRITERIA
Physical Examination

- The eyelids, eyelid margins, and external eye are assessed for the presence of edema, redness, itching, and discharges using a penlight, ophthalmoscopy, or a slit lamp.
- The conjunctiva of the lower lid is examined by pulling downward on the lid as the patient looks upward.
- The conjunctiva of the upper lid is examined by everting the lid. To do this, as the patient looks down, the examiner grasps the eyelashes and gently pulls down and forward while pushing on the upper lid border with an applicator or tongue blade.

Laboratory Tests

Diagnostic tests are usually not indicated. However, various laboratory tests facilitate differential diagnosis when initial treatment fails, when the condition is severe, or when infection with gonorrhea or chlamydia is suspected. Table 24-2-1 lists specific diagnostic tests.

 INTERVENTIONS

Treatment of conjunctivitis depends on the etiology of the condition. In most cases, warm compresses applied to the affected eye several times a day will help minimize discomfort. Only preparations designed for ophthalmic use may be used in the eyes. In all cases, precautions should be taken to prevent the spread of infection to others. Such precautions include disposing of any eye discharge or materials that touch the infected eye in a sanitary manner.

Acute/Chronic Bacterial Conjunctivitis
- The lids and lashes are cleansed using a washcloth and baby shampoo. Firm, adherent crusts may be softened with hot compresses.
- Broad-spectrum antibiotic eyedrops are administered; agents include sodium sulfacetamide (Sulamyd), 10% ophthalmic solution or ointment for 2 to 3 days; Polytrim (polymyxin B and trimethoprim), 1 drop four times a day for 10 days; topical fluoroquinolones, such as ofloxacin (Ocuflox) or ciprofloxacin (Ciloxan); and aminoglycoside eyedrops.

Hyperacute Bacterial Conjunctivitis (*Neisseria gonorrhoeae*)
- Pharmacologic therapy includes topical bacitracin, 500 U/g 8 times daily for 2 to 3 weeks, or topical erythromycin, *plus c*eftriaxone (Rocephin), a

Table 24-2-1. Determining the Differential Diagnosis of Conjunctivitis

ETIOLOGY OF CONJUNCTIVITIS	DIAGNOSTIC TESTS
Acute/chronic bacterial conjunctivitis	Examination of stained conjunctival scrapings and culture studies recommended in severe cases
Hyperacute bacterial conjunctivitis	Stained smear, Gram's stain, and cultures of the discharge on Thayer-Martin and chocolate agar
Chlamydial keratoconjunctivitis: Trachoma or adult inclusion conjunctivitis	Giemsa-stained conjunctival scrapings (cytologic examination), direct fluorescent antibody assay, or an enzyme immunoassay
Viral conjunctivitis	Clinical signs: cultures, Gram's stain, or immunofluorescent techniques rarely used
Conjunctivitis neonatorum: • Bacterial	Culture media: reduced blood agar, thioglycolate broth, chocolate agar in CO_2, Thayer-Martin media
• Chlamydial	Culture media: McCloy cell culture
• Herpetic	Culture media: viral cultures

single 1-g dose intramuscularly or 1 to 2 g every 24 hours for 5 days if the cornea is involved.

- The infected person's sexual partner(s) should also be treated with systemic antibiotics.

Chlamydial Keratoconjunctivitis
Trachoma

- Pharmacologic therapy may include oral antibiotics: tetracycline, erythromycin, or doxycycline. A single dose of azithromycin may also be effective. (Note that tetracycline is contraindicated during pregnancy and breast-feeding.)
- A topical antibiotic ointment—erythromycin (Ilotycin) one or two times daily—may be applied.
- Surgical treatment may include correction of eyelid deformities or corneal transplantation.
- The infected person's sexual partner(s) should also be treated with systemic antibiotics.

Adult Inclusion Conjunctivitis

- Oral antibiotic therapy may include tetracycline or erythromycin, 250 to 500 mg four times daily, or doxycycline, 300 mg initially followed by 100 mg once a day for 2 weeks.

Viral Conjunctivitis

- Supportive treatment includes artificial tears, topical decongestants, prophylactic topical antibiotics to prevent secondary infections, or warm compresses applied to the affected eye.
- Topical steroids and antiviral therapy (e.g., intravenous acyclovir [Zovirax]) are often prescribed.

Allergic Conjunctivitis

- Cold compresses are applied to the affected eye(s) to relieve itching.
- Prophylactic treatment may be provided with a mast cell stabilizer, which can be used before exposure to offending allergens. One mast cell stabilizer, topical lodoxamide (Alomide), four times daily, is recommended for

mild and moderately severe allergic disease. Other mast cell stabilizers include cromolyn sodium 4% (Crolom) and olopatadine (Patanol), which has antihistamine properties.

- Topical vasoconstrictors and antihistamines are occasionally used in persons with hay fever conjunctivitis to relieve the overall allergic reaction, but are of limited efficacy.
- A topical antihistamine-decongestant may be administered four times daily to treat acute symptoms. Levocabastine (Livostin) is a newer, very effective antihistamine.
- Oral antihistamines, such as diphenhydramine hydrochloride (Benadryl), may help relieve itching.
- Topical steroids can be very effective in controlling the symptoms, but should be used with the supervision of an ophthalmologist because of the risk of cataract and secondary glaucoma.
- A nonsteroidal anti-inflammatory drug, such as ketorolac (Acular), may be given to relieve itching.
- Cold compresses are applied as needed.
- The offending allergen(s) should be identified and avoided when possible.

Irritative Conjunctivitis

- The eye is irrigated with normal saline solution or plain water as soon as possible after exposure.
- Artificial tears may be administered.
- The causative agent must be identified and removed.

COMMUNITY CARE

Assessment

Patient history should focus on identifying risk factors, including:

- Exposure to others with conjunctivitis (i.e., direct or indirect contact, swimming pools)
- History of systemic disease, such as diabetes mellitus, arthritis, hypertension, thyroid disease, and multiple sclerosis
- History of ocular disease, such as cataracts, acute angle closure glaucoma, strabismus, ambylopia, and retinal detachment
- History of allergies
- Exposure to irritants, such as overwear of contact lenses, overexposure to infrared or ultraviolet light, or mechanical trauma (e.g., surgical procedure)

Assess for signs and symptoms of conjunctivitis: red, inflamed conjunctiva and discharge, itching or discomfort of the eye. Evaluate the patient's ability to self-administer eyedrops and assess compliance with prescribed oral and topical medications.

Monitoring

Teach persons who have had close contact with the patient with conjunctivitis to report any redness, itching, discomfort, or discharge from their eyes to their health care provider. Assess for complications of conjunctivitis:

- Visual impairment
- Conjunctival scarring
- Keratitis
- Blindness
- Corneal ulcers or perforation, infiltrates, or endophthalmitis in the neonate

Instruct the patient to report any of the following to health care provider:
- No relief of symptoms in 48 to 72 hours
- Moderate to severe eye pain
- Changes in vision
- Suspicion that the conjunctivitis is caused by herpes simplex

Prevention

Reinforce patient teaching regarding the importance of:
- Washing the hands often using antibacterial soap, and using single-use towels while infected to prevent the spread of conjunctivitis
- Using a clean tissue to remove discharge from the eyes, discarding the tissue in a sanitary manner, and then thoroughly washing the hands
- Finishing the course of antibiotics as prescribed, to make sure that the infection is resolved
- Avoiding contact, including swimming, vigorous physical activities, and "toy-sharing" activities, with other persons until symptoms resolve
- Avoiding known allergens and chemical irritants
- Using proper protective eyewear and screens to prevent eye damage when in areas where welding occurs

It is not necessary to isolate persons with eye infections if standard precautions are followed. Appropriate cleansing, handling, and wearing of contact lenses (soft or hard) are important in preventing eye infections.

 PROGNOSIS

With proper treatment, conjunctivitis has a favorable prognosis. With delayed treatment or lack of treatment, visual impairment, conjunctival scarring, corneal involvement, or blindness can occur.
- Acute bacterial conjunctivitis is usually self-limiting, resolving in 10 to 14 days.
- In *hyperacute bacterial conjunctivitis*, the gonococcal organism, *Neisseria gonorrhoeae,* may occasionally affect the eye and cause blindness if not treated. This is an ophthalmologic emergency because corneal involvement may rapidly lead to perforation.
- In *chlamydial keratoconjunctivitis, trachoma* can be arrested in the early stages with topical and oral antibiotics. If treatment is delayed or absent, trachoma can result in conjunctival scarring, keratitis, and blindness.
- *Adult inclusion conjunctivitis* is arrested in the early stages with topical and oral antibiotics.
- In *viral conjunctivitis*, visual loss is more likely to be a complication of one common type of viral conjunctivitis, epidemic keratoconjunctivitis, because of corneal subepithelial infiltrates. The disease usually lasts for 1 to 2 weeks.
- *Allergic conjunctivitis* generally resolves itself with symptomatic treatment and removal of the allergen.
- *Irritative conjunctivitis* generally resolves itself with removal of the irritative agent, irrigation of the eye, and instillation of artificial tears.

 CLINICAL PEARLS

○ In conjunctivitis, scrupulous hand washing before and after touching the eyes is imperative.

○ For a patient scheduled to receive frequent eyedrops, it may be necessary to identify one or more family members or friends to assist with administration.

○ Check the availability of fortified eyedrops if the patient lives in a small community. Fortified medications are not usually commercially available and must be prepared by a pharmacist. These preparations usually expire within days or weeks of preparation.

○ To prevent skin breakdown in older adults, apply a thin layer of petroleum jelly on the skin under the eyelid. Leave a margin at the eyelid so that the jelly does not accidentally enter the eye. This protects the thin, delicate skin of older adults from irritation owing to constant tearing and application of frequent eyedrops.

NURSING PROBLEM/ DIAGNOSIS	NURSING INTERVENTIONS CLASSIFICATION (NIC)
Eye inflammation/infection	Eye care
	Infection control
	Medication administration: topical
Risk for contagion	Infection prevention

Glaucoma

Section 3   Gigi Robison

 OVERVIEW

Glaucoma is a common eye disease that affects almost 3 million persons in the United States. The risk of glaucoma increases dramatically with age. Glaucoma is the third-leading cause of blindness in the United States and is the leading cause of blindness in African Americans.

Approximately 80% of persons in the United States with glaucoma have primary open-angle glaucoma. The other 20% may have juvenile open-angle glaucoma (which occurs in persons younger than age 40) or acute angle-closure glaucoma.

 PATHOPHYSIOLOGY

Glaucoma, a condition where the optic nerve is damaged, is thought to be due to excessively high IOP. Normally, aqueous humor is continuously produced by the ciliary body. It flows between the iris and lens around the pupil's edge and into the anterior chamber. From there, it exits the eye through the trabecular meshwork, where it is filtered, and drains into Schlemm's canal, where it moves out into venous circulation through scleral veins. Two primary mechanisms can cause increased IOP: excessive production of aqueous humor by the ciliary body and an obstruction that blocks the drainage of aqueous humor from the eye into the bloodstream. The increased pressure distorts the shape of optic nerve fibers, causing indentation ("cupping") and then atrophy (pallor) of the optic nerve.

Vision loss begins with blind spots in the peripheral field of vision, which is usually not noticed and progresses to the loss of central vision.

Risk factors for glaucoma include:

- Myopia (near-sightedness). Persons with myopia have a twofold to three-fold increased risk of developing glaucoma compared with persons without myopia.
- Diabetes mellitus. Persons with diabetes have an increased incidence of glaucoma.
- Family history. Prevalence among first-degree relatives may be as high as 40%.
- Genetics. A research study located the first glaucoma gene (a mutation in the CYP1B1 gene) in persons with primary infantile glaucoma.
- Race. The prevalence of glaucoma in African Americans aged 45 to 65 years is three to five times higher than that in whites in the same age range.
- Age-related changes. The incidence is several times higher in people older than 60 years of age.

Glaucoma is actually a group at least 20 different forms of ocular disease. These can be classified as:

- Primary, which occurs spontaneously, or *secondary*, which occurs as a result of another disease or trauma (e.g., postoperative complication, hemorrhage into the anterior chamber, lens displacement, laceration)
- *Acute* (rapid onset) or *chronic* (insidious onset)
- *Open* (or wide)-*angle* or *angle-closure* (or narrow), based on the width of the anterior chamber angle
- *Congenital*, occurring in infants
- *Low-tension*, which resembles primary open-angle glaucoma and develops in the presence of a statistically normal IOP

Primary Open-Angle Glaucoma

Primary open-angle glaucoma (POAG) is the most common form of glaucoma in adults. In POAG, the anterior chamber angle is wide open, and IOP is elevated because of decreased aqueous humor outflow through the trabecular meshwork. POAG usually affects both eyes, has a subtle onset, and has a slowly progressive course. It produces no symptoms at first, and half of affected persons are unaware that they have it. Symptoms occur late in the disease.

Juvenile Open-Angle Glaucoma

Juvenile open-angle glaucoma (JOAG) is similar to POAG in terms of pathophysiology, signs and symptoms, and treatment. JOAG differs from POAG in that it may present in the third or fourth decade of life, and most patients with JOAG have a genetic abnormality and a strong family history of the disease. Patients with JOAG respond very poorly to medicine and often require surgery to control the disease.

Normal-Tension Glaucoma

Optic nerve damage and narrowed peripheral vision occur unexpectedly in persons with normal IOP. The cause of optic nerve damage in this type of glaucoma is unknown. Treatment for normal-tension glaucoma is the same as for open-angle glaucoma.

Acute Angle-Closure Glaucoma

In acute angle-closure glaucoma (AACG), the anterior chamber angle is narrow, and sudden obstruction of the drainage channels of the eye blocks aqueous humor from exiting the anterior chamber. This type of glaucoma produces a sudden, large increase in IOP, which can cause damage to the optic nerve in only 1 day. AACG usually has a rapid onset and represents a *medical emergency*. Immediate treatment (e.g., prompt laser surgery) is needed to clear the blockage and improve the flow of fluid. Without treatment, blindness can occur in as little as 1 or 2 days.

Chronic Angle-Closure Glaucoma

In chronic angle-closure glaucoma (CACG), the anterior chamber angle is narrow, and there is a gradual onset of obstruction of the drainage channels of the eye. CACG usually produces no symptoms, although the person may experience blurred vision and visual perception of halos around lights. If untreated, this type of glaucoma progresses to absolute glaucoma.

Secondary Glaucoma

This type of glaucoma can develop as a complication of other medical conditions. It may be associated with eye surgery or advanced cataracts, certain eye tumors, eye injuries, uveitis (eye inflammation), corticosteroid drugs, or diabetes ("neovascular glaucoma").

Absolute Glaucoma

This is the final stage of the glaucoma disease process, producing pain and blindness.

SIGNS AND SYMPTOMS

Primary and Juvenile Open-Angle Glaucoma

No symptoms occur initially; these appear late in the disease. Onset is insidious in older persons, with a gradual loss of peripheral vision fields over several years, resulting in tunnel vision. Reduced visual acuity, especially at night, is uncorrectable with glasses. The visual perception of "halos around lights" is present if IOP is severely elevated. Mild aching in the eyes may occur. Elevated IOP is associated with pathologic cupping of the optic disk.

Normal-Tension Glaucoma

Signs and symptoms are the same as in POAG, except that the IOP is within the normal range.

Acute Angle-Closure Glaucoma

AACG has a rapid onset in older persons, which constitutes a medical emergency. Profound visual changes occur, including blurred or decreased vision, visual perception of halos around lights, and sensitivity to light. Severe pain and inflammation occur unilaterally. The eye appears red and hard with a feeling of pressure over the eye. A cloudy cornea obscures the view inside the eye. The pupils are moderately dilated and nonreactive to light. No ocular discharge is present. Nausea and vomiting occur related to the increased IOP, and pain occurs occasionally. IOP is significantly increased (40 to 80 mm Hg).

Chronic Angle-Closure Glaucoma

CACG usually produces no symptoms. Blurred vision and perception of halos around lights are possible.

Absolute Glaucoma

This final stage of glaucoma is characterized by pain and blindness.

 DIAGNOSTIC CRITERIA

Glaucoma is diagnosed when two of the following three characteristics are present:

- Increased IOP
- Indentation and atrophy of the optic nerve head
- Progressive loss of peripheral vision fields

Various instruments and tests are used to diagnose glaucoma.

Tonometer. This instrument is used to measure IOP by assessing the amount of pressure necessary to depress the cornea. Types of tonometers include those that actually contact the cornea, requiring the instillation of an anesthetizing solution, and those that do not make direct contact, such as the "air puff" test, which measures pressure using a jet of air.

Ophthalmoscope. This instrument is used to view the lens, the vitreous body, the retina, and the optic nerves. Results may show atrophy (pale yellowish color instead of a healthy pink color) and cupping (indentation) of the optic nerve head in glaucoma.

Visual Field (Perimetry) Testing. This test determines the extent of peripheral vision loss. It detects blind spots in the field of vision before the person with glaucoma is aware of them. In POAG, a small crescent-shaped scotoma (blind spot) appears early in the course of the disease. In AACG, the peripheral fields show larger areas of significant vision loss.

Gonioscope. This instrument, consisting of a magnifier and a lens equipped with mirrors, is placed on the cornea to examine the depth of the anterior chamber angle. It is used to differentiate between narrow-angle and wide-angle glaucoma. It is also used to examine the entire circumference of the angle for any abnormal changes in the trabecular meshwork.

Slit Lamp. This instrument is used to examine the depth of the eye's anterior chamber. It may be used to screen persons for predisposition to AACG.

 INTERVENTIONS

Medical Management

Medications that decrease IOP work by increasing the outflow of aqueous humor or by decreasing the rate of aqueous humor production. In most cases, glaucoma can be effectively controlled with medications, usually in the form of eyedrops. Topically applied medications are more site specific and are associated with a decreased incidence of systemic side effects. Some persons may also require medications in pill or capsule form.

Glaucoma medications include:

- Beta-adrenergic antagonists (beta-blockers)

- Prostaglandin (PG) agonists
- Alpha-2 adrenergic agonists
- Carbonic anhydrase inhibitors
- Cholinergic drugs (miotics)

Table 24-3-1 summarizes these drugs.

Several medications are contraindicated in glaucoma. Anticholinergic and adrenergic agents used to dilate the pupils for ophthalmoscopic exams, including *mydriatics* (which dilate the pupil) and *cycloplegics* (which dilate the pupil and block accommodation by paralyzing the ciliary muscles), may cause an acute attack of angle-closure glaucoma in persons with narrow angles by impeding the outflow of aqueous humor.

The effectiveness of medical therapy is monitored by assessing IOP. Usually, the target IOP is 15 to 18 mm Hg, or a reduction of the pretreatment level by 25% to 30%.

Medical treatment of AACG requires prompt lowering of IOP, usually with hyperosmotic agents (i.e., intravenous mannitol, oral isosorbide, or glycerin) and topical pilocarpine until surgical interventions can be initiated.

Surgical Treatment

Surgical treatment may be indicated in open-angle or closed- angle glaucoma. In POAG and JOAG, surgery is needed when medical therapy fails. In AACG and CACG, surgery is almost always required.

Laser Iridectomy. Argon or a krypton laser is used to create an opening in the iris that allows for the outflow of aqueous humor. This simple, painless procedure is usually performed in the doctor's office. It usually produces a permanent cure in patients with primary AACG (Fig. 24-3-1).

Laser Trabeculoplasty. In this minor operation, a laser beam is focused onto the clogged trabecular meshwork to create an opening. This fast, painless procedure is well tolerated by patients. It can be performed in the doctor's office or in a hospital clinic. It is used both as primary therapy for persons with POAG and as an adjunct to topical therapy.

Trabeculectomy. This procedure creates a small opening in the sclera that allows aqueous humor to drain. It is usually performed under local anesthesia and may require 1 or 2 days of hospitalization. Trabeculectomy is indicated when IOP remains elevated despite medical and laser therapy. It is about 80% effective in reducing IOP, and carries a 5% to 10% risk of diminished vision or the need for reoperation because of complications. Occasionally, the small opening in the sclera heals over, and IOP again increases.

Complications of trabeculectomy include cataract development, corneal problems, inflammation or infection inside the eye, and swelling of blood vessels behind the eye. Effective treatments for these complications are readily available.

 COMMUNITY CARE

Assessment

The patient history focuses on risk factors that can cause transient increases in IOP: smoking, ingestion of caffeine or large amounts of fluids, alcohol, illicit drugs, corticosteroids, altered hormone levels, posture, and eye movements.

Assessment also includes signs of disease progression and associated factors,

Table 24-3-1. Medications to Treat Glaucoma

CLASSES OF GLAUCOMA MEDICATION	ACTION OF MEDICATIONS	COMMENTS/NURSING CONSIDERATIONS
1st-Line Drugs: Beta blockers (beta-adrenergic antagonists) Timolol maleate (Timoptic) Betaxolol Carteolol Levobunolol	Beta-receptor stimulation decreases the production of aqueous humor and reduces intraocular pressure (IOP)	• Use: open-angle glaucoma • Contraindication: severe cardiovascular disease • Evaluate pulse and blood pressure during initial therapy. If pulse <80, hold drug and notify MD. If the person is hypotensive, place the person in the recumbent position until his/her blood pressure stabilizes. • Contraindicated in clients with asthma and COPD • Space out the administration of eyedrops.
Prostaglandin (PG) agonists (or analogues) • Latanoprost (Xalatan) • Unoprostone	Increases the uveoscleral outflow of aqueous humor	• Use: open-angle glaucoma • New class of ocular hypotensive drugs • Drug has rare systemic side effects; potent at very low concentrations; well tolerated • Latanoprost has a greater ocular hypotensive effect when combined with beta-blockers, adrenergic and cholinergic agonists, or carbonic anhydrase inhibitors. • Permanent increases in iris pigmentation
2nd-Line Drugs: Alpha-2 adrenergic agonists Brimonidine	Alpha-receptor stimulation inhibits formation of aqueous humor	• Use: open-angle glaucoma • Brimonidine may be used in addition to a beta-blocker or as initial therapy when beta-blockers are contraindicated.
Carbonic anhydrase inhibitor Dorzolamide Brinzolamide	• Decreases production of aqueous humor • Diuretic effects • May reduce IOP	• Use: open-angle glaucoma. • Dorzolamide is useful in patients resistant to beta-blockers, as adjunctive therapy, or when beta-blockers are contraindicated.
3rd-Line Drugs: Alpha-2 adrenergic agonist Apraclonidine	Decreases the production of aqueous humor	Uses: control/prevent postsurgical increases in IOP (e.g., after laser surgery), and postpone the need for surgery in patients receiving maximal medical therapy.
Miotics (direct-acting cholinergic drugs) Pilocarpine HCl (Pilocar)	• Constricts the pupil by contracting sphincter muscles to produce miosis • Decreases the production of and increases outflow of aqueous humor	• Used in open-angle glaucoma, angle closure glaucoma including during or after iridectomy, secondary glaucoma. • Also used to produce miosis, thus reversing the effects of cycloplegic and mydriatic drugs. • Contraindicated in glaucoma associated with acute inflammatory processes.

Indirect-acting cholinergic drugs:
Short acting
Physostigmine salicylate (Isopto Eserine)
• Physostigmine sulfate (Eserine sulfate)

• Produces miosis, increased accommodation, and a decrease in IOP with decreased resistance to outflow of aqueous humor.
• Opens intratrabecular spaces by ciliary muscles contraction and facilitates aqueous humor outflow

• Due to its side effects (i.e., induced myopia in younger patients and pupillary constriction that compromises vision in persons with cataracts), pilocarpine is most often used as adjuvant therapy.
• Pilocarpine is not effective until the IOP is lowered below 50 mm Hg.
• Use: for open-angle glaucoma
• The drug is a reversible acetylcholinesterase inhibitor. (Increases concentration of acetylcholine at nerve endings, which can antagonize anticholinergic drugs.)
• Assess for side effects.
• Warn the patient about blurred vision; conjunctivitis may occur with chronic use.
• Persons who experience side effects may have poor compliance.
• Antidote for overdose: administer atropine.

Indirect-acting cholinergic drugs:
• Long-acting drugs:
Demecarium bromide
Isoflurophate
Echothiophate iodide

• Opens intertrabecular spaces by ciliary muscle contraction and facilitates aqueous humor outflow
• Allows prolonged action of acetylcholine to contract the sphincter muscle, causing miosis

• Used for resistant/chronic open-angle glaucoma, when shorter acting agents have been unsuccessful
• Used in angle-closure glaucoma after iridectomy
• Contraindicated in narrow-angle glaucoma
• Potent acetylcholinesterase inhibitor
• Redness around the cornea may be a side effect. Epinephrine or phenylephrine HCl (10%) may also be ordered to minimize this reaction.

Oral carbonic anhydrase inhibitors
Acetazolamide (Diamox)

• Decreases production of aqueous humor
• Diuretic effects
• May reduce IOP

• Use: open-angle glaucoma
• Oral carbonic anhydrase inhibitors are used if topical therapy is inadequate but are used less frequently with the availability of dorzolamide.

Adrenergic agonists, alpha and beta
Epinephrine (Epifrin, Glaucon)

• Alpha receptor stimulation increases outflow of aqueous humor.
• Beta receptor stimulation decreases the production of aqueous humor.

• Use: open-angle glaucoma and ocular surgery (mydriatic and antihemorrhagic effects).
• Contraindications: predisposition to closed-angle glaucoma or severe cardiovascular disease.
• Warn person of possible ocular side effects: discomfort, burning, stinging, tearing, pain, redness, eye ache, headache, mydriasis, macular edema.

Drugs for Acute Attacks:
Hyper-osmotic agents
Isosorbide (oral) (Ismotic)
• Mannitol

• Reduces water volume from intraocular structures (i.e., vitreous humor) to circulation via plasma osmolarity
• Decreases IOP
• Osmotic diuresis

• Keep an emesis basin nearby.
• Monitor input and output.
• Monitor vital signs closely throughout the administration of mannitol.

821

Complete Iridectomy   Peripheral Iridectomy

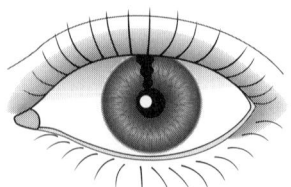 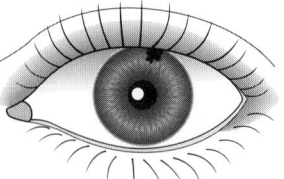

Figure 24-3-1. The appearance of the eye after an iridectomy.

including noncompliance with medical treatment, lack of follow-up care, and ineffectiveness of medical or surgical treatment.

Monitoring

Tonometric and ophthalmoscopic examinations should be performed every 3 to 5 years in all persons over age 40. Eye examinations are indicated every 1 to 2 years in persons at high risk for glaucoma, including African Americans older than 40 years of age, all persons older than age 60, persons with diabetes, and those with a family history of glaucoma. Persons who are experiencing signs and symptoms of chronic or acute glaucoma should see an ophthalmologist. Slit lamp examination may be used to screen for a predisposition to AACG.

Assess for complications of glaucoma, including vision changes, halos around lights, and eye pain. Teach the patient to report any of the following: changes in vision, halos around lights, eye pain, or medication side effects that affect how the person feels or limit his or her ability to perform normal activities.

Teach the patient guidelines for living with glaucoma:

- Take your medicine exactly as your doctor has ordered. These medicines are needed to prevent changes in vision that could lead to blindness.
- Wear a Medic-Alert bracelet or carry identification that states that you have glaucoma.
- Inform your eye doctor about other medicines that you are taking, because many drugs may be ordered for purposes other than eye disorders and they may cause or aggravate glaucoma.
- Inform any new doctor about your diagnosis of glaucoma.
- Contact community resources to learn more about glaucoma, so that you can deal with this disease in the best way that you can.

Prevention

Reinforce teaching to the patient and his or her significant others regarding the following:

- Keep a reserve bottle of eyedrops at home, and always carry eyedrops when away from home.
- Avoid activities that may increase IOP, for example, carrying heavy objects, weight-lifting, shoveling, moving furniture, mopping floors, opening stuck windows or jar lids, karate, water skiing, prolonged bending, Valsalva's

maneuver, and so forth. If in doubt, the patient should discuss the activity with the doctor and obtain approval before performing a particular activity.

Community Resource	Address	Phone Numbers/ Web Sites
American Academy of Ophthalmology	655 Beach Street P.O. Box 7424 San Francisco, CA 94120-7424	(415) 561-8500 Glaucoma 2001 Information and Referral Line (toll-free): (800) 391-EYES http://www.eyenet.org
American Health Assistance Foundation (AHAF)	15825 Shady Grove Road, Suite 140 Rockdale, MD 20850	(800) 437-2423 (301) 948-3244 sbarnard@ahaf.org
American Optometric Association	243 N. Lindbergh Blvd. St. Louis, MO 63141-7881	(888) 396-EYES (toll-free) (314) 991-4100 AmOptNEWS@aol.com
The Glaucoma Foundation	33 Maiden Lane, 7th Floor New York, NY 10038	1-800-GLAUCOMA (Toll-free) (212) 504-1900
Glaucoma Research Foundation	490 Post Street, Suite 830 San Francisco, CA 94102	(800) 826-6693 (toll-free) (415) 986-3162 info@glaucoma.org http://www.glaucoma.org
National Eye Institute, National Institutes of Health	2020 Vision Place Bethesda, MD 20892-3655	(301) 496-5248 2020@b31.nei.nih.gov http://www.nei.nih.gov
Prevent Blindness America	500 East Remington Road Schaumburg, IL 60173	(800) 331-2020 (toll-free) (847) 843-2020 http://www.prevent-blindness.org

 PROGNOSIS

The prognosis for persons with treated glaucoma is excellent. In most cases, glaucoma can be successfully controlled with early detection and proper monitoring and treatment. Persons with untreated chronic glaucoma that begins at age 40 to 45 will probably become blind by age 60 to 65. Vision loss from glaucoma cannot be restored.

AACG that is treated within a few hours of an acute attack can be effectively cured. Untreated AACG will result in severe and permanent visual loss within 2 to 5 days after the onset of symptoms.

CLINICAL PEARLS

○ Teach the patient to place only one drop at a time into each eye. If the patient needs to apply two or more different drops, instruct him or her to wait at least 5 minutes between eyedrops. This allows time for the eyes to absorb the medication adequately, for tearing to decrease, and to prevent the second drops from washing out the first drops.

○ Iridectomy leaves a "keyhole" appearance (see Fig. 24-3-1).

○ Legal blindness is defined as vision in the better eye less than 20/200 with corrective lenses. However, a limited amount of vision may remain.

○ A person with 20/200 vision can see at 20 feet what a person with normal vision can see from 200 feet.

○ A legally blind person can receive magnifying glasses, books on tape, assistance with walking, assistance with organization, and other resources.

NURSING PROBLEM/ DIAGNOSIS	NURSING INTERVENTIONS CLASSIFICATION (NIC)
Decreased visual perception	Communication enhancement: visual deficit
	Environmental management
	Surveillance: safety
Risk for blindness	Medication administration: topical
	Teaching: disease process
	Teaching: prescribed medication

Meniere's Disease

Section 4　　　　　　　　　　　　　　　　　　　　　　　　Linda Krebs

OVERVIEW

Meniere's disease is a disorder of inner ear function characterized by loss of hearing, tinnitus, and vertigo. The disorder typically follows a course of multiple acute attacks and prolonged remissions. A typical attack includes a feeling of fullness in the ear, decreased hearing, and tinnitus, followed by nausea and vomiting, rotational vertigo, postural imbalance, and nystagmus. Attacks may last from 20 to 30 minutes to more than 24 hours. A sense of imbalance may last from 1 day to 2 weeks following the attack, whereas hearing rapidly returns to normal. Over time and with repeated attacks, hearing diminishes and eventually is destroyed. Spontaneous remission has been noted and may occur up to 10 years after the disease was diagnosed.

Incidence of Meniere's disease is higher in caucasians than in other races, with a high incidence in the United Kingdom. Incidence in the United States is approximately 46 new cases per 100,000 population each year. It occurs equally in men and women and most commonly between age 20 and 60, with most cases occurring in the fifth decade.

It generally begins as unilateral disease, but over time bilateral involvement occurs in more than 40% of all affected individuals. Because 15% of all affected persons have a relative with the disease, a genetic component is assumed. Contributing factors include serious otitis media, head trauma, exposure to loud noise, stress, allergies, and a high salt intake.

 PATHOPHYSIOLOGY

The vestibular system of the inner ear is designed to maintain body and head stability and prevent falls. It is responsible for sensing and perceiving motion and position. It has three main components: the peripheral sensory apparatus, a central processor, and a mechanism for motor output. The peripheral sensory apparatus consists of structures in the inner ear and includes the bony and membranous labyrinths and hair cells. The bony labyrinth is filled with perilymphatic fluid, whereas the membranous labyrinth is filled with endolymphatic fluid. Impaired resorption of endolymphatic fluid in the endolymphatic sac results in hydrops. Periodic ruptures of the membranes between the cerebrospinal fluid-like perilymph and the intracellular-like endolymph produce episodes of vertigo.

Although the exact cause of Meniere's disease is unknown, various etiologic factors have been suggested:

- Anatomic. Abnormalities of the temporal bone are common.
- Genetic. Autosomal dominant genetic familial predisposition is seen in 7% to 15% of affected persons.
- Immunologic. Immune complex deposition has been noted in those with Meniere's disease.
- Metabolic. Endolymph is potassium rich; rupture of membranes or distention of the endolymphatic sac allows potassium in the endolymph to affect inner ear structures, resulting in vertigo and deafness.
- Psychological. Increased incidence of psychological disorders is associated with Meniere's disease.
- Viral. Controversy exists with conflicting reports of a viral etiology.
- Vascular. There is a correlation between Meniere's disease and migraine headache, with one in three persons diagnosed with Meniere's disease having a history of migraine headaches.

 SIGNS AND SYMPTOMS

Meniere's disease is a disease of exclusion, characterized by a triad of symptoms: tinnitus, vertigo, and fluctuating hearing loss. All three symptoms must be present for the diagnosis to be made. Differential diagnosis includes benign recurrent vertigo, vestibular paroxysms, viral and bacterial vestibular infections, acoustic neuroma, multiple sclerosis, vascular insufficiency, and syphilitic labyrinthitis, among others.

Spontaneous nystagmus always precedes an attack, with eye movements beating away from the affected ear. Episodes are acute with sudden onset and include pallor, diaphoresis, dizziness, nausea, vomiting, roaring tinnitus, vertigo, and hearing loss.

Meniere's disease is generally considered to consist of three stages:

- Stage I. The main symptom is vertigo, associated with nausea and vomiting, pallor, and sweating. This stage is associated with a sense of pressure or fullness in the ear or side of the head. The attack usually lasts between

20 minutes and 3 to 4 hours. Hearing fluctuates but returns to baseline during remission. Remissions often are prolonged with negative physical findings.

- Stage II. This stage is associated with increased hearing loss, particularly at the lower frequencies. The vertigo becomes more pronounced, but as deafness increases, vertigo diminishes as hair cells in inner ear are destroyed. Remissions are of progressively shorter duration.
- Stage III. Hearing loss becomes progressively worse and begins to involve both ears. Episodes of vertigo cease; however, imbalance, particularly in the dark, continues.

Lermoyez's syndrome is a variant of Meniere's disease in which hearing loss and tinnitus precede the first episode of vertigo by months to years. In many cases, both improve as vertigo increases in severity.

Tumarkin's ortholitic crisis (vestibular drop attacks) occur from a standing or sitting position. Without warning, the patient feels as if he or she were being shoved or pushed to ground or as if the earth were suddenly moving or tilting, resulting in a fall to the ground. These episodes may occur at any time following the diagnosis of Meniere's disease, often occur in a flurry of attacks, and are associated with spontaneous remissions.

 DIAGNOSTIC CRITERIA

Diagnosis of Meniere's disease is difficult, because it is a diagnosis of exclusion.

- The triad of symptoms—tinnitus, vertigo, and fluctuating hearing loss—must be present.
- An audiogram shows low-frequency sensorineural hearing loss with impaired speech discrimination.
- Electronystagmography (ENG) tests ocular motion and positioning as a method to quantify vestibular function. The ENG shows abnormal functioning on affected side.
- Electrocochleography (EcoG) determines whether there is an increased buildup of fluid in the inner ear.
- MRI and CT scans are used to rule out benign or neoplastic tumors or other abnormalities.
- A tuning fork is applied to bony prominence of the toe or ankle to assess proprioception.
- Blood pressure is measured with the patient lying and standing to rule out orthostatic hypotension.
- Serum chemistries may be obtained to help rule out other abnormalities.

 INTERVENTIONS

Management of Acute Attacks

Pharmacologic Management

Drug therapy for Meniere's disease is aimed at managing symptoms and may include:

- Droperidol for severe nausea and vomiting
- Promethazine for mild to moderate nausea and vomiting
- Meclizine for mild dizziness

- Diazepam to decrease anxiety
- A mild diuretic to decrease endolymphatic pressure
- A potassium supplement to combat hypokalemia resulting from diuretic use

Physical Management
- Provide a calm environment.
- Maintain the patient on bed rest.
- Instruct the patient to keep the eyes closed.
- Protect the patient from falls.

Surgical Management
Some 5% to 10% of patients with Meniere's disease undergo surgery; surgical management remains controversial, however.
- For patients with normal hearing, surgery may include decompression of the endolymphatic sac or intracranial transection of the vestibular nerve.
- For patients with unsalvageable hearing, decompression of the cochlea (cochleocentesis) or labyrinthectomy (considered radical, because it ablates vestibular function) may be indicated.
- Surgical intervention is almost never indicated for those with bilateral disease.

Other
- Focused ultrasound is an external approach to partially ablating vestibular function without invasive surgery.
- Lasers or endoscopy may be used to decrease endolymph accumulation.

Education
The patient should be taught to:
- Avoid driving, climbing ladders, and working in or around hazardous equipment.
- Obtain assistance when walking.
- Minimize reading, and avoid looking at glaring lights.
- Decrease food intake to minimize nausea and vomiting.

Management of Remission/Maintenance Treatment

This aspect of treatment is aimed at decreasing the frequency of attacks and maintaining hearing without increasing tinnitus. Measures include maintaining a low-salt diet and administering a mild diuretic, such as a combination of hydrochlorothiazide and triamterene or furosemide. Other drugs may include:
- Vasodilators to prevent hydrops
- Betahistine to prevent vertigo
- Propranolol to minimize migraine headache in patients with a history of these
- Fentanyl or droperidol to minimize drop attacks

Long-Term Management

Diet
Controversy exists about the benefits of dietary modifications. Nonetheless, the following general guidelines hold:
- Decrease water intake.
- Decrease salt intake.
- Eliminate alcohol, nicotine, and caffeine-containing products.

Pharmacologic Management
- Instillation of an ototoxic drug, such as gentamycin or streptomycin, via a plastic tube into the inner ear eliminates vertigo but, with repeated doses, may cause total hearing loss.
- Dexamethasone may be instilled to decrease inflammation and stabilize balance and hearing.

Surgical Management
- An endolymphatic sac shunt may be implanted to decrease hydrops.
- Vestibular nerve section may be performed in patients who have nonresponsive vertigo and no salvageable hearing; this surgery eliminates vertigo.

Other
- Vestibular exercises are of no known benefit unless vestibular function has been ablated.

 COMMUNITY CARE

Assessment
- Assess for spontaneous nystagmus.
- Assess for sudden attacks of whirling or rotary vertigo.
- Assess for sensation of fullness or pressure in ear.
- Assess for the triad of hearing loss, vertigo, and tinnitus.

Monitoring
- Assess hearing loss for progression, which may be a sign of an acoustic neuroma that mimics Meniere's disease.
- Evaluate long-term sequelae of Meniere's disease, including chronic tinnitus, deafness, injuries as a result of vertigo, and impaired ability to function at work or at home.

Prevention
- Encourage a patient who smokes to stop.
- Decrease salt intake to less than 1 g/day.
- Protect the ears from loud noise.
- Minimize the use of ototoxic drugs.

 PROGNOSIS

Meniere's disease is characterized by a pattern of recurrent acute attacks and remissions. Resolution of symptoms without recurrence has been reported, usually within 10 years of diagnosis. Approximately 75% of affected patients respond to medical treatment, whereas the remaining 25% require surgery to minimize effects of vertigo. In most patients, the disease progresses over 10 to 20 years to a total deterioration of hearing and cessation of vertigo.

 CLINICAL PEARLS

- Meniere's disease involves the triad of tinnitus, vertigo, and fluctuating hearing loss.
- Primary management is aimed at minimizing symptoms rather than curing the disease.

- Spontaneous remission may occur even after the disease has been present for many years.
- Protecting the patient from falls is an essential aspect of management.

NURSING PROBLEM/ DIAGNOSIS	NURSING INTERVENTIONS CLASSIFICATION (NIC)
Risk for falls	Environmental enhancement: safety Fall prevention Teaching: disease process Positioning
Progressive hearing loss	Communication enhancement: hearing deficit

chapter 25

Urinary

Neurogenic Bladder

Section 1   Mikel Gray

OVERVIEW

A neurogenic bladder occurs whenever a neurologic lesion affects the function of the lower urinary tract structures (i.e., bladder, urethra, and pelvic floor muscles). Various voiding dysfunctions can result.

Although the epidemiology of neurogenic bladder is not known, its prevalence can be appreciated by considering the epidemiology of the various neurologic diseases associated with neurogenic bladder dysfunction. For example, cerebrovascular accidents occur in approximately 83 per 100,000 Americans, and 51% to 70% experience subsequent neurogenic bladder dysfunction and incontinence. Parkinson's disease affects approximately 20 per 100,000 Americans, and approximately 71% experience neurogenic bladder dysfunction. Multiple sclerosis affects approximately 10 per 100,000 Americans between the ages of 20 and 50. Most experience neurogenic bladder dysfunction during their illness. Spinal lesions including traumatic injuries (3 per 100,000) and spina bifida (1 per 1000 live births) are associated with neurogenic bladder dysfunction in approximately 90% of cases, and 80% of patients with disk disease affecting the lumbar spine have evidence of abnormal bladder function on urodynamic assessment. In addition to these disorders of the central nervous system, various other disorders may lead to neurogenic bladder dysfunction through their effects on the peripheral nerves. For example, diabetes mellitus affects 1% to 2% of the population and is known to cause both peripheral and autonomic polyneuropathies, and 27% to 85% of diabetic patients experience bladder dysfunction as one component of this significant disorder.

PATHOPHYSIOLOGY

Neurogenic bladder requires the nurse to understand the progressive effects of: (1) obstruction, (2) hostile neurogenic bladder dysfunction, and (3) the natural history of the underlying neurologic disorder.

Obstruction

Obstruction can be defined as an anatomic lesion or functional disorder of the lower urinary tract that increases urethral resistance to urinary outflow. Although it seems desirable to define obstruction as a dichotomous variable in the clinical setting (i.e., obstruction versus no obstruction), this condition is more accurately classified as occurring along a continuum ranging from normal urethral resistance to severe obstruction causing complete retention of urine. Based on this understanding, the goal of clinical evaluation of obstruction in the patient with neurogenic bladder shifts from merely identifying its presence to understanding its magnitude and the associated risks of additional bladder dysfunction or upper urinary tract distress.

Prolonged obstruction causes various long-term negative effects on lower urinary tract function, including decompensation of the detrusor muscle; deposition of collagen in the bladder wall, causing trabeculation and an increased risk of low bladder wall compliance; and further neurogenic changes in the spinal reflexes affecting bladder function. It is also associated with a risk of upper urinary tract distress, particularly when associated with low bladder wall compliance.

Hostile Neurogenic Bladder Function

The history of neurogenic bladder management in patients with spinal cord injuries illustrates the importance of determining the potential for a neurogenic bladder to create upper urinary tract distress. Historically, most patients who experienced spinal cord injuries died of urinary system complications related to neurogenic bladder dysfunction. However, with the advent of indwelling and intermittent catheterization, early mortality associated with neurogenic bladder dysfunction has declined sharply, owing in large part to increasing awareness that maintenance of low intravesicular pressures during bladder filling and the relief of clinically relevant obstruction are critical to long-term preservation of renal function and general health.

Two aspects of neurogenic bladder dysfunction are associated with a risk of upper urinary tract distress: low bladder wall compliance and obstruction. Compliance can be defined as the distensibility of the bladder wall in response to urine filling and storage. Two aspects of bladder function—detrusor muscle tone and the passive distensibility of the bladder wall—determine its compliance. Normally, bladder wall compliance is high, indicating low bladder filling pressure despite filling with 300 to 600 mL of urine. However, in the case of a patient with a neurogenic bladder, low bladder wall compliance causes high bladder filling pressure, which compromises kidney function and increases the risk of upper urinary tract distress.

 SIGNS AND SYMPTOMS

Lower Urinary Tract

- Detrusor hyperreflexia: diurnal frequency (urination more than every 2 hours while awake), nocturia (awakening three or more times to urinate), enuresis, urge or reflex urinary incontinence
- Detrusor areflexia: diurnal frequency, nocturia, inability to urinate (urinary retention) or dribbling, overflow urinary incontinence
- Sphincter incompetence: urine loss with physical exertion, coughing, laughing, transfers in and out of wheelchair (stress incontinence)
- Detrusor sphincter dyssynergia: interrupted or stuttering urinary stream, often associated with diminished or absent sensations of bladder filling

Upper Urinary Tract

Symptoms of upper urinary tract distress include febrile urinary tract infection (UTI) or a new onset of UTI without fever.

 DIAGNOSTIC CRITERIA

The diagnostic evaluation of a neurogenic bladder typically includes urinalysis, urine culture and sensitivities when indicated, serum creatinine and blood urea nitrogen (BUN), and in selected cases urodynamics and an imaging study of the upper urinary tract. Urinalysis identifies evidence of clinically relevant UTI. For many patients with neurogenic bladder, particularly those managed by indwelling or intermittent catheterization, asymptomatic bacteriuria does not indicate a clinically significant infection and does not justify a course of antibiotics, because treatment has been shown to provide no substantial benefit to the patient and actually may cause long-term harm by promoting colonization with antibiotic resistant pathogens. However, when a patient has a symptomatic infection (associated with urinary incontinence, fever, hematuria, autonomic dysreflexia, or an exacerbation of spasticity that interferes with activities of daily living), a urine culture is completed and sensitivity-guided antibiotic therapy is used to eradicate the infection.

Urodynamic testing accomplishes the following goals: it characterizes the causes of urinary incontinence and retention, and it can be used to predict hostile neurogenic bladder function before the onset of upper urinary tract distress.

Upper urinary tract imaging is used to determine the presence and extent of upper urinary tract distress and renal calculi and to assess renal function. An ultrasound is usually preferred when establishing a baseline of renal anatomy or when following patients with serial images over time. Intravenous pyelography (IVP) or computed tomography (CT) may be used when more detailed anatomic images are needed. The use of intravenous contrast also allows evaluation of renal function. When a detailed analysis of renal function is indicated, a radionuclide study is preferred.

INTERVENTIONS

Treatment decisions regarding the neurogenic bladder are influenced by the characteristics of the voiding dysfunction, the risk of upper urinary tract distress, functional or cognitive impairments associated with the underlying disorder, and the patient's preferences. From the nursing perspective, treatment of a neurogenic bladder focuses on establishing a bladder management program that is acceptable to the patient, prevents upper urinary tract distress, and corrects or contains urinary incontinence or retention. The management options of neurogenic bladders are associated with the following nursing diagnoses: urge incontinence, reflex urinary incontinence related to detrusor hyperreflexia, urinary retention related to detrusor sphincter dyssynergia, urinary retention related to detrusor areflexia, and stress incontinence related to sphincter incompetence.

Spinal Cord Injury

During the initial period of spinal shock, the neurogenic bladder is typically managed by an indwelling catheter or intermittent catheterization. An indwelling catheter is usually selected because high volume urinary output typically occurs during the immediate postinjury phase, particularly when the patient requires a ventilator. While prolonged indwelling catheterization is reserved as a last resort for long-term management of neurogenic bladder in the patient with a neurogenic bladder, it has proved effective and safe when limited to the immediate postinjury phase.

As spinal shock subsides and urine output normalizes, the rehabilitation team consults with the patient and family concerning long-term bladder management. Table 25-1-1 provides an overview of the various bladder management programs used for patients with spinal cord injuries, as well as the associated risk of incontinence and upper urinary tract distress, and nursing implications.

Whenever possible, spinal injured patients prefer to spontaneously urinate. Most patients who can be managed by spontaneous urination after a spinal cord injury have detrusor hyperreflexia and striated sphincter dyssynergia but they also have preserved sensations and minimal motor deficits. The nursing management of these patients focuses on prevention of incontinence and urinary tract infection. Patients are taught to void on a routine schedule; usually every 2 hours while awake. They are advised to continue to drink adequate fluids (approximately 1/2 oz/lb (30 ml/kg) in the active adult) and to avoid bladder irritants, such as caffeine or alcohol, which increase sensory urgency and reduce functional bladder capacity. Because of the presence of detrusor hyperreflexia, they are educated that they will have a limited time between the perception of urgency and the onset of voiding. Therefore, they are advised to rapidly heed the urge to urinate.

Many patients require an antispasmodic agent, such as tolterodine or long-acting oxybutynin. They are taught the dosage of the medication (long-acting antispasmodics are administered once daily) and side effects including dry mouth and a risk of constipation. Patients are also advised of the relationship between UTI and acute urinary incontinence. Specifically, they are taught that a sudden exacerbation of urgency and urge incontinent episodes is often caused by a UTI compared with a change in bladder function. Therefore, they should consult their physician or nurse practitioner about obtaining a urine specimen for urinalysis and culture before changing their medication regimen or other aspects of their bladder management program.

In contrast, patients with more complete injuries and severe motor deficits usually require a more aggressive bladder management program. Those with injuries above the sacral micturition center typically have detrusor hyperreflexia, striated sphincter dyssynergia but no sensation of bladder filling. They can be managed by intermittent catheterization or a reflex voiding program. Intermittent catheterization is preferred because it is associated with a low risk of upper urinary tract distress and a moderate risk of incontinence.

Instruction in intermittent catheterization should involve the patient and at least one significant other willing to provide care if the patient is unable to perform self-catheterization. Quadriplegics or others with impaired upper extremities are taught to verbally instruct someone to perform a catheterization procedure and multiple significant others are also taught to catheterize the patient every 4 to 6 hours as directed.

The patient and family members are taught to wash the hands, preferably with soap and water, although a cleansing towelette or similar cleansing agent may be used when a sink is not available. The nurse teaches the patients and family to handle the catheter in a clean fashion, then apply water-soluble lubricant to identify the urethral meatus by visualization or palpation and to gently insert the catheter until urine flows. Adult men are typically taught to catheterize using a 14 French straight catheter, and women are typically taught to use a 12–14 French catheter. Children are taught to use an 8–10 French straight catheter, depending on their age and the size of the urethra. The patient

Table 25-1-1. Options for Managing the Patient with Spinal Cord Injury and Neurogenic Bladder

BLADDER MANAGEMENT PROGRAM	RISK OF INCONTINENCE	RISK OF UPPER URINARY TRACT DISTRESS	NURSING IMPLICATIONS
Spontaneous voiding	30%	0%	Limited to patients with preserved sensations of bladder filling, detrusor hyperreflexia, and mild to moderate obstruction from detrusor sphincter dyssynergia.
Intermittent catheterization	55%	8%	Preferred for patients with intact upper extremity dexterity (paraplegics) who are willing to regularly catheterize the bladder. Quadriplegics are good candidates only if they have care providers able to perform procedure throughout the day. Often must be combined with chronic pharmacotherapy for detrusor hyperreflexia.
Reflex voiding with condom catheter	30% achieve "wet continence" (urine consistently contained by a condom catheter)	29%	Condom catheter increases risk of penile skin problems, and urinary tract infection. Often must be combined with chronic pharmacotherapy for dyssynergia or transurethral sphincterotomy or placement of urethral stent.
Indwelling catheter	45% (15 years and older)	75%	Often seen as an attractive alternative to intermittent catheterization, but this convenience must be weighed against increased risk for long-term complications.

and family are taught to gently apply suprapubic pressure to ensure maximal bladder emptying while the catheter is in place and to slowly withdraw the catheter to achieve optimal urine drainage. When the catheter is completely withdrawn, the patient or care provider is taught to pinch the tube to avoid dribbling leakage from the catheter.

Cleansing of the catheter begins with immediate rinsing with cold tap water, whenever feasible. The catheter is then cleansed with soap and water, including the lumen, and reused. The nurse emphasizes that the catheters are stored clean and dry, but they are never stored in a solution.

Alternatively, a microwave cleansing technique may be used. Several catheters are cleansed as described previously and placed while moist in the microwave next to an 8-oz container filled with water, which serves as a heat bath to prevent catheter melting. One minute is allowed for each catheter. This alternative method may be preferred, because it provides superior killing of bacteria compared with cleansing with soap and water only.

Unfortunately, an intermittent catheterization program is not realistic for many because of impaired upper extremity dexterity or a lack of availability of a care provider to perform the procedure. Men who are unable to catheterize may be managed by reflex voiding. Urine is contained by a condom catheter and the nurse teaches the patient to fit a condom in a manner that prevents urine loss but does not impede local blood flow. He is also taught to change the condom, and perform routine checks for penile skin integrity. This program may be more realistic for quadriplegic men, because the condom requires changing on a daily or every-other-day basis. Because most men managed with reflex voiding and condom catheter containment have detrusor sphincter dyssynergia, it is often necessary to reduce obstruction by pharmacologic means (using an alpha-adrenergic blocking agent) or through surgical methods (through either transurethral sphincterotomy or insertion of a urethral stent).

Although reflex voiding is a realistic alternative for men, it is not feasible for women because of the lack of adequate condom devices (despite multiple attempts to develop such a product). Therefore, women who are unable to manage their bladder by intermittent catheterization may require an indwelling catheter. This strategy may also be used for men who are not adequately managed by reflex voiding or intermittent catheterization. Nevertheless, placement of an indwelling catheter should be reserved as a final alternative, because it is associated with both a significant risk of upper urinary tract distress, urinary incontinence, and bladder cancer when worn for 5 to 10 years or longer.

Nursing management of a patient with an indwelling catheter focuses on adequate containment of urine and prevention or prompt management of complications. Whereas the decision to place a catheter is made by the entire rehabilitation team, many aspects of catheter care are managed by the nurse. The size and material of the catheter are important considerations. For men, a 14 to 16 French catheter should provide adequate drainage and a 12 to 14 French catheter is adequate for most women. When managing a patient with a long-term catheter, a silicone or lubricious coated catheter is selected. A leg bag that holds at least 500 mL is used during waking hours, and a bedside bag that holds at least 2000 mL is used during sleep. Elastic leg straps may be used, but latex straps are avoided. Alternatively, the bag may be secured to the thigh using a cloth pocket manufactured to hold a urine drainage bag. The patient and family are taught to empty the leg bag and bedside bag regularly and to reduce bacterial overgrowth and disagreeable odors by routine cleansing with a vinegar solution.

Patients are taught that bacteriuria is inevitable with a long-term indwelling catheter, but only symptomatic urinary tract infections should be treated with antibiotic medications. Symptomatic infections cause hematuria, detrusor hyperreflexia and catheter bypassing (leakage around the catheter), autonomic dysreflexia, a fever, or a marked worsening of skeletal muscle spasticity. Although no intervention will prevent bacteriuria, patients are advised to ensure adequate fluid intake, to routinely cleanse the urethral meatus, and to use clean technique when changing from a leg bag to a bedside bag or when emptying either bag.

Multiple Sclerosis

Multiple sclerosis is characterized by multiple lesions affecting the central nervous system. It is a chronic disease with symptom flares (exacerbations) and remissions. Therefore, the characteristics of the associated neurogenic bladder also change frequently, and conservative management of the neurogenic bladder is preferred.

In patients who have preserved mobility (i.e., who are able to walk independently or who need minimal assistance), urge incontinence caused by detrusor hyperreflexia and minimal or no dyssynergia can be managed by scheduled voiding, regulation of fluid intake, and avoidance of bladder irritants, including caffeine and alcohol. In addition, many require antispasmodic medications, and the nurse should teach medication dosage, administration, and side effects.

Intermittent catheterization is often used for the patient with detrusor hyperreflexia, detrusor sphincter dyssynergia, and greater physical impairment. This is usually combined with an antispasmodic medication. In more severe cases, particularly when multiple sclerosis has advanced and the patient's upper extremity strength and dexterity are severely limited, an indwelling catheterization may be warranted.

Nursing care of patients with multiple sclerosis who require an indwelling or intermittent catheterization is described in the spinal cord injury section (see Chapter 19, Section 9). In addition to the teaching described earlier, patients are educated about the relationship between a UTI and an exacerbation of multiple sclerosis and the need to seek immediate treatment when signs of a clinically relevant infection occur.

Parkinsonism

Most patients (approximately 90%) with Parkinson's disease and a neurogenic bladder have detrusor hyperreflexia, preserved sensations, and a coordinated sphincter response to micturition. Nevertheless, their neurogenic bladder dysfunction is often complicated by prostate outlet obstruction in men or stress urinary incontinence in women. In addition, Parkinson's disease may be confused with Shy-Drager syndrome (i.e., multisystem atrophy), which is associated with pelvic floor muscle weakness, compared with the hypertonicity that is often seen in parkinsonism.

Initial management includes scheduled voiding, regulation of fluid intake, and avoidance of bladder irritants as described previously. The nurse also teaches the family and patient strategies to maximize rapid access to the toilet.

For example, the patient may require a bedside toilet or hand-held urinal if nocturia is a problem. Hand-held urinals are often used for men; the nurse should consult with medical supply companies or a wound, ostomy, and continence nurse specialist about urinal devices for women. For some patients with parkinsonism and a neurogenic bladder, an antispasmodic medication, such as tolterodine or long-acting oxybutynin, may be added. In addition to the education described previously, the nurse should teach the family to remain alert for side effects (particularly in an elderly patient), including short-term memory loss, confusion, nightmares, and hallucinations.

A few patients with Parkinson's disease (~10%) experience urinary retention owing to detrusor areflexia. Although intermittent catheterization is preferred for these patients, an indwelling catheter is often required when severe physical limitations or an enlarged prostate render catheterization excessively difficult.

Cerebrovascular Accident

Detrusor areflexia is common during the acute phase immediately after a stroke that is managed by a short-term indwelling catheter. This brief phase is followed by detrusor hyperreflexia with preserved sensations and a coordinated sphincter response to micturition. Fortunately, bladder function spontaneously improves during the first 3 to 12 months after a stroke, and conservative management of urge urinary incontinence is indicated.

Nursing management focuses on scheduled toileting, fluid regulation, and avoidance of bladder irritants. A relatively frequent voiding schedule of every 1 to 1.5 hours may be necessary during the initial recovery period. These patients also may be taught urge suppression techniques. Urge suppression requires the patient to identify and contract the pelvic floor muscles. Mastering this skill usually requires biofeedback, particularly for the patient with neuromuscular impairment after a stroke and referral to a continence nurse specialist is indicated. In addition, antispasmodic medications are often prescribed.

Although most patients experience improvement in voiding function while they recover from a stroke, others have persistent voiding problems. Persistent voiding difficulties may arise from urinary retention related to prostatic outlet obstruction, compromised detrusor contraction strength caused by prolonged diabetes mellitus, premorbid urinary incontinence, advanced age, and institutionalization at the time of the stroke. These patients are typically managed by referral to a urologist for complex urodynamic testing.

Diabetes Mellitus

Despite its prevalence, surprisingly little is known about neurogenic bladder dysfunction associated with diabetes mellitus. Traditionally, diabetes mellitus has been associated with impaired bladder sensations caused by a combination of peripheral polyneuropathy and chronic overdistension from polyuria. As a result, the bladder becomes increasingly overdistended, ultimately impairing detrusor contractility and leading to chronic urinary retention and an increased risk for episodes of acute urinary retention. To interrupt this sequence of events leading to urinary retention, the nurse teaches the patient to void on a timed schedule of every 3 to 4 hours while awake, regardless of the desire to urinate.

Although most patients with diabetes mellitus experience impaired sensations and a large bladder capacity, some develop urge incontinence. They are managed by scheduled urination, urge suppression, fluid regulation, and avoidance of bladder irritants. Pharmacologic agents also may be used for these patients; but they are prescribed with caution when detrusor contraction strength is often impaired and administration of antispasmodics may cause urinary retention.

Spina Bifida

Neurogenic bladder dysfunction in the patient with spina bifida varies according to the level and extent of the spinal lesion. In addition to this variability, bladder dysfunction changes as the child grows. In neonates, detrusor hyperreflexia with or without detrusor sphincter dyssynergia is common. However, as the child ages and the spinal column grows, there is an increasing risk of spinal cord tethering, which affects bladder as well as musculoskeletal function. In older children, detrusor areflexia with a fixed, denervated sphincter is common. Low bladder wall compliance is also more common, greatly increasing the risk for upper urinary tract distress.

Urine leakage is expected during infancy. The nurse explains the need for intermittent catheterization in order to prevent kidney problems as the infant grows rather than to prevent urinary leakage. A 5 to 6 French catheter may be selected for catheterization, and a schedule of 4 hours is often prescribed. The parents are taught to visualize the meatus and insert the catheter using a clean technique. Mastery of this technique may be particularly challenging in the infant girl, and multiple return demonstrations are recommended. Care and cleansing of catheters are similar to those reviewed in the spinal cord injury section.

As the child ages, clean intermittent catheterization remains the cornerstone of bladder management. In addition to catheterization, antispasmodic medications are frequently prescribed. The nurse teaches the parents the proper dosage, administration, and side effects. In addition to dry mouth, children may experience behavior changes or flushing and heat intolerance as a result of antispasmodic medications. Parents are taught to monitor their child for such effects and to contact their physician or nurse practitioner should they occur.

Surgical Management

When conservative management fails to adequately control continence or prevent upper urinary tract distress and renal damage, surgical reconstruction of the lower urinary tract or urinary diversion may be required.

 COMMUNITY CARE

Assessment

Assess the patient for compliance with the bladder management program, frequency of catheterization, intake of antispasmodic or other medications used to alter lower urinary tract function, and self-monitoring for signs and symptoms of urinary tract infection.

Assess for upper urinary tract distress when the patient reports a history of a febrile urinary tract infection, a new onset of recurrent urinary tract infections, increasing residual urine volumes, or changes on upper urinary tract imaging studies.

Assess for signs and symptoms of a current UTI (e.g., fever), hematuria, new onset or acute exacerbation of urinary incontinence, exacerbation of autonomic dysreflexia, or skeletal muscle spasticity. Signs of a current infection include nitrites and leukocytes on dipstick urinalysis or pyuria and bacteriuria on microscopic examination.

Monitoring

Neurogenic bladders with upper urinary tract distress should be monitored on an annual or biannual basis with an ultrasound. All patients with a neurogenic bladder should be screened for a UTI through urinalysis. All patients with a neurogenic bladder should be monitored routinely for continence and referred to a urologist if urinary incontinence is present. Patients managed by spontaneous voiding should be monitored for changes in urinary residual volumes.

Prevention

Teach the patient and family to monitor for symptomatic UTI and reassure them that asymptomatic bacteriuria is expected and should not be treated.

Instruct the patient and family about the relationship between bladder management and kidney health. Advise them to seek care from the urologist if a febrile UTI occurs or if changes in upper urinary tract anatomy are noted on routine imaging studies.

Educate the family of the importance of compliance with bladder management programs including use of medications to lower bladder pressures during filling or micturition, regular intermittent catheterization, and management of an indwelling catheter.

 PROGNOSIS

Without proper management, urinary system–related complications can lead to death for the patient with a neurogenic bladder and upper urinary system distress. Refer to Table 25-1-1 for the relative risk of upper urinary tract distress associated with bladder programs used to manage patients with neurogenic bladder caused by spinal cord injuries.

 CLINICAL PEARLS

- A sudden onset or acute exacerbation of urinary incontinence in the patient managed by clean intermittent catheterization usually indicates urinary tract infection.
- Prevention of upper urinary tract distress in the patient with a spinal cord injury, multiple sclerosis, or spina bifida usually requires annual or biannual ultrasonography of the kidneys.
- A change in bladder behavior or an onset of recurrent urinary tract infections may indicate upper urinary tract distress and requires further evaluation by the patient's physician.
- A finding of detrusor sphincter dyssynergia on urodynamic testing indicates an increased risk for a UTI and upper urinary tract distress.

NURSING PROBLEM/ DIAGNOSIS	NURSING INTERVENTIONS CLASSIFICATION (NIC)
Urinary incontinence	Urinary habit training Urinary retention care Urinary catheterization Urinary incontinence care
Risk for urinary tract infection	Infection protection
Impaired comfort/bladder spasms	Pain management Analgesic administration

Renal Calculi

Section 2   Jan Addy

OVERVIEW

Commonly called kidney stones, renal calculi (or urolithiasis) affect approximately 240,000 to 720,000 Americans annually. Incidence is greater in men than in women by a ratio of 4:1. Renal calculi can affect all age groups, but incidence is highest in the third and fourth decades of life. By the sixth and seventh decades of life, women and men are affected equally.

Geographic factors contribute to the development of stones. High humidity and elevated temperature appear to be contributing factors, and the incidence of symptomatic ureteral stones is greatest during hot summer months.

Factors that have been identified as contributing to the development of stone formation include:

- High-sodium diet
- Low water intake
- High-protein diet
- Excess intake of oxalates and purines in the diet
- Genetic disorders, such as hereditary cystinuria and distal renal tubular acidosis
- Metabolic risk factors, such as hypercalcemia
- Urinary retention
- Immobilization
- Medications

Most patients with kidney stones do not need to seek medical attention primarily owing to passage of a small stone. Of the patients who do seek medical attention, most experience recurrent episodes necessitating acute medical care.

PATHOPHYSIOLOGY

Five types of stones affect the urinary tract: (1) calcium phosphate, (2) calcium oxalate, (3) uric acid, (4) cystine, and (5) struvite (magnesium-ammonium). The exact mechanism of stone formation remains unclear. A primary factor in stone formation is a process called crystallization. Crystallization occurs when the urine is supersaturated with elements such as calcium, phosphate, and oxalate, which precipitate and unite to form stones.

High urine pH also contributes to stone formation. Uric acid and cystine stones are more likely to precipitate in acid urine, whereas, calcium phosphate and struvite stones are more common in alkaline urine. It is known that a mucoprotein, a matrix for the stone, which is formed in the kidney, can initiate stone development.

Each type of stone has its own unique characteristics. *Calcium oxalate stones,* the most common type, are small but can be trapped in the ureter. Factors predisposing to the development of these stones include hypercalcemia, hyperoxaluria, and hereditary factors.

Calcium phosphate stones are typically mixed with oxalate or struvite. Alkaline urine and primary hyperparathyroidism contribute to their development.

Struvite stones result from a UTI with proteus (most common), *Klebsiella, pseudomonas*, and staphylococci. These stones are usually large and form a staghorn type appearance.

Uric acid stones are seen in patients with gout. These occur predominately in men of Jewish heritage. Heredity plays a large role in the development of uric acid stones.

Cystine stones result from a genetic autosomal recessive defect or poor absorption of cysteine in the gastrointestinal tract and kidney. Excessive concentrations of cysteine in the presence of acid urine can cause stone development.

 ## SIGNS AND SYMPTOMS

Urine flow may be obstructed, especially at the ureteropelvic junction. Severe flank pain, called *renal colic*, begins in the region of the affected kidney and radiates over the abdomen and into the groin. As the stone moves down the ureter, excruciating and intermittent pain is caused by a muscular spasm of the ureter. The pressure of the stone on the ureter causes a lack of oxygen supply (anoxia) to this area, resulting in pain. A patient commonly has two or three attacks of acute renal colic before a stone passes. Stones that are too large to pass require surgical intervention.

Nausea and vomiting are often associated with the presence of renal colic. Hematuria may be gross if the stone edges are rough. Hematuria may also be occult.

Frequency, dysuria, and other signs of a UTI can be present, especially when the stone reaches the bladder.

Renal stones can sometimes be "silent," causing no symptoms for years. This is especially true of large stones that develop over a long period. In addition, very small smooth stones can be passed without the patient's knowledge.

 ## DIAGNOSTIC CRITERIA

A flat and upright abdominal radiograph of the kidneys, ureters, and bladder (KUB) may reveal radiopaque stones, especially if they are large. Uric acid stones are not radiopaque.

IVP shows filling defects at the site of the stone. A CT scan shows the presence and location of the stone.

Urograms are helpful in identifying urinary tract obstructions. Renal ultrasonography is used to produce images from the sound waves. Structures that are very dense, like stones, can be seen easily in this type of diagnostic test.

Urinalysis may show the presence of red blood cells (RBCs), white blood cells (WBCs), and bacteria. The presence of RBCs indicates trauma of the lining of the ureter, bladder, or urethra. WBCs and bacteria indicate the presence of urinary stasis. WBC count is elevated in infection. The differential count can detect an increase in the number of immature WBCs. Urine culture and sensitivity will identify any organisms present.

Microscopic examination of the urine may identify crystals. Urine pH will determine whether the urine is acid or alkaline.

Elevated serum phosphate, calcium, or uric acid levels indicate the presence of minerals that can form stones.

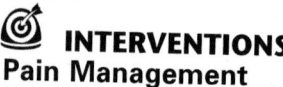# INTERVENTIONS
Pain Management

Management of pain begins with assessing the location, characteristics, and rating scale of the patient's perception of pain. The pain is often described as severe or excruciating not relieved by over-the-counter medications. Morphine or Demerol is usually prescribed. Dosage and route depends on the patient and care provider. It is not uncommon for maximum dosages of these drugs to be used. The nurse must continually assess the patient's pain threshold and tolerance level throughout an acute attack. Reassessment of the patient's pain provides the nurse with valuable information about how well the medication is working for the patient. Pain medications are more effective when they are given at regularly scheduled intervals or through a constant delivery system instead of as needed. Spasmolytic agents, such as oxybutynin chloride (Ditropan) and propantheline bromide (Pro-Banthīne) have been shown to be effective in the relief and control of renal colic. Other methods used to control pain include relaxation, hypnosis, guided imagery, therapeutic touch, and acupuncture.

Hydration

For years it was believed that patients in acute distress from renal stones should have at least 3 L/day of fluid to help flush the stone through the urinary tract. Massive diuresis has been shown to be more harmful than beneficial for the patient. Ureter peristalsis becomes ineffective or even nonexistent as a result of severe spasms owing to increased pressure exerted within the ureter, resulting in anoxia of the ureter. This creates more intense pain and unnecessary discomfort for the patient. However, patients with a history of kidney stones and not experiencing an acute episode should drink at least 2 to 4 L/day of fluid to help prevent stone formation.

Dietary Considerations

Patients with recurrent renal stones should be instructed to adhere to a prescribed diet. Through the reduction and elimination of known causative agents, subsequent attacks can be minimized or prevented.

Calcium Phosphate Stones

- Maintain a low calcium intake (400 mg/day); avoid calcium supplements and milk and dairy products, and limit intake of leafy vegetables and whole grains.

Table 25-2-1. Acid and Alkaline Ash Food Groups

ACID ASH	ALKALINE ASH	NEUTRAL
Meat	Milk	Beverages (e.g., coffee, tea)
Whole grains	Vegetables	
Eggs	Fruits (except cranberries,	
Cheese	prunes, and plums)	
Cranberries		
Prunes		
Plums		

From Williams SR: Essentials of Nutrition and Diet Therapy, 7th ed. St. Louis, CV Mosby, 1999, p 465.

- Maintain a low phosphorus intake (1000 to 1200 mg/day) by limiting dairy products.
- If urinary pH is alkaline, an acid ash diet (Table 25-2-1) is recommended.

Calcium Oxalate Stones. Follow a low-oxalate diet; oxalate food sources, such as beer, cocoa, tea, beets, chocolate, nuts, berries, most vegetables, tofu, and soy products.

Uric Acid Stones
- Maintain a low-purine diet by avoiding meat and meat sources, whole grains, and legumes.
- Follow an alkaline ash diet (see Table 25-2-1).

Cystine Stones
- Increase vegetables in the diet, maintain a high fluid intake, and follow an alkaline ash diet.
- Limit methionine (an essential amino acid).

Struvite Stones
- Follow an acid ash diet (see Table 25-2-1).
- Limit phosphorous intake (1000 to 1200 mg/day).

Infection Prevention

The patient should be assessed for signs and symptoms of urinary tract infection, including frequency, urgency, dysuria, chills, and fever (temperature above 101°F [38.8°C]). Infection can occur from stasis of urine in the urinary system, stone perforation through the urinary tract mucosa, or invasive procedures, tubes, or surgery.

Intake and Output Monitoring

The urine should be strained in all patients suspected of an acute kidney stone episode. A specialized strainer cup is used for this purpose. Any suspicious-looking material should be sent to the laboratory for analysis. Intake and output should be approximately equal unless bladder irrigations are ordered.

Pharmacologic Therapy

Despite concerted effort to adhere to dietary regimens, many patients are unable to eliminate stone reformation necessitating pharmacologic interventions. Medications commonly prescribed for the different types of renal stones follow.

Calcium Stones
- Furosemide (Lasix) inhibits sodium and chloride reabsorption in the loop, thus causing calcium elimination through the urine. Monitor potassium levels.
- Thiazide diuretics (e.g., hydrochlorothiazide) inhibit tubular resorption of sodium and chloride in ascending renal tubule also causing a loss of calcium in the urine. Do not use in patients with hyperparathyroidism.
- Cellulose sodium phosphate (Calcibind) binds calcium exchange in the intestines. Give medication with meals.
- Orthophosphate decreases the excretion of urinary calcium and increases inhibitor activity. Give 1 g vitamin C four times a day to acidify urine.

Oxalate Stones
- Pyridoxine (vitamin B_6) reduces the excretion of oxalates in the urine.
- Cholestyramine (Questran) binds oxalate in the gastrointestinal tract.

Uric Acid Stones
- Allopurinol (Zyloprim) reduces urinary excretion of uric acid.
- Sodium citrate or sodium bicarbonate is given to increase urinary pH. Urinary pH should be maintained at 7 to dissolve existing uric acid calculi.

Cystine Stones
- Penicillamine (Cuprimine) binds cystine to make a more soluble form.

Struvite Stones
- Acetohydroxamic acid inhibits urea-splitting organisms.
- Renacidin solution is a chemolysis agent that dissolves stones.

Surgical Interventions

Approximately 90% of renal stones are passed spontaneously. If there is no infection or obstruction, the stone may be left in the ureter for several months. Patients experiencing renal stones that are unable to pass through the urinary system (obstructing stones) require either open or closed surgical intervention. Common minimally invasive procedures include stenting, retrograde ureteroscopy, percutaneous antegrade nephroureterolithotomy, and laparoscopic ureterolithotomy. Open surgical procedures such as ureterolithotomy, pyelolithotomy, and nephrolithotomy can also be done.

Invasive (Endourologic) Procedures

Cystoscopy. Direct examination of the bladder with a cystoscope is used to remove small stones from the bladder.

Lithotripsy (Ultrasonic, Electrohydraulic, Laser, Extracorporeal Shock Wave). These procedures are usually done percutaneously. The most common types are laser and extracorporeal shock wave lithotripsy (ESWL). Laser probes are used to smash lower ureteral and large bladder stones. ESWL requires conscious sedation or general anesthesia to help keep the patient still during the procedure. Common problems after these procedures include hematuria and ecchymoses on the flank of the affected side. All urine should be strained for stone fragments.

Stenting. A stent is inserted to dilate the ureter and provide a passageway for stones or fragments. An indwelling (Foley) catheter may be used to facilitate passage of stone fragments.

Retrograde Ureteroscopy. This endoscopic procedure can visualize stones in the ureter. Stones can be extracted using grasping baskets, forceps, or loops. ESWL can also be done if stones cannot be retrieved.

Laparoscopic Ureterolithotomy. This procedure provides laparoscopic visualization of the ureters, allowing removal of stones or fragments.

Percutaneous Antegrade Nephrostoureterolithotomy. Using fluoroscopy, the physician passes a needle into the collecting system of the kidney. Stone and fragments are removed. This procedure requires general anesthesia. The patient usually has a nephrostomy tube in place postoperatively. Possible complications include bleeding at the site, hematuria, pneumothorax, and infection.

Open Surgical Procedures

Ureterolithotomy. An incision is made into the ureter through the lower abdominal wall. The most common complication is bleeding. Management includes care of ureteral tubes, drains, and urinary catheter as appropriate. Monitor intake and output, strain urine, provide wound care, and monitor for infection.

Pyelolithotomy. An incision is made through the flank of the affected side and extending into the renal pelvis. The most common complication is bleeding. Management is the same as for ureterolithotomy with a nephrostomy tube.

Nephrolithotomy. An incision is made through the flank of the affected side and extends into the kidney. The most common complication is bleeding. Management is the same as for ureterolithotomy with a nephrostomy tube.

COMMUNITY CARE

Assessment

Obtain a thorough nursing history to identify patients at increased risk for the development of renal calculi. A patient with a personal and family history of stones should be asked whether cysteine stones were identified, because these stones can be genetically inherited. A patient with a history of stones should be asked whether chemical analysis of the stone was performed and, if so, what type of stone was identified.

Assess the patient's compliance with the prescribed dietary and medication regimens. Instruct the patient to keep a daily log of food and fluid intake. Count the number of pills in the medication container to ensure compliance. Have the patient explain the actions and major side effects of the medications taken.

Assess for signs and symptoms of complications such as oliguria, increasing pain, anuria, or extremely bloody urine. Assess the patency and output of any postsurgical drains or tubes (e.g., nephrostomy tubes, Foley catheters, Jackson-Pratt or Hemovac drains) that were left in place from the acute care setting.

Assess the current medication regimen. Protease inhibitors have been associated with the development of renal stones.

Monitoring

Monitor urinalysis and urine culture results at periodic intervals as ordered. Monitor serum electrolyte levels for abnormal calcium, phosphorus, uric acid, alkaline phosphate, and parathyroid hormone levels. Dipstick the urine to determine pH. Monitor serum creatinine and BUN levels for adequate renal function.

Evaluate the incision site in a patient who has undergone an open surgical procedure. Monitor for signs and symptoms of infection.

Teach the patient how to care for the surgical wound, catheters, and drainage tubes. Teach the patient how to strain the urine if the stone has not been passed.

Prevention

Teach the patient how to prevent stone recurrence through dietary control. Reinforce teaching about the purpose of medications.
Teach the patient to maintain hydration by drinking 3 L/day of water.

 PROGNOSIS

The prognosis for patients with renal calculi is good with prompt and adequate treatment, although recurrence may occur.

 CLINICAL PEARLS

○ The location of pain depends on the location of the renal stone. If the stone is in the kidney pelvis, pain is caused by hydronephrosis (collection of urine in the kidney pelvis due to obstructed outflow) and is characterized as a consistent dull pain that occurs mostly in the costovertebral angle. Severe pain that occurs lower in the urinary tract is caused by spasms and pressure exerted in the ureter. Pain medications should be given around the clock to ensure adequate control.

○ Patients with history of renal stones should be taught to drink 2 to 4 L/day to prevent stone formation or dissolve present stones. Instruct the patient to get up once during the night to drink a glass of water to help keep the urine dilute and help prevent new stone formation. There is no research data that supports the use of high intake of cranberry juice to prevent stone formation.

○ The patient who is ambulatory is more likely to pass a renal stone than the patient who is sedentary. Encourage ambulation. Assist the patient with ambulation when necessary.

○ Strain all urine in the case of a patient who is suspected of having a renal stone. Instruct the patient how to do this at home.

○ Patients with renal insufficiency, renal failure, or fluid excretion problems should be limited in fluid intake. Consult with the physician regarding the amount of fluid intake needed.

○ ESWL should not be used in patients with pacemakers and cautiously used in women of childbearing age (because of potential ovarian damage). Instruct the patient receiving ESWL that redness or bruising at the site is common and that pain may persist for up to 3 days after the procedure.

NURSING PROBLEM/ DIAGNOSIS	NURSING INTERVENTIONS CLASSIFICATION (NIC)
Acute pain/impaired comfort (urinary)	Pain management Analgesic administration Fluid management
Deficient knowledge	Teaching: disease process Nutrition counseling

Renal Failure

Section 3 Veronica P. S. Njie

OVERVIEW

Renal failure is destruction of the renal tubules to the extent that they are unable to perform normal functions of excretion of metabolic wastes; regulation of fluid and electrolytes, and acid-base balance; production of hormones (erythropoietin, prostaglandins, and renin); and conversion of vitamin D to its active form, 1,25 dihydroxycholecalciferol. Renal failure is classified as acute or chronic. It is estimated that 5% of individuals hospitalized develop acute renal failure (ARF). The incidence increases to 30% in critical and special care units. Although ARF can be reversed, the mortality rate can be as high as 90%.

ARF can lead to chronic renal failure (CRF) if interventions are not undertaken early. CRF develops over years. It affects males more than females and African Americans and Native Americans more than whites.

PATHOPHYSIOLOGY

In renal failure, nephrons are damaged to the extent that they are unable to perform normal functions. In ARF, there is sudden insult to the nephrons leading to imbalances and the inability of the nephrons to function effectively, resulting in fluid and electrolyte imbalances and elevations in BUN and creatinine levels. This condition is reversible with prompt intervention.

CRF is progressive, with few or no symptoms until irreversible damage occurs. The kidneys cannot then perform normal functions, and alternate methods must be used.

Acute Renal Failure

There are three etiologic categories of ARF, each of which has different causes (Table 25-3-1) and requires different interventions.

Prerenal. Renal hypoperfusion directly relates to decreased blood circulation

---

Table 25-3-1. Causes of Acute Renal Failure

Prerenal Failure
Renal hypoperfusion from:
Volume depletion from dehydration, hemorrhage, gastrointestinal losses (e.g., vomiting, diarrhea), or excessive diuresis (diuretics)
Impaired cardiac function seen in cardiogenic shock, congestive heart failure, myocardial infarction, and dysrhythmias
Vasodilation due to sepsis or anaphylaxis

Intrarenal Failure
Parenchymal damage caused by:
Nephrotoxins: Medications, contrast dye, or heavy metals (see Chapter 6, Section 1)
Prolonged renal ischemia from myoglobinuria, hemolytic anemia, transfusion reactions, trauma
Infectious processes, including acute glomerulonephritis and acute pyelonephritis

Postrenal Failure
Urinary tract obstructions due to calculi, tumors, or strictures

and perfusion of the renal tissue. Decreased blood volume to the kidneys results in decreased glomerular filtration rate. The prerenal form accounts for 40% to 80% of cases of ARF.

Intrarenal. There is damage to the renal parenchyma (interstitium). Intrarenal ARF may be further classified by the specific site of damage: tubular damage, glomerular damage, or interstitial damage.

Tubular damage is clinically referred to as *acute tubular necrosis* (ATN). It is the most common cause of intrarenal failure. Injury to the tubules can be ischemic or toxic in origin or may result from obstruction. Ischemic injury is most commonly due to untreated prerenal failure (as the perfusion leads to ischemia). Toxic injury occurs from nephrotoxic drugs such as aminoglycosides and contrast agents (contrast nephropathy) (see Table 25-3-1). Obstruction from cellular debris and casts can cause further ischemia and increase pressure in the tubules. *Rhabdomyolysis* is the breakdown of muscle due to systemic infection or major trauma. It causes myoglobin (a protein released from muscle when injury occurs) and hemoglobin to be liberated in the blood, resulting in renal toxicity and ischemia from clogging of the tubules. Myoglobulin is not normally found in either serum or urine. Large quantities of hemoglobin may also enter the tubules because of massive hemolysis, as occurs in hemolytic reactions. Both myoglobin and hemoglobin cause urine color to change to "tea," red, brown, or black.

Direct *glomerular* parenchymal damage from glomerulonephritis can also lead to intrarenal failure. Glomerulonephritis can cause both ARF and CRF. The specific types that cause ARF are the rapidly progressive glomerulonephritis and acute proliferative glomerulonephritis.

Interstitial pyelonephritis may result from allergic reactions to drugs such as nonsteroidal anti-inflammatory drugs, allopurinol (Zyloprim), autoimmune disease, or infection. Urine stain positive for eosinophils suggests presence of the disease.

Postrenal. In this type, the least common cause of intrarenal ARF, results from an obstruction beyond the renal tubules that causes backflow of urine to the nephrons, leading to damage. Causes of obstruction include renal calculi, tumors, and trauma. Bladder outlet obstruction from tumors or neurogenic bladder or prostatic hypertrophy is the most common cause of postrenal failure. The obstruction can be bilateral or unilateral. Bilateral obstructions may be due to ureteral obstruction related to renal calculi or stricture; or unilateral if the patient has only one kidney.

Regardless of the etiology, ARF involves three phases (Table 25-3-2). These phases sometimes overlap, making it difficult to determine where one phase ends and the other begins.

Chronic Renal Failure

In CRF, the etiologic factors are prolonged and occur over a period of many years. Any chronic renal disease (e.g., recurrent renal calculi, chronic glomerulonephritis) can lead to CRF. Diabetic nephropathy is the leading cause of end-stage renal disease (ESRD) in the United States, accounting for 36% of cases. This is due to glycosylation of glomerular proteins. Hypertension is the second most common cause, accounting for 30% of cases. CRF caused by hypertension is due to direct nephron injury leading to impaired renal perfusion.

Table 25-3-2. Phases in Acute Renal Failure and Assessment Findings

PHASE	TIME PERIOD	ASSESSMENT FINDINGS
Onset	Initial insult to kidneys	Immediate intervention may result in preventing renal damage
Oliguric	Starts within hours and lasts 8–14 days If prolonged, uremia develops	• Oliguria <400 mL/day urine output • Fluid retention leading to edema,
Nonoliguric	Milder form, but seen more often Common in toxic tubular necrosis	hypertension, and pulmonary edema • Electrolyte imbalance such as hyperkalemia (>6.0) • Elevated BUN, creatinine (azotemia) Urine output is >400 mL/day Less azotemia present
Diuretic	End of the oliguric phase Lasts 10 days	• Tissues regenerate and healing starts • Gradual increase in urine output • Some azotemia and electrolyte imbalances remain • GFR improves but tubular transport mechanisms are still abnormal thus the urine is dilute
Recovery	Starts from 3 months and lasts up to 1 year	BUN and creatinine to normal levels Kidney function fully recovers but may have some residual renal impairment

BUN, blood urea nitrogen; GFR, glomerular filtration rate.

CRF progresses through four stages if the process is not halted:
- Decreased renal reserve. In this stage, 50% of the nephrons are destroyed. The body compensates, and the individual is usually asymptomatic.
- Renal insufficiency. In this stage, 20% to 35% of normal kidney function remains. Anemia, hypertension, polyuria or isosthenuria (due to the kidneys' inability to concentrate urine), azotemia, and uremia may be present.
- Renal failure. In this stage, 5% to 20% of normal kidney function remains. The person continues to exhibit anemia, azotemia, hypertension, and polyuria. Uremia with signs and symptoms indicating elevated serum levels of BUN, creatinine, and potassium is present.
- ESRD. By this stage of CRF, only 5% to 10% of normal kidney function remains. All of the signs and symptoms seen in renal failure worsen. Oliguria, which may lead to anuria, occurs. All normal kidney functions are severely compromised. When the patient reaches this stage of the disease, dialysis is indicated.

 SIGNS AND SYMPTOMS

Renal failure affects all body systems. Table 25-3-3 lists and compares the signs and symptoms of ARF and CRF/ESRD. Azotemia is an early sign of renal failure. Uremia with overt signs and symptoms is present in ESRD. Uremic syndrome is the term used to describe the results or manifestations from a total loss of renal function. As uremia progresses and the waste products accumulate, other organ systems become affected. Without intervention, coma and death occur.

Table 25-3-3. Signs and Symptoms of Acute Renal Failure and Chronic Renal Failure/End-Stage Renal Disease

	ACUTE RENAL FAILURE	CHRONIC RENAL FAILURE/ESRD
Urinary/renal	• Oliguria	• Oliguria/anuria, decreased creatinine clearance—due to the kidneys' inability to excrete the urine • Proteinuria; hematuria—damage to the interstitial tissues
Electrolytes	• Elevated K$^+$ level • Elevated BUN and creatinine	• Elevated K$^+$, phosphorus, magnesium, and pH—the kidneys' inability to excrete them • Elevated BUN and creatinine—retention of the wastes • Decreased CA$^+$—due to the elevated phosphorus levels and reduced vitamin D for calcium absorption • Metabolic acidosis—the retention of hydrogen ions in the blood
Cardiovascular	• Hypertension; peripheral edema	• Peripheral edema, hypertension—sodium and water retention from the kidneys' inability to excrete them and the rennin—angiotensen-aldosterone system, which compounds the retention • Coronary artery disease and arrhythmias—due to altered lipid and carbohydrate metabolism • Congestive heart failure—as a result of fluid overload • Pericarditis—from the uremic toxin buildup
Gastrointestinal	• Nausea, vomiting, anorexia, diarrhea	• Uremic fetor, stomatitis, gingivitis—due to the breakdown of saliva urea to ammonia • Nausea and vomiting, anorexia—toxins in the system • Gastrointestinal bleeding—as a result of platelet dysfunction • Constipation—from fluid restriction and low-fiber intake. High-fiber foods are restricted in ESRD because of their high potassium and phosphorus content. Phosphate-binding agents and decreased activity also cause constipation.

System		
Respiratory	• Crackles (rales)	• Crackles, pulmonary edema—from fluid overload • Kussmaul respirations, pleural effusion, dyspnea, orthopnea—secondary to metabolic acidosis as the lungs compensate for the increased hydrogen ions in the blood
Musculoskeletal	• Muscle weakness	• Potential for fractures, joint pain, and swelling—due to the elevated phosphorus and low calcium levels
Hematologic	• Anemia	• Anemia, clotting dysfunction, easy bruising—the kidneys are not producing erythropoietin, which is essential for blood cell production.
Integumentary	• Pale skin/edema	• Pale—due to anemia • Dry skin, poor skin turgor—decreased perspiration and inactive sweat glands • Pruritus—due to uremic crystals and calcium deposited in the skin • Edema—fluid retention • Hyperpigmentation—deposition of waste • Uremic frost—the deposition of uremic crystals (rare now because of treatment interventions)
Neurologic	• Headache, lethargy, confusion	• Altered mental status, lethargy, headache, change in behavior—from the toxins crossing the blood-brain barrier, excess cerebral fluid, and electrolyte imbalances • Peripheral neuropathy—from demyelinization and atrophy of the nerves from the toxins in the blood
Endocrine		• Glucose intolerance—due to impaired peripheral insulin use • Elevated parathyroid hormones—response to low calcium levels
Reproductive		• Amenorrhea, impotence—from low estrogen and testosterone levels from the high levels of uremic toxins
Immunologic	Risk for infection—leading cause of death	• White blood cell decrease—suppression of blood cell production

BUN, blood urea nitrogen; ESRD, end-stage renal disease.

DIAGNOSTIC CRITERIA

Laboratory Tests (see also Chapter 11, Section 5)

- Urinalysis may show low or fixed specific gravity because the kidneys are unable to concentrate and dilute urine. There is oliguria or anuria. Casts and cells are present in the urine. Urine protein is elevated.
- Creatinine clearance is a urine test done to determine the kidney's ability to clear the blood of creatinine. Creatinine clearance decreases as kidney function diminishes. Urine is collected for a 24-hour period for this test.
- Serum creatinine level is elevated. This is the most significant and reliable test for kidney function.
- Complete blood count reveals decreased hemoglobin and hematocrit due to the kidney's inability to produce erythropoietin.
- Potassium, phosphorus, and BUN levels are elevated. Calcium level is low.
- The BUN–creatinine ratio may be greater than 20:1, depending on the stage of the disease.

Arterial Blood Gas Analysis. This test reveals metabolic acidosis, which can occur because the kidneys cannot eliminate hydrogen ions and waste substances.

Radiographs. KUB radiographs can reveal an obstruction or problems in the renal tract.

Intravenous Pyelography. This test evaluates the structure of the kidneys. A contrast dye is injected in the individual's veins, and radiographs of the kidneys and pelvis are taken. The patient must be restricted from ingesting anything by mouth for at least 6 to 8 hours before the test. The nurse must check for allergy to iodine or shellfish. If patient is allergic, premedication with Benadryl and corticosteroids is usually done to desensitize the patient. After the test, extra oral and intravenous fluids should be given to facilitate excretion of the dye. The contrast medium may precipitate ARF.

Cystoscopy with Brush Biopsy. The bladder is visualized using a cystoscope, and then a ureteral catheter with a biopsy brush is introduced to obtain tissue fragments for analysis. After the procedure, the patient is given fluids to prevent clots. The patient must be told to expect mild hematuria for about 48 hours after the procedure but is instructed to report excessive bleeding.

Renal Biopsy. Renal biopsy is performed for a definitive diagnosis of kidney damage and to differentiate between ARF and CRF. Coagulation studies must be within normal limits before biopsy is performed. In this procedure, a piece of tissue is aspirated from the individual's kidney through a needle. The percutaneous needle biopsy technique requires manual pressure for 20 minutes, followed by a pressure dressing because of the kidneys' high vascularity. The patient is positioned on the side of the puncture site to help prevent bleeding. The site is checked for bleeding. Serial urine collection is done to evaluate bleeding. The patient is advised to avoid heavy lifting and other strenuous activities for 1 to 2 weeks and to increase fluid intake to flush the kidneys.

Renal Ultrasonography and Computed Tomography. These studies reveal obstruction and determine the size of the kidneys. In ARF, the kidneys are enlarged from inflammatory processes of the acute insult; in CRF, the kidneys are shrunken because of atrophic changes from long-term damage.

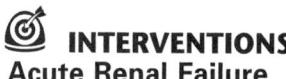

INTERVENTIONS
Acute Renal Failure

Generally, treatment of ARF depends on the etiology of the disease. The goal is to eliminate the cause and to prevent irreversible kidney damage.

Prerenal. A fluid challenge is performed to increase vascular fluid volume, thus increasing systemic blood pressure and pressure in the kidneys to stimulate renal function.

Intrarenal. Interventions focus on eliminating toxins or treating the causative factor. Depending on the patient's laboratory values, temporary dialysis may be needed to remove waste substances. Approximately 20% to 60% of patients with BUN levels exceeding 100 mg/dL or creatinine levels of 5 to 10 mg/dL require dialysis.

Postrenal. The focus is on relieving the cause of obstruction through conservative or surgical means and on repairing damage to tissues due to trauma.

Chronic Renal Failure

The goal of treatment is to retard progression and prevent complications. If the patient is already in ESRD, then the goals are to maintain homeostasis through artificial means and make plans for kidney transplant.

Nutritional Management

Nutritional management of the renal patient depends on whether the patient is on dialysis. The goal of nutritional management is to decrease levels of the metabolic end products of urea, potassium, phosphate, and hydrogen by decreasing the intake of protein. Urea is formed in the liver from ammonia and is the chief nitrogenous component of urine. Under normal circumstances, urea is excreted through the kidneys. *Protein intake* can affect the amount of urea excreted. For patients not undergoing dialysis, protein is generally restricted to 0.6 to 0.8 g/kg of ideal body weight if creatinine clearance is below 20 mL/min. Once dialysis is started, the patient can then tolerate 1 to 1.5 g/kg of ideal body weight of protein when creatinine clearance is below 20 mL/min. This rule does not apply to patients on peritoneal dialysis (PD), because of the large amount of protein lost during PD. The protein intake for these patients can be as high as 1.2 to 2 g/kg of ideal body weight. *Sufficient carbohydrates* are needed to prevent the breakdown of body protein. Generally, 100 g of carbohydrate and an adequate amount of fat are needed to maintain an intake of 35 kcal/kg/day.

Sodium and potassium restrictions are based on the patient's ability to excrete these electrolytes. When serum potassium level exceeds 6 mEq/L, measures must be taken to lower this level because of the potential for cardiac dysrhythmias. Sodium restriction can range from 1 to 4 g/day; potassium restrictions, from 1.5 to 4 g/day. Potassium restrictions are not as essential for patients undergoing PD. The clinical term "renal diet" refers to restrictions on protein, sodium, and potassium. Ensure that the patient has enough information to adhere to the dietary restrictions. A nutritionist should be consulted.

Nursing Interventions

- Carefully monitor intake and output to prevent fluid overload. The patient is usually on fluid restriction of 500 mL to 1.5 L/day, depending on clinical status.

- Weigh the patient daily to monitor for fluid imbalance.
- Provide meticulous skin care to relieve dryness and pruritus.
- Monitor laboratory values and report significant results of electrolyte and blood tests.
- If serum potassium level is below 6 mEq/L, obtain an electrocardiogram, which will show tall, tented, or peaked T waves, and notify the physician.
- Dialysis (see Chapter 6, Sections 2 and 3).

Pharmacologic Therapy

- Diuretics are used to control edema, potassium elevations, and hypertension. Lasix may be given for fluid overload and for ascites.
- Antihypertensive agents, particularly angiotensin-converting enzyme (ACE) inhibitors, are used to lower blood pressure if diuretics alone prove ineffective.
- Kayexalate or insulin is given when serum potassium level exceeds 5.5 mEq/L to reduce these levels. When insulin is used, the patient may need glucose (D50W) owing to the potential for hypoglycemia as the glucose is driven into the cells with potassium.
- Antihistamines are administered to relieve pruritus.
- Erythropoietin (Epogen) is used to stimulate production of RBCs by the bone marrow. This drug stimulates erythropoiesis in the bone marrow and induces the release of reticulocytes. Increased production of RBCs is important also because uremic toxins decrease RBC survival.
- Calcium and vitamin D are often prescribed to prevent hyperparathyroidism or bone disease. Calcijex is an injectable form of the kidney-produced hormone calcitriol. Calcitriol activates vitamin D.
- Phosphate-binding antacids (e.g., PhosLo, calcium acetate [Calphron]) are often prescribed because of impaired phosphate excretion in renal failure. These act by increasing fecal losses of phosphate. Caution must be used to avoid antacids that contain magnesium (e.g., Gelusil, Maalox, Mylanta), because the kidneys are responsible for magnesium excretion. Aluminum-based antacids increase the risk for bone diseases or possible encephalopathy due to excessive aluminum intake. Elevated levels of phosphorus (hyperphosphatemia) can lead to the formation of metastatic calcifications that are deposited throughout the body (e.g., joints, arteries, skin, kidneys, and cornea). Antacids are not given to treat heartburn.
- Iron supplements are given to correct anemia.
- Histamine-2 antagonists are used to prevent gastrointestinal bleeding from platelet dysfunction and stress.
- Sodium bicarbonate is given to correct metabolic acidosis.
- Patients with renal insufficiency may need decreased dosages of drugs, because target organs have increased sensitivity owing to uremic changes.

Surgical Intervention

Dialysis, either PD or hemodialysis, involves filtering blood through a semipermeable membrane to eliminate waste products. In PD, the patient's peritoneal membrane acts as the semipermeable membrane. In hemodialysis, the semipermeable membrane is an external machine.

Continuous venovenous hemofiltration (CVVH) is a slow hemodialysis process (usually 100 mL to 1 L/hr) used instead of fast conventional hemodialysis

(2 L or more in 2 to 3 hours). CVVH is used mainly in patients who are clinically unstable and cannot tolerate the rapid fluid withdrawal in conventional hemodialysis.

Transplantation of a kidney from a donor (cadaver or live person) is done to replace the failed kidney in the recipient.

For more information on hemodialysis and various surgical interventions, see Chapter 6, Section 2.

 COMMUNITY CARE

- Provide patient teaching about the disease, medications, activity, diet, and posthospital care.
- Assess the need for home care.
- Advise a patient with ESRD to avoid strong soaps, to shower rather than bathe, and to rinse the body thoroughly to minimize pruritus.
- Determine the availability of dialysis centers and monetary funds and provide appropriate information.
- Check the dialysis access site and teach the patient how to do so at home.
- Monitor for complications related to dialysis (see Chapter 6, Sections 2 and 3, for potential complications).
- Provide information on the National Kidney Foundation and the American Association of Kidney Patients and other available resources.
- Maintain infection prevention precautions at all times.

 PROGNOSIS

Each year, approximately 42,000 people in the United States die of renal failure. The mortality rate for ARF can be as high as 90%, depending on the severity. The top two causes of mortality in ARF include infection, accounting for 75% of deaths, and cardiopulmonary complications. Elderly patients are at highest risk because of their multisystem problems and diminished renal reserves.

Patients who have progressed to irreversible CRF need to undergo dialysis (PD or hemodialysis) for life. The 1-year mortality rate for long-term dialysis is approximately 20%.

 CLINICAL PEARLS

- Close monitoring of fluid volume, BUN, and creatinine level is essential to prevent ARF, especially in persons at increased risk: the elderly, postoperative individuals, and those who have lost a lot of blood from trauma.
- One liter of fluid is equal to 1 kg (2.2 lb) of body weight.
- Include oral intake at night when computing 24-hour fluid restriction.
- Prepare the patient for dialysis if BUN level is above 100 mg/dL, serum creatinine is 5 to 10 mg/dL, or serum potassium level is above 6 mEq/L and is not decreased with medications.
- Detecting infection in patients with ESRD is difficult because of their inability to develop fever.
- Do not ignore subtle increases in serum creatinine, especially with concurrent abnormal urinalysis or with hypertension.
- Measure and record the patient's vital signs and weight before and after dialysis.

NURSING PROBLEM/ DIAGNOSIS	NURSING INTERVENTIONS CLASSIFICATION (NIC)
Excess fluid volume	Fluid management
	Fluid monitoring
	Nutrition therapy
Acid-base imbalance	Acid-base management
Anemia	Energy management
Risk for infection	Infection protection
	Teaching: disease process

Urinary Tract Infection

Section 4   Selma Brophy

 OVERVIEW

UTIs result from various causative agents invading the lower urinary tract. UTI is one of the most common causes for seeking health care, accounting for an estimated 7 to 9.6 million ambulatory health care visits each year. UTI is the most common nosocomial infection; at an incidence of 40%, it affects approximately 600,000 patients per year.

Lower UTIs are very common. Women younger than 50 years of age are more commonly affected than men of that age group. As many as 20% or more of women develop a UTI during their lifetime. After age 50, the incidence increases for men, mainly due to prostatic hyperplasia, strictures of the urethra, and neurogenic or neuropathic bladder. UTIs in men involving the prostate most commonly result from an obstruction (e.g., renal calculi or enlarged prostate).

 PATHOPHYSIOLOGY

Damage to the integrity of the mucosal lining of the urinary tract can lead to bacteria invasion. When organisms invade the lining of the urinary tract, inflammation occurs, as does cellular damage. Any change in the mucosal lining that produces decreased resistance to invading organisms increases the potential for infection. Infection of the lower urinary tract can be present in the ureter, the urethra, bladder (most common), or prostate (e.g., urethritis, cystitis, prostatitis). Pyelonephritis (i.e., infection of the renal parenchyma and pelvis), either acute or chronic, may be a complication of repeated or untreated UTIs caused by the infecting organism ascending from the bladder to the kidney.

The most common causative organisms in UTI are enteric gram negative with *Escherichia coli* accounting for more than 90% of all cases. Gram-positive organisms may account for a minority of cases. Most organisms are normal flora of the gastrointestinal system. Most infecting organisms are bacterial; however, occasionally, fungi and viruses may cause an infection.

Common predisposing or risk factors include:
- Poor hygiene
- Sexual intercourse (irritation to the urethra)

- Urinary stasis (due to obstruction/congenital anomalies)
- Urinary sphincter stricture
- Tight clothing (which irritates the urethra in women)
- Diabetes (owing to high glucose content of the urine)
- Indwelling catheter
- Failure to empty the bladder completely
- Urinary retention
- Neurologic disorders (e.g., spinal cord injury, multiple sclerosis, stroke)
- Atrophy of the urethral epithelium with aging
- Debilitating illness
- Delay in responding to the urge to void
- Any invasive diagnostic procedure of the urinary tract
- Diaphragm use with foam spermicide
- Age over 65 and institutionalized

UTI is a common medical complication in persons with neurologic problems (e.g., multiple sclerosis). Untreated UTIs can lead to urinary incontinence, especially in elderly persons. Institutionalized elderly persons are at increased risk for UTIs because of frequent use of antimicrobial agents, chronic diseases, and immobility.

 ## SIGNS AND SYMPTOMS

The most common signs and symptoms of UTI are frequent pain and burning (dysuria) on urination, sometimes accompanied by lower back or suprapubic pain. Urgency, frequency, nocturia and, in some cases, incontinence may also occur. Elderly persons may exhibit confusion or anorexia as the initial symptom.

Urine may be malodorous and cloudy. Pyuria (presence of WBCs in the urine) and hematuria often accompany UTIs. As many as 50% of persons who have bacteria in the lower urinary tract exhibit no symptoms of infection. Fever and flank pain are generally considered signs of upper UTI (pyelonephritis).

 ## DIAGNOSTIC CRITERIA

Urinalysis and urine cultures (see Chapter 11, Section 5), with samples obtained by the clean-catch, midstream method, are the primary tests for suspected UTI. Testing for sexually transmitted diseases, which produce similar symptoms, may be performed. Urethritis caused by *Chlamydia trachomatis*, *Neisseria gonorrhoeae*, or herpes simplex virus mimics UTIs. Vaginitis may also cause dysuria.

For a patient with frequently recurring UTIs, the following tests may also be ordered:
- Voiding cystoureterography
- Intravenous urogram
- IVP if urinary tract obstruction or anomaly is suspected

 ## INTERVENTIONS
Antimicrobial Therapy

Options for antimicrobial treatment of uncomplicated UTIs include:
- Single dose of an antimicrobial

- Short-course regimen (3 to 4 days of therapy)
- 7- to 10-day therapy

The distinct trend is toward short-course therapy for females with uncomplicated lower UTIs. As many as 80% of such cases are cured after 3 days of therapy. Longer therapy (7 to 10 days) is prescribed for men, especially those with prostatitis, and patients over 65. Persons with pyelonephritis require a 10- to 14-day course of therapy and may need to be hospitalized.

Antimicrobials should be low cost with few side effects. The therapeutic goal is minimal effect on vaginal and fecal flora. It is important to monitor for gastric upset, which may lead persons to discontinue medication prematurely.

Commonly used medications include:
- Sulfisoxazole (Gantrisin)
- Trimethoprim/sulfamethoxazole (Bactrim, Septra)
- Nitrofurantoin (Macrodantin) (not to be used in patients with renal insufficiency)
- Quinolones (ciprofloxacin, norfloxacin, ofloxacin)
- Nalidixic acid (NegGram)
- Amoxicillin (frequently used in pregnant women)

Relieving Pain and Fever

Medications that may be used to relieve pain include:
- Aspirin, acetaminophen, ibuprofen
- Pyridium (urinary tract analgesic), an Azo dye with an incompletely understood mechanism of action that changes the color of urine
- Propantheline bromide (Pro-Banthine) to reduce spasm

Apply heat to the perineum with sitz baths or using warm, moist compresses.

Patient Education

Hygiene
- Showers are preferable to baths; avoid bubble baths.
- Cleanse the perineum after each bowel movement in a front-to-back fashion.
- Avoid douches and feminine sprays, which can irritate the urinary mucosa.

Voiding Habits
- Void every 2 to 3 hours and empty the bladder completely.
- Void immediately after intercourse.

Drug Therapy. Take medications as prescribed. Promptly report any problems, such as fatigue, nausea, vomiting, or pruritus.

Fluids. Restrict caffeinated beverages and alcohol. Drink 1500 to 2000 mL/day of clear fluids.

Self-Management

Preventive measures include maintaining long-term therapy of antimicrobial agents for repeated infections as prescribed. Teach the patient to self-test urine as directed, using dipsticks that measure nitrates (see Chapter 4, Section 2). Emphasize the need to consult with a health care provider if an infection recurs.

Reinforce dietary considerations. Point out that a balanced diet helps to maintain normal body function and healthy, intact skin and mucosa.

Promote adequate fluid intake. Recommend fluids with acid ash, such as cranberry juice, which acidifies the urine and reduces the risk of bacterial growth. Recent investigations are trying to determine how much cranberry juice is necessary to achieve this effect. An alternative to cranberry juice may be oral vitamin C, 1000 mg/day, except when taking Bactrim/Septra or any sulfa drug. (Sulfa drugs tend to crystallize in an acid environment.)

Collaborative interventions include surgery to relieve obstruction or other anomalies. Other collaborative interventions are long-term antimicrobial therapy, usually with complicated UTIs or other problems.

Possible complications of UTIs include recurrent UTIs and renal failure due to kidney damage. Patients with indwelling catheters are at greater risk for gram-negative sepsis with up to a 50% mortality rate.

Expected outcomes of interventions for UTIs include pain relief, understanding of treatment regimen, and few or no complications.

 ## COMMUNITY CARE

Patient education focuses on hygiene, fluid intake, voiding habits, and self-monitoring for episodes of reinfection. Issues related to voiding habits in the workplace include making sure that the patient has sufficient opportunities to void during the workday.

UTIs in men and complicated UTIs in women require repeat culture after treatment.

 ## PROGNOSIS

Simple UTIs are usually managed and treated with antimicrobials. Chronic and/or untreated or undertreated UTIs can lead to chronic problems. If the UTI progresses to gram-negative sepsis, mortality rate can be as high as 50%, especially in elderly patients.

 ## CLINICAL PEARLS

○ Repeated UTIs suggest the need for consultation with a urologist.
○ Not all UTIs produce overt symptoms. Careful assessment, especially in elderly patients, is essential. In the elderly, confusion or anorexia may be the only presenting symptoms.
○ Many patients with voiding problems may be reluctant to increase fluid intake, which exacerbates the problem. Much encouragement may be necessary to get them to drink the recommended 8 to 10 glasses of fluid daily.
○ Instruct the patient to avoid cranberry juice when taking trimethoprim/sulfamethoxazole (Bactrim, Septra).

NURSING PROBLEM/ DIAGNOSIS	NURSING INTERVENTIONS CLASSIFICATION (NIC)
Infection	Medication management
	Fluid management
Impaired comfort (urinary)	Analgesic administration
	Pain management
Prevention of recurrence	Teaching: prescribed medication
	Perineal care
	Infection protection

Chapter 26

Reproductive

Benign Prostatic Hypertrophy

Section 1   Cecilia Tiller

OVERVIEW

Benign prostatic hypertrophy (BPH), a noncancerous enlargement of the prostate gland, is a common condition in older men. About 50% of all men age 60 and older develop BPH; 25% of men in the United States are treated for BPH by age 80. Approximately 50% of men over age 50 and 90% of men ages 70 to 90 have symptoms of BPH.

PATHOPHYSIOLOGY

The cause of age-related prostatic hyperplasia is unknown. The degree of hypertrophy appears to be the result of endocrine changes associated with aging. Recent studies indicate that androgenic changes at the cellular level may be the influencing factor. The accumulation of dehydrotestosterone and increased estrogen levels may influence the hyperplasia.

BPH develops from nodular hyperplasia of the prostate. This begins in periurethral glandular tissue and exerts inward pressure on the urethra. As the prostate enlarges, urethral resistance to urine flow increases, and muscular hypertrophy of the urinary bladder develops. The narrowing urethra hinders the ability to empty the bladder adequately, leading to residual urine and predisposition to bladder infection.

The enlarged prostate pushes upward into the bladder, causing the internal urethral orifice to become elevated. Sometimes the enlarged prostate forms a valve-like stricture at the urethral orifice. Straining to urinate only makes the condition worse.

Increased bladder pressure can lead to urethral dilation, hydronephrosis, and renal deterioration. Bladder failure occurs when the detrusor (the external longitudinal muscular coat of the urinary bladder) cannot exert sufficient pressure to overcome urethral obstruction, resulting in urinary retention. The hyperplastic prostate is very vascular, and painless hematuria often occurs.

SIGNS AND SYMPTOMS

Symptoms of BPH may be nonspecific, but a weak urine stream and hesitancy are frequently reported. Other common symptoms include frequency, nocturia, hematuria, a sense of incomplete voiding, stream interruption, and dribbling. Symptoms often come and go, with gradual deterioration over a period of several years.

Urinary tract infections (UTIs) may be the first sign of BPH; hematuria can also be an early sign. The severity of symptoms does not correlate with the size of the prostate, and some men may be completely asymptomatic. Stress, environmental factors, exposure to cold, and use of medications such as sympathomimetics may influence the severity of symptoms.

Because symptoms and the patient's tolerance levels vary, the therapeutic approach is designed to meet the patient's needs. Close monitoring is necessary to prevent further complications. Severe BPH can lead to hydronephrosis, profuse hematuria, urinary retention, and UTIs. Prolonged urinary retention may lead to renal failure and azotemia.

Symptom Assessment

A voiding diary or completion of the American Urological Association (AUA) symptom index is helpful in determining how troublesome the symptoms are to the patient. The AUA index is important to identify baseline symptom severity and guide treatment. The index comprises seven questions regarding BPH symptoms. The symptoms are evaluated on a scale of mild (0 to 7), to moderate (8 to 19), to severe (20 to 35). The AUA symptom index must be used with caution, however, because the symptoms are not specific for BPH.

 DIAGNOSTIC CRITERIA

Because symptoms vary and some men may be embarrassed to discuss urinary tract problems, the health care provider may need to specifically ask the older patient if he is having problems. Vague symptoms may be reported; however, nocturia and dysuria are often the most common symptoms causing the patient to seek care.

The initial evaluation should include a detailed medical history focusing on the urinary tract, previous surgical procedures, general health issues, and current health status. Specific attention should be paid to any medications that the patient is taking, to determine if these medications may be contributing to the problem. It is important to rule out other medical conditions, especially diabetes.

A thorough physical examination should be conducted, including palpation of the bladder and a digital rectal exam (DRE). An enlarged prostate is easily palpated; however, prostate size does not correlate with symptom severity or the degree of obstruction. An enlarged prostate feels harder and larger than a normal prostate, which is soft, pliable, and about the size of a walnut. Absence of the median furrow and a rubbery consistency also indicate enlargement. Not all prostate enlargement is caused by BPH; thus, other conditions (e.g., prostatitis, cancer, calculi, sexually transmitted diseases) must be ruled out.

Laboratory Studies

Urinalysis by dipstick or microscopic examination is indicated to rule out infection, hematuria, and bladder cancer. Serum creatinine and blood urea nitrogen (BUN) levels are evaluated to detect renal insufficiency.

Measurement of prostate-specific antigen (PSA) is optional in the initial evaluation. PSA is a glycoprotein found in prostate tissue that does not demonstrate diurnal variations. It is considered a more specific marker for metastatic tumor of prostate origin than acid phosphatase (an enzyme also found in prostate tissue). The PSA test does not discriminate well between patients with symptomatic BPH and those with prostate cancer. A large number of false-positives and false-negatives occur among PSA values, and there is a lack of consensus about the significance of minimal evaluations. PSA levels normally increase with age and in patients taking finasteride (Proscar), an androgen inhibitor. This medication adversely affects the PSA test. The test measures the percentage of free PSA in the total serum PSA. A free PSA below 25% and a total PSA of 4.0 to 10.0 ng/mL indicate high risk for prostate cancer. A free PSA above 25% and a total PSA of 4.0 to 10.0 ng/mL with a normal-feeling prostate on DRE, regardless of prostate size or the patient's age, are consistent with BPH.

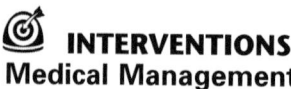

INTERVENTIONS
Medical Management

If the patient's AUA symptom index score is in the mild range and he is not troubled by the symptoms, then "watchful waiting" may be the most appropriate approach. Annual monitoring is advised, and lifestyle changes are encouraged. Limiting alcohol, table salt, caffeine, spicy foods, and after-dinner fluids, along with not eating less than 4 hours before bedtime, may help decrease mild symptoms. Saw palmetto I (*Serenoa repens*), a natural herbal product, may provide benefits to men with BPH. Saw palmetto berries contain *B*-sitosterol, which acts like a 5∝-reductase-inhibitor, preventing the conversion of testosterone to the potent metabolic 5∝-dihydrotestosterone, a substance that is partially responsible for BPH. Another alternative therapy is an extract derived from the bark of the *Pygeum africanum* tree. Both of these alternative therapies are currently under study and show promise for use in treating BPH.

A patients with AUA symptom index scores in the moderate range whose symptoms are bothersome, but not severe enough to warrant surgery, may be treated with medications. Three classes of medications may be used to treat uncomplicated BPH.

Reductase Inhibitors

The most commonly used medication in this group is finasteride. This drug hinders the conversion of testosterone to the more active dihydrotestosterone without affecting testosterone plasma levels or sexual function. Finasteride helps reduce prostate size, alleviating urinary symptoms. Results vary from study to study, and it may take at least 6 months for the full effects of finasteride to occur. This drug affects the results of PSA testing; however, it is possible to continue PSA testing to detect and monitor cancer. The PSA level must be multiplied by two to obtain a true reading.

Blockers

Selective agents such as doxazosin, tamsulosin, and terazosin relax the smooth muscle of the prostate and bladder neck, thereby reducing urethral obstruction. Symptom relief, especially increased urine flow rate, often occurs within hours, but the full effects may not be felt for 4 to 6 weeks.

Muscarinic Receptor Antagonists

Tolterodine tartrate helps increase bladder control. It can be given alone or with the aforementioned two classes of drugs. Tolterodine has a good safety profile, but it should be used with caution in patients with narrow-angle glaucoma, gastrointestinal obstructive disorders, or clinically significant bladder outflow obstruction.

Patient Teaching

The patient should be instructed to avoid drugs that can exacerbate symptoms or increase retention, including sedatives, alcohol, and over-the-counter cold, allergy, or sleeping pills. The patient should also be taught to report any signs and symptoms of UTI, hematuria, and worsening of retention.

Surgical Interventions

Prostate surgery provides the best chance for symptom improvement. New, less invasive procedures are being used. Data are not sufficient to predict the safety and efficacy of some of the newer procedures.

Balloon dilatation of the prostatic urethra may provide temporary relief. Symptoms often recur within 2 years. This procedure is simple, short, and less expensive than the others. It can be done on an outpatient basis with topical or local anesthesia.

Laser prostatectomy shows promise, but its benefits, risks, and long-term effectiveness are unclear. Laser probes are inserted into the urethra to ablate or vaporize prostatic tissue. This quick procedure has few side effects, but significant urinary tract irritation may occur.

Electrovaporization of the prostate (EVP) is a radiofrequency technique. A generator delivers energy to a roller at the end of a catheter. Once inserted into the urethra, the roller vaporizes and desiccates the prostate tissue. Self-limiting light hematuria is the most common complication, but this typically resolves within 24 hours.

Transurethral needle ablation (TUNA) uses needles selectively deployed from a catheter's shielded tip into prostatic tissue. Low-level radio frequency energy sent to the needles produce necrotic lesions that reduce prostate mass. Self-limiting transient mild hematuria and dysuria have been reported, but urinary flow rate is greatly improved.

Other laser surgeries include transurethral ultrasound-guided laser-induced prostatectomy (TULIP), transurethral laser ablation of the prostate (TULAP), visual laser ablation of the prostate (VLAP), and endoscopic laser ablation of the prostate (ELAP). These techniques are associated with shorter procedure time and shorter hospitalization than some of the other procedures. Very little bleeding has been reported.

Transurethral microwave thermotherapy (TUMT) is one of the newest procedures and is frequently used in emergency situations. TUMT uses high- or low-energy thermotherapy and can be performed as an outpatient procedure with no anesthesia. The procedure results in a significant increase in urine flow rate, decreased postvoid residual, and decreased nocturia. Mild side effects include occasional bladder spasms, self-limiting hematuria, dysuria, and retention.

Transurethral resection of the prostate (TURP) is the standard BPH surgical procedure. A resectoscope is passed through the urethra to the bladder neck, and an electric cutting loop is used to resect the enlarged tissue. After resection, a large (18–22 French) three-way indwelling catheter with a 30-mL balloon containing 30 to 60 mL of sterile water is placed to provide hemostasis and facilitate urinary drainage. The bladder is irrigated, either continuously or intermittently, for the first 24 hours to prevent obstruction from mucus and blot clots. TURP does not remove all prostatic tissue, and thus hyperplasia may recur. Self-limiting hematuria and urinary incontinence are common side effects. Most men experience retrograde ejaculation and some may have erectile dysfunction.

Transurethal incision of the prostate (TUIP) is similar to TURP but instead of removing tissue, small incisions are made in the prostate to relieve urethral pressure. TUIP tends to be underused even though it has lower morbidity and ejaculatory dysfunction rates than TURP. There is a short operating time, no fluid absorption, shorter hospitalization, and little self-limiting bleeding with this procedure.

Open prostatectomy is the most invasive procedure and is used in patients with very large prostates (more than 30 grams). This procedure involves removal of the entire prostate through a low abdominal incision. The risks are the same as for any patient undergoing major surgery. A prophylactic vasectomy may be done to decrease the risk of epididymitis.

Postsurgical Management

After surgery, the patient is monitored closely for complications, such as hemorrhage, infection, deep vein thrombosis, urinary catheter obstruction, and urinary bladder spasm. After any prostatectomy, the three-way urinary catheter is left in place until the urine appears clear. Continuous irrigation facilitates drainage and is maintained to keep urine pink-tinged. The catheter and drainage tube are checked frequently to prevent kinking. Additional irrigation of the catheter may be necessary if blockage occurs.

Inability to irrigate the catheter, blood or urine expressed from the catheter–eatal junction, and patient restlessness are usually signs of bladder spasm related to irrigation, clots, presence of the catheter, and/or the surgical procedure. If gentle irrigation is needed, 50 mL of irrigating fluid is used at a time. The amount of fluid recovered in the drainage bag must equal the amount of fluid injected. To relieve pain and decrease spasms, instruct the patient in relaxation techniques such as deep breathing exercises and distraction therapy or visual imagery and give prescribed belladonna and opium suppositories or other pain medications as ordered.

Discharge Teaching

Discharge instructions are very important to prevent complications. The patient needs to know that he may have bloody urine for up to 2 weeks. Frank bleeding, decreased urinary stream, difficulty voiding, elevated temperature, chills, or flank pain must be reported to the health care provider. Home care should include taking showers instead of baths to reduce the possibility of infection. The patient should be instructed to avoid strenuous exercise or heavy lifting (anything over 20 pounds). He should refrain from intercourse for at least 3 weeks or as directed. Likewise, he should avoid straining at stool by increasing fiber, water intake, and mild exercise to prevent constipation. A follow-up visit should be scheduled at the time of discharge.

COMMUNITY CARE
Assessment

Conduct digital rectal examinations of the prostate as part of an annual physical checkup every year after age 40.

The PSA blood screening test is recommended annually for men beginning at age 50. The PSA can be elevated in men with prostate cancer and symptomatic BPH; therefore, it should not be used without other diagnostic methods.

Monitoring

Monitor symptoms and evaluate the patient's tolerance of symptoms when treated with medications. Monitor blood pressure closely in patients receiving blocker drugs.

Evaluate the AUA symptom index periodically to follow the patient's progress and to detect evidence of increased symptoms.

If the patient is discharged with a catheter in place, assist him with postoperative catheter care.

Prevention

Educate elderly men about the possibility of BPH as they age, and encourage them to seek medical attention. Stress the importance of annual DREs for early detection of BPH and to rule out cancer.

 PROGNOSIS

Because BPH is a progressive disease, the patient must be evaluated annually. Continual review of treatment modalities and side effects of medications or treatment is necessary. Most patients respond well to surgery and experience relief from symptoms. With the exception of open prostatectomy, some prostate tissue remains and may continue to grow. Thus, about 10% of patients may require repeat surgery if regrowth leads to urethral strictures or if bladder neck contractures develop.

 CLINICAL PEARLS

○ A three-way catheter is used for closed bladder irrigation; one lumen is for inflation of the retention balloon, one lumen is for urine drainage, and one lumen is for infusing irrigant.

○ Do not slow a continuous irrigation without specific orders, signs of bladder distention, or a plugged catheter.

○ Always record, on an intake and output record, the amount of irrigant infused and the amount of drainage. Subtract the infused amount from the output to determine the urine output. The drainage must always equal or exceed the amount of output.

○ The bladder normally feels full when it contains 300 mL of urine. If a prescribed amount of irrigant is not ordered, do not infuse more than 150 mL of irrigant.

○ A confused patient may interpret the feeling of bladder irrigation as the need to urinate. Instruct the patient about the purpose of a catheter and warn him not to pull it out.

○ Be sure the irrigant is at least room temperature, preferably body temperature, to prevent bladder spasm.

○ Inform the patient that because some prostatic tissue remains after all surgical procedures except open prostatectomy, and this tissue can possibly regenerate and become malignant, annual prostatic examinations must be continued.

NURSING PROBLEM/ DIAGNOSIS	NURSING INTERVENTIONS CLASSIFICATION (NIC)
Risk for postsurgical hemorrhage	Bleeding precautions Bladder irrigation Fluid monitoring
Risk for postsurgical infection Risk for postsurgical bladder spasms	Infection protection Analgesic administration Bladder irrigation Urinary retention care Tube care: urinary

Pelvic Inflammatory Disease

Section 2   Cecilia Tiller

 OVERVIEW

PID is the most severe complication of STDs in women. More than 1 million cases of PID occur each year, making it one of the most prevalent debilitating diseases in women. Patients at highest risk are young non-white women of lower socioeconomic status who have multiple sexual partners. Short-term complications include tubo-ovarian abscess and perihepatitis (Fitz-Hugh-Curtis syndrome); long-term sequelae include chronic pelvic pain, infertility, and ectopic pregnancy. Some cases of PID can be treated in a health care provider's office, but other cases require immediate hospitalization and possible surgical intervention. The increasing incidence of STDs in adolescents has put this age group at high risk for PID.

 PATHOPHYSIOLOGY

PID describes any combination of upper genital tract infections, including endometritis (uterus), salpingitis (fallopian tubes), and oophoritis (ovaries). The disease can be acute, recurrent, or chronic. The infection results from organisms that ascend from the vagina or cervix. Commonly implicated organisms include alpha streptococci, *Chlamydia trachomatis, Escherichia coli, Neisserian gonorrhea,* mycoplasma, and anaerobic organisms such as bacteroides (gram-negative, anaerobic, pleomorphic rods). The two most commonly identified causative organisms continue to be chlamydia and *N. gonorrhoeae.*

PID usually results from a vaginal infection that was either not treated or inadequately treated, or from an antibiotic-resistant strain of microorganism. Severe pelvic pain does not occur until the infection has spread from the cervix through the lymphatics into the parametria and fallopian tubes. This process may not develop until weeks or months after initial exposure to an infection. Once a woman has experienced an initial episode of PID, she is at increased risk for recurrent or chronic disease, even without reinfection with a sexually transmitted pathogen.

Acute salpingitis (infection of the fallopian tube) is often bilateral; however, one side may be more involved than the other. The infection causes scarring of the fallopian tubes, which increases the risk of infertility and ectopic pregnancy. Investigators have found the presence of chlamydia DNA in the fallopian tubes of infertile women who have never had a clinical episode of PID; thus asymptomatic PID may be caused by chlamydia.

Along with ectopic pregnancy and infertility, a woman with PID is at risk for recurrent PID and chronic pelvic or back pain. About 25% of patients with PID experience a subsequent pelvic infection. An episode of PID increases a woman's chance of having an ectopic pregnancy by a factor of 7 to 10. Recurrent infections increase the risk of infertility. Pelvic infections also result in chronic pelvic pain.

 ## SIGNS AND SYMPTOMS

The symptoms that usually bring the woman to a health care provider include acute pelvic pain; vague, nonspecific pelvic pain; or lower back pain. The pain may be mild and intermittent, increasing slowly over a period of weeks or severe and debilitating with an abrupt onset of a few hours or days. Women with endometritis may complain of increased vaginal discharge and intermenstrual bleeding and have uterine tenderness only on bimanual examination. In a woman with more severe pain, systemic symptoms, such as constipation, nausea, vomiting, diarrhea, flank pain, dyspareunia (painful intercourse), menometrorrhagia (excessive uterine bleeding at and between menstrual periods), and dysuria may occur. She may or may not have vaginal discharge. If discharge occurs, she may also report vaginal tenderness, itching, burning on urination, and/or vulvar pain.

 ## DIAGNOSTIC CRITERIA

The clinical diagnosis of PID is challenging because the upper reproductive tract structures are difficult to palpate. A thorough patient history, including a sexual history and inquiry about previous STD, is necessary. A physical examination with a complete pelvic examination is imperative. The pelvic exam may reveal purulent cervical discharge, friability of the cervix, cervical motion tenderness, or adnexal tenderness (pain in the area of the uterus on palpation). There may also be edema, erythema, and excoriation of the perineal area. Pap smear and cultures should be taken. A vaginal wet smear and endocervical Gram stain should be done. Tests for chlamydia and gonorrhea should be taken from the cervix. There is poor correlation between cervical and fallopian tube sampling and PID; however, a negative gonorrhea or chlamydia test result does not rule out the possibility of sexually transmitted PID. If an intrauterine device (IUD) is in place, it should be removed. Care should be taken to rule out other processes, such as appendicitis, acute pyelonephritis, or ureteral stones. All young sexually active women who present with lower abdominal pain must be tested for STDs and evaluated for PID with a thorough speculum and bimanual examination.

The clinical examination and history provide the basis for the diagnosis of PID. The health care provider should be aware that misdiagnosis is likely, and the woman should be reexamined within 48 to 72 hours after initial treatment. Criteria for a presumptive diagnosis for PID include:

- Recent history of lower abdominal pain
- Pain reproduced by palpation of the endometrium and/or fallopian tubes
- Cervical motion tenderness
- Evidence of lower genital tract infection

Systemic signs such as elevated temperature, elevated ESR, and leukocytosis increase the specificity of the diagnosis but are not found in many cases of PID.

INTERVENTIONS

Because PID is a polymicrobial syndrome and the results of cervical sampling are not highly predictive of microbiologic etiology, all women with PID must be treated with a regimen that covers all the major STD pathogens as well as the anaerobic bacteria.

PID may be treated on an outpatient basis if the patient is nontoxic and reliable. These women should be advised to rest for 2 to 3 days until the pain subsides. Sexual intercourse should be avoided for at least 2 weeks. Pain medications may be necessary; however, acetaminophen (Tylenol) or ibuprofen (Motrin) may be just as effective as narcotics.

Infertility specialists recommend that women who desire future pregnancies be hospitalized for PID treatment. Adolescents, patients with nausea and vomiting, or those who have adnexal masses should be hospitalized. Women who do not show significant improvement within 48 to 72 hours should also be hospitalized for further evaluation and treatment.

Women with PID need to be educated about the potential risk of infertility. It is critical that they comply with full treatment and avoid reinfection. The male partner, although often asymptomatic, also should be treated with a regimen effective against gonorrhea and chlamydia. Patients and their partners should be educated about safe sex practices and consequences of PID. All patients with vaginitis or pelvic pain should be advised to avoid douches, irritating soaps, bubble baths, and genital deodorants because they are irritating to the vaginal mucosa which increases the risk for STDs and/or masks STD symptoms. Table 26-2-1 lists medications used to treat PID.

Table 26-2-1. Medications for Pelvic Inflammatory Disease

LIKELY MICROBIOLOGY	THERAPY	COMMENTS
Gonococcus (gram-negative diplococcus) Chlamydia (gram-negative bacterium) Bacteroides (gram-negative, anaerobic, rod-shaped bacteria) Enteric gram-negative (found in the small intestine)	Outpatient: Ceftriaxone 250 mg IM plus 100 mg doxycycline PO bid for 14 days or azithromycine 500 mg for 1 day, then 250 mg for 4 days Inpatient: Cefotetan 2 g every 12 hours IV plus 100 mg doxycycline bid for 14 days	Candidates for outpatient therapy are those with temperature <38°C, WBC <11,000 mm^3, and no indication of peritonitis.

COMMUNITY CARE

Assessment

Screen at-risk groups for gonorrhea, chlamydia, HIV, and other STDs. Individuals who test positive should be referred for further services and should be counseled about risky behaviors and safer sex practices.

Inquire about sexual practices, use of condoms, and number of sexual partners.

Monitoring

Perform follow-up examinations to determine clinical improvement and evaluate effectiveness of treatment for STDs. Screen sexual partners for STDs.

Teach women to follow the treatment regimen, to avoid sexual activity during treatment, and to return immediately if other symptoms develop.

Prevention

Teach safe sex practices to all females age 9 and older in a realistic and nonjudgmental way. Encourage the use of condoms or suggest that women use a diaphragm and nonoxynol-9 spermicidal jelly, which offers some protection from gonorrhea and chlamydia if used correctly; remember, however, this does not prevent HIV.

Inform sexually active individuals that screening is done for public protection as well as early treatment.

 PROGNOSIS

Of an average of 1.2 million visits to a private physician's office each year, about 34% are for PID. Nearly all of the visits (95%) are made by women of childbearing age. Despite all the public awareness of STDs, some women continue to place themselves at increased risk for infection. Education about the risks and early diagnosis and treatment for an STD may prevent the development of PID. PID may be prevented if an STD is detected early, fully treated, and the patient does not become reinfected. If she does develop PID, early diagnosis and treatment is essential. Even with treatment, the damage to the fallopian tubes may result in infertility and/or ectopic pregnancy. Patient education is critical, and health care providers must be aggressive in educating patients about safe sex practices to decrease the risk for STDs that could lead to PID.

Untreated PID can be life threatening. PID causes adhesions and strictures of the fallopian tubes. Ectopic pregnancy may result from the inability of a fertilized egg to travel through the scarred tube. Pelvic, tubal, and ovarian abscesses may rupture, leading to pelvic or generalized peritonitis. Embolic episodes may follow thrombophlebitis of pelvic veins. Bacterial endotoxin coming from infected areas could result in septic shock.

 CLINICAL PEARLS

○ A recent history of acute lower genital tract infection with pain and tenderness in both lower quadrants, especially with cervical motion, is often indicative of PID.

○ Leukocyte count and erythrocyte sedimentation rates are usually elevated, indicating the presence of an infection.

○ A complete STD workup should be completed, with cultures for gonorrhea and chlamydia and Gram stains for other bacteria taken from the vagina and cervix.

○ Instruct the patient to take all medications, avoid intercourse and douching, restrict general activities, get adequate rest and nutrition, and return to the health care provider in 48 to 72 hours if symptoms persist or increase.

○ If outpatient treatment is not successful or if the patient is acutely ill or in severe pain, hospital admission is needed for intravenous antibiotic therapy and evaluation for surgery.

○ Surgery is indicated in the advent of residual masses or abscesses that can rupture and cause peritonitis, failure of the patient to respond to conservative treatment, and a history of frequent recurrences. The extent of disease and the age and overall health of the patient guide the choice of surgery.

NURSING PROBLEM/ DIAGNOSIS	NURSING INTERVENTIONS CLASSIFICATION (NIC)
Acute pain	Pain management
Deficient knowledge regarding disease process and treatment	Teaching: disease process Teaching: prescribed medication Teaching: safe sex
Risk for infertility, pelvic abscess, ectopic pregnancy, or septic shock	Infection protection

Sexually Transmitted Diseases

Section 3   Cecilia Tiller

 OVERVIEW

Sexually transmitted disease (STD) is a term used to cover all diseases transmitted through sexual activity. These diseases can be caused by more than 25 infectious bacterial or viral organisms. The incidence of STDs has increased over the last few years despite the emphasis on safe sex practices to prevent human immunodeficiency virus (HIV). The Centers for Disease Control reported that people under age 25 account for two-thirds of the estimated 13 million people in the United States who acquire an STD each year. As many as 3 million adolescents acquire an STD, which means that one of every eight adolescents age 13 to 19 years will have an STD. Estimates indicate that 25% of adolescents will develop an STD by the time they graduate from high school. Despite decreased incidence of some STDs, other STDs are showing increases to the point where the United States once again has epidemics of STDs—everything from genital herpes to HIV to human papillomaviruses. A complicating factor is that today, health care providers are faced with antibiotic-resistant strains of organisms causing STDs.

 PATHOPHYSIOLOGY

The pathology of STDs depends on the causative organism (Table 26-3-1). Each organism has an incubation period before symptoms become apparent; *Text continued on page 875*

Table 26-3-1. Sexually Transmitted Diseases: Causative Organisms, Signs and Symptoms, and Treatments

DISEASE/DESCRIPTION	CAUSATIVE ORGANISM	SIGNS AND SYMPTOMS	TREATMENTS
Chancroid a soft nonsyphilitic venereal sore	*Hemophilus ducreyi*	Painful ulcer with tender inguinal adenopathy	Single dose therapy with azithromycin orally or ceftriaxone IM, or 7-day therapy with erythromycin base or amoxicillin. Ciprofloxacin orally for 3 days is an alternative.
Herpes **Genital Herpes** herpes simplex	Herpes virus hominis (HSV-1 and HSV-2); most genital herpes are caused by HSV-2	Viral disease that may be recurrent and has no cure. Painful red ulcers that eventually scab and heal. Highly contagious when vesicles rupture. Accompanying symptoms include dysuria, pain, fever, edema, and bilateral inguinal lymphadenopathy.	Acyclovir orally for 7–10 days or until clinical resolution is attained. Oral analgesics may be required.
Lymphogranuloma Venereum an STD that affects genital lymph glands	Chlamydia trachomati	Small vesicle that progresses to ulceration and lymphatic involvement. May have proctocolitis or inflammatory involvement of perirectal or perianal lymphatic tissue resulting in fistulas and strictures.	Doxycycline orally, or sulfisoxazole orally for 21 days.
Primary and Secondary Syphilis a highly contagious STD. Formerly called lues.	*Treponemia pallidum*	Primary: Chancre—a painless ulcer. May have painless swelling of lymph glands near the ulceration. Symptoms appear 9 days to 3 months after exposure. Secondary: Maculopapular rash, mucocutaneous lesions, and adenopathy. Large elevated plaques (Condylomata lata) may develop. Flu-like symptoms. Symptoms 2 to 6 months after primary sores disappear.	Benzathine penicillin G, IM in a single dose Doxycycline orally for 2 weeks for penicillin allergy. Secondary syphilis should be treated with doxycycline or tetracycline orally for 2 weeks.

Table continued on following page

871

Table 26-3-1. Sexually Transmitted Diseases: Causative Organisms, Signs and Symptoms, and Treatments *Continued*

DISEASE/DESCRIPTION	CAUSATIVE ORGANISM	SIGNS AND SYMPTOMS	TREATMENTS
Nongonococcal Urethris inflammation of the urethra not caused by gonorrhea	*Chlamydia trachomatis* (23%–55% of cases) *Ureaplasma urealyticum* (20%–40% of cases) *Trichomonas vaginalis* (2%–5% of cases)	May be asymptomatic, mucoid, or purulent urethral discharge. Signs and symptoms of a urinary tract infection.	Doxycycline orally for 7 days with erythromycin base or erythromycin ethylsuccinate orally for 7 days as alternatives.
Chlamydia a widespread, gram-negative nonmotile bacteria	*Chalmydia trachomatis*	Frequently asymptomatic. May have a yellowish mucopurulent cervicitis. Cervix may be erythematous and edematous. May have symptoms of vaginal irritation, pruritus, and burning with urination.	Doxycycline orally for 7 days, or azithromycin orally in a single dose. Alternatives include: Ofloxacin, erythromycin base, erythromycin ethylsuccinate, or sulfisoxazole.
Uncomplicated Gonococcal Infections a highly contagious bacterial infection	*Neisseria gonorrhoeae*	May be asymptomatic. Greenish, purulent discharge with symptoms of dysuria, urinary frequency, pruritus, burning and pain, swelling, and in women, abnormal uterine bleeding. Often found with chlamydia. At risk for PID.	Single dose therapy with ceftriaxone IM, or cefixime orally, or ciprofloxacin orally, or ofloxacin orally. Plus, doxycycline orally for possible coinfection with C trachomatis.
Bacterial Vaginosis any variety of nonspecific bacterial infections	Nonspecific. Likely pathogens: *Gardnerella* vaginalis, *Bacteroides*, *Streptococcus*-related gram-positive cocci, *Mycoplasma homonis*, or changes in normal *Lactobacillus*	Vaginal odor that increases with sexual intercourse. May be asymptomatic. May have mild to moderate clear to gray thin, bubbly discharge. Rarely complains of dysuria or dyspareunia. May not be a true STD but number of cases becoming epidemic. Only treat symptomatic women.	Metronidazole orally in a single dose or for 7 days (note: patients should be advised to avoid using alcohol during treatment with metronidazole and for 24 hours thereafter to avoid a disulfiram-type reaction) The following alternatives have been effective in clinical trials, although experience is limited. Clindamycin cream or orally. Metronidazole gel, 0.75%.

Condition	Organism / Clinical Features	Treatment
Trichomoniasis a genus of flagellated protozoan parasite	*Trichomonas vaginalis* Profuse, thin, frothy, gray to yellowish discharge, with a fishy odor. Causes pruritus, dyspareunia, and dysuria. Female may have vaginal wall erythema, vaginal erosions, and occasionally a "strawberry cervix." Both partners must be treated.	Recommended regimen Metronidazole 2 g orally in a single dose Alternative regimen Metronidazole 500 mg twice daily for 7 days
Vulvovaginal Candidiasis infection by a fungi (yeast)	*Candida albicans* Marked itching, watery to cottage cheese-thick discharge. Vaginal erythema, dyspareunia, erythema, and swelling of labia and vulva. Symptoms may exacerbate week before menses. Males: transient rash, erythema, pruritus or burning. Balanitis. Frequent recurrence and unresolved cases are suspicious of HIV and/or diabetes.	Therapy involves intravaginal formulations from the azole family. Butoconazole, Clotrimazole, Miconazole, Tioconazole, Terconazole, or Fluconazole (Diflucan), the only azole that is taken orally for the treatment of VVC.
Pelvic Inflammatory Disease	See Chapter 26, Section 2	
Epididymitis inflammation of the epididymis	Men <35 years old; *Neisseria gonorrhoeae, Chlamydia trachomatis,* or *Escherichia coli* Men >35 years old; gram-negative enteric organisms. Unilateral testicular pain and tenderness, and palpable swelling of the epididymis. Chills, fever and malaise with scrotal swelling so great that it interferes with ambulation.	Ceftriaxone IM in a single dose, plus doxycycline orally for 10 days. Alternative regimen—ofloxacin orally for 10 days

Table continued on following page

873

Table 26-3-1. Sexually Transmitted Diseases: Causative Organisms, Signs and Symptoms, and Treatments *Continued*

DISEASE/DESCRIPTION	CAUSATIVE ORGANISM	SIGNS AND SYMPTOMS	TREATMENTS
Genital, Perianal or Oral Warts any subgroup of the papouaviruses causing papiflomata (warts). They may appear on the perineum, in the vagina, in the urethral meatus, on the penis, on and in the rectum and anus, or in the mouth.	Human Papillomavirus (HPV). HPV types 6 or 11 most common. Other types (16, 18, 31, 33, and 35) more associated with genital dysplasia and carcinoma	Benign growths that cause minor or no symptoms aside from their cosmetic appearance. Whitish, pinkish, or brownish papules with a characteristic verraceous, cauliflower-like surface. No therapy completely eradicates HPV. May have recurrences. Some may have itching and tenderness of tissue around lesion. Women with history of HPV should have regular Pap smears because HPV is associated with cervical dysplasia and cancer.	Cryotherapy with liquid nitrogen or cryoprobe, or podofilox 0.5% solution for self-treatment (genital warts only). Applied with a cotton swab to warts twice daily for 3 days, followed by 4 days of no therapy. This cycle may be repeated as necessary for a total of 4 cycles. Contraindicated during pregnancy. or Podophyllin 10%–25%, in compound tincture of benzoin. The use of podophyllin is contraindicated during pregnancy. or Trichloracetic acid (TCA) 80%–90%
Genital Herpes Herpes simplex of the genitals	Herpes simplex virus 1 or 2 (HSV-1 or HSV-2) HSV-2 most common	Asymptomatic shedding to multiple, painful ulcers or atypical, minor lesions. Primary infections most severe. Severe vulvar pain and dysuria. Shallow ulcers with a pink base have clear and watery exudate, and an erythematous border. Will have painful, unilateral, inguinal lympadenopathy, fever, headaches, myalgia, photophobia, and meningismus. Recurrent HSV is similar, may start with a tingling feeling. Men are usually asymptomatic	Both primary HSV and recurrent HSV are treated with acyclovir. Oral analgesics may be required.
Human Immunodeficiency Virus (HIV)	See Chapter 12, Section 1.		

however, many diseases are easily transmitted to others before they become noticed in the individual. The stigma associated with STDs makes them difficult to talk about with a partner or a health care provider. Because many of the diseases develop without causing outward symptoms, millions of carriers may not know that they are infected. Although most of the STDs are not fatal, they can cause significant morbidity from secondary and more complicated problems, such as PID, infertility, and increased risk for cancer. Most STDs are curable with timely diagnosis and treatment.

 SIGNS AND SYMPTOMS

The signs and symptoms depend on the causative organism (see Table 26-3-1). Vulvar or penile itching with or without a discharge may be the main symptom bringing the patient to the health care provider. Characteristic vaginal or penile discharge and odor help classify the disease. Many STDs are asymptomatic, but even when symptoms occur, distinguishing among the different infections may be difficult.

Bacterial vaginosis, formerly known as *Haemophilus* and *Gardnerella*, and vaginal candidiasis are not classified as STDs, although they are both considered the most common causes of vaginitis. Both infections can be found in male sexual partners, and a contributing factor is intercourse with an uncircumsized male. For recurrent or resistant infections, the sexual partner should be evaluated and treated.

 DIAGNOSTIC CRITERIA

History should include the onset of the discharge, its appearance, amount, odor (if any), and any associated symptoms. The relation of the discharge to phase of the menstrual cycle, coitus, and use of medications (especially antibiotics) should be noted. Details about associated symptoms, such as dysuria, pruritus, pain, dyspareunia (painful intercourse), and skin rash provide additional information.

A detailed sexual history is necessary to determine the risk for STDs. The greater the patient's number of sexual partners, the greater the risk for STDs. Questions should be asked about possible exposure to STDs and whether the patient's partner has a complaint of itching, discharge, or lesion(s).

The patient should be asked about the use of foreign bodies, bubble baths, soaps, or genital deodorants. Known allergies need to be reviewed in conjunction with the use of spermicidal preparations and douches. A history of previous infection, diabetes, or recent use of antibiotics or corticosteroids should be considered in a search for alterations in vaginal flora or host defenses. Any self-treatment should be carefully investigated, because antifungal medications are now readily available without prescription.

Physical examination begins with careful inspection of the penis or vulva and vaginal canal for evidence of lesions, discharge, erythema, atrophy, or prolapse. During vaginal speculum examination, the surface of the cervix should be carefully examined for lesions, erosion, erythema, or friability. The color, consistency, pH, and odor of discharge can provide useful clues to the etiology. The bimanual examination on the female should be used to check for tenderness on cervical motion and for adnexal and uterine masses. Palpation for bilateral inguinal nodes should be conducted on both genders. Males need to have testicular examinations.

Laboratory Studies

Wet mount examination of discharge is simple and potentially diagnostic. This examination is about 25% effective in detecting trichomonads (trichomonas), 90% effective for clue cells (bacterial vaginosis), 40% to 80% for hyphe (candida), and about 85% effective in detecting increased number of lactobacilli (chlamydia).

Gram stains are more sensitive than wet mounts in detecting up to 95% for trichomonads. Gram stains also help to more clearly identify the lactobacilli of chlamydia. It is considered positive for gonorrhea when biscuit-shaped gram-negative diplococci are seen within polymorphonuclear leukocytes. The sensitivity is greater than 95% in symptomatic males and 50% to 60% in those with asymptomatic urethral infection.

Complete blood count is indicated if pelvic pain or dysuria is present, to rule out other infection or concurrent condition.

Screening tests for syphilis are the Venereal Disease Research Laboratories test (VDRL), the rapid plasma reagin test (RPR), and the automated reagin test (ART). These tests are readily available, fast, inexpensive, and sensitive. A positive result should be confirmed by the fluorescent treponemal antibody absorption (FTA-ABS) test or the microhemagglutination assay for antibodies to *T. pallidum* (MHA-TP). When an STD is suspected, blood should be drawn and tested for syphilis and to rule out hepatitis B, syphilis, and/or AIDS/HIV. A fasting blood sugar may be necessary, because women with diabetes are more prone to candida.

Urinalysis should be obtained to check for pyuria and bacteriuria, especially if there is concurrent dysuria or flank pain. Rapid urine tests have been developed to test for chlamydia and gonorrhea. Their sensitivity ranges from 46% to 100% and specificity ranges from 85% to 100%. These tests are quick, noninvasive, and useful for screening patients.

Cultures remain the gold standard for identifying gonorrhea and chlamydia. In all individuals with suspected sexual abuse, cultures must be obtained for gonorrhea and chlamydia. Chlamydia cultures have a sensitivity of 70% to 90% and a specificity nearing 100%. DNA probes, including the Gen-Probe PACE system (direct chemiluminescent DNA probe test), has a sensitivity of 90% to 97%. A distinct advantage of the Gen-Probe PACE system is the ability to test simultaneously using the same swab for both chlamydia and gonorrhea. Polymerase chain reaction tests are also useful and have a 79% sensitivity and 96% specificity for gonorrhea. Diagnosis of chancroid can be made from cultures (80% sensitivity) as can herpes simplex virus (HSV), which has a 27% to 94% sensitivity depending on the stage of vesicles.

A *Papanicolaou (Pap) smear* should be done on all women although it will most likely be abnormal in the presence of inflammation. It is very important to rule out cervical cancer, especially since human papilloma virus (HPV) has been linked with cervical cancer. The Pap smear is also 40% to 50% sensitive for HSV. In patients with obvious infection, it may be reasonable to defer the Pap test until the vaginitis or cervicitis has been treated.

 INTERVENTIONS

Once the causative organism has been identified, the patient is treated with specific antibiotics. It is best to go ahead and begin treating the patient before definitive results are back than to try to get the patient to return for treatment. Some of the dosages are one-time-only, which makes treatment effective and efficient. See Table 26-3-1 for more information on medical management.

Over-the-counter (OTC) medications for vaginal yeast infections are now available. Their labels clearly state that if the woman has never been diagnosed with a yeast infection, then she should consult a health care provider first. OTC treatments give women some control and relief and they can effectively treat several yeast infections in 1 year, yet the underlying cause may go undiagnosed. This can occur in HIV infection or in diabetes. Women should not self-treat yeast infections more than twice a year without seeking advice from a health care provider for diagnosis of underlying causes. The immediate danger to an incorrect self-diagnosis is the risk of PID, pyelonephritis, or other STDs. Yeast can be resistant to OTC medications, and the woman's partner may require treatment.

 ## COMMUNITY CARE

Safe sex education for adolescents and every patient treated for an STD is critical. However, the incidence of STDs continues to increase despite the emphasis placed on safe sex as a precaution. Some of the contraceptive foams provide some protection from STDs. Young women taking oral contraceptives must be encouraged to continue to use condoms for STD protection. Condoms generally provide fairly good protection; however, they are not entirely fool-proof.

Diagnoses of gonorrhea, syphilis, and HIV/AIDS must be reported to the public health department. Other STDs are not yet reported, but probably should be. STDs do not discriminate; one cannot tell if another person is infected by how clean or nice he or she appears. Any individual having unprotected sex needs to be tested for STDs.

 ## PROGNOSIS

With early diagnosis and treatment, most STDs can be cured with a single dose of antibiotics. A delay in diagnosis and treatment can increase the risk of complications and transmission of the disease to others. Infection with one STD suggests the possibility of concurrent infections with others. The possibility of HIV infection should be investigated with any STD diagnosis.

If left untreated, STDs can lead to serious complications. One example is tertiary syphilis, a slowly progressive inflammatory disease that affects multiple organs. The most common sequelae are aortitis and neurosyphilis, which leads to dementia, psychosis, paresis, stroke, or meningitis. STDs in women are especially serious, because many can develop into PID, which contributes to infertility. Recurrent, nonresponding candida is frequently found with AIDS, and vaginal warts are associated with cervical dysplasia and cancer.

Underreporting and undertreating of STDs is a problem. Explicit patient education is critical for anyone diagnosed with an STD. Because chlamydia has become the most common STD, experts recommend that sexually active women age 20 or younger be screened every 6 months and older women with multiple partners be screened once a year. Work continues to improve diagnosis, vaccines, and topical agents to protect against STDs. Until these are developed, safe sex and good screening provide the best protection.

CLINICAL PEARLS

○ Instill erythromycin (0.5%) eye ointment into the eyes of all newborns after delivery to prevent permanent blindness from gonorrheal eye infections (ophthalmia neonatorum) that may be transmitted by an infected mother.

○ Patients taking metronidazole (Flagyl) should avoid alcohol during treatment and for at least 1 day after treatment to prevent a disulfiram-like reaction (flushing, nausea, vomiting, headache, abdominal cramps).

○ Sexual abstinence is encouraged during treatment for all STDs. Condoms may prevent the spread of infection and reinfection if abstinence cannot be maintained.

○ Health care providers have a legal obligation to maintain patient confidentiality unless required by law to report those who pose a risk to the health or life of others.

○ Certain STDs are mandated by law to be reported to the Public Health Departments, including gonorrhea, syphilis, and HIV/AIDS.

NURSING PROBLEM/ DIAGNOSIS	NURSING INTERVENTIONS CLASSIFICATION (NIC)
Deficient knowledge regarding disease process and treatment	Teaching: disease process Teaching: prescribed medication Teaching: safe sex
Risk for HIV and other STDs	Infection protection

Bibliography

1–1

American Nurses Association. (1998a). *Standards of clinical nursing practice* (2nd ed.). Washington, DC: American Nurses Publishing.

American Nurses Association. (1998b). *Legal aspects of standards and guidelines for clinical nursing practice.* Washington, DC: American Nurses Publishing.

Anonymous. (1999). Getting wired to defensive documentation. *Massachusetts Nurse, 69*(8), 12.

Brown, S. M. (1999). Good Samaritan laws: Protections and limits. *RN, 62*(11), 65–68.

Catalano, J. T. (2000). *Nursing now: Today's issues, tomorrow's trends* (2nd ed.). Philadelphia: FA Davis.

Cherry, B., & Jacob, S. R. (1999). *Contemporary nursing: Issues, trends and management.* St. Louis, MO: CV Mosby.

Guido, G. W. (1997). *Legal issues in nursing* (2nd ed.). E. Norwalk, CT: Appleton & Lange.

Iyer, P. W., & Camp, N. H. (1999). *Nursing documentation: A nursing process approach* (3rd ed.). St. Louis, MO: CV Mosby.

Lancaster, J. (1999). *Nursing issues in leading and managing change.* St. Louis, MO: CV Mosby.

Mastering documentation (2nd ed.). (1999). Springhouse, PA: Springhouse Corporation.

Nursing Practice Guideline Documentation. (2000). (Online). Available at: *http://www.rnabc.bc.ca/practice/334.htm.*

Sullivan, E. J. (1999). *Creating nursing's future: Issues, opportunities and challenges.* St. Louis, MO: CV Mosby.

Twiname, B. G., & Boyd, S. M. (1999). *Student nurse handbook: Difficult concepts made easy.* E. Norwalk, CT: Appleton & Lange.

1–2

Kennedy, M. S., & Zolot, Z. S. (2000). New focus on systolic blood pressure. *American Journal of Nursing, 100* (8), 18.

Leahy, J., & Kizalay, P. (1998). *Foundations of nursing practice: A nursing process approach.* Philadelphia: WB Saunders.

Potter, P. A., & Perry, A. G. (1997). *Fundamentals of nursing: Concepts, process and practice* (4th ed.). St. Louis, MO: CV Mosby.

Seidel, H. M., et al. (1999). *Mosby's guide to physical examination* (4th ed.). St. Louis, MO: CV Mosby.

Sixth Joint National Committee on Prevention. (1997). Detection, evaluation and treatment of high blood pressure. *Archives of Internal Medicine, 157,* 2413–2446.

Taylor, C., Lillis, C., & LeMone, P. (1997). *Fundamentals of nursing: The art and science of nursing care* (3rd ed.). Philadelphia: JB Lippincott.

1–3

Black, J. M., & Matassarin-Jacobs, S. E. (1997). *Medical-surgical nursing: Clinical management for continuity of care* (5th ed.). Philadelphia: WB Saunders.

Brooks-Brunn, J. A. (1997). *Expert 10-minute physical examinations.* St. Louis, MO: CV Mosby.

Knudston, M. D. (1998). *Assessment made incredibly easy.* Springhouse, PA: Springhouse Corporation.

Langan, J. (1998). Abdominal assessment in the home: From A to Z. *Home Healthcare Nurse, 16*(1), 50–57.

Ludwig, L. (1998). Cardiovascular assessment for home healthcare nurses, part II: Assessing blood pressure and cardiac function. *Home Healthcare Nurse, 16*(8), 547–554.

McCance, K., & Huether, S. (1998). *Pathophysiology: The biologic basis for disease in adults and children* (3rd ed.). St. Louis, MO: CV Mosby.

O'Hannon-Nichols, T. (1998). Basic assessment series: Gastrointestinal system. *American Journal of Nursing, 98*(4), 48–53.

O'Hannon-Nichols, T. (1998). Basic assessment series: The adult pulmonary system. *American Journal of Nursing, 98*(2), 29–45.

1–4

American College of Emergency Physicians. (1997). In P. Pons & D. Cason (Eds.), *Paramedic field care: A complaint-based approach* (pp. 542–544, 586). St. Louis, MO: Mosby-Year Book.

Bledsoe, B. E., Porter, R. S., Shade, B. R. (1997). In R. A. Cherry, B. E. Bledsoe, R. S. Porter, et al., *Brady paramedic emergency care* (3rd ed., pp. 546, 821–828, 874–879). Englewood Cliffs, NJ: Prentice-Hall.

Henry, M. C., & Stapleton, E. R. (1997). In M. C. Henry & E. R. Stapleton, *EMT: Prehospital care* (2nd ed., pp. 386–390). Philadelphia: WB Saunders.

Prehospital Trauma Life Support Committee of the National Association of Emergency Medical Technicians in Cooperation with the Committee on Trauma of the American College of Surgeons. (1999). In J. Roche (Ed.). *PHTLS* (4th ed., pp. xxiv–xxvii, 38–45, 196–199, 243). St. Louis, MO: CV Mosby.

2–1

Anonymous. (2000). Critical care procedures: A guide to pediatric fluid replacement and maintenance. *DCCN—Dimensions of Critical Care Nursing, 19*(4), 24.

Fabian, B. (2000). Intravenous complication: Infiltration. *Journal of Intravenous Nursing, 23*(4), 229–231.

Fox, N. (2000). Managing the risks posed by intravenous therapy. *Nursing Times, 96*(30), 37–39.

Moureau, N., & Zonderman, A. (2000). Does it always have to hurt? Premedications for adults and children for use with intravenous therapy. *Journal of Intravenous Nursing, 23*(4), 213–219.

Seemann, S., Soukup, M., & Adams, P. (2000). Hospital-wide intravenous initiative. *Nursing Clinics of North America, 35*(2), 361–373.

Skokal, W. (2000). IV push at home? *RN, 63*(10), 26–30.

Workman, B. (1999). Peripheral intravenous therapy management. *Nursing Standard, 14*(4), 53–60, 62.

York, J., Arrillaga, A., Graham, R., & Miller, R. (2000). Fluid resuscitation of patients with multiple injuries and severe closed head injury: Experience with an aggressive fluid resuscitation strategy. *Journal of Trauma-Injury, Infection, and Critical Care, 48*(3), 376–380.

2–2

Kim, D. K., Gottesman, M. H., Forero, A., et al. (1998). The CVC removal distress syndrome: An unappreciated complication of central venous catheter removal. *The American Surgeon, 64*, 344–347.

Macklin, D. (2000). Basic IV therapy. Available at: *http://www.ceuzone.com.*

Macklin, D. (2000). Basic IV therapy complications. Available at: *http://www.ceuzone.com.*

Maki, D. G. (1998). *Infusion care strategies across the continuum of care in the new millenium.* Philadelphia: The Jefferson Health System.

Maki, D. G., & Mermel, L. A. (1998). Infections due to infusion therapy. In J. V. Bennett & P. S. Brachman (Eds.), *Hospital infections* (4th ed., pp. 687–724). Philadelphia: Lippincott-Raven.

Mermel, L. A. (2000). Prevention of intravascular catheter-related infections. *Annals of Internal Medicine, 132,* 391–402.

2–3

American Association of Blood Banks. (2000). Circular of information for the use of human blood and blood components. America's blood centers and American Red Cross. ARC Publication No. 1751.

Boley, R. B., & Polaski, A. L. (1997). Structure and function of the hematologic system. In J. M. Black & E. Matassarin-Jacobs (Eds), *Medical surgical nursing clinical management for continuity of care* (5th ed., pp. 1455–1456). Philadelphia: WB Saunders.

Dailey, J. F. (1998). *Blood self-teaching hematology, immunology, and transfusion therapy.* Arlington, MA: Medical Consulting Group.

Hansen, M. (1998). Inflammation, immunity, and related disorders. In M. Hansen, *Pathophysiology, foundations of disease and clinical intervention.* Philadelphia: WB Saunders.

Kaye, J. (1997). Nursing assessments and common hematologic interventions. In L. O. Burrell, M. J. Gerlach, & B. S. Pless (Eds.), *Adult nursing acute and community care* (2nd ed., pp. 555–556). E. Norwalk, CT: Appleton & Lange.

Wright, P. A. (1999). Donor selection and component preparation. In D. M. Harmening (Ed.), *Modern blood banking and transfusion practices.* Philadelphia: FA Davis. Available at: *http://www.cc.nih.gov/nursing/bldprodp.html,* 2000

3–1

Baranoski, S. (2000). Skin tears: The enemy of frail skin. *Advances in skin and wound care. Journal for Prevention and Healing, 13,* 123–126.

Calianno, C. (2000). Assessing and preventing pressure ulcers. *Advances in skin and wound care. Journal for Prevention and Healing, 13*(5), 244–246.

Cuzzell, J. (1999) Interventions for clients with skin problems. In D. D. Ignatavicius, M. L. Workman, & M. A. Mishler (Eds.), *Medical-surgical nursing across the health-care continuum* (3rd ed.). Philadelphia: WB Saunders.

Davies, C. (1999). Cleansing rites and wrongs. *Nursing Times, 95*(43), 71–75.

Groves, R. W., & Schmidt-Lucke, J. A. (2000). Recombinant human GM-CSF in the treatment of poorly healing wounds. *Advances in Skin and Woundcare. The Journal for Prevention and Healing, 13,* 107–112.

Hess, C. T. (2000). When to use alginate dressings. *Advances in Skin and Woundcare. The Journal for Prevention and Healing, 13,* 131.

Hess, C. T. (2000). When to use hydrogel dressings. *Advances in Skin and Woundcare. The Journal for Prevention and Healing, 13,* 42.

Hess, C. T. (2000). When to use transparent films. *Advances in Skin and Woundcare. The Journal for Prevention and Healing, 13,* 202.

Kane, L. H. (2000). Postoperative nursing management. In S. C. Smeltzer & B. G. Bare (Eds.), *Medical-surgical nursing* (9th ed.). Philadelphia: JB Lippincott.

Nayduck, D. A. (1999). Trauma wound management. *Nursing Clinics of North America, 34*(4), 895–906.

Stotts, N. A. (2001). Wound and skin care. In P. L. Swearingen & J. H. Keen (Eds.), *Manual of critical care nursing* (4th ed.). St. Louis: CV Mosby.

3–2

Hak, D. J. (2000). Retained broken wound drains: A preventable complication. *Journal of Orthopedic Trauma, 14*(3), 212–213.

3–3

Brunner, S. C., & Bare, B. G. (2000). *Textbook of medical-surgical nursing* (9th ed., pp. 875–915). Philadelphia: JB Lippincott.

Burrell, L. O., Gerlach, M. J., & Pless, B. S. (1997). Disorders of the small and large intestines and anorectal disorders. In M. J. Gerlach, *Adult nursing: Acute and community care* (Vol. VII, 2nd ed., p. 1419). E. Norwalk, CT: Appleton & Lange.

ConvaTec. (January 1998). A professional's guide for counseling ostomy patients. Internet source.

Handbook of clinical skills. (1997). Colostomy and ileostomy care (pp. 230–237). Springhouse, PA: Springhouse Corporation.

Hollister Incorporated. Ostomy supply pamphlet. January, 1999.

Kozier, B., Erb, G., Blasis, K., & Wilkinson, J. M. (1998). Fecal elimination and urinary elimination. In E. Mulligan, *Fundamentals of nursing: Concepts, process, and practice* (5th ed. pp. 1179 and 1222). Menlo Park, CA: Addison Wesley Longman.

Swearingen, P. L., & Ross, D. G. (1999). *Manual of medical surgical nursing care* (4th ed., pp 457–464). St. Louis: CV Mosby.

United Ostomy Association Internet. Available at: *http://www.uoa.org/chapc1.html*

3–4

Burrell, L. O., Gerlach, M. J. M., & Pless, B. S. (1997). *Adult nursing: Acute and community care* (2nd ed., pp. 1337–1385; 1531–1554). E. Norwalk, CT: Appleton & Lange.

Interventional Radiology. Vascular procedures/non-vascular procedures. Available at: *http://www.ddc.musc.edu/public/test/ir.htm* (7-20-99)

Kozier, B., Erb, G., Blasis, K., & Wilkinson, K. (1998). Nutrition and perioperative nursing. In E. Mulligan & W. Earl, *Fundamentals of nursing: Concepts, process, and practice* (5th ed., pp. 1014–1056; 1397–1421). Menlo Park, CA: Addison Wesley Longman.

Lewis, S., Heitkemper, M., & Dirksen, S. (2000). Medical-surgical nursing: Assessment and management of clinical problems (5th ed., pp. 1136–1190). St. Louis, MO: CV Mosby.

McPhee, A. T. (1997). Handbook of clinical skills (pp. 551–554; 560–566; 878–882). Springhouse, PA: Springhouse Corporation.

O'Brien, B., Davis, S., & Erwin-Toth, P. (1999). G-tube site care: A practical guide. *RN, 62*(2), 52–56.

4–1

Brzana, R. J., & Kock, K. L. (1997). Gastroesophageal reflux disease presenting with intractable nausea. *Annals of Internal Medicine, 126*(9), 704–708.

Cavanaugh, B. M. (1999). Analysis of gastric and duodenal secretions. In B. M. Cavanaugh *Nurses' manual of laboratory and diagnostic tests* (3rd ed., pp. 445–460). Philadelphia: FA Davis.

Clinical toxicology: Position paper (1997). Gastric lavage (AACT/EAPCCT). *Journal of Toxicology, 35*(7), 711–720.

Fischbach, F. (2000). *A manual for laboratory and diagnostic tests* (6th ed.). Philadelphia: JB Lippincott.

Henry, J., & Hoffman, J. R. (1998). Continuing controversy on gut decontamination. *The Lancet, 352* (9126), 420–422.

Jaffe, M. S., & McVan, B. F. (1997). *Laboratory and diagnostic test handbook* (pp. 818–820). Philadelphia: FA Davis.

Knies, R. C. (2000). Research applied to clinical practice: Confirming safe placement of nasogastric tubes. Available at: *Emergency Nursing World, www.enw.org/Research-NGT.html* (Web article).

Perry, A. G., & Potter, P. A. (1998). *Clinical nursing skills and techniques* (4th ed., pp. 1228–1231; 1244–1246). St. Louis: CV Mosby.

Thorsby, S. (1997). Methods of gastric decontamination. *Nursing Times, 93*(21), 49–52.

4–2

Bell, G. D., & Chow, E. (1997). Double take: A case of drug-induced green urine? *Consultant, 37*(1), 70.

Burr, R. G., & Nusebeh, I. M. (1997). Urinary catheter blockage on urine pH, calcium and rate of flow. *Spinal Cord, 35*(8), 521–525.

Capon, D. (1997). Urinalysis and the practice of herbal medicine. *Journal of Australia-Traditional Medical Society, 3*(1), 11–14.

Chernecky, C., & Berger, B. (2000). *Laboratory tests and diagnostic procedures* (3rd ed.). Philadelphia: WB Saunders.

Jackson, B., & Hicks, L. E. (1997). Effect of cranberry juice on urinary pH in old adults. *Home Healthcare Nurse, 15*(3), 198–202.

Labuhn, K., Valanis, B., Schoeny, R., et al. (1998). Nurses' and pharmacists' exposure to antineoplastic drugs: Findings from industrial hygiene scan and urine mutagenicity tests. *Cancer Nursing, 21*(2), 79–89.

Lewis, J. (1998). Clean-catch versus urine collection pads: A prospective trial. *Pediatric Nurse, 10*(1), 15–16.

Urine Culture Contamination. A College of American Pathologists' Q-Probes Study of Contaminated Urine Cultures in 906 Institutions. *Archives of Pathology and Laboratory Medicine, 122*(2), 123–129.

4–3

Chernecky, C., & Berger, B. (2000). *Laboratory tests and diagnostic procedures* (3rd ed.). Philadelphia: WB Saunders.

Fujimoto, K., Kubo, K., Matsuzawa, Y., & Sekiguchi, M. (1997). Eosinophilic cationic protein levels in induced sputum correlate with the severity of bronchial asthma. *Chest, 112*(5), 1241–1247.

Keatings, V. M., Evans, D. J., O'Connor, B. J., & Barnes, P. J. (1997). Cellular profiles in asthmatic airways: A comparison of induced sputum, bronchial washings, and bronchoalveolar lavage fluid. *Thorax, 52*(4), 372–374.

4–4

Abrams, A. C. (1998). *Clinical drug therapy: Rationales for nursing practice* (5th ed.). Philadelphia: JB Lippincott.

American Diabetes Association. (1998). Position statement: Insulin administration. *Diabetes Care, 21*(Suppl. 1), S11–16, 69–78.

Capriotti, T., & McLaughlin, S. (1998). A revitalized battle against diabetes mellitus for the new millenium. *Medical-Surgical Nursing, 7*(6), 323–340.

Dietz, P. W. (1999). Slide into better control. *Diabetes Forecast, 52*(7), 52.

Guitterrez, K. (1999). *Pharmacotherapeutics: Clinical decision making in nursing.* Philadelphia: WB Saunders.

Guven, S., & Kuenzi, J. (1998). Diabetes mellitus. In C. Porth (Ed.) *Pathophysiology: Concepts of altered health states* (5th ed., pp. 803–829). Philadelphia: JB Lippincott.

Hirsch, I. B. (1999). Type 1 diabetes and the use of flexible insulin regimens. *American Family Physician, 60*(8), 2343.

Ignatavicius, D. D., Workman, M. L., & Mishler, M. A. (Eds.). (1999). *Medical-surgical nursing across the health care continuum* (3rd ed.). Philadelphia: WB Saunders.

Monahan, F. D., & Neighbors, M. (1998). *Medical-surgical nursing: Foundations for clinical practice* (2nd ed.). Philadelphia: WB Saunders.

Porth, C. M. (1998). *Pathophysiology: Concepts of altered health states* (5th ed.). Philadelphia: Lippincott-Raven.

Sommers, M. S., & Johnson, S. A. (Eds). (1997). *Davis's manual of nursing therapeutics for diseases and disorders.* Philadelphia: FA Davis.

Thompson, J., McFarland, G., Hirsch, J., & Tucker, S. (1997). *Mosby's clinical nursing* (4th ed.). St. Louis, MO: Mosby Year-Book.

Wilson, D. (1999). *Nurses' guide to understanding laboratory and diagnostic tests.* Philadelphia: JB Lippincott.

5–1

Buck, E. (1998). Fluids, electrolytes and acid-base balance. In P. Beare & J. Myers (Eds.), *Adult health nursing* (3rd ed., pp. 52–59). St. Louis, MO: CV Mosby.

Calianno, C., Clifford, D., & Titano, K. (1995). Oxygen therapy. *Nursing, 25*(12), 33–38.

Carroll, P. (1997). Pulse oximerty at your fingertips. *Registered Nurse, 60*(2), 22–27

Czekaj, L. A. (1998). Promoting acid-base balance. In M. R. Kinney, S. B. Dunbar, J. A. Brooks-Brunn, N. Molter, & J. M. Vitello-Cicciu (Eds.), *AACN clinical reference for critical care nursing* (pp. 135–144). St. Louis, MO: CV Mosby.

Grap, M. J. (1998). Protocols for practice: Applying research at the bedside. Pulse oximetry. *Critical Care Nurse, 11*(1), 94–99.

Jensen, L., Onyskiw, J., & Prasad, N. (1998). Ventilatory assistance. In J. Hartshorn, M. L. Sole, & M. Lamborn (Eds.), *Introduction to critical care nursing* (2nd ed., pp. 122–169). Philadelphia: WB Saunders.

LeGrand, D. T., & Peteres, J. (1999). Pulse oximetry: Advantages and pitfalls. *Journal of Respiratory Diseases, 20*(3), 195–206.

Thelan, L., Urden, L., Lough, M., & Stacy, K. (Eds.). (1998). *Critical care nursing: Diagnosis and management* (3rd ed., pp. 661–688). St. Louis, MO: CV Mosby.

5–2

Dunn, L., & Chishlom, H. (1998). Oxygen therapy. *Nursing Standard, 13*(7), 57–60.

Funderburg Wilmoth, D. (1998). Patient management: Respiratory system. In C. M. Hudak, B. M. Gallo, & P. G. Morton (Eds.), *Critical care nursing: A holistic approach* (7th ed.) Philadelphia: JB Lippincott.

Hansen, M. (1998). *Pathophysiology: Foundations of disease and clinical intervention* (p. 515). Philadelphia: WB Saunders.

Hartshorn, J., Sole, M. L., & Lamborn, M. (Eds.). (1997). *Introduction to critical care nursing (*2nd ed., pp. 140–142). Philadelphia: WB Saunders.

Thelan, L., Urden, L., Lough, M., & Stacy, K. (1998). *Critical care nursing: Diagnosis and management* (3rd ed., pp. 689–695). St. Louis: CV Mosby.

Weilitz, P. B. (1998). Oxygen therapy. In A. Potter & P. Perry (Eds.), *Clinical nursing skills and techniques* (pp. 422–443). St. Louis, MO: CV Mosby.

5–3

Brook, A. D., Sherman, G., Malen, J., & Kollef, B. F. (2000). Early versus late tracheostomy in patients who require prolonged mechanical ventilation. *American Journal of Critical Care, 9*(5), 352–352.

Chulay, M., Guzzetta, C., & Dossey, B. (1997) *AACN Handbook of critical care nursing.* E. Norwalk, CT: Appleton & Lange.

Dixon, L. (2000). Tracheostomy: Postoperative recovery. *Perspectives in Nursing, 1*(1). Available at: *http://www.perspectivesinnursing.org/v1n1* (Web article)

Effects of the Passy-Muir tracheostomy speaking valve on pulmonary aspiration in adults. *Heart and Lung: The Journal of Acute and Critical Care, 29*(4), 287–293.

George-Gay, B. (1997). Pulmonary diseases. Part 3: Tracheostomy care. *Health and Sciences Television Network*, EDA CNE 201–271.

Mishler, M. A. (1999). Interventions for clients with oxygen or tracheostomy. In D. D. Ignatavicius, M. L. Workman, & M. A. Mishler (Eds.), *Medical-surgical nursing: A nursing approach* (3nd ed.). Philadelphia: WB Saunders.

Tuiri, J. (1997). Disorders of the larynx and tracheobronchial tree. In L. O. Burrell, M. J. Gerlach, & B. Pless (Eds.), *Adult nursing acute and community care* (2nd ed., pp. 730–740). E. Norwalk, CT: Appleton & Lange.

5–4

Atrium Medical Corporation. *Managing chest drainage and postoperative autotransfusion: Product information.* Hudson, NH: Author.

Becton Dickinson AcuteCare. *Heimlich chest drain valve: Product information.* Franklin Lakes, NJ: Author.

Gallon, A. (1998). Pneumothorax. *Nursing Standard, 13*(10), 35–39.

Geeks, G. J., & Firmin, R. K. (1997). Reducing morbidity from insertion of chest drains: Patients must be disconnected from positive airways pressure before insertion of drains. *British Medical Journal, 315*(7103), 313.

Genzyme Surgical Products.(1997). *Fluid management systems: Product information* (No. 25–0715). Tucker, GA: Author.

Hayden, A. M. (1998). Thoracic surgery. In M. R. Kinney, S. B. Dunbar, J. Brooks-Brunn, et al. (Eds.), *AACN: Clinical reference for critical care nurses* (4th ed.). St. Louis: CV Mosby.

Lynn-McHale, D., & Dorozinsky, C. (1999). Cardiac surgery and heart transplantation. In L. Bucher & S. Melander (Eds.), *Critical care nursing.* Philadelphia: WB Saunders.

Maloney, J. P., & Anderson, F. D. (1997). Common respiratory interventions. In L. O. Burrell, M. J. Gerlach, & B. S. Pless (Eds.), *Adult nursing: Acute and community care* (2nd ed., pp. 684–691). E. Norwalk, CT: Appleton & Lange.

Munnell, E. R. (1997). Thoracic drainage. *Annals of Thoracic Surgery, 63,* 1497–1502.

Pettinicchi, T. A. (1998). Troubleshooting chest tubes. *Nursing, 28*(3), 58–59.

Porth, C. M. (1998). *Pathophysiology: Concepts of altered health states* (5th ed.). Philadelphia: JB Lippincott.

St. John, R. E., & Reichert, P. (1998). Nursing intervention common to respiratory disorders. In P. G. Beare & J. L. Myers (Eds.), *Adult health nursing* (3rd ed.). St. Louis, MO: CV Mosby.

Wilmonth, D. F. (1997). Patient management: Respiratory system. In C. M. Hudak, B. M. Gallo, & P. G. Morton (Eds.), *Critical care nursing: A holistic approach* (7th ed.). Philadelphia: JB Lippincott.

6–1

Black, J., & Matassarin-Jacobs, E. (1997). *Medical-surgical nursing: Clinical management for continuity of care* (5th ed., pp. 1636–1647). Philadelphia: WB Saunders.

Cotran, R. S., Kumar, V., & Collins, T. (1999). *Pathologic basis of disease* (6th ed., p. 935). Philadelphia: WB Saunders.

Hansen, M. (1998). *Pathophysiology. Foundations of disease and clinical intervention* (pp. 517–541). Philadelphia: WB Saunders.

Jaffe, M., & McVan, B. (1997). *Davis's laboratory and diagnostic test handbook* (pp. 351–357). Philadelphia: FA Davis.

Jarvis, C. (2000). *Physical examination and health assessment* (3rd ed., p. 606). Philadelphia: WB Saunders.

Tasota, F., & Tate, J. Eye on diagnostics: Assessing renal function. *Nursing 2000, 30*(5), 20.

Watson, C. (1999). Categorizing the response to epoetin alfa therapy: Case Study of the anemic patient. *American Nephrology Nurses Association, 26*(2), 629–632.

6–2

Breckenridge, D. M., & Locking-Cusolito, H. (1997). Patient's perceptions of why, how, and by whom dialysis treatment modality was chosen. *ANNA Journal, 24*(3), 313.

Chernecky, C. I., & Berger, B. (2000). *Laboratory tests and diagnostic procedures* (3rd ed.). Philadelphia: WB Saunders.

Corea, A. L., Smolka-Hill, S., Christensen, L. S., et al. (1999). Patient and machine monitoring and assessment. In C. F. Gutch, M. H. Stoner, & A. L. Corea (Eds.), *Review of hemodialysis for nurses and dialysis personnel* (6th ed., p. 113). St. Louis: CV Mosby.

Degroot, P. J., Rubes-Kenler, S., & Dwyer, J. T. (1997). Optimizing dialysis past present and future. *Nutrition Today, 32*(1), 30.

Gutch, C. F. (1999). Principles of hemodialysis. In C. F. Gutch, M. H. Stoner, A. L. Corea (Eds.), *Review of hemodialysis for nurses and dialysis personnel* (6th ed., p. 35). St. Louis, MO: CV Mosby.

Ismail, N., & Hakim, R. M. (1997). Hemodialysis. In D. Z. Levine (Ed.), *Caring for the renal patient* (3rd ed.). Philadelphia: WB Saunders.

Johnson, C. A., & Simmons, W. D. (1998). *Dialysis of drug*. New York: McMahon Publishing Group.

Pepper, G. (1999). Medication problems and dialysis. In C. F. Gutch, M. H. Stoner, & A. L. Corea (Eds.), *Review of hemodialysis for nurses and dialysis personnel* (6th ed., p. 142). St. Louis, MO: CV Mosby.

Rolston, M., Gardner, P. W., Peterson, P., & Gutch, C. F. (1999). Dialyzers, dialysate, and delivery systems. In C. F. Gutch, M. H. Stoner, A. L. Corea (Eds.), *Review of hemodialysis for nurses and dialysis personnel* (6th ed., p. 46). St. Louis, MO: CV Mosby.

United States Renal Data System Annual Report.(1999). The National Institutes of Health, The National Institutes of Diabetes and Digestive and Kidney Disease, Division of Kidney, Urologic, and Hematologic disease. Bethesda, MD. Available at: *http://www.med.umich.esrds/chapters/adr.html*

Vogel, S. C. (1999). Access to the bloodstream. In C. F. Gutch, M. H. Stoner, & A. L. Corea (Eds.), *Review of hemodialysis for nurses and dialysis personnel* (6th ed., p. 96). St. Louis, MO: CV Mosby.

6–3

Breckenridge, D. M., & Locking-Cusolito, H. (1997). Patient's perceptions of why, how, and by whom dialysis treatment modality was chosen. *ANNA Journal, 24*(3), 313.

Chernecky, C. I., & Berger, B. (2000). *Laboratory tests and diagnostic procedures* (3rd ed.). Philadelphia, WB Saunders.

Corea, A. L., Smolka-Hill, S., Christensen, L. S., et al. (1999). Patient and machine monitoring and assessment. In C. F. Gutch, M. H. Stoner, & A. L. Corea (Eds.), *Review of hemodialysis for nurses and dialysis personnel* (6th ed., p. 113). St. Louis, MO: CV Mosby.

Degroot, P. J., Rubes-Kenler, S., & Dwyer, J. T. (1997). Optimizing dialysis past present and future. *Nutrition Today, 32*(1), 30.

Dombros, N. V., Digenis, G. E., & Oreopoulos, D. G. (1997). Peritoneal dialysis. In D. Z. Levine (Ed.), *Caring for the renal patient* (3rd ed., pp. 250–288). Philadelphia, WB Saunders.

Gutch, C. F. (1999). Principles of hemodialysis. In C. F. Gutch, M. H. Stoner, & A. L. Corea (Eds.), *Review of hemodialysis for nurses and dialysis personnel* (6th ed., p. 35). St. Louis, MO: CV Mosby.

Johnson, C. A., & Simmons, W. D. (1998). Dialysis of drug. New York: McMahon Publishing Group.

Miller, S. (1995). Renal diseases. In G. A. Ewald & C. R. McKenzie (Eds.), *The Washington manual. Manual of medical therapeutics* (28th ed., p. 262). Boston: Little, Brown.

Pepper, G. (1999). Medication problems and dialysis. In C. F. Gutch, M. H. Stoner, A. L. Corea (Eds.), *Review of hemodialysis for nurses and dialysis personnel* (6th ed., p. 142). St. Louis, MO: CV Mosby.

Rolston, M., Gardner, P. W., Peterson, P., & Gutch, C. F. (1999). Dialyzers, dialysate, and delivery systems. In C. F. Gutch, M. H. Stoner, & A. L. Corea (Eds.), *Review of hemodialysis for nurses and dialysis personnel* (6th ed., p. 46). St. Louis, MO: CV Mosby.

United States Renal Data System Annual Report. The National Institutes of Health, The National Institutes of Diabetes and Digestive and Kidney

Disease, Division of Kidney, Urologic, and Hematologic disease. Bethesda, MD, 1999. Available at: *http://www.med.umich.esrds/chapters/adr.html*

Vogel, S. C. (1999). Access to the bloodstream. In C. F. Gutch, M. H. Stoner, & A. L. Corea (Eds.), *Review of hemodialysis for nurses and dialysis personnel* (6th ed., p. 96). St. Louis, MO: CV Mosby.

6–4

McCann, J. (1999). Can skin cancers be minimized or prevented in organ transplant patients? *Journal of the National Cancer Institute, 11*(91), 991.

New monoclonal antibodies to prevent transplant rejection. (1998). *Medical Letter on Drugs & Therapeutics, 40*(1036), 93.

United Network for Organ Sharing. (1998). UNOS Critical Data. Richmond, VA. Available at: *http://www.unos.org*.

USRDS Patient Database. USRDS 1999 Annual Data Report. Health Care Finance Administration.

Wunsch, H. (1998). Predicting the fate of transplanted kidneys. *Lancet, 351*, 963.

7–1

Crigger, N., & Forbes, W. (1997). Assessing neurologic function in older patients. *American Journal of Nursing, 97*(3), 37–40.

Downey, D. L., & Leigh, R. J. (1998). Eye movements: Pathophysiology, examination and clinical importance. *Journal of Neuroscience Nursing, 30*(1), 15–22.

Goetx, C. G., & Pappert, E. J. (1999). *Textbook of clinical neurology.* Philadelphia: WB Saunders.

Hickey, J. (1997) *The clinical practice of neurological and neurosurgical nursing* (4th ed.). Philadelphia: JB Lippincott.

Luckman, J. (Ed.). (1997). *Saunders manual of nursing care.* Philadelphia: WB Saunders.

Neatherlin, J. S. (1999). Foundation for practice: Neuroassessment for neuroscience nurses. *Nursing Clinics of North America, 34*(3), 573–592.

7–2

Arbour, R. (1998). Aggressive management of intracranial dynamics. *Critical Care Nurse, 18*(3), 30–40.

Brain Trauma Foundation. (1995). *Guidelines for the management of severe head injury.* Chicago, IL: Brain Trauma Foundation.

Hickey, J. (1997) *The clinical practice of neurological and neurosurgical nursing* (4th ed.). Philadelphia: JB Lippincott.

McNair, N. D. (1999). Traumatic brain injury. *Nursing Clinics of North America, 34*(3), 637–658.

Wong, F. (2000). Prevention of secondary brain injury. *Critical Care Nurse, 20*(5), 18–27.

7–3

Boss, B. J. (1998). Alterations of neurologic function. In K. L. McCance & S. E. Huether (Eds.), *Pathophysiology: The biologic basis for disease in adults and children* (3rd ed.). St. Louis, MO: CV Mosby.

Hickey, J. (1997). *The clinical practice of neurological and neurosurgical nursing* (4th ed.). Philadelphia: JB Lippincott.

Stewart-Amidei, C. (1998). The 1998 neuro-oncology symposium: New horizons, new hope. *Journal of Neuroscience Nursing, 30*(6), 361–368.

8–1

Criley, J. M., Criley, D., & Zalace, C. (1997). Multimedia instruction of cardiac auscultation. *Trans America Clinical Association, 108*, 271–285.

Erickson, B. A. (1997). *Heart sounds and murmurs: A practical guide* (3rd ed.). St. Louis, MO: CV Mosby.

Hartshorne, J. C., Sole, M. L., & Lamborne, M. L. (1997). *Introduction to critical care nursing* (2nd ed., pp. 232–268). Philadelphia: WB Saunders.

Keen, J. H., & Swearingen, P. L. (1997). *Critical care nursing consultant* (pp. 40–42; 272). St. Louis, MO: CV Mosby.

Mangione, S., & Nieman, L. Z. (1997). Cardiac auscultatory skills of internal medicine and family practice trainees. *Journal of the American Medical Association, 278*, 712–722.

8–2

Pless, B. S. (1997). Nursing assessment and common vascular interventions. In L. O. Burrell, M. J. Gerlach, & B. S. Pless (Eds.), *Adult nursing: Acute and community care* (2nd ed., pp. 477–493). E. Norwalk, CT: Appleton & Lange.

Turner, J. (1997). Caring for people with peripheral vascular and lymphatic disorders. In J. Luckmann (Ed.), *Manual of nursing care.* Philadelphia: WB Saunders.

8–3

Burrell, L. O., & Streit, L. A. (1997). Cardiac arrhythmias. In L. O. Burrell, M. J. Gerlach, & B. S. Pless (Eds.), *Nursing management of adults with cardiovascular and hematologic problems* (2nd ed.). E. Norwalk, CT: Appleton & Lange.

Walraven, G. (1999). *Basic arrhythmias* (5th ed.). Englewood Cliffs, NJ: Prentice Hall.

8–4

Burrell, L. O., & Streit, L. A. (1997). Cardiac arrhythmias. In L. O. Burrell, M. J. Gerlach, & B. S. Pless (Eds.), *Nursing management of adults with cardiovascular and hematologic problems* (2nd ed.). E. Norwalk, CT: Appleton & Lange.

Knight, L., Livingston, N., & Gawlinski, A. (1997). Caring for patients with third-generation implantable cardioverter defibrillators: From decision to implant to patient's return home. *Critical Care Nurse, 17*(5), 46–61.

Morton, P. (1997). The pacemaker and defibrillator codes: Implications for critical care nursing. *Critical Care Nurse, 17*(1), 50–59.

Zimetbaum, P. J., & Josephson, M. E. (1999). The evolving role of ambulatory arrhythmia monitoring in general clinical practice. *Annals of Internal Medicine, 130*, 848–856.

8–5

Kinney, M. R., Dunbar, S. B., Brooks-Brun, J., et al. (1998). *AACN's clinical reference for critical care nursing* (4th ed., pp. 329–334). St. Louis, MO: CV Mosby.

Moccia, J. M. (1997). How to use serial and expanded ECGs. *Nursing 97, 27*(9), 32cc1–2, 32cc4–5.

Warner, C. D. (1997). Triaging and interpreting chest pain. *Journal of Cardiovascular Nursing, 12*(1), 84–92.

8–6

Beare, P. G., & Myers, J. L. (1998). *Adult health nursing.* St. Louis, MO: CV Mosby.

Cataldo, C. B., DeBruyne, L. K., & Whitney, E. N. (1999). *Nutrition and diet therapy: Principles and practice.* Belmont, CA: Wadsworth Publishing Company.

Dudek, S. G. (2000). Malnutrition in hospitals: Who's assessing what patients eat? *American Journal of Nursing, 100*(4), 36–43.

Dudek, S. G. (1997). *Nutrition handbook for nursing practice* (3rd ed.). Philadelphia: JB Lippincott.

Hensrud, D. D. (1998). Nutrition screening and diet assessment. *Medical Clinics of North America, 83*(6), 1540.

Ignatavicius, D. L., Workman, M. L., & Mishler, M. A. (1999). *Medical surgical nursing across the health care continuum* (3rd ed.). Philadelphia: WB Saunders.

Lusky, K. (1999). Herbal medicines: Some caution required. *Tennessee Nurse, 62*(1), 17–19.

McClave, S. A., Snider, H. L., & Spain, D. A. (1999). Preoperative issues in clinical nutrition. *Chest, 115*(5), 64–70.

Mitchell, M. K. (1997). *Nutrition across the lifespan.* Philadelphia: WB Saunders.

Ogawa, A. M. (1997). Macronutrient requirements. In S. A. Shikora, & G. L. Blackburn (Eds.), *Nutrition support: Theory and therapeutics* (pp. 54–65). New York: Chapman & Hall.

Pleuss, J. (1998). Alterations in nutritional status. In C. M. Porth (Ed.), *Pathophysiology concepts of altered health states* (5th ed.). Philadelphia: JB Lippincott.

Rahman, M., & Smith, M. C. (1998). Chronic renal insufficiency: A diagnostic and therapeutic approach. *Archives of Internal Medicine, 156*(16), 1743–1752.

Smeltzer, S. C., & Bare, B. C. (2000). *Textbook of medical surgical nursing.* Philadelphia: JB Lippincott.

Taylor, C., Lillis, C., & LeMone, P. (1997). *Fundamentals of nursing: The art and science of nursing care* (3rd ed.). Philadelphia: JB Lippincott.

9–1, 9–2, and 9–3

Atkins, R. C. (1992). *Dr. Atkins new diet revolution.* New York: M. Evans & Co.

Beare, P. G., & Myers, J. L. (1998). *Adult health nursing.* St. Louis: CV Mosby.

Cataldo, C. B., DeBruyne, L. K., & Whitney, E. N. (1999). *Nutrition and diet therapy: Principles and practice.* Belmont, CA: Wadsworth Publishing.

Dudek, S. G. (2000). Malnutrition in hospitals: Who's assessing what patients eat? *American Journal of Nursing, 100*(4), 36–43.

Dudek, S. G. (1997). *Nutrition handbook for nursing practice* (3rd ed.). Philadelphia: JB Lippincott.

Hensrud, D. D. (1998). Nutrition screening and diet assessment. *Medical Clinics of North America, 83*(6), 1540.

Ignatavicius, D. L., Workman, M. L., & Mishler, M. A. (1999). *Medical surgical nursing across the health care continuum* (3rd ed.). Philadelphia: WB Saunders.

Institute of Medicine. (1995). *Weighing the options: Criteria for evaluating weight management problems.* Washington, DC: Food and Nutrition Board.

Lusky, K. (1999). Herbal medicines: Some caution required. *Tennessee Nurse, 62*(1), 17–19.

McClave, S. A., Snider, H. L., & Spain, D. A. (1999). Preoperative issues in clinical nutrition. *Chest, 115*(5), 64–70.

Mitchell, M. K. (1997). *Nutrition across the lifespan.* Philadelphia: WB Saunders.

Ogawa, A. M. (1997). Macronutrient requirements. In S. A. Shikora, G. L. Blackburn (Eds.), *Nutrition support: Theory and therapeutics* (pp. 54–65). New York: Chapman and Hall.

Pate, R. R. (1995). Physical activity and public health: A recommendation from the Centers for Disease Control and Prevention and the American College of Sports Medicine. *Journal of the American Medical Association, 273*:402–407.

Pleuss, J. (1998). Alterations in nutritional status. In C. M. Porth (Ed.), *Pathophysiology concepts of altered health states* (5th ed.). Philadelphia: JB Lippincott.

Rahman, M., & Smith, M. C. (1998). Chronic renal insufficiency: A diagnostic and therapeutic approach. *Archives of Internal Medicine, 156*(16), 1743–1752.

Smeltzer, S. C., & Bare, B. C. (2000). *Textbook of medical surgical nursing.* Philadelphia: JB Lippincott.

Taylor, C., Lillis, C., & LeMone, P. (1997). *Fundamentals of nursing: The art and science of nursing care* (3rd ed.). Philadelphia: JB Lippincott.

Thompson, J. M., & Wilson, S. F. (1996). *Health assessment for nursing practice.* St. Louis: CV Mosby.

Williams, S. R. (1995). *Basic nutrition and diet therapy* (10th ed.). St. Louis: CV Mosby.

9–4

American Society for Parenteral and Enteral Nutrition. (2000). *Guidelines for the use of parenteral and enteral nutrition in adult and pediatric patients.* Section IV: Nutritional support for adults with specific disease and conditions. Available at: *http://www.nutritioncare.org/publications/Guidelines/SectionIV.html* (24 October, 2000).

Anderson, K. N., Anderson, L. E., & Glanze, W. D. (1998). *Mosby's medical, nursing, and allied health dictionary* (5th ed.). St. Louis, MO: CV Mosby.

Bender, C. M., Yasko, J. M., & Stohl, R. A. (2000). Nursing management: Cancer. In S. M. Lewis, M. M. Heitkemper, & S. R. Dirksen (Eds.), *Medical-surgical nursing: Assessment and management of clinical problems* (5th ed.). St. Louis, MO: CV Mosby.

Charney, P. J. (1998). Nutritional screening and assessment. In A. Skipper (Ed.), *Dietitian's handbook of enteral and parenteral nutrition* (2nd ed., pp. 3–24). Gaithersburg: Aspen.

Colagiovanni, L. (1997). Parenteral nutrition. *Nursing Standard, 12*(9), 39–45.

Dudeck, S. G. (1997). *Nutrition handbook for nursing practice* (3rd ed.). Philadelphia: JB Lippincott.

Evans-Stoner, N. (1997). Nutrition. In N. Evans-Stoner & L. K. Lysen (Eds.), *The Nursing Clinics of North America, 32*(4), 637–650.

Galica, L. A. (1997). Parenteral nutrition. In N. Evans-Stoner & L. K. Lysen (Eds.), *Nursing Clinics of North America, 32*(4), 705–717.

Ishibashi, N., Plank, L. D., Sando, K., & Hill, G. (1998). Optimal protein requirements during the first 2 weeks after the onset of critical illness. *Critical Care Medicine, 26*(9), 1529–1535.

Lenseen, P. (1998). Management of total parenteral nutrition. In A. Skipper (Ed.), *Dietitian's handbook of enteral and parenteral nutrition* (2nd ed., pp. 25–46). Gaithersburg: Aspen.

McConnell, E. A. (1998). Clinical do's and don'ts: Administering parenteral nutrition. *Nursing, 28*(7), 18.

The Merck Manual. (2000). Nutritional Support. *http://www.merck.com/pubs/mmanual/section1/1c.htm* (24 October, 2000).

Montgomery, J. W. (1999). Overview of parenteral nutrition support. *US Pharmacist, 24*(5), 21–30.

National Advisory Group on Standards & Practice Guidelines for Parenteral Nutrition. (1998). Safe practices for parenteral nutrition formulations. *JPEN, Journal of Parenteral and Enteral Nutrition, 22*(2), 54–59.

National Cancer Institute. (2000). Nutrition. Available at: *http://imsdd.meb.uni-bonn.de/cancernet/304467.html* (24 October, 2000).

Pleuss, J. (1998). Alterations in nutritional status. In C. M. Porth (Ed.), *Pathophysiology concepts of altered health states* (5th ed.). Philadelphia: JB Lippincott.

Steinhart, A. H., Baker, J. P., & Detsky, A. S. (1998). Nutritional therapeutics. In E. B. Larson & P. G. Ramsey (Eds.), *Medical therapeutics* (3rd ed.). Philadelphia: WB Saunders.

Westfall, U. E. (2000). Nursing management: Nutritional Problems. In S. M. Lewis, M. M. Heitkemper, & S. R. Dirksen (Eds.), *Medical-surgical nursing: Assessment and management of clinical problems* (5th ed.). St. Louis, MO: CV Mosby.

www.cdc.gov/ncidod/hip/iv/iv.html

9–5

Bliss, D. Z., & Lehmann, S. (1999). Tube feeding: Administration tips. *Registered Nurse, 62*(8), 29–32.

Guenter, P., Jones, S., & Ericson, M. (1997). Enteral nutrition therapy. *Nursing Clinics of North America, 32*(4), 651–668.

Kennedy, J. F. (1997). Enteral feeding for the critically ill. *Nursing Standard, 11*(33), 39–43.

Lord, L. M. (1997). Enteral access devices. *Nursing Clinics of North America, 32*(4), 651–668.

McAthie, M. (1999). Nutrition and fluids. *Fundamentals of contemporary nursing practice.* Philadelphia: WB Saunders.

Morrissey, N. A. (2000). Gastrointestinal intubation and special nutritional modalities. In S. C. Smeltzer & B. G. Bare (Eds.), *Brunner & Suddarth's textbook of medical-surgical nursing* (9th ed., pp. 834–856). Philadelphia: JB Lippincott.

Orr, M. E. (1998). Enteral nutrition. In A. G. Perry & P. A. Potter (Eds.), *Clinical nursing skills and techniques* (4th ed., pp. 762–765). St. Louis, MO: CV Mosby.

Skipper, A., & Ratz, N. B. (1998). Enteral nutrition. In A. Skipper (Ed.), *Dietitian's handbook of enteral and parenteral nutrition* (2nd ed.). Gaithersburg: Aspen.

Steinhart, A. H., Baker, J. P., & Detsky, A. S. (1998). Nutritional therapeutics. In Larson, E. B., & Ramsey P. G. (Eds.), *Medical therapeutics* (3rd ed.). Philadelphia: WB Saunders.

Thelan, L., Urden, L., Lough, M., & Stacy, K. (1998). Nutritional alterations and management. In *Critical care nursing: Diagnosis and management* (3rd ed., pp. 156–159). St. Louis, MO: CV Mosby.

10–1

Chernecky, C., & Berger, B. J. (1997). *Laboratory tests and diagnostic procedures* (pp. 391–393, 453–456). Philadelphia: WB Saunders.

Copstead, L., & Banasik, J. (2000). *Pathophysiology: Biological and behavioral perspectives*. Philadelphia: WB Saunders.

Cotran, R. S., Kumar, V., & Collins, T. (1999). *Pathologic basis of disease* (pp. 188–195). Philadelphia: WB Saunders.

Guyton, A., & Hall, J. (1997). *Human physiology and mechanisms of disease* (pp. 288–295). Philadelphia: WB Saunders.

Hansen, M. (1998). *Pathophysiology: Foundations of disease and clinical interventions* (pp. 287–311). Philadelphia: WB Saunders.

Huether, S., & McCance, K. (2000). *Understanding pathophysiology* (pp. 125–150). St. Louis, MO: CV Mosby.

Kee, J. L. (1999). *Laboratory diagnostic tests with nursing implications* (pp. 454–455). E. Norwalk, CT: Appleton & Lange.

Nowak, T. J., & Handford, A. G. (1999). *Essentials of pathophysiology* (pp. 74–85). Boston: McGraw-Hill.

Sparks, S., & Camp-Sorrell, D. C. (1997). Assessing the myelosuppressed patient. *American Journal of Nursing Supplement,* E22–E28.

Witek-Janusek, L., Stoddard, J., & Mathets, H. L. (1998). Trauma-induced immune dysfunction: A challenge for critical care. *Dimensions of Critical Care Nursing, 17*(4), 187–198.

10–2

Camp-Sorrell, D. (1998). In J. K. Itano & K. N. Taoka, *Core curriculum for oncology nursing* (3rd ed., pp. 207–211). Philadelphia: WB Saunders.

Dix, S. P., & Yee, G. C. (1997). In M. B. Whedon & D. Wujcik, *Blood and marrow stem cell transplantation: Principles, practice and nursing insights* (2nd ed., pp. 125–135). Boston: Jones & Bartlett.

Ellerhorst-Ryan, J. M. (1997). Infection. In S. L. Groenwald, M. H. Frogge, M. Goodman, & C. H. Yarbro, *Cancer nursing: Principles and practice* (4th ed., p. 595). Boston: Jones & Bartlett.

10–3

Bhorade, S. M., Christenson, J., Pohlman, A. S., et al. (1999). The incidence of and clinical variables associated with vancomycin-resistant enterococcal colonization in mechanically ventilated patients. *Chest, 115*(4), 1085–1091.

Dembek, Z. F., Kellerman, S. E., Ganley, L., et al. (1999). Reporting of vancomycin-resistant enterococci in Connecticut: Implementation and validation of a state-based surveillance system. *Infection Control and Hospital Epidemiology, 20*(10), 671–675.

Evenson, W. (2000). Occupational exposure to *Mycobacterium tuberculosis*:

Legal issues in workers' compensation. *Journal of the American Association of Occupational Health Nurses* [On-line]. Available at: *http://www.aaohn.org/cemodules/aug99art.htm*

Garner, J. S. (1997). *Guidelines for isolation precautions in hospitals.* Centers for Disease Control and Prevention, Hospital Infection Control Practices Advisory Committee. Published by the Public Health Service, US Department of Health and Human Services, Centers for Disease Control and Prevention, Atlanta, Georgia.

Goetz, A., Posey, K., Fleming, J., Jacobs, S., Boody, L., Wagener, M. M., & Muder, R. R. (1999). Concise communication: Methicillin-resistant *Staphylococcus aureus* in the community: A hospital-based study. *Infection Control and Hospital Epidemiology, 20*(10), 689–691.

Hoffman, K. K., & Kittrell, I. P. (1997). North Carolina guidelines for control of antibiotic resistant organisms, specifically methicillin-resistant *Staphylococcus aureus* (MRSA) and vancomycin-resistant *Enterococcus* (VRE). Available at: *http://www.unc.edu/depts/spice/guide2.html*

Kuehnert, M. J., Jernigan, J. A., Pullen, A. L., et al. (1999). Association between mucositis severity and vancomycin-resistant enterococcal bloodstream infection in hospitalized cancer patients. *Infection Control and Hospital Epidemiology, 20*(10), 660–663.

Lee, Y., Cesario, T., Tran, C., et al. (2000). Nasal colonization of methicillin-resistant coagulase-negative *Staphylococcus* in community skilled nursing facility patients. *American Journal of Infection Control, 28*(3), 269–272.

Palmer, R. (1999). Bacterial contamination of curtains in clinical areas. *Nursing Standard, 14*(2), 33–35.

11–1

Carroll, P. (1997). Clarifying the CBC. *RN, 60*(9), 29–33.

Chernecky, C. C., & Berger, B. J. (1997). *Laboratory tests and diagnostic procedures* (2nd ed.). Philadelphia: WB Saunders.

Dailey, J. F. (1998). *Blood* (pp. 445–446, 462–463). Arlington, MA: Medical Consulting Group.

George-Gay, B. (2000). Understanding the CBC with differential: Long-term care network *EDA* 318–373. (Available from Primedia Health Care, Carrollton, TX.)

Uthman, E. (1998). *Understanding anemia.* Jackson: University Press of Mississippi.

11–2

Black, J. M., & Matassarin-Jacobs, E. (1997). *Medical-surgical nursing: Clinical management for continuity of care* (5th ed.). Philadelphia: WB Saunders.

Carroll, R. (1997). Clarifying the CBC. *RN, 60*(9), 29–34.

Chernecky, C., & Berger, B. J. (1997). *Laboratory tests and diagnostic procedures* (pp. 391–393, 453–456). Philadelphia: WB Saunders.

Hansen, M. (1998). Pathophysiology: Foundations of disease and clinical intervention (pp. 287–311). Philadelphia: WB Saunders.

Kee, J. L. (1999). Laboratory diagnostic test with nursing implications (pp. 454–455). E. Norwalk, CT: Appleton & Lange.

McCance, K., & Huether, S. (1998). *Pathophysiology: The biologic basis for disease in adults and children* (3rd ed.). St. Louis, MO: CV Mosby.

11–3

Felver, L. (2000). Fluid and electrolyte homeostasis and imbalances. In L. C. Copstead & J. L. Banasik (Eds.), *Pathophysiology: Biological and behavioral perspectives* (2nd ed.). Philadelphia: WB Saunders.

Gahart, B. L., & Nazareno, A. R. (2001). *2001 Intravenous medications* (17th ed.). St. Louis, MO: CV Mosby.

11–4

Carroll, P. (1997). Clarifying the CBC. *RN, 60,* 29–32.

Cavanugh, B. M. (1999). *Nurses' manual of laboratory tests* (3rd ed.). Philadelphia: FA Davis.

Chernecky, C. C., & Berger, B. J. (1997). *Laboratory tests and diagnostic procedures* (2nd ed.). Philadelphia: WB Saunders.

Doern, G. V., Brueggemann, A., Huynh, H. (1999). Antimicrobial resistance with *Streptococcus pneumoniae* in the United States 1997–1998. *Emerging Infections, 6*(2), 757–765.

Forbes, B., Sahm, S., & Weissfeld, A. (1998) *Bloodstream infections in diagnostic microbiology* (10th ed.). St. Louis, MO: CV Mosby.

Forbes, B., Sahm, S., & Weissfeld, A. (1998). *Role of microscopy in the diagnosis of infectious disease in diagnostic microbiology* (10th ed.). St. Louis, MO: CV Mosby.

Pagana, K., & Pagana, T. (1997). *Diagnostic and laboratory test reference* (3rd ed.). St. Louis, MO: CV Mosby.

Robson, M. C. (1997). Wound infection: A failure of wound healing caused by an imbalance of bacteria. *Surgical Clinics of North America, 77,* 637–650.

Stotts, N., & Whitney, J. (1999). Wound care: Identifying and evaluating wound infection. *Home Healthcare Nurse, 17*(3), 159–165.

11–5

Albright, R. (2001). Acute renal failure: A practical update. *Mayo Clin Updates, 76,* 67–74.

Bates, P. (1999). Nursing assessment: Urinary system. In S. M. Lewis, M. Heitkemper, S. Dirksen, et al. *Medical surgical nursing: Assessment of clinical problems* (5th ed.). St. Louis, MO: CV Mosby.

Cavanaugh, B. M. (1999). *Nurses' manual of laboratory tests* (3rd ed.). Philadelphia: FA Davis.

Pagana, K., & Pagana, T. (1997). *Diagnostic and laboratory test reference* (3rd ed.). St. Louis, MO: CV Mosby.

12–1

Abbott Laboratories, Actiq: Product overview. Online 1999 [May 29, 2000]. Available at: *http://www.abbotthosp.com/Prod/PAIN/actiqprod/act002.htm*

Anesta Products, Oralet: product. Online 1999 [May 29, 2000]. Available at: *http://www.anesta.com/products/prods.html*

Bennett, P. P. (1999). Pain management: State of the art nursing guidelines. Seminar conducted by the American Healthcare Institute, Philadelphia, PA, August 1999.

Coyne, P. (1997). Pancreatic cancer: Pain treatment and interventions. *American Society of Pain Management Nurses Pathways, 6*(1), 14.

Hain, R. D. W. (1997). Pain scales in children: A review. *Palliative Medicine, 11,* 341–350.

Jacob, E., & Puntillo, K. A. (1999). A survey of nursing practice in the assessment and management of pain in children. *Pediatric Nursing, 25*(3), 278–286.

Jedlinsk, B. P., McCarthy, C. F., & Michel, T. H. (1999). Validating pediatric pain measurement: Sensory and affective components. *Pediatric Physical Therapy, 11*, 83–88.

Joint Commission on Accreditation of Health Care Organizations. (1999). Design, education and change programs to manage pain consistently. Joint Comm Benchmark, *1*(3), 4–5.

Kitzes, J. A. (1999). Chronic/intractable pain management: Opioid therapy. *HIS Primary Care Provider, 24*(7), 115–117.

Kozier, B., Erb, G., Blias, K., et al. (2000). *Fundamentals of nursing* (6th ed.). Menlo Park, CA: Addison-Wesley.

McCaffery, M., & Pasero, C. (1999). *Pain: Clinical manual for nursing practice*. St. Louis, MO: CV Mosby.

McKenry, L. M., & Salerno, E. (1998). *Pharmacology in nursing* (20th ed.). St Louis, MO: CV Mosby.

Pasero, C. L. (1998). Assessing and treating the pain of pancreatitis. *American Journal of Nursing, 98*(11), 14–15.

Pasero, C. L. (1999). JCAHO on assessing and managing pain. *American Journal of Nursing, 99*(7), 22.

Pasero, C. L. (1998). Teaching patients how to use PCA. *American Journal of Nursing, 98*(9), 14–15.

Pasero, C. L., & McCaffery, M. (2000). Reversing respiratory depression with naloxone. *American Journal of Nursing, 100*(2), 26.

Vanegas, G., Ripamonti, C., Sbanotto, A., & De Conno, F. (1998). Side effects of morphine administration in cancer patients. *Cancer Nursing, 21*(4), 289–297.

Wessman, A. C., & McDonald, D. D. (1999). Nurses' personal pain experiences and their pain management knowledge. *Journal of Continuing Education in Nursing, 30*(4), 152–157.

12–2

American Heart Association: Anticoagulants, 2000. Available at: *http://www.americanheart.org/Heart_and_Stroke_A_Z_Guide/antico.html*

Arrants, J., Willis, M. E., Stevens, B., et al. (1999). Reliability of an intravenous intermittent access port (saline lock) for obtaining blood samples for coagulation studies. *American Journal of Critical Care, 8*, 344–348.

Carr, N. (1999). A nurse-led initiative on anticoagulation. *Practitioner Nurse, 17*, 605–608.

Cohen, M., Demer, C., Gurfinkel, E. P., et al. (1997). A comparison of low-molecular-weight heparin with unfractionated heparin for unstable coronary artery disease: Efficacy and safety of subcutaneous enoxaparin in Non-Q-Wave Coronary Events Study Group. *New England Journal of Medicine, 337*, 447–452.

The Columbus Investigators. (1997). Low-molecular weight heparin in the treatment of patients with venous thromboembolism. *New England Journal of Medicine, 337,* 657–662.

Corbett, J. V. (2000). *Laboratory tests and diagnostic procedures* (5th ed.). Englewood Cliffs, NJ: Prentice Hall.

Coyne, N. R. (1997). Current concepts in anticoagulant therapy. *Journal of Care Management, 3*, 28–46.

Dellinger, R. P. (1997). Effective thromboembolic prophylaxis for high-risk patients. *Journal of Critical Illness, 12,* 547–556.

Glaser, V. (1999). Platelet inhibitors: Old and new uses. *Patient Care, 33,* 111–112, 114–117.

Guyton, A. C., & Hall, J. E. (2000). *Textbook of medical physiology* (10th ed.). Philadelphia: WB Saunders.

Hospital Focus. (2000). TIA guidelines will change how you treat patients. *Registered Nurse, 63,* 24hf1–24hf4.

Kuhn, M. (1998). *Pharmacotherapeutic nursing process approach* (4th ed.). Philadelphia: FA Davis.

Kupecz, D. (1998). Low molecular weight heparins: The future of thromboembolic therapy. *Nurse Practitioner, 23,* 98–107.

Kupecz, D. (1999). Using clopidogrel bisulfate: A new antiplatelet drug. *Nurse Practitioner, 24,* 100–110.

Pagana, K. D., & Pagana, T. J. (1999). *Diagnostic testing and nursing implications* (5th ed.). St. Louis, MO: CV Mosby.

Sellman, J. S., & Holman, R. L. (2000). Thromboembolism during pregnancy. *Postgraduate Medicine, 108.* Available at: *http://www.postgradmed.com/issues/2000/09_00/sellman.html*

Simonneau, G., Sors, H., Charbonnier, B., et al. (1997). A comparison of low-molecular-weight heparin with unfractionated heparin for acute pulmonary embolism. *New England Journal of Medicine, 337,* 663–669.

Turpie, A. G., Weart, C. W., & White, R. (1998). Anticoagulation promises and pitfalls. *Patient Care, 4,* 106–125.

Warfarin complications in pregnancy. (1999). *Nurses' Drug Alert, 23,* 62.

12–3

Adams, M. H., Lammon, C. B., & Stover, L. M. (1998). Applied pharmacology: Responding to tricyclic antidepressant overdose. *Dimensions of Critical Care Nursing, 17*(2), 67–74.

Anonymous (1999). Antidepressants. In M. R. Riley, S. K. Hebel, T. Burnham, et al. (Eds.), *Facts and comparisons* (pp. 262j–264z). St. Louis, MO: Facts and Comparisons.

Cohen, L. J. (1997). Rational drug use in the treatment of depression. *Pharmacotherapy, 17*(1), 45–61.

Davis, K. M., & Mathew, E (1998). Pharmacologic management of depression in the elderly. *Nurse Practitioner, 23*(6), 16, 18, 26.

Grimsley, S. R. (1998). Mood disorders. In B. L. Carter, K. D. Lake, M. A. Raebel, et al. (Eds.), *Pharmacotherapy self-assessment program. Module 4: Neurology and psychiatry,* (3rd ed., pp. 119–143). St. Louis, MO: American College of Clinical Pharmacy.

Kelsey, J. E. (1998). The use of antidepressants in long-term care and the geriatric patient. *Geriatrics, 53*(Suppl. 4):S4–S43.

Thapa, P. B., Gideon, P., Cost, T. W., Milam, A. B., & Ray, W. A. (1998). Antidepressants and the risk of falls among nursing home residents. *New England Journal of Medicine, 339*(13), 875–882.

Wells, B. G., Mandos, L. A., & Hayes, P. E. (1997). Depressive disorders. In J. T. DiPiro, R. L. Talbert, G. C. Yee, et al. (Eds.), *Pharmacotherapy: A pathophysiologic approach* (3rd ed., pp. 1395–1418). E. Norwalk, CT: Appleton & Lange.

Wintz, C. J. B. (1998). Nursing management of psychotropic drug reactions. *Nursing Clinics of North America, 33*(1), 217–231.

12–4

Clayton, B. D., & Stock, Y. N. (1997). *Basic pharmacology for nurses* (11th ed.). St. Louis, MO: CV Mosby.

Cleveland, L., Aschenbrenner, D. S., Venable, S. J., & Yensen, J. A. P. (1999). *Nursing management in drug therapy.* Philadelphia: JB Lippincott.

Eisenhauer, L. A., Nichols, L. W., Spencer, R. T., & Bergan, F. W. (1998). *Clinical pharmacology and nursing management* (5th ed.). Philadelphia: JB Lippincott.

Gutierrez, K. (1999). *Pharmacotherapeutics: Clinical decision-making in nursing.* Philadelphia: WB Saunders.

Ignatavicius, D. D., Workman, M. L., & Mishler, M. A. (1999). *Medical-surgical nursing across the health care continuum* (3rd ed.). Philadelphia: WB Saunders.

Kee, J. L., & Hayes, E. R. (1997). *Pharmacology: A nursing process approach* (2nd ed.). Philadelphia: WB Saunders.

Kuhn, M. (1998). *Pharmacotherapeutics: A nursing process approach* (4th ed.). Philadelphia: FA Davis.

Smeltzer, S. C., & Bare, B. G. (2000). *Brunner and Suddarth's textbook of medical-surgical nursing* (9th ed.). Philadelphia: JB Lippincott.

Williams, B. R., & Baer, C. L. (1998). *Essentials of clinical pharmacology in nursing* (3rd ed.). Springhouse, PA: Springhouse Corporation.

Wilson, B. A., & Shannon, M. T., & Stang, C. L. (2000). *Nurses' drug guide.* E. Norwalk, CT: Appleton & Lange.

12–5

Bartlett, J. G. (1998). *Pocket book of infectious disease therapy.* Baltimore: Williams & Wilkins.

12–6

Dambro, M. R. (2000). *Griffith's 5-minute consult.* Philadelphia: Lippincott Williams & Wilkins.

Drugs of Choice from the Medical Letter (revised ed.). (1997). *The medical letter on drugs and therapeutics.* New Rochelle, NY: Medical Letter.

McCance, K. L., & Huether, S. E. (1998). *Pathophysiology: The biologic basis for disease in adults and children* (3rd ed.). St. Louis, MO: CV Mosby.

Mladenovic, J. (1999). *Primary care secrets* (2nd ed.). Philadelphia: Hanley & Belfus.

Monthly Prescribing Reference, February 2000.

Wells, B. G., DiPiro, J. T., Schwinghammer, T. L., & Hamilton, C. W. (1998). *Pharmacotherapy handbook.* E. Norwalk, CT: Appleton & Lange.

12–7

Cohen, R. M. (1997). Transdermal nicotine for ulcerative colitis. *Internal Medicine World Report, 12*(10), 10.

Foster, S., & Tyler, V. E. (1998). *Tyler's honest herbal* (p. 141). Binghamton, NY: Hayworth Press.

Gastrointestinal tract drugs. (1999). *Nursing99 drug handbook.* Springhouse, PA: Springhouse Corporation.

Gerlach, M. J. (1997). Common gastrointestinal interventions. In L. O. Burrell,

M. J. M. Gerlach, & B. S. Pless (Eds.). *Adult nursing: Acute and community care* (Vol. VII, 2nd ed., p. 1368). E. Norwalk, CT: Appleton & Lange.

Hunt, R. H. (1999). Importance of pH control in the management of GERD. *Archives of Internal Medicine, 159*(7), 649.

Lehne, R. A. (1998). *Laxatives: Pharmacology for nursing care* (3rd ed., p. 787). Philadelphia: WB Saunders.

Lehne, R. A. (1998). *Other gastrointestinal drugs: Pharmacology for nursing care* (3rd ed., p. 794). Philadelphia: WB Saunders.

Lilley, L. L., & Aucker, R. S. (1999). *Antacids and antiflatulents: Pharmacology and the nursing process* (2nd ed., p. 660). St. Louis, MO: CV Mosby.

Lilley, L. L., & Aucker, R. S. (1999). *Antidiarrheals and laxatives: Pharmacology and the nursing process* (2nd ed., p. 675). St. Louis, MO: CV Mosby.

Lilley, L. L., & Aucker, R. S. (1999). *Antiemetic (antinausea) agents: Pharmacology and the nursing process* (2nd ed., p. 692). St. Louis, MO: CV Mosby.

Loren, D. E., & Peppercorn, M. A. (1998). Crohn's disease in the elderly. Part II: Medical and surgical therapies. *Clinical Geriatrics, 6*(3), 53.

McQuaid, K. R. (1998). Alimentary tract. In L. M. Tierney, J. McPhee, & M. A. Papadakis (Eds.), *Current medical diagnosis and treatment* (37th ed.). E. Norwalk, CT: Appleton & Lange.

12–8

Lehne, R. A. (1998). *Pharmacology for nursing care* (3rd ed., p. 395). Philadelphia: WB Saunders.

Lilly, L., & Aucker, R. (1999). *Pharmacology and the nursing process* (2nd ed., pp. 319–334). St. Louis, MO: CV Mosby.

Skidmore-Roth, L., & McKenry, L. (1999). *Mosby's drug guide for nurses* (4th ed., pp. 1351–1353). St. Louis, MO: CV Mosby.

Spratto, G. R., & Woods, A. L. (2000). *PDR nurse's drug handbook* (pp. 114–118). Montvale, NJ: Delmar Publishers and Medical Economics Company.

12–9

Abrams, A. C. (1998). *Clinical drug therapy: Rationales for nursing practice* (5th ed.). Philadelphia: JB Lippincott.

American Diabetes Association. (1998). Position statement: Insulin administration. *Diabetes Care, 21*(Suppl. 1), S72–S75.

Drug facts and comparisons. (1999). St. Louis, MO: Facts and Comparisons.

Guitterrez, K. (1999). *Pharmacotherapeutics: Clinical decision making in nursing.* Philadelphia: WB Saunders.

Ignatavicius, D. D., Workman, M. L., & Mishler, M. A. (Eds.). (1999). *Medical-surgical nursing across the health care continuum* (3rd ed.). Philadelphia: WB Saunders.

Lewis, S. M., Heitkemper, M. M., & Dirksen, S. R. (2000). *Medical-surgical nursing: Assessment and management of clinical problems* (5th ed.). St. Louis, MO: Mosby-Year Book.

Monahan, F. D., & Neighbors, M. (1998). *Medical-surgical nursing: Foundations for clinical practice* (2nd ed.). Philadelphia: WB Saunders.

Spratto, G. R., & Woods, A. L. (1999). *PDR nurse's handbook.* Montage, NJ: Delmar.

Wilson, B. A., Shannon, M. T., & Stang, C. L. (2000). *Nurses' drug guide 2000.* E. Norwalk, CT: Appleton & Lange.

12–10

Abrams, A. C. (1998). *Clinical drug therapy: Rationales for nursing practice* (5th ed.). Philadelphia: JB Lippincott.

Drug facts and comparisons. (1999). St. Louis, MO: Facts and Comparisons.

Guitterrez, K. (1999). *Pharmacotherapeutics: Clinical decision making in nursing.* Philadelphia: WB Saunders.

Hansen, M. (1998). *Pathophysiology: Foundations of disease and clinical intervention.* Philadelphia: WB Saunders.

LeMone, P., & Burke, K. M. (2000). *Medical-surgical nursing: Critical thinking in client care.* (2nd ed.). Menlo Park, CA: Addison-Wesley Nursing.

Lewis, S. M., Heitkemper, M. M., & Dirkson, S. R. (2000). *Medical-surgical nursing: Assessment and management of clinical problems* (5th ed.). St. Louis, MO: Mosby-Year Book.

Monahan, F. D., & Neighbors, M. (1998). *Medical-surgical nursing: Foundations for clinical practice* (2nd ed.). Philadelphia: WB Saunders.

Spratto, G. R., & Woods, A. L. (1999). PDR nurse's handbook. Montage, NJ: Delmar.

Wilson, B. A., Shannon, M. T., & Stang, C. L. (2000). *Nurses' drug guide 2000.* E. Norwalk, CT: Appleton & Lange.

12–11

Ahonen, J., Olkkola, K. T., Takala, A., & Neuvonen, P. J. (1999). Interaction between fluconazole and midazolam in intensive care patients. *Acta Anaesthesiologica Scandinavica, 43*(5), 509–514.

Anonymous (1999). Antianxiety agents. In M. R. Riley, S. K. Hebel, T. Burnham, et al. (Eds.), *Facts and comparisons* (pp. 260–262). St. Louis, MO: Facts and Comparisons.

Anonymous (1998). Guidelines mailed to physicians on proper use of hypnotic sedatives can reduce inappropriate prescribing. *Research Activities, 222,* 16.

Anonymous (1999). Sedatives and hypnotics, barbiturates. In M. R. Riley, S. K. Hebel, T. Burnham, et al. (Eds.), *Facts and comparisons* (pp. 274–280). St. Louis, MO: Facts and Comparisons.

Borchardt, M. (1999). Review of the clinical pharmacology and use of the benzodiazepines. *Journal of Perianesthesia Nursing, 14*(2), 65–72.

Elliott, R., & Wright, L. (1999). Verbal communication: What do critical care nurses say to their unconscious or sedated patients? *Journal of Advanced Nursing, 29*(6), 1412–1420.

Hales, R. E., Hilty, D. A., & Wise, M. G. (1997). A treatment algorithm for the management of anxiety in primary care practice. *Journal of Clinical Psychiatry, 58*(Suppl. 3), 41–47.

Kendler, K. S., Karkowski, L., & Prescott, C. A. (1999). Hallucinogen, opiate, sedative and stimulant use in a population-based sample of female twins. *Acta Psychiatrica Scandinavica, 99*(5), 368–376.

Kirkwood, C. K., & Hayes, P. E. (1997). Anxiety disorders. In J. T. DiPiro, R. L. Talbert, G. C. Yee, et al. (Eds.), *Pharmacotherapy: A pathophysiologic approach* (3rd ed., pp. 1443–1462). E. Norwalk, CT: Appleton & Lange.

Kirkwood, C. K., & Sood, R. K. (1997). Sleep disorders. In J. T. DiPiro, R. L. Talbert, G. C. Yee, et al. (Eds.), *Pharmacotherapy: A pathophysiologic approach* (3rd ed., pp. 1477–1488). E. Norwalk, CT: Appleton & Lange.

Kirkwood, C. K. (1998). Anxiety Disorders. In B. L. Carter, K. D. Lake, M. A. Raebel, et al. (Eds.), *Pharmacotherapy self-assessment program. Module 4: Neurology and psychiatry* (3rd ed., pp. 165–1196). St. Louis, MO: American College of Clinical Pharmacy.

Moore, P. A. (1999). Adverse drug interactions in dental practice: Interactions associated with local anesthetics, sedatives and anxiolytics. Part IV of a series. *Journal of the American Dental Association, 130*(4), 541–554.

Piraino, A. J. (1997). Drug use in the elderly: Tips for avoiding adverse effects and interactions. *Consultant, 37*(11), 2825–2827, 2830–2834.

12–12

Black, J. M., & Matassarin-Jacobs, E. (1997). *Medical-surgical nursing: Clinical management for continuity of care* (5th ed., pp. 321, 665, 670, 874, 885, 1172, 1389, 2048t, 2049t, 2201, 2199t). Philadelphia: WB Saunders.

Lehne, R. A. (1998). *Pharmacology for nursing care* (3rd ed., pp. 616–623; 709–719). Philadelphia: WB Saunders.

Lilly, L., & Aucker, R. (1999). *Pharmacology and the nursing process* (2nd ed., pp. 421–429). St. Louis, MO: CV Mosby.

Skidmore-Roth, L., & McKenry, L. (1997). *Mosby's drug guide for nurses* (2nd ed., pp. 1349–1351). Philadelphia: CV Mosby.

13–1

Abramowicz, M. (Ed.). (2000). Drugs for asthma. *The Medical Letter on Drugs and Therapeutics, 42*(1073), 19–24.

Abramowicz, M. (Ed.). (1999). Drugs for asthma. *The Medical Letter on Drugs and Therapeutics, 41*(1044), 5–10.

Burrell, L. O., Gerlach, M. J., & Pless, B. S. (1997). *Adult nursing: Acute and community*. E. Norwalk, CT: Appleton & Lange.

Chambers, C. V., Smith, L. J., & Weinberger, M. (2000). Asthma: Getting the priorities straight. *Patient Care, 34*(8), 56–81.

Fenstermacher, K., & Hudson, B. T. (1997). Practice guidelines for family nurse practitioners. Philadelphia: WB Saunders.

Hayden, M. L. (2000). Asthma in the elderly: A diagnostic and management challenge. *Advance for Nurse Practitioners, 8*(7), 30–35.

Hayden, M. L. (2000). Leukotriene modifiers: Expanded role may be on the horizon. *Advance for Nurse Practitioners, 8*(10), 42–46.

Henderson, S. O., Acharya, P., Kilaghbian, T., et al. (1999). Use of heliox-driven nebulizer therapy in the treatment of acute asthma. *Annals of Emergency Medicine, 33*, 141–146.

Jowers, J., Corsello, P. R., Shafer, A. L., et al. (2000). Partnering specialist care with nurse case management: A pilot project for asthma. *Journal of Clinical Outcomes Management, 7*(5), 17–22.

Kosseim, L. M., & Neuman, W. R. (2000). Exercise-induced asthma. *Patient Care, 34*(13), 55–61.

McCance, K. L., & Heuther, S. E. (1998). *Pathophysiology: The biologic basis for disease in adults and children* (3rd ed.). St. Louis, MO: CV Mosby.

Mellins, R. B., Evans, D., Clark, N., et al. (2000). Developing and communicating a long-term treatment plan for asthma. *American Family Physician, 61*(8), 2419–2426.

Mladenovic, J. (1999). *Primary care secrets* (2nd ed.). Philadelphia: Hanley & Belfus.

Monthly Vital Statistics Report, August 14, 1997, *46*(11).

Petty, T. L. (2000). Toward "quiet" asthma: Keys to preventing life-threatening attacks. *Consultant, 40*(6), 1152–1160.

Plaut, T. F. (1998). *One minute asthma: What you need to know.* Amherst, MA: Pedipress.

Reicin, A., White, R., Weinstein, S. F., et al. (2000). Montelukast: A leukotriene receptor antagonist, in combination with Loratadine, a histamine receptor antagonist, in the treatment of chronic asthma. *Archives of Internal Medicine, 160*(16), 2481–2488.

Sloan, P. D., Slatt, L. M., Curtis, P., & Ebell, M. H. (1998). *Essentials of family medicine* (3rd ed.). Baltimore: Williams & Wilkins.

Uphold, C. R., & Graham, M. V. (1998). *Clinical guidelines in family practice* (3rd ed.). Gainesville, FL: Barmarrae Books.

Wells, B. G., DiPiro, J. T., Schwinghammer, T. L., & Hamilton, C. W. (1998). *Pharmacotherapy handbook.* E. Norwalk, CT: Appleton & Lange.

13–2

Ball, P., Chodosh, S., Grossman, R., et al. (2000). Causes, epidemiology, and treatment of bronchial infections. *Infections in Medicine, 17*(3), 186.

Carey, C. F., Lee, H. H., & Woeltje, K. F. (1998). *Washington manual of medical therapeutics.* Philadelphia: Lippincott Williams & Wilkins.

Fenstermacher, K., & Hudson, B. T. (1997). Practice guidelines for family nurse practitioners. Philadelphia: WB Saunders.

Gross, N. J., Payne, D. K., & Petty, T. L. (2000). Optimal treatment for COPD. *Patient Care, 34*(10), 60–73.

Larimore, W. L., Hartman, J. R., Shupe, T. B., et al. (1999). Diary from a week in practice. *American Family Physician, 59*(5), 1157.

McCance, K. L., & Heuther, S. E. (1998). *Pathophysiology: The biologic basis for disease in adults and children* (3rd ed.). St. Louis, MO: CV Mosby.

Mladenovic, J. (1999). *Primary care secrets* (2nd ed.). Philadelphia: Hanley & Belfus.

Sloan, P. D., Slatt, L. M., Curtis, P., & Ebell, M. H. (1998). *Essentials of family medicine* (3rd ed.). Baltimore: Williams & Wilkins.

Uphold, C. R., & Graham, M. V. (1998). *Clinical guidelines in family practice* (3rd ed.). Gainesville, FL: Barmarrae Books.

Wells, B. G., DiPiro, J. T., Schwinghammer, T. L., & Hamilton, C. W. (1998). *Pharmacotherapy handbook.* E. Norwalk, CT: Appleton & Lange.

13–3

Fenstermacher, K., & Hudson, B. T. (1997). *Practice guidelines for family nurse practitioners.* Philadelphia: WB Saunders.

Gross, N. J., Payne, D. K., & Petty, T. L. (2000). Optimal treatment for COPD. *Patient Care, 34*(10), 60–73.

Larimore, W. L., Hartman, J. R., Shupe, T. B., et al. (1999). Diary from a week in practice. *American Family Physician, 59*(5), 1157.

McCance, K. L., & Heuther, S. E. (1998). *Pathophysiology: The biologic basis for disease in adults and children* (3rd. ed.). St. Louis, MO: CV Mosby.

Mladenovic, J. (1999). *Primary care secrets* (2nd ed.). Philadelphia: Hanley & Belfus.

Schumann, L. (2000). Obstructive pulmonary disorders. In L. C. Copstead & J. L. Banasik (Eds.), *Pathophysiology: Biological and behavioral perspectives* (2nd ed.). Philadelphia: WB Saunders.

Sloan, P. D., Slatt, L. M., Curtis, P., & Ebell, M. H. (1998). *Essentials of family medicine* (3rd ed.). Baltimore: Williams & Wilkins.

Uphold, C. R., & Graham, M. V. (1998). *Clinical guidelines in family practice* (3rd ed.). Gainesville, FL: Barmarrae Books.

Wells, B. G., DiPiro, J. T., Schwinghammer, T. L., & Hamilton, C. W. (1998). *Pharmacotherapy handbook.* E. Norwalk, CT: Appleton & Lange.

13–4

Fenstermacher, K., & Hudson, B. T. (1997). Practice guidelines for family nurse practitioners. Philadelphia: WB Saunders.

Larimore, W. L., Hartman, J. R., Shupe, T. B., et al. (1999). Diary from a week in practice. *American Family Physician. 59*(5), 1157.

McCance, K. L., & Heuther, S. E. (1998). *Pathophysiology: The biologic basis for disease in adults and children* (3rd ed.). St. Louis, MO: CV Mosby.

Mladenovic, J. (1999). *Primary care secrets* (2nd ed.). Philadelphia: Hanley & Belfus.

Newman, D. C. (1998). Pulmonary diseases. In U. B. Prakash (Ed.), *Mayo internal medicine board review.* Philadelphia: Lippincott Williams & Wilkins.

O'Brien, M. E. (2000). Pneumonia. In R. E. Rakel (Ed.), *Saunders manual of medical practice* (2nd ed., p. 200). Philadelphia: WB Saunders.

Sloan, P. D., Slatt, L. M., Curtis, P., & Ebell, M. H. (1998). *Essentials of family medicine* (3rd ed.). Baltimore: Williams & Wilkins.

Uphold, C. R., & Graham, M. V. (1998). *Clinical guidelines in family practice* (3rd ed.). Gainesville, FL: Barmarrae Books.

Wells, B. G., DiPiro, J. T., Schwinghammer, T. L., & Hamilton, C. W. (1998). *Pharmacotherapy handbook.* E. Norwalk, CT: Appleton & Lange.

13–5

Department of Health and Human Services. (2000). *Core curriculum on tuberculosis* (4th ed.). Atlanta, GA: Centers for Disease Control and Prevention.

14–1

American Heart Association. (1999). *1999 heart and stroke statistical update.* Available at: *http://www.americanheart.org*

Braunwald, E., & Ganz, P. (1997). Coronary blood flow and myocardial ischemia. In E. Braunwald (Ed.), *Heart disease: A textbook of cardiovascular medicine* (5th ed.). Philadelphia: WB Saunders.

Dambro, M. R. (2000). *Griffith's 5 minute clinical consult.* Baltimore: Williams & Wilkins.

Graham-Garcia, J., & Raines, T. (2000). Acute coronary syndromes. *Advance for Nurses, 2*(10), 20–21.

Heger, J. W. (1998). *Cardiology* (4th ed.). Baltimore: Williams & Wilkins.

Lefkovits, J., Plow, E. F., & Topol, E. J. (1997). Platelet glycoprotein IIb/IIIa receptors in cardiovascular medicine. *New England Journal of Medicine, 332,* 1553–1559.

Steckel, L. (1999). Antiplatelet agents in acute coronary syndromes. *Advance for Nurse Practitioners, 7*(12), 41–46.

Yun, D. D., & Alpert, J. S. (1997). Acute coronary syndromes. *Cardiology, 88,* 223–237.

14–2

Antman, E. M. (1997). Medical management of the patient undergoing cardiac surgery. In E. Braunwald (Ed.), *Braunwald's heart disease: A textbook of cardiovascular medicine* (5th ed.). Philadelphia: WB Saunders.

Gawlinski, A., McCloy, K., Caswell, D., & Quinones-Baldrich, W. J. (1999). Cardiovascular disorders. In A. Gawlinski & D. Hamwi (Eds.), *Acute care nurse practitioner: Clinical curriculum and certification review.* Philadelphia: WB Saunders.

14–3

Albert, N. (1999a). Heart failure: The physiologic basis for current therapeutic concepts. *Critical Care Nurse, June Supplement,* 2–15.

Albert, N. (1999b). Manipulating survival and life quality outcomes in heart failure through disease state management. *Critical Care Nursing Clinics of North America, 11,* 121–141.

Baig, M., McKenna, C., Bonow, F., et al. (1999). The pathophysiology of advanced heart failure. *Heart and Lung, 28,* 87–101.

Chase, S. L. (1999). New strategies in the management of patients with heart failure. *Pharmacy and Therapeutics,* Feb., 84–96.

Frantz, A., Bolin, C., Gibbs, K., et al. (1998). Consensus panel of home care nurses. Summary of the nursing practice guidelines for the cardiac home care patient. *Home Healthcare Nurse, 16,* 743–752.

Lehne, R. A. (1998). Drug therapy of CHF. In *Pharmacology for nursing care* (pp. 416, 475–489). Philadelphia: WB Saunders.

McKinney, B. C. (1999). Solving the puzzle of heart failure. *Nursing 99, May,* 29(5), 33–39.

Packer, M., & Cohn, J. N. (1999). Consensus recommendations for the management of chronic heart failure. *American Journal of Cardiology, 83*(2A), 1A–38A.

Paul, S. (1997). Implementing an outpatient congestive heart failure clinic: The nurse practitioner role. *Heart and Lung 26*(6), 486–491.

Pitt, B., Zannad, F., Remme, W. J., et al. (1999). The effect of spironolactone on morbidity and mortality in patients with severe heart failure. *New England Journal of Medicine, 341*(10), 709–717.

14–4

Dambro, M. R. (Ed.). (1998). *Griffith's 5-minute clinical consult.* Baltimore: Williams & Wilkins.

Gawlinski, A., & Hamwi, D. (Eds.). (1999). *Acute care nurse practitioner: Clinical curriculum and certification review.* Philadelphia: WB Saunders.

Luckman, J. (Ed.). (1997). *Manual of nursing care.* Philadelphia: WB Saunders.

Passmore, J. M. (Ed.). (1997). Practical prevention of coronary heart disease. *Adult Health: Multidisciplinary Approaches to Wellness, 1*(3).

Thompson, D., & Ferris, L. (1997). Coronary heart disease. In L. O. Burrell, M. J. Gerlach, & B. S. Pless (Eds.), *Adult nursing: Acute and community care* (pp. 425–447). E. Norwalk, CT: Appleton & Lange.

Uphold, C. R., & Graham, M. V. (1998). *Clinical guidelines in family practice* (3rd ed.). Gainesville, FL: Barmarrae Books.

14–5

American Heart Association. (1999). *1999 heart and stroke statistical update.* Available at: *http://www.americanheart.org*

Gylys, K., & Gold, M. (2000). Acute coronary syndromes: New developments in pharmacological treatment strategies. *Critical Care Nurse,* April 2000 (Suppl.).

Hill, B., & Geraci, S. A. (1998). A diagnostic approach to chest pain based on history and ancillary evaluation. *The Nurse Practitioner, 23*(4), 20–47.

Kahn, M. G. (1997). *On call cardiology.* Philadelphia: WB Saunders.

Woods, S. L., Sivarajan-Froelicher, E. S., & Underhill-Motzer, S. (Eds.). (1999). *Cardiac nursing* (4th ed.). Philadelphia: Lippincott Williams & Wilkins.

Yun, D. D., & Alpert, J. S. (1997). Acute coronary syndromes. *Cardiology, 88,* 223–237.

14–6

Dajani, A. S. (1997). Rheumatic fever. In E. Braunwald (Ed.), *Braunwald's Heart Disease: A textbook of cardiovascular medicine* (5th ed.). Philadelphia: WB Saunders.

15–1

Gawlinski, A., McCloy, K., Caswell, D., & Quinones-Baldrich, W. J. (1999). Cardiovascular disorders: Abdominal aortic aneurysm. In A. Gawlinski & D. Hamwi (Eds.), *Acute care nurse practitioner: Clinical curriculum and certification review* (pp. 272–277). Philadelphia: WB Saunders.

Jones, M. A., Hoffman, L. A., & Makaroun, M. S. (2000). Endovascular grafting for repair of abdominal aortic aneurysm. *Critical Care Nurse, 20*(4), 38–51.

Kristt, A. M. (1999). The peripheral vascular surgical patient. In K. Litwack, (Ed.), *Core curriculum for perianesthesia nursing* (4th ed., pp. 306–334). Philadelphia: WB Saunders.

Lessig, M. L., & Lessig, P. M. (1998). The cardiovascular system. In J. G. Alspach (Ed.), *Core curriculum for critical care nursing* (5th ed., pp. 137–337). Philadelphia: WB Saunders.

Liston, S. M. (1997). Stent-graft placement procedures for descending thoracic aortic aneurysms. *AORN Journal, 66,* 433–444.

Thomas, C. L. (Ed.). (1998). *Taber's cyclopedic medical dictionary.* Philadelphia: FA Davis.

Thompson, M. M., & Bell, P. R. F. (2000). Arterial aneurysms: Clinical review: ABC or arterial and venous disease. *British Medical Journal, 320,* 1193–1196.

Turner, J. (1997). Caring for people with peripheral vascular and lymphatic disorders. In J. Luckmann (Ed.), *Saunders manual of nursing care* (pp. 1091–1126). Philadelphia: WB Saunders.

15–2

Creager, M., & Hiatt, W. (1999). Management of peripheral artery disease. Online Coverage from the American College of Cardiology 48th Annual Scientific Session, March 7–10, 1999.

Fauci, A. S., Braunwalk, E., Isselbacher, K. J., et al. (1998). *Harrison's principles of internal medicine* (14th ed.). New York: McGraw-Hill.

Hansen, M. (1998). *Pathophysiology: Foundations of disease and clinical intervention* (pp. 359–361). Philadelphia: WB Saunders.

Ignatavicius, D. D., Workman, M. L., & Mishler, M. A. (1999). *Medical-surgical nursing across the health care continuum* (3rd ed., pp. 870–871). Philadelphia: WB Saunders.

Monahan, F. D., & Neighbors, M. (1998). *Medical-surgical nursing: Founda-*

tions for clinical practice (2nd ed., pp. 351–355). Philadelphia: WB Saunders.

Phipps, W. J., Sands, J. K., & Marek, J. F. (1999). *Medical-Surgical nursing: Concepts and clinical practice* (pp. 760–761). St. Louis, MO: CV Mosby.

Porth, C. M. (1998). *Pathophysiology: Concepts of altered health states* (5th ed., p. 347). Philadelphia: JB Lippincott.

Price, S. A., & Wilson, L. M. (1997). *Pathophysiology: Clinical concepts of disease processes* (5th ed., p. 529). St. Louis, MO: CV Mosby.

Smeltzer, S. C., & Bare, B. G. (2000). *Brunner and Suddarth's textbook of medical-surgical nursing* (9th ed.). Philadelphia: JB Lippincott.

Szuba, A., & Cooke, J. P. (1998). Thromboangiitis obliterans: An update on Buerger's disease. *The Western Journal of Medicine, 168*(4), *255*(6). Infotrac Searchbank.

Thompson, J. M., McFarland, G. K., Hirsch, J. E., & Tucker, S. M. (1997). *Mosby's clinical nursing* (4th ed., pp. 87–89). St. Louis, MO: CV Mosby.

15–3

Dupvy, D. E. (2000). Venus ultrasound of lower-extremity deep venous thrombosis—when is ultrasound insufficient? *Radiographics, 20,* 1195–1200.

Elliott, C. G. (2000). The diagnostic approach to deep venous thrombosis. *Seminars in Respiratory and Critical Care Medicine, 21*(6), 511–519.

Emerson, R. J. (2000). Alterations in blood flow. In L. C. Copstead, & J. L. Banasik (Eds.), *Pathophysiology: Biological and behavioral perspectives* (2nd ed.). Philadelphia: WB Saunders.

Goll, C. A. (2001). Pulmonary emboli. In P. L. Swearingen & J. H. Keen (Eds.), *Manual of critical care nursing* (4th ed.). St. Louis, MO: CV Mosby.

Leclerc, J. R. (1998). DVT prophylaxis–pharmacologic prophylaxis and treatment of venous thromboembolism after lower extremity arthroplasty. *Medscape Orthopaedics and Sports Medicine, 2*(6).

Ofri, D. (2000). Diagnosis and treatment of deep vein thrombosis. *Western Journal of Medicine, 173*(3), 194–197.

Robertson, K. A., Bertot, A. J., Wolfe, M. W., & Barrack. R. L. (2000). Patient compliance and satisfaction with mechanical devices for preventing deep venous thrombosis after joint replacement. *Journal of the Southern Orthopedic Association, 9*(3), 182–186.

Tillman, D. J., Charland, S. L., & Witt, D. M. (2000). Effectiveness and economic impact associated with a program for outpatient management of acute deep vein thrombosis in a group model health maintenance organization. *Archives of Internal Medicine, 160*(19), 2926–2932.

15–4

Chung, E., & Tighe, D., (Eds.). (1999). *Systemic hypertension: Pocket guide to cardiovascular diseases*. Malden, MA: Blackwell Science.

Cotran R., Kumar, V., & Collins, T. (1999). *Blood vessels. Robbins' pathologic basis of disease*. Philadelphia: WB Saunders.

Dumas, M. (1999). Cardiovascular disease: Hypertension in primary care. *The American Journal for Nurse Practitioners, 3*(2), 7–32.

Guyton, A., & Hall, J. (1997). *Physics of blood, blood flow and pressure: Hemodynamics: Human physiology and mechanisms of disease* (6th ed.). Philadelphia: WB Saunders.

Guyton, A., & Hall, J. (2000). *The textbook of medical physiology* (pp. 195–207). Philadelphia: WB Saunders.

Herrera, C. Hypertension. (2000). In R. E. Rakel (Ed.), *Saunders manual of medical practice* (5th ed., p. 220). Philadelphia: WB Saunders.

Macfarlane, P., Reid, R., & Callander, R. (2000). *Cardiovascular disease: Pathology illustrated* (5th ed.). Edinburgh, Scotland: Churchill Livingstone.

National high blood pressure evaluation program. (1997). *The sixth report of the joint national committee on prevention, detection, evaluation and treatment of high blood pressure.* Bethesda, MD: US Department of Health and Human Services, National Heart, Lung, and Blood Institute. NIH pub. no. 98–4080.

Ray, J. (1997). Hypertension and vasculitis syndrome. In L. Burrell, M. Gerlach, & B. Pless (Eds.), *Nursing management of adults with cardiovascular and hematologic problems* (2nd ed.). E. Norwalk, CT: Appleton & Lange.

Tierney, L., Saint, S., Thompson, C., & Whooley, M. (1997). *Cardiovascular disease: Pocket guide to the essentials of diagnosis and treatment* (p. 32). E. Norwalk, CT: Appleton & Lange.

15–5

Granger, B. B. (1997). Cardiovascular system. In M. Chulay, C. Guzzetta, & B. Dossey (Eds.), *AACN handbook of critical care nursing* (pp. 264–267). E. Norwalk, CT: Appleton & Lange.

Kolecki, P., & Menckhoff, C. (2000). Shock, hypovolemic. Available at: *http://www.emedicine.com/EMERG/topic532.htm*

McKinley, M. G., Robinson, C. F., & Sole, M. L. (1997). Shock. In J. C. Hartshorn, M. L. Sole, & M. L. Lamborn (Eds.), *Introduction to critical care nursing* (pp. 205–230). Philadelphia: WB Saunders.

15–6

Browse, N. L., Brunand, K. G., Irvine, A. T., & Wilson, N. M. (1999). *Diseases of the veins* (2nd ed.). London: Arnold.

Bryant, J. L., & Turkowski, B. B. (1999). Relieving intermittent claudication: A nursing approach. *Journal of Vascular Nursing, 17,* 81–85.

Cantwell-Gab, K. (1996). Identifying chronic peripheral arterial disease. *American Journal of Nursing, 96,* 40–46.

Fahey, V. A. (1999). *Vascular nursing* (3rd ed.). Philadelphia: WB Saunders.

Gibson, J., & Kenrick, M. (1998). Pain and powerlessness: The experience of living with peripheral vascular disease. *Journal of Advanced Nursing, 27,* 737–745.

Kelly, J. (1999). Peripheral vascular disorders. In L. M. Hektor Dunphy (Ed.), *Management guidelines for adult nurse practitioners* (pp. 404–407). Philadelphia: FA Davis.

Pless, B. S. (1997). Disorders of the venous and lymphatic system. In L. O. Burrell, M. M. Gerlach, & B. S. Pless (Eds.), *Adult nursing, acute and community care* (2nd ed., pp. 531–547). E. Norwalk, CT: Appleton & Lange.

Ray, J. (1997). Disorders of the aorta and its branches. In L. O. Burrell, M. M. Gerlach, & B. S. Pless (Eds.), *Adult nursing, acute and community care* (2nd ed., pp. 508–530). E. Norwalk, CT: Appleton & Lange.

Summer, D. S., & van Bemmelin, P. S. (1997). Hemodynamics of the venous system: Calf pump and valve function. In S. Raju & J. L. Villavicencio

(Eds.), *Surgical management of venous disease* (pp. 16–59). Baltimore: Williams & Wilkins.

Turner, J. (1997). Caring for people with peripheral vascular and lymph disorders. In J. Luckmann (Ed.), *Saunders manual of nursing care* (pp. 1091–1126). Philadelphia: WB Saunders.

15–7

Apgar, B. (1998). Outcomes in patients with primary Raynaud phenomenon. *American Family Physician, 58*(1), 206. Infotrac Searchband (2 pages).

Bullock, B. L. (1996). *Pathophysiology: Adaptations and alterations in function* (4th ed., pp. 534–535). Philadelphia: JB Lippincott.

Copstead, L. E. (1995). Perspectives on pathophysiology. Philadelphia: WB Saunders.

Fauci, A. S., Braunwalk, E., Isselbacher, K. J., et al. (1998). *Harrison's principles of internal medicine* (14th ed.). New York: McGraw-Hill.

Hansen, M. (1998). *Pathophysiology: Foundations of disease and clinical intervention* (pp. 359–363). Philadelphia: WB Saunders.

Ignatavicius, D. D., Workman, M. L., & Mishler, M. A. (1999). *Medical-surgical nursing across the health care continuum* (3rd ed., p. 872). Philadelphia: WB Saunders.

Mallipeddi, R., & Mathis, C. J. (1998). Raynaud's phenomenon after sympathetic denervation in patients with primary autonomic failure: Questionnaire survey. *British Medical Journal, 316*(7129), 438. Infotrac Searchbank (4 pages).

Monahan, F. D., & Neighbors, M. (1998). *Medical-surgical nursing: Foundations for clinical practice* (2nd ed., pp. 355–360). Philadelphia: WB Saunders.

Phipps, W. J., Sands, J. K., & Marek, J. F. (1999). *Medical-surgical nursing: Concepts and clinical practice* (pp. 761–762). St. Louis, MO: CV Mosby.

Porth, C. M. (1998). *Pathophysiology: Concepts of altered health states* (5th ed., pp. 347–348). Philadelphia: JB Lippincott.

Price, S. A., & Wilson, L. M. (1997). *Pathophysiology: Clinical concepts of disease processes* (5th ed., pp. 529). St. Louis, MO: CV Mosby.

Prouty, H. (1997). The cold war: Battling to keep your fingers and toes warm? Your digital deep freeze could signal Raynaud's phenomenon. *Women's Sports and Fitness, 19*(9), 59(2). Infotrac Searchbank (4 pages).

Smeltzer, S. C., & Bare, B. G. (2000). *Brunner and Suddarth's textbook of medical-surgical nursing* (9th ed.). Philadelphia: JB Lippincott.

Thompson, J. M., McFarland, G. K., Hirsch, J. E., & Tucker, S. M. (1997). *Mosby's clinical nursing* (4th ed., pp. 89–90). St. Louis, MO: CV Mosby.

15–8

Angeles, T. (1997). How to prevent phlebitis. *Nursing 27*(1), 26.

Creager, M. A., & Dzau, V. J. (1998). In A. S. Fauci, E. Braunwald, K. J. Isselbacher, J. D. Wilson, J. B. Martin, D. L. Kasper, S. L. Hauser, & D. L. Longo (Eds.), *Harrison's principles of internal medicine* (14th ed., p. 1403). New York: McGraw-Hill.

Ferrari, E., Chevallier, Y., Chapelier, A., & Baudouy, M. (1999). Travel as a risk factor for venous thromboembolic disease: A case control study. *Chest, 115*(2), 440–444.

Hansen, M. (1998). *Pathophysiology: Foundations of disease and clinical intervention*. Philadelphia: WB Saunders.

Monahan, F. D., & Neighbors, M. (1998). *Medical-surgical nursing: Foundations for clinical practice* (2nd ed.). Philadelphia: WB Saunders.

National Center for Infectious Diseases: Centers for Disease Control and Prevention. *Guideline for Prevention of Intravascular Device-Related Infections.* (Updated 06/02/99). Atlanta, GA. Available at: *http://www.cdc.gov/ncidod/hip/iv/iv.htm*

Porth, C. M. (1998). *Pathophysiology: Concepts of altered health states* (5th ed.). Philadelphia: Lippincott-Raven.

Thompson, J., McFarland, G., Hirsch, J., & Tucker, S. (1997). *Mosby's clinical nursing* (4th ed.). St. Louis, MO: Mosby Year-Book.

Weinstein, S. M. (1997). *Plumer's principles and practice of intravenous therapy* (6th ed.). Philadelphia: Lippincott-Raven.

Wilson, D. D. (1999). *Nurses' guide to understanding laboratory and diagnostic tests.* Philadelphia: JB Lippincott.

15–9

Browse, N. L., Burnand, K. G., Levine, A. T., & Wilson, N. M. (1999). *Diseases of the veins* (2nd ed.). London: Arnold.

Hahn, T. L., & Dalsing, M. C. (1999). Chronic venous disease. In V. A. Fahey. *Vascular nursing* (3rd ed., pp. 364–387). Philadelphia: WB Saunders.

Villavicencio, J. L., Gillespie, D., Pikoulis, E., & Rich, N. M. (1999). Superficial varicose veins: Therapeutic options. In S. Raju & J. L. Villavicencio (Eds.), *Surgical management of venous disease* (pp. 373–390). Baltimore: Williams & Wilkins.

16–1

Beare, P. G., & Myers, J. L. (1998). *Adult health nursing* (3rd ed.). St Louis, MO: CV Mosby.

Groonroos, J., & Groonroos, P. (1999). Leukocyte count and C-reactive protein in the diagnosis of acute appendicitis. *British Journal of Surgery, 86*(4), 501–504.

Ignatavicius, D. D., Workman, M. L., & Mishler, M. A. (1999). *Medical surgical nursing across the health care continuum* (3rd ed.). Philadelphia: WB Saunders.

McColl, I. (1998). More precision in diagnosing appendicitis. *New England Journal of Medicine, 338*(3), 190–191.

Smeltzer, S. C., & Bare, B. G. (2000). *Textbook of medical surgical nursing* (9th ed.). Philadelphia: JB Lippincott.

16–2

Cirrhosis. Available at: *http://www.cdc.gov/nchs/fastats/liverdis.htm*

Cirrhosis. Available at: *http://www.gastro.org/cirrhosis.html*

Cirrhosis of the liver. Available at: *http://www.niddk.nih.gov/health/digest/pubs/cirrhosi/cirrhosi.htm*

Elrod, R. (2000). Cirrhosis. In S. Lewis, M. M. Heitkemper, & S. R. Dirksen (Eds.), M*edical-surgical nursing: Assessment and management of clinical problems* (pp. 1203–1218). Baltimore, MD: CV Mosby.

Haycraft, L. (1998). Cirrhosis. In P. G. Beare & J. L. Myers (Eds.), *Adult health nursing* (pp. 1574–1586). St. Louis, MO: CV Mosby.

Lemone, P., & Burke, K. (2000). *Medical-surgical nursing: Critical thinking in client care* (2nd ed., pp. 526–539). Upper Saddle River, NJ: Prentice-Hall.

McMaster, P. (2000). Transplantation for alcoholic liver disease in an era of organ shortage. *The Lancet, 355,* 424–427.

Sadovsky, R. (2000). Management challenges of liver cirrhosis. *American Family Physician, 61,* 1127–1128.

Smolen, D. (1997). Cirrhosis. In J. M. Black & E. Matassarin-Jacobs (Eds.), *Medical-surgical nursing: Clinical management for continuity of care* (pp. 1872–1895). Philadelphia: WB Saunders.

Trevillyan, J., & Carroll, P. J. (1997). Management of portal hypertension and esophageal varices in alcoholic cirrhosis. *American Family Physician, 55*(5), 1851–1861.

16–3

Centers for Disease Control and Prevention. CDC: Foodborne Infections. On line: March 2000a. Available at: *www.cdc.gov*

Centers for Disease Control and Prevention. CDC: Foodnet. On line: March 2000b. Available at: *http://www.cdc.gov*

Cerrato, P. L. (1999). When food is the culprit. *Registered Nurse, 62*(6), 52–56.

International Food Information Council. (IFIC). Backgrounder-Food Safety and Foodborne Illness. On Line: August 1998a. Available at: *http://ificinfo. health.org/backgrnd/bkgr10.html*

International Food Information Council. (IFIC). A consumer's guide to micro-biological risks to food safety. On Line: August 1998b. Available at: *http:// ificinfo.health.org/resource/microbiorisks.html*

Keene, W. E. (1999). Lessons from investigating food outbreaks. *Journal of the Medical Association, 281*(19), 1845–1847.

Morris, K. (1999). A danger at my table? *The Lancet, 354*(9189), 1565.

Potter, P., & Perry, A. (1999). *Basic nursing: A critical thinking approach* (4th ed.). St. Louis, MO: CV Mosby.

Sanders, T. A. (1999). Food production and food safety. *British Medical Journal, 318*(7199), 1689–1693.

Smeltzer, S. C, & Bare, B. G. (2000). *Textbook of medical surgical nursing* (9th ed.). Philadelphia: JB Lippincott.

16–4

Centers for Disease Control and Prevention (CDC). Hepatitis. Available at: *http://www.cdc.ncidod/diseases/hepatitis/index.htm*

Heathcote, J. (2000). Antiviral therapy in patients with chronic hepatitis C. *Seminars in Liver Disease, 20*(2), 185–199.

Hepatitis Fact Sheets From John Hopkins. Available at: *http://www.hopkins-id.edu/diseases/hepatitis*

Marcos, A., Ham, J. M., Fisher, R. A., et al. (2000). Emergency adult to adult living donor liver transplantation for fulminant hepatic failure. *Transplantation, 69,* 2202–2205.

Morbidity and Mortality Weekly Report. (1998). U.S. Department of Health and Human Services. CDC, *47*(RR-19).

Silverman, A. L., Sekhon, J. S., Saginaw, S. J., et al. (2000). Tattoo application is not associated with an increased risk for viral hepatitis? *American Journal of Gastroenterology, 95,* 1312–1315.

Wong, J. B., Poynard, T., Ling, M. H., et al. (2000). Cost-effectiveness of 24 or 48 weeks of interferon alpha-2b alone or with ribaviron as initial treatment of chronic hepatitis C. *American Journal of Gastroenterology, 95,* 1524–1530.

16–5

DiPiro, J., Talbert, R., Yee, G., Posey, L. M., et al. (Eds.). *Pharmacotherapy: A pathophysiologic approach* (pp. 571–583). E. Norwalk, CT: Appleton & Lange.

Feagan, B. G., Fedorak, R., Irvine, J., et al. (2000). A comparison of methotrexate with placebo for the maintenance of remission in Crohn's disease. *New England Journal of Medicine, 342*, 1627–1632.

Gerlach, M. (1997). Disorders of the small and large intestines and anorectal disorders. In L. Burrell, M. Gerlach, & B. Pless (Eds.), *Nursing management of adults with gastrointestinal problems* (pp. 1443–1448). E. Norwalk, CT: Appleton & Lange.

Ginsberg, C. (2000). Inflammatory bowel disease. In R. E. Rakel (Ed.), Conn's current therapy (pp. 482–488). Philadelphia: WB Saunders.

Greenwald, B. (2000). Ulcerative colitis. In R. E. Rakel (Ed.), *Saunders manual of medical practice* (pp. 344–346). Philadelphia: WB Saunders.

Hanauer, S. (2000). Medical therapy for ulcerative colitis. In J. Kirsner (Ed.), Inflammatory bowel disease (6th ed., pp. 529–556). Philadelphia: WB Saunders.

Iber, F. L. (2000). *Crohn's disease. Griffith's 5 minute clinical consultation* (pp. 1124–1125). Philadelphia: Lippincott William & Wilkins.

James, S. (2000). Crohn's disease. In R. E. Rakel (Ed.), *Saunders manual of medical practice* (pp. 341–343). Philadelphia: WB Saunders.

Lang, K., & Peppercorn, M. (2000). Medical therapy for Crohn's disease. In J. Kirsner (Ed.), *Inflammatory bowel disease* (6th ed., pp. 557–577). Philadelphia, WB Saunders.

McCance, K., & Huether, S. *The digestive system: Alteration of digestive function. Pathophysiology: The biologic basis for disease in adults and children* (3rd ed., pp. 1342–1344). St. Louis, MO: Mosby Year-Book.

Miller, S. (1999). In P. Rosen, R. Barkin, S. R. Hayden, et al. (Eds.), *Inflammatory bowel disease: The 5-minute emergency medicine consult* (pp. 592–593). Philadelphia: Lippincott Williams & Wilkins.

Physician Desk Reference Electronic Library. (2000). Montvale, NJ: Medical Economics Company.

Porth, C. (1998). *Alterations in gastrointestinal function. Pathophysiology concepts of altered health states* (4th ed.). Philadelphia: JB Lippincott.

16–6

Bailey, M. E., & Jourdan, I. C. (1998). Randomized placebo-controlled trial of local anesthetic infusion in day-case inguinal hernia repair. *British Journal of Surgery, 85*(10), 1451.

Gurleyik, E., Gurleyik, G., & Cetinkaya, F. (1998). The inflammatory response to open tension-free inguinal hernioplasty versus conventional repairs. *American Journal of Surgery, 175*(3), 179–182.

Ignatavicius, D. D., Workman, M. A., & Mishler, M. A. (1999). *Medical surgical nursing across the health care continuum* (3rd ed.). Philadelphia: WB Saunders.

Kark, A. E., Kurzer, M. N., & Belsham, P. A. (1999). Laparoscopic versus open mesh repair of inguinal hernia. *British Medical Journal, 318*(7177), 189–190.

16–7

Bass, K. N., Jones, B., & Bulkley, G. B. (1998). Current management of small bowel obstruction. *Advances in Surgery, 31*, 1.

Beck, D. E., Opelka, F. G., Bailey, H. R., et al. (1999). Incidence of small bowel obstruction and adhesiolysis after open colorectal and general surgery. *Diseases of the Colon and Rectum, 42*(2), 241.

Braumrucker, S. J. (1998). Management of intestinal obstruction in hospice care. *The American Journal of Hospice & Palliative Care, 15,* 232–235.

Bungard, T. J., & Kale-Pradhan, P. B. (1999). Prokinetic agents for the treatment of postoperative ileus in adults: A review of the literature. *Pharmacotherapy, 15*(4), 416.

Chen, H. S., & Sheen-Chen, S. M. (2000). Obstruction and perforation in colorectal adenocarcinoma: An analysis of prognosis and current trends. *Surgery, 127*(4), 370.

Ellis, H., Moran, B. J., Thompson, J. N., et al. (1999). Adhesion-related hospital readmissions after abdominal and pelvic surgery: A retrospective cohort study. *The Lancet, 353,* 1476.

Kinney, M. R., Brooks-Brunn, J. A., Molter, M., et al. (1998). *AACN's clinical reference for critical care nursing* (4th ed., p. 1037). St. Louis, MO: CV Mosby.

Martin, R. F., & Rossi, R. L. (1997). Management and causes of acute large bowel obstruction. *Surgical Clinics of North America, 77*(6), 1265.

Mauro, M. A., Koehler, R. E., & Baron, T. H. (2000). Advances in gastrointestinal intervention: The treatment of gastroduodenal and colorectal obstructions with metallic stents. *Radiology, 215,* 659.

Ripamonti, C., Mercadante, S., Groff, L., et al. (2000). Role of octreotide, scopolamine butylbromide, and hydration in symptom control of patients with inoperable bowel obstruction and nasogastric tubes: A prospective randomized trial. *Journal of Pain and Symptoms Management, 19*(1), 23.

Shelton, B. K. (1999). Intestinal obstruction. *AACN Clinical Issues, 10*(4), 487.

Soetikno, R. M., & Carr-Locke, D. L. (1999). Expandable metal stents for gastric-outlet, duodenal, and small-intestinal obstruction. *Gastrointestinal Endoscopy Clinics of North America, 9*(3), 447.

Turnage, R. H., & Bergan, P. C. (1998). Intestinal obstruction and ileus. In M. Feldman, B. F. Scharschmidt, & M. H. Sleisenger (Eds.), *Gastrointestinal and liver disease* (Vol. II, 6th ed., p. 1799). Philadelphia: WB Saunders.

Ulrich, S. P., Canale, S. W., & Wendell, S. A. (1998). *Medical surgical nursing care planning guides* (4th ed., p. 577). Philadelphia: WB Saunders.

16–8

Clinical guidelines on the identification, evaluation, and treatment of overweight and obesity in adults. (1998). *Obesity Research, 6*(Suppl.), 51S–209S.

Dudek, S. G. (1997). *Nutrition handbook for nursing practice* (3rd ed.). Philadelphia: JB Lippincott.

Ignatavicius, D. D., Workman, M. L., & Mishler, M. A. (1999). *Medical surgical nursing across the health care continuum* (3rd ed.). Philadelphia: WB Saunders.

Leahy, J. M., & Kizilay, P. E. (1998). *Foundations of nursing practice: A nursing process approach.* Philadelphia: WB Saunders.

Smeltzer, S. C., & Bare, B. G. (2000). *Textbook of medical surgical nursing* (9th ed.). Philadelphia: JB Lippincott.

Sorensen, T. I., Holst, C., & Stunkard, A. J. (1998). Adoption study of environmental modifications of the genetic influences on obesity. *International Journal of Obesity and Related Metabolic Disorders, 22*(1), 73–81.

Thompson, J. M., & Wilson, S. F. (1996). *Health assessment for nursing practice.* St. Louis, MO: CV Mosby.

Willett, W. C., Dietz, W. H., & Colditz, G. A. (1999). Primary care: Guidelines for healthy weight. *New England Journal of Medicine, 341*(6), 427–434.

Yanovski, J. A., & Yanovski, S. Z. (1999). Recent advances in basic obesity research. *Journal of the American Medical Association, 282*(16), 1504–1506.

16–9

Breitfeller, J. M. (1999). Peritonitis: Can you recognize the classic signs of this life-threatening complication of dialysis? *American Journal of Nursing, 99*(4), 33.

Hillebrand, D. J., & Runyon, B. A. (2000). Spontaneous bacterial peritonitis: Keys to management. *Hospital Practice, 35*(5), 87–90, 96–98.

Huether, S. E. (1998). Structure and function of the digestive system. In K. L. McCance & S. E. Huether (Eds.), *Pathophysiology: The biologic basis for disease in adults and children* (3rd ed., p. 1297). St. Louis, MO: CV Mosby.

O'Toole, M. T. (1997). *Miller-Keane encyclopedia and dictionary of medicine, nursing, and allied health* (6th ed., pp. 1227–1228.). Philadelphia: WB Saunders.

Shry-Chyr, C., Fang-Yue, L., Yeu-Sheng, H., & Wei-Jao, C. (2000). Accuracy of ultrasonography in the diagnosis of peritonitis compared with the clinical impression of the surgeon. *Archives of Surgery, 135*, 170–173.

Smeltzer, S. C., & Bare, B. G. (1999). *Brunner & Suddarth's textbook of medical surgical nursing* (9th ed., pp. 886–888). Philadelphia: JB Lippincott.

17–1

Abbott, S. A. (1998). The benefits of patient education. *Gastroenterological Nursing (United States), 21*(5), 207–209.

Ahmed, A., Cheung, R. C., & Keeffe, E. B. (2000). Management of gallstones and their complications. *American Family Physician (United States), 61*(6), 1673–1680, 1687–1688.

Coleman, J. (1999). Bile duct injuries in laparoscopic cholecystectomy: Nursing perspective. *AACN Clinical Issues* (United States), *10*(4), 442–454.

Dill, B., Dill, J. E., Berkhouse, L., Palmer, S. T. (1999). Endoscopic ultrasound for chronic abdominal pain and gallbladder disease. *Gastroenterological Nursing (United States)*, *22*(5), 209–212.

Feldman, M. (1998). *Sleisenger & Fordtran's gastrointestinal and liver disease* (6th ed., pp. 973–991). Philadelphia: WB Saunders.

George-Gay, B. (1997). Disorders of the biliary tract and exocrine pancreas. In L. Burrell, *Adult nursing in hospital and community settings* (pp. 1467–1558). E. Norwalk, CT: Appleton & Lange.

LeMone, P., & Burke, K. M. (2000). *Medical-surgical nursing: Critical thinking in client care* (2nd ed.). Upper Saddle River, NJ: Prentice Hall Health.

Porth, C. (1998). *Pathophysiology: Concepts of altered health states* (5th ed.). Philadelphia: JB Lippincott.

Rosen, C. L., Brown, D. F., Chang, Y., et al. (2001). Ultrasonography by emergency physicians in patients with suspected cholecystitis. *American Journal of Emergency Medicine (United States), 19*(1), 32–36.

Thijs, C., Knipschild, P. (1998). Abdominal symptoms and food intolerance related to gallstones. *Journal of Clinical Gastroenterology (United States)*, *27*(3), 223–231.

17–2

Beckmann, K. R., & Nozicka, C. A. (1999). Congenital diaphragmatic hernia with gastric volvulus presenting as an acute tension gastrothorax. *American Journal of Emergency Medicine, 17*(1), 35–37.

Critchlow, J. F. (1997). Diaphragmatic hernias and gastric volvulus. In Taylor, M. B. (Ed.), *Gastrointestinal emergencies* (2nd ed., pp 209–218). Baltimore: Williams & Wilkins.

Evans, R. T., & Shabahang, M. (1997). Anatomic variants: Diaphragmatic hernias, gastric volvulus and diverticula. In A. J. DiMarino Jr., & S. B. Benjamin (Eds.), *Gastrointestinal disease: An endoscopic approach* (pp. 366–373). Malden, MA: Blackwell Science.

Hawasli, A., & Zonca, S. (1999). Laparoscopic repair of paraesophageal hiatal hernia. *American Surgery, 64*(8), 703–710.

Horgan, S., Eubanks, T. R., Jacobsen, G., et al. (1999). Repair of paraesophageal hernias. *American Journal of Surgery, 177*(5), 354–358.

Mittal, R. K. (1998). The spectrum of diaphragmataic hernia. *Hospital Practice, 33*(11), 65–66, 69–70, 73–75.

Mittal, R. K., & Balaban, D. H. (1997). Mechanisms of disease: The esophagogastric junction. *New England Journal of Medicine, 336*(13), 924–932.

Murray, J., Demetriades, D., & Ashton, K. (1997). Acute tension diaphragmatic herniation: Case report. *Journal of Trauma, Injury, and Critical Care*, *43*(4), 698–700.

Oddsdottir, M. (2000). Paraesophageal hernia. *Surgical Clinics of North America, 80*(4), 1243–1252.

Pearson, F. G. (1997). Hiatus hernia and gastroesophageal reflux: Indication for surgery and selection of operation. *Seminars in Thoracic Cardiovascular Surgery, 9*(2), 163–168.

Rogers, M. A., & Cox, J. A. (1998). Laparoscopic paraesophageal hernia repair with Nissen fundoplication. *AORN Journal, 167*(3), 536, 538–540.

Sands, J. K. (1999). Management of persons with problems of the mouth and esophagus. In W. J. Phipps, J. K. Sands, & J. F. Marek (Eds.), *Medical-surgical nursing: Concepts and clinical practice* (6th ed., pp. 1253–1276). Philadelphia: WB Saunders.

Sontag, S. J. Gastroesophageal reflux disease. In J. B. Lawrence (Ed.), *Clinical practice of gastroenterology* (Vol. I, pp. 21–33). Philadelphia: Churchill Livingstone.

17–3

George-Gay, B. (2001). Acute pancreatitis. In P. Swearingen & J. Hicks Keen, *Manual of critical care nursing* (4th ed., pp. 526–536). St. Louis, MO: CV Mosby.

George-Gay, B. (1997). Disorders of the biliary tract and exocrine pancreas. In L. Burrell, *Adult nursing in hospital and community settings* (pp. 1467–1558). E. Norwalk, CT: Appleton & Lange.

17–4

Centers for Disease Control and Prevention. (1998). Economics of peptic ulcer disease and *H. pylori* infection (Document 313003). Atlanta, GA: Centers for Disease Control and Prevention.

Clinical update: Preventing and treating NSAID-induced ulcers: ACG guidelines. (1999). *Journal of Critical Illness, 14*(2), 73.

Culter, A. F., Prasad, V. M., & Santogade, P. (1998). Four trends in *Helicobacter pylori* IgG serology following successful eradication. *American Journal of Medicine, 105*, 18.

Eastwood, G. L. (1997). Is smoking still important in the pathogenesis of peptic ulcer disease? *Journal of Clinical Gastroenterology, 25*(Suppl. 1), S1.

Gerlach, M. J. M. (1997). Disorders of the stomach. In L. O. Burrell, M. J. M. Gerlach, & B. S. Pless (Eds.), *Adult nursing: Acute and community care* (Vol. VII, 2nd ed., p. 1403). E. Norwalk, CT: Appleton & Lange.

Graham, D. Y., Rakel, R. E., Fendrick, A. M., et al. (1999). Practical advice on eradicating *Helicobacter pylori* infection. *Postgraduate Medicine, 105*(3), 137.

Graham, D. Y., Rakel, R. E., Fendrick, A. M., et al. (1999). Recognizing peptic ulcer disease. *Postgraduate Medicine, 105*(3), 113.

Graham, D. Y., Rakel, R. E., Fendrick, A. M., et al. (1999). Scope and consequences of peptic ulcer disease: How important is asymptomatic *Helicobacter pylori* infection? *Postgraduate Medicine, 105*(3), 100.

Greenberger, N. J. (1998). Update in gastroenterology. *Annals of Internal Medicine, 129*(4), 309.

Helicobacter pylori: Fact sheet for health care providers. Centers for Disease Control and Prevention, July, 1998.

Heslin, J. M. (1997). Peptic ulcer disease: Making a case against the prime suspect. *Nursing 97, 97*(1), 34.

Kamen, B. J. (1999). Combating upper GI bleeding. *Nursing 99, 29*(7), 32hn1.

Lehne, R. A. (1998). *Drugs for peptic ulcer: Pharmacology for nursing care* (3rd ed., p. 773). Philadelphia: WB Saunders.

Levenstein, S., Ackerman, S., & Kiecolt-Glaser, J. K. (1999). Stress and peptic ulcer disease. *Journal of the American Medical Association, 281*(1), 10.

McQuaid, K. R. (1998). Alimentary tract. In L. M. Tierney, J. McPhee, M. A. Papadakis (Eds.), *Current medical diagnosis and treatment* (37th ed.). E. Norwalk, CT: Appleton & Lange.

Sontag, S. J. (1997). Guilty as charged: Bugs and drugs in gastric ulcer. *American Journal of Gastroenterology, 92*(8), 1255.

18–1

American Diabetes Association. (1998). Diagnosis and classification. In J. S. Skyler (Ed.), *Medical management of type 1 diabetes* (3rd ed., pp. 5–11). Alexandria, VA: American Diabetes Association.

American Diabetes Association. (1998). Diagnosis and classification. In B. R. Zimmerman (Ed.), *Medical management of type 2 diabetes* (4th ed., pp. 1–18). Alexandria, VA: American Diabetes Association.

American Diabetes Association. (1998). Major chronic complications. In B. R. Zimmerman (Ed.), *Medical management of type 2 diabetes* (4th ed., pp. 100–122). Alexandria, VA: American Diabetes Association.

American Diabetes Association. (1998). Diabetes self-management education. In J. S. Skyler (Ed.), *Medical management of type 1 diabetes* (3rd ed., pp. 34–48). Alexandria, VA: American Diabetes Association.

American Diabetes Association. (1999). Nutrition recommendations and principles for people with diabetes mellitus (Position Statement). *Diabetes Care, 22*(Suppl. 1), S42–S45.

American Diabetes Association. (2000). Standards of medical care for patients with diabetes mellitus. *Diabetes Care, 23,* S32–S42.

Diabetes Control and Complications Trial/Epidemiology of Diabetes Interventions and Complications Research Group. (2000). Retinopathy and nephropathy in patients with type 1 diabetes four years after a trial of intensive therapy. *New England Journal of Medicine, 342,* 381–389.

Horton, E. S. (1998). Exercise. In H. E. Lebovitz (Ed.), *Therapy for diabetes mellitus and related disorders (*3rd ed., pp. 150–159). Alexandria, VA: American Diabetes Association.

Lebovitz, H. E. (1998). Diagnosis and classification of diabetes mellitus. In H. E. Lebovitz (Ed.), *Therapy for diabetes mellitus and related disorders* (3rd ed., pp. 5–7)). Alexandria, VA: American Diabetes Association.

United Kingdom Prospective Diabetes Study Group. (1998). Intensive blood-glucose control with sulphonylureas or insulin compared with conventional treatment and risk of complications in patients with type 2 diabetes (UKPDS 33). *Lancet, 352,* 837–853.

18–2

Greenspan, F. S. (1997). *Basic and clinical endocrinology* (5th ed.). New York: McGraw-Hill.

Huether, S. E., & McCance, K. L. (2000). *Understanding pathophysiology* (2nd. ed., p. 482). St. Louis, MO: CV Mosby.

Nowak, T. J., & Handford, A. G. (2000). *Essentials of pathophysiology* (2nd ed., pp. 418–419). Boston: McGraw-Hill.

18–3

Anderson, L. (1998). *Mosby's medical surgical nursing and allied health dictionary* (3rd ed., p. 768). St. Louis, MO: CV Mosby.

Hansen, M. (1998). *Pathophysiology: Foundations of disease and clinical intervention.* Philadelphia: WB Saunders.

Huether, S. E., & McCance, K. L. (2000). *Understanding pathophysiology* (2nd ed., p. 482.). St. Louis, MO: CV Mosby.

Nowak, T. J., & Handford, A. G. (2000). *Essentials of pathophysiology* (2nd ed., pp. 418–419). Boston: McGraw-Hill.

18–4

Copstead, L. C., & Banasik, J. L. (2000). *Pathophysiology: Biological and behavioral perspectives* (2nd ed.). Philadelphia: WB Saunders.

18–5

Anderson, L. (1998). *Mosby's medical surgical nursing and allied health dictionary* (3rd ed., p. 768). St. Louis, MO: CV Mosby.

Huether, S. E., & McCance, K. L. (2000). *Understanding pathophysiology* (2nd ed., p. 482). St. Louis, MO: CV Mosby.

Nowak, T. J., & Handford, A. G. (2000). *Essentials of pathophysiology* (2nd ed., pp. 418–419). New York: McGraw-Hill.

Porth, C. M. (1998). *Pathophysiology: Concepts of altered health* (5th ed., pp. 789–796, 1072–1073). Philadelphia: JB Lippincott.

19–1

Alzheimer's Association. (1998). *Alzheimer's disease: statistics.*

Eliopoulos, C. (1997). *Gerontological nursing.* Philadelphia: JB Lippincott.

Tyson, S. (1999). *Gerontological nursing care.* Philadelphia: WB Saunders.

19–2

Banasik, J. L. (2000). Acute disorders of brain function. In L. C. Copstead & J. L. Banasik (Eds.), *Pathophysiology: Biological and behavioral perspectives* (2nd ed.). Philadelphia: WB Saunders.

Barker, E. (1999). Brain attack! A call to action. *RN, 62*(5), 54–57.

Bratina, P., Rapp, K., Barch, C., Kongdale, G., Donnarumma, R., Spilker, J., Daley, S., Braimah, J., Sailor, S., & the NINDS rt-PA Stroke Study Group. (1997). Pathophysiology and mechanisms of acute ischemic stroke. *Journal of Neuroscience Nursing, 29*(6), 356–360.

Chung, C., & Caplan, L. R. (1999). Neurovascular disorders. In C. G. Goetz & E. J. Pappert (Eds.), *Textbook of clinical neurology.* Philadelphia: WB Saunders.

Daley, S., Braimah, J., Sailor, S., et al., & the NINDS rt-PA Stroke Study Group. (1997). Education to improve stroke awareness and emergent response. *Journal of Neuroscience Nursing, 29*(6), 393–396.

Hickey, J. (1997). Stroke and other cerebrovascular diseases. In J. V. Hickey (Ed.), *The clinical practice of neurological and neurosurgical nursing* (4th ed.). Philadelphia: JB Lippincott.

Hock, N. H. (1999). Brain attack: The stroke continuum. *Nursing Clinics of North America, 34*(3), 689–723.

Rapp, K., Bratina, P., Barch, C., et al., & the NINDS rt-PA Stroke Study Group. (1997). Code stroke: Rapid transport, triage and treatment using rt-PA therapy. *Journal of Neuroscience Nursing, 29*(6), 361–366.

Wechsler, L. R., & Barch, C. A. (2000). Management of acute ischemic stroke. In W. C. Shoemaker, S. M. Ayres, A. Grenvik, and P. R. Holbrook (Eds.), *Textbook of critical care* (4th ed.). Philadelphia: WB Saunders.

Wojner, A. W. (1998). Neurovascular disease. In M. R. Kinney, S. B. Dunbar, J. Brooks-Brunn, N. Molter, J. M. Vitello-Cicciu (Eds.), *AACN clinical reference for critical care nursing* (4th ed.). St. Louis, MO: CV Mosby.

19–3

Chelimsky, T. C. (1998). Pain. In J. Corey-Bloom (Ed.), *Mosby's neurology psychiatry access series adult neurology.* St. Louis, MO: CV Mosby.

Ferraro-Herrera, A. S., Kern, H. B., & Nagler, W. (1997). Autonomic dysfunction as the presenting feature of Guillain-Barré syndrome. *Archives of Physical Medicine and Rehabilitation, 78,* 777–779.

Lindsay, K. W., & Bone, I. (1998). *Neurology and neurosurgery illustrated* (3rd ed.). Philadelphia: Churchill Livingstone.

Luckmann, J. (1997). *Caring for people with neurologic disorders: Saunders manual of nursing care.* Philadelphia: WB Saunders.

Shields, R. W., & Wilbourn, A. J. (1999). Demyelinating disorders of the peripheral nervous system. In C. G. Goetz & E. J. Pappert (Eds.), *Textbook of clinical neurology.* Philadelphia: WB Saunders.

19–4

Banasik, J. L. (2000). Acute disorders of brain function. In L. C. Copstead & J. L. Banasik (Eds.), *Pathophysiology: Biological and behavioral perspectives* (2nd ed.). Philadelphia: WB Saunders.

Jay, C. (1998). Infections of the nervous system. In J. Corey-Bloom (Ed.), *Mosby's neurology.* Psychiatry Access Series: Adult neurology. St. Louis, MO: CV Mosby.

King, D. S. (1999). Central nervous system infections. *Nursing Clinics of North America, 34*(3), 761–771.

Lindsay, K. W., & Bone, I. (1998). *Neurology and neurosurgery illustrated* (3rd ed.). Philadelphia: Churchill Livingstone.

Luckmann, J. (1997). *Caring for people with neurologic disorders: Saunders manual of nursing care.* Philadelphia: WB Saunders.

Quagliarello, V. J., & Schield, W. M. (1997). The treatment of bacterial meningitis. *New England Journal of Medicine, 336*(10), 708–715.

Roos, K. (1999). Viral infections. In C. G. Goetz & E. J. Pappert (Eds.), *Textbook of clinical neurology.* Philadelphia: WB Saunders.

Roos, K. (1999). Nonviral infections. In C. G. Goetz & E. J. Pappert (Eds.), *Textbook of clinical neurology.* Philadelphia: WB Saunders.

19–5

Duijnstee, M. S. H., & Boeije, H. R. (1998). Home care by and for relatives of MS patients. *Journal of Neuroscience Nursing, 30*(6), 356–360.

Frozena, C. (1997). Multiple sclerosis. *American Journal of Nursing, 97*(11), 48–49.

Halper, J., & Holland, N. (1997). *Comprehensive nursing care in multiple sclerosis.* New York, NY: Demos Vermande.

Hickey, J. (1997). Selected degenerative diseases of the nervous system. In J. V. Hickey (Ed.), *The clinical practice of neurological and neurosurgical nursing* (4th ed.). Philadelphia: JB Lippincott.

Hogancamp, W. E., & Noseworthy, J. H. (1999). Demyelinating disorders of the central nervous system. In C. G. Goetz & E. J. Pappert (Eds.), *Textbook of clinical neurology.* Philadelphia: WB Saunders.

Koopman, W., & Schweitzer, A. (1999). The journey to multiple sclerosis: A qualitative study. *Journal of Neuroscience Nursing, 31*(1), 17–26.

Luckmann, J. (1997). *Caring for people with neurologic disorders: Saunders manual of nursing care.* Philadelphia: WB Saunders.

Mass, M. K., & Bourdette, D. N. (1998). Demyelinating diseases. In J. Corey-Bloom (Ed.), *Mosby's neurology psychiatry access series: Adult neurology.* St. Louis, MO: CV Mosby.

Nortvedt, M. W, Riise, T., Myhr, K., & Nyland, H. I. (1999). Quality of life in multiple sclerosis: measuring the disease effects more broadly. *Neurology, 53*(5), 1098–1103.

Ross, A. P. (1999). Neurologic degenerative disorders. *Nursing Clinics of North America, 34*(3), 725–741.

Stuifbergen, A., Becker, H., Rogers, S., et al. (1999). Promoting wellness for women with multiple sclerosis. *Journal of Neuroscience Nursing, 31*(2), 73–79.

19–6

Augustus, L. (2000). Crisis: Myasthenia gravis. *American Journal of Nursing, 100*(1), 24AA–24HH.

Bartt, R., & Shannon, K. M. (1999). Autoimmune and inflammatory disorders. In C. G. Goetz & E. J. Pappert (Eds.), *Textbook of clinical neurology.* Philadelphia: WB Saunders.

Boss, B. J. (1997). Alterations of neurologic function. In K. L. McCance & S. E. Huether (Eds.). *Pathophysiology: The biologic basis for disease in children and adults.* St. Louis, MO: CV Mosby.

Hart, J. J. (2000). Myasthenia gravis. In R. E. Rakel (Ed.), *Saunders manual of medical practice* (2nd ed.). Philadelphia: WB Saunders.

Hickey, J. (1997). Selected degenerative disease of the nervous system. In J. V. Hickey (Ed.), *The clinical practice of neurological and neurosurgical nursing* (4th ed.). Philadelphia: JB Lippincott.

Luckmann, J. (1997). *Caring for people with neurologic disorders: Saunders manual of nursing care.* Philadelphia: WB Saunders.

Ross, A. P. (1999). Neurologic degenerative disorders. *Nursing Clinics of North America, 34*(3), 725–741.

19–7

Copstead, L. C. (2000). Acute disorders of brain function. In L. C. Copstead, & J. L. Banasik, *Pathophysiology: Biological and behavioral perspectives* (2nd ed.). Philadelphia: WB Saunders.

Fahn, S. (1999). Hypokinesia and hyperkinesia. In C. G. Goetz & E. J. Pappert (Eds.), *Textbook of clinical neurology.* Philadelphia: WB Saunders.

Herndon, C. M., Young, K., Herdon, A. D., & Dole, E. J. (2000). Parkinson's disease revisited. *Journal of Neuroscience Nursing, 32*(4), 216–221.

Jankovic, J., & Stacy, M. (1999). Movement disorders. In C. G. Goetz & E. J. Pappert (Eds.), *Textbook of clinical neurology.* Philadelphia: WB Saunders.

Luckmann, J. (1997). *Caring for people with neurologic disorders: Saunders manual of nursing care.* Philadelphia: WB Saunders.

Olanow, C. W., & Koller, W. C. (1998). An algorithm for the management of Parkinson's disease: Treatment guidelines. *Neurology, 50*(3)(Suppl. 3), 51–57.

Ross, A. P. (1999). Neurologic degenerative disorders. *Nursing Clinics of North America, 34*(3), 725–741.

Stacy, M., & Jankovic, J. (1998). Movement disorders. In J. Corey-Bloom (Ed.), *Mosby's neurology.* Psychiatry access series: Adult neurology. St. Louis, MO: CV Mosby.

19–8

Folvary, N., & Wyllie, E. (1999). Epilepsy. In C. G. Goetz & E. J. Pappert (Eds.), *Textbook of clinical neurology.* Philadelphia: WB Saunders.

Hickey, J. (1997). *Selected degenerative diseases of the nervous system: The clinical practice of neurological and neurosurgical nursing* (4th ed.). Philadelphia: JB Lippincott.

Lindsay, K. W., & Bone, I. (1998). *Neurology and neurosurgery illustrated* (3rd ed.). Philadelphia: Churchill Livingstone.

Luckmann, J. (1997). *Caring for people with neurologic disorders: Saunders manual of nursing care.* Philadelphia: WB Saunders.

Shafer, P. O. (1999). Epilepsy and seizures: Advances in seizure assessment, treatment, and self-management. *Nursing Clinics of North America, 34*(3), 743–759.

Sirven, J. I., & Sperling, M. R. (1998). The epilepsies. In J. Corey-Bloom (Ed.), *Adult neurology.* St. Louis, MO: CV Mosby.

19–9

Boss, B. J. (1998) Alterations of neurologic function. In K. I. McCance & S. E. Huether (Eds.), *Pathophysiology: The biologic basis for disease in adults and children* (3rd ed., p. 521). St. Louis, MO: CV Mosby.

Buckley, D. A., & Guanci, M. M. (1999). Spinal cord trauma. *Nursing Clinics of North America, 34*(3), 661–686.

Copstead, L. C. (2000). Chronic disorders of neurologic function. In L. C. Copstead, & J. L. Banasik (Eds.), *Pathophysiology biological and behavioral perspectives* (2nd ed.). Philadelphia: WB Saunders.

Curtis, R., & McDonald, S. (1998). Alterations in motor function. In C. M. Porth (Ed.), *Pathophysiology concepts of altered health states* (5th ed.). Philadelphia: JB Lippincott.

Evans, R. W., & Wilberger, J. F. (1999). Traumatic disorders. In C. G. Goetz & E. J. Pappert (Eds.), *Textbook of clinical neurology*. Philadelphia: WB Saunders.

20–1

Mayo-Smith, M. F. (1997). Pharmacological management of alcohol withdrawal: A meta-analysis and evidence-based practice guideline. *Journal of the American Medical Association, 278*, 144–151.

Patch, P. B., Phelps, G. L., & Cowan, G. (1997). Alcohol withdrawal in a medical-surgical setting: The 'too little, too late' phenomenon. *Medical-Surgical Nursing, 6*(2), 79–89.

Schumacher, L., Pruit, J. N., & Phillips, M. (2000). Identifying patients 'at risk' for alcohol withdrawal syndrome and a treatment protocol. *Journal of Neuroscience Nursing, 32*(3), 158–163.

Segatore, M., Adams, D., & Lange, S. (1999). Managing alcohol withdrawal in the acutely ill hospitalized adult. *Journal of Neuroscience Nursing, 31*(3), 129–141.

20–2

Fuller, M. A., & Sajatovic, M. (1999). *Drug information handbook for psychiatry 1999–2000*. Hudson, OH: Lexi-Comp.

Gabbard, G. O. (1998). The cost effectiveness of treating depression. *Psychiatric Annals, 28*(2), 98–101.

Glod, C. J. (1998). *Contemporary psychiatric mental health nursing—the brain-behavior connection* (pp. 345–362). Philadelphia: FA Davis.

Isaacs, A. (1998). Depression and your patient. *American Journal of Nursing, 98*(7), 26–32.

Kaplan, H. I., & Saddock, B. J. (1998). *Synopsis of psychiatry: Behavioral sciences, clinical psychiatry* (8th ed., pp. 538–571).

Keltner, N., Folks, D. G., Palmer, C. A., & Powers, R. E. (1998). *Psychobiological foundations of psychiatric care* (pp. 97–100). St. Louis, MO: CV Mosby.

Nelson, C. J. (1998). Combined drug treatment strategies for major depression. *Psychiatric Annals, 28*(4), 197–203.

Pearson, J. B. (1998). Indications for psychotherapy in the treatment of depression. *Psychiatric Annals, 22*(2), 80–83.

20–3

American Association of Poison Control Centers (AAPCC). Available at: *http://www.aapcc.org/*

Caliva, M. V. (1999). The telephone as lifeline in poison information. *American Journal of Nursing, 99*(7), 24F&H.

Criddle, L. A. (1998). Toxicologic emergencies. In S. B. Sheehy & L. Newberry (Eds.), *Sheehy's emergency nursing principles and practice* (pp. 647–663). St Louis, MO: Mosby Year Book.

Heroin. Available at: *http://www.nida.nih.gov/Infofax/heroin.html*

Lisanti, P. (1998). Barbiturate overdose. *American Journal of Nursing, 98*(10), 38.

Methamphetamine. Available at: *http://www.nida.nih.gov/Infofax/methamphetamine.html*

Sommers, M. S. (1998). Multisystem. In J. G. Alspach (Ed.), *Core curriculum for critical care nursing* (pp. 774–795). Philadelphia: WB Saunders.

Zimmermann, P. G. (1997). Tricyclic antidepressant overdose. *American Journal of Nursing, 97*(10), 39.

20–4

Doenges, M., & Moorhouse, M. (1998). *Nurse's pocket guide: Diagnoses, interventions, and rationales* (6th ed., pp. 397–406). Philadelphia: FA Davis.

Ladewig, P., London, M., & Olds, S. (1998). *Maternal-newborn nursing care* (4th ed., pp. 115–117). Menlo Park, CA: Addison Wesley Longman.

Shives, L. (1998). *Basic concepts of psychiatric-mental health nursing* (4th ed., pp. 547–558). Philadelphia: JB Lippincott.

Stanhope, M., & Lancaster, J. (2000). *Community and public health nursing* (5th ed., pp. 757–778). St. Louis, MO: CV Mosby.

Townsend, M. (2000). *Psychiatric mental health nursing concepts of care* (3rd ed., pp. 187–223, 739–757). Philadelphia: FA Davis.

Varcarolis, E. (1998). *Foundations of psychiatric mental health nursing* (3rd ed., pp. 387–416). Philadelphia: WB Saunders.

20–5

American Psychiatric Association. (2000). *Diagnostic and statistical manual of mental disorders IV–text revision* (4th ed.). Washington, DC: Author.

Chernecky, C., & Berger, B. (1997). *Laboratory tests and diagnostic procedures* (2nd ed., pp. 448–469). Philadelphia: WB Saunders.

Eliopoulos, C. (1997). *Gerontological nursing* (4th ed., pp. 401–403). Philadelphia: JB Lippincott.

Evangelical Lutheran Church in America. (1999). *A message on suicide prevention* (Order code 69–6602). Chicago: Author.

Fortinash, K., & Holoday-Worret, P. (2000). *Psychiatric mental health nursing* (2nd ed., pp. 652–676). St. Louis: CV Mosby.

Keltner, N., Schwecke, L., & Bostrom, C. (1999). *Psychiatric nursing* (3rd ed., pp. 413–421). St. Louis, MO: CV Mosby.

McElroy, A. (1999). The assessment and management of self-harming patients in an accident and emergency department: An action research project. *Journal of Clinical Nursing, 8*(1), 66–72.

National Alliance for the Mentally Ill. (2000). Special research section. *NAMI Advocate, 21*(4), 1–5.

Repper, J. (1999). A review of the literature on the prevention of suicide through interventions in accident and emergency departments. *Journal of Clinical Nursing, 8*(1), 3–12.

Robie, D., Edgemon-Hill, E., Phelps, B., Schmitz, C., & Laughlin, J. (1999). Suicide prevention protocol. *American Journal of Nursing, 99*(12), 53–57.

Stanhope, M., & Lancaster, J. (2000). *Community and public health nursing* (5th ed, pp. 714–778). St. Louis: CV Mosby.

Suicide Prevention Advocacy Network. (March 2000). U.S. Senate hearing on suicide. *SPANUSA, 11*.

Townsend, M. (2000). *Psychiatric mental health nursing concepts of care* (3rd ed., pp. 49–74, 225–233). Philadelphia: FA Davis.

U.S. Public Health Service (1999). *The Surgeon General's call to action to prevent suicide*. Washington, DC: Author.

Varcarolis, E. (1998). *Foundations of psychiatric mental health nursing* (3rd ed., pp. 728–735). Philadelphia: WB Saunders.

21–1

Bush, M. (2000). Arthritis and other rheumatic disorders. In S. M. Lewis, M. Heitkemper, & S. Dirksen (Eds.), *Medical surgical nursing assessment and management of clinical problems* (5th ed.). St. Louis, MO: CV Mosby.

CDC (1999). *Targeting arthritis: The nation's leading cause of disability.*

CDC Media Relations (1997). *Facts about arthritis*. Available at: *http://www.cdc.gov/od/oc/media/fact/arthriti/htm*

Corbett, J. V. (2000). *Laboratory tests and diagnostic procedures* (5th ed.). Upper Saddle River: Prentice Hall.

LeMone, P., & Burke, K. M. (2000). *Medical-surgical nursing: Critical thinking in client care* (2nd ed.). Upper Saddle River: Prentice Hall.

Liddel, D. B. (2000). Musculoskeletal care modalities. In S. C. Smeltzer & B. G. Bare (Eds.), *Textbook of medical surgical nursing*. Philadelphia: JB Lippincott.

Mengal, B., Aebi, J., Rodriguez, A., & Lemaire, R. (2001). A prospective randomized study of wound drainage versus non-drainage in primary total hip or knee arthroplasty. *Revue de Chirurgie Orthopédique et Reparatrice de l'Appareil Moteur, 87*(1), 29–39.

Potter, M. L. (2000). Spirituality, resourcefulness and arthritis impact on health perception of elders with rheumatoid arthritis. *Journal of Holistic Nursing, 18*(4), 311–332.

Shmerling, R. H. (December 2000). Harvard commentary: 10 misconceptions about arthritis. Available at: *http://www.intelihealth.com*

Schoen, D. C. (2000). *Adult orthopedic nursing*. Philadelphia: JB Lippincott.

21–2

AORN Journal. (1999). Recommendations for care of hip fracture patients. *AORN Journal, 69*(i2), 386(1).

Byrne, T. (1999). The setup and care of a patient in Buck's. *Orthopaedic Nursing, 18*(i2), 79.

Doenges, M. E., Moorhouse, M. F., & Geissler, A. C. (1997). *Nursing care plans: Guidelines for individualizing patient care* (4th ed.). Philadelphia: FA Davis.

Fauci, A. S., Braunwald, E., Isselbacher, K. J., et al. (1998). *Harrison's principles of internal medicine* (14th ed.). New York: McGraw-Hill.

Harvey, C. V. (1998). Challenges of traction in critical care: A case study. *Critical Care Nursing Quarterly, 21*(2), 1(13).

Ignatavicius, D. D., Workman, M. L., & Mishler, M. A. (1999). *Medical-surgical nursing across the health care continuum* (3rd ed.). Philadelphia: WB Saunders.

Lewis, S. M., Heitkemper, M. M., & Dirksen, S. R. (2000). *Medical-surgical nursing: Assessment and management of clinical problems* (5th ed.). St. Louis, MO: CV Mosby.

Maher, A. B., Salmond, S. W., & Pellino, T. A. (1998). *Orthopaedic nursing* (2nd ed.). Philadelphia: WB Saunders.

Monahan, F. D., & Neighbors, M. (1998). *Medical-surgical nursing: Foundations for clinical practice* (2nd ed.). Philadelphia: WB Saunders.

Phipps, W. J., Sands, J. K., & Marek, J. F. (1999). *Medical-Surgical nursing: Concepts and clinical practice* (6th ed.). St. Louis, MO: CV Mosby.

Shands, P. A., & Jansson, K. A. (1998). Compartment syndrome in the thigh as a complication of arthroscopy: A case report and review of the literature. *Medscape Orthopedics and Sports Medicine, 2*(2).

Smeltzer, S. C., & Bare, B. G. (2000). *Brunner and Suddarth's textbook of medical-surgical nursing* (9th ed.). Philadelphia: JB Lippincott.

Ulrich, S. P., Canale, S. W., & Wendell, S. A. (1998). *Medical-surgical nursing: Care planning guides* (4th ed.). Philadelphia: WB Saunders.

Walsh, C. R., & McBryde, A. M. Jr. (1997). A joint protocol for home skeletal traction. *Orthopaedic Nursing, 16*(3), 28.

21–3

Cavanaugh, B. M. (1999). *Nurse's manual of laboratory and diagnostic tests* (3rd ed.). Philadelphia: FA Davis.

Executive Health Report. (1998). Gout: Many sufferers don't know about treatments. *Executive Health's Good Health Report, 34*(11), 6(1).

Gutierrez, K. (1999). *Pharmacotherapeutics: Clinical decision-making in nursing* (pp. 275–280). Philadelphia: WB Saunders.

Harris, M. D., Siegel, L. B., Alloway, J. A. (1999). Gout and hyperuricemia. *American Family Physician, 59,* 925–934.

Ignatavicius, D. D., Workman, M. L., & Mishler, M. A. (1999). *Medical-surgical nursing across the health care continuum.* (3rd ed., pp. 434–436). Philadelphia: WB Saunders.

Jaffe, M. S., & McVan, B. F. (1997). *Davis's laboratory and diagnostic test handbook.* Philadelphia: FA Davis.

Lewis, S. M., Heitkemper, M. M., & Dirksen, S. R. (2000). *Medical-surgical nursing: Assessment and management of clinical problems* (5th ed.). St. Louis, MO: CV Mosby.

Maher, A. B., Salmond, S. W., & Pellino, T. A. (1998). *Orthopaedic nursing* (2nd ed.). Philadelphia: WB Saunders.

Monahan, F. D., & Neighbors, M. (1998). M*edical-surgical nursing: Foundations for clinical practice* (2nd ed., pp. 899–901). Philadelphia: WB Saunders.

Phipps, W. J., Sands, J. K., & Marek, J. F. (1999). *Medical-Surgical nursing: Concepts and clinical practice* (pp. 1989–1991). St. Louis, MO: CV Mosby.

Porth, C. M. (1998). *Pathophysiology: Concepts of altered health states* (5th ed., pp. 1138–1140). Philadelphia: JB Lippincott.

Price, S. A., & Wilson, L. M. (1997). *Pathophysiology: Clinical concepts of disease processes* (pp. 1056–1059). St. Louis, MO: CV Mosby.

Reeves, C. J., Roux, G., & Lockhart, R. (1999). *Medical-surgical nursing* (pp. 261–263). New York: McGraw-Hill.

Saunders, C. S. (1998). Gout: Applying current knowledge. *Patient Care, 32*(10), 125–139.

Smeltzer, S. C., & Bare, B. G. (2000). *Brunner and Suddarth's textbook of medical-surgical nursing* (9th ed.). Philadelphia: JB Lippincott.

Varner, L. (1999). Gout and its treatment through medications and lifestyle intervention. Wellness Web Homepage.

Wilson, B. A., Shannon, M. T., & Stang, C. L. (1999). *Nurses' drug guide*. E. Norwalk, CT: Appleton & Lange.

Wortmann, R. L. (1998). Effective management of gout: An analogy. *American Journal of Medicine, 105,* 513–514.

21–4

Barbieri, R. L. (1998). A step-by-step approach to osteoporosis treatment. *Patient Care, 12,* 138–142, 146–147, 151–152.

Depree, P. (2000). Building bone. Osteoporosis treatment options in lieu of hormone replacement therapy. *Advance for Nurse Practitioners, 8*(1), 36–38.

Hendler, A., & Hershkop, M. (1998). When to use bone scintigraphy: It can reveal things other studies cannot. *Postgraduate Medicine, 104*(5), 54–56, 59–61, 65–66.

Meiner, S. E. (1999). An expanding landscape. Osteoporosis treatment options today. *Advances for Nurse Practitioners, 1*(7), 27–28, 30–31, 80.

Raab, C. A., Gregerson, D., Shaw, J. M., & Snow, C. (1999). Postmenopausal women take steps to reduce their osteoporosis risk. *Women's Health Issues, 9*(4), 211–218.

Wasnich, R. D. (1998). Don't wait for a fracture. Identifying osteoporosis. *The Female Patient, 23,* 11–12, 19–22, 25–26.

Youngkin, E. Q., Sawin, K. J., Kissinger, J. F., & Israel, D. S. (1999). *Pharmacotherapeutics. A primary care clinical guide* (pp. 127–150). E. Norwalk, CT: Appleton & Lange.

21–5

Burrell, L. O., Gerlach, M. J., & Pless, B. (1997). *Foundations of contemporary nursing practice.* E. Norwalk, CT: Appleton & Lange.

Cotran, R., Kumar, V., & Collins, T. (1999). *Pathologic basis of disease* (6th ed.). Philadelphia: WB Saunders.

Davis, F. A. (1997). *Taber's cyclopedic medical dictionary* (18th ed.). Philadelphia: FA Davis.

Huether, S. E., & McCance, K. L. (2000). *Understanding pathophysiology* (2nd ed.). St. Louis, MO: CV Mosby.

Johnson, B. (1999). Systemic lupus erythematosus. *American Journal of Nursing, 99*(1), 40–41.

Kelley, W. N., Ruddy, S., Harris, E. D., & Sledge, C. B. (1997). *Textbook of rheumatology* (Vol. 12, 5th ed.). Philadelphia: WB Saunders.

Lahita, R. G. (1999*). Systemic lupus erythematosus* (3rd ed.). San Diego: Academic Press.

Lahita, R. G., Pisetsky, D. S., & Wallace, D. J. (1998). Lupus: High stakes diagnosis, broad treatment options. *Patient Care 32*(4), 101–123.

Leach, M. (1998). Signs and symptoms of systemic lupus erythematosus. *Nursing Times, 94*(13), 58–59.

Leach, M. (1998). Managing systemic lupus erythematosus. *Nursing Times, 94,* 18.

Lewis, S., Heitkemper, M., & Dirksen, S. R. (2000). *Medical surgical nursing* (5th ed.). St. Louis, MO: CV Mosby.

Maher, A.B., Salmond, S. W., & Pellino, T. A. (1998). *Orthopaedic nursing* (2nd ed.). Philadelphia: WB Saunders.

McCance, K. L., & Huether, S. E. (1998). *Pathophysiology: The biologic basis for disease in adults and children* (3rd ed.). St. Louis, MO: CV Mosby.

Petri, M. (1998). Treatment of systemic lupus erythematosus: An update. *American Family Physician, 57*(11), 2753–2760.

Roberts, W. N. (1997). Keys to managing systemic lupus. *Hospital Practice, 32*(2), 113–126.

Smeltzer, S. C., & Bare, B. G. (2000). *Brunner & Suddarth's textbook of medical-surgical nursing* (9th ed.). Philadelphia: JB Lippincott.

Wallace, D. J., & Hahn, B. H. (1997). *Dubbois' lupus erythematosus* (5th ed.). Baltimore: Williams & Wilkins.

Wernick, R., & Coyle, C. (1999). Systemic lupus erythematosus: A streamlined, rational approach to diagnosis. *Hospital Medicine, 35*(4), 16–22.

Wilson, B. A., Shannon, M. T., & Stang, C. L. (1997). *Nurses' drug guide.* E. Norwalk, CT: Appleton & Lange.

22–1

Bartlett, J. G. (1999). *Medical management of HIV infection.* Baltimore: Johns Hopkins University Department of Infectious Disease.

Centers for Disease Control (CDC). (1999). Appendix: Revised surveillance report case definition for HIV infection (On-line), *48*(RR13), 29–31. Available at: *http://www.cdc.gov/epo/mmwr/preview/mmwrhtml/rr4813e2.htm*

Centers for Disease Control and Prevention (CDC). (2001). Basic statistics-international statistics (On-line). National Center for HIV, STD, & Tb Prevention, Division of HIV/AIDS Prevention. Available at: *http://www.cdc.gov/hiv/stats/internet.htm*

Centers for Disease Control and Prevention (CDC). (2000). *HIV/AIDS surveillance report, 12*(1), 1–44.

Gawenda, D. D. (1997). *Manual of medical surgical nursing.* Boston: Little, Brown.

Henkel, J. (1999). Attacking AIDS with cocktail therapy (On-line). U. S. Food and Drug Administration. Available at: *http://www.fda.gov/fdac/features/1999/499_aids.html*

HIV/ATIS Treatment Information Service (HIVATIS). (1997). Understanding viral load (On-line). Available at: *http://www.hivatis.org/viral.html*

Murphy, S. L. (2000). Deaths: Final data for 1998. National Vital Statistics Report (Vol. 48[11]). Hyattsville, MD: National Center for Health Statistics.

National Institute of Allergy and Infectious Diseases and National Institute of Health (NIAID/NIH). (2000). HIV/AIDS statistics fact sheet (On-line), Bethesda, MD. Available at: *http://www.niaid.nih.gov/factsheets/aidsstat.html*

National Institute of Allergy and Infectious Diseases (NIAID). (2001). HIV infection and AIDS (On-line). Available at: *http://www.content.health.msn.com/content.dmk/dmk_article_5462568*

National Institute of Allergy & Infectious Diseases & National Institute of Health (NIAID/NIH). (2000). HIV infection and AIDS: an overview fact sheet (On-line), Bethesda: U.S. Department of Health & Human Services. Available at: *http://www.niaid.nih.gov/factsheets/hivinf.html*

National Institute of Allergy & Infectious Diseases and National Institute of Health (NIAID/NIH). (1998). How HIV causes AIDS fact sheet (On-line) Bethesda: U.S. Department of Health & Human Services. Available at: *http://www.niaia.nih.gov/factsheets/howhiv.html*

Phair, J. P., & Murphy, R. L. (1997). *Contemporary diagnosis and management of HIV/AIDS infections*. Newtown, PA: Handbooks in Healthcare.

Ungvarski, P. J., & Flaskerud, J. H. (1999). *HIV/AIDS: A guide to primary care management* (4th ed.). Philadelphia: WB Saunders.

22–2

AAAI parameters for diagnosis and management of anaphylaxis. (1998). *Journal of Allergy and Clinical Immunology, 101*, S465–S528.

Lieberman, P., & Wasserman, S. I. (1998). Anaphylaxis and anaphylactoid reactions. In E. Middleton, C. Reed, E. F. Ellis, et al. (Eds.), *Allergy principles and practice* (5th ed.). St. Louis, MO: CV Mosby.

Meltzer, E. O., Nathan, R. A., Selner, J. C., & Storms, W. J. (1997). Quality of life and rhinitic symptoms: Results of a nationwide survey with the SF-36 and RQLQ questionnaires. *Allergy and Clinical Immunology, 99*, S15–S19.

Task force on Allergic Disorders. (1998). Raising the standard of care for patients with allergic disorders. *Executive summary report.*

22–3

Yarbro, J. M. (1997). *Cancer nursing: Principles and practice* (4th ed., pp. 42–55). Sudbury, MA: Jones & Bartlett.

23–1

Andes, E., Goichot, B., & Schlienger, J. (2000). Food cobalamin malabsorption: A usual cause of vitamin B_{12} deficiency. *Archives of Internal Medicine, 160*(13), 2061–2062.

Chulay, M., Guzzettta, C., & Dossey, B. (1997), *AACN handbook of critical care nursing*. E. Norwalk, CT: Appleton & Lange.

Gawlinski, A., & Hamwi, D. (1999). *Acute care nurse practitioner: Clinical curriculum and certification review*. Philadelphia: WB Saunders.

Kaye, J. (1997). Disorders of the erythrocytes. In L. Burrell, M. J. Gerlach, & B. Pless (Eds.), *Adult nursing acute and community care* (2nd ed.). E. Norwalk, CT: Appleton & Lange.

McCance, K., & Huether, S. (1998). *Pathophysiology: The biologic basis for disease in adults and children* (3rd ed.). St. Louis: CV Mosby.

Snow, C. (1999). Laboratory diagnosis of Vitamin B_{12} and folate deficiency: A guide for the primary care physician. *Archives of Internal Medicine, 159*(12), 1289–1298.

Yen, P. K. (2000). Nutritional anemia. *Geriatric Nursing, 21*(2), 111–112.

23–2

Gawlinski, A., & Hamwi, D. (1999) *Acute care nurse practitioner: Clinical curriculum and certification review*. Philadelphia: WB Saunders.

Kaye, J. (1997) Disorders of leukocytes, thrombocytes, and blood-forming organs. In L. Burrell, M. J. Gerlach, & B. Pless (Eds.), *Adult nursing, acute and community care*. E. Norwalk, CT: Appleton & Lange.

McCance, K., & Huether, S. (1998). *Pathophysiology: The biologic basis for disease in adults and children* (3rd ed.). St. Louis: CV Mosby.

Ritsuro, S., Massao, S., & Morishima, Y. (1999). Treatment of acute myeloid leukemia. *New England Journal of Medicine, 340*(18), 1436–1439.

Shusterman, S., & Meadows A. (2000). Long-term survivor of childhood leukemia. *Current Opinion in Hematology, 7*(4), 217–222.

Tsiodas, S., Samonis, G., Keating, M., & Kontoyiannis, D. (2000). Infection and immunity in chronic lymphocytic leukemia. *Mayo Clinic Proceedings, 75*(10), 1039–1054.

23–3

Fenstermacher, K., & Hudson, B. T. (1997). *Practice guidelines for family nurse practitioners.* Philadelphia: WB Saunders.

Gawlinski, A., & Hamwi, D. (1999). *Acute care nurse practitioner: Clinical curriculum and certification review.* Philadelphia: WB Saunders.

Logan, P. (1999) *Principles of practice for the acute care nurse practitioner.* E. Norwalk, CT: Appleton & Lange.

McCance, K., & Hueter, S. (1998). *Pathophysiology: The biologic basis for disease in adults and children* (3rd ed). St. Louis, MO: CV Mosby.

24–1

Ebersole, P., & Hess, P. (1997). *Toward healthy aging.* St. Louis, MO: CV Mosby.

Klein, R., Klein, B. E., Moss, S. E., & Cruickshanks, K. J. (1999). Association of ocular disease and mortality in a diabetic population. *Archives of Ophthalmology, 117*(11), 1487–1495.

Koop, C. E. (1998). Cataracts. Available at: *http://www.Drkoop.com,Inc*

Lueckenotte, A. G. (2000). *Gerontologic nursing.* St. Louis, MO: CV Mosby.

National Eye Institute. (1999). Cataract information for patients (NIH Publication No 99–201). Bethesda, MD: Author unknown.

Nettina, S. M. (2000). *The Lippincott manual of nursing.* Philadelphia: JB Lippincott.

Professional guide to diseases: General medical reference. (1998). Springhouse, PA: Springhouse Corporation.

Smeltzer, S. C., & Bare, B. G. (1999). *Textbook of medical surgical nursing.* Philadelphia: JB Lippincott.

24–2

Friedlander, M. H. (1999) Conjunctivitis. In R. E. (Ed.), *Conn's current therapy,* (pp. 69–71). Philadelphia: WB Saunders.

McCance, K. L., & Huether, S. E. (Eds.). (1997). Pain, temperature regulation, sleep, and sensory function. In *Pathophysiology: The biologic basis for disease in adults and children* (3rd ed., pp. 443, 828). St. Louis, MO: CV Mosby.

Nakagawa, H. (1997) Treatment of chlamydial conjunctivitis. *Ophthalmologica, 211*(Suppl. 1), 25.

Olendorf, D., Jeryan, C., & Boyden, K. (Eds.). (1999). Conjunctivitis. In *The Gale encyclopedia of medicine* (Vol. 2, C–F; pp. 800–803). Detroit, MI: Gale Research Company.

Riordan-Eva, P., & Vaughan, D. G. (1999). Eye. In L. M. Tierney, S. J. McPhee, & M. A. Papadakis (Eds.), *Current medical diagnosis and treatment 1999* (38th ed., pp. 181–191, 207, 1281, 1506). E. Norwalk, CT: Appleton & Lange.

24–3

Black, J. M., & Matassarin-Jacobs, E. (Eds.). (1997). *Medical-surgical nursing: Clinical management for continuity of care* (5th ed., pp. 952–958, 999). Philadelphia: WB Saunders.

Epstein, D. L., Allingham, R. R., & Schuman, J. S. (1997). *Chandler and Grant's glaucoma* (4th ed.). Baltimore, MD: Wilkins & Wilkins.

Harper, R. A., & Reeves, B. C. (1999). Glaucoma screening: the importance of combining test data. *Optometry and Vision, 76*(8), 537–543.

Kakiuchi, T., Isashiki, Y., Nakao, K., et al. (1999). A novel truncating mutation of cytochrome P4501B1 (CYP1B1) gene in primary infantile glaucoma. *American Journal of Ophthalmology, 128*(3), 370–372.

Kee, J., LeFever, J., & Hayes, E. R. (1997). Drugs for disorders of the eye and the ear. In J. LeFever, J. Kee, & E. R. Hayes (Eds.), *Pharmacology: A nursing process approach* (2nd ed., pp. 581–591). Philadelphia: WB Saunders.

Lewis, P. R., Phillips, T. G., & Sassani, J. W. (1999). Topical therapies for glaucoma: What family physicians need to know. *American Family Physician, 59*(7), 1871–1879.

Linden, C., & Alm, A. (1999). Prostaglandin analogues in the treatment of glaucoma. *Drugs and Aging, 14*(5), 387–398.

Luckmann, J. (Ed.). (1997). *Caring for people with visual disorders: Saunders manual of nursing care* (pp. 769–776). Philadelphia: WB Saunders.

Merck Pharmaceuticals. *Preserving vision: Questions and answers about glaucoma.* (Publication no. L2236–1096).

Mitchell, P., Hourihan, F., Sandbach, J., & Wang, J. J. (1999). The relationship between glaucoma and myopia: The Blue Mountains Eye Study. *Ophthalmology, 106*(10), 2010–2015.

Olendorf, D., Jeryan, C., & Boyden, M. (Eds.). (1999). Glaucoma. In *The Gale Encyclopedia of Medicine* (Vol. 3: G–M). Detroit, MI: Gale Research Company.

Perkins, T. W. (1999). Glaucoma. In R. E. Rakel's (Ed.), *Conn's current therapy* (pp. 951–954). Philadelphia: WB Saunders.

Tierney, L. J., McPhee, S. J., & Papadakis, M. A. (Eds.). (1999). Eye. In *Current medical diagnosis and treatment 1999* (38th ed., pp. 183–185, 192–194, 198, 209–210). E. Norwalk, CT: Appleton & Lange.

24–4

Arts, H. A., Kileny, P. R., & Telian, S. A. (1997). Diagnostic testing for endolymphatic hydrops. *Otolaryngologic Clinics of North America, 30,* 987–1005.

Baloh, R. W. (1998). *Dizziness, hearing loss, and tinnitus.* Philadelphia, FA Davis.

Beers, M. H., & Berkow, R. (Eds.). (1999). *The Merck manual of diagnosis and therapy.* Whitehouse Station, NJ: Merck Research Laboratories.

Brandt, T. (1999). *Vertigo* (2nd ed.). London: Springer.

Fetter, M. (2000). Vestibular system disorders. In S. J. Herdman (Ed.), *Vestibular rehabilitation* (2nd ed., pp. 91–102). Philadelphia, FA Davis.

Gibson, W. P. R., & Arenberg, I. K. (1997). Pathophysiologic theories in the etiology of Menière's disease. *Otolaryngologic Clinics of North America, 30,* 961–967.

Hain, T. C., Ramaswamy, T. S., & Hillman, M. A. (2000). Anatomy and physiology of the normal vestibular system. In S. J. Herdman (Ed.), *Vestibular rehabilitation* (2nd ed., pp. 3–24). Philadelphia: FA Davis.

Hector Dunphy, L. M. (1999). *Management guidelines for adult nurse practitioners.* Philadelphia: FA Davis.

Leo, J., & Huether, S. E. (1998). Pain, temperature regulation, sleep and sensory function. In K. L. McCance & S. E. Huether (Eds.), *Pathophysiology: The biologic basis for disease in adults and children* (pp. 422–458). St. Louis, MO: Mosby-Year Book.

Saeed, S. R. (1998). Fortnightly review: Diagnosis and treatment of Menière's disease. *British Medical Journal, 316*, 368–372.

Weber, P. C., & Adkins, W. Y. (1997). The differential diagnosis of Menière's disease. *Otolaryngologic Clinics of North America, 30*, 977–986.

Wilson, P. (1999). Menière's disease information page. Available at: *http://www.geocities.com/HotSprings/Spa/3143/info.htm*

Younkin, E. Q., & Davis, M. S. (1998). *Women's health: A primary care clinical guide* (2nd ed.). E. Norwalk, CT: Appleton & Lange.

25–1

Bauer, S. B. (1998). Neurogenic dysfunction of the lower urinary tract in children. In P. C. Walsh, A. B. Retik, E. D. Vaughan, & A. J. Wein (Eds.), *Campbell's urology* (pp. 2019–2054). Philadelphia: WB Saunders.

Brittain, K. R., Peet, S. M., Optter, J. F., & Castleden, C. M. (1999). Prevalence and management of urinary incontinence in stroke survivors. *Age and Ageing, 28*, 509–511.

Chai, T. C., Gray, M. L., & Steers, W. D. (1998). The incidence of a positive ice water test on bladder outlet obstructed patients: Evidence for altered innervation. *Journal of Urology, 160*, 34–38.

Chancellor, M. B., Bennet, C., Simoneau, A. R., et al. (1999). Sphincteric stent versus external sphincterotomy in spinal cord injured men: prospective randomized multicenter trial. *Journal of Urology, 161*, 1893–1898.

Di Carlo, A., Lamassa, M., Pracucci, G., et al. (1999). Stroke in the very old: clinical presentation and determinants of 3 month functional outcome: A European perspective. European BIOMED study of stroke. *Stroke, 30*, 2313–2319.

Giannantoni, A., Scivoletto, G., Di Stasi, S. M., et al. (1999). Lower urinary tract dysfunction and disability status in patients with multiple sclerosis. *Archives of Physical Medicine and Rehabilitation, 80*, 437–442.

Gray, M. (2000). Urodynamics in the clinical management of urinary incontinence in men and women. *Topics in Geriatric Rehabilitation, 15*, 42–60.

Gray, M. (2000). Reflex urinary incontinence. In D. B. Doughty (Ed.), *Urinary and fecal incontinence: Nursing management* (pp. 105–143). St. Louis, MO: CV Mosby.

Jawad, S. H., Ward, A. B., & Jones, P. (1999). Study of the relationship between premorbid urinary incontinence and stroke functional outcome. *Clinical Rehabilitation, 13*, 447–452.

Killorin, W. K., Gray, M. L., & Steers, W. D. (1998). The incidence of a positive ice water test on bladder outlet obstructed patients: Evidence for altered innervation. *Journal of Urology, 160*, 34–38.

Levin, R. M., Levin, S. S., Zhao, Y., & Buttyan, R. (1997). Cellular and molecular aspects of bladder hypertrophy. *European Urology, 32*(Suppl. 1), 15–21.

Madersbacher, S., Pycha, A., Klingler, C. H., et al. (1999). Interrelationships of bladder compliance with age, detrusor instability and obstruction in elderly men with lower urinary tract symptoms. *Neurourology and Urodynamics, 18,* 3–15.

Mauroy, B. (1997). Bladder consequences of prostatic obstruction. *European Urology, 32*(Suppl. 1), 3–8.

Metz, L. M., McGuinness, S. D., & Harris, C. (1998). Urinary tract infection may trigger relapse in multiple sclerosis. *Axone, 19,* 67–70.

Morioka, A., Miyano, T., Ando, K., et al. (1998). Management of vesicoureteral reflux secondary to neurogenic bladder. *Pediatric Surgery International, 13,* 584–586.

Pozolli, C., Gherardi, M., Patrucco, L., et al. (1999). Clinical measures of disease activity in multiple sclerosis. *Electroencephalography and Clinical Neurophysiology, 50,* 560–564.

Smith, D. A. (2000). Urge incontinence. In D. B. Doughty (Ed.), *Urinary and fecal incontinence: Nursing management* (pp. 105–143). St. Louis, MO: CV Mosby.

Wein, A. J. (1998). Neuromuscular dysfunction of lower urinary tract. In P. C. Walsh, A. B. Retik, E. D. Vaughan, & A. J. Wein (Eds.), *Campbell's urology* (pp. 967–968). Philadelphia: WB Saunders.

25–2

Bates, P. (2000). Nursing management of renal and urologic problems. In S. M. Lewis, M. L. Heitkemper, & S. R. Dirksen (Eds.), *Medical-surgical nursing: Assessment and management of clinical problems* (5th ed., pp. 1274–1279). St. Louis. MO: CV Mosby.

Einhorn, C. J. (1997). Urolithiasis. In D. Daly-Gawenda (Ed.), *Manual of medical-surgical nursing: A med-surg fact finder* (pp. 253–262). Boston, MA: Little, Brown.

Marantides, D. K, Marek, J. F., & Morgan, J. (1999). Management of persons with problems of the kidney and urinary tract. In W. Phipps, J. Sands, & Marek J. (Eds.), *Medical-surgical nursing: Concepts and clinical practice* (6th ed., pp. 1428–1434). St. Louis, MO: CV Mosby.

Matassarin-Jacobs, E. (1997). Nursing care of clients with disorders of the ureters, bladder, and urethra. In J. M. Black & E. Matassarin-Jacobs (Eds.), *Medical-surgical nursing: Clinical management for continuity of care* (5th ed., pp. 1595–1598). Philadelphia: WB Saunders.

Pierson, C. A., & Mishler, M. A. (1999). Interventions for clients with urinary problems. In D. Ignatavicius, M. Workman, & M. Mishler (Eds.), *Medical-surgical nursing across the health care continuum* (3rd ed., pp. 1838–1844). Philadelphia: WB Saunders.

Presti, J. C., Stoller, M. L., & Carroll, P. R. (1997). Urinary stone disease. In L. M. Tierney, S. J. McPhee, & M. A. Papadakis (Eds.), *Current medical diagnosis and treatment* (pp. 866–880). E. Norwalk, CT: Appleton & Lange.

Williams, S. R. (1999). *Essentials of nutrition and diet therapy* (7th ed., pp. 462–466). St. Louis, MO: CV Mosby.

25–3

Agrawal, M., & Swartz, R. (2000). Acute renal failure. *American Family Physician, 61,* 2077–2091.

Brunier, G., & Bartucci, M. (2000) Renal failure. In S. Lewis, M. Heitkemper, & S. Dirksen (Eds.), *Medical-surgical nursing: Assessment and management of clinical problems* (pp. 1299–1339). St. Louis, MO: CV Mosby.

Dirkes, S. M. (1997). A dialysis alternative more nurses can run: Continuous venovenous hemofiltration offers a safer, easier alternative to conventional hemodialysis for your sickest patients. *Registered Nurse, 60,* 20–26.

End-stage renal disease. Available at: *http://4woman.gov/faq/esrd.htm*

Kripke, C. C. (1999). Guidelines for managing chronic renal failure. *American Family Physician, 59,* 3207–3208.

Lewis, S., Heitkemper, M., & Dirksen, S. (2000). Acute and chronic renal failure. In S. Lewis, M. Heitkemper, & S. Dirksen (Eds.), *Medical-surgical nursing: Assessment and management of clinical problems* (5th ed., pp. 1299–1341). St. Louis, MO: CV Mosby.

Lucas, B. (1999). Chronic renal failure: Slowing the onset, changing the course. *Patient Care, 33,* 76–79.

Porth, C. M. (1998). Renal failure. *Pathophysiology: Concepts of altered health status* (5th ed., pp. 667–677). Philadelphia: JB Lippincott.

Tran, M., & Rutecki, G. W. (2000). Renal disease: Tips on prevention and early recognition. *Consultant, 40,* 222–231.

25–4

Evidence report/technology assessment. No 6. Prevention and management of urinary tract infections in paralyzed persons. Rockville, MD: AHCPR. Available at: *http://www.ahcpr.gov/clinic/utisumm.htm*

National Kidney and Urologic Diseases Information Clearinghouse. Urinary tract infection in adults. Available at: *http://www.niddk.nih.gov/health/urolog/pubs/utiadult* (Updated March 2000).

Smeltzer, S. C., & Bare, B. G. (2000). *Brunner and Suddarth's textbook of medical-surgical nursing* (9th ed.). Philadelphia: Lippincott-Raven.

26–1

Mosier, W. A., Schymanski, T. J., & Walgren, K. D. (1998). Benign prostatic hyperplasia. Focusing on primary care. *Clinical Reviews, 8*(7), 55–58, 63–66, 68–70, 73–75.

Nelson, D. A., & Schumann, L. (1998). Differentiating prostate disorders. *Journal of the American Academy of Nurse Practitioners, 10*(9), 415–424.

Pfeiffer, G. M., & Giacomarra, M. (1999). Benign prostatic hyperplasia: A review of diagnostic and treatment options. *Advance for Nurse Practitioners 3,* 31–38.

Reilly, N. J. (1997). Benign prostatic hyperplasia in older men. *Lippincott's primary care practice, 1*(4), 421–430.

26–2

Centers for Disease Control and Prevention. (1998). Sexually transmitted diseases treatment guidelines. *MMWR Morbidity and Mortality Weekly Report, 47*(RR–1), 70–74.

Chandra, A., & Stephen, E. H. (1998). Impaired fecundity in the United States: 1982–1995. *Family Planning Perspectives, 30*(1), 34–42.

Hoar, S. (1998). Protocols. Pelvic inflammatory disease. *Lippincott's Primary Care Practice, 2*(3), 307–311.

Igra, V. (1998). Pelvic inflammatory disease in adolescents. *AIDS Patient Care and STDs, 12*(2), 109–124.

Quiroz, F. A. (1999). Pelvic inflammatory disease. *Applied Radiology, 28*(10), 30–35.

Salzer, E. A. J. (1997). Pelvic inflammatory disease: Management update. *Physician Assistant, 21*(4), 36, 38–40, 43–44.

Smith, C. B. (1997). Acute pelvic pain: When prompt diagnosis is vital. *Consultant, 37*(2), 404–406, 411–412.

Wolner-Hanssen, P. (1999). Pelvic inflammatory disease: Diagnosis. *Contemporary Obstetrics/Gynecology, 44*(8), 108, 113–114, 116.

26–3

Center for Disease Control and Prevention (CDC). (1998). Guidelines for treatment of sexually transmitted diseases. *MMWR Morbidity and Mortality Weekly Report, 47*(RR–1), 1–111.

Clark, J. R. (1997). Sexually transmitted diseases: Detection, differentiation, and treatment. *Physician and Sportsmedicine, 25*(1), 76–80.

Dull, P., & Miller, K. E. (1997). STDs in women: An update. *Family Practice Recertification, 19*(8), 13–16, 19–20, 22, 24, 27–28.

Erbelding, E., & Quinn, T. C. (1997). The impact of antimicrobial resistance on the treatment of sexually transmitted diseases. *Infectious Disease Clinics of North America, 11*(4), 889–903.

Gonen, J. (1999). Confronting STDs: A challenge for managed care. *Women's Health Issues, 9*(2, Suppl. 1), 36S–46S.

Kirsten, V. L., & Whipple, B. (1998). Treating HIV disease: Hope on the horizon. *Nursing 98, 28*(11), 34–40.

Reid, J. (1999). Sexually transmitted disease in the U.S. An overview of treatment guidelines. *Advance for Nurse Practitioners, 6,* 45–46, 49–50.

Rome, E. S. (1998a). Sexually transmitted diseases in the adolescent. Part I: Chlamydia and gonorrhea. *The Female Patient, 23,* 11–12, 18, 20, 23–25.

Rome, E. S. (1998b). Sexually transmitted diseases in the adolescent. Part II: Syphilis, chancroid, and herpes. *The Female Patient, 23,* 67–70, 72–73.

Index

Note: Page numbers followed by the letter f refer to figures; those followed by the letter t refer to tables.

A

AAA. *See* Abdominal aortic aneurysm (AAA).

AACG. *See* Acute angle-closure glaucoma (AACG).

AB. *See* Acute bronchitis (AB).

Abacavir. *See* Ziagen (Abacavir, 1592U89).

ABCDEF mnemonic, in first aid for injuries, 25, 26t

Abciximab (ReoPro)
  as antiplatelet drug, 330, 331t
  for myocardial infarction, 479

Abdomen, in gastrointestinal assessment, 21

Abdominal aortic aneurysm (AAA), 487. *See also* Aortic aneurysm.

Abdominal distention, in intestinal obstruction, 582

Abdominal pain
  in intestinal obstruction, 582
  in pancreatitis, 610

Abdominal radiography
  for inflammatory bowel disease, 571
  for intestinal obstruction, 583
  for pancreatitis, 611
  for renal calculi, 841

Abdominal ultrasonography
  for aortic aneurysm, 489
  for pancreatitis, 612

ABG analysis. *See* Arterial blood gas (ABG) analysis.

ABI. *See* Ankle-brachial index (ABI).

ABO blood group, 65, 66t, 67

Absence seizures, 685, 686t

Absent breath sounds, 19–20

Absolute glaucoma, 817

Absorption atelectasis, from oxygen therapy, 125

Abuse, 709

Acarbose (Precose), 385t

Accupril. *See* Quinapril (Accupril).

ACE inhibitors. *See* Angiotensin-converting enzyme (ACE) inhibitors.

Acetaminophen, for analgesia, 319

Acetazolamide (Diamox)
  for glaucoma, 821t
  pharmacology of, 378, 379t, 383t

Acetohexamide (Dymelor), 385t

Acetylcysteine (Mucomyst), 402t

Acetylsalicylic acid (ASA), 317, 318t. *See also* Aspirin.

Acid-base disturbance, in renal failure, 145

Acid-fast bacillus (AFB), 439–440

Acid-fast smear, in infection, 303

Acidosis, in hyperkalemia, 294

Acquired immunity, 263

Acquired immunodeficiency syndrome (AIDS), 764. *See also* Human immunodeficiency virus (HIV) infection.

ACTH. *See* Adrenocorticotropic hormone (ACTH).

Actigall. *See* Ursodiol (Actigall).

Activated charcoal, for drug overdose and poisoning, 706–707

Activated partial thromboplastin time (APTT), 324t, 325
  in hepatitis, 565

Active tuberculosis, 438
  drug therapy for, 441
  sputum testing for, 439

Activity
  after renal transplantation, 164
  in human immunodeficiency virus infection, 769
  progression of, for fractures, 736–738, 737t

Actos. *See* Pioglitazone (Actos).

Actron. *See* Ketoprofen (Actron, Orudis).

Acute angle-closure glaucoma (AACG), 817–818

Acute bacterial bronchitis, 423

Acute bacterial conjunctivitis
  interventions for, 811
  pathophysiology of, 809
  signs and symptoms of, 810

Acute bacterial exacerbations of chronic bronchitis (AECB), 423

Acute bronchitis (AB), 422–423
Acute exacerbations, in heart failure, 460–461
Acute fulminant hepatitis, 561
Acute lymphocytic leukemia (ALL), 794. *See also* Leukemia.
Acute myeloblastic leukemia (AML), 794. *See also* Leukemia.
Acute pain, 312
Acute pancreatitis, 610
Acute rejection, in renal transplant, 162, 164–165
Acute renal failure (ARF), 142
  interventions for, 853
  pathophysiology of, 847t, 847–848
  signs and symptoms of, 849, 850t–851t
Acute transmural ischemia, 474–475
Acute tubular necrosis (ATN), 848
Acute viral bronchitis, 423
Acyclovir, 357
Adalat CC. *See* Nifedipine (Adalat CC, Procardia XL).
Addiction, to opioids, 317
Adefavir dipivoxil (Preveon), for human immunodeficiency virus infection, 766–767, 767t
Adrenal insufficiency, in hyperkalemia, 294
Adrenalin. *See* Epinephrine (Adrenalin, Bronkaid).
Adrenergic blockers. *See* Alpha-adrenergic blockers; Beta-adrenergic blockers.
Adrenergic bronchodilators, inhaled, 393
Adrenocorticosteroids, 408–415
  categories of, 408–413, 410t, 411t
  decision-making for, 412t–415t, 413–415
  physiology of, 408
Adrenocorticotropic hormone (ACTH)
  glucocorticoids and, 409
  in hypovolemic shock, 520
Adsorbents, for diarrhea, 371–372
Adult inclusion conjunctivitis
  interventions for, 812
  pathophysiology of, 809
  prognosis for, 814
  signs and symptoms of, 810
Adventitious breath sounds, in respiratory assessment, 20

Advil. *See* Ibuprofen (Advil, Motrin).
AECB. *See* Acute bacterial exacerbations of chronic bronchitis (AECB).
Afrin. *See* Oxymetazoline (Afrin, Allerest).
Agenerase. *See* Amprenavir (Agenerase).
Aggression
  in Alzheimer's disease, 647
  medications for, 405, 405t
Agitation, in Alzheimer's disease, 647
Agranulocytes, 283, 284–286, 285t
Agranulocytosis, 289
Air embolism, with venous access device, 58t, 61
Air humidification, for bronchitis, 425
Air leak, in tracheostomy care, 132
Airborne precautions, 271
Airiness. *See* Tolbutamide (Airiness).
Airway, in meningitis, 664, 665t
Albumin
  for hypovolemic shock, 524
  in sputum smear, 108, 108t
Albuterol (Proventil), 393, 394t
Alcohol
  blood, concentration of, 693–694, 694t
  hypertension and, 516
  in peptic ulcer disease, 616
Alcohol withdrawal syndrome (AWS), 693–696, 694t
Alcohol-induced hepatitis, 560
Aldactone. *See* Spironolactone (Aldactone).
Aldomet. *See* Methyldopa (Aldomet).
Aldosterone, in hypovolemic shock, 520
Aldosterone blockers, for chronic heart failure, 462t, 464
Aldosterone-inhibiting diuretics, 375, 377t, 379
Aleve. *See* Naproxen sodium (Anaprox, Aleve).
Alginate dressings, 83
Alkaline phosphatase
  for biliary disease, 597
  in intestinal obstruction, 583
Alkylating agents, for cancer, 783, 784t
ALL. *See* Acute lymphocytic leukemia (ALL).
Allegra. *See* Fexofenadine (Allegra).
Allerest. *See* Oxymetazoline (Afrin, Allerest).

Allergic asthma, 417
Allergic conjunctivitis
  interventions for, 812–813
  pathophysiology of, 810
  prognosis for, 814
  signs and symptoms of, 811
Allergic reaction, to blood transfusion, 68t
Allergic rhinitis, 774–775
Allergies, 773–779
  community care for, 778–779
  diagnostic criteria for, 776–777
  interventions for, 777–778
  pathophysiology of, 773–774
  prognosis for, 779
  signs and symptoms of, 774–776
Allodynia, from opioids, 314, 315t
Allopurinol, for gout, 745
Alpha-2 adrenergic agonists, for glaucoma, 820t
Alpha-adrenergic blockers, 338–339, 345t
Alpha-beta blockers, 339–340, 346t
Alpha-glucosidase inhibitors, 385t, 386–387
Alpha interferons, for immunologic alterations, 264
Alprazolam (Xanax), 404t
Altace. See Ramipril (Altace).
Altered mental status
  first aid for, 25–27, 26t, 27t
  in renal failure, 144
Aluminum-based antacids, 365–366
Alupent. See Metaproterenol (Alupent, Metaprel).
Amantadine (Symmetrel), for Parkinson's disease, 677, 678t
Amaryl. See Glimepiride (Amaryl).
Ambenonium, for myasthenia gravis, 673t
Ambien. See Zolpidem (Ambien).
American Nurses Association (ANA) standards of practice, 2–4
Amikacin, 354
Amiloride (Midamor), 379
Aminoglycosides
  for pneumonia, 435
  pharmacology of, 354
Aminophylline, 393, 395t
Aminosalicylates, for inflammatory bowel disease, 571–572

5-Aminosalicylic acid agents, for irritable bowel disease, 373–374
Aminotransferases, in hepatitis, 565
Amiodarone (Cordarone), for chronic heart failure, 464
Amitriptyline (Elavil), 333, 333t
AML. See Acute myeloblastic leukemia (AML).
Amlodipine (Norvasc), 344t
Ammonia, in liver cirrhosis, 552, 553
Amoxapine (Asendin), 333, 333t
Amoxicillin, 350–351
Amphotericin B, 356–357
Ampicillin, 350–351
AMPLE mnemonic, 704
Amprenavir (Agenerase), for human immunodeficiency virus, 767, 767t
Amrinone, for cardiogenic shock, 454
Amylase
  in biliary disease, 597
  in intestinal obstruction, 583
  in pancreatitis, 611
ANA. See American Nurses Association (ANA).
Anacobin, for inflammatory bowel disease, 573
Anafranil. See Clomipramine (Anafranil).
Analgesia, 312–320
  acetaminophen for, 319
  for fractures, 738
  for pneumonia, 435
  nonsteroidal anti-inflammatory drugs for, 317–319, 318t
  opioids for, 314–317, 315t, 316t
  principles of care for, 312–314
  World Health Organization ladder for, 319–320
Anaphylactic reaction, to blood transfusion, 68t
Anaphylaxis
  first aid for, 26t, 27–28
  interventions for, 777–778
  signs and symptoms of, 775
Anaprox. See Naproxen sodium (Anaprox, Aleve).
Androgens, 408
Anemia, 275–276, 276t, 790–794, 791t
  differentiation of, by red blood cell indices, 277, 278t
  in renal failure, 144

Aneurysm, aortic. *See* Aortic aneurysm.
Angina, 446–451
  community care for, 449–450
  diagnostic criteria for, 447
  interventions for, 447–449
  pathophysiology of, 446
  prognosis for, 450
  signs and symptoms of, 446–447
Angina pectoris, 468–469
Angioedema, 775
Angiography
  for angina, 447
  for deep vein thrombosis, 504
  for peripheral vascular disease, 528
Angiotensin II, in hypovolemic shock, 520
Angiotensin receptor blockers (ARBs), 337–338, 344t
Angiotensin-converting enzyme (ACE) inhibitors
  for chronic heart failure, 461, 462t
  pharmacology of, 336–337, 343t
Anisocytosis, 279
Ankle circles, for deep vein thrombosis, 505
Ankle-brachial index (ABI)
  for Buerger's disease, 496
  for peripheral vascular disease, 529
Anorexia
  in anemia, 792
  in renal failure, 145
Antacids
  for liver cirrhosis, 554
  pharmacology of, 365–366
Anterior carotid artery syndrome, 652t
Anterior cord syndrome, 688
Anterior inferior cerebellar artery syndrome, 653t
Antianxiety drugs, 403–408. *See also* Sedatives.
Antibacterial(s)
  aminoglycosides as, 354
  carbapenems as, 351
  cephalosporins as, 352
  clindamycin as, 353
  fluoroquinolones as, 353–354
  macrolides as, 353
  metronidazole as, 356
  monobactams as, 351–352
  penicillins as, 350–351

Antibacterial(s) *(Continued)*
  sulfonamides as, 354–355
  tetracyclines as, 352–353
  vancomycin as, 355–356
Antibiotics
  for arthritis, 724
  for bronchitis, 425
  for cancer, 783, 784t
  for gallstones, 599
  for inflammatory bowel disease, 573
  for pneumonia, 435
  peak and trough levels for, 349, 349t
Antibodies
  in immune system, 260
  in inflammation, 261
Anticholinergics
  for diarrhea, 372
  for Parkinson's disease, 677, 678t
  pharmacology of, 369–370
Anticholinesterase agents, for myasthenia gravis, 673
Anticoagulant(s), 320–332
  antiplatelet drugs in, 330, 331t
  coagulation testing for, 323–325, 324t
  for chronic heart failure, 464
  heparin as, 325–327, 326t
  low molecular weight heparin in, 328, 329t
  patient education for, 328
  principles of care for, 321–323, 322f, 323t
  warfarin as, 327–328
Anticoagulation, for deep vein thrombosis, 506–507
Antidepressants
  for depression, 700
  pharmacology of, 332t–335t, 332–335
Antidiarrheal agents
  for inflammatory bowel disease, 573
  for irritable bowel disease, 373
Antidiuretic hormone, in hypovolemic shock, 520
Antidysrhythmia agents, for chronic heart failure, 464
Antiemetics, for hepatitis, 566
Antifungals, pharmacology of, 356–357
Antihistamines
  for nausea and vomiting, 370
  for renal failure, 854
  for rhinitis, cough, and colds, 397, 398t–399t

Antihypertensives, 336–348
administration of, 342
alpha-adrenergic blockers as, 338–339, 345t
alpha-beta blockers as, 339–340, 346t
angiotensin-converting enzyme inhibitors as, 336–337, 343t
angiotensin receptor blockers as, 337–338, 344t
beta-adrenergic blockers as, 339, 345t
calcium channel blockers as, 338, 344t
central alpha-adrenergic agonists as, 340, 346t
choice of, 341–342
direct vasodilators as, 340–341, 347t
diuretics in, 341
for hemodialysis, 152, 152t
for renal failure, 854
patient teaching for, 342
peripheral adrenergic neuron antagonists as, 340, 347t
principles of care for, 336
Anti-infectives, 348–358
antibacterials as, 350–356. See also Antibacterial(s).
antifungals as, 356–357
antivirals as, 357–358
for diarrhea, 373
principles of care for, 348–350, 349t
Antimalarial drugs, for systemic lupus erythematosus, 761
Antimetabolites, for cancer, 783, 784t
Antimicrobials
for rheumatic heart disease, 485–486
for urinary tract infection, 857–858
Antimitotic agents, for gout, 746
Antinuclear antibody
in rheumatoid arthritis, 722
in systemic lupus erythematosus, 757
Antiplatelets
for myocardial infarction, 478–479
pharmacology of, 330, 331t
Antipsychotic agents, for aggressive/combative behavior, 405t
Antirheumatic drugs, for arthritis, 723–724
Antiseizure medications, 358–364
for precipitating factors and events, 359
patient and caregiver education for, 364

Antiseizure medications (Continued)
principles of care for, 359, 360t–361t
use of, 359, 362t–363t
Antiseptics, for wound cleansing, 81
Antispasmodic agents, for irritable bowel disease, 373
Antithyroid drugs, for hyperthyroidism, 636, 636t
Antituberculin medication, 439t, 441, 441t, 442t
Antitumor antibiotics, for cancer, 783, 784t
Antitussives, for rhinitis, cough, and colds, 397, 400t
Antivirals
for hepatitis, 566
pharmacology of, 357–358
Antrectomy, for peptic ulcer disease, 619
Anturane. See Sulfinpyrazone (Anturane).
Anuria, 17
Anxiety
in asthma, 421
in emphysema, 430
medications for, 404, 404t. See also Sedatives.
Anxiolytic drugs, 403–408. See also Sedatives.
Aortic aneurysm, 487–494
diagnostic criteria for, 488–490
interventions for, 490–493
pathophysiology of, 487–488
signs and symptoms of, 488
Aortocoronary bypass, for angina, 449
Apathetic hyperthyroidism, 635
Apical rate, measurement of, 12
Aplastic anemia, 790, 791t
Aplastic crisis, 799–800
Appendectomy, 548
Appendicitis, 547–549
Apraclonidine, for glaucoma, 820t
Apresoline. See Hydralazine (Apresoline).
APTT. See Activated partial thromboplastin time (APTT).
Arachidonic acid derivatives, in allergies, 774
Arachidonic acid metabolites, in inflammation, 262t, 262–263
ARBs. See Angiotensin receptor blockers (ARBs).

Ardeparin (Normiflo), 329t
Areflexia, detrusor, 831
ARF. *See* Acute renal failure (ARF).
Aristocort. *See* Prednisone (Aristocort, Deltasone).
Arrhythmias, 476–477
Artane. *See* Trihexyphenidyl (Artane).
Arterial blood gas (ABG) analysis
    for emphysema, 429
    for intestinal obstruction, 583
    for oxygenation, 120–123, 121t–123t
    for renal failure, 852
Arterial elasticity, blood pressure and, 9
Arterial ulcers, 79
Arteriography
    for aortic aneurysm, 489
    for Buerger's disease, 496
    for deep vein thrombosis, 504
Arteriosclerosis, 467–468, 468f
Arteriovenous (AV) fistula, in hemodialysis, 148–149, 150f
Arteriovenous (AV) graft, in hemodialysis, 149, 150f
Arthralgia, in inflammatory bowel disease, 570
Arthritis, 720–729
    community care for, 728
    diagnostic criteria for, 722–723
    gouty, 743
    in inflammatory bowel disease, 570
    maintenance of functional status in, 725
    nutrition for, 725
    pain and symptom management in, 723–725
    pathophysiology of, 720
    prevalence of, 720, 721f
    prognosis for, 728
    rheumatoid, 262, 262t
    signs and symptoms of, 720–722
    surgical intervention for, 726–728
Arthrodesis, for arthritis, 726
Arthroplasty
    hip, 726–727
    knee, 727–728
ASA. *See* Acetylsalicylic acid (ASA); Aspirin.
Asacol. *See* Mesalamine (Asacol, Pentasa, Rowasa).
Ascending colostomy, 89t

Asendin. *See* Amoxapine (Asendin).
Aspergillosis, in human immunodeficiency virus infection, 766, 770t
Aspiration pneumonia, 432–434
Aspirin
    as antiplatelet drug, 330, 331t
    for angina, 447–448
    for myocardial infarction, 477
    for rheumatic heart disease, 484
    in peptic ulcer disease, 616
    pharmacology of, 317, 318t
Astemizole (Hismanal), 399t
Asthma, 417–422
    community care for, 421
    diagnostic criteria for, 419
    interventions for, 419–421, 420t
    pathophysiology of, 417–418
    prognosis for, 421–422
    signs and symptoms of, 418–419, 776
Atacand. *See* Candesartan cilexetil (Atacand).
Atelectasis
    from immobilization, 737t
    from oxygen therapy, 125
Atenolol (Tenormin), 345t
Ativan. *See* Lorazepam (Ativan).
ATN. *See* Acute tubular necrosis (ATN).
Atopic dermatitis, 775–776
Atrial flutter and fibrillation, 476
Atrioventricular block, 476–477
Atropine, for diarrhea, 372
Atrovent. *See* Ipratropium bromide (Atrovent).
Attapulgite (Kaopectate), 371–372
Atypical depression, 332, 332t
Aura, in seizures, 681
Auscultation, in respiratory assessment, 19–20
Autoimmune disorders, 262, 262t
Autologous blood, administration of, 70t
Autolytic débridement, 81
Autonomic dysfunction, in Guillain-Barré syndrome, 658, 659, 659t, 660
Autonomic dysreflexia, in spinal cord injury, 688–690
Autonomy, definition and rules of care for, 6t
Autoregulation
    definition of, 178t

Autoregulation *(Continued)*
  in increased intracranial pressure, 179
AV fistula. *See* Arteriovenous (AV)
  fistula.
Avandia. *See* Rosiglitazone (Avandia).
Avapro. *See* Irbesartan (Avapro).
Avascular necrosis, from fractures,
  739–740
Avonex. *See* Interferon beta-1a (Avonex).
AWS. *See* Alcohol withdrawal syndrome
  (AWS).
Axid. *See* Nizatidine (Axid).
Axillary temperature, measurement of, 16
Azatadine maleate (Optimine), 399t
Azathioprine (Imuran)
  for inflammatory bowel disease, 572
  for irritable bowel disease, 374
  for myasthenia gravis, 673t
  for renal transplantation, 163t
Azithromycin
  for pelvic inflammatory disease, 868t
  pharmacology of, 353
AZT. *See* Zidovudine (Retrovir, AZT).
Aztreonam, pharmacology of, 351–352
Azulfidine. *See* Sulfasalazine
  (Azulfidine).

B

B lymphocytes, 260, 285, 286
Bacampillin, 350–351
Bacille Calmette-Guérin (BCG) vaccine,
  442
Bacteremia
  blood culture for, 300–301
Bacteria
  in food poisoning, 556–558
  in urinalysis, 308
Bacterial bronchitis, 423
Bacterial conjunctivitis
  interventions for, 811
  pathophysiology of, 809
  prognosis for, 814
  signs and symptoms of, 810
Bacterial endocarditis prophylaxis, for
  rheumatic heart disease, 486
Bacterial meningitis
  clinical manifestations of, 663, 663t
  pathophysiology of, 662
Bacterial peritonitis, in liver cirrhosis,
  550

Bacterial pneumonia, 432
Bacterial vaginosis, 870, 872t
Bactericidal agents, 349
Bacteriostatic agents, 349
Bacteroides, in pelvic inflammatory
  disease, 868t
Bainbridge reflex, 8
Balanced suspension traction, for
  fractures, 734
Balloon dilatation, for benign prostatic
  hypertrophy, 863
Balloon tamponade, for liver cirrhosis,
  554
Bands, 284
  elevated levels of, 286
Barbiturates
  drug interactions with, 407t
  for sleep disorders, 405t
Barium enema, in inflammatory bowel
  disease, 571
Baroreceptors, heart rate and, 8
Basal metabolic rate (BMR), 10
Basilar artery syndrome, 652t
Basopenia, 289
Basophilia, 287
Basophils, 283, 284
  peripheral smear of, 286, 287f
BCG vaccine, 442
Bed rest, for deep vein thrombosis, 507
Bedside specimen collection, 98–114
  and blood glucose monitoring, 109–
    114. *See also* Blood glucose speci-
    men collection and monitoring.
  of gastrointestinal specimens, 98–101
  of sputum, 105–108, 107t, 108t
  of urine, 101–105, 102t
Behavioral problems, in Alzheimer's
  disease, 647
Benadryl. *See* Diphenhydramine
  (Benadryl).
Benazepril (Lotensin), 343t
Beneficence, definition and rules of care
  for, 6t
Benemid. *See* Probenecid (Benemid).
Benign hypertension, 510–511. *See also*
  Hypertension (HTN).
Benign prostatic hypertrophy (BPH),
  860–866
  community care for, 864–865
  diagnostic criteria for, 861–862

Benign prostatic hypertrophy (BPH)
    (Continued)
    interventions for, 862–864
    pathophysiology of, 860
    prognosis for, 865
    signs and symptoms of, 860–861
Benylin DM. *See* Dextromethorphan
    (Benylin DM).
Benzodiazepines
    drug interactions with, 407t
    pharmacology of, 405t
Benzonatate (Tessalon Perles), 400t
Benzothiazepines, 338, 344t
Benztropine (Cogentin), for Parkinson's
    disease, 678t
Beta-adrenergic blockers
    for angina, 448
    for chronic heart failure, 462t, 463–
        464
    for glaucoma, 820t
    for hyperthyroidism, 636, 636t
    for liver cirrhosis, 554
    for myocardial infarction, 477
    pharmacology of, 339, 345t
Betalin, for inflammatory bowel disease,
    573
Betamethasone dipropionate, for systemic
    lupus erythematosus, 760
Betaseron. *See* Interferon beta-1b
    (Betaseron).
Betaxolol (Kerlone)
    for glaucoma, 820t
    pharmacology of, 345t
Bicadren. *See* Timolol (Bicadren).
Biguanides, 385t, 386
Bile
    in gallstone formation, 595
    in liver cirrhosis, 551
Biliary drainage tubes, 93–95, 94f
Biliary surgery, for liver cirrhosis, 554
Biliary/pancreatic stents, 97
Bilirubin
    in biliary disease, 597
    in hepatitis, 564–565
    in liver cirrhosis, 552, 553
    in urinalysis, 102, 102t
Biochemical markers, for osteoporosis,
    750
Biofeedback, for Raynaud's disease,
    534–535

Biopsy
    for liver cirrhosis, 553
    for peptic ulcer disease, 618
    for renal failure, 852
Biot's respirations, 14
Bisacodyl (Dulcolax), 368
Bismuth subsalicylate (Pepto-Bismol),
    371–372
Bisoprolol (Zebeta), 345t
Bites and stings, 26t, 28, 29t, 30t
Bladder
    in multiple sclerosis, 667, 668t
    neurogenic. *See* Neurogenic bladder.
    radiography of, in renal function, 309
Blasts, on peripheral smear, 286, 287f
Bleeding
    from hemodialysis, 153, 154t
    in anemia, 792
    in hepatitis, 565
    in renal failure, 145
    in stoma assessment, 89
Bleeding time, 325
Bleeding time test, 281
Blood
    in culture report, 302
    in hepatitis, 571
    in urinalysis, 102, 102t
    isolation of, 270
Blood alcohol concentration, 693–694,
    694t
Blood and blood product administration,
    64–69
    decision-making for, 67–69, 68t, 70t–
        75t
    principles of care for, 65–67, 66t
Blood cell count, complete. *See*
    Complete blood count (CBC).
Blood chemistry, for hypertension, 514
Blood cultures
    for infection, 300–301
    for pneumonia, 434
    for thrombophlebitis, 539
Blood flow
    in neurologic assessment, 166
    in wound care, 84
Blood glucose specimen collection and
    monitoring, 109–114
    false values in, 111, 113t
    fasting, 111, 112t
    glucose tolerance test in, 111, 112t

Blood glucose specimen collection and monitoring *(Continued)*
  glycosylated hemoglobin test in, 111, 112t
  insulin coverage formula in, 111, 113t
  principles of care for, 109–110
  self-monitoring, 110, 110t
  urine testing for ketones in, 111–114
Blood loss, during surgery, for arthritis, 726, 727
Blood pressure
  in hypertension, 514
    assessment of, 515
    classification schema of, 513, 513t
  in hypovolemic shock, 521, 522t, 523
  in renal failure, 144
  measurement of, 14–15
  principles of care for, 8–9
Blood samples, for prothrombin time, 324
Blood-streaked sputum, 108
Blood tests
  for allergies, 776–777
  for hepatitis, 570–571
Blood transfusion reactions, 67, 68t
Blood typing, 65–67, 66t
Blood urea nitrogen (BUN)
  in intestinal obstruction, 583
  in renal function, 305
Blood vessels, in heart failure, 457–458
Blood viscosity, blood pressure and, 9
Blood volume
  blood pressure and, 8–9
  increased, 179
Bloody diarrhea, in inflammatory bowel disease, 569
Blue bloater, in chronic bronchitis, 424
BMI. *See* Body mass index (BMI).
BMR. *See* Basal metabolic rate (BMR).
Body fat, body temperature and, 11
Body fluids, isolation of, 270
Body mass index (BMI), in obesity, 586, 587
Body temperature, 10–11
  measurement of, 15–16
Bone healing, of fractures, 730, 730f
Bone marrow, radiation effects on, 785, 785t
Bone mass density, for osteoporosis, 750
Bone pain, in renal failure, 145

Bounding pulse, 13t
Bowel function
  in gastrointestinal assessment, 21
  in human immunodeficiency virus, 769
  in multiple sclerosis, 667, 668t
Bowel sounds
  in gastrointestinal assessment, 21
  in intestinal obstruction, 582
BPH. *See* Benign prostatic hypertrophy (BPH).
Bradycardia, arterial pulse in, 13t
Bradypnea, respiration in, 14
Brain death, in increased intracranial pressure, 182t, 182–183
Brain lesions, in neurologic alterations, 183–187, 184t, 185t, 187t
Brain volume, increased, 179
Breath sounds
  in respiratory assessment, 19–20
  in tracheostomy care, 132
Breath test, in peptic ulcer disease, 617
Breathing exercises, for asthma, 421
Breathing techniques, for emphysema, 430
Brethine. *See* Terbutaline sulfate (Brethine).
Brimonidine, for glaucoma, 820t
Brinzolamide, for glaucoma, 820t
Bromocriptine (Parlodel), for Parkinson's disease, 678t
Brompheniramine, 398t
Bronchial obstruction, 392–396, 394t–396t
Bronchitis, 422–427
  community care for, 425–426
  diagnostic criteria for, 424–425
  interventions for, 425
  pathophysiology of, 423
  prognosis for, 426
  signs and symptoms of, 423–424, 424t
Bronchodilators
  anticholinergic, 393
  for bronchitis, 425
  inhaled, 393
    for emphysema, 429
  pharmacology of, 392–393, 394t–395t
Bronchoscopic aspiration, for sputum samples, 106, 107t
Bronkaid. *See* Epinephrine (Adrenalin, Bronkaid).

Brown-Séquard syndrome, 688
Bruit, arteriovenous fistula and, 148
Brush biopsy, for renal failure, 852
Buck's traction, for fractures, 734
Buerger-Allen exercises, for Buerger's disease, 497, 498f
Buerger's disease, 494–500
    community care for, 499
    diagnostic criteria for, 496
    interventions for, 496–499, 498f
    pathophysiology of, 494–495
    prognosis for, 500
    signs and symptoms of, 495–496
Bullectomy, for emphysema, 430
Bumetanide (Bumex), 378
BUN. See Blood urea nitrogen (BUN).
Bupropion, adverse effects of, 333, 334t
Burns, first aid for, 30t, 31, 31t
Buspirone (BuSpar), 404t
Bypass
    aortocoronary, 449
    carotid, 651
    coronary artery. See Coronary artery bypass graft surgery.
    gastric, 588, 589f

C

CACG. See Chronic angle-closure glaucoma (CACG).
CAD. See Coronary artery disease (CAD).
CAGE screening questionnaire, 694
CAIs. See Carbonic anhydrase inhibitors (CAIs).
Calan. See Verapamil (Calan, Calan SR, Covera-HS, Isoptin, Verelan).
Calan SR. See Verapamil (Calan, Calan SR, Covera-HS, Isoptin, Verelan).
Calcijex, for renal failure, 854
Calcitonin, in hypothyroidism, 636t, 641–642
Calcium, 294–296
    for osteoporosis, 751
    for renal failure, 854
    for systemic lupus erythematosus, 760
    in hyperparathyroidism, 632–633
    in pancreatitis, 611
    in renal failure, 144, 310, 310t
Calcium channel blockers (CCBs)
    for angina, 448

Calcium channel blockers (CCBs) *(Continued)*
    for hyperthyroidism, 636, 636t
    pharmacology of, 338, 344t
Calcium oxalate stones, 840
Calcium phosphate binder, for hemodialysis, 152, 152t
Calcium phosphate stones, 840
Calcium stones, in hyperparathyroidism, 632
Calcium-based antacids, 365–366
Calculi, renal. See Renal calculi.
Calf pump, in thrombophlebitis, 542, 543
Callus formation, in bone healing, 730, 730f
Callus ossification, in bone healing, 730, 730f
Camphorated paregoric, for diarrhea, 372
Camptothecins, for cancer, 783, 784t
Campylobacter, in food poisoning, 556
Cancer, 780–789
    community care for, 786–788
    diagnostic criteria for, 782
    from inflammatory bowel disease, 569
    from renal transplantation, 162
    hepatocellular, 550
    interventions for, 782–786, 784t, 785t, 787t
    pathophysiology of, 780t, 780–781
    prognosis for, 788–789
    signs and symptoms of, 781–782
Candesartan cilexetil (Atacand), 344t
Candidiasis
    oropharyngeal, 766, 770t
    vulvovaginal, 870, 873t
Cannabinoids, for nausea and vomiting, 370
CAPD. See Continuous ambulatory peritoneal dialysis (CAPD).
Capillary colloid osmotic pressure (CCOP), in intravenous fluid therapy, 40
Capillary hydrostatic pressure, in intravenous fluid therapy, 40
Capoten. See Captopril (Capoten).
Capreomycin, for tuberculosis, 441, 442t
Captopril (Capoten), 343t
Carbamazepine (Tegretol), 360t, 361t, 362t
Carbapenems, 351

Carbenicillin, 351
Carbohydrates
  for renal failure, 853
  in liver cirrhosis, 551
  regulators of, 409–413
Carbonic anhydrase inhibitors (CAIs)
  for glaucoma, 820t, 821t
  pharmacology of, 375, 376t, 378, 380t,
    383t
Cardene. See Nicardipine (Cardene,
  Cardene SR).
Cardiac angiography, for cardiogenic
  shock, 453
Cardiac. See also Heart entries.
Cardiac catheterization
  for angina, 447
  for myocardial infarction, 475–476
Cardiac dysfunction, in hemorrhagic
  stroke, 655, 656t
Cardiac dysrhythmias, in Guillain-Barré
  syndrome, 659t
Cardiac output
  blood pressure and, 8
  heart rate and, 8
  in heart failure, 457
Cardiac pacing, for cardiogenic shock,
  455
Cardiac rhythm, in drug overdose and
  poisoning, 705
Cardiac tamponade, 453, 454
Cardiogenic shock, 451–456
  community care for, 455
  diagnostic criteria for, 452–453, 453t
  interventions for, 454–455
  pathophysiology of, 451–452
  prognosis for, 455
  signs and symptoms of, 452, 453t
Cardiovascular system, 446–486
  angina and, 446–451
  cardiogenic shock and, 451–456. See
    also Cardiogenic shock.
  coronary artery disease and, 467–471,
    468f, 470t, 471t
  heart failure and, 456–467. See also
    Heart failure (HF).
  in expedited physical assessment, 20t,
    20–21
  in hyperkalemia, 294
  in hyperparathyroidism, 632
  in hypertension, 513

Cardiovascular system (Continued)
  in hyperthyroidism, 635
  in hypokalemia, 293
  in hypomagnesemia, 298
  in hypoparathyroidism, 638–639
  in increased intracranial pressure, 181
  in renal failure, 144, 850t
  in spinal cord injury, 691
  in systemic lupus erythematosus, 756
  myocardial infarction and, 472–481.
    See also Myocardial infarction
    (MI).
  rheumatic heart disease and, 481–486.
    See also Rheumatic heart disease
    (RHD).
Carditis, rheumatic, 483
Cardizem CD. See Diltiazem (Cardizem
  CD, Cardizem SR, Dilacor XR,
  Diltia XT, Tiamate, Tiazac).
Cardura. See Doxazosin (Cardura).
Carotid bypass surgery, 651
Carotid endarterectomy, 651
Carteolol, for glaucoma, 820t
Carvedilol (Coreg)
  for chronic heart failure, 462t, 463
  pharmacology of, 346t
Cast(s), in urinalysis, 308
Casting, of fractures, 733
Catapres. See Clonidine (Catapres).
Cataracts, 804–808
Catatonic depression, 332, 332t
Catecholamines, in heart failure, 457
Catheter(s). See also Catheterization.
  damage to, with venous access device,
    62
  for blood product administration, 67
  for fluid therapy, 49–51, 50t–53t, 54f,
    55f
  for hemodialysis, 149–151
  for intravenous therapy, 48, 49
  for peritoneal dialysis, 156
  for spinal cord injury, 834t, 835–836
Catheter embolism, with venous access
  device, 58t
Catheter encrustation, in urine collection,
  104–105
Catheter manipulation, with venous
  access device, 63
Catheter migration/malposition, with
  venous access device, 62–63

Catheter occlusion, with venous access device, 59t, 62
Catheter tip cultures, in infection, 301–302, 302t
Catheterization
  cardiac, for angina, 447
    for myocardial infarction, 475–476
  intermittent, spinal cord injury and, 833–835, 834t
CAVH. See Continuous arteriovenous hemofiltration (CAVH).
CB. See Chronic bronchitis (CB).
CBC. See Complete blood count (CBC).
CCBs. See Calcium channel blockers (CCBs).
CCOP. See Capillary colloid osmotic pressure (CCOP).
CCPD. See Continuous cycling peritoneal dialysis (CCPD).
CD. See Crohn's disease (CD).
CD4+ cells, in human immunodeficiency virus, 764, 765
Cecostomy, 89t
Cefotetan, for pelvic inflammatory disease, 868t
Ceftriaxone, for pelvic inflammatory disease, 868t
Cellular phase, of inflammation, 261–263, 262t
Cellular proliferation, in bone healing, 730, 730f
Central alpha-adrenergic agonists, 340, 346t
Central cord syndrome, 688
Central nervous system (CNS)
  in hyperparathyroidism, 632
  in hyperthyroidism, 635
  in hypoparathyroidism, 639
Central venous catheters
  in fluid therapy, 49–51, 51t–53t, 54f, 55f
  in hemodialysis, 149
Centrax. See Prazepam (Centrax).
Centriacinar emphysema, 428
Centrilobular emphysema, 428
Cephalosporins
  for pneumonia, 435
  pharmacology of, 352
Cephulac. See Lactulose (Cephulac, Chronulac).

Cerebellar hemorrhage, 653t
Cerebral edema, 178t
Cerebral perfusion pressure (CPP), 178t
Cerebrospinal fluid (CSF)
  in culture report, 302
  in meningitis, 663, 664t
  in multiple sclerosis, 667
  increased, 179
Cerebrovascular accident (CVA), 649–657
  community care for, 655
  diagnostic criteria for, 650–651
  interventions for, 651–655, 654t, 656t
  pathophysiology of, 649–650
  prognosis for, 656
  risk factors for, 649, 650t
  signs and symptoms of, 650, 652t–653t
  spinal cord injury and, 837
Cerebyx. See Fosphenytoin (Cerebyx).
Cervical spine injury, 31–32, 32t, 33t
Cervical spine protection, in first aid, 25
Cetirizine (Zyrtec), 399t
CFUs. See Colony-forming units (CFUs).
Chancroid, 870, 871t
Charcoal, activated, 706–707
Charting, methods of, 6, 7t
Chemical compensation, in hypovolemic shock, 520–521
Chemical débridement, 81
Chemical solvent dissolution, for gallstones, 599
Chemoreceptors, in respiration, 9
Chemotactic factors, in allergies, 774
Chemotherapy, for cancer, 783–784, 784t
  side effects of, 786, 787t
Chenodiol, for gallstones, 598–599
Chest drainage systems, 135–141
  decision-making for, 138–140
  principles of care for, 136–138, 137t
Chest pain, in coronary artery disease, 468–469
Chest physiotherapy, for bronchitis, 425
Chest radiography
  for cardiogenic shock, 453
  for emphysema, 429
  for heart failure, 459
  for hiatal hernia, 605
  for myocardial infarction, 475
  for pneumonia, 434

Chest radiography *(Continued)*
  for rheumatic heart disease, 484
  for tuberculosis, 440
Cheyne-Stokes respirations, 14
Chlamydia, 870, 872t
  in pelvic inflammatory disease, 868t
  in pneumonia, 432
Chlamydial keratoconjunctivitis
  interventions for, 812
  pathophysiology of, 809
  prognosis for, 814
  signs and symptoms of, 810
Chloral hydrate (Noctec), for sleep
    disorders, 405t
Chlordiazepoxide (Librium)
  for aggressive/combative behavior,
      405t
  for diagnostic procedures, 406t
  pharmacology of, 404t
Chlorpheniramine (Chlortrimeton), 398t
Chlorpromazine (Thorazine), for
    aggressive/combative behavior, 405t
Chlorpropamide (Diabinese), 385t
Chlortrimeton. *See* Chlorpheniramine
    (Chlortrimeton).
Cholangiography, 598
Cholangitis, from gallstones, 596
Cholecystectomy, 599–600
Cholecystitis, 595–602. *See also*
    Gallstones.
Cholecystogram, oral, for biliary disease,
    597
Choledocholithiasis, 596
Choledochostomy, for gallstones,
    600–601
Cholelithiasis, 595–602. *See also*
    Gallstones.
Cholesterol
  in coronary artery disease, 468, 469–
      470
  in gallstone formation, 595
Cholestyramine, for inflammatory bowel
    disease, 573
Choline magnesium trisalicylate
    (Trilisate), 317, 318t
Cholinergic crisis, anticholinesterase
    agents and, 673–674
Cholinergic drugs, for glaucoma, 821t
Chronic angina, 446
Chronic angle-closure glaucoma (CACG)
  pathophysiology of, 817

Chronic angle-closure glaucoma (CACG)
    (Continued)
  signs and symptoms of, 818
Chronic asthmatic bronchitis, 423
Chronic bacterial conjunctivitis
  interventions for, 811
  pathophysiology of, 809
  signs and symptoms of, 810
Chronic bronchitis (CB), 422–423
  signs and symptoms of, 423–424, 424t
Chronic fatigue, in renal failure, 144
Chronic heart failure, 461–464, 462t
Chronic hepatitis, 561
Chronic lymphocytic leukemia (CLL),
    794. *See also* Leukemia.
Chronic myelocytic leukemia (CML),
    794. *See also* Leukemia.
Chronic obstructive pulmonary disease
    (COPD), 422–423, 427
Chronic pain, 312
Chronic pancreatitis, 610
Chronic persistent hepatitis, 563
Chronic rejection, in renal
    transplantation, 162
Chronic renal failure (CRF), 142
  interventions for, 853–855
  pathophysiology of, 848–849
  signs and symptoms of, 849, 850t–
      851t
Chronic venous insufficiency, from deep
    vein thrombosis, 502
Chronulac. *See* Lactulose (Cephulac,
    Chronulac).
Chvostek's sign, in hypoparathyroidism,
    639
Chylothorax, with venous access device,
    59t, 61–62
Cigarette smoking. *See* Smoking.
Ciguatera, in food poisoning, 558
Cilastatin sodium. *See* Imipenem.
Cimetidine (Tagamet), 366–367
Ciprofloxacin, 353–354
Circulatory overload, with venous access
    device, 57t
Cirrhosis, 549–555
  community care for, 554–555
  diagnostic criteria for, 552–553
  interventions for, 553–554
  pathophysiology of, 550, 551t
  prognosis for, 555

Cirrhosis *(Continued)*
   signs and symptoms of, 550–552
Citrate of magnesia. *See* Magnesium
   citrate (Citrate of magnesia).
Citrucel. *See* Methylcellulose (Citrucel).
CIWA-A. *See* Clinical Institute
   Withdrawal Assessment for Alcohol
   (CIWA-A).
CK. *See* Creatine kinase (CK).
Claritin. *See* Loratadine (Claritin).
Clarity, in urinalysis, 307
Classic angina, 446
Clean surgical wounds, 78
Cleansing, pouch, 91
   wound, 81
Clemastine fumarate (Tavist), 398t
Clindamycin, pharmacology of, 353
Clinical Institute Withdrawal Assessment
   for Alcohol (CIWA-A), 695
CLL. *See* Chronic lymphocytic leukemia
   (CLL).
Clobetasol propionate, for systemic lupus
   erythematosus, 760
Clomipramine (Anafranil), 333, 333t
Clonazepam (Klonopin), 360t, 361t
Clonidine (Catapres), 346t
Clopidogrel (Plavix), 330, 331t
Clorazepate (Tranxene), 404t
Closed drains, 85
Closed fracture, 729
Closed reduction, of fractures, 732
Clostridium, in food poisoning, 557, 558
Clot destruction, in hemostasis, 323
Clot retraction, in hemostasis, 323
Clotting cascade, 321–323, 322f, 323t
Clotting factors, in liver cirrhosis, 551
CML. *See* Chronic myelocytic leukemia
   (CML).
CNS. *See* Central nervous system (CNS).
Coagulation, 320
Coagulation cascade, 321–323, 322f,
   323t
Coagulation phase, of hemostasis,
   321–323, 322f, 323t
Coagulation testing, 323–325, 324t
   in liver cirrhosis, 552
Coccidioidomycosis, in human
   immunodeficiency virus infection,
   766, 770t
Codeine
   dosages of, 315, 316t

Codeine *(Continued)*
   for gout, 747
   for rhinitis, cough, and colds, 397,
      400t
Cogentin. *See* Benztropine (Cogentin).
Cognitive dysfunction, in stroke patients,
   654t
Colchicine, for gout, 746
Cold [common], respiratory drugs for,
   397–403, 398t–402t
Cold [therapy], for arthritis, 724
Cold intolerance, in anemia, 792
Colectomy, for inflammatory bowel
   disease, 573, 574
Colic, renal, from renal calculi, 841
   in renal dysfunction, 143
Colitis, ulcerative, 568. *See also*
   Inflammatory bowel disease (IBD).
Colloids
   for hypovolemic shock, 524
   in intravenous therapy, 39, 39t
Colon cancer, from inflammatory bowel
   disease, 569
Colonized bacteria, in infection, 299
Colonoscopy, in inflammatory bowel
   disease, 570–571
Colony-forming units (CFUs), in culture
   report, 302
Colony-stimulating factors (CSFs), for
   immunologic alterations, 264
Color
   in integumentary assessment, 18
   in stoma assessment, 89
   in urinalysis, 307, 308t
Colostomy, principles of care for, 88
Colostomy irrigation, 90
Colyte. *See* Polyethylene glycol (PEG)
   (Colyte, GoLYTELY).
Combative behavior, medications for,
   405, 405t
Commercially prepared plastic units, for
   chest drainage, 138
Comminuted fracture, 729
Common pathway, in coagulation, 321,
   322f
Communicating veins, in
   thrombophlebitis, 542
Communication
   in Alzheimer's disease, 647
   in tracheostomy care, 133

Communication deficit, in stroke patients, 654t
Community-acquired pneumonia, 432, 433t
  interventions for, 435
  pathophysiology of, 432
Community care
  for angina, 449–450
  for cardiogenic shock, 455
  for myocardial infarction, 479–480
  for rheumatic heart disease, 484–485
Compartment syndrome, from fractures, 738
Compazine. See Prochlorperazine (Compazine).
Complement fixation, 304
Complement level, in systemic lupus erythematosus, 757–758
Complement system, in inflammation, 262
Complete blood count (CBC), 274
  in hepatitis, 565
  in hypertension, 514
  in immunologic alterations, 264
  in inflammatory bowel disease, 570
  in intestinal obstruction, 583
  in liver cirrhosis, 552
  in peritonitis, 592
  in renal failure, 852
  in rheumatoid arthritis, 723
Complete fracture, 729
Complete spinal cord injury, 687, 687t
Completed stroke, 649
Compliance
  definition of, 178t
  in increased intracranial pressure, 179
Complicated appendectomy, 548
Compound fracture, 729
Compression
  for thrombophlebitis, 539–540
  in spinal cord injury, 687
Compression devices, for deep vein thrombosis, 505–506
Compression dressings, 83
Compression stockings, for thrombophlebitis, 540
Computed tomography (CT)
  for aortic aneurysm, 489
  for biliary disease, 598
  for cerebrovascular accident, 651

Computed tomography (CT) (Continued)
  for deep vein thrombosis, 505
  for inflammatory bowel disease, 571
  for intestinal obstruction, 583
  for pancreatitis, 612
  for renal calculi, 841
  for renal failure, 852
  for spinal cord injury, 690
Computer, documentation issues with use of, 6, 7t
Condom catheter, in spinal cord injury, 834t, 835
Conduction, in heat loss, 10–11
Congestive heart failure, 458
Conjunctivitis, 809–815
  community care for, 813–814
  diagnostic criteria for, 811, 812t
  interventions for, 811–813
  pathophysiology of, 809–810
  prognosis for, 814
  signs and symptoms of, 810–811
Conscious patient, neurologic assessment of, 22
Consciousness, in neurologic assessment, 166–170, 167t
Consolidation, with remodeling, in bone healing, 730, 730f
Constipation, 365
  from immobilization, 737t
  from opioids, 314, 315t
  in intestinal obstruction, 582
  medications for, 367–369
Contac. See Phenylpropanolamine HCl (Contac, Triaminic).
Contact isolation, 270
Continent ileostomy, for inflammatory bowel disease, 573
Continuous ambulatory peritoneal dialysis (CAPD), 157
Continuous arteriovenous hemofiltration (CAVH), 147
Continuous bacteremia, blood culture for, 300–301
Continuous cycling peritoneal dialysis (CCPD), 157
Continuous infusion, of opioids, 315
Continuous renal replacement therapy (CRRT), 147
Continuous supplemental oxygen, for emphysema, 429–430

Continuous venovenous hemofiltration (CVVH), 147
  for renal failure, 854
Contraception, in systemic lupus erythematosus, 759
Contrast studies, in intestinal obstruction, 583
Conus medullaris syndrome, 688
Convection, in heat loss, 10–11
Coombs' test, for systemic lupus erythematosus, 758
Copaxone. *See* Glatiramer acetate (Copaxone).
COPD. *See* Chronic obstructive pulmonary disease (COPD).
Cor pulmonale, 423
Cordarone. *See* Amiodarone (Cordarone).
Coreg. *See* Carvedilol (Coreg).
Corgard. *See* Nadolol (Corgard).
Coronary angiography
  cardiac catheterization with, for angina, 447
  for coronary artery disease, 470
  for heart failure, 460
  for myocardial infarction, 475–476
Coronary artery bypass graft surgery
  for angina, 449
  for cardiogenic shock, 454
  for coronary artery disease, 470
Coronary artery disease (CAD), 446, 467–471, 468f, 470t, 471t
Corrigan's pulse, 13t
Cortical cataract, 804
Corticosteroids, 408–413
  for arthritis, 724
  for emphysema, 429
  for gout, 746
  for irritable bowel disease, pharmacology of, 374
  for systemic lupus erythematosus, 760–761
  inhaled, 393
  pharmacology of, 408
Corticotropin-releasing factor (CRF), 409
Cough
  in bronchitis, 425
  in chronic bronchitis, 423–424
  in emphysema, 428
  respiratory drugs for, 397–403, 398t–402t

Cough reflex, in gastrointestinal assessment, 21
Coumadin. *See* Warfarin (Coumadin).
Countertraction, for fractures, 735
Covera-HS. *See* Verapamil (Calan, Calan SR, Covera-HS, Isoptin, Verelan).
COX-2 inhibitors. *See* Cyclooxygenase-2 (COX-2) inhibitors.
Cozaar. *See* Losartan (Cozaar).
CPP. *See* Cerebral perfusion pressure (CPP).
Crackles, in respiratory assessment, 20
Cranial nerves
  in Guillain-Barré syndrome, 658
  in neurologic assessment, 171, 172t–175t
C-reactive protein
  in appendicitis, 548
  in immunologic alterations, 264
Creatine kinase (CK)
  in intestinal obstruction, 583
  in myocardial infarction, 474
Creatinine, serum, in renal function, 305–306
Creatinine clearance
  in renal failure, 852
  in renal function, 306–307
CRF. *See* Chronic renal failure (CRF); Corticotropin-releasing factor (CRF).
Crixivan. *See* Indinavir (Crixivan).
Crohn's disease (CD), 568. *See also* Inflammatory bowel disease (IBD).
  antidiarrheals for, 373
CRRT. *See* Continuous renal replacement therapy (CRRT).
Cryoprecipitate, administration of, 72t
Cryptococcal meningitis, in human immunodeficiency virus infection, 766, 770t
Cryptococcosis, in human immunodeficiency virus infection, 766, 770t
Crystalloids
  for hypovolemic shock, 523–524
  in intravenous therapy, 39, 39t. *See also* Intravenous (IV) fluids.
Crystals, in urinalysis, 308
C&S. *See* Culture and sensitivity (C&S).
CSF. *See* Cerebrospinal fluid (CSF).

CSFs. *See* Colony-stimulating factors (CSFs).
CT. *See* Computed tomography (CT).
Cuff pressure measurements, in tracheostomy care, 132
Cullen's sign, in pancreatitis, 610
Culture(s)
  for sexually transmitted diseases, 876
  for tuberculosis, 440
Culture and sensitivity (C&S)
  in anti-infective therapy, 348
  in infection, 300–304, 302t
  in urine collection, 103
Curschmann's spiral structures, in sputum smear, 108, 108t
Cushing's response, 178t
Cushing's triad, 178t
Cutaneous lupus erythematosus, 753–754
CVA. *See* Cerebrovascular accident (CVA).
CVVH. *See* Continuous venovenous hemofiltration (CVVH).
Cyanocobalamin, for inflammatory bowel disease, 573
Cyanosis
  in chronic bronchitis, 424
  in peripheral vascular disease, 527
Cyclooxygenase-2 (COX-2) inhibitors, for arthritis, 724
Cyclophosphamide (Cytoxan), for myasthenia gravis, 673t
Cycloplegics, for glaucoma, 819
Cycloserine, for tuberculosis, 441, 442t
Cyclosporine (Sandimmune)
  for inflammatory bowel disease, 572–573
  for renal transplantation, 163t
Cyproheptadine (Periactin), 399t
Cystine stones, 840
Cystopaz. *See* Hyoscyamine (Cystopaz, Gastrosed).
Cystoscopy
  for renal calculi, 844
  for renal failure, 852
  for renal function analysis, 310
Cytokines, in inflammation, 261, 262
Cytomegalovirus retinitis, in human immunodeficiency virus infection, 766, 771t
Cytotoxic T cells, 260

Cytoxan. *See* Cyclophosphamide (Cytoxan).

D

Dalmane. *See* Flurazepam (Dalmane).
Dalteparin (Fragmin), 329t
Danaparoid (Organan), 329t
DASH diet. *See* Dietary Approaches to Stop Hypertension (DASH) diet.
Dawn phenomenon, from insulin therapy, 391
D-Dimer tests, 325
  for deep vein thrombosis, 504
Débridement, wound, 81
Decadron. *See* Dexamethasone (Decadron).
Decannulation, in tracheostomy care, 133
Decompression, intestinal, 583–584
Decongestants, for rhinitis, cough, and colds, 397, 401t
Deep brain stimulation, for Parkinson's disease, 678
Deep tendon reflexes (DTRs), in neurologic assessment, 177
Deep vein thrombosis (DVT), 500–509
  community care for, 508
  diagnostic criteria for, 503t, 503–505
  in arthritis, 727, 728
  interventions for, 505–508
  pathophysiology of, 501–502
  prognosis for, 488
  signs and symptoms of, 502–503
Deep veins, in thrombophlebitis, 542
Degenerative joint disease. *See* Osteoarthritis (OA).
Dehydration, in peritonitis, 592
Delavirdine (Rescriptor), for human immunodeficiency virus, 767t, 767–768
Delayed primary closure, 78
Delayed union, of fractures, 740
Deltasone. *See* Prednisone (Aristocort, Deltasone).
Demadex. *See* Torsemide (Demadex).
Demecarium bromide, for glaucoma, 821t
Demeclocycline, 352–353
Demerol. *See* Meperidine (Demerol).
Deontologic theories, 4
Deoxyribonucleic acid (DNA), recombinant, for immunologic alterations, 264

Depakote. *See* Valproic acid (Depakote).
Depression, 332, 332t, 696–702
    community care for, 701–702
    diagnostic criteria for, 698
    from immobilization, 737t
    interventions for, 698–701
    pathophysiology of, 696–697
    poststroke, 654t
    prognosis for, 702
    signs and symptoms of, 697–698
Dermatitis, atopic, 775–776
Descending colostomy, 89t
Desipramine (Norpramin), 333, 333t
Desyrel. *See* Trazodone (Desyrel).
Detrusor areflexia, 831
Detrusor hyperreflexia, 831
Detrusor sphincter dyssynergia, 831
Dexa scan. *See* Dual-energy x-ray
        absorptiometry (Dexa) scan.
Dexamethasone (Decadron)
    for nausea and vomiting, 371
    pharmacology of, 414t
Dexamethasone suppression test, for
        depression, 696
Dexchlorpheniramine (Polaramine), 398t
Dextromethorphan (Benylin DM), 400t
Dextrose
    for drug overdose and poisoning, 705
    in intravenous therapy, 43
Diabeta. *See* Glyburide (Diabeta,
        Micronase).
Diabetes mellitus (DM), 262, 262t,
        624–631
    community care for, 627
    diagnostic criteria for, 626, 630t
    hyperglycemia in, 109
    insulin for, pharmacology of, 384
    interventions for, 626–627
    pathophysiology of, 624–625
    prognosis for, 627–630
    renal transplantation in, 160
    signs and symptoms of, 625–626,
        628t–629t
    spinal cord injury and, 837–838
Diabetic ketoacidosis (DKA), 625
    hyperglycemia in, 109
Diabetic nephropathy, 142
Diabetic ulcers, 79–80
Diabinese. *See* Chlorpropamide
        (Diabinese).

Dialysate
    for hemodialysis, 146
    for peritoneal dialysis, 156, 158
Dialysate leakage, during peritoneal
        dialysis, 159t
Dialysis
    for renal failure, 854
    peritoneal. *See* Peritoneal dialysis
        (PD).
Dialyzable pharmacology
    for hemodialysis, 151–153, 152t, 153t
    for peritoneal dialysis, 158–159
Dialyzer, in hemodialysis, 146
Diamox. *See* Acetazolamide (Diamox).
Diaphoresis, from opioids, 314, 315t
Diaphragmatic breathing, for
        emphysema, 430
Diarrhea, 365
    in inflammatory bowel disease, 569
    medications for, 371–373
Diastolic heart failure, 464–465
Diastolic pressure, 9
    measurement of, 15
Diazepam (Valium)
    for aggressive/combative behavior,
        405t
    for diagnostic procedures, 406t
    pharmacology of, 361t, 404t
Diazoxide (Hyperstat), 347t
Dibenzyline. *See* Phenoxybenzamine
        (Dibenzyline).
Dicloxacillin, 351
Didanosine (Videx), for human
        immunodeficiency virus infection,
        766–767, 767t
Diet
    after renal transplantation, 164
    for gallstones, 601
    for hemodialysis patient, 148
    for hiatal hernia, 606, 606t
    for hypertension, 517–518
    for osteoporosis, 751
    for parkinsonism, 678
    for renal calculi, 842–843
Dietary Approaches to Stop Hypertension
        (DASH) diet, 517
Dietary intake, hypertension and, 517
Diffusion, in respiration, 9
Diflunisal (Dolobid), 317, 318t
Digestive tract medications, 365–375
    for constipation, 367–369

Digestive tract medications *(Continued)*
  for diarrhea, 371–373
  for heartburn, 365–367
  for irritable bowel disease, 373–374
  for nausea and vomiting, 369–371
  principles of care for, 365, 366f
Digital subtraction angiography, for
    peripheral vascular disease, 528
Digitalis, for chronic heart failure, 462t,
    463
Dihydropyridines, 344t
Dilacor XR. *See* Diltiazem (Cardizem
    CD, Cardizem SR, Dilacor XR,
    Diltia XT, Tiamate, Tiazac).
Dilantin. *See* Phenytoin (Dilantin).
Diltia XT. *See* Diltiazem (Cardizem CD,
    Cardizem SR, Dilacor XR, Diltia
    XT, Tiamate, Tiazac).
Diltiazem (Cardizem CD, Cardizem SR,
    Dilacor XR, Diltia XT, Tiamate,
    Tiazac)
  for hyperthyroidism, 636, 636t
  pharmacology of, 344t
Dilution, for blood and blood product
    administration, 69
Dilutional hyponatremia, 292
Dimenhydrinate (Dramamine), for nausea
    and vomiting, 370
Diminished breath sounds, in respiratory
    assessment, 19–20
Diovan. *See* Valsartan (Diovan).
Dipentum. *See* Olsalazine (Dipentum).
Diphenhydramine (Benadryl)
  for aggressive/combative behavior,
      pharmacology of, 405t
  for rhinitis, coughs, and colds, 400t
  pharmacology of, 398t, 404t
Diphenoxylate (Lomotil)
  for diarrhea, 372
  for inflammatory bowel disease, 573
Diphenylalkylamines, 338, 344t
Diprivan. *See* Propofol (Diprivan).
Dipyridamole (Persantine), 330, 331t
Direct antiglobulin test, for systemic
    lupus erythematosus, 758
Direct ophthalmoscopy, for cataracts, 805
Direct vasodilators, pharmacology of,
    340–341, 347t
Directly observed therapy (DOT), for
    tuberculosis, 442

Disalcid. *See* Salsalate (Disalcid).
Discoid lupus erythematosus, 753–754
Disequilibrium syndrome (DS), from
    hemodialysis, 153, 154t
Disk diffusion method, for antimicrobial
    sensitivity, 302–303
Dislocation, in arthritis, surgery and,
    727–728
Dissecting aortic aneurysm, 488
  diagnosis of, 489–490
  pathophysiology of, 487
Diuretics, 375–384
  decision-making for, 376t–377t, 379,
      380t–383t
  for cardiogenic shock, 454
  for chronic heart failure, 461–463,
      462t
  for renal failure, 854
  loop, 375, 376t, 378
  osmotic, 375, 377t, 378
  pharmacology of, 341
  principles of care for, 375–379, 376t–
      377t
Diving accidents, first aid for, 34t,
    34–35, 35t
DKA. *See* Diabetic ketoacidosis (DKA).
DM. *See* Diabetes mellitus (DM).
DMP-266. *See* Efavirenz (Sustiva, DMP-
    266).
DNA. *See* Deoxyribonucleic acid (DNA).
Dobutamine (Dobutrex)
  for cardiogenic shock, 454
  for chronic heart failure, 462t, 464
Documentation
  decision-making and, 6, 7t
  in nursing practice, 4
Dolobid. *See* Diflunisal (Dolobid).
Dopamine
  for cardiogenic shock, 454
  for hypovolemic shock, 524
Dopamine agonists, for Parkinson's
    disease, 678t
Dopamine antagonists, for nausea and
    vomiting, 370–371
Dopaminergic agents, for Parkinson's
    disease, 677, 678t
Doppler flowmeter, for blood pressure
    measurement, 15
Doppler ultrasonography
  for Buerger's disease, 496

Doppler ultrasonography *(Continued)*
for intestinal obstruction, 583
for peripheral vascular disease, 528
for varicose veins, 544
Doral. *See* Quazepam (Doral).
Dorzolamide, for glaucoma, 820t
DOT. *See* Directly observed therapy (DOT).
Double-barreled colostomy, 88
Double-lumen Silastic catheters, in hemodialysis, 149–151
Doxazosin (Cardura), 345t
Doxepin (Sinequan), 333, 333t
Doxycycline
for pelvic inflammatory disease, 868t
pharmacology of, 352–353
Doxylamine (Unisom), for sleep disorders, 405t
Dramamine. *See* Dimenhydrinate (Dramamine).
Dressings, 82–83
wound drainage, 86
Drift, evidence of, in neurologic assessment, 170–171
Drixoral. *See* Pseudoephedrine (Drixoral, Sudafed, Sudafed SA).
Dronabinol (Marinol), for nausea and vomiting, 370
Droperidol (Inapsine), for diagnostic procedures, 406t
Drug overdose and poisoning, 703–709
community care for, 707–708, 708t
diagnostic criteria for, 704
interventions for, 704–707
pathophysiology of, 703
prognosis for, 708
signs and symptoms of, 703–704
Drug-induced asthma, 417
Drug-induced hepatitis, 560
Drug-induced lupus erythematosus, 754, 755t
Drug-resistant organisms, isolation of, 271–272
DS. *See* Disequilibrium syndrome (DS).
d4T. *See* Stavudine (d4T, Zerit).
DTRs. *See* Deep tendon reflexes (DTRs).
Dual-energy x-ray absorptiometry (Dexa) scan, for osteoporosis, 750
Dulcolax. *See* Bisacodyl (Dulcolax).
Duodenal juice, 98–99

Duplex ultrasonography
for deep vein thrombosis, 504
for thrombophlebitis, 539
Dymelor. *See* Acetohexamide (Dymelor).
DynaCirc. *See* Isradipine (DynaCirc, DynaCirc CR).
Dyrenium. *See* Triamterene (Dyrenium).
Dysfunctional voiding, in renal dysfunction, 143
Dysphagia
in Guillain-Barré syndrome, 659t
in stroke patients, 654t
Dyspnea, 14
on exertion, in emphysema, 428
Dysrhythmias, in Guillain-Barré syndrome, 659t
Dysuria, in renal dysfunction, 143

E

Echocardiography
for angina, 447
for aortic aneurysm, 489
for cardiogenic shock, 452–453
for coronary artery disease, 470
for heart failure, 460
for hypertension, 514
for myocardial infarction, 475
for rheumatic heart disease, 483–484
Echothiophate iodide, for glaucoma, 821t
ECT. *See* Electroconvulsive therapy (ECT).
Edecrin. *See* Ethacrynic acid (Edecrin).
Edema
cerebral, 178t
in cardiovascular assessment, 20, 20t
in chronic bronchitis, 424
in deep vein thrombosis, 502
in intravenous fluid therapy, 40
in peripheral vascular disease, 527
in renal failure, 145
in varicose veins, 543
Edrophonium chloride test, for myasthenia gravis, 672
EEG. *See* Electroencephalogram (EEG).
Efavirenz (Sustiva, DMP-266), for human immunodeficiency virus infection, 767t, 767–768
Effector cells, 285
Effusion, pleural, in renal failure, 145
ELAP. *See* Endoscopic laser ablation of prostate (ELAP).

Elastance, definition of, 178t
Elastic stockings, for deep vein thrombosis, 505, 507
Elavil. *See* Amitriptyline (Elavil).
Eldepryl. *See* Selegiline (Eldepryl).
Elderly, hypertension and, 512–513
Electrocardiography (ECG)
    for angina, 447
    for cardiogenic shock, 452, 453t
    for coronary artery disease, 470
    for heart failure, 459
    for hypertension, 514
    for myocardial infarction, 474–475
    for rheumatic heart disease, 483
Electroconvulsive therapy (ECT), for depression, 334, 700–701
Electroencephalogram (EEG), for depression, 696
Electrohydraulic lithotripsy, for renal calculi, 844
Electrolyte(s), 290–299
    calcium as, 294–296
    in cardiogenic shock, 454
    in hepatitis, 571
    in inflammatory bowel disease, 570
    in intestinal obstruction, 582–583
    in intravenous therapy, 43
    in liver cirrhosis, 552
    in renal failure, 850t
    in renal function testing, 309t, 310
    phosphate as, 296–298
    potassium as, 292–294
    principles of care for, 290–291
    sodium as, 291–292
Electronic thermometer, 15, 16
Electrovaporization of prostate (EVP), for benign prostatic hypertrophy, 863
Elevation, for thrombophlebitis, 539
ELISA. *See* Enzyme-linked immunosorbent assay (ELISA).
Embolic stroke, 649
Embolism
    air, 58t, 61
    catheter, 58t
    from deep vein thrombosis, 502
    pulmonary, 502
Emetics, for drug overdose and poisoning, 706
Emollient agents, pharmacology of, 369

Emotional abuse. *See* Mental/emotional abuse.
Emotional depression. *See* Depression.
Emphysema, after tracheostomy, 134
Empiric therapy, for anti-infective therapy, 348
Enalapril (Vasotec), 343t
Encephalopathy, hepatic, 550, 551t
Endarterectomy, carotid, 651
Endocarditis, 483
Endocrine disease, secondary hypertension and, 510, 510t
Endocrine system, 624–643
    diabetes mellitus and, 624–631. *See also* Diabetes mellitus (DM).
    hyperparathyroidism and, 631–634
    hyperthyroidism and, 634–637, 636t
    hypoparathyroidism and, 638–640
    hypothyroidism and, 640–643, 642t
    in renal failure, 851t
Endoscopic laser ablation of prostate (ELAP), 863
Endoscopic laser lithotripsy, of gallstones, 599
Endoscopic retrograde cholangiography (ERC), 597, 598
Endoscopic retrograde cholangiopancreatography (ERCP), 597, 612
Endoscopic ultrasound, for biliary disease, 597
Endoscopy
    for inflammatory bowel disease, 571
    for peptic ulcer disease, 617
Endotracheal (ET) tube aspiration, for sputum samples, 106, 107t
Endovascular care, for aortic aneurysm, 492–493
End-stage renal disease (ESRD), 142
    signs and symptoms of, 849, 850t–851t
Enema, barium, in inflammatory bowel disease, 571
Energy conservation, for emphysema, 430
Enoxaparin (Lovenox), 329t
Enteral stenting, for intestinal obstruction, 584
Enterococci, vancomycin-resistant, 271–272

Environmental temperature, body temperature and, 11
Enzyme(s), liver
  in hepatitis, 565
  in liver cirrhosis, 552–553
  in pancreatitis, 611
Enzyme-linked immunosorbent assay (ELISA), 304
  for human immunodeficiency virus, 766
  for immunologic alterations, 264
Eosinopenia, 289
Eosinophilia, 287
Eosinophilic cationic protein (ECP), 108, 108t
Eosinophils, 283, 284
  in inflammation, 261
  in sputum smear, 108, 108t
  peripheral smear of, 286, 287f
Ephedrine sulfate (Ephedsol, Vantronol)
  for rhinitis, coughs, and colds, 401t
  pharmacology of, 393, 394t
Epididymitis, 870, 873t
Epidural analgesia, with opioids, 315
Epifrin. See Epinephrine (Epifrin, Glaucon).
Epigastric pain, in peptic ulcer disease, 617
Epilepsy, 680
Epinephrine (Adrenalin, Bronkaid), 393, 394t
Epinephrine (Epifrin, Glaucon), for glaucoma, 821t
Epipodophyllotoxins, for cancer, 783, 784t
Episcleritis, in inflammatory bowel disease, 570
Epithelial cells, in urinalysis, 308
Epivir. See Lamivudine (3TC, Epivir).
EPO. See Erythropoietin (EPO, Epogen).
Epogen. See Erythropoietin (EPO, Epogen).
Epsom salts. See Magnesium sulfate (Epsom salts).
Equianalgesia, 315, 316t
ERC. See Endoscopic retrograde cholangiography (ERC).
ERCP. See Endoscopic retrograde cholangiopancreatography (ERCP).
Erythema nodosum, in inflammatory bowel disease, 570

Erythrocyte(s), 274, 275f
Erythrocyte sedimentation rate (ESR), 280t, 280–281
  in immunologic alterations, 264
  in inflammatory bowel disease, 570
  in myocardial infarction, 474
  in rheumatoid arthritis, 722
Erythrocytosis, 276, 276t
Erythromycin, pharmacology of, 353
Erythropoiesis, 274
Erythropoietin (EPO, Epogen)
  administration of, 74t
  in hemodialysis, 152, 152t
  in renal failure, 144, 854
Eschar, 78, 78t
Escherichia coli O157:H7, in food poisoning, 557
Eserine Sulfate. See Physostigmine sulfate (Eserine Sulfate).
Esophageal manometry, for hiatal hernia, 605
Esophagoscopy, in liver cirrhosis, 553
ESR. See Erythrocyte sedimentation rate (ESR).
ESRD. See End-stage renal disease (ESRD).
Essential hypertension, 509–510. See also Hypertension (HTN).
Estazolam (ProSom), for sleep disorders, 405t
Estrogen, for osteoporosis, 751
ESWL. See Extracorporeal shock wave lithotripsy (ESWL).
Ethacrynic acid (Edecrin), 378
Ethambutol, for tuberculosis, 441, 441t
Ethanolamines, 398t
Ethical issues, 4, 5–6, 6t
Ethionamide, for tuberculosis, 441, 442t
Ethosuximide (Zarontin), 360t, 363t
Ethylenediamines, 398t
Etodolac (Lodine), 317, 318t
Evidence of drift, in neurologic assessment, 170–171
EVP. See Electrovaporization of prostate (EVP).
Exercise
  after renal transplantation, 164
  body temperature and, 11
  for bronchitis, 425
  for Buerger's disease, 497, 498f

Exercise *(Continued)*
 for deep vein thrombosis, 505, 507
 for diabetes mellitus, 627
 for hypertension, 516, 518
 for osteoporosis, 751
 for systemic lupus erythematosus, 758
Exercise testing
 for angina, 447
 for heart failure, 460
 for peripheral vascular disease, 529
Exercise therapy, for arthritis, 725
Exercise tolerance, in heart failure, 459
Exercise-induced asthma, 417
Exertional angina, 446
Exophthalmos, in hyperthyroidism, 635
Expectorants
 for pneumonia, 435
 for rhinitis, cough, and colds, 397,
  402t
Expectorated sample, of sputum, 106
Expedited physical assessment, 17–23
 decision-making for, 18–23
  cardiovascular system in, 20t, 20–21
  environment in, 23
  gastrointestinal system in, 21
  general appearance in, 18, 18t
  genitourinary system in, 21–22
  integumentary system in, 18–19
  neurologic system in, 22–23
  respiratory system in, 19–20
 principles of care in, 17–18
External fixation, for fractures, 735
External standards, of practice, 4
Extracapsular cataract extraction, 806
Extracerebral tumors, 184–185
Extracorporeal shock wave lithotripsy
  (ESWL)
 for gallstones, 599
 for renal calculi, 844
Extravasation, with venous access device,
  56t, 61
Extrinsic asthma, 417
Extrinsic pathway, in coagulation, 321,
  322f
Eye(s)
 in inflammatory bowel disease, 570
 radiation effects on, 785, 785t
Eye opening, in Glasgow Coma Scale,
  167t, 167–168

F

Face shields, protective, 270
False aneurysm, pathophysiology of, 487
False values, in blood glucose specimen
  collection and monitoring, 111, 113t
False-negative results, of skin tests, 439
False-positive results, of skin tests, 439
Famciclovir, 357
Family violence, 709
Famotidine (Pepcid), 366–367
FANA. *See* Fluorescent antinuclear
  antibody (FANA) test.
Fasting blood glucose test, 111, 112t
Fasting plasma glucose, in diabetes
  mellitus, 626
Fat, body temperature and, 11
Fat embolus, from fractures, 738–739
Fat metabolism
 in liver cirrhosis, 551
 regulators of, 409–413
Fatigue
 in diabetes, 625
 in multiple sclerosis, 667, 668t
 in renal failure, 144
 reduction of, for arthritis, 724–725
Fatty stools, in cholecystitis, 596
Fax, documentation issues for, 6, 7t
Febrile nonhemolytic reaction, to blood
  transfusion, 68t
Fecal occult test, 100
Feces, 99
 in stoma assessment, 89, 89t
Felbamate (Felbatol), 361t
Felodipine (Plendil), 344t
Femoral hernia, 577
Fenestrated tube, in tracheostomy care,
  131t, 134
Fenprofen calcium (Nalfon), 317, 318t
Fentanyl (Sublimaze), for diagnostic
  procedures, 406t
Fetal nigra transplantation, for
  Parkinson's disease, 678
Fever
 definition of, 15–16
 in peritonitis, 592
Fexofenadine (Allegra), 399t
FFP. *See* Fresh frozen plasma (FFP).
Fiberall. *See* Psyllium (Metamucil,
  Fiberall).
Fiberglass casting, of fractures, 733

Fibrin degradation products, 325
Fibrin formation, during peritoneal
   dialysis, 159t
Fibrin split products, in clot destruction,
   323
Fibrinogen assay, 325
Fibrinogen degradation products, in clot
   destruction, 323
Fibrinogen synthesis, in liver cirrhosis,
   551
Fibrinolysis, in hemostasis, 323
Fidelity, definition and rules of care for,
   6t
Filters
   for blood and blood product adminis-
      tration, 67
   for blood product administration, 67
Filtration, in fluid therapy, 40–41
Finger stick capillary method, for blood
   glucose monitoring, 110, 110t
Fingernails
   in cardiovascular assessment, 20
   in peripheral vascular disease, 528
FIO₂. See Fraction of inspired oxygen
   (FIO₂).
First aid, for injuries, 24–36
   altered mental status in, 25–27, 26t,
      27t
   anaphylaxis in, 26t, 27–28
   bites and stings in, 26t, 28, 29t, 30t
   burns in, 30t, 31, 31t
   cervical spine injury in, 31–32, 32t,
      33t
   musculoskeletal injury in, 32–34,
      33t
   near-drowning and diving accidents
      in, 34t, 34–35, 35t
   principles of care in, 24–25, 26t
   soft tissue injury in, 35–36, 36t
FK 506. See Tacrolimus (FK 506).
Flagyl. See Metronidazole (Flagyl).
Flat-plate radiograph, for biliary disease,
   597
Fleet Babylax. See Glycerin (Fleet
   Babylax).
Fletcher's Castoria. See Senna (Senokot,
   Fletcher's Castoria).
Flomax. See Tamsulosin (Flomax).
Flowmeter, Doppler, for blood pressure
   measurement, 15

Fluconazole, 356
Fludrocortisone (Florinef Acetate), 408,
   414, 415t
Fluid(s)
   for bronchitis, 425
   for cardiogenic shock, 454
   for hepatitis, 571
   for renal transplantation, 161
   for urinary tract infection, 858–859
Fluid and electrolyte management
   in hemorrhagic stroke, 655, 656t
   in hepatitis, 565
   in increased intracranial pressure, 181t,
      181–182
   in intestinal obstruction, 582, 583
   in pancreatitis, 612
   sodium in, 291
Fluid overload, during peritoneal dialysis,
   158, 158t, 159t
Fluid restriction, for renal failure, 853
Fluid therapy, 39–76
   blood and blood product administra-
      tion in, 64–69. See also Blood
      and blood product administration.
   for hypovolemic shock, 523–524
   intravenous, 39–45. See also Intrave-
      nous (IV) fluids.
   vascular access device in, 48–64. See
      also Vascular access device
      (VAD).
Fluid underload, during peritoneal
   dialysis, 158, 158t
Fluid viscosity, in intravenous therapy,
   49
Fluorescent antinuclear antibody (FANA)
   test, for systemic lupus
   erythematosus, 756–757
Fluoroquinolones
   for pneumonia, 435
   pharmacology of, 353–354
Flurazepam (Dalmane), for sleep
   disorders, 405t
Focal seizures, 685, 686t
Folex. See Methotrexate (Folex,
   Rheumatrex).
Folic acid replacement, in anemia, 792
Food poisoning, 556–560
Foot care
   for Buerger's disease, 497–499
   for diabetes mellitus, 627

Foot pumps, for deep vein thrombosis, 506

Fortivase. See Saquinavir (SQV, Invirase, Fortovase).

Fosinopril (Monopril), 343t

Fosphenytoin (Cerebyx), 361t

Fraction of inspired oxygen (FIO₂), 115–116, 116t

Fracture(s), 729–742
  activity progression for, 736–738, 737t
  community care for, 740–741
  complications of, 738–740
  diagnostic criteria for, 731
  medical management of, 732–735
  neurovascular compromise with, 735–736
  nursing management of, 735
  pain management in, 738
  pathologic, in renal failure, 145
  pathophysiology of, 729–730, 730f
  prognosis for, 741
  signs and symptoms of, 730–731

Fragmin. See Dalteparin (Fragmin).

Frank-Starling mechanism, in heart failure, 457

Fresh frozen plasma (FFP), 71t

Full-thickness wounds, 78

Functional intestinal obstructions, 580–581, 581t

Fundoplication, Nissen, 607

Funduscopy, in hypertension, 513

Fungal meningitis, 662

Fungus, in infection, 299

Furosemide (Lasix), 378, 379t, 383t

Fusiform aortic aneurysm, 487

G

Gabapentin (Neurontin), 360t, 363t

GABHS. See Group A beta-hemolytic streptococci (GABHS).

Gag reflex, in gastrointestinal assessment, 21

Gallstones, 595–602
  community care for, 601
  diagnostic criteria for, 597–598
  interventions for, 598–601
  pathophysiology of, 595–596
  prognosis for, 601–602
  signs and symptoms of, 596–597

Ganciclovir, 357–358

Gangrene, in Buerger's disease, 495, 496

Garb, protective, 270

Gas gangrene, from fractures, 739

Gastric bypass surgery, for obesity, 588, 589f

Gastric juice, 98

Gastric lavage, 100
  for drug overdose and poisoning, 706

Gastroccult test, 99–100

Gastroesophageal reflux disease (GERD). See Hiatal hernia.

Gastrointestinal drainage systems, 92–97
  biliary/pancreatic stents in, 97
  biliary tubes in, 93–95, 94f
  gastrointestinal tube suctioning in, 95–97
  gastrostomy tubes in, 92–93, 93t
  nasogastric tubes in, 95, 95f, 96t
  principles of care for, 92

Gastrointestinal endoscopy, in inflammatory bowel disease, 571

Gastrointestinal (GI) system
  in hyperparathyroidism, 632
  in hyperthyroidism, 635
  in renal failure, 145, 850t
  in spinal cord injury, 691
  in systemic lupus erythematosus, 756
  lower. See Lower gastrointestinal tract.
  radiation effects on, 785, 785t
  review of, in expedited physical assessment, 21
  upper. See Upper gastrointestinal tract.

Gastrointestinal losses, in hypovolemic shock, 520t

Gastrointestinal pH, 99

Gastrointestinal series
  for hiatal hernia, 605
  for inflammatory bowel disease, 571
  for peptic ulcer disease, 617

Gastrointestinal specimen collection, 98–101

Gastrointestinal tube suctioning, 95–97

Gastroscopy, in inflammatory bowel disease, 571

Gastrosed. See Hyoscyamine (Cystopaz, Gastrosed).

Gastrostomy tube (G-tube), 92–93, 93t

GBS. See Guillain-Barré syndrome (GBS).

GCS. See Glasgow Coma Scale (GCS).

G-CSF. *See* Granulocyte colony-stimulating factor (G-CSF).
General appearance, in expedited physical assessment, 18, 18t
Genetics
in gallstone formation, 596
in inflammatory bowel disease, 568
Genital herpes, 870, 871t, 874t
Genital warts, 870, 874t
Genitourinary system
in spinal cord injury, 691
review of, in expedited physical assessment, 21–22
Genitourinary tract, radiation effects on, 785, 785t
Gentamicin, pharmacology of, 354
GERD (gastroesophageal reflux disease). *See* Hiatal hernia.
Geriatrics, analgesia for, 320
GFR. *See* Glomerular filtration rate (GFR).
GI. *See* Gastrointestinal (GI) system.
Glasgow Coma Scale (GCS), 167t, 167–170
Glass bottles, for chest drainage, 136–138
Glass thermometer, 16
Glatiramer acetate (Copaxone), for multiple sclerosis, 667–669, 670t
Glaucoma, 815–824
community care for, 819–823
diagnostic criteria for, 818
interventions for, 818–819, 820t–821t
pathophysiology of, 815–817
prognosis for, 823
signs and symptoms of, 817–818
Glaucon. *See* Epinephrine (Epifrin, Glaucon).
Glimepiride (Amaryl), 385t
Glipizide (Glucotrol), 385t
Glomerular filtration rate (GFR), 304–305
Glomerular parenchymal damage, in acute renal failure, 848
Glomerulonephritis, in systemic lupus erythematosus, 755
Gloves, protective, 270
Glucocorticoids
for immunologic alterations, 264
for inflammatory bowel disease, 572

Glucocorticoids *(Continued)*
for nausea and vomiting, 371
in hypovolemic shock, 520
pharmacology of, 408, 409–413, 410t, 411t
Glucophage. *See* Metformin hydrochloride (Glucophage).
Glucose
in diabetes mellitus, 626
in pancreatitis, 611
in urinalysis, 102, 102t
Glucose tolerance test (GTT), 111, 112t
Glucotrol. *See* Glipizide (Glucotrol).
Glyburide (Diabeta, Micronase), 385t
Glycerin (Fleet Babylax), 368–369
Glycerin (Osmoglyn), 378
Glycerol guaiacolate. *See* Guaifenesin (glycerol guaiacolate, Robitussin).
Glycosylated hemoglobin test, 111, 112t
Glyset. *See* Miglitol (Glyset).
GM-CSF. *See* Granulocyte-macrophage-colony stimulating factor (GM-CSF).
Goggles, protective, 270
Goiter, in hyperthyroidism, 635
GoLYTELY. *See* Polyethylene glycol (PEG) (Colyte, GoLYTELY).
Gonads, radiation effects on, 785, 785t
Gonioscope, for glaucoma, 818
Gonococcal infection, 870, 872t
in pelvic inflammatory disease, 868t
Good Samaritan law, 3–4
Goodpasture's syndrome, 262, 262t
Gout, 742–749
community care for, 747–748
diagnostic criteria for, 744
interventions for, 745–747
pathophysiology of, 742–744
prognosis for, 748
signs and symptoms of, 744
Gowns, protective, 270
GP IIb/IIIa platelet inhibitors
for angina, 449
for myocardial infarction, 478–479
Grafts, synthetic, in hemodialysis, 149, 150f
Gram-negative bacilli, in pneumonia, 432, 433t
Gram-positive bacilli, in pneumonia, 432, 433t

Gram stain
  in anti-infective therapy, 348
  in infection, 303
  in pneumonia, 434
  in sexually transmitted diseases, 876
Granulocyte(s), 283, 283f, 283–284
  in inflammation, 262
  peripheral smear of, 286, 287f
Granulocyte colony-stimulating factor
    (G-CSF), 74t
Granulocyte count, 266, 266t
Granulocyte-macrophage-colony
    stimulating factor (GM-CSF), 75t
Granulocytopenia, 288
Granulocytosis, 286
Graves' disease, 262, 262t, 634–637,
    636t
Grayish-black sputum, 108
Greenstick fracture, 729
Grey Turner's sign, in pancreatitis, 610
Gross examination, of urine, 307–308,
    308t
Group A beta-hemolytic streptococci
    (GABHS), 482–483
Growth factors, in wound care, 83
GTT. See Glucose tolerance test (GTT).
G-tube. See Gastrostomy tube (G-tube).
Guaifenesin (glycerol guaiacolate,
    Robitussin), 402t
Guanabenz (Wytensin), 346t
Guanadrel (Hylorel), 347t
Guanethidine (Ismelin), 347t
Guanfacine (Tenex), 346t
Guided imagery, for Raynaud's disease,
    535
Guidelines, for practice, 5, 5t
Guillain-Barré syndrome (GBS),
    657–661, 659t, 661t

H

HAART. See Highly active antiretroviral
    therapy (HAART).
Haemophilus influenzae, in pneumonia,
    432, 433t
Hair, in peripheral vascular disease, 528
Halazepam (Paxipam), 404t
Halcion. See Triazolam (Halcion).
Haloperidol (Haldol), for aggressive/
    combative behavior, 405t
Hashimoto's thyroiditis, 641

Hb. See Hemoglobin (Hb).
HCTZ. See Hydrochlorothiazide (HCTZ,
    HydroDIURIL).
HDL cholesterol, in coronary artery
    disease, 468, 469–470
Head trauma, seizures and, 680
Healing
  of fractures, 730, 730f
  wound, 77
Heart. See also Cardiac; Cardio- entries.
  ultrasonography of, 475
Heart disease, rheumatic. See Rheumatic
    heart disease (RHD).
Heart failure (HF), 456–467
  community care for, 465–466
  diagnostic criteria for, 459–460
  interventions for, 460–465
    in acute exacerbations, 460–461
    in chronic heart failure, 461–464,
      462t
    in diastolic heart failure, 464–465
  pathophysiology of, 456–458
  prognosis for, 466
  signs and symptoms of, 458–459, 459t
Heart rate
  in hypovolemic shock, 521, 522t
  measurement of, 12, 13t
  principles of care for, 7–8
Heart rhythm, in cardiovascular
    assessment, 21
Heart sounds, in cardiovascular
    assessment, 21
Heart transplantation, for cardiogenic
    shock, 455
Heartburn, medications for, 365–367
Heat, for arthritis, 724
Heat conservation, for Raynaud's
    disease, 534
Heat loss, mechanisms of, 10–11
Heel pumping, for deep vein thrombosis,
    505
Helicobacter pylori infection, 615, 616
  testing for, 617–618
Heliox, for asthma, 419
Helper T cells, 260
  human immunodeficiency virus and,
    764, 765
Hematocrit (Hct), 279–280, 280t
  in pancreatitis, 611
Hematologic disorders, in systemic lupus
    erythematosus, 755

Hematologic system, 790–803
anemia and, 790–794, 791t
in renal failure, 851t
leukemia and, 794–799. *See also* Leukemia.
sickle cell disease and, 799–803, 800t
Hematoma, in bone healing, 730, 730f
Hematopoietic changes, in liver cirrhosis, 551
Hematopoietic growth factors, administration and management of, 69, 74t–75t
Hematopoietic system, in renal failure, 144
Hematuria, in renal dysfunction, 143–144
Hemifiltration, for drug overdose and poisoning, 707
Hemoccult test, 100
Hemodialysis, 145–154
complications of, 153, 154t
for drug overdose and poisoning, 707
for renal failure, 854
pharmacology for, 151–153, 152t, 153t
physical examination for, 151
principles of care for, 146–148, 147t, 148t
procedure of, 151
vascular access for, 148–151, 150f
Hemodynamic monitoring
for cardiogenic shock, 452–453, 453t
for myocardial infarction, 475
Hemoglobin (Hb), 279, 279t
Hemolytic crisis, 799–800
Hemolytic reaction, to blood transfusion, 68t
Hemoperfusion, for drug overdose and poisoning, 707
Hemorrhage
after tracheostomy, 134
from fractures, 740
in hypovolemic shock, 520t
Hemorrhagic stroke
interventions for, 655, 656t
pathophysiology of, 650
Hemostasis, phases of, 321–323, 322f, 323t
Hemothorax, with venous access device, 59t, 61–62
Heparin
for angina, 449

Heparin *(Continued)*
for deep vein thrombosis, 506
for hemodialysis, 152, 152t
for myocardial infarction, 477
low molecular weight, 328, 329t
pharmacology of, 325–327, 326t
Hepatic. *See also* Liver *entries.*
Hepatic encephalopathy, in liver cirrhosis, 550, 551t
Hepatitis, 560–567
community care for, 566–567
diagnostic criteria for, 564–565
epidemiology of, 552t, 560t, 560–561
interventions for, 565–566
pathophysiology of, 561–563
prognosis for, 567
signs and symptoms of, 563–564
Hepato-iminodiacetic acid (HIDA) scans, for biliary disease, 597
Hepatocellular cancer, in liver cirrhosis, 550
Hepatorenal syndrome, in liver cirrhosis, 550
Hepatotoxic agents, 560, 560t
Hernia, 576–580
hiatal, 602–609. *See also* Hiatal hernia.
Herpes, 870, 871t, 874t
in human immunodeficiency virus infection, 766, 771t
HF. *See* Heart failure (HF).
Hiatal hernia, 602–609
community care for, 607–608
diagnostic criteria for, 605–606
interventions for, 606t, 606–607
pathophysiology of, 602–604, 603f
prognosis for, 608
signs and symptoms of, 604–605
HIDA scans. *See* Hepato-iminodiacetic acid (HIDA) scans.
High-flow systems, for oxygen therapy, 125–128, 126t–127t
Highly active antiretroviral therapy (HAART), 768
Hip arthroplasty, 726–727
Hip replacement, 726
Hismanal. *See* Astemizole (Hismanal).
Histamine, in allergies, 774
Histamine-2 antagonists, for renal failure, 854

Histamine-2 receptor antagonists, for
    liver cirrhosis, 554
    pharmacology of, 366–367
Histoplasmosis, in human
    immunodeficiency virus infection,
    766, 770t
HIV. *See* Human immunodeficiency virus
    (HIV) infection.
Hives, signs and symptoms of, 775
Hivid. *See* Zalcitabine (Hivid).
HMG-CoA (hydroxymethyl glutaryl
    coenzyme A) reductase inhibitors,
    for angina, 448
HNKC. *See* Hyperosmolar nonketotic
    coma syndrome (HNKC).
HNKS. *See* Hyperosmolar nonketotic
    syndrome (HNKS).
Home blood pressure monitoring, for
    hypertension, 518
Home health care, for emphysema,
    430–431
Hormonal agents, for cancer, 783, 784t
Hormonal compensation, in hypovolemic
    shock, 520
Hormone metabolism, in liver cirrhosis,
    552
Hormone replacement therapy,
    hypertension and, 512
Hospice care, for Alzheimer's disease,
    648
Hospital-acquired pneumonia,
    interventions for, 435
Hospitalization, for pneumonia, 435
Host factors, in anti-infective therapy,
    348
HTN. *See* Hypertension (HTN);
    Hypertensive nephropathy (HTN).
Huber needle, in intravenous therapy,
    53t, 54f
Human immunodeficiency virus (HIV)
    infection, 764–772, 870, 874t
    community care for, 772
    diagnostic criteria for, 766
    nursing care for, 768–769
    pathophysiology of, 764–765
    pharmacologic management for, 766–
        768, 767t, 770t–771t
    prognosis for, 772
    screening for, 264
    signs and symptoms of, 765–766

Humidification, air, for bronchitis, 425
Hunger, diabetes and, 625
Hycodan. *See* Hydrocodone (Hycodan).
Hydantoin. *See* Fosphenytoin (Cerebyx).
Hydralazine (Apresoline), 347t
Hydration, for bronchitis, 425
    for renal calculi, 842
Hydrocephalus, in hemorrhagic stroke,
    655, 656t
Hydrochlorothiazide (HCTZ,
    HydroDIURIL), 379, 381t, 383t
Hydrocodone (Hycodan)
    dosages of, 316t
    for rhinitis, cough, and colds, 397,
        400t
Hydrocolloids, for wound dressings, 83
Hydrocortisone, 414t
HydroDIURIL. *See* Hydrochlorothiazide
    (HCTZ, HydroDIURIL).
Hydrogels, for wound dressings, 83
Hydromorphone, dosages of, 316t
Hydrostatic pressure
    in intravenous fluid therapy, 40
    in thrombophlebitis, 542
Hydrothorax, with venous access device,
    59t, 61–62
Hydroxymethyl glutaryl coenzyme A
    (HMG-CoA) reductase inhibitors,
    448
Hydroxyzine (Vistaril), 404t, 405t
Hylorel. *See* Guanadrel (Hylorel).
Hyoscine, for diarrhea, 372
Hyoscyamine (Cystopaz, Gastrosed),
    372, 373
Hyperacute bacterial conjunctivitis
    interventions for, 811–812
    pathophysiology of, 809
    prognosis for, 814
    signs and symptoms of, 810
Hyperalgesia, from opioids, 314, 315t
Hypercalcemia, 296
    in hyperparathyroidism, 632, 633
Hypercarbia, in increased intracranial
    pressure, 180–181
Hyperchromic cells, 279
Hypercoagulability
    in deep vein thrombosis, 501–502
    in thrombophlebitis, 537
Hyperglycemia, 624
    blood glucose monitoring in, 109–110

Hyperglycemia *(Continued)*
  from insulin therapy, 391
  signs and symptoms of, 626, 628t
Hyperkalemia, 294
Hypermagnesemia, 298
Hypermature segmented neutrophils,
    286–287
Hypernatremia, 291–292
Hyperosmolar nonketotic coma syndrome
    (HNKC), 625
Hyperosmolar nonketotic syndrome
    (HNKS), hyperglycemia in, 109
Hyperosmotic agents, 368–369
  for glaucoma, 821t
Hyperoxia, in oxygenation, 116–117
Hyperparathyroidism, 631–634
Hyperpnea, 14
Hyperreflexia, 831
  in spinal cord injury, 688–690
Hypersensitivity, to blood transfusion,
    68t
Hyperstat. *See* Diazoxide (Hyperstat).
Hypertension (HTN), 509–519
  aneurysm formation and, 488
  community care for, 517–518, 518t
  diagnostic criteria for, 513t, 514
  in Guillain-Barré syndrome, 659t
  interventions for, 514–517, 516t
  pathophysiology of, 509–513, 510t
  portal, in liver cirrhosis, 550
  prognosis for, 518
  signs and symptoms of, 513t, 513–514
Hypertensive crises, 511
Hypertensive nephropathy (HTN), 142
Hypertensive urgency, 511
Hyperthyroidism, 634–637, 636t
Hypertonic solutions
  for hypovolemic shock, 524
  in fluid therapy, 42
  in intravenous therapy, 43–45, 47t
Hyperuricemia, in gout, 742
Hyperventilation, respiration in, 14
Hypnotics, 403–408. *See also* Sedatives.
Hypoaldosteronism, 294
Hypocalcemia, 295–296
  in hypoparathyroidism, 638
Hypochromic cells, 277
Hypoglycemia
  blood glucose monitoring in, 109
  from insulin therapy, 391

Hypoglycemia *(Continued)*
  interventions for, 626–627
  signs and symptoms of, 626, 628t
Hypoglycemic agents, oral, 384–387,
    385t
Hypokalemia, 293–294
Hypomagnesemia, 297–298
  in hypoparathyroidism, 638
Hyponatremia, 292
Hypoparathyroidism, 638–640
Hypophosphatemia, 296–297
Hypostatic pneumonia, from
    immobilization, 737t
Hypotension
  assessment for, 15
  from hemodialysis, 153, 154t
  in Guillain-Barré syndrome, 659t
Hypothalamus, in temperature regulation,
    10
Hypothyroidism, 640–643, 642t
Hypotonic solutions
  in fluid therapy, 42
  in intravenous therapy, 45, 47t
Hypoventilation, from oxygen therapy,
    125
Hypovolemia, from hemodialysis, 153,
    154t
Hypovolemic shock, 519–525
  community care for, 525
  diagnostic criteria for, 521–523
  interventions for, 523–525
  pathophysiology of, 519–521
  prognosis for, 525
  signs and symptoms of, 521, 522t
Hypoxemia, in oxygenation, 116, 117t
Hytrin. *See* Terazosin (Hytrin).

I

^{125}I fibrinogen scan, for thrombophlebitis,
    539
IABP. *See* Intra-aortic balloon pump
    (IABP) counterpulsation.
IBD. *See* Inflammatory bowel disease
    (IBD).
Ibuprofen (Advil, Motrin), 317, 318t
ICP. *See* Intracranial pressure (ICP).
Ictal phase, of seizures, 681
Icteric phase, of hepatitis, 564
IFA. *See* Indirect fluorescent antibody
    (IFA).

IICP. *See* Increased intracranial pressure (IICP).
Ileoanal reservoir, for inflammatory bowel disease, 574
Ileoconduit, 88
Ileostomy, 88, 89t
 for inflammatory bowel disease, 573
IM. *See* Intramuscular (IM) administration.
Imaging. *See also specific imaging modality, e.g.,* Magnetic resonance imaging (MRI).
 for coronary artery disease, 470
 for intestinal obstruction, 583
 for myocardial infarction, 475
 for neurogenic bladder, 832
Imidazole agents, 356
Imipenem, 351
Imipramine (Tofranil), 333, 333t
Immobilization, fracture, 733–738, 737t
Immune system, components of, 259–260
Immunity
 as protective mechanism, 259, 260t
 types of, 263
Immunizations. *See also* Vaccine.
 in emphysema, 431
 in systemic lupus erythematosus, 759
Immunocompromised host, 265–269, 266t, 268t
Immunocytes, 283, 285–286
Immunoglobulins
 administration of, 73t
 for Guillain-Barré syndrome, 660
 for inflammation, 261
 for myasthenia gravis, 674
 for rheumatoid arthritis, 723
Immunologic alterations, 259–273
 assessment of, 259–265
  components in, 259–260
  immunity types in, 263
  inflammation in, 261–263, 262t
  protective mechanisms in, 259, 260t
 decision-making for, 263–264
 immunocompromised host in, 265–269, 266t, 268t
 isolation precautions for, 269–273
Immunologic factors, in inflammatory bowel disease, 568
Immunology, 764–789
 allergies and, 773–779. *See also* Allergies.

Immunology *(Continued)*
 cancer and, 780–789. *See also* Cancer.
 human immunodeficiency virus and, 764–772. *See also* Human immunodeficiency virus (HIV) infection.
 in renal failure, 851t
Immunomodulating drugs, for irritable bowel disease, 374
Immunosuppressants
 for arthritis, 724
 for inflammatory bowel disease, 572–573
 for myasthenia gravis, 673
Immunosuppression
 for immunologic alterations, 264
 for renal transplantation, 162–164, 163t
 for systemic lupus erythematosus, 761
Imodium. *See* Loperamide (Imodium, Imodium A-D).
Impedance plethysmography, for deep vein thrombosis, 504
Implantation, intraocular lens, 806
Implanted ports, in intravenous therapy, 53t, 54f
Imuran. *See* Azathioprine (Imuran).
Inapsine. *See* Droperiderol (Inapsine).
Incarcerated hernia, 577
Incisional hernia, 577
Incomplete fracture, 729
Incomplete spinal cord injury, 687, 687t
Incontinence
 in Alzheimer's disease, 647
 in stroke patients, 654t
Increased intracranial pressure (IICP), 177–183
 brain death in, 182t, 182–183
 definition of, 178t
 in stroke patients, 654t
 monitoring of, 180
 overview of, 177–178, 178t
 principles of care for, 179–180
 systemic interventions for, 180–182, 181t
Inderal. *See* Propranolol (Inderal).
Indinavir (Crixivan), for human immunodeficiency virus infection, 767, 767t
Indirect fluorescent antibody (IFA) testing, 304

Indirect ophthalmoscopy, for cataracts, 805

Indwelling catheter
  in spinal cord injury, 834t, 835–836
  specimen collection with, 104

Infarctive crisis, 799–800

Infection
  after renal transplantation, 164
  after tracheostomy, 134–135
  culture and sensitivity in, 300–304, 302t
  during peritoneal dialysis, 159t
  from chemotherapy, 786, 787t
  from hemodialysis, 153, 154t
  from renal transplantation, 162
  in arthritis, 727, 728
  in bronchitis, 425
  in conjunctivitis, 809–810
  in emphysema, 429
  in human immunodeficiency virus infection, 769
  in meningitis, 664, 665t
  in neurologic assessment, 166
  in wound care, 82
  pin tract, 735
  principles of care for, 299
  renal calculi and, 843
  with venous access device, 56t, 61

Infectious hepatitis, 561

Infiltration, with venous access device, 56t, 60–61

Inflammation, 261–263, 262t
  as protective mechanism, 259, 260t
  in wound healing, 77

Inflammatory bowel disease (IBD), 568–576
  antidiarrheals for, 373
  community care for, 574–575
  diagnostic criteria for, 570–571
  interventions for, 571–574
  pathophysiology of, 568–569
  prognosis for, 575
  signs and symptoms of, 569–570

Infliximab (Remicade), for inflammatory bowel disease, 572

Infusion, continuous, of opioids, 315

Inguinal hernia, 576–577

INH. See Isoniazid (INH).

Inhalant medications, for bronchial obstruction, 393–396, 396t

Inhaled bronchodilators, for emphysema, 429

Injury(ies)
  first aid for, 24–36. See also First aid, for injuries.
  head, post-traumatic, 680
  peritonitis from, 591
  tissue, 78, 78t

Inotropes, for chronic heart failure, 462t, 464

INR. See International normalization ratio (INR).

Insulin
  administration of, 389
  complications of, 391
  coverage by, 389–391, 390t
  drug interactions with, 391–392
  for renal failure, 854
  mixing of, 389, 390t
  principles of care for, 384
  snacks and, 391

Insulin coverage formula, 111, 113t

Insulin reaction, from insulin therapy, 391

Integrity, in integumentary assessment, 19

Integumentary system
  in expedited physical assessment, 18–19
  in renal failure, 144, 851t

Interferon(s), for immunologic alterations, 264

Interferon beta-1a (Avonex), for multiple sclerosis, 667–669, 670t

Interferon beta-1b (Betaseron), for multiple sclerosis, 667–669, 670t

Intermittent bacteremia, blood culture for, 300–301

Intermittent catheterization, spinal cord injury and, 833–835, 834t

Intermittent claudication
  in Buerger's disease, 495
  in peripheral vascular disease, 527

Intermittent peritoneal dialysis (IPD), 157

Internal bleeding, peritonitis from, 591

Internal carotid artery syndrome, 652t

Internal standards, of practice, 4–5

International normalization ratio (INR)
  for deep vein thrombosis, 507

International normalization ratio (INR)
(*Continued*)
prothrombin time and, 324, 325
International Sensitivity Index (ISI),
prothrombin time and, 324
Interstitial colloid osmotic pressure, 41
Interstitial fluid hydrostatic pressure, 40
Interstitial pneumonitis, 432
Interstitial pyelonephritis, in acute renal
failure, 848
Interstitial space, body water in, 39, 40f
Intestinal decompression, 583–584
Intestinal flora modifiers, 372
Intestinal obstructions, 580–586
community care for, 585–586
diagnostic criteria for, 582–583
interventions for, 583–585, 584t
pathophysiology of, 580–581, 581t
prognosis for, 586
signs and symptoms of, 581–582
Intoxication, water, 43
Intra-aortic balloon pump (IABP)
counterpulsation, for cardiogenic
shock, 454–455
Intracapsular cataract extraction, 806
Intracellular space, body water in, 39,
40f
Intracerebral tumors, 184, 185t
Intracranial pressure (ICP)
definition of, 178t
increased. *See* Increased intracranial
pressure (IICP).
Intramuscular (IM) administration, of
opioids, 315
Intraocular lens (IOL) implantation, for
cataracts, 806
Intravenous (IV) administration, of
opioids, 315
Intravenous catheter
for blood and blood product administration, 67
for blood product administration, 67
Intravenous dipyridamole thallium stress
test, for coronary artery disease, 470
Intravenous (IV) fluids, 39–45
management of, 45, 46t–47t
movement of water in, 39–42, 40f, 42f
properties of, 42–43, 44t
tonicity of, 43–45
Intravenous immunoglobulin (IVIg)
administration of, 73t

Intravenous immunoglobulin (IVIg)
(*Continued*)
for Guillain-Barré syndrome, 660
Intravenous pyelography (IVP)
in renal failure, 852
in renal function testing, 309–310
Intravenous therapy, with vascular access
device, 48–64. *See also* Vascular
access device (VAD).
Intrinsic asthma, 417
Intrinsic pathway, in coagulation, 321,
322f
Intussusception, 580
Invirase. *See* Saquinavir (SQV, Invirase,
Fortovase).
Iodine, radioactive, for hyperthyroidism,
636–637, 636t
IOL implantation. *See* Intraocular lens
(IOL) implantation.
IPD. *See* Intermittent peritoneal dialysis
(IPD).
Ipratropium bromide (Atrovent)
for rhinitis, coughs, and colds, 401t
pharmacology of, 393
Irbesartan (Avapro), 344t
Iridectomy, laser, for glaucoma, 819,
822f
Iron
for hemodialysis, 152, 152t
for renal failure, 854
Irreducible hernia, 577
Irrigation
colostomy, 90
whole bowel, 707
Irritable bowel disease, medications for,
373–374
Irritative conjunctivitis
interventions for, 813
prognosis for, 814
signs and symptoms of, 811
Ischemic rest pain
in Buerger's disease, 495
in peripheral vascular disease, 527
Ischemic stroke
interventions for, 651–655
pathophysiology of, 649–650
Ischemic ulcer, in peripheral vascular
disease, 528
ISI. *See* International Sensitivity Index
(ISI).

Ismelin. *See* Guanethidine (Ismelin).
Ismotic. *See* Isosorbide (Ismotic).
Isoflurophate, for glaucoma, 821t
Isolation
  for tuberculosis, 440–441
  precautions of, 269–273
  requirements of, 265–266
  reverse, 267–268
Isoniazid (INH), for tuberculosis, 441, 441t
Isoptin. *See* Verapamil (Calan, Calan SR, Covera-HS, Isoptin, Verelan).
Isopto Eserine. *See* Physostigmine salicylate (Isopto Eserine).
Isosorbide (Ismotic)
  for glaucoma, 821t
  pharmacology of, 378
Isotonic solutions
  in fluid therapy, 42
  in intravenous therapy, 45, 46t–47t
Isotopep studies, in myocardial infarction, 475
Isradipine (DynaCirc, DynaCirc CR), pharmacology of, 344t
Itraconazole, 356
IV fluids. *See* Intravenous (IV) fluids.
IVIg. *See* Intravenous immunoglobulin (IVIg).
IVP. *See* Intravenous pyelography (IVP).

J

Jackson-Pratt drain, for renal transplantation, 161
Jaundice, in cholecystitis, 596
JCAHO. *See* Joint Commission on Accreditation of Healthcare Organizations (JCAHO).
JOAG. *See* Juvenile open-angle glaucoma (JOAG).
Joint Commission on Accreditation of Healthcare Organizations (JCAHO), on standards of practice, 4
Joint contractures, from immobilization, 737t
Joint fluid, in culture report, 302
Joint replacement, for arthritis, 726
Justice, definition and rules of care for, 6t
Juvenile open-angle glaucoma (JOAG), 816–817

K

Kanamycin, for tuberculosis, 441, 442t
Kaolin with pectin, 371–372
Kaopectate. *See* Attapulgite (Kaopectate).
Kayexalate, for renal failure, 854
Keppra. *See* Levetiracetam (Keppra).
Kerlone. *See* Betaxolol (Kerlone).
Ketoconazole, pharmacology of, 356
Ketones
  in urinalysis, 102, 102t
  urine testing for, 111–114
Ketoprofen (Actron, Orudis), 317, 318t
Ketorolac (Toradol), 317, 318t
Kidney, radiography of, in renal function assessment, 309
Kidney disease, secondary hypertension and, 510, 510t
Kidney pain, in renal dysfunction assessment, 143
Kidney stones. *See* Renal calculi.
Kidney transplantation. *See* Renal transplantation.
Kidneys, ureters, and bladder (KUB), 309
Klebsiella pneumoniae, 432, 433t
Klonopin. *See* Clonazepam (Klonopin).
Knee arthroplasty, 727–728
Knee replacement, 727–728
Kock pouch, for inflammatory bowel disease, 573
Korotkoff sounds, in blood pressure measurement, 14
KUB. *See* Kidneys, ureters, and bladder (KUB).
Kussmaul's respirations, 14
  in renal failure, 145

L

Labetalol (Normodyne, Trandate), 339–340, 346t
Labile pulse, 13t
Lactate dehydrogenase
  in intestinal obstruction, 583
  in myocardial infarction, 474
Lactated Ringer's solution, for hypovolemic shock, 524
Lactulose (Cephulac, Chronulac)
  for liver cirrhosis, 554
  pharmacology of, 368–369
Lamictal. *See* Lamotrigine (Lamictal).

Lamivudine (3TC, Epivir), for human immunodeficiency virus, 766–767, 767t
Lamotrigine (Lamictal), 360t, 361t
Lansoprazole (Prevacid), 367
Laparoscopic cholecystectomy, for gallstones, 599–600
Laparoscopic surgery, for hernias, 578
Laparoscopic ureterolithotomy, for renal calculi, 845
Large bowel obstruction, 581
Laser angioplasty, for coronary artery disease, 470
Laser iridectomy, for glaucoma, 819, 822f
Laser lithotripsy, for gallstones, 599
Laser prostatectomy, for benign prostatic hypertrophy, 863
Laser trabeculoplasty, for glaucoma, 819
Lasix. *See* Furosemide (Lasix).
Latent tuberculosis infection (LTBI), 438
drug therapy for, 441
Lavage, peritoneal, 592
Laxatives, 367–369
LDL cholesterol, in coronary artery disease, 468, 469–470
Left ventricular assist device, for cardiogenic shock, 455
Left ventricular failure, in cardiogenic shock, 452
Legal issues
decision-making and, 5, 6t
in nursing practice, 2–4
Legal regulation, of nursing practice, 3
Legionella, in pneumonia, 432, 433t
Lermoyez's syndrome, 826
Leukemia, 794–799
community care for, 796–797
diagnostic criteria for, 796
interventions for, 796, 797t
pathophysiology of, 794–795
prognosis for, 797–798
signs and symptoms of, 795–796
Leukocytes. *See also* White blood cells (WBCs).
classification of, 283
development of, 282–283
in appendicitis, 548
in myocardial infarction, 474
in urinalysis, 102, 102t

Leukocytes *(Continued)*
origin, development, and structure of, 274, 275f
Leukocytosis, 286
Leukopenia, 288
Leukotrienes, in inflammation, 262
Level of consciousness (LOC)
in first aid for injuries, 25, 26t
in hypovolemic shock, 521, 522t
in neurologic assessment, 166–170, 167t
Levetiracetam (Keppra), 360t
Levin tube, 95, 95f
Levobunolol, for glaucoma, 820t
Levodopa, for Parkinson's disease, 678t
Levofloxacin, pharmacology of, 353–354
Levorphanol, dosages of, 316t
Librium. *See* Chlordiazepoxide (Librium).
Lipase
in biliary disease, 597
in pancreatitis, 611
Lisinopril (Prinivil, Zestril), 343t
Listeria, in food poisoning, 557
Lithotripsy
for gallstones, 599
for renal calculi, 844
Liver, inflammatory disease of. *See* Hepatitis.
Liver biopsy, in liver cirrhosis, 553
Liver cirrhosis, 549–555. *See also* Cirrhosis.
Liver enzymes
in hepatitis, 565
in liver cirrhosis, 552–553
in pancreatitis, 611
Liver function tests, in inflammatory bowel disease, 570
Liver transplantation, for hepatitis, 566
Liver ultrasound, in liver cirrhosis, 553
LMWH. *See* Low-molecular-weight heparin (LMWH).
LOC. *See* Level of consciousness (LOC).
Lodine. *See* Etodolac (Lodine).
Lomotil. *See* Diphenoxylate (Lomotil).
Long-acting nitrates, for angina, 448
Long-term acute central catheters, in fluid therapy, 49, 50–51, 52t–53t, 54f, 55f
Loniten. *See* Minoxidil (Loniten).

Loop colostomy, principles of care for, 88
Loop diuretics, pharmacology of, 341, 375, 376t, 378, 379t, 383t
Loperamide (Imodium, Imodium A-D) for diarrhea, 372
    for inflammatory bowel disease, 573
Lopinavir, for human immunodeficiency virus, 767, 767t
Lopressor. *See* Metoprolol (Lopressor).
Loratadine (Claritin), pharmacology of, 399t
Lorazepam (Ativan)
    for diagnostic procedures, 406t
    pharmacology of, 361t, 404t
Losartan (Cozaar), pharmacology of, 337, 344t
Lotensin. *See* Benazepril (Lotensin).
Lovenox. *See* Enoxaparin (Lovenox).
Low self-esteem, abuse and, 711–712
Lower gastrointestinal tract, 547–594
    appendicitis and, 547–549
    cirrhosis and, 549–555. *See also* Cirrhosis.
    food poisoning and, 556–560
    hepatitis and, 560–567. *See also* Hepatitis.
    hernias and, 576–580
    inflammatory bowel disease and, 568–576. *See also* Inflammatory bowel disease (IBD).
    intestinal obstructions and, 580–586. *See also* Intestinal obstructions.
    obesity and, 586–590, 589f
    peritonitis and, 590–594
Low-flow systems, for oxygen therapy, 125, 126t–127t
Low-molecular-weight heparin (LMWH)
    for angina, 449
    for deep vein thrombosis, 507
    pharmacology of, 328, 329t
LTBI. *See* Latent tuberculosis infection (LTBI).
Lubricant agents, 369
Luminal. *See* Phenobarbital (Luminal).
Lung(s). *See also* Pulmonary; Respiratory *entries*.
    in hypertension, 513
    radiation effects on, 785, 785t
Lung scan, for deep vein thrombosis, 504–505

Lung sounds, in respiratory assessment, 19–20
Lymphocyte(s), 259–260, 285–286, 287f
Lymphocyte subsets, for immunologic alterations, 264
Lymphocytopenia, 289
Lymphocytosis, 288
Lymphogranuloma venereum, 870, 871t

M

Macrocytic cells, 277
Macrocytic normochromic anemia, 790, 791t
Macrocytosis, 279
Macrolides
    for pneumonia, 435
    pharmacology of, 353
Macrophages, 284–285, 285t
    in inflammation, 261
Magnesium, 297–298
    in renal failure, 310, 310t
Magnesium citrate (citrate of magnesia), 368
Magnesium phosphate, 368
Magnesium salicylate, 317, 318t
Magnesium sulfate (Epsom salts), 368
Magnesium-ammonium stones, 840
Magnesium-based antacids, 365–366
Magnetic resonance cholangiography (MRC), for biliary disease, 598
Magnetic resonance imaging (MRI)
    for angina, 447
    for aortic aneurysm, 489
    for Buerger's disease, 496
    for deep vein thrombosis, 504
    for multiple sclerosis, 667
    for pancreatitis, 612
    for peripheral vascular disease, 529
    for spinal cord injury, 690
Malecot drain, 85
Malignant hypertension, 511. *See also* Hypertension (HTN).
Malignant pain, 312
Malpractice, 3
Mannitol (Osmitrol)
    for glaucoma, 821t
    pharmacology of, 378, 381t, 383t
Manometry, esophageal, for hiatal hernia, 605
Mantoux skin test, for tuberculosis, 438–439, 439t

Manual traction, for fractures, 735
MAOIs. *See* Monoamine oxidase inhibitors (MAOIs).
MAP. *See* Mean arterial pressure (MAP).
Maprotiline, adverse effects of, 333, 334t
Marinol. *See* Dronabinol (Marinol).
Masks, protective, 270
Mass lesions, in neurologic assessment, 166
Massage, for arthritis, 724
Mast cell(s), 284
  in sputum smear, 108, 108t
Mast cell stabilizers, 393–396
Mavik. *See* Trandolapril (Mavik).
McBurney's point, in appendicitis, 547
MCH. *See* Mean corpuscular hemoglobin (MCH).
MCHC. *See* Mean corpuscular hemoglobin concentration (MCHC).
MCV. *See* Mean corpuscular volume (MCV).
MDI. *See* Metered-dose inhaler (MDI).
Mean arterial pressure (MAP), measurement of, 15
Mean corpuscular hemoglobin concentration (MCHC), 277–279
Mean corpuscular hemoglobin (MCH), 277
Mean corpuscular volume (MCV), 277, 278t
Mechanical débridement, 81
Mechanical intestinal obstructions, 580, 581t
Mechanical therapy, for hypovolemic shock, 524–525
Meclofenamate sodium (Meclomen), 317, 318t
Mefenamic acid (Ponstel), 317, 318t
Megacolon, toxic, 569
Meglitinides, 385t, 387
Melancholic depression, 332, 332t
Meniere's disease, 824–829
  community care for, 828
  diagnostic criteria for, 826
  interventions for, 826–828
  pathophysiology of, 825
  prognosis for, 828
  signs and symptoms of, 825–826
Meningitis, 662–666, 663t–665t
  in human immunodeficiency virus, 766, 770t

Mental/emotional abuse, 709–714
  community care for, 713
  diagnostic criteria for, 712
  interventions for, 712–713
  pathophysiology of, 710–711
  prognosis for, 713
  signs and symptoms of, 711–712
Mental status
  in human immunodeficiency virus infection, 769
  in neurologic assessment, 22
  in renal failure, 144
Meperidine (Demerol)
  dosages of, 316t
  for gout, 747
Mercaptopurine (Purinethol)
  for inflammatory bowel disease, 572
  for irritable bowel disease, 374
Meropenem, 351
Mesalamine (Asacol, Pentasa, Rowasa)
  for inflammatory bowel disease, 572
  for irritable bowel disease, 373–374
Mestinon. *See* Pyridostigmine (Mestinon).
Metabolic acidosis, in renal failure, 145
Metabolic disorders, in neurologic assessment, 166
Metabolic syndrome, 624–625
Metallic taste, in renal failure, 145
Metamucil. *See* Psyllium (Metamucil, Fiberall).
Metaproterenol (Alupent, Metaprel), 393, 394t
Metastatic brain tumors, 185
Metered-dose inhaler (MDI), 396, 396t
  for asthma, 420–421
Metformin hydrochloride (Glucophage), 385t
Methadone, 316t
Methicillin, 351
Methicillin-resistant *Staphylococcus aureus* (MRSA), 271, 272
Methimazole (Tapazole), for hyperthyroidism, 636, 636t
Methotrexate (Folex, Rheumatrex)
  for arthritis, 724
  for inflammatory bowel disease, 572
Methylcellulose (Citrucel), 367–368, 371–372
Methyldopa (Aldomet), 340, 346t

Methylprednisolone
for multiple sclerosis, 667
for spinal cord injury, 690
Methylprednisolone (Solu-Medrol), for gout, 746
Methylxanthines, 393, 395t
Metoclopramide (Reglan), 367
Metoprolol (Lopressor), 345t
Metronidazole (Flagyl)
for inflammatory bowel disease, 573
pharmacology of, 356
MG. See Myasthenia gravis (MG).
Micardis. See Telmisartan (Micardis).
Microbial resistance, to anti-infective therapy, 350
Microcytic cells, 277
Microcytic hypochromic anemia, 790, 791t
Microcytosis, 279
Micronase. See Glyburide (Diabeta, Micronase).
Microorganisms, in infection, 299
Microscopic examination, of urine, 308–309
Microscopic hematuria, in renal dysfunction, 144
Midamor. See Amiloride (Midamor).
Midazolam (Versed), for diagnostic procedures, 406t
Middle carotid artery syndrome, 652t
Midstream clean-catch specimens, 102, 103
Miglitol (Glyset), 385t
Military antishock trouser, for hypovolemic shock, 525
Milk-alkali syndrome, 619
Milrinone (Primacor)
for cardiogenic shock, 454
for chronic heart failure, 462t, 464
Mineral salts, regulators of, 408
Mineralocorticoids, 408
Minipress. See Prazosin (Minipress).
Minocycline, 352–353
Minoxidil (Loniten), 347t
Miosis, from opioids, 314, 315t
Miotics, for glaucoma, 820t
Mirtazapine, adverse effects of, 333, 334t
Mixed adrenergic antagonists, 339–340, 346t
Mixed-anxiety disorder, 332, 332t

MMF. See Mycophenolate mofetil (MMF).
Mobilization, for deep vein thrombosis, 505, 507
Moexipril (Univasc), 343t
Moist-to-moist dressings, 82
Moisture, in integumentary assessment, 19
Monoamine oxidase inhibitors (MAOIs)
for depression, 699–700
for Parkinson's disease, 678t
pharmacology of, 333, 334, 334t, 335t
Monobactams, 351–352
Monoctanoin, for gallstones, 599
Monocytes, 284–285, 285t
in inflammation, 261
peripheral smear of, 286, 287f
Monocytopenia, 289
Monocytosis, 287–288
Monopril. See Fosinopril (Monopril).
Morbid obesity, 586–587
Morphine
dosages of, 315, 316t
for myocardial infarction, 477
Moss tube, 95
Motor function
in Guillain-Barré syndrome, 658
in neurologic assessment, 170–171
Motor response, in Glasgow Coma Scale, 167t, 167–168, 169–170
Motrin. See Ibuprofen (Advil, Motrin).
MRC. See Magnetic resonance cholangiography (MRC).
MRI. See Magnetic resonance imaging (MRI).
MRSA. See Methicillin-resistant Staphylococcus aureus (MRSA).
MS. See Multiple sclerosis (MS).
MTB. See Mycobacterium tuberculosis bacilli (MTB).
Mucoid sputum, 106
Mucolytics
for pneumonia, 435
for rhinitis, cough, and colds, 402t, 403
Mucomyst. See Acetylcysteine (Mucomyst).
Mucopurulent sputum, 106–108
Mucosal biopsy, in peptic ulcer disease, 618
Mucosal ulcerations, in renal failure, 145

Mucous membranes
administration to, of opioids, 315
in cardiovascular assessment, 20
Multiple sclerosis (MS), 666–671
community care for, 669
diagnostic criteria for, 667
interventions for, 667–669, 668t, 670t
pathophysiology of, 666
prognosis for, 669
signs and symptoms of, 666–667
spinal cord injury and, 836
Murmur of valvulitis, 483
Murphy sign, in cholecystitis, 597
Muscarinic receptor antagonists, for
benign prostatic hypertrophy, 862
Muscle atrophy, from immobilization,
737t
Muscle cramps, from hemodialysis, 153,
154t
Musculoskeletal injury, first aid for,
32–34, 33t
Musculoskeletal system, 720–763
arthritis and, 720–729. See also Arthritis.
fractures and, 729–742. See also Frac-
ture(s).
gout and, 742–749. See also Gout.
in peripheral vascular disease, 528
in renal failure, 144–145, 851t
in systemic lupus erythematosus, 755
osteoporosis and, 749–753, 750t
systemic lupus erythematosus and,
753–763. See also Systemic lupus
erythematosus (SLE).
Myasthenia gravis (MG), 262, 262t,
671–675, 672t, 673t
Myasthenic crisis, 671–672, 672t
Mycobacterium tuberculosis
acid-fast smear for, 303
in human immunodeficiency virus infection, 766, 771t
Mycobacterium tuberculosis bacilli
(MTB), 437–438
sputum testing for, 439–440
Mycophenolate mofetil (MMF), in renal
transplantation, 163t
Mycoplasma pneumoniae, 432, 433t
Mydriatics, for glaucoma, 819
Myeloproliferative disorders, 286
Myocardial infarction (MI), 472–481
community care for, 479–480

Myocardial infarction (MI) *(Continued)*
diagnostic criteria for, 473–476
interventions for, 476–479
pathophysiology of, 472–473
prognosis for, 480
signs and symptoms of, 473
Myocardial ischemia, 469
Myoclonic seizures, 685, 686t
Mysoline. *See* Primidone (Mysoline).
Myxedema, in hypothyroidism, 641

N

Nadolol (Corgard), 345t
Nafcillin, 351
Nails
in cardiovascular assessment, 20
in peripheral vascular disease, 528
Nalfon. *See* Fenprofen calcium (Nalfon).
Naloxone (Narcan)
for drug overdose and poisoning, 705
for opioid reversal, 317
Naphazoline (Privine), for rhinitis,
coughs, and colds, 401t
Naproxen (Naprosyn), 317, 318t
Naproxen sodium (Anaprox, Aleve), 317,
318t
Nasogastric tubes, 95, 95f, 96t
Nasointestinal tubes, for intestinal
obstruction, 584
Nasotracheal/orotracheal aspiration, for
sputum samples, 106, 107t
Natural immunity, 263
Natural killer (NK) cells, 260, 285, 286
Nausea and vomiting, 365
from chemotherapy, 786, 787t
from opioids, 314, 315t
in peritonitis, 592
in renal failure, 145
medications for, 369–371
Near-drowning, first aid for, 34t, 34–35,
35t
Neck, in hypertension, 513
Necrotic tissue, 78, 78t
Nefazodone, adverse effects of, 333, 334t
Negligence, 3
Neisseria gonorrhoeae, in conjunctivitis,
809
Nelfinavir (Viracept), for human
immunodeficiency virus infection,
767, 767t

Nembutal. *See* Pentobarbital (Nembutal, Tuinal).
Neo-Synephrine. *See* Phenylephrine HCl (Neo-Synephrine, Sinex).
Neomycin
    for liver cirrhosis, 554
    pharmacology of, 354
Neostigmine, for myasthenia gravis, 673t
Nephritis, in systemic lupus erythematosus, 755
Nephrolithotomy, for renal calculi, 845
Nephron, diuretic actions in, 375
Nephropathy, 142
Nephrostoureterolithotomy, for renal calculi, 845
Nephrotoxic drugs, 143, 143t
Nerve assessment, in fractures, 736
Neural compensation, in hypovolemic shock, 520
Neurogenic bladder, 830–840
    cerebrovascular accident and, 837
    community care for, 838–839
    diabetes mellitus and, 837–838
    diagnostic criteria for, 831–832
    multiple sclerosis and, 836
    Parkinson's disease and, 836–837
    pathophysiology of, 830–831
    prognosis for, 839
    signs and symptoms of, 831
    spina bifida and, 838
    spinal cord injury and, 832–836, 834t
    surgical management of, 838
Neurogenic shock, in spinal cord injury, 688
Neurologic alterations, 166–188
    assessment of, 166–177
        cranial nerves in, 171, 172t–175t
        deep tendon reflexes in, 177
        level of consciousness in, 166–170, 167t
        motor function in, 170–171
        principles of care in, 166
        pupillary signs in, 171
        Rancho Los Amigos scale in, 177
        vital signs in, 171–177, 176t
    brain lesions in, 183–187, 184t, 185t, 187t
    from opioids, 314, 315t
    increased intracranial pressure in, 177–183. *See also* Increased intracranial pressure (IICP).

Neurologic system, 644–692
    Alzheimer's disease and, 644–649, 645f
    cerebrovascular accident and, 649–657. *See also* Cerebrovascular accident (CVA).
    Guillain-Barré syndrome and, 657–661, 659t, 661t
    heart rate and, 8
    in hypertension, 513
    in increased intracranial pressure, 180
    in liver cirrhosis, 552
    in meningitis, 664, 665t
    in renal failure, 144, 851t
    in systemic lupus erythematosus, 756
    meningitis and, 662–666, 663t–665t
    multiple sclerosis and, 666–671. *See also* Multiple sclerosis (MS).
    myasthenia gravis and, 671–675, 672t, 673t
    parkinsonism and, 675–679, 677t, 678t
    review of, in expedited physical assessment, 22–23
    seizures and, 680–686. *See also* Seizures.
    spinal cord injury and, 686–692. *See also* Spinal cord injury (SCI).
Neuromuscular activity, sodium in, 291
Neuromuscular system
    in hyperkalemia, 294
    in hypocalcemia, 295
    in hypokalemia, 293
    in hypomagnesemia, 297–298
    in hypoparathyroidism, 638
Neurons, in Alzheimer's disease, 644, 645f
Neurontin. *See* Gabapentin (Neurontin).
Neuropathic syndrome, 624, 625
Neurotransmitters, in depression, 696
Neurovascular assessment, for arthritis, 726
Neurovascular compromise, in fractures, 735–736
Neutropenia, 288–289
Neutropenic precautions, 266t, 266–267
Neutrophil(s), 283, 284
    in inflammation, 261
    peripheral smear of, 286, 287f
Neutrophil count, 266, 266t
Neutrophilia, 286

Nevirapine (Viramune), for human immunodeficiency virus infection, 767t, 767–768

Nicardipine (Cardene, Cardene SR), 344t

Nicotine transdermal system (Nicotrol), for irritable bowel disease, 374

Nicotrol. *See* Nicotine transdermal system (Nicotrol).

Nifedipine (Adalat CC, Procardia XL), 344t

90–90 traction, for fractures, 734

Nipride. *See* Nitroprusside (Nipride).

Nisoldipine (Sular), 344t

Nissen fundoplication, for hiatal hernia, 607

Nitrates
   for angina, 448
   for myocardial infarction, 477–478

Nitrites, in urinalysis, 102, 102t

Nitrogenous waste products, in renal function, 305–306

Nitroglycerin
   for angina, 448
   for cardiogenic shock, 454
   for myocardial infarction, 478

Nitroprusside (Nipride)
   for cardiogenic shock, 454
   pharmacology of, 347t

Nizatidine (Axid), 366–367

NK cells. *See* Natural killer (NK) cells.

NNRTIs. *See* Nonnucleoside reverse transcriptase inhibitors (NNRTIs).

Nociception, 312

Noctec. *See* Chloral hydrate (Noctec).

Nocturia, in renal dysfunction, 143

Nonadherent dressings, 82

Nonantibody tests, for human immunodeficiency virus infection, 766

Nonatopic asthma, 417

Nongonococcal urethritis, 870, 872t

Nongranulocytes, 284–286, 285t
   peripheral smear of, 286, 287f

Nonmaleficence, definition and rules of care for, 6t

Nonnucleoside reverse transcriptase inhibitors (NNRTIs), 767t, 767–768

Nonopioid analgesics, 317–319, 318t

Nonsteroidal anti-inflammatory drugs (NSAIDs)

Nonsteroidal anti-inflammatory drugs (NSAIDs) *(Continued)*
   for analgesia, 317–319, 318t
   for arthritis, 723
   for gout, 745
   for peptic ulcer disease, 616
   for systemic lupus erythematosus, 760

Nonunion, of fractures, 740

Nonviable tissue, 78, 78t

NOPQRSTUV mnemonic, in myocardial infarction, 474

Norepinephrine, for cardiogenic shock, 454

Norfloxacin, pharmacology of, 353–354

Normal saline, for hypovolemic shock, 524

Normal-tension glaucoma, 816, 817

Normiflo. *See* Ardeparin (Normiflo).

Normochromic cells, 277

Normocytic cells, 277

Normocytic normochromic anemia, 790, 791t

Normodyne. *See* Labetalol (Normodyne, Trandate).

Norpramin. *See* Desipramine (Norpramin).

Norvasc. *See* Amlodipine (Norvasc).

Norvir. *See* Ritonavir (Norvir).

Norwalk virus, in food poisoning, 558

Nosocomial aspiration pneumonia, 432–434

NRTIs. *See* Nucleoside reverse transcriptase inhibitors (NRTIs).

NSAIDs. *See* Nonsteroidal anti-inflammatory drugs (NSAIDs).

Nuclear cataract, 804

Nucleation, in gallstone formation, 596

Nucleoside analogs, 766–767, 767t

Nucleoside reverse transcriptase inhibitors (NRTIs), 766–767, 767t

Nursing practice, regulation of, 2–3

Nursing standards. *See* Standards of nursing.

Nursing's Social Policy Statement, 2–3

Nutrition
   in arthritis, 725
   in bronchitis, 425
   in deep vein thrombosis, 508
   in emphysema, 429, 430
   in hemodialysis, 148

Nutrition *(Continued)*
  in hepatitis, 565–566, 574
  in human immunodeficiency virus infection, 769
  in inflammatory bowel disease, 570
  in meningitis, 664, 665t
  in peptic ulcer disease, 618–619
  in peritoneal dialysis, 156
  in pneumonia, 435
  in renal failure, 853–854
  in systemic lupus erythematosus, 758
  in tuberculosis, 442
  in wound care, 84

O

OA. *See* Osteoarthritis (OA).
Obesity, 586–590, 589f
Objective behaviors, of pain, 313
Oblique fracture, 729
Obstruction, in neurogenic bladder, 830–831
Obstructive chronic bronchitis, 423
Occlusion, catheter, 59t, 62
Occupational Safety and Health Administration (OSHA), 4
Odor, in urinalysis, 307–308
Ofloxacin, 353–354
OGTT. *See* Oral glucose tolerance test (OGTT).
OKT, in renal transplantation, 163t
Oliguria, 17
Olsalazine (Dipentum), for inflammatory bowel disease, 572
Omeprazole (Prilosec), 367
Ondansetron (Zofran), for nausea and vomiting, 371
Open appendectomy, 548
Open cholecystectomy, 600
Open drains, 85
Open fracture, 729
Open heart surgery, 449
Open prostatectomy, 864
Open reduction, of fractures, 732
Ophthalmoscopy
  for cataracts, 805
  for glaucoma, 818
Opiates, for diarrhea, 372
Opioids
  for analgesia, 314–317, 315t, 316t
  for gout, 747

Opioids *(Continued)*
  for rhinitis, cough, and colds, 397, 400t
Opium tincture, for diarrhea, 372
Optimine. *See* Azatadine maleate (Optimine).
Oral administration, of opioids, 314
Oral cholecystogram, for biliary disease, 597
Oral contraceptives, hypertension and, 512
Oral glucose tolerance test (OGTT), for diabetes mellitus, 626
Oral hypoglycemic agents, 384–387, 385t
Oral solubilizing agents, for gallstones, 598–599
Oral temperature, 15–16
Oral warts, 870, 874t
Organan. *See* Danaparoid (Organan).
Orogastric lavage, for drug overdose and poisoning, 706
Oropharyngeal candidiasis, 766, 770t
Orthopnea, 14
Orthostatic hypotension
  assessment of, 15
  from immobilization, 737t
Orudis. *See* Ketoprofen (Actron, Orudis).
OSHA. *See* Occupational Safety and Health Administration (OSHA).
Osmitrol. *See* Mannitol (Osmitrol).
Osmoglyn. *See* Glycerin (Osmoglyn).
Osmolality
  in fluid therapy, 41
  in intestinal obstruction, 583
Osmosis, in fluid therapy, 40, 41–42, 42f
Osmotic diuretics, 375, 377t, 378, 381t, 383t
Osteoarthritis (OA)
  diagnostic criteria for, 722
  pathophysiology of, 720
  signs and symptoms of, 721
Osteodystrophy, renal, 145
Osteoporosis, 749–753, 750t
  from immobilization, 737t
  in systemic lupus erythematosus, 760
Osteotomy, for arthritis, 726
Ostomies, 87–92
  assessment of, 89, 89t
  irrigation of, 90
  pouching systems for, 90t, 90–91

Ostomies *(Continued)*
  principles of care for, 88
Otrivin. *See* Xylometazolin (Otrivin).
Over-the-needle catheters, in intravenous
    therapy, 49, 50t
Overhead traction, for fractures, 734
Overweight, 587
Oxacillin, pharmacology of, 351
Oxazepam (Serax), 404t
Oxcarbazepine (Trileptal), 360t
Oximetry, pulse, 119t, 119–120, 120t
Oxycodone, 316t
Oxygen
  complications of, 124–125
  for cardiogenic shock, 455
  for deep vein thrombosis, 507
  for emphysema, 429–430
  for pneumonia, 435
  in oxygenation, 115
Oxygen delivery devices, 124–128,
    126t–127t
Oxygen toxicity, 116–117, 125
Oxygenation, 115–141
  assessment of, 115–123
    arterial blood gas analysis in, 120–
        123, 121t–123t
    fraction of inspired oxygen in, 115–
        116, 116t
    hypoxemia in, 116, 117t
    oxygen in, 115
    oxygen toxicity in, 116–117
    pulse oximetry in, 119t, 119–120,
        120t
    respiratory failure in, 117–118, 118t
  chest drainage systems in, 135–141.
      See also Chest drainage systems.
  for hypovolemic shock, 523
  for increased intracranial pressure,
      180–181
  for meningitis, 664, 665t
  for tracheostomy care, 132
  for wound care, 84
  oxygen delivery devices for, 124–128,
      126t–127t
  tracheostomy care for, 128–135. *See
      also* Tracheostomy care.
Oxymetazoline (Afrin, Allerest), for
    rhinitis, coughs, and colds, 401t
Oxymorphine, 316t

P
Packed red blood cells, 71t
Pain
  assessment of, 313–314
  fracture, 730–731, 738
  from renal calculi, 842
  from varicose veins, 543
  in arthritis, 723–727, 728
  in Buerger's disease, 495
  in coronary artery disease, 468–469
  in deep vein thrombosis, 507
  in intestinal obstruction, 582
  in meningitis, 664, 665t
  in multiple sclerosis, 667, 668t
  in pancreatitis, 610, 612–613
  in peptic ulcer disease, 617
  in peripheral vascular disease, 526–
      527
  in peritoneal dialysis, 159t
  in peritonitis, 592
  in renal dysfunction, 143
  in renal failure, 145
  physiology of, 312
  types of, 312
Painful stimuli, response to, 171
Pallidus pallidotomy, for Parkinson's
    disease, 678
Panacinar emphysema, 428
Pancreatitis, 609–615
  community care for, 613–614
  diagnostic criteria for, 611–612
  interventions for, 612–613
  pathophysiology of, 609–610
  prognosis for, 614, 614t
  signs and symptoms of, 610–611
Panlobular emphysema, 428
Pap smear, for sexually transmitted
    diseases, 876
Para-aminosalicylic acid, for tuberculosis,
    441, 442t
Paracentesis, for liver cirrhosis, 554
Paraesophageal hiatal hernia
  pathophysiology of, 603f, 603–604
  signs and symptoms of, 604–605
Paralytic ileus, in Guillain-Barré
    syndrome, 659t
Paraplegia, 686, 687
Parasites
  in food poisoning, 556, 558
  in infection, 299

Parasympathetic nervous system, heart
    rate and, 8
Parathyroid hormone (PTH)
    in hyperparathyroidism, 631–632
    in hypoparathyroidism, 638
    in renal failure, 144–145
Paregoric. *See* Camphorated paregoric.
Parkinsonism, 675–679, 677t, 678t
    spinal cord injury and, 836
Parkinson's disease (PD), 675–679, 677t,
    678t
Parlodel. *See* Bromocriptine (Parlodel).
Partial thromboplastin time (PTT), 324t,
    325
Partial-thickness wounds, 78
PASG. *See* Pneumatic antishock garment
    (PASG).
Passy-Muir valve, 134
Paste, in pouching principles, 91
Patency, drain, 86
Pathogenic bacteria, 299
Pathologic brain lesions, 183–187, 184t,
    185t, 187t
Pathologic fractures, in renal failure, 145
Patient-controlled analgesia (PCA), with
    opioids, 315
Paxipam. *See* Halazepam (Paxipam).
PCA. *See* Patient-controlled analgesia
    (PCA).
PCI. *See* Percutaneous coronary
    interventions (PCIs).
PCP. *See* Pneumocystis carinii
    pneumonia (PCP).
PCR test. *See* Polymerase chain reaction
    (PCR) test.
PD. *See* Parkinson's disease (PD);
    Peritoneal dialysis (PD).
PE. *See* Pulmonary embolism (PE).
Peak expiratory flow (PEF), in asthma,
    418, 419
Peak flow meter (PFM), for asthma, 421
Peak level, of antibiotics, 349, 349t
PEF. *See* Peak expiratory flow (PEF).
PEG. *See* Polyethylene glycol (PEG)
    (Colyte, GoLYTELY).
PEG tubes. *See* Percutaneous endoscopic
    gastrostomy (PEG) tubes.
Pelvic inflammatory disease (PID),
    866–870, 868t, 873t
Penicillin(s), 350–351

Penicillinase, 351
Penrose drain, 85
Pentasa. *See* Mesalamine (Asacol,
    Pentasa, Rowasa).
Pentobarbital (Nembutal, Tuinal), for
    sleep disorders, 405t
Pentoxifylline, for peripheral vascular
    disease, 530
Pepcid. *See* Famotidine (Pepcid).
Peptic ulcer disease (PUD), 615–623
    community care for, 619–622
    diagnostic criteria for, 617–618
    interventions for, 618–619, 620t–621t
    pathophysiology of, 615–617
    prognosis for, 622
    signs and symptoms of, 617
Pepto-Bismol. *See* Bismuth subsalicylate
    (Pepto-Bismol).
Percussion, for pneumonia, 435
Percutaneous antegrade nephrosto-
    ureterolithotomy, 845
Percutaneous coronary interventions
    (PCIs)
    for angina, 449
    for cardiogenic shock, 454
    for myocardial infarction, 479
Percutaneous endoscopic gastrostomy
    (PEG) tubes, 93
Percutaneous endoscopic laser lithotripsy,
    599
Percutaneous transhepatic cholan-
    giography (PTC), 597
Percutaneous transluminal coronary
    angioplasty, 470
Perforation
    from inflammatory bowel disease, 569
    peritonitis from, 591
Pergolide, for Parkinson's disease, 678t
Periactin. *See* Cyproheptadine (Periactin).
Perianal warts, 870, 874t
Pericardiocentesis, for cardiogenic shock,
    455
Pericarditis
    in renal failure, 144
    in systemic lupus erythematosus, 756
Perimetry
    for cataracts, 805
    for glaucoma, 818
Perineum, in genitourinary assessment,
    22

Peripheral adrenergic neuron antagonists, 340, 347t
Peripheral arterial disease, 526. *See also* Peripheral vascular disease (PVD).
Peripheral catheters, in fluid therapy, 49, 50t
Peripheral pulses, in hypovolemic shock, 521, 522t
Peripheral smear, of white blood cells, 286, 287f
Peripheral vascular disease (PVD), 526t, 526–531
    community care for, 531
    diagnostic criteria for, 528–529
    interventions for, 529–531
    pathophysiology of, 526
    prognosis for, 531
    signs and symptoms of, 526–528
Peripheral vascular resistance, 8
Peripheral venous disease, 526. *See also* Peripheral vascular disease (PVD).
Peripherally inserted central catheter (PICC), 53t, 54f
Peristomal skin, protection of, 91
Peritoneal dialysis (PD), 154–160
    access for, 156
    complications of, 159t, 159–160
    for peritonitis, 593
    for renal failure, 854
    pharmacology for, 158–159
    principles of care for, 155–156
    procedure of, 156–158, 158t, 159t
Peritoneal lavage, for peritonitis, 592
Peritonitis, 590–594
    during peritoneal dialysis, 158, 158t, 159t, 160
    in liver cirrhosis, 550
Perm-a-Cath catheters, in hemodialysis, 149–151
Permanent colostomy, 88
Persantine. *See* Dipyridamole (Persantine).
PFM. *See* Peak flow meter (PFM).
pH
    gastrointestinal, 99
    hiatal hernia and, 605–606
    in urinalysis, 309
Phacoemulsification, for cataracts, 806
Phagocytes, 283f, 283–286, 285t
Phagocytic cells
    in inflammation, 261

Pharmacology, 312–416
    dialyzable, for hemodialysis, 151–153, 152t, 153t
        for peritoneal dialysis, 158–159
    for immunocompromised host, 268, 268t
    of adrenocorticosteroids, 408–415. *See also* Adrenocorticosteroids.
    of analgesia, 312–320. *See also* Analgesia.
    of anti-infectives, 348–358. *See also* Anti-infectives.
    of anticoagulants, 320–332. *See also* Anticoagulant(s).
    of antidepressants, 332t–335t, 332–335
    of antihypertensives, 336–348. *See also* Antihypertensives.
    of antiseizure medications, 358–364. *See also* Antiseizure medications.
    of digestive tract medications, 365–375. *See also* Digestive tract medications.
    of diuretics, 375–384. *See also* Diuretics.
    of insulins, 384, 387–392, 388t. *See also* Insulin.
    of oral hypoglycemic agents, 384–387, 385t
    of respiratory drugs, 395–403. *See also* Respiratory drugs.
    of sedatives, 403–408. *See also* Sedatives.
Phenergan. *See* Promethazine (Phenergan).
Phenobarbital (Luminal), 360t, 361t, 363t
Phenothiazines, 399t
Phenoxybenzamine (Dibenzyline), 345t
Phentolamine mesylate (Regitine), 345t
Phenylephrine HCl (Neo-Synephrine, Sinex), for rhinitis, coughs, and colds, 401t
Phenylpropanolamine HCl (Contac, Triaminic), for rhinitis, coughs, and colds, 401t
Phenytoin (Dilantin), 360t–362t
Phlebitis, with venous access device, 56t, 61
Phlebography, for thrombophlebitis, 538–539
Phlebothrombosis, 537

Phlegmasia alba dolens, in deep vein thrombosis, 502
Phlegmasia cerulea dolens, in deep vein thrombosis, 502
Phone, documentation issues for, 6, 7t
Phosphate, 296–298
Phosphate-binding antacids, for renal failure, 854
Phosphodiesterase inhibitors, for chronic heart failure, 462t, 464
Phosphorus, in renal failure, 310, 310t
Phototherapy, for depressive disorders, 334
Physical abuse, 709–710
Physical activity. *See* Exercise.
Physical examination
    expedited. *See* Expedited physical assessment.
    for heart failure, 459
    for hemodialysis, 151
    for immunologic alterations, 263
    for peritoneal dialysis, 158, 158t, 159t
Physical therapy, for arthritis, 725
Physiotherapy, chest, 425
Physostigmine salicylate (Isopto Eserine), for glaucoma, 821t
Physostigmine sulfate (Eserine Sulfate), for glaucoma, 821t
PICC. *See* Peripherally inserted central catheter (PICC).
PID. *See* Pelvic inflammatory disease (PID).
Pilocarpine hydrochloride, for glaucoma, 820t
Pin tract infection, 735
Pink eye. *See* Conjunctivitis.
Pink puffer, in emphysema, 428
Pioglitazone (Actos), 385t
Piperacillin, 351
Piperazines, 399t
Piperidines, 399t
Plasma, body water in, 39, 40f
Plasma glucose, in diabetes mellitus, 626
Plasma protein fraction (Plasmanate), for hypovolemic shock, 524
Plasmapheresis
    for Guillain-Barré syndrome, 659t, 659–660, 661t
    for myasthenia gravis, 674
Plasmin, in clot destruction, 323

Plasminogen, in clot destruction, 323
Plaster casting, of fractures, 733
Platelet(s), 274, 281
    administration of, 72t
    in coagulation testing, 323, 324t
    in hemostasis, 321
    in myocardial infarction, 472
    laboratory tests related to, 281, 282t
    origin, development, and structure of, 274, 275f
Platelet count, 281, 325
Plavix. *See* Clopidogrel (Plavix).
Plendil. *See* Felodipine (Plendil).
Plethysmography
    for Buerger's disease, 496
    for deep vein thrombosis, 504
    for peripheral vascular disease, 529
    for thrombophlebitis, 539
Pleural effusion, in renal failure, 145
Pleural friction rub, in respiratory assessment, 20
Pluripotent stem cells, 274, 275f
PMNs. *See* Polymorphonuclear neutrophils (PMNs).
Pneumatic antishock garment (PASG), for hypovolemic shock, 525
Pneumocystis carinii pneumonia (PCP)
    in human immunodeficiency virus infection, 766, 770t
    interventions for, 435
    pathophysiology of, 434
Pneumomediastinum, after tracheostomy, 134
Pneumonia, 431–437
    community care for, 435–436
    diagnostic criteria for, 434–435
    interventions for, 435
    organisms in, 433t
    pathophysiology of, 432–434
    prognosis for, 436
    signs and symptoms of, 434
Pneumothorax
    after tracheostomy, 134
    with venous access device, 59t, 61–62
POAG. *See* Primary open-angle glaucoma (POAG).
Poikilocytosis, 279
Poisoning, food, 556–560
Polaramine. *See* Dexchlorpheniramine (Polaramine).

Polycystic disease of kidneys, 142

Polycythemia, 276

Polydipsia, diabetes and, 625

Polyethylene glycol (PEG) (Colyte, GoLYTELY), 368–369

Polymerase chain reaction (PCR) test, for hepatitis, 564

Polymorphonuclear neutrophils (PMNs), 284

in sputum smear, 108, 108t

Polyphagia, diabetes and, 625

Polys. *See* Polymorphonuclear neutrophils (PMNs).

Polytetrafluoroethylene (PTFE) graft, in hemodialysis, 149, 150f

Polyurea, 625

Polyurethane foams, for wound dressings, 83

Polyuria, 17

in renal dysfunction, 143

Ponstel. *See* Mefenamic acid (Ponstel).

Pontine hemorrhage, 653t

Portal hypertension, in liver cirrhosis, 550

Positioning, for arthritis, 724

Posterior cerebral artery syndrome, 653t

Posterior inferior cerebellar artery syndrome, 653t

Posterior subcapsular cataract, 804–805

Postictal phase, of seizures, 681

Posticteric phase, of hepatitis, 564

Postoperative care

for aortic aneurysm surgery, 491–492

for cataract surgery, 806

for hepatitis, 574

Postpartum depression, 332, 332t

Poststroke depression, in stroke patients, 654t

Post-thrombotic syndrome, from deep vein thrombosis, 502

Post-traumatic head trauma, seizures and, 680

Postural drainage, for pneumonia, 435

Postural hypotension, assessment for, 15

Potassium, 292–294

in hypertension, 517

in pancreatitis, 611

in renal failure, 310, 310t, 853

Potassium-sparing diuretics, 341, 375, 377t, 379, 381t, 383t

Pouching systems, for ostomies, 90t, 90–91

Powder, in pouching principles, 91

PPD skin test. *See* Purified protein derivative (PPD) skin test.

PQRST mnemonic, for pain assessment, 18, 18t

Practice standards, 2

Prandin. *See* Repaglinide (Prandin).

Prazepam (Centrax), 404t

Prazosin (Minipress), 345t

Precose. *See* Acarbose (Precose).

Prednisone (Aristocort, Deltasone)

for gout, 746

for inflammatory bowel disease, 572

for myasthenia gravis, 673t

for renal transplantation, 163t

for rheumatic heart disease, 484

pharmacology of, 414t

Preeclampsia, 512

Pregnancy

human immunodeficiency virus infection and, 764

hypertension and, 512

Preictal phase, of seizures, 681

Preicteric phase, of hepatitis, 563

Premenstrual dysphoric disorder, 332, 332t

Preoperative care, for aortic aneurysm, 491

Preservatives, for blood product administration, 69

Pressure, avoidance of, in wound care, 82

Pressure ulcers, 80

Prevacid. *See* Lansoprazole (Prevacid).

Preveon. *See* Adefavir dipivoxil (Preveon).

Priapism, in sickle cell disease, 802

Prilosec. *See* Omeprazole (Prilosec).

Primacor. *See* Milrinone (Primacor).

Primary intention, in wound closure, 78

Primary open-angle glaucoma (POAG)

pathophysiology of, 816

signs and symptoms of, 817

Primidone (Mysoline), 360t, 361t, 363t

Principalism, 4

Prinivil. *See* Lisinopril (Prinivil, Zestril).

Prinzmetal's angina, 446–447

in coronary artery disease, 468–469

Priscoline. *See* Tolazoline (Priscoline).
Privine. *See* Naphazoline (Privine).
Pro-Banthine. *See* Propantheline bromide (Pro-Banthine).
Probenecid (Benemid), for gout, 745–746
Procardia XL. *See* Nifedipine (Adalat CC, Procardia XL).
Prochlorperazine (Compazine), for nausea and vomiting, 370–371
Proctocolectomy, for inflammatory bowel disease, 573
Professional regulation, 2–3
Progressive stroke, 649
Prokinetics, 367, 371
Proliferative phase, in wound healing, 77
Promethazine (Phenergan), 399t
Propantheline bromide (Pro-Banthine), 373
Prophylaxis
  for deep vein thrombosis, 505
  for immunocompromised host, 268, 268t
Propofol (Diprivan)
  for aggressive/combative behavior, 405t
  for diagnostic procedures, 406t
Propranolol (Inderal)
  for hyperthyroidism, 636, 636t
  pharmacology of, 345t, 404t
Propylthiouracil, for hyperthyroidism, 636, 636t
ProSom. *See* Estazolam (ProSom).
Prostaglandin agonists, for glaucoma, 820t
Prostaglandins, in inflammation, 262
Prostatectomy
  laser, 863
  open, 864
  transurethral ultrasound-guided laser-induced, 863
Prostate-specific antigen (PSA), for benign prostatic hypertrophy, 861–862
Prostatic pain, in renal dysfunction, 143
Protease inhibitors, for human immunodeficiency virus infection, 767, 767t
Protection, barrier, 270
Protein
  in liver cirrhosis, 551

Protein *(Continued)*
  in renal failure, 853
  in renal function testing, 309
  in urinalysis, 102, 102t
  regulators of, 409–413
Prothrombin, in liver cirrhosis, 551
Prothrombin time (PT), 324t, 324–325
  in hepatitis, 565
Proton pump inhibitors, 367
Proventil. *See* Albuterol (Proventil).
Pruritus
  in hepatitis, 566
  from opioids, 314, 315t
Pseudoaneurysm, 487
Pseudoephedrine (Drixoral, Sudafed, Sudafed SA), for rhinitis, coughs, and colds, 401t
Pseudohypertension, in older individuals, 512
Pseudomonas aeruginosa, in pneumonia, 432, 433t
Psychosocial health, 693–719
  alcohol withdrawal syndrome in, 693–696, 694t
  depression in, 696–702. *See also* Depression.
  drug overdose and poisoning in, 703–709. *See also* Drug overdose and poisoning.
  mental/emotional abuse in, 709–714. *See also* Mental/emotional abuse.
  suicidal ideation in, 714–719. *See also* Suicidal ideation.
Psychosocial isolation, in human immunodeficiency virus infection, 769
Psychotic depression, 332, 332t
Psyllium (Metamucil, Fiberall), 367–368, 371–372
PT. *See* Prothrombin time (PT).
PTC. *See* Percutaneous transhepatic cholangiography (PTC).
PTH. *See* Parathyroid hormone (PTH).
PTT. *See* Partial thromboplastin time (PTT).
Pulmonary. *See also* Lung(s).
Pulmonary arteriography, for deep vein thrombosis, 504
Pulmonary artery catheter monitoring
  in cardiogenic shock, 452–453, 453t

Pulmonary artery catheter monitoring (*Continued*)
  in myocardial infarction, 475
Pulmonary edema, in renal failure, 145
Pulmonary embolism (PE)
  from deep vein thrombosis, 502, 503
  from immobilization, 737t
Pulmonary function testing, for emphysema, 428–429
Pulmonary pressure, in heart failure, 459
Pulmonary system
  in increased intracranial pressure, 180–181
  in systemic lupus erythematosus, 756
  in tuberculosis, 441
Pulse
  in cardiovascular assessment, 21
  in hypovolemic shock, 521, 522t, 523
  in peripheral vascular disease, 528
  measurement of, 12, 13t
    principles of care in, 7–8
Pulse deficit, 12
Pulse oximetry
  for Buerger's disease, 496
  for cardiogenic shock, 453
  for oxygenation, 119t, 119–120, 120t
Pulsed lavage, in wound débridement, 81
Pulsus alternans, 13t
Pulsus biferiens, 13t
Pulsus bigeminus, 12, 13t
Pulsus differens, 13t
Pulsus paradoxus, 13t
Pupil dilatation, for cataracts, 805
Pupillary signs, in neurologic assessment, 171
Purified protein derivative (PPD) skin test, 438–439, 439t
Purinethol. *See* Mercaptopurine (Purinethol).
Pursed-lip breathing
  for bronchitis, 425
  for emphysema, 430
Putaminal hemorrhage, 653t
PVD. *See* Peripheral vascular disease (PVD).
Pyelography, intravenous
  in renal failure, 852
  in renal function testing, 309–310
Pyelolithotomy, for renal calculi, 845
Pyelonephritis, pathophysiology of, 856

Pyloroplasty, for peptic ulcer disease, 619
Pyoderma gangrenosum, in inflammatory bowel disease, 570
Pyrazinamide (PZA), for tuberculosis, 441, 441t
Pyridostigmine (Mestinon), for myasthenia gravis, 673t
P8Z. *See* Tripelennamine (P8Z).
PZA. *See* Pyrazinamide (PZA).

Q

Quazepam (Doral), for sleep disorders, 405t
Quinapril (Accupril), 343t
Quinton catheters, in hemodialysis, 149–151

R

RA. *See* Rheumatoid arthritis (RA).
RAA mechanism. *See* Renin-angiotensin-aldosterone (RAA) mechanism.
Racial population, hypertension and, 511–512
Radiation therapy
  for cancer, 784–786, 785t
  for hyperthyroidism, 636, 636t
  for immunologic alterations, 264
Radioactive iodine, for hyperthyroidism, 636–637, 636t
Radiography
  abdominal. *See* Abdominal radiography.
  chest. *See* Chest radiography.
  for peritonitis, 592
  for renal failure, 852
  for rheumatoid arthritis, 723
  for spinal cord injury, 690
Radioisotopes, for angina, 447
Radiology
  for pancreatitis, 611–612
  for renal function testing, 309–310
Radionuclide studies, in myocardial infarction, 475
Ramipril (Altace), 343t
Rancho Los Amigos scale, 177
Random specimens, in urinalysis, 102
Randon's prognostic signs, for pancreatitis, 614, 614t
Ranitidine (Zantac), 366–367

Rapid sequence magnetic resonance imaging, for angina, 447
Raynaud's disease, 531–537
  community care for, 535–536
  diagnostic criteria for, 533–534
  interventions for, 534–535
  pathophysiology of, 532–533
  prognosis for, 536
  signs and symptoms of, 533
RBCs. See Red blood cells (RBCs).
Reactivated tuberculosis, 438
Reagent strips, for urine testing, 102t, 102–103
Rebound tenderness, in intestinal obstruction, 582
Recombinant DNA, for immunologic alterations, 264
  for deep vein thrombosis, 507
  for stroke patients, 655
Rectal temperature measurement, 16
Recurrent brief depression, 332, 332t
Red blood cell (RBC) count, 275–276, 276t
Red blood cells (RBCs), 274–282
  decreased levels of, 275–276, 276t
  erythrocyte sedimentation rate in, 280t, 280–281
  hematocrit in, 279–280, 280t
  hemoglobin in, 279, 279t
  in urinalysis, 308
  increased levels of, 276, 276t
  indices of, 277–279, 278t
  morphology of, 279
  principles of care in assessment of, 274, 275f
  reticulocytes in, 276–277, 277t
Red eye. See Conjunctivitis.
Reducible hernia, 577, 578
Reductase inhibitors, for benign prostatic hypertrophy, 862
Reduction, fracture, 732
Reflex voiding, 834t, 835
Regitine. See Phentolamine mesylate (Regitine).
Reglan. See Metoclopramide (Reglan).
Regulation, of nursing practice, 2–3
Regulator cells, 285
Rejection, of renal transplantation, 162, 164–165
Relaxation techniques, for arthritis, 724

Remicade. See Infliximab (Remicade).
Remodeling
  in bone healing, 730, 730f
  in wound healing, 77
Renal. See also Kidney entries.
Renal activity, sodium in, 291
Renal alterations, 142–165
  assessment of, 142–145, 143t
  hemodialysis for, 145–154. See also Hemodialysis.
  peritoneal dialysis for, 154–160. See also Peritoneal dialysis (PD).
  transplantation for, 160–165. See also Renal transplantation.
Renal biopsy, for renal failure, 852
Renal calculi, 840–846
  community care for, 845–846
  diagnostic criteria for, 841–842
  from immobilization, 737t
  in hyperparathyroidism, 632
  interventions for, 842–845, 843t
  pathophysiology of, 840–841
  prognosis for, 846
  signs and symptoms of, 841
Renal colic
  renal calculi and, 841
  renal dysfunction and, 143
Renal failure, 142, 847–856
  community care for, 855
  diagnostic criteria for, 852
  hyperkalemia in, 294
  interventions for, 853–855
  pathophysiology of, 847t, 847–849, 849t
  prognosis for, 855
  signs and symptoms of, 849, 850t–851t
Renal function
  in systemic lupus erythematosus, 755
  laboratory data in, 304–311
    nitrogenous waste products in, 305–306
    principles of care for, 304–305
    radiologic procedures in, 309–310
    serum electrolytes in, 310, 310t
    urine tests in, 306–309, 307t, 308t
Renal losses, in hypovolemic shock, 520t
Renal osteodystrophy, 145
Renal studies, for hypertension, 514
Renal transplantation, 160–165
  complications of, 161–162

Renal transplantation *(Continued)*
  diet and lifestyle for, 164–165
  immunosuppression for, 162–164, 163t
  management of, 161
  principles of care for, 160–161
  procedure of, 161
Renin-angiotensin-aldosterone (RAA)
      mechanism
  in heart failure, 457
  in hypovolemic shock, 520
ReoPro. *See* Abciximab (ReoPro).
Repaglinide (Prandin), 385t
Reproductive system, 860–878
  benign prostatic hypertrophy and, 860–
      866. *See also* Benign prostatic
      hypertrophy (BPH).
  in renal failure, 851t
  pelvic inflammatory disease and, 866–
      870, 868t
  sexually transmitted diseases and,
      870–878. *See also* Sexually trans-
      mitted disease (STD).
Rescriptor. *See* Delavirdine (Rescriptor).
Reserpine (Serpasil, Serpalan), 347t
Respiration
  assessment of, 19
  measurement of, 13–14
  principles of care for, 9–10
Respiratory depression, from opioids,
      314, 315t
Respiratory distress, after tracheostomy,
      134
Respiratory drugs, 395–403
  for bronchial obstruction, 392–396,
      394t–396t
  for rhinitis, cough, and colds, 397–
      403, 398t–402t
  principles of care for, 395
Respiratory failure, in oxygenation,
      117–118, 118t
Respiratory isolation, 271
Respiratory rate, in hypovolemic shock,
      521, 522t
Respiratory support, for Guillain-Barré
      syndrome, 659–660
Respiratory system, 417–444
  asthma and, 417–422. *See also*
      Asthma.
  bronchitis and, 422–427. *See also*
      Bronchitis.

Respiratory system *(Continued)*
  emphysema and, 427–431
  in expedited physical assessment,
      19–20
  in Guillain-Barré syndrome, 658
  in renal failure, 145, 851t
  in spinal cord injury, 691
  pneumonia and, 431–437. *See also*
      Pneumonia.
  tuberculosis and, 437–444. *See also*
      Tuberculosis (TB).
Respite care, in Alzheimer's disease, 647
Rest
  for hepatitis, 565
  for systemic lupus erythematosus, 758
Rest pain
  in Buerger's disease, 495
  in peripheral vascular disease, 527
Restless legs syndrome, in renal failure,
      144
Restoril. *See* Temazepam (Restoril).
Reticulocyte count, 276–277, 277t
Retinitis, cytomegalovirus, 766, 771t
Retrograde filling test, in thrombo-
      phlebitis, 543–544
Retrograde ureteroscopy, for renal
      calculi, 844
Retrovir. *See* Zidovudine (Retrovir,
      AZT).
Reverse isolation, for immunocom-
      promised host, 267–268
Reversible ischemic neurologic deficit,
      650
Rh blood group, 65
Rhabdomyolysis, in acute renal failure,
      848
Rheumatic heart disease (RHD), 481–486
  community care for, 484–486
  diagnostic criteria for, 483–484
  interventions for, 484
  pathophysiology of, 482–483
  prognosis for, 486
  signs and symptoms of, 483
Rheumatoid arthritis (RA), 262, 262t
  diagnostic criteria for, 722
  pathophysiology of, 720
  signs and symptoms of, 721–722
Rheumatoid factor (RF), 722
Rheumatrex. *See* Methotrexate (Folex,
      Rheumatrex).

Rhinitis
  allergic, 774–775
  drugs for, 397–403, 398t–402t
Rhonchi, in respiratory assessment, 20
Rifampin, for tuberculosis, 441, 441t
Right ventricular failure, in cardiogenic shock, 452–453, 454
Ritonavir (Norvir), for human immunodeficiency virus, 767, 767t
Robitussin. *See* Guaifenesin (glycerol guaiacolate, Robitussin).
Roentgenography, for rheumatic heart disease, 484
Rosiglitazone (Avandia), 385t
Rowasa. *See* Mesalamine (Asacol, Pentasa, Rowasa).
rt-PA. *See* Recombinant tissue plasminogen activator (rt-PA).
Rubor, in peripheral vascular disease, 527
Ruptured aortic aneurysm, 488, 489–490
Russell's traction, for fractures, 734

S

Saccular aortic aneurysm, 487
SAD PERSONS scale, 716–717
Safety
  for Alzheimer's disease, 647
  for Buerger's disease, 497–499
Salem sump tube, 95, 95f
Salicylates
  for arthritis, 724
  for rheumatic heart disease, 484
Saline
  for hypovolemic shock, 524
  pharmacology of, 368
Salmonella, in food poisoning, 556–557
Salsalate (Disalcid), 317, 318t
Sample collection, for tuberculosis, 440
Sandimmune. *See* Cyclosporine (Sandimmune).
Saquinavir (SQV, Invirase, Fortovase), for human immunodeficiency virus, 767, 767t
Scene size-up, in first aid for injuries, 24
Schistocytes, 279
SCI. *See* Spinal cord injury (SCI).
Scintigraphy, for osteoporosis, 750
Sclerotherapy
  for liver cirrhosis, 554

Sclerotherapy *(Continued)*
  for thrombophlebitis, 544–545
Scopolamine (Transderm Scop), 369–370
Sealants, skin, in pouching principles, 91
Seasonal depressive disorder, 332, 332t
Secobarbital (Seconal), for sleep disorders, 405t
Secondary glaucoma, 817
Secondary hypertension, 510, 510t. *See also* Hypertension (HTN).
Secondary intention, in wound closure, 78
Secretions, in tracheostomy care, 132–133
Sedatives, 403–408
  decision-making for use of, 404–406, 405t–407t
  for diagnostic procedures, 405, 406t
  principles of care for use of, 404
Sediment, urinary, in renal function, 309
Segmental colectomy, for inflammatory bowel disease, 573
Segmental plethysmography, for peripheral vascular disease, 529
Segmented neutrophils, 284
  elevated levels of, 286–287
Segs. *See* Segmented neutrophils.
Seizures, 680–686
  community care for, 685–686
  diagnostic criteria for, 681–684
  in hemorrhagic stroke, 655, 656t
  interventions for, 684–685, 685t
  pathophysiology of, 680–681
  prognosis for, 686
  signs and symptoms of, 681, 682t–683t
Selective serotonin reuptake inhibitors (SSRIs), 333, 334t
Selegiline (Eldepryl), for Parkinson's disease, 678t
Self-monitoring of blood glucose (SMBG), 110, 110t
Self-regulation, of nursing practice, 3
Semipermeable membrane, in fluid therapy, 41–42, 42f
Senile cataracts, 804
Senna (Senokot, Fletcher's Castoria), 368
Sensorimotor disability/immobility, in stroke patients, 654t
Sensory dysfunction, in Guillain-Barré syndrome, 658

Sensory function, 804–829
    cataracts and, 804–808
    conjunctivitis and, 809–815. See also
        Conjunctivitis.
    glaucoma and, 815–824. See also Glau-
        coma.
    Meniere's disease and, 824–829. See
        also Meniere's disease.
SEP testing. See Somatosensory evoked
    potential (SEP) testing.
Sepsis, with venous access device, 57t,
    61
Septicemia, blood culture for, 300, 301
Sequestration crisis, 799–800
Serax. See Oxazepam (Serax).
Serology
    in immunologic alterations, 264
    in infection, 303–304
    in peptic ulcer disease, 617
Serotonin blockers, for nausea and
    vomiting, 371
Serotonin reuptake inhibitors (SSRIs), for
    depression, 699
Serpalan. See Reserpine (Serpasil,
    Serpalan).
Serpasil. See Reserpine (Serpasil,
    Serpalan).
Serum albumin, administration of, 72t
Serum amylase
    in biliary disease, 597
    in intestinal obstruction, 583
    in pancreatitis, 611
Serum bilirubin, for biliary disease, 597
Serum calcium
    in hyperparathyroidism, 632–633
    in pancreatitis, 611
Serum creatinine
    for renal failure, 852
    in renal function, 305–306
Serum electrolytes, in renal function,
    309t, 310
Serum glucose, in pancreatitis, 611
Serum hepatitis, 561
Serum lipase, in pancreatitis, 611
Serum lipid profile, for hypertension, 514
Serum potassium, in pancreatitis, 611
Serum transaminases, in hepatitis, 565
Sexual activity, after renal
    transplantation, 164
Sexually transmitted disease (STD),
    870–878

Sexually transmitted disease (STD)
        (Continued)
    community care for, 877
    diagnostic criteria for, 875–876
    interventions for, 876–877
    pathophysiology of, 870–875, 871t–
        874t
    prognosis for, 877
    signs and symptoms of, 875
Sharp débridement, 81
Shift to the left, of bands, 286
Shift to the right, of segs, 286–287
Shigella, in food poisoning, 557
Shock, cardiogenic. See Cardiogenic
        shock.
    hypovolemic. See Hypovolemic shock.
    neurogenic, 688
    spinal, 688
Short-term acute central catheters, in
        fluid therapy, 49–50, 51t
Shy-Drager syndrome, spinal cord injury
        and, 836
SIADH. See Syndrome of inappropriate
        antidiuretic hormone (SIADH).
Sickle cell anemia, 279
Sickle cell disease, 799–803, 800t
Side-arm traction, for fractures, 734
Sigmoid colostomy, 89t
Sigmoidoscopy, in inflammatory bowel
        disease, 570
Silastic catheters, in hemodialysis,
        149–151
Simple chronic bronchitis, 423
Simple fracture, 729
Sinequan. See Doxepin (Sinequan).
Sinex. See Phenylephrine HCl (Neo-
        Synephrine, Sinex).
Sinus bradycardia, 476
Skeletal traction, for fractures, 733–734
Skin
    fractures and, 739
    in cardiovascular assessment, 20
    in human immunodeficiency virus in-
        fection, 769
    in hypovolemic shock, 520t, 521, 522t
    in meningitis, 664, 665t
    in peripheral vascular disease, 527,
        528
    in pouching principles, 91
    in spinal cord injury, 691

Skin *(Continued)*
  in systemic lupus erythematosus, 755,
    759
  in varicose veins, 543
  peristomal, 91
  radiation effects on, 785, 785t
  tears of, 79
  wound drainage systems and, 86
Skin cancer, from renal transplantation,
    162
Skin test
  for allergies, 776
  tuberculin, 438–439, 439t
Skin traction, for fractures, 733
SLE. *See* Systemic lupus erythematosus
    (SLE).
Sleep disorders, medications for, 405,
    405t
Sliding hiatal hernia
  pathophysiology of, 602–603, 603f
  signs and symptoms of, 604
Slit-lamp examination
  for cataracts, 805
  for glaucoma, 818
Slo-bid. *See* Theophylline (Slo-bid, Slo-
    phyllin, Somaphyllin, Theo-Dur,
    Theolair-SR).
Slo-phyllin. *See* Theophylline (Slo-bid,
    Slo-phyllin, Somaphyllin, Theo-Dur,
    Theolair-SR).
Slough, 78, 78t
Small bowel obstruction, 581
SMBG. *See* Self-monitoring of blood
    glucose (SMBG).
Smoking
  bronchitis and, 425
  Buerger's disease and, 494
  emphysema and, 428, 429, 430
  hypertension and, 516
  peptic ulcer disease and, 616
Snellen visual acuity test, for cataracts,
    805
Social services, for emphysema, 431
Sodium, 291–292
  in intravenous therapy, 43
  in renal failure, 310, 310t, 853
  urinary, 309
Sodium bicarbonate
  for hypovolemic shock, 524
  for renal failure, 854

Sodium depletion hyponatremia, 292
Sodium heparin, for hemodialysis, 152,
    152t
Sodium intake, hypertension and, 517
Sodium salicylate (Urasel-5), 317, 318t
Soft tissue injury, first aid for, 35–36, 36t
Solu-Medrol. *See* Methylprednisolone
    (Solu-Medrol).
Solubilizing agents, for gallstones,
    598–599
Somaphyllin. *See* Theophylline (Slo-bid,
    Slo-phyllin, Somaphyllin, Theo-Dur,
    Theolair-SR).
Somatosensory evoked potential (SEP)
    testing, 690
Somogyi phenomenon, from insulin
    therapy, 391
Sonata. *See* Zaleplon (Sonata).
Spasm, venous, 56t, 61
Spasticity, in multiple sclerosis, 667,
    668t
Speaking valve, 134
Specific gravity, in urinalysis, 308–309
Specimen collection, bedside, 98–114.
    See also Bedside specimen
    collection.
Sphincter incompetence, in neurogenic
    bladder, 831
Spider veins, in thrombophlebitis, 543
Spina bifida, 838
Spinal cord injury (SCI), 686–692
  community care for, 690–692
  diagnostic criteria for, 690
  interventions for, 690, 691t
  neurogenic bladder and, 832–836, 834t
  pathophysiology of, 687t, 687–688
  signs and symptoms of, 688–690, 689t
Spinal shock, 688
Spine injury, cervical, 31–32, 32t, 33t
Spiral fracture, 729
Spironolactone (Aldactone)
  for chronic heart failure, 462t, 464
  pharmacology of, 379, 381t, 383t
Spontaneous bacterial peritonitis, in liver
    cirrhosis, 550
Spontaneous voiding, spinal cord injury
    and, 833, 834t
Sputum
  bedside specimen collection of, 105–
    108, 107t, 108t

Sputum *(Continued)*
  in chronic bronchitis, 423–424
  in culture report, 302
  in pneumonia, 434
  in tuberculosis, 439–440
SQV. *See* Saquinavir (SQV, Invirase, Fortovase).
SSRIs. *See* Serotonin reuptake inhibitors (SSRIs).
Stable angina, 446
  in coronary artery disease, 468–469
Stabs, 284
Standards of Clinical Nursing Practice, 2
Standards of nursing, 2–7
  decision-making in, 4–6, 5t–7t
  principles of care in, 2–4
Standards of practice, 2
  decision-making and, 4–5, 5t
Staphylococcus
  in food poisoning, 557
  in pneumonia, 432, 433t
  methicillin-resistant, 271, 272
Stasis, in deep vein thrombosis, 501
Stasis ulcer, in peripheral vascular disease, 528
Status asthmaticus, 417
Status epilepticus, 681
Stavudine (d4T, Zerit), for human immunodeficiency virus, 766–767, 767t
STD. *See* Sexually transmitted disease (STD).
Steatorrhea, in cholecystitis, 596
Steel needles, in intravenous therapy, with venous access device, 49, 50t
Stelazine. *See* Trifluoperazine (Stelazine).
Stenosis, tracheal, after tracheostomy, 135
Stenting
  biliary/pancreatic, 97
  for intestinal obstruction, 584
  for renal calculi, 844
Steroids
  for bronchitis, 425
  monocytes and, 275
Stoma assessment, 89, 89t
Stoma irrigation, 90
Stomach stapling, for obesity, 588, 589f
Stomatitis, in renal failure, 145
Stool(s), fatty, in cholecystitis, 596

Stool examination, in inflammatory bowel disease, 570
Stool softeners, pharmacology of, 369
Straight catheter specimen collection, 104
Straight skeletal traction, for fractures, 734
Strangulated hernia, 577
Streptococcus pneumoniae, 432, 433t
Streptomycin, for tuberculosis, 441, 441t
Stress
  body temperature and, 11
  in systemic lupus erythematosus, 760
Stress echocardiography, for angina, 447
Stress electrocardiography, for coronary artery disease, 470
Stress thallium test
  for angina, 447
  for coronary artery disease, 470
Stress ulcers, gastric pH in, 99
Stretch receptors, heart rate and, 8
Stroke. *See also* Cerebrovascular accident (CVA).
Stroke volume, heart rate and, 8
Struvite stones, 840
Subcutaneous emphysema, after tracheostomy, 134
Subendocardial ischemia, 474
Sublimaze. *See* Fentanyl (Sublimaze).
Sublingual nitroglycerin, for angina, 448
Subsyndromal symptomatic depression, 332, 332t
Sudafed. *See* Pseudoephedrine (Drixoral, Sudafed, Sudafed SA).
Suicidal ideation, 714–719
  community care for, 718–719
  diagnostic criteria for, 716–717
  interventions for, 717–718
  pathophysiology of, 715–716
  prognosis for, 719
  signs and symptoms of, 716
Sular. *See* Nisoldipine (Sular).
Sulfadoxine, 354–355
Sulfamethoxazole, 354–355
Sulfasalazine (Azulfidine)
  for inflammatory bowel disease, 571
  for irritable bowel disease, 373–374
Sulfinpyrazone (Anturane), for gout, 745–746
Sulfisoxazole, 354–355

Sulfonamides, 354–355
Sulfonylureas, 385t, 385–386
Sunlight, for systemic lupus
    erythematosus, 758–759
Superficial thrombophlebitis, 538
Superficial veins, in thrombophlebitis,
    542
Superinfection, 349–350
Suppressor T cells, 260
Suppurative thrombophlebitis, 538
Suprapubic area, in genitourinary
    assessment, 22
Suprapubic catheter specimen collection,
    104
Surgical débridement, 81
Susphrine, 393, 394t
Sustiva. See Efavirenz (Sustiva, DMP-
    266).
Swallowing reflex, in gastrointestinal
    assessment, 21
Symmetrel. See Amantadine
    (Symmetrel).
Sympathetic nervous system
  heart rate and, 8
  in heart failure, 456–457
Sympatholytics, 340, 346t
Sympathomimetics, for chronic heart
    failure, 462t, 464
Syndrome of inappropriate antidiuretic
    hormone (SIADH), 292
  in Guillain-Barré syndrome, 659t
Synovectomy, for arthritis, 726
Synovial fluid, in rheumatoid arthritis,
    722
Synthetic grafts, in hemodialysis, 149,
    150f
Syphilis, 870, 871t
  screening tests for, 876
Systemic lupus erythematosus (SLE),
    262, 262t, 753–763
  community care for, 761–762
  diagnostic criteria for, 756–758, 757t
  interventions for, 758–761
  pathophysiology of, 753–754, 755t
  prognosis for, 762–763
  signs and symptoms of, 754t, 754–756
Systemic vascular congestion, in liver
    cirrhosis, 551–552
Systolic pressure, 9
  measurement of, 15

T

T cells, 260, 285
Tachycardia, 13t
Tachypnea, 14
Tacrolimus (FK 506), in renal
    transplantation, 163t
Tagamet. See Cimetidine (Tagamet).
Talking tracheostomy, 134
Tamsulosin (Flomax), 345t
Tapazole. See Methimazole (Tapazole).
Tavist. See Clemastine fumarate (Tavist).
Taxanes, for cancer, 783, 784t
TB. See Tuberculosis (TB).
T&C. See Type and crossmatch (T&C).
3TC. See Lamivudine (3TC, Epivir).
TCAs. See Tricyclic antidepressants
    (TCAs).
TE fistula. See Tracheoesophageal (TE)
    fistula.
Tears, skin, 79
TEDS. See Thromboembolic disease
    stockings (TEDS).
Tegretol. See Carbamazepine (Tegretol).
Teleologic theories, 4
Telmisartan (Micardis), 344t
Temazepam (Restoril), for sleep
    disorders, 405t
Temperature
  in integumentary assessment, 19
  measurement of, 15–16
  of blood and blood products, 67
  principles of care for, 10–11
Temporary colostomy, 88
Temporary tracheostomy, 130–132
Tenckhoff catheter, for peritoneal
    dialysis, 156
Tenex. See Guanfacine (Tenex).
Tenormin. See Atenolol (Tenormin).
Tenosynovectomy, for arthritis, 726
Tensilon test, for myasthenia gravis, 672
Terazosin (Hytrin), 345t
Terbutaline sulfate (Brethine), 393, 394t
Tertiary intention, in wound closure, 78
Tessalon Perles. See Benzonatate
    (Tessalon Perles).
Tetanus, from fractures, 739
Tetany, in hypoparathyroidism, 639
Tetracyclic antidepressants, 333, 334t
Tetracyclines, 352–353
Tetrahydrozoline (Tyzine), for rhinitis,
    coughs, and colds, 401t

Tetraplegia, 686–687

Thalamectomy, for Parkinson's disease, 678

Thalamic hemorrhage, 653t

Thalassemia, in anemia, 792

Thallium test
for angina, 447
for coronary artery disease, 470

Theophylline (Slo-bid, Slo-phyllin, Somaphyllin, Theo-Dur, Theolair-SR), 393, 395t

Thermometers, for temperature measurement, 15–16

Thiamine, for drug overdose and poisoning, 705

Thiazides, 341, 375, 377t, 379, 381t, 383t

Thiazolidinediones, 385t, 387

Thirst, diabetes and, 625

Thoracentesis, for sputum samples, 106, 107t

Thoracic aortic aneurysm, 487. See also Aortic aneurysm.

Thorazine. See Chlorpromazine (Thorazine).

Thrill, arteriovenous fistula and, 148

Thrombocytes. See Platelets.

Thrombocytopenia, 281, 282t

Thrombocytosis, 281

Thromboembolic disease stockings (TEDS)
for deep vein thrombosis, 505
for thrombophlebitis, 540

Thromboembolus, from deep vein thrombosis, 502

Thrombolysis, for cardiogenic shock, 454

Thrombolytic therapy
for deep vein thrombosis, 507
for myocardial infarction, 478
for strokes, 651–655

Thrombophlebitis, 537–541, 538t

Thrombopoietin (TPO), 75t

Thromboprophylaxis, for deep vein thrombosis, 505

Thrombosis
of arteriovenous grafts and fistulas, 149
with venous access device, 57t, 61

Thrombotic stroke, 649

Thromboxane, in inflammation, 262

Thrombus
from immobilization, 737t
pathophysiology of, 501

Thrush, 766, 770t

Thymectomy, for myasthenia gravis, 674

Thyroid hormones, in hyperthyroidism, 634

Thyroid-releasing hormone (TRH), 640

Thyroid-stimulating hormone (TSH), 636t, 640, 641–642

Thyroid storm, 635
treatment for, 637

Thyroidectomy, for hyperthyroidism, 636, 636t

L-Thyroxine, in hypothyroidism, 636t, 641–642

TIA. See Transient ischemic attack (TIA).

Tiamate. See Diltiazem (Cardizem CD, Cardizem SR, Dilacor XR, Diltia XT, Tiamate, Tiazac).

Tiazac. See Diltiazem (Cardizem CD, Cardizem SR, Dilacor XR, Diltia XT, Tiamate, Tiazac).

Ticarcillin, 351

Ticlopidine (Ticlid), 330, 331t

Tidal volume, 10

Timolol (Bicadren), 345t

Timolol maleate (Timoptic), for glaucoma, 820t

Tissue damage, hyperkalemia in, 294

Tissue injury, 78, 78t

Tissue macrophages, 285, 285t

Tissue perfusion, in heart failure, 458

Tissue plasminogen activator (t-PA), in clot destruction, 323

Tissue-specific macrophages, in inflammation, 261

Tissue thromboplastin, prothrombin time and, 324

TMP-SMX. See Trimethoprim-sulfamethoxazole (TMP-SMX).

TMS. See Transcranial magnetic stimulation (TMS).

Tobramycin, pharmacology of, 354

Todd's paralysis, in seizures, 681

Tofranil. See Imipramine (Tofranil).

Tolazamide (Tolinase), 385t

Tolazoline (Priscoline), 345t

Tolbutamide (Airiness), 385t

Tolinase. *See* Tolazamide (Tolinase).
Tonic-atonic seizures, 685, 686t
Tonic-clonic seizures, 685, 686t
Tonicity
  in fluid therapy, 42
  of intravenous fluids, 43–45
Tonometry
  for cataracts, 805
  for glaucoma, 818
Tonsillopharyngitis, 482–483
Topamax. *See* Topiramate (Topamax).
Tophaceous gout, 742, 743
Topiramate (Topamax), 360t, 361t
Toradol. *See* Ketorolac (Toradol).
Torsemide (Demadex), 378
Total hip arthroplasty, 726–727
Total hip replacement, 726
Total knee arthroplasty, 727–728
Total knee replacement, 727–728
Toxic agent–induced hepatitis, 560, 560t
Toxic megacolon, from inflammatory
    bowel disease, 569
Toxicity
  from oxygen therapy, 125
  in oxygenation, 116–117
t-PA. *See* Tissue plasminogen activator
    (t-PA).
Trabeculectomy, for glaucoma, 819
Trabeculoplasty, for glaucoma, 819
Tracheal stenosis, after tracheostomy,
    135
Tracheoesophageal (TE) fistula, after
    tracheostomy, 136
Tracheomalacia, after tracheostomy, 136
Tracheostomy care, 128–135
  assessment of, 132–133
  communication in, 133–134
  complications in, 134–135
  decannulation in, 133
  principles of, 128–132, 129t, 131t
Trachoma
  interventions for, 812
  pathophysiology of, 809
  prognosis for, 814
  signs and symptoms of, 810
Traction, 732, 733–735
Traditional open appendectomy, 548
Trandate. *See* Labetalol (Normodyne,
    Trandate).
Trandolapril (Mavik), 343t

Transaminases, in hepatitis, 565
Transcellular space, 39, 40f
Transcranial magnetic stimulation (TMS),
    for depressive disorders, 334–335
Transderm Scop. *See* Scopolamine
    (Transderm Scop).
Transdermal administration, of opioids,
    315
Transesophageal echocardiography, for
    aortic aneurysm, 489
Transfusion reactions, blood, 67, 68t
Transient bacteremia, blood culture for,
    300–301
Transient ischemic attack (TIA)
  interventions for, 651–655
  pathophysiology of, 649–650
Transmural myocardial necrosis, 475
Transparent adhesive films, 82
Transplantation
  for hepatitis, 566
  for liver cirrhosis, 554, 555
Transthoracic echocardiography, for
    aortic aneurysm, 489
Transtracheal aspiration, for sputum
    samples, 106, 107t
Transurethral laser ablation of prostate
    (TULAP), 863
Transurethral microwave thermotherapy
    (TUMT), 863
Transurethral needle ablation (TUNA),
    863
Transurethral resection of prostate
    (TURP), 863
Transurethral ultrasound-guided laser-
    induced prostatectomy (TULIP), 863
Transverse colostomy, 89t
Transverse fracture, 729
Tranxene. *See* Clorazepate (Tranxene).
Trauma. *See* Injury(ies).
Traveling clot, from deep vein
    thrombosis, 502
Trazodone (Desyrel)
  adverse effects of, 333, 334t
  for sleep disorders, 405t
Trendelenburg test, for varicose veins,
    543–544
TRH. *See* Thyroid-releasing hormone
    (TRH).
Triaminic. *See* Phenylpropanolamine HCl
    (Contac, Triaminic).

Triamterene (Dyrenium), 379

Triazolam (Halcion), for sleep disorders, 405t

Trichomoniasis, 870, 873t

Tricyclic antidepressants (TCAs)
    adverse effects of, 333, 334t
    dosages of, 333, 333t
    for depression, 699

Trifluoperazine (Stelazine), for aggressive/combative behavior, 405t

Triglycerides, in coronary artery disease, 468, 469–470

Trihexyphenidyl (Artane), for Parkinson's disease, 678t

Triiodothyronine (T₃), in hypothyroidism, 636t, 641–642

Trileptal. See Oxcarbazepine (Trileptal).

Trilisate. See Choline magnesium trisalicylate (Trilisate).

Trimethoprim-sulfamethoxazole (TMP-SMX)
    for human immunodeficiency virus, 768
    pharmacology of, 354–355

Tripelennamine (P8Z), 398t

Troponin I, in myocardial infarction, 474

Trough level, of antibiotics, 349, 349t

Trousseau's sign, in hypoparathyroidism, 639

Trovafloxacin, pharmacology of, 353–354

Truss, for hernias, 577–578

TSH. See Thyroid-stimulating hormone (TSH).

T-tubes, 93–95, 94f
    for gallstones, 600

Tuberculin skin test, 438–439, 439t

Tuberculosis (TB), 437–444
    community care for, 442–443
    diagnostic criteria for, 438–440, 439t
    interventions for, 439t, 440–442
    isolation of, 271
    Mycobacterium, 766, 771t
    pathophysiology of, 437–438
    prognosis for, 443
    signs and symptoms of, 438

Tubular damage, in acute renal failure, 848

Tuinal. See Pentobarbital (Nembutal, Tuinal).

TULAP. See Transurethral laser ablation of prostate (TULAP).

TULIP. See Transurethral ultrasound-guided laser-induced prostatectomy (TULIP).

Tumarkin's ortholytic crisis, 826

Tumors, 780–789. See also Cancer.
    brain, 183–187, 184t, 185t, 187t

TUMT. See Transurethral microwave thermotherapy (TUMT).

TUNA. See Transurethral needle ablation (TUNA).

Tunneled catheters, in intravenous therapy, 52t, 54f

Turgor, in integumentary assessment, 19

TURP. See Transurethral resection of prostate (TURP).

12-hour urine collection, 103

12-lead electrocardiogram
    for angina, 447
    for hypertension, 514
    for myocardial infarction, 474–475

24-hour urine collection, 103

2-hour urine collection, 104

Tympanic membrane thermometer, 16

Type and crossmatch (T&C), 65–67

Tyzine. See Tetrahydrozoline (Tyzine).

U

1592U90. See Ziagen (Abacavir, 1592U89).

UC. See Ulcerative colitis (UC).

UDCA. See Ursodeoxycholic acid (UDCA).

UKM. See Urea kinetic modeling (UKM).

Ulcer(s)
    arterial, 79
    diabetic, 79–80
    in Buerger's disease, 495–496
    in peripheral vascular disease, 528
    mucosal, in renal failure, 145
    peptic, 615–623. See also Peptic ulcer disease (PUD).
    pressure, 80
    venous, 80
        in thrombophlebitis, 543

Ulcerative colitis (UC), 568. See also Inflammatory bowel disease (IBD).

Ulcerogenesis, in peptic ulcer disease, 615

Ultrasonic lithotripsy, for renal calculi, 844
Ultrasonography
  Doppler. *See* Doppler ultrasonography.
  for aortic aneurysm, 489
  for biliary disease, 597
  for deep vein thrombosis, 504
  for liver cirrhosis, 553
  for myocardial infarction, 475
  for pancreatitis, 612
  for peritonitis, 592
  for renal calculi, 841–842
  for renal failure, 852
Ultraviolet light, for systemic lupus erythematosus, 758–759
Umbilical hernia, 577
Uncomplicated laparoscopic appendectomy, 548
Unilateral neglect, in stroke patients, 654t
Unisom. *See* Doxylamine (Unisom).
Univasc. *See* Moexipril (Univasc).
Universal donor, 65
Universal recipient, 65
Unstable angina, 446
  in coronary artery disease, 468–469
  treatment for, 448–449
Upper gastrointestinal tract, 595–623
  cholelithiasis and cholecystitis and, 595–602. *See also* Gallstones.
  hiatal hernia and, 602–609. *See also* Hiatal hernia.
  pancreatitis and, 609–615. *See also* Pancreatitis.
  peptic ulcer and, 615–623. *See also* Peptic ulcer disease (PUD).
Urasel-5. *See* Sodium salicylate (Urasel-5).
Urea kinetic modeling (UKM), in dialysis assessment, 148
Urea (Ureaphil), 378
Uremia, 792
Uremic factor, 145
Uremic frost, 144
Ureter(s), radiography of, 309
Ureterolithotomy, for renal calculi, 845
Ureteroscopy, for renal calculi, 844
Uric acid
  in gout, 742
  in renal function, 306

Uric acid stones, 840
Uricosuric agents, for gout, 745–746
Urinalysis, 102
  in benign prostatic hypertrophy, 861
  in neurogenic bladder, 832
  in renal calculi, 842
  in renal failure, 852
  in renal function testing, 307t, 307–309, 308t
  in sexually transmitted diseases, 876
Urinary diversion, principles of care for, 88
Urinary frequency, in renal dysfunction, 143
Urinary retention
  from opioids, 314, 315t
  in Guillain-Barré syndrome, 659t
Urinary sediment and sodium, in renal function, 309
Urinary tract, 830–859
  infection of, 856–859
    from immobilization, 737t
  neurogenic bladder and, 830–840. *See also* Neurogenic bladder.
  renal calculi and, 840–846. *See also* Renal calculi.
  renal failure and, 847–856. *See also* Renal failure.
Urination, in diabetes, 625
Urine
  bedside specimen collection of, 101–105, 102t
  in genitourinary assessment, 21–22
Urine amylase, in pancreatitis, 611
Urine output
  in hypovolemic shock, 521, 522t
  measurement of, 16–17
  principles of care in, 11–12
Urine protein, in renal function, 309
Urine sedimentation, in urine collection, 105
Urine testing
  for ketones, 111–114
  of renal function, 306–309, 307t, 308t
Urobilinogen, in urinalysis, 102, 102t
Urodynamic testing, for neurogenic bladder, 832
Urogram, for renal calculi, 841
Urokinase, for deep vein thrombosis, 507
Urokinase plasminogen activator, in clot destruction, 323

Urolithiasis. *See* Renal calculi.
Ursodeoxycholic acid (UDCA), for gallstones, 598–599
Ursodiol (Actigall), for gallstones, 598–599
Urticaria, 775
Utilitarianism, 4
Uveitis, in inflammatory bowel disease, 570

V

Vaccine. *See also* Immunizations.
  bacille Calmette-Guérin, 442
  for hepatitis, 567
Vacuum reservoir, in wound drainage, 85
VAD. *See* Vascular access device (VAD).
Vagal nerve stimulation (VNS), for seizures, 685
Vaginitis, in human immunodeficiency virus, 766, 770t
Vagotomy, for peptic ulcer disease, 619
Valacyclovir, 357
Valium. *See* Diazepam (Valium).
Valproic acid (Depakote), 360t, 363t
Valsartan (Diovan), 344t
Valvular insufficiency, in thrombophlebitis, 542
Valvulitis, murmur of, 483
Vancomycin, 355–356
Vancomycin-resistant enterococci (VRE), 271–272
Vantronol. *See* Ephedrine sulfate (Ephedsol, Vantronol).
Variant angina, 446–447
Varicose veins, 541–546
  community care for, 545
  diagnostic criteria for, 543–544
  interventions for, 544–545
  pathophysiology of, 542–543
  prognosis for, 545
  signs and symptoms of, 543
Vascular access, in hemodialysis, 148–151, 150f
Vascular access device (VAD), 48–64
  care and maintenance of, 60
  central venous catheters in, 49–51, 51t–53t, 54f, 55f
  complications of, 58t–59t, 60–63, 62t, 63t
  peripheral catheters in, 49, 50t

Vascular access device (VAD) *(Continued)*
  principles of care for, 48–49
  selection of, 51–60
  site care and maintenance for, 63–64
Vascular assessment, in fractures, 736
Vascular brain tumors, 185
Vascular congestion, in liver cirrhosis, 551–552
Vascular device–related infection, 302
Vascular endothelial injury, in thrombophlebitis, 537
Vascular phase, of hemostasis, 321
  of inflammation, 261
Vascular stent, for coronary artery disease, 470
Vascular syndrome, in diabetes, 624, 625
Vascular system, 487–546
  aortic aneurysm and, 487–494. *See also* Aortic aneurysm.
  Buerger's disease and, 494–500. *See also* Buerger's disease.
  deep vein thrombosis and, 500–509. *See also* Deep vein thrombosis (DVT).
  hypertension and, 509–519. *See also* Hypertension (HTN).
  hypovolemic shock and, 519–525. *See also* Hypovolemic shock.
  peripheral vascular disease and, 526–531. *See also* Peripheral vascular disease (PVD).
  Raynaud's disease and, 531–537. *See also* Raynaud's disease.
  thrombophlebitis and, 537–541, 538t
  varicose veins and, 541–546. *See also* Varicose veins.
Vasoconstriction, in Buerger's disease, 496
Vasodilation, in Buerger's disease, 496–497, 498f
Vasodilators
  for chronic heart failure, 464
  pharmacology of, 340–341, 347t
Vasopressin, for liver cirrhosis, 554
Vasopressors, for hypovolemic shock, 524
Vasospasm
  in hemorrhagic stroke, 655, 656t
  in hemostasis, 321

Vasotec. *See* Enalapril (Vasotec).
Vein ligation and stripping, for thrombophlebitis, 544
Venipuncture, for blood culture, 301
Venlafaxine, adverse effects of, 333, 334t
Venography
  for deep vein thrombosis, 504
  for thrombophlebitis, 508–509
  for varicose veins, 544
Venous obstruction, in thrombophlebitis, 542
Venous spasm, with venous access device, 56t, 61
Venous stasis, in thrombophlebitis, 537, 543
Venous thrombosis. *See* Thrombophlebitis.
Venous ulcers, 79
Ventilation
  for hypovolemic shock, 523
  in meningitis, 664, 665t
  in respiration, 9
Ventilation/perfusion scan, for deep vein thrombosis, 504–505
Ventral hernia, 577
Ventricular fibrillation, 476
Ventricular remodeling, in heart failure, 457
Ventricular tachycardia, 476
Veracity, definition and rules of care for, 6t
Verapamil (Calan, Calan SR, Covera-HS, Isoptin, Verelan), 344t
Verbal response, in Glasgow Coma Scale, 167t, 167–169
Verelan. *See* Verapamil (Calan, Calan SR, Covera-HS, Isoptin, Verelan).
Vermiform appendix, 547
Vertebral artery syndrome, 652t–653t
Vertical banded gastroplasty, for obesity, 588, 589f
Vessel shunts, for liver cirrhosis, 554
Vestibular drop attacks, 826
Videx. *See* Didanosine (Videx).
Vinca alkaloids, for cancer, 783, 784t
Violence, 709
Viracept. *See* Nelfinavir (Viracept).
Viral bronchitis, acute, 423
Viral conjunctivitis
  interventions for, 812

Viral conjunctivitis *(Continued)*
  pathophysiology of, 809–810
  prognosis for, 814
  signs and symptoms of, 810–811
Viral hepatitis, 560–561, 562t
  classifications of, 561–563
Viral load testing, in hepatitis, 565
Viral meningitis
  clinical manifestations of, 663, 663t
  pathophysiology of, 662
Viral pneumonia, interventions for, 435
Viramune. *See* Nevirapine (Viramune).
Virchow's triad, in thrombophlebitis, 537
Virologic tests, for human immunodeficiency virus infection, 766
Virus
  in food poisoning, 556, 558
  in infection, 299
  in pneumonia, 432, 433t
Viscous sputum, 108
Vision, diabetes and, 625
Vistaril. *See* Hydroxyzine (Vistaril).
Visual field testing, for glaucoma, 818
Vital signs, 7–17
  decision-making for, 12–17
    blood pressure in, 14–15
    heart rate in, 12, 13t
    respiration in, 13–14
    temperature in, 15–16
    urine output in, 16–17
  in meningitis, 664, 665t
  in neurologic assessment, 171–177, 176t
  principles of care in assessment of, 7–12
    blood pressure in, 8–9
    heart rate/pulse in, 7–8
    respiration in, 9–10
    temperature in, 10–11
    urine output in, 11–12
Vitamin B_{12}
  in anemia, 792
  in inflammatory bowel disease, 573
Vitamin D
  in osteoporosis, 751
  in renal failure, 144, 854
Vitamin K, in liver cirrhosis, 551, 554
VNS. *See* Vagal nerve stimulation (VNS).

Voiding, in renal dysfunction, 143
Volkmann's contracture, from fractures, 738
Volume expansion, for hypovolemic shock, 523–524
Volume overload, in heart failure, 458
Volvulus, 580
Vomiting, 365. *See also* Nausea and vomiting.
  in intestinal obstruction, 582
  medications for, 369–371
VRE. *See* Vancomycin-resistant enterococci (VRE).
Vulvovaginal candidiasis, 870, 873t

W

Wafers, skin barrier, in pouching principles, 91
Walking, for Buerger's disease, 497
Wandering, in Alzheimer's disease, 647
Warfarin (Coumadin)
  for chronic heart failure, 464
  for deep vein thrombosis, 506
  pharmacology of, 327–328
Water
  in intravenous therapy, 43
  movement of, 39–42, 40f, 42f
Water deficit, 291–292
Water intoxication, 292
  in intravenous therapy, 43
Water-hammer pulse, 13t
WBCs. *See* White blood cells (WBCs).
Weakness, in diabetes, 625
Weight loss
  for emphysema, 429
  for hypertension, 516
  for obesity, 589
  in diabetes, 625
Western blot analysis, 304
  for human immunodeficiency virus infection, 766
Wet mount examination, for sexually transmitted diseases, 876
Wheezing
  in bronchitis, 425
  in respiratory assessment, 20
White blood cell (WBC) count
  in biliary disease, 597
  in infection, 304
  in meningitis, 663

White blood cell (WBC) count
  (Continued)
  in pancreatitis, 611
White blood cells (WBCs), 282–290
  analysis of, 286–289, 287f, 288t
  classification of, 283
  development of, 282–283
  in inflammation, 261, 262
  in urinalysis, 308
  phagocytes in, 283f, 283–286, 285t
WHO. *See* World Health Organization (WHO).
Whole blood administration, 70t
Whole bowel irrigation, for drug overdose and poisoning, 707
Winged steel butterfly needles, in intravenous therapy, 49, 50t
Women, hypertension and, 512
World Health Organization (WHO), analgesic ladder of, 319–320
Wound(s), traumatic, 79
Wound care, 77–84
  after renal transplantation, 164
  assessment in, 80
  avoiding pressure in, 82
  blood flow and oxygenation in, 84
  cleansing in, 81
  débridement in, 81
  dressings for, 82–83
  growth factors in, 83
  infection management in, 82
  normal healing in, 77
  nutrition in, 84
  tracheostomy and, 133
  wound classification in, 77–78, 78t
  wound types in, 78–80
Wound cultures, in infection, 300
Wound drainage systems, 84–87
Wytensin. *See* Guanabenz (Wytensin).

X

Xanax. *See* Alprazolam (Xanax).
Xanthine oxidase inhibitors, for gout, 745
Xanthines. *See* Methylxanthines.
Xerostomia, from opioids, 314, 315t
Xylometazolin (Otrivin), for rhinitis coughs, and colds, 401t

Y

Yellow-green sputum, 108

Z

Zalcitabine (Hivid), for human
immunodeficiency virus infection,
766–767, 767t
Zaleplon (Sonata), for sleep disorders,
405t
Zantac. *See* Ranitidine (Zantac).
Zarontin. *See* Ethosuximide (Zarontin).
Zebeta. *See* Bisoprolol (Zebeta).
Zerit. *See* Stavudine (d4T, Zerit).
Zestril. *See* Lisinopril (Prinivil, Zestril).

Ziagen (Abacavir, 1592U89), for human
immunodeficiency virus, 766–767,
767t
Zidovudine (Retrovir, AZT), for human
immunodeficiency virus infection,
766–767, 767t
Zofran. *See* Ondansetron (Zofran).
Zollinger-Ellison syndrome, in peptic
ulcer disease, 616
Zolpidem (Ambien), for sleep disorders,
405t
Zone of inhibition, for antimicrobial
sensitivity, 303
Zyrtec. *See* Cetirizine (Zyrtec).